2950

Psychiatric/Mental Health Nursing

Giving Emotional Care

Psychiatric Nursing

Mental Health

Giving Emotional Care

RUTH BECKMANN MURRAY, R.N., M.S.N.
Professor of Psychiatric Nursing
St. Louis University School of Nursing
St. Louis, Missouri

M. MARILYN WILSON HUELSKOETTER, R.N., M.S.N.
Associate Professor of Psychiatric Nursing
St. Louis University School of Nursing
St. Louis, Missouri

PRENTICE-HALL, INC., ENGLEWOOD CLIFFS, N.J. 07632

Library of Congress Cataloging in Publication Data

Murray, Ruth.
    Psychiatric/mental health nursing.

    Includes bibliographies and index.
    1. Psychiatric nursing. I. Huelskoetter, M.
Marilyn Wilson. II. Title. [DNLM: 1. Psychiatric
nursing. WY 160 M983p]
RC440.M87   1983   610.73'68   82–16143
ISBN 0–13–731851–0

Editorial/production supervision: Karen J. Clemments
Interior design: Karen J. Clemments
Cover design: Edsal Enterprises
Manufacturing buyer: John Hall

Psychiatric/Mental Health Nursing: Giving Emotional Care
Ruth Beckmann Murray and M. Marilyn Wilson Huelskoetter

Printed in the United States of America

10 9 8 7 6 5 4 3 2 1

ISBN 0-13-731851-0

Prentice-Hall International, Inc., *London*
Prentice-Hall of Australia Pty. Limited, *Sydney*
Editora Prentice-Hall do Brasil, Ltda., *Rio de Janeiro*
Prentice-Hall Canada Inc., *Toronto*
Prentice-Hall of India Private Limited, *New Delhi*
Prentice-Hall of Japan, Inc., *Tokyo*
Prentice-Hall of Southeast Asia Pte. Ltd., *Singapore*
Whitehall Books Limited, *Wellington, New Zealand*

About the Authors

Ruth Beckmann Murray, R.N., M.S.N., doctoral candidate in education and counseling, is Professor of Psychiatric Nursing and Assistant Dean, Continuing Nursing Education, at St. Louis University School of Nursing, St. Louis, Missouri. She has had nursing service and teaching experience in psychiatric, medical-surgical, gerontological, and obstetrical/gynecological nursing, and experience as a school nurse in a college setting. She has taught all levels of nursing students and is well-known as a speaker on psychosocial topics in continuing education and as a curriculum consultant. She is the primary author of three other nursing texts and author of numerous articles in nursing periodicals on topics related to psycho-social nursing and development of the person.

M. Marilyn Wilson Huelskoetter, R.N., M.S.N., is an Associate Professor of Psychiatric Nursing and Chairperson of the Psychiatric Nursing Section at St. Louis University School of Nursing, St. Louis, Missouri. She has taught in all three types of nursing programs, has had experience in community, medical-surgical, and gerontological nursing and has many years of experience in psychiatric nursing. She is a consultant to hospitals and other agencies in the area of psychiatric/mental health concerns and a frequent speaker at professional conferences.

Sandra L. Blaesing, R.N., M.S.N., doctoral candidate in family counseling, is Assistant Director, Undergraduate Program, for the Registered Nurse Curriculum at St. Louis University School of Nursing, St. Louis, Missouri. Her graduate degree is in child psychiatric nursing, and she has had extensive experience in working with children and their families as a clinician, educator, consultant, and administrator in a variety of health care and school settings.

Joyce Dees Brockhaus, R.N., Ph.D., is an Adjunct Associate Professor in the Graduate Program, Psychiatric/Mental Health Nursing at St. Louis University School of Nursing, St. Louis, Missouri. She maintains an active practice in child and family counseling, and is a frequent speaker at professional conferences. She earned her doctorate degree in counselor education from St. Louis University, and holds a master's degree in child psychiatric nursing. She is certified in marital and family therapy. She is very active in local, state, and national levels in the area of adoption of older children and children with handicaps. She has published in both journals and textbooks on the topics of adoption, values clarification, adolescents, family therapy, and stress management.

Margaret Ederer, R.N., M.S.N., Communications Coordinator, St. Joseph Hospital, St. Charles, Missouri, and formerly Adjunct Instructor of Psychiatric Nursing, St. Louis University School of Nursing, St. Louis, Missouri. She has extensive experience in psychiatric nursing and in counseling nurses and other health professionals to resolve conflictual issues related to employment, and she is a frequent speaker for professional conferences.

Doris M. Edwards, R.N., M.S.N., is an Associate Professor in Psychiatric Nursing and Acting Director, Graduate Program, Psychiatric/Mental Health Nursing at St. Louis University School of Nursing, St. Louis, Missouri. She has had extensive experience in psychiatric nursing at several mental health centers and has taught all levels of undergraduate baccalaureate students. Her current major focus is on graduate education directed toward providing effective mental health services to underserved individuals/families. She was Assistant Coordinator, Midwest Regional Project, to study nursing distribution, sponsored by the Western Interstate Commission on Higher Education.

Wayne D. Hooker, R.N., Ph.D., is Psychiatric/Mental Health Instructor at Angelina College, Department of Nursing, at Lufkin, Texas. He has a special interest in community mental health, has studied and worked with people of Spanish-speaking cultures, and has many years of experience in psychiatric nursing and nursing education. He has taught all levels of professional nursing students and has been a director of a diploma school of nursing.

Phyllis M. Jacobs, R.N., M.S.N., is an Adjunct Assistant Professor in Psychiatric Nursing at St. Louis University School of Nursing, St. Louis, Missouri. Her clinical interests are in the emotional needs of hospitalized clients in medical/surgical settings, and in nonhospital care settings for psychiatric clients. She has taught in both baccalaureate and diploma schools of nursing.

Patricia Kaufmann, R.N., M.S.N., is an Adjunct Instructor in Nursing of Children at St. Louis University School of Nursing, St. Louis, Missouri. Her graduate degree is in nursing of children. She has been a clinical specialist working with developmentally disabled children and their families in a demonstration child development center. Another primary clinical interest is child abuse prevention.

Marcea E. Kjervik, R.N., M.S., is a clinical nursing specialist at Hennepin County Mental Health Center in Minneapolis, Minnesota. Her graduate studies in psychiatric nursing focused on sex differences of personal space preferences with two cultures. She is an adjunct faculty member of the University of Minnesota School of Nursing. She is also the chairperson of the Council of Advanced Practitioners in Psychiatric/Mental Health Nursing in Minnesota.

Virginia M. Luetje, R.N., M.S.N., is an Adjunct Assistant Professor in Psychiatric Nursing at St. Louis University School of Nursing, St. Louis, Missouri, in addition to doing consultation and education in psychosocial nursing for other local institutions. She has ten years' experience in hotline telephone counseling and has been an instructor for crisis intervention and suicide prevention at many continuing education conferences. She served as nursing consultant and researcher for Counsel to Plaintiff in a lengthy class action lawsuit regarding level of care rendered in a public hospital and has an active interest in nursing advocacy for the client.

Dorothy O'Driscoll, R.N., M.S.N., J.D., is Attorney at Law at Legal Services of Eastern Missouri and is Adjunct Associate Professor, Medical-Surgical Nursing at St. Louis University School of Nursing, St. Louis, Missouri. She has had experience in all areas of hospital nursing and has taught all levels of professional nursing students. She has served on various boards and committees related to health care, including being a member of the Nursing Home Ombudsman Advisory Committee, St. Louis, and the Elderly Committee of the Young Lawyers Section, Metropolitan St. Louis Bar Association. She is editor of *The Senior Citizens Handbook*, 4th ed., published by the Missouri Division of Aging and the Metropolitan St. Louis Bar Association.

Evelyn Romano, R.N., M.S.N., is Instructor in Psychiatric Nursing, Catholic University, Washington, D.C. She was formerly Director of Nursing at St. Louis State Hospital, St. Louis, Missouri, and an Instructor of Psychiatric Nursing, St. Louis University School of Nursing. She has extensive experience in nursing service administration as well as in nursing education.

Gail Stringer, R.N., M.S.N., Clinical Nurse Specialist, Alcohol Treatment Unit, Veterans Administration Medical Center, and Adjunct Instructor, St. Louis University School of Nursing, St. Louis, Missouri. She has extensive experience in both individual and group counseling of clients who suffer substance abuse as well as in counseling other psychiatric clients.

Brief Contents

Contents

To the Reader

Principles and practices of psychiatric/mental health nursing (providing emotional care) are applicable in every health care setting and to each person, family, or group that you touch as a nurse.

The authors believe that the humanistic framework is appropriate, in fact essential, for giving emotional care to any client. The humanistic framework is introduced in Chapter 2 with the Third Force Theorists, after First and Second Force Theories/Theorists are described. Consequently, you can better compare theories and realize how the humanistic approach undergirds the nursing process throughout the book.

The goals of this book are to help you look at both yourself and your client(s) (the people you work with), as well as to present specific assessment data and intervention skills to help you work with people who have emotional needs. The content is organized around five steps of the nursing process: assessment, nursing diagnosis, goal-setting for planning care, intervention related to the goals, and evaluation. A comprehensive, in-depth perspective is taken throughout the book to assist you in your understanding of people and your use of the nursing process.

The emphasis of the book is twofold: Psychosocial processes are discussed as a basis for emotional (psychiatric) illness, although biological processes are also indicated, and the importance of the nurse–client relationship in care is emphasized. This approach is intentional. Our society and profession are becoming increasingly more mechanized and scientific, while the feelings of people are being minimized. Although the scientific process is useful to life and nursing, the authors believe that feelings, attitudes, values, and beliefs—the psychological or emotional component of the person—are important to life, to keeping our humanness, to being a social being, and to the nursing process. Social groups and processes are equally important.

You are in a special position to play a unique but vital role in the lives of those you care for and work with. You can bring your love, in the *agape* sense, your humanness, your health, and your understanding, based upon principles and practices of psychiatric/mental health nursing, to touch those in need.

The essence of emotional care is to fully perceive the humanness of the person, your own as well as the people with whom you work. As you gain heightened awareness of your own feelings and behaviors, you will understand more fully some of the feelings and behaviors of your clients.

In turn, you will be better able to encourage others to look more closely at their feelings and behavior and to move toward greater self-acceptance and more effective interpersonal and social relationships. As you gain knowledge of and experience with people, you will understand more fully the pain, loneliness, terror, and defensive maneuvers of another human being. The better you know your client, the more you will be able to care for and love your client.

We believe that emotional care, which involves close interaction and relationship, is one of the unique roles of the nurse. This involves giving of self without obligation on the part of another. You must, however, learn what this relationship means, what can make it helpful to the person you work with, and what can provide a climate of growth for you as well as another. You must provide nurturing for the clients and staff you work with, as well as for yourself.

Emotional care covers a wide range of behaviors: Conveying acceptance and warmth, providing protection for expression of feelings, encouraging trust, cherishing the self, being a catalyst for expansion of others, and "letting go" at appropriate times. Emotional care means to stand back sometimes so another can try new skills, to move in sometimes with physical intervention or problem-solving attitudes, to work as a professional to improve health care delivery, and to be involved as a citizen to improve social situations. Always, emotional care means to grapple with facing yourself realistically; accepting your strengths and limits; staying empathic and compassionate in a technological and fast changing society; understanding the unique values, feelings, and needs of another; and using the nursing process based on your self-awareness and understanding of and compassion for the other person. Thus, to give emotional care —to use the principles of psychiatric/mental health nursing—is not easy. It is rewarding.

The five parts of this book are written to promote your development as a professional nurse. *Part I, The Developing Person*, explores insights about you, the nurse, and the individual client. *Chapter 1* is *devoted to you*, the student. The chapter introduces the student to psychiatric nursing and explores normal feelings and concerns of the student in the health care system, especially when caring for psychiatric clients. Myths and stereotypes are explored, along with ways to enhance coping in the student experience. *Chapter*

2 gives an in-depth *description of theories* pertinent to understanding people. The reason for the emphasis on psychological theories was previously mentioned. The psychological theorists are divided into the First, Second, and Third Force as a way to group similar theories and theorists, for comparison, and to enhance your understanding. You will find aspects of all of the theories useful in explaining and understanding people at some point in their life development and on health-illness continuum. The Humanistic Framework of this book utilizes knowledge from other disciplines —the biological, psychological, behavioral, and social sciences—for an eclectic theory base. *Chapter 3* gives an *overview of the individual* and influences upon the development and health of the person.

Part II, Nursing Behaviors in the Psychiatric/Mental Health Setting, describes what every psychiatric/mental health nurse will be doing, in any setting, with any client. *Chapter 4 relates the nursing process to psychiatric/mental health nursing*. The author describes five steps of the nursing process in detail as a basis for discussion of the nursing process in the rest of the book. The Humanistic Model is referred to, and the philosophy of nursing shared by the authors reflects the Humanistic Framework, as well as application of selected Second and Third Force Theories. *Chapter 5* discusses *communication* for in-depth emotional care. *Chapter 6* explains the *nurse–client relationship* in depth as a basis for nursing intervention throughout the book. *Chapter 7* describes the *change process* as it applies to the individual, group, and setting. As a nurse, you will be a change agent in the lives of individual people, families, or groups, as well as in the system in which you work. Insights about what is involved in change is necessary if you are to persist in the role of change agent. *Chapter 8* describes the effects of *crisis* and principles of crisis intervention. As a nurse, you will always be working with actual or potential crises. Even the chronically ill or tertiary-care client has crises points in life, as does the family. You will also encounter crises in your life and profession. An understanding of the processes involved can help you cope.

Part III, The Nursing Process with Special Systems in Psychiatric/Mental Health Nursing, covers three client systems that you must understand and will work with in nursing. *Chapter 9* describes the *importance of culture* to the client and of considering selected cultural variables in emotional care. *Chapter 10* describes the *family as a client*, and family interactions and dynamics that affect health and your nursing process. You will be caring for the family as a unit as well as relating to the family of each client, as is described in Part IV. *Chapter 11* describes the *group as a client* and the dynamics and processes within a group that you must consider when you work with a group.

Part IV, Nursing Diagnoses and the Nursing Process, is devoted to a comprehensive view of the person who is responding to stress and anxiety, and demonstrating behavior that reflects unmet needs, feelings of alienation from self and others, and ineffective coping with the environment. The content is organized around assessment, formulation of nursing diagnosis and client-care goals, nursing therapy and other intervention measures, and evaluation of care related to common nursing diagnoses. These nursing diagnoses refer to behaviors that are hurtful to the person or contribute to ineffective or dysfunctional relations with others. While nursing responsibilities related to drugs and other modalities are included, emphasis under nursing intervention will be of use in therapy skills. Nurse therapy (psychotherapy) is an infinitely human process, and drugs and machines cannot take the place of the nurse. In this book we shall speak to specific behaviors appropriate for the emotional care of specific illness. Never forget that these specific behaviors are not to be used as a recipe. Consider first the client and his/her needs, environment, and life situation; then consider your strengths and the resources available to you, and arrive at a plan of care, involving the client and family to the fullest extent possible. At times you will need the caring behaviors of others—instructor, colleague, supervisor, family, friends. The chain process of giving and receiving is necessary for continued development.

Medical diagnostic categories are spoken to as they relate to nursing diagnoses. Although there are limitations to the diagnostic categories, we believe that the historically derived syndromes do lend themselves to study of the human dimension. In addition, there can be no interdisciplinary collaboration between nursing and other professions without knowledge of these syndromes. We have included both nursing and medical knowledge as well as our own insights and experiences in order to help you synthesize and use the depth and breadth of scientific knowledge and experimental insight that this combined approach permits.

Chapter 12 covers content on response to *stressors and the stress syndrome*; feelings and behaviors pertinent to each of the four levels of anxiety; the mind-body relationship (including psychosomatic or physiological illnesses); emotional reactions to illness, the sick role, and impaired role behavior; and specific goals and intervention for management of stress and anxiety, including in illness. *Chapter 13* further describes the feelings and behaviors as well as care of the person with *chronic, dysfunctional anxiety* (selected neuroses). *Chapter 14* discusses needs, feelings, and care of the person who *overuses or abuses various substances*, including alcohol, various drugs, and food. *Chapter 15* describes dynamics and the nursing process with the *depressed client*. *Chapter 16* discusses dynamics and the nursing process with the *withdrawn (schizophrenic) client*. *Chapter 17* relates information on dynamics and nursing process pertinent to the *suspicious person*. *Chapter 18* describes types of *cognitive impairment*, relates various medical diagnoses to the phenomenon of impaired cognition or confusion, and differentiates the disease processes and care for reversible and nonreversible brain disease. *Chapter 19* is innovative in formulating nursing diagnoses pertinent to *abusive, aggressive behavior* in its various forms. This chapter describes dynamics, behavior, and the nursing process pertinent to each nursing diagnosis. *Chapter 20* discusses *sexual role conflicts*, a topic of increasing concern to nurses both in relation to yourself and the client. The content about developmental theories adds to the discussion of theories begun in Chapter 2. Variables contributing to sexual role conflicts and the nurse's role are discussed. *Chapter 21* presents information about various *conditions of childhood and adolescence* that you may encounter in a family unit. Your understanding of these disorders is important for case finding and referral purposes, even if you are not directly caring for a child or adolescent client.

Part V, Realities in Comprehensive Mental Health Nursing, presents information that will help you adjust to and carry out your responsibilities in the health care system. In *Chapter 22*, pertinent, general, *legal* information for the psychiatric client and nurse is presented. *Chapter 23* discusses the need for *client advocacy* in psychiatric/mental health settings and the role of the nurse in advocacy. *Chapter 24* discusses *feelings, conflicts, and adjustment of the nurse* in the practice setting. You are presented with practical information on how to work with others and cope with job stresses, as well as considerations for making a choice about changing the work setting. The reader who is already a practicing nurse will better understand the constraints of the work system and ways to handle them after reading this chapter. *Chapter 25* emphasizes the importance of and approach to *primary prevention* in various settings, and gives an *overview of secondary and tertiary care approaches.*

We hope to stimulate you to look at the person, family, or group in emotional pain, in any setting, with a more positive, yet realistic attitude. We want to stimulate your sense of empathy and compassion through an understanding of people as well as of psychiatric illness, so that you can intervene and thus contribute to changes in the lives of people. Through knowledge of and practice with specific skills, you will be able to work with the troubled person, rather than to reinforce society's traditional way of coping with the emotionally and mentally ill.

We use the term *you* throughout the text in order to speak to you and involve you as an active reader. We hope that this will stimulate the integration of this information into your nursing so that your care will be more knowledgeable, compassionate, and practical.

We believe the knowledge and skills presented in this text will help you provide emotional care with love and genuine caring. We also believe that as your love is channeled through assessment skills, undergirded by your intervention skills, and challenged by your evaluation skills, you will be emerging stronger than when you began study and care of the emotionally ill person.

Acknowledgments

The authors appreciate the support and assistance from many friends.

We are especially grateful to Sally Lehnert for her conscientious assistance in preparing most of the manuscript, as well as to Barbara Groneck, Kathy Imbs, and Karen Deubler for their typing assistance. A special thanks to our husbands, C. Edwin Murray and Frank Huelskoetter, for their support; to Ann Becker, R.N., M.S.N., for review of selected nursing diagnoses; and to Frances Bruner, M.A., for proofing assistance.

We thank Prentice-Hall, Inc., especially Dudley Kay, college editor, and Karen J. Clemments, production editor, for their guidance during preparation of the text.

In addition, the following persons are acknowledged for reviewing the manuscript, partially or totally: Joan E. Bowers, R.N., Ed.D., Assistant Professor, School of Nursing, University of Washington; Beatrice Carruth, Associate Professor, School of Nursing, University of Texas—Austin; Clare Delaney, Associate Professor, University of Oklahoma—Health Science Center; Priscilla Ebersole, Field Director, Geriatric Nurse Practitioner Project, Funded by the Kellogg Foundation, on leave from San Francisco State University; Karolyn Gadbey, R.N., A.R.N.P., Associate Professor, University of Florida—Gainesville; Mildred Gottdank, Professor and Department Chairperson, Psychiatric Mental Health Nursing Department, Wayne State College of Nursing; Mary Lou Komarek, R.N., M.S., Assistant Professor, College of Nursing, Alfred University; Martha McNiff, Coordinator for Staff Development, Clinical Resource Division, Mt. Sinai Hospital, New York; and Delores Swan, R.N., M.Ed., Director of Nursing, College of Lake County.

Ruth Beckmann Murray
M. Marilyn Wilson Huelskoetter

The Developing Person

1

Feelings and Adjustment of the Student in the Psychiatric/ Mental Health Care Setting

Study of this chapter will assist you to:

1. Identify and discuss your feelings, concerns, and needs as a student in the psychiatric/ mental health nursing experience.

2. Compare and contrast the goals of your psychiatric/mental health course with your personal goals for this experience.

3. Examine myths and stereotypes about psychiatric clients, settings, and workers.

4. Explore how the clinical laboratory can help you to achieve your course and personal goals.

5. Determine support systems and ways to obtain support from others during your psychiatric/mental health experience.

6. Examine your established coping skills and those new skills that are developing during this experience.

7. Evaluate special strengths you have brought to the psychiatric/mental health experience.

8. Evaluate whether or not your goals for the course are met.

This chapter contributed by Margaret Ederer, R.N., M.S.N.

You may begin your psychiatric/mental health course with eager anticipation, joy, anxiety, or hesitation. You may feel ready, or you may wish you could delay the course. Students approach this experience with a variety of feelings and concerns. Your previous contacts with a mentally ill person, your own feelings of uncertainty or fear in dealing with the mentally ill, the stereotypes and myths you bring, and your concerns about success in the course all may combine to shake your self-confidence.

The purpose of this chapter is to consider some of these common concerns and to explore ways of handling them. Factors over which you have no control, as well as ways of accepting or "letting go" in order to conserve energy and time and avoid frustration, will be discussed. Constructive ways of working through your feelings and finding creative, helpful approaches to your education, your behavioral change, and nursing practice will be explored. You are a developing person during this educational experience.

VARIETY IN CLINICAL EXPERIENCES FOR THE STUDENT

Influence of the Educational Program

Understanding the goals and objectives of the psychiatric/mental health experience is an essential first step in helping you to feel comfortable and able to cope with the situation. In some programs, the main goal may be observation and analysis. Although a great deal can be learned from observation, your wanting to do something may cause you to feel uncomfortable during observation and frustrated that you cannot attempt direct intervention in the situation.

In programs where student participation in patient care is expected, you may have the opportunity to practice beginning psychiatric nursing skills in addition to critical observation. Here the focus is often on the words *acquaint* and *beginning*. Although you may initially feel that you do not know how to talk when you begin your clinical experience, you are probably more competent in communications than you realize. Remember that no one expects perfection. If you could perform expertly, there would be no need for this experience. Furthermore, you can learn from your errors.

Rather than wasting time and energy hoping that magically you will not make mistakes, you should try to anticipate situations, think of how to avoid communication barriers, and learn from the communication process with your client. The more readily you accept the reality that you are human and will make some mistakes, the freer you will be to experiment with new behaviors, seek constructive criticism, and accept appropriate support.

The emphasis in the clinical experience will be determined by your particular nursing school's philosophy and its conceptual framework and curriculum plan; the instructor's expectations; and the available clinical laboratory experiences. The best way to determine expectations is to listen carefully and to ask questions. Students often spend so much time trying to determine what will please the instructor that they have little energy or time to learn and practice. Once expectations are clarified, you can see how they relate to your own educational and personal goals and can then make the most of the learning experience.

Influence of the Clinical Setting

Students may have little or no choice in the selection of the setting for their clinical experience. A setting where the philosophy and principles of the educational program are put into practice is ideal. Contact with psychiatric nursing staff members who model therapeutic behaviors and who are interested in the student's professional and personal growth is the ultimate learning experience. However, the ideal therapeutic environment does not always exist.

As M. Kramer and C. Schmalenberg point out, you can waste much energy in bemoaning the fact that things are not what they "should" be (1). Although you need ideals and standards to guide and serve as a basis for evaluation, if you demand that the situation be perfect before you associate yourself with it, your ideals can never be achieved to any degree.

Plan on using to the best advantage the situation in which you find yourself. It is far more constructive to view the clinical setting, regardless of its attributes, as a place where learning is possible as long as you are willing to make the appropriate adjustments. Negative aspects of the situation can increase your awareness of obstacles that affect nursing care, whether they relate to the agency's policies, to the physical environment, or to the client and staff population. Observe what seems ineffective in nursing care and plan alternatives. Investigate ways to avoid similar obstacles in the future.

Positive components of the clinical setting include opportunities to observe and work with a variety of clients, to practice and evaluate a variety of approaches and interventions, to share feelings and ideas with proficient professionals, to identify the characteristics of the environment that enhance nursing care, and to experience learning in other ways.

Whether the positive factors outweigh the negative in the clinical setting, or vice versa, you will learn the most by accepting the realities and using them to augment your understanding of theoretical concepts.

Educational and Personal Goal Setting

Insights about human behavior can be gained and interventions practiced in any program or setting. The very fact that you are where you are now is evidence that you have been relating successfully on some levels. You have a history of interacting with a variety of people. Interactions that were caring and helpful can be designated as therapeutic. Other actions that would not be classified as growth-enhancing may still have been useful in learning about yourself and others. Since people generally are more alike than different (2), you cannot claim total inexperience as you approach clients in the psychiatric/mental health nursing experience.

Deliberate goal-setting may be a new experience for you, but it is a method that is constantly used by nurses. Goal setting begins with asking a series of questions: What do I need to learn? How can I best learn? How can I best prepare myself for learning? How can I come to the experience open to involvement? What have others suggested that might be beneficial? What other things are happening in my life that might affect the goals I set now?

Goals cannot be set in a vacuum. Both identified and felt needs must be considered. Demands and responsibilities outside the educational program will influence your direction. Your own expectations are important. However, because expectations so often distort the overall view of things, it is advantageous first to write down all expectations specifically and then determine which are reality-based and which are wishful thinking or distortions of past experiences.

It is not always possible or desirable to separate educational and personal goals into discrete categories. If you are dealing with a personal crisis, you may have to use your available energy for that situation and set only modest educational goals. If you feel the need for an intellectual challenge because of lack of stimulation in other areas, you may set goals that reflect this. If the course's objectives and the instructor's expectations stress theory or observation and your past success has been in practical application of concepts, it may be wise to study intensely and wait to apply new knowledge in another setting. If the emphasis is on therapeutic interaction and you are more comfortable working with concepts, it may be appropriate to concentrate first on what is comfortable —the concepts—and then gradually practice the therapeutic skills that are required.

Talk with the instructor about your feelings and difficulties. Often the instructor can help you select learning experiences appropriate to your level of maturity and skill. The instructor can also validate your observations and practice and in the process help you gain new insights and maturity. View the instructor as a helpful colleague rather than as a person who gives grades. You may have begun the course fearing a low grade because of your perceived lack of knowledge or skill. As you work with others in the course—instructor and peers—you can learn a great deal about yourself, the clients, and mental health nursing. The final grade you earn will accurately reflect your efforts and learning.

The essential thing to remember about goal setting is that you do have choices. Passing the course is a primary objective, but there are instances when a grade of C will suffice because of extenuating circumstances. Facilitating your own development is also a primary goal, and you can make decisions about how and in what areas to proceed. Your goals should be flexible. There are times when it is necessary and appropriate to redefine and modify a goal, especially when the goal is not realistic. Although goals should encourage stretching and risk taking, they must be attainable and not "setups" for failure.

Regardless of the educational program or clinical setting, you have a choice about how to approach the experience and on which aspects to focus attention. You also have a responsibility to base these choices on all available data: your intellectual and behavioral strengths and weaknesses, your cultural background, your past educational and life experiences, and current circumstances. Goals assist in planning for constructive change and growth. They can also keep you aware of your strengths and limitations and, used wisely, can be a source of support and affirmation.

MYTHS AND STEREOTYPES ABOUT PSYCHIATRIC CLIENTS, SETTINGS, AND WORKERS

Just as you come to the psychiatric experience with already learned interpersonal patterns, you also bring myths, stereotypes, or ghosts from the past. Your anticipations may interfere with choosing a client for interaction and relationship during this experience as well as with your effective use of the nursing process.

Everyone has seen movies and television shows depicting various kinds of mental aberrations. For example, people portrayed as "perfectly normal" may suddenly take screaming flight into insanity because of one traumatic incident. Mental illness and violence are shown as inseparable. The focus is on the pain the ill person inflicts rather than on the pain he experiences. Or there may be a desperate search to find the one childhood event that is responsible for all of a person's subsequent difficulties.

Once that incident is identified, the person is "cured" and the movie ends. These representations are usually very dramatic but they are unrealistic.

Psychiatric settings are also presented more for dramatic effect than realism. M. I. Ward's book, *Snake Pit* (3), lives in the minds of many, as do the sterile, gleaming rooms of the so-called scientific institutions. Violence occurs in the form of terror-inspiring machines, leather restraints, locks, and barred windows.

The imaginary individuals who work in these psychiatric settings receive similarly fictionalized treatment. Either they are selfless, saintlike people who go to any lengths, including risking all personal and professional investment, for the sake of the client, or they are sadistic, inhumane staff members who use their positions to demean and damage.

In addition to movies and television, each individual draws from personal experience to create unique, personal myths. What comes to mind when you think of mental illness may be the old man from your childhood who wore strange clothes and mumbled to himself. Although your parents may have assured you that he was harmless, you may also have been warned to stay away from him. "Double" messages are confusing. Or maybe there was a neighbor or relative who "suffered from nerve trouble," was alcoholic, or made periodic trips to the "funny farm." The particular words chosen to describe a situation will have their own impact. Whoever your ghosts are, you may know them well, or they may be hidden from your recall. You may also have learned something about causation if Mom ever said, "You kids are driving me crazy."

In your adult life, you will also have encountered stereotypes. Not only do you hear about people who are "a little strange" or "odd" but also about psychiatrists and psychiatric nurses who "act like they need more help than their patients." These very people might contribute to this misconception by stating, "You have to be crazy to stay in this business."

What do you do with all this negative input? You may have been taught, directly or indirectly, to fear, avoid, look down on, and possibly to laugh at people associated with emotional problems, either victims or helpers.

As with most myths and stereotypes learned early, your role models did not intentionally give misinformation or mean harm. You were taught some things because your "teachers" truly believed them; i.e., ignorance rather than knowledge was passed on. Other information might have been offered in an honest effort to protect you. Those who molded your attitudes in childhood were doing the best they could with the information available to them.

As a child, you undoubtedly received misinformation in many areas of life. Most of it was discarded when you got more accurate information or when the stereotypes and fantasies were no longer useful. The myths that persist usually do so because of lack of access to the facts (this has been the case until recently in the area of human sexuality) or because they continue to serve a necessary function.

Believing that people with emotional problems are quite different from everyone else can seem protective. Dividing people into "crazy" and "noncrazy" categories is very comforting as long as you are in the "noncrazy" group. Emotions, however, are not so conveniently classified. Although each of us is a unique, one-of-a-kind individual, we are all more alike than we are different. There are no "new" emotions. Rather there are questions of intensity, appropriateness, and sequence. These are the factors with which psychiatric nursing is involved. Feelings are not right or wrong, good or bad, but existing and valid or real for the person. Since all people experience feelings, deviance is determined not by what is felt but by the reaction to those feelings. In mental health there are no absolutes, no black or white, only shades of gray. Specifics of psychopathology are discussed elsewhere in this book. It is sufficient now that you recognize deviance as a subjective designation. Viewing clients as people like yourself, with many healthy as well as maladaptive coping patterns, is most conducive to establishing satisfying relationships in and out of the clinical setting. Remember, the person responds in the best way possible for that person, at that time. Even the emotionally ill person is doing the best that he or she can do.

REACTIONS OF THE STUDENT TO THE PSYCHIATRIC CLIENT AND SETTING

As mentioned above, a wide range of feelings about and reactions to the psychiatric/mental health experience is normal. Fear of the unknown is to be expected. However, many of the previously learned coping mechanisms used to decrease feelings of inadequacy with medical-surgical clients are not appropriate in this new situation. Observing for specific, clearly defined signs and symptoms often is not a suitable behavior. High-visibility nursing functions are seldom indicated. You may have been taught that talking with clients is what you do after the "real work" is finished. Now it *is* your *real work*. Students report amazement at being exhausted after having done "nothing but talk and listen." Granted, the student's anxiety contributes to this feeling of fatigue, but even experienced psychiatric nurses confess they would be less tired after digging ditches than after some therapeutic sessions. The amount of energy needed to listen and concentrate is significant.

You may also experience some of the following concerns and needs along with their accompanying feelings during your learning experience.

You may be concerned about either being assigned or having to choose a client. Often instructors arrange for students to choose the client rather than assigning a client. You should choose someone to whom you can respond with warmth, interest, and concern. Your feelings toward the person can be the basis for much learning. The medical or nursing diagnoses, in and of themselves, are not adequate predictors of the learning experience. Choice of client allows the student to work with someone who is perceived positively; both student and client benefit. In most agencies, nurses have a choice as to at least some of the clients with whom they will work.

You may be concerned that the client will not talk or will try to avoid you. It is natural but unrealistic for you to assume responsibility for a client's behavior. A client's reasons for avoiding interaction may not be obvious. Some simply lack the energy necessary to carry on a conversation. This is especially true of the depressed person, and sitting silently with him/her is an appropriate intervention. Other clients may be so preoccupied with their own feelings that they consider any interruption an intrusion. A person may also decline to interact with you because of factors beyond your control, such as your age or physical resemblance to someone else in the past, or the client's current psychological state (fear, withdrawal, or anger), or past experience with other students. Taking silence as a personal rebuke is not useful to either the client or yourself. Clients, just like anyone else, sometimes do not want to talk.

Review your behavior and discuss your approach with the instructor to determine what alternate approaches might be tried. Then return to the client and try again to establish contact. You cannot depend entirely on the individual's responses to validate your professional performance. For evaluation you also need a frank critique of your own efforts, appraisal from instructors, and input from peers. Use this data as a basis for changing and moving ahead rather than indulging in self-recriminations and feelings of helplessness.

Clients may sometimes decide to discuss social or superficial topics unrelated to their deeper feelings. This can be upsetting because you may feel that unless you are pursuing deep, dark secrets, you are not being therapeutic. However, there may be many reasons why the client chooses to relate superficially. Perhaps he/she has just done some hard mental work on personal problems and needs to relax. Or it may have been decided by the client, with or without physician input, that only the client-physician relationship is suitable for discussing problems. Also practice in social interaction may be a goal for the client who feels that unless a social or pleasant situation is discussed, no one will be interested. Furthermore the client may want some time to test you, with the idea that if the two of you relate well on a superficial level, a more indepth relationship can develop. Superficial interactions or conversations about general or social concerns can also afford opportunities to build self-esteem and to affirm the sense of being a person. Your interest and willingness to make related comments and ask questions will help to validate the client as a unique human being. This is no small accomplishment and in some cases may be a new and meaningful experience for the person.

The client who does share significant thoughts and feelings may be frightening to you. You may assume that because the person offers such information you have to do something about it. Indeed, clients often directly or indirectly place the student in the role of rescuer, and you may, because of a need to be actively helpful, accept that role, which can be anxiety-producing. To feel the responsibility for "making it all better" is uncomfortable even for the most experienced nurse. Accept the idea that the nurse does not "make" anyone better. Just as you cannot "make" a tree grow (although you can provide it with sunlight, moisture, soil nutrients, and protect it from insects and severe weather), you cannot "make" people grow. When it seems that the person expects more than you can possibly deliver in terms of effecting a cure, it is helpful to remember this analogy. You can do many things to promote and support growth-producing behaviors, but the actual growing is the client's province and will be done at a pace consistent with his/her available energy and potential.

Clients are sometimes concrete or specific in their demands. Asking you to provide candy, cigarettes, or money is not an unusual behavior. The client may be testing you to see if you really care, or to keep from talking about real feelings. You can best prepare for such requests by considering your feelings prior to the event. You may feel eager to give, or you may feel you are being used by the person. Or you might like to give but really do not have money to spend this way. The key in making this and many other decisions about nursing care is to determine whose needs will actually be met. If you give what is requested as a substitute for relating, the client's needs are ignored. And if you refuse to give what is requested when your giving would signify something much deeper, the client's needs may also be ignored. Sometimes something small and inexpensive might meet the client's needs and help him/her to feel nourished emotionally and physically. Such items could be a stick of gum, a glass of juice, a cup of coffee, or an ice cream bar. The decision should be pertinent to the situation. If you resent the giving or deny all requests automatically just to demonstrate authority or control, then your personal needs rather than the client's needs are guiding the interaction. Discuss your feelings with your instructor in order to determine their significance. Students may sometimes decide to deny requests for items in order to avoid complications in the therapeutic process. When this is the case, a clear, honest response to the first request lets the client know what to expect. Statements could include: "No, I won't be giving you candy," or "Money isn't one of the things I can give you."

Saying the wrong thing to the client is another common fear. For some reason we believe there is one right thing that should be said and anything else might be harmful. It is doubtful that any relationship, in or out of the clinical setting, is sustained without some ups and downs. It is the feeling, more than the words, that determines the effectiveness of the relationship. When there is true caring and a sincere desire to be helpful, people will readily overlook a few awkward remarks. Clients will survive your inexperience, lack of sophistication, or any inappropriate interventions when it is obvious that the motive underlying these behaviors is concern for them as unique human beings. Rather than becoming preoccupied with responses that did not work or with missed opportunities, focus on alternatives and be willing to try again. Careful attention to the client's reactions to what you are saying, feeling, and doing will give valuable information about the most effective way to deal with that particular person. Approaches that do not work immediately are not always wrong. You do not know what will work for a specific client until you try and see what happens.

You may be concerned that you do not know what to talk about with the client. After the initial greeting, you may select a topic related to the client's family, occupation, or past history, but the conversation is likely to remain on a social level unless the topic is significant for the client. A principle to follow is to allow the person to initiate the topic and lead the conversation at his/her pace. Use the principles and techniques of communication described in Chapter 5. Observe the person's reaction to what you say and modify your approach as necessary. Remember, silence can be productive. Learn to be comfortable with silence when the client is not ready to talk. When the person senses your interest, comfort, and empathy, he/she will talk about what is important. Avoid having a rigid plan. You do not always have to select or initiate topics for conversation.

The fear of being physically harmed by a client may be experienced by you and by your family. Attributing these fears to myths and ghosts rather than to the here-and-now reality makes the fear no less real. It takes time to become comfortable in the setting, to know the clients and staff, and to become confident with your own skills. Discussing fears prior to the experience is the first step. You may feel embarrassed about being frightened and hesitant to express these feelings to peers or instructors. Open sharing will enable you to discover that you are not alone with your feelings and will promote group problem solving. Although physical violence is rare in most psychiatric settings, it is not impossible. Therefore recognizing the fear and discussing it with supportive people are essential. Discover what procedures are used in the setting to deal with violence in order to increase your feelings of security. When fears persist, decide how the setting can be changed to allay anxiety. For example, talking with a client in a large room where others are available, but not so close as to interfere with privacy, might be easier than talking in a secluded conference room or office. If accompanying a client to other areas in the hospital is frightening, arrangements can be made for a group of clients and staff to travel together. Even adding one other person can be a support. If fear becomes the predominant feeling with a client or in the setting in general, the instructor must be consulted. No one can relate therapeutically when overwhelmed by concern for personal physical safety.

Being harmed psychologically by the client is another common concern of the student. Emotionally ill persons are often sensitive to and frightened by the vulnerabilities of others. They can be very blunt in verbalizing the feelings that they sense from another. As the person becomes anxious, he/she may lash out with anger and yell at you. No one wants to be yelled at or ridiculed. If this does occur, it is helpful to remember that this is the client's way of coping with fear, confusion, or some other painful emotion—although realizing this does not necessarily make the event more comfortable for you. It is appropriate when you feel very threatened, either physically or psychologically, to leave the situation. Immediate support will decrease your feelings of inadequacy. Also immediate review of the circumstances surrounding the event will help put it in perspective and allow for realistic evaluation. We all sometimes miss clues that a client is becoming upset. Going over the interaction helps to identify contributing factors and to plan more effective interventions.

Clients may sometimes engage in power struggles with the staff. Students unfamiliar with this behavior can be caught off guard. The therapy-sophisticated client often is more familiar with psychiatric terminology and with the mental health care system than you are. Such a client seems to delight in setting traps by making statements and then critiquing responses. For example, the client may say, "You weren't supposed to say what you thought. You were supposed to ask how I felt about it." Or the client asks questions to test you rather than to obtain information. If you assume that you should know more about the client and the illness than he/she does, you become very vulnerable to these behaviors. The client has had more experience with his/her unique responses and needs than anyone else. Remember, such behavior and responses may be an attempt to hide fear, anger, or loneliness. The client may sound like an expert on self, but usually such insight is limited. Try to understand the person's feelings from his/her words and behavior. Discuss the treatment plan with staff members so that the approach is consistent. Avoid a psychological battle with the client to determine who knows more or who is right since both you and the client will lose. Graciously accepting the client's critical remarks and continuing the interaction may be enough to extinguish the behavior. Acknowledging the person's interest in obtaining quality care may help to build trust and enhance self-esteem.

At some point, focusing on such feelings and behavior may be appropriate. If the client persists in correcting you, you might say, "I notice that you often correct me. Let's talk about that." However, if you confront the client too early about such critical responses, the individual may deny the behavior, especially if he/she is anxious or mistrustful. Only if you and the client have a firm relationship and feel comfortable will such a confrontive approach be appropriate. For example, you might say, "It seems very important to you to let me know when I make a mistake. Can you tell me more about that?" Whatever approach is chosen, you need support in dealing with the feelings evoked. If the client can realize you are authentic and have a sincere desire to learn how best to help, the testing will decrease. Validate your approaches with your instructor. Honesty in asking for assistance, in recognizing your feelings, and in approaching the client is the most effective coping behavior.

Most students at some time during the psychiatric/mental health experience will have concerns about the staff's responses and their own behavior and mental health. You may fear that the instructor or staff (as well as the client) can read your mind. At times they may make statements that come close to what you were actually thinking. You may feel uncomfortable about or resent having to discuss your feelings, and you may feel your privacy is being invaded. Be assured that although others may be insightful about your behavior, they will not focus on reading your thoughts or changing your identity. It is natural that your instructor and clinical staff may ask you to discuss your feelings. Although there will be some areas of your life that you do not want to share with anyone, in other areas, share as much as you can in order to learn more about the reasons for your behavior.

Exploring the whys of behavior can make you more alert to your own variances, just as studying about the cardiovascular system made you more aware of your own pulse rates and irregularities. Students who developed physical symptoms consistent with whatever disease they were studying are sometimes disconcerted to find the same things happening when they study psychiatric nursing. Remember, there is no sharp line between mental health and illness. No matter how sick a person appears, there are many healthy aspects to the personality. Nor is the healthy person always completely without illness. Accepting yourself as a unique, worthwhile person includes accepting that you also have dimensions of illness as well as health.

As with other fears, honestly acknowledging and discussing your feelings, seeking support, and experimenting with coping behaviors will provide the answer.

Various concerns and feelings of students and ways of dealing with them have been considered. However, we would be remiss if we did not emphasize that the psychiatric/mental health experience can be one of the most exciting and fulfilling opportunities available to you. Witnessing the courage and determination with which clients attack problems, the genuineness and gentleness with which the staff assist, and the energy generated and growth produced for all involved by this intense sharing can be inspiring. Not every student will enjoy the psychiatric experience, but each can learn a great deal about how people grow and about how life works. You may also find that your own emotional health improves during the psychiatric nursing experience.

BUILDING SUPPORT SYSTEMS

Every person needs support and nurturance at times. It is a part of the human condition to have many needs met through other people. Therefore you have a responsibility to build a personal support system. However, others cannot support you unless they know what you feel and need. Much of the interpersonal pain you experience can be attributed to your failure to ask for assistance. You may expect that the people around you will somehow guess what you would like and will provide it, while you remain passive. Such expectations are unrealistic and lead to disappointment if not depression. Granted, it is risky to ask. The other person may not produce. However, you will at least know where you stand. Most people can cope better when they have the facts. Is it better to know that something is not available or to wait and hope for it? Neither is satisfying, but knowing is faster. The sooner you realize something is not effective, the sooner you can make other arrangements. Being supported is vital to your existence, personally and professionally. Therefore, evaluate what support systems are currently available and determine what further development you must undertake.

Your instructor can be a significant support person. She/he knows the specific details of your situation and can offer specific feedback, validations, and suggestions for the nursing process. View your instructor as a friend and mentor as well as a supervisor and evaluator.

Family and friends who are not directly involved in the educational situation have special gifts to offer. Usually they will sympathize, affirm, and offer unquestioning reassurance. Everyone can benefit at times from unconditional support. It is nice to hear, "Don't worry. You can do it. Just do your best and you'll be fine. Don't let them upset you." Although this kind of caring and love feels good and is very necessary, it does have limitations. The deficiency is apparent when you have the urge to respond with, "But you don't understand! I am doing my best and it isn't fine. I can't relax." Often students are also disappointed by the matter-of-fact way friends and family react to their success. This may be because it never occurred to anyone but the student that failure was possible.

When you feel that supportive people do not really understand, you may need to turn to someone who has gone through a similar situation successfully for additional help. The course instructor, or another instructor who was helpful in the past, is a good resource since either one is familiar with the system and the demands involved. The instructor can offer objective opinions of your nursing strengths and limits with specific suggestions for improvement. You will benefit most from contact with people who are kind and courageous enough to tell the truth.

Nurses who have completed their educational programs and whose professional performances you admire are also excellent resources. It is a real comfort to discover that the nurse who seems to function so effectively originally had the same anxieties, made the same mistakes, and felt the same inadequacies and misgivings that you are now experiencing. Practicing nurses are often eager to provide support because they remember how needful they were at times.

Peers can also be a tremendous source of support. The friends you have made in school, the people who have "suffered through" the same things, can give valuable feedback. Sharing fears and reactions provides an opportunity for discovering that you are not alone, that your responses are not unique or bizarre. You can talk in "shorthand" to people who are sitting in the same class or who are experiencing the same clinical situation. Feedback from those who have actually observed an incident is usually more profitable than that offered by those to whom you have to describe what you believe happened.

The trap to avoid when sharing with other students is letting attempts at support deteriorate into destructive gripe sessions. Griping does have some positive aspects. It can help to establish a common frame of reference or to identify and clarify problem areas, and sometimes it just feels good to moan and groan. However, there are limits. Self-pity is contagious. The focus of any truly supportive interaction is problem solving. The peer group can address the following questions: What can I change to make things better? What creative ways can I discover to help me live with the things I cannot change? What worked for you that I might try? What was your experience with the behavior and the consequences of it? Any relationships that increase self-esteem and decrease feelings of helplessness will aid in survival. But gathering together only to ruminate about how impossible, unfair, or horrible things are will result in mutual misery and damage to all involved.

One type of support frequently overlooked is that which we give ourselves. Each person has an obligation to be kind to and to affirm the self. To discover how well you are doing in this pursuit, ask yourself the following questions:

1. Do I acknowledge the positive things I did today? (Initially these might be hard to recognize, but they are there. Acknowledge the little things such as going to class, giving attention to someone who seemed to need it, reading this chapter.)

2. Am I realistic in my expectations of myself? (I'm not perfect. I don't have unlimited energy. I can't do everything well. I can enjoy my successes and be comfortable with my limitations.)

3. Do I look at problematic situations in terms of how they can be improved in the future? (I can moan about the low grade I got, or I can look at my study habits, outside activities, and other factors and decide if I want to make changes.)

4. Do I take some time just for myself to do what feels good to me? (If there's never any free time, use a little time that isn't free. Take a long bath. Read an article that has nothing to do with school. Take a short walk. What you do isn't as important as the fact that you decide to do something for yourself and do it, rather than just wishing you had the time.)

5. Am I as kind to and understanding of myself as I would be with a friend in the same situation? (If I can accept, empathize with, and love others, I have the capacity to do that for myself. Maybe I was just waiting for permission.)

6. Do I ask clearly and specifically for what I need? (There's no advantage to sitting around feeling sorry for myself because no one is guessing correctly about what I want. I can't expect to get what I need if I don't ask for it, including the support and encouragement I'd like from other people.)

When you determine you need help, be honest with yourself and the person(s) you seek out. Let them know your feelings, concerns, and needs.

DEVELOPING COPING SKILLS

As a nurse, you offer psychiatric clients the most valuable gifts you have to give: sincere concern and caring, ability to see beyond the maladaptive behavior to the pain that caused it, and your desire to be helpful while remaining intact yourself. Realize you will not "make" anyone well, but that you will do everything possible to provide an environment in which wellness can happen. In such an environment the client can experience an authentic relationship, can have access to a consistent view of reality, and can feel secure enough to try more effective behavior.

You can develop coping skills to help you be effective in the psychiatric/mental health experience. *Coping involves facing and adjusting to reality.* Increase coping behaviors by *first working through feelings about yourself.* Being human means you have things in common with other humans. You are aware of the feelings and needs of others to the degree that you are self-aware. You can accept differences in others to the degree that you are able to accept positive and negative characteristics in yourself.

Psychiatric clients are people in pain. You may

not immediately understand the origins or complexities of that pain, but you have had similar feelings, and you are now developing specialized skills. Therefore, you can help, not as an expert, but as a caring, eager, sincere beginner. Because your self and personality are the most important equipment you use in psychiatric nursing, it is essential that you *keep yourself in top condition physically and emotionally.* Tools available to keep yourself in top condition emotionally include: self-awareness and values clarification exercises, group discussions, a sound theoretical framework, practical life experiences, reflection, religious or cultural practices, observation, and experimentation with new behaviors. Guidance and support are necessary for developing skills and must be sought if not readily accessible.

You want to pass the course, meet the requirements, and still have opportunities to pursue your individual goals. This requires self-knowledge, an openness to yourself and others, an understanding of the system, and guidance from someone familiar with you and the process. *Expressing fears, concerns, and feelings about the experiences to people who can be supportive and who can offer suggestions and evaluate responses are necessary steps in your adjustment to the psychiatric setting.*

Accept the psychiatric/mental health experience, the setting, and the predetermined objectives as they are and make choices and decisions about how you will expend your energies. You will undoubtedly see and hear things that will disturb and concern you. Some situations will be amenable to change. Others will not. Obviously you are well advised to *focus on what can be altered and let the rest go.*

You will encounter professionals, paraprofessionals, and nonprofessionals whose attitudes and behaviors are different from yours. Again, determine what you can change and what you cannot. Observing others interacting with clients and coworkers can yield vast amounts of information, sometimes more than you can deal with comfortably. *The trap to avoid in this situation is judging what you see before you have thoroughly investigated the situation.* Each person develops a unique style of therapeutic interaction. There are so many variables, such as length and type of relationship, experiences lived through together, present therapeutic goals, and current circumstances, that you cannot hastily evaluate another's approach or the client outcome. It is fine to make judgments

about what you might like to imitate, retain, or reject as you observe others but merely labeling another's performance as "good" or "bad" is usually counterproductive.

Another trap to avoid is assuming that the techniques others use successfully will work for you. Joking with a client is sometimes very effective, but certainly not for every client at all times. You will develop a feel for what works best for you through trial and error as well as through instruction, supervision, and feedback. Some of the approaches you observe, consider, and reject now may be useful later. *As your comfort level and skills increase, you will be able to experiment more and can choose the best from what you have observed for integration into your own style.*

Members of the health care team are often eager to offer their attitudes and opinions about clients to the students. Caution is essential. Often their intent is to protect. Statements such as "You won't get anywhere with him," or "She'll manipulate you if you're not careful" are warnings, but they can interfere with your ability to be helpful. You do not want to alienate coworkers (part of that very important support system) by saying, "That's a terrible attitude," but *you should try* to keep an open mind. What others have experienced with a client is not necessarily what you will experience. So many factors are involved that you can rarely predict exactly how anyone will react in a given situation. *Approaching the client without preconceived ideas gives the relationship a better chance of working.*

Occasionally others in the setting may criticize your performance. Usually this is done in an effort to help. Since you are designated a learner, others may automatically assume the role of teacher in order to balance the situation. Some may even offer advice on matters not related to clinical performance. It is important to *acknowledge criticism positively and evaluate it in terms of appropriateness to you.* There is no point in becoming defensive. Neither is it wise to accept without analysis every criticism offered. If the comments seem valid, use them to plan change. If they do not fit, discard them. If in doubt, check with the instructor or a student whose opinion you value.

Coping with criticism, regardless of the source, is not easy. It seems we are always running into people who are eager to tell us what is wrong with us. If the message consists only of pointing out shortcomings, it is not very valuable. *When some-*

one criticizes what you are doing, you have a right to ask what behaviors would be acceptable as alternatives. It is also your right to explain your rationale for what you are doing. At first you may feel uneasy about being assertive. It is easy to walk away from a negative remark with nothing but a bad feeling about yourself. However, you must find out specifically what the complaint is. You have to take the responsibility and ask. You can make better decisions when you know what is expected. Criticism, like other kinds of input, has to be weighed and discussed and then incorporated or discarded.

Goal setting, along with clarifying your own expectations and asking others to clarify theirs, are *effective coping strategies.* Asking for what you need, rejecting help that is not really helpful, and then asking again will help you through all kinds of stressful situations. Your carefully built support system will assist you.

Applying these coping skills will not only serve you well during the psychiatric/mental health experience, but they will also enable you to appreciate yourself and those around you to a much greater degree. Other methods to manage stress and other coping skills are described in Chapter 12. Those strategies can be as useful to you as to your clients. Chapter 6 also describes other concerns involved in the therapeutic relationship and ways to work through these concerns.

REFERENCES

1. Kramer, M., and C. Schmalenberg, *Path to Biculturalism.* Wakefield, Mass.: Contemporary Publishing, Inc., 1977.

2. Sullivan, H. S., *Conceptions of Modern Psychiatry.* New York: W. W. Norton Co., Inc., 1940.

3. Ward, M. J., *Snake Pit.* New York: The New American Library, Inc., 1946.

2

Theoretical Foundations for Understanding the Developing Person

Study of this chapter will assist you to:

1. Identify major theoretical perspectives for understanding the developing person and his/her behavior and emotional health and illness.

2. Describe some physiological theories about causation of behavior and emotional illness.

3. Compare and contrast the basic frameworks and major concepts of First, Second, and Third Force theorists.

4. Apply ecological theories to a discussion of the role of community factors in the causation of behavior and emotional illness.

5. Compare each of the theories discussed to your own ideas about development of the person and behavior.

6. Apply concepts from the First, Second, and Third Force theorists to nursing practice.

7. Formulate a personal theoretical framework for nursing practice.

This chapter contributed by Ruth Murray, R.N., M.S.N.

AN OVERVIEW OF THEORY DEVELOPMENT

Definitions

A *theory* *is a systematic explanation of events useful to the purposes one has in view.* A theory is *a set of assumptions, facts, concepts, or variables that are systematically connected, can be interpreted, and are used to explain and predict a relatively wide variety of empirical events and actions* (14, 16, 60). A theory interprets what is. However, a theory that holds for one frame of reference may be totally inadequate or misleading for another (27).

Theory can be constructed on many levels, and the amount of data included in a theory will vary. In the study of human behavior and personality, a theory may range from a comprehensive, holistic, molar level to a minute or atomic level. However, no theory of development, behavior, or learning will totally explain all aspects of the person (27, 110, 127), although theories that are more inclusive or molar tend to be more useful to the health professional (27).

Historical Perspectives

People have always tried to explain their environment, themselves, and the events that happened to them. In some areas we have progressed from the magical or pragmatic to complex and scientific explanations. In other areas so little is known that future generations will probably consider our current scientific explanations to be magical or fanciful.

Table 2-1 outlines: (1) the historical progression through the Pre-Modern period of theories about causation of mental illness, (2) causative agent/factor in mental illness and the proponent or theorist, and (3) the treatment methods that have been used because of the beliefs about mental illness. As you read Table 2-1 you may be surprised that some current ideas on causation and treatment strategies were common thousands of years ago. For example, causation of mental illness has been attributed to psychological processes and brain disease both currently and historically. Therapeutic milieu, relaxation methods, and exploration of feelings are treatment methods as old as history itself. You may note that some people still hold some of the ideas that were held in ancient times, for example, that mental illness is caused by the devil or is God's punishment. Some of our ideas on treatment are ancient also, for example, using exorcism and shock so that the person learns better behavior. The table

TABLE 2-1.   Historical Review of Theories about and Treatment of Mental Illness

HISTORICAL ERA	CAUSATIVE AGENT/FACTOR IN MENTAL ILLNESS AND CONTRIBUTIONS OF THEORIST	CONTRIBUTIONS OF THEORY/THEORIST TO TREATMENT
Prehistoric and throughout history, including present preliterate societies and some religious cultural groups.	Supernatural and magical forces, evil spirits, devil, gods, ancestors. Animism—world alive with supernatural spirits that cause illness and evil. Simplistic explanation given.	Shaman, medicine man, voodoo healer, or priest exorcised or removed evil forces. Skull trephining allowed escape of evil (used 2000 B.C.–A.D. 1000). Witch burning to remove evil and save soul. Confined the possessed person in dungeon.
Golden Age Ancient Greece	Punishment for offending gods. Some diseases divine, such as epilepsy; victims granted priesthood.	Mental healing through walking and sleeping in group of temples dedicated to god of healing/medicine, Aesculopius. Religious ceremonies by priests. Medical advice from oracles.
Hippocrates (460–377 B.C.) "Father of Medicine"	Body events, diseased brain, and natural phenomena cause illness. Denied divine causes. Believed body humors basis of personality. First attempt to classify mental illness.	Emphasized doctor–patient relationship. Used warm, humane approach. Concerned for physical comfort: rest, baths, diet, aesthetic environment.
Plato (427–347 B.C.) Philosopher	Organismic view: conflicts between emotion and reason. Believed behavior product of total psychologic process.	Utilized reason and teaching to promote good life and happiness.
Aristotle (384–322 B.C.) Philosopher	Injustice and wrongdoing. Expectation of loss, defeat, or rejection. Imbalance of pain and pleasure.	Emphasized use of reason.
Ancient Rome Asclepiades (first century B.C.) Physician	Emotional imbalance. Distinguished between acute and chronic disease process.	Concerned for physical comfort: baths, massage, music therapy, diets, quiet environment, rest. Objected to bloodletting, purging, and imprisonment.
Aretaeus (first century B.C.) Physician	Emotional factors. Brain affected even if disease elsewhere. Inaccurate description of hysteria: believed caused by wandering uterus. Accurate description of manic-depression. Classi-	Emphasized more humane approach.

TABLE 2-1. Continued

HISTORICAL AREA	CAUSATIVE AGENT/FACTOR IN MENTAL ILLNESS AND CONTRIBUTIONS OF THEORIST	CONTRIBUTIONS OF THEORY/THEORIST TO TREATMENT
	fication of abnormal behavior based on prognosis.	
Celsus (A.D. 14–37) Physician	Flaw in intelligence or understanding.	Emphasized punishment by hunger and chains and fetters and simultaneous teaching through coercion or shock to learn better behavior. Rationale for brutal treatment.
Galen (130–200) Physician	Brain directly involved or affected by other organ disturbances.	Emphasized treatment of total person; believed could not separate mind, body, and environment.
Early Christianity St. Augustine (354–430)	Feelings, mental anguish, and human conflicts. Through written self-analysis, laid groundwork for modern psychodynamic theories. Earliest forerunner of psychoanalysis.	Used introspection and exploration of inner emotional life.
Middle Ages	Supernatural forces. Demons. Disease epidemics believed to cause group hysteria. Combination of demon possession, superstition, and early Christian theology used for explanation.	Monks only medical practitioners of Middle Ages. Monasteries were places of refuge for sick and confinement of insane.
400–600	Person considered a saint or disciple.	In early Middle Ages, believed in sprinkling with holy water; visiting shrines; contact with relics; using herbs.
		Institution in Gheel, Belgium, for retarded and psychotic children, with later family placement.
	Remainder of Middle Ages— abnormal behavior equated with sin; person possessed by devil.	Mentally ill regarded as heretics or traitors. Barbaric treatment: person's body considered an unpleasant habitat for demons, forced to confess to heresy. Witchcraft trials organized by

TABLE 2-1. Continued

HISTORICAL AREA	CAUSATIVE AGENT/FACTOR IN MENTAL ILLNESS AND CONTRIBUTIONS OF THEORIST	CONTRIBUTIONS OF THEORY/THEORIST TO TREATMENT
		church in 1484, by Papal permission, followed by witch burning.
Paracelsus (1493–1541) Physician	Astrological phenomenon— stars and planets.	Argued for rational approach and more humane treatment.
Renaissance Johann Weyer (1515–1576) Physician and first psychiatrist	Rational cause rather than superstition and demons. Inner experiences and disturbed interpersonal relationships. Considered witches to be mentally ill, not caused by the devil. Clinical and descriptive work resulted in separation of medical psychology from theology and resulted in formation of psychiatry as medical specialty.	Emphasized humane medical treatment rather than theological treatment. Argued that treatment should meet needs of people, not rules of institution. Theory on custodial care was corrupted into inhumane care in Bethlem Hospital, London, with result of bedlam.
Wm. Shakespeare (1564–1616)	Unconscious and neurotic conflicts; problems of human motivation and emotions referred to in literature. Described psychotic behavior.	Used drama as mode of understanding.
Age of Reason (17th century) and *Age of Enlightment* (18th century)	Scientific approach to study of mental illness; recorded case studies and attempted to find patterns to abnormal behavior. Concerned with classification.	Gradual increase in tolerance. York Retreat, Quaker custodial facility, established where treatment relied on moral permission and kindness rather than on coercion.
Wm. Harvey (1578–1657)	Interrelationship between psychological and physiological aspects.	
Spinoza (1632–1677)	Mind and body inseparable. Emphasized role of emotions, ideas, desires, and unconcious and conscious mechanisms.	
Wm. Cullen (1712–1790)	Regarded physical defects in nervous system as cause of neurotic behavior.	Cold baths. Bloodletting. Diet. Exercise. Physical therapy.
Anton Mesmer (1734–1815)	Animal magnetism and planets.	Equalization of magnetic field. Used power of suggestion. Basis for later hypnosis (mesmerism).

TABLE 2-1. Continued

HISTORICAL AREA	CAUSATIVE AGENT/FACTOR IN MENTAL ILLNESS AND CONTRIBUTIONS OF THEORIST	CONTRIBUTIONS OF THEORY/THEORIST TO TREATMENT
Romantic Reaction to Age of Reason and Enlightment	Recognized whole person and inner life and mental stresses that underlie behavior.	Emphasized self-awareness.
Reform Movement Philippe Pinel (1745–1826)	Hereditary defect or nervous system lesion. Believed mentally ill should have full status as individuals. Documented observations scientifically and classified illness according to observable characteristics.	Proponent for humane care rather than punishment. Removed chains from male patients and freed female patients in French hospitals. Opened asylum doors. Devised specific treatment for different behaviors.
Moral Treatment Johann Heinroth (1773–1843)	Psychological and moral. Unconscious conflicts between unacceptable impulses and resulting guilt feelings.	Believed hard work, good food, healthy atmosphere, good frame of mind, and firm convictions would resolve problems and help mental illness.
William Hone George Cruikshank V. Chiarugi John Conolly Amariah Brigham Cesare Lombroso Valentine Magnan William Tuke (early 1800s)	Descriptions of mental illness followed medical model; extended to more conditions. Attempted systematic classifications. Mental illness included mental defective, paresis, criminal, and variety of conditions.	Protested inhumane conditions. Fixed schedule. Pleasant surroundings. Diet. No restraints. Physical and mental activities. Rallied public support for enlightened legislation. Establishment of mental hospitals emphasized to ensure proper care.
Benjamin Rush (1745–1813) "Father of American Psychiatry"	Wrote first systematic book on mental illness in America.	Emphasized treatment to occur in hospitals rather than in custodial institution.
Dorothea Dix (1802–1887)		Efforts aimed at building mental hospitals. Worked to abolish cruel treatment.
Clifford Beers (late 1800s–early 1900s)		Ex-mental patient who wrote book, *Mind That Found Itself,* c. 1908; gathered support for citizens' reform group that later became National Association for Mental Hygiene.
Pre-Modern Era Organic View (19th century)	Organic and biological. Classified all abnormal behavior under	Custodial care because of fatalistic belief about progno-

TABLE 2-1.   Continued

HISTORICAL AREA	CAUSATIVE AGENT/FACTOR IN MENTAL ILLNESS AND CONTRIBUTIONS OF THEORIST	CONTRIBUTIONS OF THEORY/THEORIST TO TREATMENT
Emil Kraepelin (1800s)	dementia praecox (schizophrenia) or manic-depressive psychosis. Classified mental illness on basis of behavior; description still used today.	sis.
Wilhelm Griesinger (1817–1868)	Believed disease of brain caused all psychologic disorders; symptoms a clinical sign of underlying disease process. Manifest behavior considered less important than underlying pathology.	Treated as a disease.
Psychologic View— Medical Model		
Jean Martin Charcot (1825–1893)	Hysterical symptoms caused by psychological factors and related to mental abnormalities.	Hypnosis.
Pierre Janet (1859–1947)	Extended Charcot's work on hysteria. Hysteria due to splitting off certain ideas, into unconsciousness, that still influenced behavior.	Hypnosis.
Jean Pierre Falret (1774–1870)		Early attempts at psychotherapy.
Leonardo Branchi Walter Fernald C. Floyd Haviland Isaac Ray Thomas Salmin Elmer Southard (late 1800s– early 1900s)		Early pioneers in mental hygiene movement.

Note: This table purposefully ends in the late 1800s. The rest of this chapter discusses other theorists of the Pre-Modern and Modern eras, beginning with Pavlov and Freud. Chapter 25 and other chapters throughout this book discuss current treatment programs and treatment trends.

also shows that periods of enlightenment were often followed by periods of regressive or harsh ideas.

Throughout your nursing career you will probably continue to see theories come and go, and then be revived again, since a study of medical and nursing history shows such a pattern. Thus, knowing the historical beliefs about causation, disease, treatment, and care is important. Such a study can provide both inspiration and prediction.

CURRENT BIOLOGICAL THEORIES
ABOUT HUMAN DEVELOPMENT AND BEHAVIOR

Research on the physiological basis for behavior has gained sophistication with our advancing technology in studying the brain and nervous system, endocrine functions, and physiological responses in a variety of situations. These findings are having an impact on current beliefs about health, normality, development, and emotional illness. In the following discussion, theories related to genetic, biochemical, and neurophysiological factors as well as to biological deficiencies in emotional illness will be briefly covered. For comprehensive study, you are referred to the text by C. Levinthal (81) and to other references listed at the end of this chapter (45, 95, 96, 136, 138).

Genetic Factors

Understanding of the role of genetic factors has been derived historically from studies focusing on pedigree descriptions, incidence of abnormalities in generations of families, and more recently in direct visual examination of chromosomes and biochemical analyses of genetic material and enzymatic processes (32).

The Mendelian Law of Inheritance states that a dominant gene for disorder in at least one parent will cause, on the average, one-half of the children to inherit the disorder. If both parents have the dominant gene, three-fourths of their children will inherit the disorder. When the disorder is attributed to a recessive gene, the offspring does not inherit the disorder unless the gene was received from both parents. If the gene was received from only one parent, the offspring is not affected by the disorder but will probably pass the gene on to his child (the grandchild), who may or may not inherit the disorder, depending on the genes received from the other parent. If the spouses are *heterozygous* for a recessive gene (*both received the same kind of gene from only one of their parents*), then one-fourth of the children will probably be affected by the disorder. If the spouses are *homozygous* for the recessive gene (*the same kind of gene was received from both of their parents*), then all of the children will probably inherit the disorder (56, 81, 119).

The Mendelian Law is the exception rather than the rule in behavioral disorders. If behavioral defects occur, geneticists feel the defects depend on a combination of many genes acting together to produce a behavioral characteristic (polygenic inheritance). Finding the genetic cause is difficult because environmental effects all contribute to the person's development of genetic potential from the moment of conception on (55, 118, 122, 128).

To isolate environmental factors from genetic effects, researchers have used several methodological designs, such as the family resemblance method, the twin study method, and a combination of the two. The family resemblance method looks for similarity between a person with a disorder and his/her relatives. The twin study method relies on differences between *monozygotic twins* (*from a single ovum and therefore identical*) and between *dizygotic twins* (*from two ova fertilized by two sperm and therefore not identical, i.e., fraternal twins.*) Supposedly, differences in monozygotic twins would be environmental, whereas differences between dizygotic twins could be either environmental or hereditary. Research is also being done on identical and fraternal twins reared apart (56, 81).

Studies have been done on schizophrenic patients to try to prove a biological basis for mental illness. The incidence of schizophrenia is higher in monozygotic twins than in dizygotic twins of the same sex; however, dizygotic twins of opposite sex are rarely both affected by schizophrenia when reared by the same parents. Although the incidence of schizophrenia in dizygotic twins is the same as in siblings, the incidence in monozygotic twins is over 60 percent whether the twins are reared together or apart. It is unknown whether the inheritance of schizophrenia results from a single gene pair, many genes, or the cumulative effects of many genes. Inequality in the twins' prenatal environment may also be a factor. Monozygotic twins do not show 100 percent incidence of schizophrenia, which suggests that environmental influences and other factors play a role along with genetic factors in emotional illness. Generalizations to all people from data of twin studies may be inaccurate since twins differ from the general population in many ways: preterm birth, lower birth weight, older parental age, and different societal response (32, 119). Family studies reveal that parents of schizophrenic children have a 2 to 5 percent rate of schizophrenia, and siblings have a 6 to 10 percent chance of developing the illness. It is unclear whether this incidence results from genetic or interpersonal and environmental causes (128).

Early studies on children born to schizophrenic mothers but reared in an institution or adoptive foster homes showed more psychopathology in these children than in children born to normal mothers. However, the researchers did not account for the effects of antipsychotic medication given to the mothers during pregnancy, effects of institutionalization, lack of relationships found in foster home care, and negative attitudes toward the children of adoptive parents who knew the mothers had been schizophrenic (119).

Genes determine a foundation for reaction or predisposition; the exact behavioral expression depends on many prenatal, parental, and postnatal influencing factors. For example, a specific chromosomal aberration like the presence of an extra chromosome is directly related to Down's Syndrome, with resultant limited intellectual function. Yet the intellectual achievement may be lower than the inherited capacity if the person receives inadequate education, and the achievement may be somewhat higher than indicated by early testing when a loving family and appropriate education coexist to develop fully the inherited potential (123).

Research indicates that heredity is an element in some affective disorders. Twin studies for affective disorders show that monozygotic twins have a 69 percent chance of the illness, compared to a 13 percent chance of dizygotic twins developing an affective disorder. The mode of inheritance is hypothesized to be a dominant gene on the X chromosome, but data are inconsistent from different research centers (45). People who alternate between depression and mania usually have two generations of relatives who have shown similar behavior. Many researchers are looking at hereditary factors along with events and experiences in the person's life to determine what combination of inherited predisposition and stressors produce depressive behavior (119).

In summary, there are two principles that explain how differences in heredity may exert influence. (1) The **Principle of Differential Susceptibility** suggests that *individual differences in heredity exist that make people susceptible to the influence of certain environments.* Given different experiences, a person with certain hereditary potential would develop in different ways. For example, the person with hereditary predisposition to schizophrenia would be likely to develop the disease if raised in a certain kind of environment. (2) The **Principle of Differential Exposure** suggests *inherited*

characteristics cause differing reactions from people, which in turn affect or shape the personality of the individual. For example, body build, facial structure, and presence or absence of overall physical attractiveness result primarily from inheritance. People perceive, judge the actions, and react more favorably to physically attractive children than to less attractive children. Over time, reactions of others contribute to formation of the self-concept, positive or negative feelings about self, and a sense of competency or incompetency that may affect behavior toward others or general performance. Excessive negative reaction from others may predispose to abnormal behavior and even mental illness if the stress is great enough (128).

There is much yet unknown about the manner and extent to which early individual differences result in later personality differences. Many variables are environmental in nature; even early transactions between mother and child tend to obscure genetic characteristics (128).

Biochemical Factors

The research on relationship between biochemical factors and behavior involves three areas: neurochemistry, hormones, and blood components.

Neurochemistry

Neurochemistry is implicated in some affective disorders. The amount of biogenic amines, especially the *neurotransmitters, chemicals involved in transfer or modulation of nerve impulses from one cell to another*, appear to be related to mood disorders. Catecholamines, including adrenalin, nonadrenalin, dopamine, and serotonin, are important neurotransmitters in the brain and are involved in emotional states such as arousal, fear, rage, pleasure, motivation, exhilaration, sleep, and wakefulness. Although a deficiency of one neurotransmitter, norepinephrine, in certain areas of the brain appears to be a causal factor in depression, the evidence is inconclusive. Deficiency of another neurotransmitter, serotonin, is found in both depressed and manic persons (81, 103, 119).

Dopamine, another neurotransmitter, may contribute to schizophrenia in one of three ways: (1) increased sensitivity of dopamine at nerve terminals, (2) increased sensitivity of dopamine receptors, and (3) reduction of substances that reduce dopamine effects. In one study, injections of a small amount of chemical methylphenidate, which like amphetamine causes release of dopamine and prevents re-uptake of dopamine from the synaptic gap, caused increased psychotic behavior in schizophrenics but not in normal persons. When the injection of the chemical was repeated with schizophrenics who were in remission without symptoms for a month, their reaction did not differ from that of normal subjects. Apparently dopamine levels are lower in schizophrenics when they are functioning normally, and the increased dopamine level was not enough to push them to psychosis (119). Other variables contributing to psychosis were not explored in this study.

Studies are being done on monoamine oxidase (MAO) neurotransmitters in relation to synthesis, secretion, transport, reabsorption, and degradation. People with chronic schizophrenia have half the normal level of MAO in their platelets, but normal levels are found in people with acute schizophrenia (132).

Biochemical differences between schizophrenic, depressed, and sociopathic persons suggest that their maladjustment may be linked to biochemical imbalances. Biochemical theories for schizophrenia suggest a blocked metabolic pathway, and the resultant accumulation of chemical byproducts appears responsible for the increased abnormal behavior (132). Families with affective disorders show variations in conversion of tyrosine to catecholamines and increased enzyme activity in conversion of norepinephrine and epinephrine to metanephrine (45).

The relationships need to be clarified by further research. However, chemical imbalances appear to be improved by various medications. Pharmacology texts explain these drug actions in detail.

Hormonal Factors

Hormonal factors, based on changes in the endocrine system during stress, or endocrine system disorders may contribute to emotional illness. Steroid hormones are increased during stress behavior. Yet physiological and psychological systems are complexly interrelated. S. Schacter and J. Singer's research involved giving adrenalin to four groups of people to stimulate anxiety (121). The first group was told the physical effects that would result. The second group was not told of the effects. The third group was told to expect effects that were incorrect for adrenalin, and the fourth group was given a placebo. The subjects in the first three groups had different reactions from the same drug, depending on the different expectations they held. This finding indicates that higher thought processes influence physiological reactions as well as the subjective experience of emotional states (80, 119, 121).

Blood Components

Blood components are also implicated in emotional illness. The orthomolecular view holds that vitamin deficiencies or food allergies may cause schizophrenia. Others claim that an abnormal blood protein, taraxein, causes schizophrenia. Yet research results are inconclusive. For example, taraxein injected into volunteers caused schizophreniclike behavior, but another researcher found the same results when salt water was injected. The crucial factor was that the subjects had expected the substance to "make them crazy." Massive doses of vitamins either improve schizophrenia or make it worse, depending on the researchers. Severe nutritional deficiencies during infancy and the preschool years have been associated with detrimental alterations in brain development, alterations that in turn retard physical growth and behavioral development. Whether abnormal physical growth and reduced intellectual development contribute to mental illness is unknown (32, 119, 136); there is no known link to specific mental illness.

Finding organic or biochemical differences between normal and emotionally ill people is not difficult. It is the explanation that accounts for these differences that is difficult to find.

Neurophysiological Factors

All behavior is mediated by the nervous system; however, neurophysiological factors in emotional illness are inconclusive. Some specific motor and speech functions and various sensations in different body parts can be traced to specific brain areas; there are also large areas of the cerebral cortex that do not have localized functions. Relationships between symptoms and organic damage cannot always be determined (119).

Biological Deficiencies

Biological Stressors

Biological stressors may change behavior. For example, severe malnutrition prenatally and during the first six months of life can contribute to low intellectual capacity, and behavior problems may result in childhood and later in adulthood. Too much or too little sugar may also have a rapid effect on behavior. Brain patterns revealed by neurological scanners show that the brains of normal, manic-depressive, and schizophrenic people appear differently and differ in the metabolism of glucose. Studies of schizophrenics show decreased metabolism of glucose in the frontal lobe; manic-depressive persons, manic phase, show increased metabolism of glucose in the brain. Medications, such as perphenazine for schizophrenics and lithium for manic patients, appear to return brain metabolic activity to normal (78). Sensory deprivation and isolation can result in perceptual and motor changes, reduced reasoning (including reduced problem-solving and learning), mood changes, and sometimes hallucinations (60, 138).

Sleep Deprivation

Sleep deprivation research shows that after 40 sleepless hours, behavior and mood changes and perceptual distortions occur. After 100 sleepless hours, psychoticlike symptoms appear. Research on the relationship of biological rhythms and emotional illness is inconclusive. Persons under stress often change living rhythms; forced changes in biological rhythms is a stressor, and mood, motor, and behavioral changes can occur (60, 138).

Biological factors are important in some, but not all, emotional and behavioral disturbances. The brain and the rest of the body constitute *one system*. Disorders of behavior may originate in the glandular system since neural function is dependent on certain hormones. Disorders of behavior may also originate in the person's perceptions and thoughts. Mental stress can contribute to emotional illness without any predisposing factor of heredity or biological deficiency. Both biology and experience are important; they may operate separately or simultaneously in causation and do not preclude one another (60).

CURRENT PSYCHOLOGICAL THEORIES ABOUT HUMAN DEVELOPMENT AND BEHAVIOR

A number of psychological theories have been formulated to explain human development, behavior, personality, and mental health and illness. This discussion is not meant to be exhaustive.

Utilization of these theories in therapy and nursing practice will be presented in Table 2-10 at the end of the chapter. Examples in this table are not comprehensive in their application but are meant to stimulate further thought and discussion.

A current model to help understand behavior and its underlying reasons and the approaches to working with people in a helping relationship is to categorize the many schools of thought (and the different theorists) under either First, Second, or Third Force theories. There are significant differences between these different theories or schools of thought (Force) in terms of their beliefs about human behavior, the perspectives from which their observations are made, and their different foci of learning and therapy. These theories are grouped together under the term *Force* because they go in the same general direction of beliefs.

The First Force is identified with the Behaviorist and Neo-Behaviorist Schools of Psychology, whose focus is the stimulus-response link. Behaviorism extends the product and input-output perspective of technology to the human. Technology is viewed as no different than the human and may be viewed as superior. The Second Force was originally identified with Psychoanalytic Theory, both Freudian and Neo-Freudian, but has been expanded to include cognitive and developmental theorists. The Third Force was first identified with humanistic psychology and now includes existential and phenomenological theorists.

Although the three Forces, and families of theorists within each Force, will be discussed separately, a theorist who considers himself in one of the families may disagree with another theorist from the same family. For example, the Behaviorists C. Hull and B. F. Skinner would disagree on some points, and followers of K. Koffka and C. Lewin would each differ in their explanation of Field Theory (14). Further, no theorist or group of theorists have all the answers about human behavior; none of them are complete in their interpretations. Yet the theorists within one Force hold certain ideas in common about personality development and behavior. This classification of theorists can assist you in synthesizing and using the main ideas of several theorists who hold similar views about the person and in realizing that often theorists who sound very different in their theory may be stating basically similar concepts.

First Force Theory

Overview

First Force theorists are Behaviorists who adhere to stimulus-response conditioning theories. This scientific approach to the study of the person began in the late 1800s, and results from animal experiments were the primary source of data until recently. These results have been generalized to people. The Neo-Behaviorist obtains data for laws of behavior by observing the human's behavioral response to stimuli. The person is considered in terms of component parts. The focus is atomistic or reductionistic in that isolated, small units of behavior or parts of behavioral patterns are objectively observed and analyzed from the perspective of nonmental, physiological associations. There is no concern with or study of other aspects of the person. Introspection or emphathic projection is not used for data collection (25, 139, 140).

View of the Human

First Force theorists define the living organism as a self-maintaining mechanism. The essence of a human machine is a system of receptors (sense organs), conductors (neurons), switching organs (brain and spinal cord), and effectors (muscles) attached to levers (bones), along with fueling and controlling organs, such as the stomach and glands. The person is seen as an object, a reactive organism responding mechanically, automatically, involuntarily, overtly, and quantitatively to past conditionings. The person is envisioned as a highly complicated machine, a collection of predictable responses programmed by various stimuli or causes. The person is regarded as neither inherently good nor evil and is a product of learning. The person is acted upon or reinforced by the environment, which causes predictable behavior (25, 60).

Because the focus is on physiological processes and identifiable aspects of the person, subjective, unobservable, unique, and inner aspects of the human are denied or dismissed as illusory. There are no concepts that explain self-concept; ideas; emotions such as love, joy, sadness, or anger; the meaning in a situation; memory; understanding; insight; empathy; the person initiating and being an active agent in his/her behalf; or variety in human behavior. The person has sensory input; he/she does not perceive. There are no biases except for past conditioning. The person simply acts to reduce a need; there is a natural tendency and drive to satisfaction. The learner or the client is considered deficient, which results in activity or behavior called *learning*. Rest or cessation of behavior follows reward (25, 60).

View of Education and Therapy

The goals of education and psychiatric treatment are to: (1) control the person's behavior; (2) help the person become more efficient and realistic, as defined by others in the environment; (3) move toward a goal set by external standards; and (4) create learning by forming bonds, connections, or associations. Responses that are appropriate are rewarded and therefore are stamped in to form habits (59, 60).

The teacher or therapist is at the center of and in control of the educational or treatment process. The learner or client is passive. Programmed learning is considered efficient education, with the teacher functioning as a reinforcement machine to help the learner achieve behavioral objectives. The teacher sets up the external situation to get the desired response and creates organized sequential steps so that the person achieves a goal and gets a reward. The therapist looks on the treatment process from the outside, controlling interchanges and diagnosing and interpreting the client's statements and problems. That which is predetermined will be accomplished. Intent or insight is not considered. Bad, superstitious, or inefficient behavior is removed from the person by *shaping, setting up the situation so that the person acts in a desired way, and then rewarding the desired behavior* (25, 119).

If education or treatment is individualized, it is as a means to an end since the emphasis is on the preconceived end product rather than on the process. The teacher or therapist sees self as part of the system, and he or she exists to carry out the rules of the institution. There is an assembly line sameness to learning, treatment, and nursing practice. Nursing as a role is an extension of a man-made structure (the institution and the law), and practice must concern itself with legal regulations and constraints (25, 119).

First Force Theorists

Early Theorists

Ivan Pavlov laid the foundations for the Behavioral School. He was a Russian physiologist and pharmacologist of the midnineteenth century who wrote about psychic processes during his study of salivation and flow of digestive juices in dogs. His experiments established *classical conditioning*. An *unconditioned or new stimulus is presented with a stimulus that is already known just prior to the response to the conditioned, familiar stimulus. The organism learns to respond to a new stimulus in the same way it responded to a familiar stimulus.* Associations are shifted from one stimulus to another, with the same response being made to the substituted stimuli. J. B. Watson's experiments showed that fears and phobias could result from classical conditioning, and could in turn be unlearned (60). Some of the present-day relaxation methods use classical conditioning. The client is trained to respond to a therapist's direction by relaxing a muscle group; then music is played while the therapist gives directions for relaxing. Later the person is able to respond automatically by relaxing when music plays (14, 60, 119). Classical conditioning is also used in the Lamaze preparation for childbirth. Emotions are believed by Behaviorists to arise from body changes or to be learned through classical conditioning. Emotions arise in the present situation, based on past learning that is associated with the present event. For example, a person likes men with beards because he/she learned this response as a result of associating beards with a kindly bearded uncle during childhood.

John B. Watson is considered the founder of Behaviorism, and Edward L. Thorndike was an early American disciple. Both emphasized physiological associations and connections in understanding psychological processes. E. Guthrie and C. Hull also contributed to Behaviorism (14).

Although contemporary psychologists do not use these theories in their original form, many psychologists have sufficiently similar orientations to be called *Neo-Behaviorists.* Leading stimulus-response conditioning theorists who are currently influential include Robert Gagne, Neal Miller, John Dollard, Robert Glaser, and B. F. Skinner. Because these theorists all focus on stimulus-response conditioning in some form to explain behavior, the terms *Behaviorism* and *S-R Conditioning Theory* are used interchangeably (14, 60).

Several leading theorists will be discussed in the following pages. Theorists frequently utilized in psychiatric nursing are discussed in detail. Other theorists of the First Force will then be presented in Table 2-2.

TABLE 2-2.   Summary of Additional First Force Theorists

THEORIST/THEORY	MAJOR HYPOTHESES/ASSUMPTIONS	IMPLICATIONS FOR EDUCATION AND THERAPY
Edwin Guthrie Theory of Continuity in Learning	1. Closeness of occurrence of stimulus and response emphasized. 2. Behavior is any complex combination of specific actions, which combine to make total act or event. 3. Learning occurs in one trial (*all or nothing*). 4. Person always learns what was presented or done last (*Postremity*).	1. Specific instructions must be given about performing any behavior rather than using abstract general instructions. 2. Everything must be taught in the smallest content units possible. 3. Specific responses in a situation are required. 4. Learner should never leave a learning situation with wrong answer or incorrect response, or will always behave in the wrong way. 5. Teacher or therapist must be in charge. Learner must be caught in the act of doing what is desired in order for a new stimulus to become associated with desirable behavior.
Clark Hull Systematic Behavior Theory	1. Behavior or learning stamped in by increments. 2. *Principle of Primary Reinforcement:* Decrease of physiological drive a motivating force; strengthens response to stim-	1. Learning affected by activity, practice, training, observation, and sensory experience. 2. Language and nonverbal behavior that accompany feeding or physical care remain powerful secondary reinforcers.

TABLE 2-2. Continued

THEORIST/THEORY	MAJOR HYPOTHESES/ASSUMPTIONS	IMPLICATIONS FOR EDUCATION AND THERAPY
	ulus so that response more likely to recur. 3. *Principle of Secondary Reinforcement:* Any stimulus supplied with drive reduction will become a secondary reinforcer. 4. *Postulate of Reactive Inhibition:* Every action results in after-effect of fatigue or a reactive inhibition preventing further response. 5. *Goal-Gradient Hypothesis:* The closer a person comes to a goal, the more active (eager) the response. Responses closest to reinforcement are most effectively learned. Sequences in activity are learned in reverse. 6. *Fractional Antedating Response:* Learning means person solves situation without help and anticipates what to do in similar situation. 7. *Habit Family Hierarchy:* Responses occur in a hierarchy; some more likely to occur in a situation than others. Learning consists of rearranging responses or habits. 8. *Continuity Hypotheses:* Learning continuous and cumulative. Reinforcement strengthens response, even if person unaware learning is occurring.	3. Avoid teaching or counseling when client is fatigued, irritable, or avoiding situation; limit amount of practice at one time. 4. Maintain reinforcement at crucial times during learning. Do not restrict or end learning session when person near goal. 5. All steps in an activity must be equally practiced or teach skill in backwards order. 6. Counseling and teaching directed to make person independent in problem solving and able to determine hierarchy of response. 7. Reinforce behavior only if it should be learned; learning may occur when neither client nor nurse is aware of or planning learning. Evoke desired response so it can be rewarded.

Robert Gagne
 	
Information Processing Theory
	1. Behavioristic eclectic approach to psychology of learning.
	
	2. Any learning requires prior learning of simpler or subordinate content.
	  a. Signal learning: Classical conditioning; person makes general response to signal.
	  b. Stimulus-response learning: Instrumental conditioning or discriminated operant response. Person discriminates which stimulus results in reinforcement and which does not; response increasingly differentiated.
	  c. Chaining: Series of connected or sequential stimuli and responses; motor or verbal associations.
	  d. Verbal association: Verbal chains.
	  e. Multiple discrimination: Discriminative learning. Person responds differently to similar stimuli.
	  f. Concept learning: Common response
		1. Theory basis for mechanistic instructional technology associated with competency-based or mastery education or behavior modification.
		
		2. Student-teacher interaction, creative or aesthetic learning, or discovery learning is ignored in theory.
		
		3. Use hierarchy of learning in teaching plan.
		
		4. As a teacher, first motivate client through creating anticipation for reward or reinforcement. Motivation or sense of striving for goal will increase attention to stimulus. Knowledge is stored in the brain and recalled in response to cues. Teaching must involve giving cues to aid recall and transferring of learning to produce observable behavior. Then teach in a way that desired learning is achieved so that person can be given feedback and be reinforced.

TABLE 2-2.   Continued

THEORIST/THEORY	MAJOR HYPOTHESES/ASSUMPTIONS	IMPLICATIONS FOR EDUCATION AND THERAPY
	to collection or class of stimuli that differ widely from each other in appearance. g. Rule learning: Chain of two or more concepts; superconcept; behavior governed by internalized state of capabilities or pattern of response. h. Problem solving: Two or more rules or principles combined to produce higher order rule by using a new capability, thinking, discovery, or learning strategy. Person constructs own solution or discovers previously learned rules to solve novel situation.	
Neal Miller and John Dollard (Utilization of theories of Pavlov, Hull, and Freud)	1. Elaborate on and formulate conflict theory, beginning with Lewin's ideas: a. Approach-approach conflicts are resolved in favor of more attractive alternative. b. Approach-avoidance conflicts cause alternating behavior toward ambivalent choices. c. Avoidance-avoidance conflicts cause ongoing unstable behavior and no positive resolutions; many conflicts related to sexual and aggressive impulses. 2. Behavior has physiological and biochemical substrates. 3. Organism can learn control of visceral responses considered involuntary. 4. Environmental stimuli influence behavior; person in turn influences environment. 5. Behavior learned and can be unlearned. 6. Four fundamentals of learning: a. Drive or motivation that is biological or secondary. b. Cue or stimulus. c. Response in thought, feeling, or action. d. Reinforcement. 7. Response hierarchy to any stimulus; person makes one of several responses. Reinforced responses most likely to reoccur and are higher in hierarchy of response.	1. Helping client work through conflicts and their basis is part of teaching and therapy. Conflict causes less anxiety, which causes less effective behavior. 2. Physiological and biochemical bases to motivation, reinforcement, and behavior result in psychologic illness; symptoms that are noticed and reinforced meet needs and are continued. Consider motivation in treatment. 3. Control of involuntary visceral responses basis for biofeedback; learning to control body processes and symptoms. 4. Use learning theories in treating mental illness so that abnormal behavior is unlearned. 5. Rearrange hierarchy response in client. 6. Extinction of behavior occurs with no reinforcement. 7. Certain responses in hierarchy prevents recall, labeling of, and ability to solve problems. Therapist is a teacher who listens, accepts, creates trusting atmosphere, reduces fear-anxiety, and reinforces so that new behavior learned and higher mental processes used for problem solving. Reward attempts at new behavior; create situations so fear-anxiety overcome.

TABLE 2-2.   Continued

THEORIST/THEORY	MAJOR HYPOTHESES/ASSUMPTIONS	IMPLICATIONS FOR EDUCATION AND THERAPY
	8. Conflict is basis for neurosis, which results from depression.	

Thorndike: S-R Bond Theory or Connectionism

E. Thorndike was the most dominant figure in American psychology for much of the twentieth century. From experiments with cats, he formulated a theory of learning called *S-R Bond Theory* or *Connectionism*, which affected every educational facility directly and many psychiatrists and mental health facilities at least indirectly. Thorndike's theory implies that through *instrumental conditioning, a specific response is linked with a specific stimulus, and the response is followed by a reward or is instrumental in bringing about reinforcement.* The reward increases the likelihood of the response recurring, thereby causing a behavioral change. These links, bonds, or connections are products of biological, synaptic changes in the nervous system. Thorndike thought that trial and error (selecting and connecting) was primarily responsible for S-R connections but that learning was a process of "stamping in" connections in the nervous system that had nothing to do with insight or understanding (14, 60). Transfer of learning was facilitated when the second situation was identical to the first.

Thorndike is best known for three laws, which are paraphrased and applied as follows (14, 60):

1. *Law of Readiness:* When the person is ready to perform or learn, it is satisfying to do so. It is annoying not to be able to act when a state of readiness exists or when action is demanded but there is no readiness. In education and therapy, the readiness level of the person toward action, learning, or behavioral change must be assessed and is considered essential for results.

2. *Law of Effect:* When a connection is made between a stimulus and response and is accompanied by a satisfying state of affairs, the connection is increased. If a person is ready to respond, the response is itself pleasurable, and the response will be fixed or learned. When working with the client, the teaching-learning situation should be satisfying, pleasurable, or harmonious, rather than boring, harsh, or conflictual, in order for the person to follow through with directions or suggestions.

3. *Law of Exercise* (Repetition): Whenever a connection is made between a stimulus and response, the connection's strength is increased. The more times a stimulus-induced response is repeated or the person performs an activity, the longer it will be retained in behavior.

Thorndike later claimed that exercise and repetition were not important other than to provide an opportunity to give reinforcement. Behavior that is not rewarded would become boring and be discontinued. Yet most people continue to apply the Law of Exercise because repetition is used in education. However, repetition may be considered excessive by the learner, and too much repetition of an idea in therapy may cause resistance to carrying out directions (60).

One of Thorndike's secondary laws, *Associative Shifting,* or *Stimulus Substitution,* is now considered important by all behaviorists. The law states that any response can be linked with any stimulus; the person's purposes or thoughts have nothing to do with learning (14, 60). This is an example of automatic behavior, which all people use in certain situations, although such behavior would be inappropriate elsewhere. The social courtesies are an example. If too much behavior undergoes associative shifting, the behavior may be inappropriate, and the person may be considered emotionally ill.

Other ideas and principles proposed by Thorndike remain in use today. He advocated reward of acceptable behavior (strengthening a connection) rather than punishment of undesirable behavior. The *Principle of Set or Attitude* states that the person's attitude or mental set guides learning and behavior change; the response is set or determined by enduring adjustment patterns that result from being reared in a certain environment or culture. The mind set or attitude will determine what will be satisfying or annoying to the person. Certainly the client who has an attitudinal set against counseling is unlikely to benefit by it (14, 60).

Skinner: Operant Conditioning Theory

B. F. Skinner is well known for his Operant Conditioning Theory, which builds on the theories of Watson and Thorndike. His animal studies with the "Skinner Box" and his espousal of Radical Behaviorism leave no place in learning theory for consciousness, awareness, sensation, drive, or any subjective, emotional, or experiential concepts. He sees psychology as a science of overt behavior and considers the purposes of psychology to be the prediction and control of the behavior of individuals. Operations of the nervous system cannot be confirmed by observation, so Skinner feels related theories make little contribution to a scientific psychology (126).

According to Skinner, *behavior is an overt response that is externally caused and is primarily controlled by its consequences.* There are no intervening variables. The environmental stimuli will determine how a person alters his/her behavior and people or objects in the environment. Feelings or emotions are, at best, the accompaniments or result, not the cause of behavior. Innate or hereditary reflexes activate the internal glands and smooth muscles, but reflexive behavior accounts for little of human behavior (14, 60, 126).

Learning is a change in the form or probability of response as a result of conditioning. *Operant conditioning is the learning process whereby a response (operant) is shaped and is made more probable or frequent by reinforcement. Transfer is an increased probability of response in the future.* Responses or a set of acts are called *operant* because they operate on the environment and generate consequences. The important stimulus is the one immediately *following* the response, not the one preceding it. Operant conditioning occurs in most everyday life activities, according to Skinner. People constantly cause others to modify their behavior by reinforcing certain behavior and ignor-

ing other behavior. People learn to balance, walk, talk, play games, and handle instruments and tools because they are reinforced after performing a set of motions, thereby increasing the repetition of these motions. Social and ethical behaviors are learned as people are reinforced to continue them through their reinforcing of others for the same behaviors. Operant reinforcement improves the efficiency of behavior. An example of operant conditioning that you may see is the typical behavior seen in patients who have been institutionalized for many years. If attention is given only when the patient talks incoherently, neglects hygiene, speaks of hallucinations, or generally "acts crazy," the attention, even if negative, reinforces the responses to the institutional environment (14, 60, 126).

Positive reinforcement occurs when the presence of a stimulus strengthens a response; negative reinforcement occurs when withdrawal of a stimulus strengthens the tendency to behave in a certain way. A positive reinforcer is food, water, or a smile. A negative reinforcer consists of removing noxious stimuli, such as an electric shock or pain. Skinner's theory emphasizes positive reinforcement. He rejects the use of negative reinforcement or aversive control, contending that this merely produces escape and/or avoidance behavior. A *reinforcement schedule is a pattern of rewarding behavior at fixed time intervals, with a fixed number of responses between reinforcements.* Reinforcement does not strengthen a specific response, but rather it tends to strengthen a general tendency to make the response, or a class of responses, in the future. Thus trial-and-error learning does not exist (14, 126).

Punishment consists of presenting a negative stimulus or removing a positive one. Experiments show that punishment does not reduce a tendency to respond. Apparently reward strengthens behavior because the response is stamped in. However, punishment does not weaken behavior because the response cannot be stamped out. *Extinction, letting a behavioral response die by not reinforcing it,* is preferred instead of punishment for breaking habits. Extinction is a slower process than reinforcement in modifying behavior (14, 60, 126).

There are two types of operant reinforcement that cover most human behavior, along with reflex conditioning: (1) stimulus discrimination and (2) response differentiation. Discrimination of stimuli involves establishing certain behavior as a result of a given stimulus preceding or accompanying the behavior and then reinforcing the behavior. Imitative behavior is an example. It arises over time because of discriminative reinforcement. You wave to someone because of the reinforcement, not because of the stimulus of the other person's hand waving. Differentiation of responses improves motor skills. The person selects a motion because it was reinforced. In this process, reinforcement must be immediate (14, 60).

Application of Skinner's theory is threefold. His theory, when applied to clinical and classroom problems, is called *behavior modification*. When applied to courses of study, this theory is called *programmed learning* and uses teaching machines. When his theory is applied to physiological problems, it is called *biofeedback* (49, 126).

***Behavior Modification** is the deliberate application of learning theory and principles of conditioning, thereby structuring different social environments to teach alternate behaviors and to help the person gain some measure of control over behavior and environment.* Shaping is also a procedure designed to achieve behavioral change. ***Shaping** refers to the gradual modification of behavior by breaking a complex behavior into small steps, and reinforcing each small step that is a closer and closer approximation to the final desired behavior.* Once the desired response has been established and maintained by a continuous reinforcement schedule (i.e., each time the desired response is seen, it is reinforced), the next step is to switch to an ***intermittent schedule of reinforcement**, whereupon reinforcement is contingent upon increasingly multiple emissions of the desired behavior.* After this, occasional reinforcement will keep the desired behavior going. In behavior modification, the behavior must first be reinforced each time it occurs, and then reinforcement can be gradually tapered off until the behavior is learned. Behavior that has been maintained by an intermittent schedule of reinforcement is highly resistant to extinction (14, 126). For example, to teach a patient to talk, you would first reward him/her, possibly with food, every time there was the slightest movement of lips. Later, the reward would be given only for an utterance. Eventually food would be given only for sounds of words, then phrases, and then meaningful sentences.

The aim of behavioral therapy is maximum benefit for the client and society, but behavioral therapy is exclusively reliant on the therapist's judgment and goals for the client. Sometimes aversive methods are used to change behavior. For example, seclusion may be used as part of behavior therapy. The purpose is not punishment but time out; for example, to allow a tantrum to run its course without accidental reinforcement and without triggering similar behavior in other people. Or punishment by a brief electric shock may be used to decrease self-destructive or autistic behaviors. These strategies are seen as no different than punishment and deprivation, which are standard techniques in child rearing (14, 126). Some parents do not question sending a child to bed without a meal as punishment, and parents may even be criticized by other parents if they do not spank their children for naughty behavior.

Before beginning a behavior modification program, the therapist must analyze the following: (1) maladaptive behavior, or the behavior to be decreased, (2) target, or desired observable outcome, (3) current repertoire of behaviors, which is a starting point to get to desired behaviors, (4) environmental factors supporting present behavior, (5) explicitly specified steps to get client from current to desired behaviors, and (6) consequences that are considered as rewards or punishment by the client and can be manipulated to alter the subject's behavior. Consequences may be: (1) material rewards (money, food, trinkets), (2) surrogate rewards (tokens, stars, or points on a chart), (3) social rewards (approval or joining in group activities), and (4) behavioral rewards (opportunity to do special activities). Presentation of each new program step or behavioral unit, contingent on meeting requirements of the preceding one, can also be viewed as challenging and intrinsically reinforcing and thus will maintain progress. Behavior therapy deals with a specific problem at a time rather than with a combination of all the perceived behavioral problems. The client is told that he/she is responsible for a certain behavior and is capable of attaining a higher degree of competence (12, 14, 80, 126, 137).

Behavior modification includes using techniques such as operant conditioning for many situations, such as to: (1) replace undesirable behaviors of autistic, retarded, or normal children; (2) reduce self-destructive behavior, such as anorexia nervosa or head banging; (3) train parents, teachers, probation officers, and nurses to be more efficient in their roles; (4) reduce specific maladaptive behaviors such as stuttering, tics, poor hygiene, or messy eating habits; (5) promote institutional control through token economies; (8) control physical symptoms through biofeedback; and (9) control behavior that is seen as a problem by others in the terminally ill person.

Wolpe: Desensitization Theory

Joseph Wolpe uses Skinner's principles in deconditioning of anxiety or desensitization of phobias or other neurotic behaviors (137). When treating symptoms of fear by desensitization, the person is helped to relax completely. Then over many sessions, the person is presented with progressively more threatening situations and is instructed to remain simultaneously relaxed. Then the person is asked to think of the feared object but to stop thinking about it if he/she feels uneasy. Step by step the person is helped to remain relaxed while thinking about all the factors that have previously been frightening. After a number of treatments, the person can face directly, with feelings of relaxation, what was frightening (137).

The major criticism of Wolpe's therapy is that only the symptom and not the underlying problem is treated. Therefore, symptom substitution, another maladaptive behavior replacing the extinguished behavior, will occur. Wolpe states that the behavior, not the symptom, is the problem. He denies symptom substitution (24). Additional information on Wolpe's techniques is available in Lebow (80).

Because behavior modification programs vary in techniques and are applicable to many situations, you are referred to M. Baltes and M. Zerbe (6), R. Bernie and W. Fordyce (12), I. Goldiamond (49), G Redmond (109), B. Rottkamp (118), M. Swanson and A. Woolson (130), and H. Whitman and S. Lukes (135).

Glaser: Reality Therapy

William Glaser is the founder of Reality Therapy, which derives its name from the insistence on dealing with behavior in the real world rather than with a client's subjective interpretation of feelings and thoughts (46). Reality Therapy can be used with people of any age and with any problem. Like problems are handled in the same manner (8, 47).

According to Reality Therapy, the two basic psychological needs of all humans are (1) to love and to be loved, and (2) to feel worthwhile to self and others. These needs are not being met in the person who needs treatment. The severity of the symptoms reflects the degree to which needs are not met (46, 47).

The reality therapist helps the client to meet these needs by teaching what is realistic, responsible, and right behavior. The therapist focuses on the present behavior rather than on interpretations of past events, feelings, attitudes, insights, or reasons. The past is discussed only if it pertains to the present. Talk during therapy centers on the client's strengths and capacities as well as on problems. The therapist elicits a commitment from the client to change behavior but avoids imposing values on the client. The therapist supports the client with personal involvement, enabling the client to face that he/she is responsible for personal behavior and change. Specific alternatives are presented by the therapist; the therapist is responsible for teaching the client better ways to fulfill needs. The client is encouraged to make a plan aimed at a desired goal and is not permitted to make excuses or place blame if the plan fails or if the commitment is not kept. The client is encouraged to make choices and live responsibly from day to day, taking into consideration consequences to self and others. However, the client is not punished or rejected as he/she struggles to change behavior, even if success is not always reached (46, 47). Belief in the client's integrity is important.

The most effective ways for the therapist to use the involvement-commitment process is to remember the following points: (1) a single experience with definition of a problem, involvement, and satisfaction of the person's needs does not guarantee responsible behavior in the next experience of a similar nature; (2) responsible behavior is not necessarily generalized by the client and applied in a cognitive way; (3) the therapist's demands for behavioral standards may be unrealistic for the client; (4) the client may find ways of satisfying his/her psychological needs without using responsible behavior; (5) behavior changes slowly; thus, the therapist or client should never give up (8, 46).

The goal of therapy is to develop a sense of responsibility defined as the ability to satisfy one's own needs without interfering with the needs of others, while behaving responsibly. The therapeutic problem is to get the client to abandon what may be called the "primitive pleasure principle" and to adopt long-term, wise pursuit of pleasure, satisfaction, joy, happiness, which the reality principle implies (8, 46).

Advocates of Reality Therapy differ from conventional psychiatry and clinical psychology in the following ways:

1. They do not believe in a concept of mental illness and its associated concepts of classification and diagnosis. Such labeling tends to relieve the individual of responsibility for behavior.

2. They work in the present and future, and do not get involved with the past, which is unchangeable.

3. They relate to clients as people, not transference figures.

4. Unconscious conflicts are considered excuses for undesirable behavior.

5. Morality of behavior is emphasized; i.e., it is important for a person to know if behavior is right or wrong.

6. Reality Therapy stresses teaching people behaviors that will help fulfill their needs rather than teaching an understanding of historical or unconscious conflicts or motivations.

Second Force Theory

Overview

Second Force theorists include those who adhere to Psychoanalytic, Neo-Analytic, Cognitive Learning, and Gestalt Field theories. These theorists generally believe data for study about the person come from within the developing person, from observation of interpersonal relationships and from knowledge of the impact of social units, norms, and laws upon the person. Data from earlier development are also used in relation to present behavior and goal direction. This group of theorists studies the person more comprehensively and as a total social being, using experimentation, objective observation, and self-report methods. Second Force theorists give us a helpful view of causation and provide a way of dealing with problems (119, 139, 140).

View of the Human

Second Force theorists add knowledge of genetics, developmental levels, effects of internal stimuli, unconscious processes, social relationships, and environmental context to understanding of the person.

Reality is external and interpersonal—what people agree on. The person is a social organism with a developmental past on which to build and a level of readiness that influences or contributes to learning and behavior. The person has social needs that affect learning and behavior, seeks social role satisfaction, and reacts to social values and symbolic processes. The person is rational, internalizes societal rules because of the approval gained, can understand cause-effect relationships and complex abstract issues, is capable of insight and emotions, and initiates action and makes choices. The person is seen as a reactive being, responding to stimuli that are usually sociosexual in nature. The goal of behavior is seen as reduction of symbolic or internal needs or tension (119, 139, 140).

View of Education and Therapy

The goal of education and psychiatric/mental health treatment is to help the person become an adaptive, effective social being, aware of and responsive to social reality and patterns. The person has to learn and follow socially prescribed values, customs, and norms in order to fit into society as an effective and well citizen. Mental health and illness are defined by what society calls "normal behavior." Learning and behavior are controlled or influenced by social forces and standards and by modeling; yet learning and behavior are also influenced strongly by the person's developmental level, personal history, cognitive processes and intellect, and intrapsychic processes (139, 140).

All of these internal and social factors must be considered in teaching or counseling. The teacher or therapist is the central figure, a social role model, who imparts or directs the client toward what is socially needed and expected by structuring the learning or therapy situation. Constraints that inhibit learning or need satisfaction are removed by the teacher/therapist. The therapist interprets and diagnoses the underlying symbolic roots of the behavior so that the client can better understand self and his/her behavior. The increased insight also promotes development and maturation. If the person is not ready to learn or change behavior, the teacher or therapist acts as an external motivator of facilitator of readiness to change. The teacher and therapist gives rewards through approval, affiliation, and various verbal and nonverbal methods. Learning and behavior change also are self-reinforcing to the person (139, 140).

Second Force Theorists

Second Force theorists are numerous and can be divided into those with a psychodynamic perspective or those with a cognitive perspective. The *psychodynamic perspective* is then divided into two theories: Psychoanalytic (Freud) and Neo-Analytic (C. Jung, A. Adler, O. Rank, K. Horney, E. Fromm, H. Sullivan, E. Erikson, and E. Berne). The Neo-Analysts can be further subdivided. Jung, Adler, Rank, Horney and Fromm reinterpreted Freud's Psychoanalytic Theory in formulating their theory. Sullivan developed a new emphasis in his Interpersonal Theory in that causation of behavior was seen as the result of dyad relationships and development continued into adulthood. Erikson, in his Epigenetic Theory, expanded understanding of normal developmental stages and tasks through the life span, emphasized sociocultural influences to a greater degree, and saw the person as capable of emotional growth throughout life. Eric Berne formulated Transactional Analysis, a Communication Theory that acknowledges the effect of past experiences and internal ego and feeling states but also studies transactions between people.

The *cognitive perspective* includes a number of theorists. Some have combined or modified concepts from behavioral and psychodynamic theories with an emphasis on cognitive processes to learn adaptive, satisfying behavior and to gain control over personal life. Such theorists are A. Bandura (Social Learning Theory) and J. Rotter (a social learning theorist). Other theorists focus more on cognition and are not concerned with therapy. J. Piaget describes stages of cognitive development and the progression of learning strategies in his Theory of Cognitive Development. J. Bruner (Cognitive Construct Theory) is a cognitive learning and developmental psychologist who is concerned with the processes of learning but integrates concepts from other disciplines in his eclectic psychology. Kurt Lewin (Cognitive Field Theory) is the best known of the Gestalt Field theorists, and he and Fritz Perls (Gestalt Therapy) are close to the Third Force theorists and their phenomenological view.

The Psychodynamic Perspective

The psychodynamic perspective is concerned with the inner and unconscious processes of the person—drives, needs, motivations, feelings, and conflicts. Behavior is described from a historical frame of reference; past developmental experiences are important in the causation of emotional illness. The approach has been useful for diagnosis of illness.

A major goal of all psychotherapies is to help the client achieve a more realistic view of self and life situations.

Freud: Psychoanalytic Theory

Sigmund Freud, a Viennese neurologist, developed Psychoanalytic Theory, the first psychological theory including a fully developed explanation of abnormal behavior. Psychoanalytic theory emphasizes intrapsychic processes; thought and emotions are considered to be important sources of behavior and the focus in treatment. Freud at first believed that eventually all behavior could be explained by bodily changes, but because so little was known about the relationship of body and mind at the time, he gave biological factors little emphasis. He did, however, use the medical model of emphasizing pathology, symptoms, and the patient as a passive recipient of professional treatment. Most of the psychoanalytic theorists who have followed him have paid little attention to biology. Not all psychoanalytic theorists emphasize the same inner events and sources of environmental stimulation, but they do agree that personality is shaped by a combination of inner and outer events, with emphasis on the inner ones. Because thoughts and feelings are not directly observable, these theorists infer them from overt behavior. They use their inferences about inner processes to account for other aspects of overt behavior (56).

Freud's theory of personality seems complicated because it incorporates many interlocking factors. Major components are psychic determinism; psychic structures of id, ego, and superego; primary and secondary process thinking; the conscious-unconscious continuum; libido or psychic energy; behavior; anxiety and defense mechanisms; and psychosexual development. Table 2-3 summarizes these concepts.

Freud believed that all behavior and symptoms are caused by internal factors and are meaningful to either the conscious or unconscious mind. Behavior is *dynamic: the person expends energy in pursuit of goals.* Psychic energy is channeled by conscious and unconscious forces that operate purposely to achieve their aims, and these forces are not always in harmony (37, 38, 41, 42). The greater the degree of intrapsychic conflict, the greater the likelihood that mental events remain unconscious. The greater the unconscious conflict, the greater the vulnerability to anxiety (39).

TABLE 2-3.   Summary of Freud's Theory of Personality

Psychic Determination	All behavior determined by prior thoughts and mental processes.
Psychic Structures	**Id**—*Unorganized reservoir of psychic energy;* furnishes energy for ego and supergo. *Consists of instinctual forces, primitive biological drives, and impulses necessary for survival.* Operates on **Pleasure Principle** *(seeking of immediate gratification and avoidance of discomfort).* Discharges **tension** *(increased energy)* through reflex physiological activity and **primary process thinking** *(image formation, drive-oriented behavior, free expression of feelings and impulses, inability to distinguish between reality and nonreality).* **Ego**—*Establishes relations with environment through conscious perception, feeling, action.* *Controls impulses from id and demands of superego.* Operates on **Reality Principle** *(external conditions considered and immediate gratification delayed for future gains that can be realistically achieved).* Controls access of ideas to conscious. Appraises environment and reality. Uses various mechanisms to help person feel emotionally safe. Guides person to acceptable behavior. Directs motor and all cognitive functions. Assists with **secondary process thinking** *(delayed or substitutive gratification; realistic thoughts; conscious processes; cognitive strategies).* **Superego**—*Represents internalized moral code based on perceived social rules and norms; restrains expression of instinctual drives; prevents disruption of society.* Active and concrete in directing person's thoughts, feelings, actions. Made up of two systems: 　　Ego Ideal—perfection to which person aspires. 　　Conscience—responsible for guilt feelings.
Conscious– Unconscious Continuum	**Conscious**—*All aspects of mental life currently in awareness or easily remembered.* **Preconscious**—*Aspects of mental life remembered with help;* not currently in awareness. **Unconscious**—*Thoughts, feelings, actions, experiences, dreams not remembered; difficult to bring to awareness; not recognized.* Existence inferred from effects on behavior.
Instincts *(Drives)*	Basic force in personality and behavior. *Inborn psychological representation or wish of inner somatic source of excitation.* Kinds of instincts: self-preservation, preservation of species, life, death. Life and death instincts in conflict.
Libido *(Sexuality)*	*Sexual or psychic energy arising from hidden drives or impulses involved in conflict.* Desire for pleasure, sexual gratification.

TABLE 2-3. Continued

	Not limited to biology or genital areas; includes capacity for loving another, parental love, and preservation of species.
Anxiety	*Response to presence of unconscious conflict, tension, or dread; perceived or anticipated danger; and stress—primary motivation for behavior.*
	Basic source is the unconscious, related to loss of self-image.
	Psychic energy accumulates if anxiety not expressed; may overwhelm ego controls; panic may result.
	Kinds of anxiety: (1) neurotic—id-ego conflict; (2) realistic—in response to real dangers in world; (3) moral anxiety—id-superego conflict.
	Managed by direct action, coping strategies, or unconscious mechanisms.

An understanding of ego defense mechanisms is an important part of Psychodynamic Theory. Anxiety alerts the person to the presence of an intense unconscious conflict or an unacceptable wish. If anxiety cannot be managed by direct action or coping strategies, the ego initiates unconscious defenses by warding off awareness of the conflict, to keep the material unconscious, to lessen discomfort, and to maintain the self-image. Since everyone experiences psychological danger, the use of defense mechanisms clearly is not a special characteristic of maladaptive behavior. Such mechanisms are used by all people, either singly or in combination, at one time or another. The level of adaptive behavior depends on the defense repertoire characteristic of the person. Table 2-4 defines and gives examples of commonly used ego adaptive/defense mechanisms.

The most important and basic of the defense mechanisms is repression, and it is the cornerstone on which psychoanalysis rests. Repression, like other defenses, is directed at external dangers, such as fear-arousing events, and at internal dangers, such as wishes, impulses, and emotions that cry out for gratification but arouse guilt. Repression reduces anxiety by keeping anxiety-laden thoughts and impulses out of awareness or by motivating forgetting of certain events. The energy to keep material repressed sometimes makes other behavior less effective. Sometimes repressions are expressed indirectly (36).

The sexual instincts provided Freud with the basis for his theories on psychosexual development.

As the person grows from infancy to adulthood, libido energy progressively centers on different body parts. Stages of development are indicated by these various areas, called *erotogenic* (erogenous) zones. Conflicts at each psychosexual stage must be resolved before the person passes on to the next stage. When a substantial part of the libido is left behind, or fixated, the individual's personality becomes dominated by less mature modes of obtaining gratification or tension reduction. Neurosis occurs when a person is unable to pass from one stage of psychosexual development to the next. The person is unable to resolve the anxieties that arise and unconsciously represses material that is too threatening to the ego. The repressed material becomes displaced into emotional and physical symptoms. The primary gain of a neurotic symptom is the keeping of the impulse from awareness. The secondary gains come from the special attention, relief from duties, or other interactions that come about because of the symptom (52, 54, 56, 119).

Freud proposed five stages of psychosexual development and contended that personality was formed by age five. The stages in psychosexual development are described as follows (5, 31, 38).

1. *The oral stage.* During the first year of life, satisfaction is obtained primarily through the erogenous zone of the mouth. Security is the greatest need. Narcissistic pleasure-seeking is through eating and sucking. Aggressive instincts are shown by biting and chewing. Weaning is a crucial conflict in this period.

TABLE 2-4.   Ego Defense Mechanisms

MECHANISM	DEFINITION/EXAMPLE
Compartmentalization	Separation of two incompatible aspects of the psyche from each other to maintain psychological comfort; behavioral manifestations show the inconsistency. *Example:* The person who attends church regularly and is overtly religious conducts a business that includes handling stolen goods.
Compensation	Overachievement in one area to offset deficiencies, real or imagined, or to overcome failure or frustration in another area. *Example:* The student who makes poor grades devotes much time and energy to succeed in music or sports.
Condensation	Reacting to a single idea with all of the emotions associated with a group of ideas; expressing a complex group of ideas with a single word or phrase. *Example:* The person says the word "crazy" as a shorthand expression for many types of mental illness and for feelings of fear and shame.
Conversion	Unconscious conflicts are disguised and expressed symbolically by physical symptoms involving portions of the body, especially the five senses and motor areas. Symptoms are frequently not related to innervation by sensory or motor nerves. *Example:* The person is under great pressure on the job; awakes at 6 A.M. and is unable to walk but is unconcerned about the symptom.
Denial	Failure to recognize an unacceptable impulse or undesirable, but obvious thought, fact, behavior, conflict, or situation, or its consequences or implications. *Example:* The alcoholic person believes that he/she has no problem with drinking even though family and work colleagues observe the classic signs.
Displacement	Release or redirection of feelings and impulses upon a safe object or person as a substitute for that which aroused the feeling. *Example:* The person punches a punching bag after an argument with the boss.
Dissociation	Repression or splitting off from awareness of a portion of a personality or of consciousness. However, the repressed material continues to affect behavior (compartmentalization). *Example:* A client discusses a conflict-laden subject and goes into a trance.
Identification	Similar to and the result of introjection. Unconscious modeling of another person so that basic values, attitudes, and behavior are similar to those of a significant person or group, but overt behavior is manifested in an individual manner. (*Imitation* is not considered a defense mechanism per se,

TABLE 2-4. Continued

MECHANISM	DEFINITION/EXAMPLE
	but imitation usually precedes identification. Imitation is consciously copying another's values, attitudes, movements, etc.) *Example:* The adolescent over time manifests the assertive behavior and states ideas similar to those that she admires in one of her instructors, although she is unaware that her behavior is similar.
Introjection	Symbolic assimilation of or process of taking in attitudes, behavior, wishes, ideals, or values of significant person into the ego and/or superego (a part of identification). *Example:* The client talks about how much he/she helps other people with their problems.
Isolation	Repression of the emotional component of a situation, although the person is able to remember the thought, memory, or event dealing with problems as interesting events that can be rationally explained but have no feelings attached. *Example:* The person talks about the spouse's death and details of the accident that caused it with an apathetic expression and without crying or signs of grieving.
Projection	Attributing one's unacceptable or anxiety-provoking feelings, thoughts, impulses, wishes, or characteristics to another person. *Example:* The person declares that the supervisor is lazy and prejudiced; work colleagues note that this person often needs help at work and frequently makes derogatory remarks about others.
Rationalization	Justification of behavior or offering a socially acceptable, intellectual, and apparently logical explanation for an act or decision actually caused by unconscious or verbalized impulses. Behavior in response to unrecognized motives precedes reasons for it. *Example:* A student fails a course but maintains that the course was not important and that the grade can be made up in another course.
Reaction Formation	Unacceptable impulses repressed, denied, and reacted to by opposite overt behavior. *Example:* A married woman who is unconsciously disturbed by feeling sexually attracted to one of her husband's friends treats him rudely and keeps him at a safe distance.
Regression	Adopting behavior characteristic of a previous developmental level; the ego returns to an immature but more gratifying state of development in thought, feeling, or behavior. *Example:* The person takes a nap, curled in a fetal position, upon arriving home after a stressful day at work.
Repression	Automatic, involuntary exclusion of a painful or conflictual feeling, thought, impulse, experience, or memory from

TABLE 2-4.   Continued

MECHANISM	DEFINITION/EXAMPLE
	awareness. The thought or memory of the event is not consciously perceived. *Example:* The mother seems unaware of the date or events surrounding her child's death and shows no emotion when the death is discussed.
Sublimation	Substitution of a socially acceptable behavior for an unacceptable sexual or aggressive drive or impulse. *Example:* The adolescent is forbidden by her parents to have a date until she is graduated from high school. She gives much time and energy to editorial work and writing for the school paper. The editor of the school paper and the faculty advisor are males.
Suppression	Intentional exclusion of material from consciousness. *Example:* The husband carries the bills in his pocket for a week before remembering to mail in the payments.
Symbolization	One object or act unconsciously represents a complex group of objects and acts, some of which may be in conflict or unacceptable to the ego; external objects or acts stand for any internal or repressed desire, idea, attitude, of feeling. The symbol may not overtly appear to be related to the repressed ideas or feelings. *Example:* The husband sends his wife a bouquet of roses, which ordinarily represents love and beauty. But roses have thorns; his beautiful wife is hard to live with, but he consciously focuses on her beauty.
Undoing	An act, communication, or thought that cancels the significance or partially negates a previous one; treating an experience as if it had never occurred. *Example:* The husband purchases a gift for his wife after a quarrel the previous evening.

Insecurity in parting with breast or bottle may cause fixation at the oral stage. Sensory discrimination and differentiation between mental images and reality and of self from others occur.

The oral personality is fixated at the oral stage and is likely to develop dependent relationships in adulthood, recreating dependency and immaturity of the oral stage. If fixated at an early stage, he/she may be unusually friendly and generous with a childish belief that the world will nurture and owes him/her a living. The person is optimistic, gullible, and will "swallow anything." The person fixated in the later aggressive oral stage may be pessimistic, cynical, competitive, and highly aggressive in adult life. This individual uses oral approaches to hurt—for example, biting sarcasm.

2. *The anal stage.* For the second and third years of life, the anus is the site of tension and sensual gratification. Excretory processes, retentive (holding back) and expulsive (forcing out), are experienced as pleasurable, particularly as these functions come under the child's control. The child uses this new skill to please

or annoy parenting adults. The Reality Principle is introduced, resulting in ego development and beginning superego development. The child exhibits motor self-control and independence through negativistic behavior.

The anal personality is fixed at the anal stage. Adult characteristics depend on whether fixation centers on the retentive or expulsive mode. The anal-retentive personality shows traits of obstinancy, parsimony, and orderliness. The adult is likely to be stingy, hoarding, stubborn, and compulsively neat. The anal-expulsive personality shows traits of generosity, an outgoing nature, and may be highly creative, expressive, and artistically inclined.

3. *The phallic stage.*   In the fourth and fifth years the libido is centered in the genital region. Masturbation, fantasy, play activities, experimentation with peers, and questioning of adults about sexual topics are indicative behaviors. This stage is labeled *phallic* because the penis is presumed to be the object of main interest: to the little girl who is envious (according to Freud), or to the little boy who is constantly fearing castration for unconscious desires to experience sexual gratification with mother. This represents the major conflict and has been termed the *Oedipal Complex*, in reference to Oedipus Rex, a figure in Greek drama who murdered his father and married his mother. Resolution occurs with the child's identification with the same-sexed parent. The girl assumes a female role, rather than desiring to become a boy. The boy relinquishes the desire to possess mother and begins to emulate traits of father. Through identification, the superego is internalized. In Freud's view, failure to resolve the Oedipal Complex is one of the most important sources of guilt in neurotic people.

The phallic personality results from fixation at the phallic stage. Adult characteristics reflect partial resolution of the Oedipal complex. Overinvolvement with sexual attractiveness and flirtatiousness result. The person may appear self-centered and narcissistic; the woman is seductive and the man adopts a "ladies' man" role. The Don Juan stereotype may appear, which results in conquests with little depth of affection. One female pattern Freud noted is the masculinity complex sometimes referred to as the "castrating woman"—

in which the woman does not accept femininity and feminine roles and pursues competitive relationships with men.

4. *The latency period.* After about the sixth year, the child's sexual urges are dormant until their reawakening at puberty. During this period, libido is channeled into school, home, and organizational activities, hobbies, and relationships with peers. This is the time for increased intellectual activity, identification with teachers and peers, and weakening of home ties.

5. *The genital stage.* At puberty, the adolescent becomes sexually mature, and libido is centered again on the genital area. Chances for nonneurotic heterosexual relationships at this stage are increased if the person has passed through the pregenital stages without major fixation of libido. The person strives for independence, gains intellectual maturity, selects a love object of the opposite sex, and settles into adult roles. In well-socialized adults, the sexuality of earlier psychosexual stages blossoms into mature love, and the person is then capable of genuine caring and adult sexual satisfaction.

Freud's ideas about psychosexual development are undoubtedly the most controversial aspect of his theory. Although many theorists agree that childhood experiences are very important in personality development, many reject Freud's assertions about childhood sexuality and the Victorian and stereotyped ideas about men and women (56, 119).

Psychoanalysis is the treatment modality based on Freudian constructs and aims at total personality reconstruction. The goal of the therapeutic relationship is to make unconscious and repressed material conscious, thereby curing the symptom. The main target of treatment is the forces that are believed to generate the symptoms. *Free association, where the patient talks about thoughts, feelings, and dreams as freely as possible,* clarification after silent listening, and interpretation are tools used to bring repressed material into consciousness and to promote insight, which is curative.

Treating only the symptom is considered dangerous because the symptom represents a delicate balance of compromise in the psychic system. Upsetting this balance by relying on a temporary solution may cause *symptom substitution, where a new symptom is generated by unconscious processes.* Also more drastic disintegration of the personality may occur. The psychodynamic cure is always directed at the historical development of the conflict rather than at the symptom that brought the patient to treatment.

During therapy, the psychoanalyst considers *fixation, arrested development in which the person retains means of gratification characteristic of an earlier phase,* transference, and resistance. Transference and resistance will be more fully described in Chapter 6.

Psychoanalytic Theory has been criticized for many reasons, and an objective critique is given by J. Graves (51). However, Freud's ideas and writings have been seminal. Although now in abundant supply, few books on personality theory existed prior to Freud's hypotheses about behavior and personality development. The amount of research generated from basic postulates of personality theory by disciples and critics of Freud has made a major contribution to the scientific community in understanding behavior. Another contribution of psychodynamic theory was psychotherapy as a treatment method. Although clinical psychoanalysis as developed by Freud is a less frequently used form of treatment today, its basic elements greatly influenced the development of the entire field of psychotherapy (56).

Major Neo-Analytic Theorists

Neo-Freudians or Neo-Analysts follow Freud's theory in general but disagree with or have modified some of the original propositions. They all maintain the medical model and share the view of intrapsychic determinism as the basis for external behavior. Some take into account the social and cultural context in which the person lives. Some therapists have moved from individual to group therapy, and from long-term to time-limited therapy. Important theorists joining Freud in this tradition are Carl Jung, Alfred Adler, Otto Rank, Karen Horney, Eric Fromm, Harry Stack Sullivan, Heinz Hartmann, and Erik Erikson.

Sullivan and Erikson are described in detail; other theorists will be described in Table 2-6.

Sullivan: Interpersonal Theory of Psychiatry

Harry Stack Sullivan formulated the Inter-

personal Theory of Psychiatry. The theory focus is on relationships between and among people, in contrast to Freud's emphasis on intrapsychic sexual phenomena and Erikson's focus on social aspects. Experiences in major life events are the result of either positive or negative interpersonal relationships.

Each person in any two-person interaction is involved as part of an interpersonal field, rather than relating as a separate entity. Thus social and not just intrapsychic experiences are important. Personality development is largely the result of mothering, childhood experiences, and interpersonal encounters. There are two basic needs: satisfaction (biological needs) and security (emotional and social needs). Biological and interpersonal needs are interrelated. How biological needs are met in the interpersonal situation will determine sense of satisfaction and security and will provide avoidance of anxiety (5, 129).

Sullivan utilized the following biological principles to understand the person's development:

1. *Principle of Communal Existence:* A living organism cannot be separated from the necessary environment in order to survive. For example, the embryo must have the correct intrauterine environment to live, and the baby must have love and human contact to become socialized or human.
2. *Principle of Functional Activity:* Functional or physiological activities and processes affect the person's interaction with the environment.
3. *Principle of Organization:* The person is systematically arranged physically and emotionally and within societies, and this organization enables function (129).

An important principle for the study of people is the **One Genus Postulate,** *which states that we are all more simply human than otherwise— hence more similar than different in basic needs, development, and behavior (129).*

Sullivan postulated that people experience events in three modes as outlined below. The differences between these modes are due to the crucial role of language in experience and development (129).

1. *Prototaxic Mode of Experiencing refers to experiences that occur in infancy before language symbols are acquired or to the first*

time a person experiences an event that is difficult to describe in words. The infant perceives self and environment as an undifferentiated whole initially, and this feeling may recur.

2. *Parataxic Mode of Experiencing refers to experiences characterized by symbols used in a private (autistic) way and encompasses fantasy, magical thinking, and lack of cause-effect thinking.* The undifferentiated whole is broken into parts that are perceived as momentary, illogical, and disconnected. Children and adults have parataxic experiences.

3. *Syntaxic Mode of Experiencing refers to experiences of preadolescence, adolescence, and adulthood, characterized by **consensual validation**, whereby persons communicate with each other using language or symbols that are mutually understood.* Perceptions form whole, logical, coherent pictures of reality that can be validated by others.

Sullivan implied that an inherent intolerance of anxiety and avoidance of anxiety along with gratification of basic needs are the primary motivations for behavior. The *Concept of Anxiety states that emotional tension or discomfort of anxiety has its origin in the prolonged dependency of infancy, urgency of biological and emotional needs, and how the mothering person meets those needs. Anxiety is the result of uncomfortable interpersonal relationships, is the chief disruptive force in interpersonal relationships, is contagious through empathic feelings, and can be relieved by being in a secure interpersonal relationship* (52, 54, 129).

The infant is highly empathic to anxiety; the anxious feelings of others, especially of the mother, during feeding, holding, diapering, or otherwise caring for the baby, are sensed. The *self-esteem is an organization of experiences that exist to defend against anxiety and to secure necessary satisfaction.* One aspect of the self-system is known as *good-me, bad-me,* and *not-me.* The *child learns those behaviors approved of by parents and identifies them as **good-me**.* A positive self-concept results if the child has consistent positive interpersonal experiences. *Behaviors receiving disapproval generate anxiety and are identified by the child as **bad-me**.* A negative self-concept results if the child has consistent bad-me experiences. *Behaviors generating an extreme level of anxiety are denied*

*and identified as **not-me**.* For example, an adult who was strongly conditioned in childhood against showing anger may say, "I never get mad; that's not me." Or the person may disregard or block out of awareness of the genital region and sexual and erotic impulses and needs if diapering was done in a rough manner and toilet training was a harsh experience. The self-system is dynamic, changeable, and positively directed; it must be reorganized if substantial personality change is to be effected (5, 54, 129).

Sullivan describes developmental stages in the following way (5, 54, 129):

1. *Infancy* is from birth to emergence of speech. The main developmental tools are: (a) the mouth, (b) the ability to cry, babble, and coo, (c) the satisfaction response (pleasure principle), (d) empathic observation and response, (e) exploration of environment, and (f) autistic invention (infant feels master of all that is seen). The infant during this stage cannot be spoiled; needs should be met promptly to lay a firm foundation for trust and to avoid anxiety of needs. The mode of experiencing is prototaxic. The infant manifests emotional reactions of fear, rage, and anxiety in times of discomfort. The developmental task is to learn to rely on others to gratify needs.

2. *Childhood* is from one and one-half years to the emergence of need for peer associations. Developmental tools are: (a) language, (b) the anus, (c) self-system and self-concept (d) experimentation with self and environment, (e) motor skills, (f) peer associations, and (g) identification. The young child must have realistic limits set consistently in order to develop a sense of reality about the environment. The mode of experiencing is parataxic. The child manifests anxiety, anger, shame, guilt, and doubt when distress is felt. The developmental task is to learn to delay gratification and accept interference with wish-fulfillment.

3. *The juvenile period* extends from six years to the emergence of the capacity for caring for another. Developmental tools are: (a) increasing intellectual abilities, (b) internal control over behavior, (c) competition, compromise, and collaboration, and (d) experimentation, exploration, and motor skills.

The child learns to attend to peers' wishes in order to have personal needs met. He/she may ignore parental rules in deference to peer ideas. The developmental task is to form a satisfactory relationship with peers of both sexes.

4. *Preadolescence* begins at about nine years and extends until evidence of puberty. The child now has the capacity to care emotionally and unselfishly for another person. The child experiences in the syntaxic mode and can engage in consensual validation. Developmental tools include: (a) collaboration, (b) experimentation, (c) exploration, and (d) manipulation of people and the environment. Allegiance to, communication with, and consensual validation from peers increase. This period is known as the **chum stage** because the developmental task is to *become interested in and relate closely to a friend of the same sex and to care about the chum as fully as oneself.* Because of mutual sharing of secrets, dreams, fantasies, and reality aspects of life, this stage offers corrective experiences to the child who previously encountered deprivation of needs or high anxiety.

5. *Early adolescence* extends from onset of puberty (about twelve years) until completion of primary and secondary sexual changes (about fourteen years). Developmental tools are: (a) sexual feelings, (b) fantasies, (c) experimentation, (d) exploration, (e) motor and interpersonal skills, and (f) heightened anxiety in interpersonal contacts. Rebellion and dependence often mark this period. Peer relations and mores are more influential than family allegiance. The developmental task is to learn to master independence and establish satisfactory relationships with peers of the opposite sex.

6. *Late adolescence* extends from about fourteen years until the establishment of a durable relationship. Developmental tools are: (a) sense of self as an integrated and sexual being, (b) ability to use logic and abstractions, (c) exploration, (d) experimentation, and (e) interpersonal skills. During this period, an initial heterosexual love relationship is formed. Other loves may follow, and deep feelings between partners may eventuate in marriage or cohabitation. The developmental task is to learn how to maintain an enduring relationship with a member of the opposite sex.

7. *Adulthood* is the period of biological maturity and when the person is able to establish an interdependent and permanent love relationship with another person of the opposite sex. A major developmental tool is the ability to **collaborate**, *to adjust personal behavior to another's behavior and needs in pursuit of mutual gratification of needs.* Other tools include feelings of lust and the genital organs as well as feelings of responsibility and caring. The person assumes a vocation, is responsible and creative, and maintains a balanced involvement with family, friends, and community. The adult reaffirms important values in life. The developmental task is to achieve feelings of love and **intimacy**, *a situation involving two people whereby each accepts all aspects of the other, and the physical needs and psychological security of another are more important than one's own needs.*

Sullivan assumed that mental illness results from inadequate communication with others. He defined **mental illness** *as inappropriate interpersonal relationships.* The appearance of anxiety indicates developmental deficits, and therapy focuses on anxiety and its cause rather than on overt symptoms. The therapist, in Sullivan's view, is a participant-observer in the relationship with the client. The therapist helps the client to identify areas of development that are incomplete and to increase self-awareness. Consensual validation is an important tool since it helps the client to develop the ability to assess reality objectively. Dynamic changes in the client-therapist relationship provide opportunities for the client to live through and to correct developmental deficits and to learn appropriate and adequate communication and interpersonal skills (129).

Hildegarde Peplau, a psychiatric nurse, developed further the Interpersonal Theory as it applied to nursing (105). Peplau will be referred to in later chapters.

Erikson: Epigenetic Theory of Personality Development

Erik Erikson formulated the Epigenetic Theory, which is based on the principle of the unfolding embryo; that is, anything that grows has a ground plan out of which parts arise. Each part has its time of special ascendancy, until all parts have arisen to form a functional whole (32).

His theory explains step-by-step unfolding of emotional development and social characteristics during encounters with the environment. His theory enlarges upon Psychoanalytic Theory because it: (1) is not limited to historical era or personality types, (2) encompasses development through the life span, and (3) acknowledges that society, as well as heredity and childhood experiences, influences the person's development (5, 33).

His studies of personality development crossculturally show that people in any society, including so-called primitive ones, have their own norms of child and adult behavior, maturation and sequential development, and their own kinds of neurosis and psychosis (5, 32).

Basic principles of his theory, based on crosscultural studies, are (32):

1. The psychosexual sequences of developmental phases are universal to people, although resolution of these phases vary from society to society.

2. Each stage of development sets the groundwork for the next stage. Things happen within the person biologically that makes him/her ready for new experiences in the environment. Innate characteristics and the environment are seen as equally important to development.

3. Each phase has a specific developmental task that is to be achieved or solved. These tasks describe the order and sequence of human development and the conditions necessary to accomplish these, but actual accomplishment is done at an individual pace, tempo, and intensity.

4. Each psychosexual stage of development is a developmental crisis because there is a radical change in the person's perspective, shift in energy, and an increased emotional vulnerability. During this peak time the potential in the personality arises or comes in contact with the whole environment, and the person has some degree of success or failure in solving the crucial developmental task of the specific era. How the person copes with the task and crisis depends on previous strengths and weaknesses.

5. Internal organization is central to development. Maturity increases as each central task is accomplished, at least in part, in its proper order. Attainment of the highest level of maturity depends on successfully mastering tasks of each prior level.

6. The potential inherent in each person evolves if given adequate chance to survive and grow. Anything that distorts the necessary environment interferes with evolvement of the personality. Society attempts to safeguard and encourage the proper rate and sequence of the unfolding of human potential so that humanity is maintained.

7. Each developmental task is redeveloped, reworked, and redefined in subsequent stages. Potential for further development always exists.

Erikson proposed eight stages of development and described the developmental task or cirsis for each stage, as outlined in Table 2-5. Although the

TABLE 2-5.   Erikson's Eight Stages of Development

CHRONOLOGICAL AGE PERIOD	STAGE DEVELOPMENT/ DEVELOPMENTAL TASK	BEHAVIOR
Infancy (0 to 12 months)	Oral-Sensory: Develops basic attitudes of trust versus mistrust.	Experiences of consistent loving and tender care from the nurturing person is foundation for trust and positive attitudes toward self and others. Mouth is source of satisfaction and means of dealing with anxiety-producing events.

TABLE 2-5. Continued

CHRONOLOGICAL AGE PERIOD	STAGE DEVELOPMENT/ DEVELOPMENTAL TASK	BEHAVIOR
Toddler (1 to 3 years)	Anal-Muscular: Develops basic attitudes of autonomy versus shame and doubt.	Learns extent to which environment can be directly manipulated to meet needs. Begins to develop self-control and independence unless excessively constrained by environment.
Preschooler (3 to 6 years)	Genital-Locomotor: Develops basic attitudes of initiative versus guilt.	Learns the extent to which initiative, assertiveness, and motor, language, and cognitive skills will influence others or manage environmental objects. Explores the environment with senses, thoughts, imagination, and motor skills. Activities demonstrate direction and purpose. Engages in first real social contacts through cooperative play. Is intrusive or receptive, based on male and female anatomy, respectively. Develops conscience. Experiences guilt feelings if significant others disapprove excessively of child and his/her behavior.
School Age (6 to 12 years)	Latency: Develops basic attitudes of industry versus inferiority.	Learns to use energy to be creative and develops physical, motor, social, and cognitive skills that can be applied to tasks in the adult world. Feels inadequate and avoids tasks if unsuccessful in initiating or completing tasks. Understands and follows rules and regulations. Involved with peers in new relationships.
Adolescence (12 to 18–20 years, or even to 25 years)	Puberty and Adolescent: Develops sense of identity and roles in life.	Integrates all life experiences into coherent unified sense of self. Begins to establish place in society and relations with opposite sex. Explores ideologies and attempts to resolve conflicts resulting from ideals versus real situations. Feels lost and confused if unable to integrate life experiences or to find meaning in existence.
Late Adolescence or Youth and Young Adulthood (18–20 to 25 years until the 40's)	Young Adulthood: Develops basic attitudes of intimacy versus isolation.	Is concerned primarily with establishing intimate relationship with another adult, independence, and a vocation.
Young Adult (25 to 45 years and beyond into middle age)	Adulthood: Develops basic attitude of generativity versus stagnation or self-absorption.	Is concerned primarily with establishing and maintaining a family and guiding the next generation. Displays creativity and interest in welfare of others and society. Devotes energy to organizations or social causes. Re-evaluates life's accomplishments and goals. Adjusts to middle age.

TABLE 2-5.   Continued

CHRONOLOGICAL AGE PERIOD	STAGE DEVELOPMENT/ DEVELOPMENTAL TASK	BEHAVIOR
Middle and Old Age (50 years to death)	Maturity: Develops basic attitudes of ego integrity versus self-despair or self-disgust.	Reminisces. Accepts life as meaningful and fulfilling. Adjusts to limitations imposed by retirement, aging, other losses, and changing family patterns, but remains optimistic and continues to develop psychologically. Accepts approaching death. If life has not been satisfying, death is feared.

general age span is given with the developmental task, there is no necessary relationship. This is the ideal sequence, but the person may be an adult before developing trust. Erikson's emphasis is that a sense of trust is essential before the person can meet any other developmental tasks; each task lays the groundwork for achieving the next. If one task is not met, the person is unable to meet the next task in the hierarchy. Motivation for behavior is anxiety, generated by failure to negotiate the steps of development successfully.

Psychoanalysis is the treatment method used with adults by Erikson and his disciples. Play Therapy is used with children to help them negotiate earlier stages and resolve crises. The goal is successful resolution of conflicts and expansion of self-awareness to achieve a strong sense of identity, a healthy body, a discerning and curious mind, and a social awareness (32).

The Cognitive Perspective

Cognitive psychology deals with the human as an information processor and problem solver. The cognitive perspective is concerned with internal processes but emphasizes how people attempt to acquire, interpret, and use information to solve life's problems and to remain normal or healthy. It emphasizes conscious processes, present thoughts, and problem-solving strategies. The cognitive perspective has grown out of new directions in learning and psychodynamic theory. Some present-day learning theorists are becoming increasingly

TABLE 2-6.   Summary of Additional Second Force Neo-Analytic Theorists

THEORIST/THEORY	MAJOR ASSUMPTIONS
Carl Jung Analytical Psychology	1. Two basic attitudes toward experience: introversion and extroversion. 2. Four personality functions: 　a. Perceiving mode of sensation. 　b. Perceiving mode of intuition. 　c. Judging function of thinking. 　d. Judging function of feeling. 3. Each person has dominant perceiving modes and judging functions and basic attitude toward experience influenced by genetic predisposition or environment. 4. Life a series of periods identified by different energy uses. Early years not emphasized and sexual drive latent until puberty. Late thirties and early forties important transi-

TABLE 2-6. Continued

THEORIST/THEORY	MAJOR ASSUMPTIONS
	tion: energy from youthful interests channeled to cultural and spiritual pursuits. 5. Collective unconscious a storehouse of memory traces of inherited past; a racial history. Possibility of reviving memories is inherited because certain ideas and behaviors occur in all cultures. If wisdom of unconscious ignored, phobias and delusions may occur. Archetypes of universal thoughts are emotion-filled: birth, death, power, earth mother, wise old man, and the animal. 6. Person needs spiritual as well as rational ideas. 7. Therapy to balance psychological functions of sensing, thinking, feeling, and intuition.

Alfred Adler
 	
Individual
Psychology
	1. Behavior has conscious and unconscious determinants.
	2. Social interest a determinant of mental health.
	3. Primary motivating force in infancy is helplessness with resulting inferiority feelings, rather than libido.
	4. Inferiority feelings from conscious and unconscious recognition of physical, psychological, or social imperfections. Inferiority complex develops when person unable to accept that some imperfection is part of being human.
	5. Striving for superiority or drive for perfection, completeness, and self-actualization inherent to overcome inferiority feelings; results in overcompensation for imperfections.
	6. Person is a social being, motivated by interpersonal needs. Thus inferiority feelings may be problem in areas of friendship, work, and family. Competency in these areas necessary for adjustment.
	7. Well-adjusted person strives for community-oriented goals. Neurotic person strives for egoistic or selfish goals: power, fame, self-love in compensation for inferiority feelings. Maladjusted person manifests discouragement, intense inferiority feelings, exaggerated goal of personal superiority, and underdeveloped social interest.
	8. Therapist is a moderately active helping person. Client:
	  a. Realizes why wrong means was chosen to solve problems; made to understand unique life style.
	  b. Overcomes low opinion of self.
	  c. Becomes interested in others.
	  d. Develops realistic, adaptive life style through improved socialization.
	9. Therapy to emphasize prevention of disorders: teaching parents effective child-rearing techniques and helping child overcome inferiority in comparison to adults.

Otto Rank Birth Anxiety	1. All anxiety and consequent behavior result from birth trauma, separation, and anxiety. 2. Neurotic anxiety a repetition of prototype-anxiety at

TABLE 2-6. Continued

THEORIST/THEORY	MAJOR ASSUMPTIONS
	birth; neurosis reflects conflict between desire to mature and regain intrauterine existence.
Karen Horney Horneyan Psychology	1. Anxiety results if absence of warm relationships in childhood, interpersonal deprivation, frustration, and disapproval. 2. Culture influences personality development. 3. Present events more important than past in influence on behavior. 4. Therapy helps person face real self, avoid idealized self-image, release potential, and adjust to culture.

Eric Fromm	1. Culture and society important in shaping character.
	2. Redefined Freud's personality types:
	  a. Oral receptive.
	  b. Oral aggressive.
	  c. Anal.
	  d. Genital, a sexually mature person with capacity for productivity and love.
	3. Defined five types of love: brother, mother, erotic, self, and supreme being.

Eric Berne
 	
Transactional Analysis
	1. All behavior, thinking, feeling, and experience categorized into three ego states: parent, adult, child.
	  a. Parent ego state contains attitudes, thoughts, feelings, and behavior learned from parents and other authority figures. Expressed in critical, directive, tradition-bound, and judgmental or nurturing behavior. Parent scolds, teaches, lectures, disciplines, cares for or comforts, passes on traditions and values, defines reality.
	  b. Adult ego state processes facts characterized by organized, adaptable, intelligent, rational behavior; thinking clearly, objectively, and without feelings. Operates on Reality Principle.
	  c. Child ego state contains all impulses, needs, desires, feelings, and behavior natural for child and memories of early experiences. Behavior expressed as adapted or natural. The adapted child is compliant, conveys self-pity, dependency, fear, anger, rebellion, sadness. The natural child is spontaneous, self-centered, impulsive, affectionate, creative, and conveys feelings of fun and caring. Includes social behaviors learned when young as well as spontaneous behavior. Operates on Pleasure Principle.
	2. Transaction, responses between people, may be complementary (getting predicted response), crossed (getting response from ego state that was unintended or unexpected), or ulterior (involving hidden message).
	3. Motivation for behavior is need for personal recognition (strokes) in form of verbal or nonverbal responses.

TABLE 2-6. Continued

THEORIST/THEORY	MAJOR ASSUMPTIONS
	4. People interact with others through intimacy or close relations, rituals, activities or work, friendship, socialization, and games (a series of responses and events).
	5. Psychological positions about worth of self and others are: a. I'm OK—you're OK. b. I'm OK—you're not OK. c. I'm not OK—you're OK. d. I'm not OK—you're not OK.
	6. Therapist analyzes ego state, transactions, games played by persons, and kinds of strokes (support) acceptable to client.

interested in what goes on in the individual between the application of a stimulus and the response, and some current psychodynamic theorists are focusing on thinking and problem solving as well as on feelings and emotions. Relationships among emotions, motivations, and cognitive processes are being increasingly studied. Overlap between the cognitive perspective and other approaches is becoming more evident (14, 119).

Several major cognitive theorists will be described in detail. Others will be presented in Table 2-7.

TABLE 2-7. Summary of Additional Second Force Cognitive Theorists

THEORIST/THEORY	MAJOR ASSUMPTIONS

Julian Rotter
 	
Cognitive Social Learning Theory
	1. Problems of maladjusted person originates in interpersonal relations.
	2. Expectations of situation greatly influence behavior; person may defend self against expected failure rather than learn how to achieve goals.
	3. Amount of perceived control over situation affects behavior.
	  a. Internal locus of control: Person believes he/she has power to affect outcome of situation; sense of autonomy.
	  b. External locus of control: Person believes he has little control in situation but is controlled by others, environmental events, or supernatural forces; sense of fatalism.

Jerome Bruner Cognitive Construct Theory	1. Eclectic approach to psychology: integrates biology, anthropology, linguistics, philosophy, sociology, and Gestalt psychology. 2. Needs for curiosity, master of knowledge, and happy life basic along with biological needs. 3. Theory emphasizes discovering learning. Person anticipates, categorizes, actively selects data, adjusts responses, and infers principles or rules that allow transfer of learning to different problems.

TABLE 2-7.   Continued

THEORIST/THEORY	MAJOR ASSUMPTIONS
	4. Person relates incoming data to previously acquired frame of reference in order to go beyond information given in learning. Details must be organized into structure and presented simply to be remembered.
	5. Learning and behavior are goal-directed.
	6. Knowledge based on perception of event or constructed model of reality—first adopted from culture, then adapted to person's use. Data may be distorted to attain valued goals. Increased amount of data allows transfer and flexibility in problem solving.
	7. Three modes of representing reality seen in normal and ill people: a. Enactive—use of motor skills, habits, conditioning, without use of words or imagery; b. Iconic—use of internal imagery, graphics, or pictures that stand for but do not define concept; predominates in ages 5 to 7. c. Symbolic—use of language and abstract, reflective, flexible thought system; learned in school.
	8. Theory recommends internal reinforcement that comes from pleasure of discovery of information and coping with problems. Deemphasizes external rewards and motivation.

Bandura: Social Learning Theory

Albert Bandura has formulated Social Learning Theory; he believes that learning occurs without reinforcement, conditioning, or trial-and-error behavior since humans can think and anticipate consequences of behavior and act accordingly. This theory emphasizes: (1) the importance of vicarious, symbolic, and self-regulatory processes in psychological functioning; (2) the capacity of the person to use symbols, represent events, analyze conscious experience, communicate with others at any distance in time and space, and plan, create, imagine, and engage in foresightful action, and (3) the central role of self-regulatory processes. The person does not simply react to external forces. He/she selects, organizes, and transforms impinging stimuli, and through self-generated inducements and consequences, exercises some influence over personal behavior. There is a continuous, reciprocal interaction between cognitive, behavioral, and environmental determinants (7).

Human nature is characterized as a vast potentiality that can be fashioned by direct and vicarious experience into a variety of forms of development and behavior, within biological limits. The level of psychological and physiological development restricts what can be acquired at any given time (7).

The person may be motivated by cognitive representation of future consequences or by personal goal-setting behavior. If the person wants to accomplish a certain goal, and there are distractions from the task, the person visualizes to the self how he/she will feel when the goal is attained. People respond evaluatively to their own behavior and tend to persist until the behavior or performance meets the goal (7, 119).

Bandura proposes that learning occurs through *modeling, imitation of other's behavior.*

According to his theory, much of our daily behavior is learned by modeling. Imitation is one of the most effective forms of learning: babies learn to speak by imitating the sounds of their parents; older children learn a number of behaviors by watching the teacher, parent, or peers. People learn how to be normal or neurotic. Maladaptive behavior may arise from modeling when the child imitates abnormal parental behavior. Or modeling may inhibit behavior in that the person does not respond as he/she normally would because of imitation. Phobic behaviors may arise, not from injurious experiences, but by watching others respond directly or indirectly to the object or situation with fear. Therefore, analysis of dysfunctional behavior should always include study of the significant adults in the person's earlier life. Bandura's research also shows the power of watching television on people's behavior, and that for some people the model of aggressive behavior will cause later acting-out behavior (7, 56).

Bandura categorizes maladaptive behavior in the following way:

Behavioral excess: Responses are made too frequently or too intensely.

Behavioral deficit: Responses that should occur do not, or are infrequent or weak. Behavior may not have been learned, or a once-learned response may decrease because of subsequent punishment or extinction.

Distortions in reinforcing stimuli: The usual reinforcers, such as a smile or verbal praise, may not be reinforcers for some people. Or inappropriate stimuli, such as scolding, may be a positive reinforcement in the form of attention, which strengthens undesirable behavior.

Distortion in discrimative stimulus control: Antecedent events that normally control behavior do not, or the person may act similarly with a number of people and show overcontrolled, rigid behavior.

Aversive behavior repertoire: The person may use aversive behaviors, such as tantrums, to control others.

Treatment involves helping the person learn new and more adaptive or normal behavior by observing and imitating others in a safe and con-trolled environment. For example, Bandura's research shows that some fears can be overcome by imitating another person who is doing what the person fears to do (7).

Piaget: Theory of Cognitive Development

Jean Piaget formulated the Theory of Cognitive Development. The bulk of his research was concerned with the child's thinking at particular periods of life and with studying differences among well children of a specific age. A great amount of empirical data was used in developing the theory. His background of biology, philosophy, mathematics, logic, psychometrics, and epistomology all contributed to his theory. He believed that development is neither maturational, an unfolding of the innate growth processes, nor learning, an accumulation of experiences, but an active process resulting from *equilibration, an internal force that is set in motion to organize thinking when the child's belief system develops sufficiently to contain self-contradictions.* Piaget emphasizes the innate, inborn processes of the person as the essential force to start the process of equilibration or cognitive growth. Cognitive development proceeds from the motor world into interaction with the wider social world and finally to abstract ideas. Development is seen as solidly rooted in what already exists, and it displays a continuity with the past. Adaptations do not develop in isolation; all form a coherent pattern so that the totality of biological life is adapted to its environment. His theory focuses on development of intellectual capacities with little reference to emotional or social development (5, 134).

Basic assumptions that underlie Piaget's work are as follows (109, 139, 140):

1. Knowledge is organized in a logical structure, and sources of this order are found in interaction between the structure of external conditions and active imposition of structure by the individual. The person structures knowledge into meaningful patterns rather than being molded by the environment entirely. Thus, Piaget is known as a *Structuralist* and a *Rationalist.*

2. Intelligence is an adaptive process by which the person modifies and structures the environ-

ment to fit his/her needs and also modifies self in response to environmental demands.

3. By interaction with the environment, the person constructs reality by assimilation, accommodation, and adaptation. Thus, Piaget is also known as an *Interactionist. Assimilation is defined as taking new content into the cognitive structure. Accommodation is defined as the revising, realigning, and readjusting of the cognitive structure to take into account the new content. Adaptation is the change that results from the first two processes.*

4. There is an innate tendency to equilibrium, which energizes the process of adaptation, or makes sense out of disequilibrium; this results from new knowledge entering existing cognitive structures by assimilation and accommodation.

5. The person has need to be competent in all environmental situations. This need generates interaction with the environment, which is the basis for forming knowledge.

Table 2-8 summarizes Piaget's Theory of Cognitive Development.

The thinking process is explained by schematic mental structures of pictures formed in response to stimuli. A *schema is a complex concept encompassing both motor behavior and internalized thought processes.* The child sees whatever is located at the spot on which his eyes are focused. A *schema involves movement of the eyeballs, paying attention, and the mental picture that is formed as a result of the sensory process.* Thinking eventually involves using combinations of mental pictures, forming concepts, internalizing use of language or subvocal speech, drawing implications, and making judgments. When these internal actions become integrated into a coherent, logical system, they are considered logical operations. The primitive concepts of the newborn gradually broaden, merge with one another, differentiate, become internal and more mobile, and acquire organization.

Piaget divides human development into four periods: infancy or sensorimotor, preoperational, concrete operations, and formal operations.

TABLE 2-8.   Summary of Piaget's Theory of Cognitive Development

PERIOD	AGE	CHARACTERISTICS
Sensorimotor Period		
Stage 1: Use of reflexes	0–1 months	Behavior innate, reflexive, specific, predictable to specific stimuli. *Example:* sucking, grasping, eye movements, startle (Moro reflex).
Stage 2: First acquired adaptations and primary circular reactions	1–4 months	Initiates, prolongs, and repeats behavior not previously occurred. Acquires response to stimulus that creates another stimulus and response. Modifies innate reflexes to more purposeful behavior; repeated if satisfying. Learns feel of own body as physiological stabilization occurs. *Example:* Looks at object, reaches for it, and continues to repeat until vision, reaching, and mouthing coordinated.
Stage 3: Secondary circular reactions	4–8 months	Learns from unintentional behavior. Motor skills and vision further coordinated as learns to prolong or repeat interesting act. Interest in environment around self. Explores world from sitting position. Assimilates new objects into old behavior pattern.

TABLE 2-8.   Continued

PERIOD	AGE	CHARACTERISTICS
		Behavior increasingly intentional. *Example:* Looks for object that disappears from sight; continues to drop object from different locations, which adult continues to pick up.
Stage 4: Acquisition of instrumental behavior, active search for vanished objects	8–12 months	Uses familiar behavior patterns in new situation to accomplish goal. Differentiates objects, including mother from stranger (stranger anxiety). Retains memory of object hidden from view. Combines actions to obtain desired, hidden object; explores object. Imitates others when behavior finished. Develops individual habits more so. Cognitive development enhanced by increasing motor and language skills.
Stage 5: Tertiary circular reactions and discovery of new means by active experimentation	12–18 months	Invent new behavior not previously performed. Uses fewer previous behaviors. Repeats action without random movements. Explores variations that occur when same act accomplished. Varies action deliberately as repeats behavior. Uses trial-and-error behavior to discover solution to problem. Differentiates self from object and object from action performed by self; increasing exploration of how objects function. Invents new means to solve problems and variation in behavior essential to later symbolic behavior and concept formation.
Stage 6: Internal representation of action in external world	18–24 months	Pictures events to self; follows through mentally to some degree. Imitates when model out of sight. Forms mental picture of external body, of body in same space with another object, and of space in limited way. Uses deliberate trial and error in solving problems.
Preoperational Period	2–7 years	Internalizes schemata of more and more of the environment, rules, and relationships. Forms memories to greater extent. Uses fantasy or imitation of others in behavior and play. Intermingles fantasy and reality. Uses words to represent objects and events more accurately; symbolic behavior increases. **Egocentric** *(self-centered in thought)* —focuses on single aspect of object and neglects other attributes because of lack of experience and reference systems, which results in false logic.

TABLE 2-8. Continued

PERIOD	AGE	CHARACTERISTICS
		Follows rules in egocentric way; rules external to self.
		Is static and irreversible in thinking; cannot transform from one state to another (e.g., ice to water).
		Develops story or idea while forgetting original idea so that final statements disconnected, disorganized. Answer not connected to original idea in monologue.
		Tries logical thinking; at times sounds logical but lacks perspective so that false logic and inconsistent, unorganized thinking result.
		Is magical, global, primitive in reasoning.
		Begins to connect past to present events, not necessarily accurate.
		Links events by sequence rather than causality.
		Deals with information by recall; begins to categorize.
		Is **anthropomorphic** *(attributes human characteristics to animals and objects).*
		Unable to integrate events separated by time, past to present.
		Lacks reversibility in thinking.
		Unable to anticipate how situation looks from another viewpoint.
Preconceptual Stage (2–4 years)		Forms images or preconcepts on basis of thinking just described.
		Lacks ability to define property or to denote hierarchy or relationships of objects.
		Constructs concepts in global way.
		Unable to use time, space, equivalence, and class inclusion in concept formation.
Intuitive Stage (4–7 years)		Forms concepts increasingly; some limitations.
		Defines one property at a time.
		Has difficulty stating definition but knows how to use object.
		Uses transductive logic (from general to specific) rather than deductive or inductive logic.
		Begins to classify in ascending or descending order; labels.
		Begins to do seriation; reverses processes and ordinality.
		Begins to note cause-effect relationships.
Concrete Operations Period	7–11 years (or beyond)	Organizes and stabilizes thinking; more rational.
		Sees interrelationships increasingly.
		Does mental operations using tangible, visible references.
		Able to decenter (sees other perspectives; associates or combines events; understands reversibility (e.g., add-subtract; ice-water transformation).
		Recognizes number, length, volume, area, weight as the same even when perception of object changes.
		Develops conservation as experience is gained with physical properties of objects.

TABLE 2-8.   Continued

PERIOD	AGE	CHARACTERISTICS
		Arranges objects in order of size and other characteristics. Fits new objects into series. Understands simpler relationships between classes of objects. Distinguishes between distances. Understands observable world, tangible situations, time, and tangible space. Retains essential idea when perceiving conflicting or unorganized data. Recognizes rules as essential; perceives mutually agreed upon standards. Is less egocentric except in social relationships.
Formal Operations Period	12 years and beyond	Manifests adultlike thinking. Not limited by own perception or concrete references for ideas. Combines various ideas into concepts. Coordinates two or more reference systems. Develops morality of restraint and cooperation in behavior. Uses rules to structure interaction in socially acceptable way. Uses probability concept. Works from definition or concept only to solve problem. Solves problem mentally and considers alternatives before acting. Considers number of variables at one time. Links variables to formulate hypotheses. Begins to reason deductively and inductively instead of solving problem by action. Relates concepts or constructs not readily evident in external world. Formulates advanced concepts of proportions, space, destiny, momentum. Increases intellectual ability to include art, science, humanities, religion, philosophy. Is increasingly less egocentric.

Lewin: Gestalt Field Psychology/ Cognitive Field Theory of Learning

Gestalt Field Psychology originated in Germany in the early twentieth century by four men who later migrated to the United States: Max Wertheimer, Wolfgang Kohler, Kurt Koffka, and Kurt Lewin. Contemporary leaders are Roger Barker, Ernest Bayles, Jerome Bruner, Donald Snygg, and Herbert Wright (14).

Wertheimer formulated the basic theory along with his followers. The central idea is that an organized whole is greater than the sum of its parts and forms a *Gestalt, an organized pattern or configuration that includes a total picture of an object or situation with parts that form a relationship.* Nothing can be understood by studying only the constituent parts. In all perception, qualities appear that represent more than the physical items sensed. The perceiver confers on the physical objects of perception a form, configuration, or meaning, and tries to organize or integrate what is seen. The total environment inside and outside is experienced as a meaningful whole, rather than as discontinuous stimuli (14).

Kurt Lewin added new concepts to Gestalt Psychology, coined a new terminology, and developed Field Psychology, also referred to as "topological and vector psychology" because he borrowed ideas from geometry and physics to explain his system of psychology. Kurt Lewin also applied Systems Theory to the individual. The person is a totality of systems. It is the way the systems are integrated that makes a person unique. Field Theory centers on the idea that all psychological activity of a person at any given moment is a function of the totality of coexisting, interdependent factors in the person and environment (82, 83).

Cognitive Field Theory of Learning is derived from Gestalt and Field psychological theories. The cognitive aspect deals with the problem of how people understand themselves and their environments and how they act in relation to their environments. The field aspect consists of concurrent interrelationships of a person and the psychological environment at any one time. Cognitive Field Theory uses the principle of relativism or interactionism: nothing is perceivable or conceivable as a thing in itself. Everything is perceived or conceived in relation to something else, as a figure against a background. Psychological reality is defined in perceptual terms rather than in objective physical terms. Cognitive Field Psychology is an interpersonal, social psychology that integrates biological and social factors with the interactive person (14).

Gestalt Field Psychology sees the person as purposely active on his/her own behalf in the environment. Learning and therefore behavior are closely related to perception. *Perception is the process by which sensory stimuli are organized and given meaning as the person identifies and describes the environment and everything in it. Perception involves sensation of, feelings about, and interpretation of or the meaning related to an object or situation in its totality.* Perception and behavior are relative; an object or behavior derives its qualities from its relationship to other things when a point of reference is used. To Gestalt Field theor-

ists there is a difference between reality and existence. Each person perceives and interprets the environment in a way that has meaning for him/her, and that interpretation is the reality on which the person designs behavior (14, 82).

The Gestalt psychologists study perception extensively in relation to figure-ground phenomena. *Figure refers to the object or event observed; ground refers to the background of the object/event or the frame of reference held by the person.* In any visual perceptual field, the figure will dominate over the background. In any situation, one object will stand out over others and will be remembered; the person may not remember the contextual, background, or other simultaneous events (14, 79). This is true whether the person is recounting a major developmental life event or a scene of a crime. Distortions of perception may account for abnormal behavior.

Laws of Perception have been formulated in Gestalt Psychology to explain factors that influence perceptions. They are as follows (14, 79, 139, 140):

1. **Law of Pragnanz:** The perceiver organizes perception of the environment so that it changes from disorganized to as simple, orderly, and predictable as possible. Pleasing or harmonious configurations, rather than complicated and irregular ones, are seen.

2. **Law of Similarity:** Similar items tend to form groups in perception when other factors are not interfering.

3. **Law of Proximity:** Elements that are near each other tend to be seen as belonging together and are grouped in the perceptual process.

4. **Law of Closure:** An incomplete figure is perceived as a complete figure; closed areas are more stable and pleasing to the eye than are open areas.

5. **Law of Good Continuation:** Elements tend to be grouped together when they appear to be continuing a directional pattern already established. Reversals and sharp changes of direction are usually avoided; straight lines are continued as straight lines and curves are continued as curves until closure.

6. **Law of Membership Character:** A single part of a whole does not have fixed characteristics; it gets its characteristics from the content in which it appears.

7. **Law of Experience or Familiarity:** Perceptions tend to be related to the familiar figures. If

familiar objects are presented in unfamiliar conditions, they tend to lose their identity.

These laws apply as much to memory and emotional phenomena as to physical objects.

Kurt Lewin was primarily interested in human motivation. His Field Theory was not developed as a learning theory but as a theory of motivation and perception that could be applied to learning situations, group dynamics, and action research. *Motivation is defined as a product of disequilibrium within the life space and refers to the instigative forces of behavior; the goals versus barriers; and experiences, interactions, tensions, purposes, consciousness, and vitalism of the person.* Success and failure do not refer to achievement but rather to the relationship or congruency between ambitions or expectancies and achievement. Lewin's comprehensive, basic concept was the *life space* or *perceptual field, the totality of the person's characteristics and psychological environment*—that is, everything that is perceived at the moment (14, 82).

Thus, *life space is a series of recurring but overlapping situations that are unique and yet related, the sum of all present facts or events at a given time.* Life space represents the total pattern of factors or influences that affect a person's behavior at any one time, including: memories; language; myths; art; cultural factors; religion; emotions; knowledge, concepts, and precepts; thoughts, beliefs, and anticipations; forward, present, and backward time perspectives; abstract ideas; family; peers; places; and concrete objects. Each person's life space and perceptual environment are unique. Two persons may appear to be in the same location in time and space but may have very different psychological environments because of different purposes and experiential backgrounds. Thus, two siblings can turn out very differently in behavior. Whenever a person has a new experience, he/she will never be able to recapture the old environment in its identical form (14, 82).

The *psychological environment surrounds the person and is everything in which, toward which, and away from which the person can make psychological movement.* Psychological environment includes memories, anticipations, and impressions of parts of the physical environment. Forces operating in a psychological field bring about reorganization of that field and provide the basis for psychological behavior (14, 82).

The life space is surrounded by a *nonpsychological foreign hull, which includes the biological organism, the physical and social environments that are not part of the life space, and potential perceptions.* Anything in the physical and social environments can become a part of the person's life space or psychological environment at any time when the person interacts with the factor. Some experiences involve the outer or peripheral area of the psychological person; other experiences involve the core or inner layer of the person. Psychologically, a person is composed of: (1) inner-personal region, which is composed of tensions and needs that move a person to a goal; and (2) a motor-perceptual region, which is divided into: (a) the motor or manipulative abilities using muscles and glands, and (b) the cognitive and sensory processes and knowledge (14, 82).

Various forces or vectors draw the person toward or away from various regions of the life space or goals in an attempt to meet needs. The degree of attraction is influential in reaching a goal. Once the tensions accompanying needs are decreased, other tensions arise, and objects in the environment take on different attraction or valences (15, 54, 82).

Behavior is a change in the psychological life space rather than in observable space and is verbal, nonverbal, symbolic, or experiential. Behavior may be a change of location in the environment, a moving toward the person affectively with feelings of warmth and desire, a cognitive reorganization or re-explanation of an event or object in the physical or social environment, or a restructuring of the self as some needs are met and tensions are reduced. Psychological behavior may be an overt, purposive act, an attitudinal shift, an emotional change, a change in the perceived value of an object or activity, or a new relationship or cognitive association between two or more events, objects, or activities (14). Present behavior is influenced by anticipation of future situations. A person must learn to delay goals in order to function effectively. The future must have some reality in the present if the person is to be motivated to delay gratification (54, 82).

Learning is reorganization of the person's perceptual or psychological world—the field. Learning is *an interactive process whereby a person attains or discovers new insights, values, meanings, attitudes, skills, expectations, thought patterns, or cognitive structures, or changes previously acquired ones.* Learning is goal-directed and occurs when the person sees new ways of utilizing elements in the environment (14, 82).

Insight is a sense of or feeling for pattern, event, or relationship, a feel about a situation that permits continued striving to meet a goal. Insights may or may not be verbalized and may change with new experiences. Learning is seen as purposive, explorative, imaginative, creative, and personal. From insightful learning comes generalizations to other situations, even though the rules or insights may not be discussed. Learning may occur without an observable change in behavior, and a change of behavior may occur without learning or insight. Some behavior is automatic, but learning is a persistent pattern (14, 82).

Outward behavior is important only insofar as it provides clues to what the person is experiencing psychologically or perceptually in relation to the life space. Physiological aspects of the person are acknowledged but are not seen to be closely associated with the development of psychological or **cognitive structures,** *the person's perception of the psychological aspects of the personal, physical, and social world.* As understanding of the person's life space increases, so does the ability to predict behavior (14, 82).

Perls: Gestalt Therapy

Gestalt Therapy, as formulated by Fritz Perls, uses the concepts of Gestalt Psychology. The most pressing figure or part of the life space is the person's needs. In therapy, the primary goal is for the person to become more self-aware and self-responsible in meeting needs. The person is under no obligation to meet the expectations of others but should be able to avoid engaging in infantile games with another. To increase maturity is to decrease personal dependency and broaden the life space and personal potential. The focus is on present feelings in a situation; the past is not analyzed but reexperienced affectively. The person is not asked "Why?" because rationalization and defensiveness follow. Instead, concern is on what the person is doing. Gestalt Therapy is holistic. Mind and body are seen as one; mental and physical activities are manifestations of a total existence (34, 35, 79, 106).

Kohlberg: Theory of Moral Development

Lawrence Kohlberg has formulated a Theory of Moral Development. Since moral development is related to cognitive and emotional development as well as to societal values and norms, Kohlberg can be identified with Second Force theorists.

Kohlberg theorizes that a person's moral reasoning process and behavior develop through six stages. Each stage is derived from a prior stage and is the basis for the next stage. No stage is missed, although the time required to move through each stage may vary. Few people progress through all six stages. Determination of the person's moral stage is dependent on the *reason* for behavior, and he/she is considered in a specific stage when the same level of reason for behavior is given at least half of the time. One criterion of moral maturity, the ability to *autonomously* decide what is right and wrong, is lacking in the Preconventional and Conventional levels because in each level the person is always doing what he/she is told to do by authority figures. Table 2-9 shows the three levels and six stages of moral development.

Third Force Theory

Overview

Third Force theorists include those who are proponents of Humanistic Psychology, Existential Psychology, and Phenomenological Psychology. Humanistic and existential psychologies acknowledge the dynamic aspect of the person but emphasize the impact of environment to a greater degree. They seek to answer the questions: What are the possibilities of the human? From these possibilities what is an optimum state for the human, and under what conditions is this state most likely to be reached? These disciplines strive to maximize the individuality and developmental potential of the human (27, 63).

Since all behavior is considered a function of the person's perceptions, data for study of the person are subjective and come completely from self-reports, including: (a) feelings at the moment about experiences, (b) meaning of the experience, (c) feelings about self and status of self-concept in the situation, (d) personal values, needs, attitudes, beliefs, behavioral norms, expectations, and (e) current experiences. Perception is synonymous with meaning. An immediate view of the person instead of an historical approach is important. The person is made up of many components: physical, physiological, cognitive, emotional, spiritual, cultural, social, and familial, and cannot be adequately understood if studied by individual components. The person is also affected by many variables, both

TABLE 2-9. Progression of Moral Development

LEVEL	STAGE
Preconventional: The person is responsive to cultural rules of labels of good and bad, right or wrong.	**I.** *Punishment and Obedient Orientation* Fear of punishment, not respect for authority, is the reason for decisions, behavior, and conformity. Good and bad are defined in terms of physical consequences to the self from parental, adult, or authority figures. The person defers to superior power or prestige of the person who dictates rules. (*"I'll do something because you tell me, and to avoid getting punished."*) Average age: Toddler to seven years. **II.** *Instrumental Relativist Orientation* Conformity is based on egocentricity and narcissistic needs. The person's decisions and behavior are usually based on concern for self: something is done in order to get something in return. Occasionally the person does something to please another for pragmatic reasons. There is no feeling of justice, loyalty, or gratitude. These concepts are expressed physically. (*"I'll do something if I get something for it or because it pleases you."*) Average age: Preschooler through school age.
Conventional: The person is concerned with maintaining expectations of the family, group, nation, or society. A sense of guilt has developed and affects behavior. The person values conformity, loyalty, and active maintenance of social order and control. Conformity means good behavior or what pleases or helps another and is approved.	**III.** *Interpersonal Concordance Orientation* A. Decisions and behavior are based on concerns about others' reactions; the person wants others' approval or a reward. The person has moved from egocentricity to consideration of others as a basis for behavior. Behavior is judged by the person's intentions. (*"I'll do something because it will please you or because it is expected."*) B. An empathic response, based on understanding of how another person feels, is a determinant for decisions and and behavior. (*"I'll do something because I know how it feels to be without; I can put myself in your shoes."*) Average age: School age through adulthood. Most American women are found to be in this stage. **IV.** *Law-and-Order Orientation* The person wants established rules from authorities, and the reason for decisions and behavior is that social and sexual rules and traditions demand the response. The person obeys the law just because it is the law or out of respect for authority. The law takes precedent over personal wishes, good intentions, and conformity to group stereotypes. (*"I'll do something because it's the law and my duty."*) Average age: Adolescence and adulthood. Most men are found in this stage; 80 percent of adults do not move past this stage.
Postconventional:	**V.** *Social Contract Legalistic Orientation* The social rules are not the sole basis for decisions and be-

TABLE 2-9.   Continued

LEVEL	STAGE
The person lives autonomously; defines moral values and principles that are distinct from his own identification with group values. He/she lives according to principles that are universally agreed upon and that the person considers appropriate for life.	havior because the person believes a higher moral principle applies, such as equality, justice, or due process. The person defines right actions in terms of general individual rights and standards that have been agreed upon by the whole society. The person believes laws can be changed as people's needs change. The person utilizes freedom of choice in living up to higher principles but believes the way to make changes is through the system. Outside the legal realm, free agreement and contract are the binding elements of obligation. (*"I'll do something because it is morally and legally right, even if it isn't popular with the group."*) Average age: Middle age or older adult. Only 20 percent, or less, of Americans achieve this stage.
	VI. *Universal Ethical Principle Orientation* Decisions and behavior are based on internalized rules, on conscience rather than on social laws, and on self-chosen ethical and abstract principles that are universal, comprehensive, and consistent. The rules are not concrete moral rules but instead encompass the Golden Rule, justice, reciprocity, and equality of human rights, and respect for the dignity of human beings as individual persons. Human life is inviolable. The person believes there is a higher order than social order, has a clear concept of civil disobedience, and will use self as an example to right a wrong. The person accepts injustice, pain, and death as an integral part of existence but works to minimize injustice and pain for others. (*"I'll do something because it is morally, ethically, and spiritually right, even if it is illegal and I get punished, and even if no one else participates in the act."*) Average age: Middle age or older adult. Few people attain or maintain this stage. Examples of this stage are seen in times of crisis or extreme situations.

objective and subjective. All behavior is pertinent to and a product of the phenomenal or perceptual field of the person at the moment of action. The phenomenal field is the frame of reference and the universe as experienced by the person at the specific moment (the existential condition). Perceptions lie within the person and are uniquely individual representations of the external forces that are continually in the process of being made consistent with the rest of the phenomenal field (25, 27, 48, 139).

The Third Force theories have the advantage of providing understanding of immediate causation and immediate guidelines for action. The disadvantage of these theories is that they use a subjective approach in observing behavior; the therapist is a participant-observer. This internal basis for behavior is not directly observable or measurable. Further, cooperation of the client is essential in order to get data about the person's perceptions (25, 48, 139).

View of the Human

The person is viewed as an unique whole individual, in dynamic interaction with the environment, and in the process of becoming. The person is seen as holistic—more than the sum of the parts and active on his/her own behalf. The person is constantly growing, changing, expanding perceptual processes, learning, developing potential, and gaining insights. Every experience affects the person, depending on the perceptual field. The person is never quite the same as he/she was even an hour or day previously since each is a product of personally unique phenomena. The goals of the creative being are growth, feeling adequate, reaching the potential, and meeting self-actualization needs. The person is active in pursuing these goals. The basic needs are the maintenance and enhancement of the phenomenal self or self-concept and a sense of adequacy and self-actualization (25, 27, 48, 139).

Reality is internal; the person's reality is his/her perception of the event rather than the actual event itself since no two people will view a situation in exactly the same way. Various factors affect perception: (1) the sensory apparatus and central nervous system of the person, (2) time for observation, (3) opportunities available to experience events, (4) the external environment, (5) interpersonal relationships, and (6) self-concept. The most important thing to the person is what is happening to the self at a given time. The person is aware of social values and norms but lives out those values and norms in a way that has been uniquely and personally defined (27, 139).

Perceptions about the self are crucial in influencing behavior. Of all the perceptions that exist for the person, none are more important than those held about the self, and the personal meaning and belief related to a situation. The self-concept is learned as a consequence of meaningful interactions with others and the world. The self-concept has a high degree of stability at its core, changing only with time and opportunity to try new perceptions of self.

The self-concept controls the phenomenal field and perceptual input; its maintenance and enhancement are the main motivating forces in life. The person always does what must be done, from a personal point of view. Thus human failures and abnormal behavior are seen as problems in faulty perception of self, others, and the world (27, 48, 139).

The truly adequate person sees self (and others) as an individual with dignity, integrity, worth, and importance. Only if he/she has a positive view of self can the person risk trying the untried or accepting the undefined situation. The person can become self-actualized only through the experience of being treated as an adequate person by significant others (27). This person is open to all experiences, develops trust in self, and dares to recognize feelings, live life fully, and express uniqueness. The person feels a sense of oneness with other people, depending on the nature of previous contacts with other people who have been important. The truly adequate, self-actualized person has a rich, varied, and available perceptual field. The person's phenomenal field is capable of change and able to make maximal use of experiences. The person does not have to defend against events or distort perceptions (27, 111, 112).

View of Education and Therapy

Education and therapy are: (1) growth-oriented rather than controlling, (2) rooted in perceptual meaning rather than facts, (3) concerned with people rather than things, (4) focused on the immediate rather than the historic view of people, and (5) hopeful rather than despairing. The goals of education and therapy are the same goals as those of the person: (1) the full functioning of the person, (2) ongoing development, (3) meeting the individual's potential, and (4) movement toward self-actualization. Education and therapy are a process, not a condition or institution, and through the process the person achieves effective behavior (27, 111, 112).

The learner or client brings to the learning or counseling situation a cluster of understandings, skills, values, and attitudes that have personal meaning and are the sum of reactions to previous experiences. The learner or client is unique, with a unique heredity and cultural and home background. He/she wants to learn that which has personal meaning and which will contribute to making a more adequate person. Therefore, the person must be fully involved, and learning involves all dimensions of the person. Learning results from experiencing. Facts are not as important as developing the perceptual field and finding the self. The learning that occurs depends on the meaning given by the person to the situation (27, 111, 112, 113).

The teacher or therapist is also a unique, whole

person with a self-concept that directly affects the philosophy and style of teaching or counseling. He/she does not consider self as central, but instead is learner- or client-centered. Each sees the self as using the personality as an instrument, acting as a permissive facilitator, and providing a warm, accepting, supportive environment that is as free from threat and obstacles as possible. The teacher or therapist provides an enriched environment and a variety of ways for the person to perceive new experiences and to learn. The teacher/therapist realizes that all people need to be perceived and related to as empathic, cooperative, forward-looking, trustworthy, and responsible. Third Force theorists reject the traditional, pessimistic, or mechanical view of people. Therefore, the central focus of learning or therapy is to develop a relationship rather than to have answers. The teacher or therapist lives in such a way as to make life as inviting and interesting as possible. The reward in living fully is the person's own feeling of adequacy, accomplishment, creativity, and meeting of self-actualization needs (25, 27, 111, 113).

One of the most positive contributions of the Third Force viewpoint is its focus on human consciousness. The Behaviorists rejected the idea of a conscious mind. Psychodynamic writers agreed that conscious mental activity was important but only as much as it reflected what was going on in the unconscious. Third Force psychologists are very much interested in consciousness as the vehicle by which we solve personal problems. For this reason, they have broadened their interests in recent years to include the study of altered states of consciousness through drugs (such as LSD), meditation, hypnosis, and yoga, to determine their effects on perception, thinking, and processes of human awareness.

Third Force Theorists

The theorists who belong to the Third Force include the humanists Abraham Maslow (Theory of Motivation and Hierarchy of Needs) and Carl Rogers (Theory on Self-Concept and Client-Centered Therapy). Other humanistic theorists include Arthur Combs (27), Donald Snygg (27), and Sidney Jourard (63). Humanistic nursing as a framework has been developed by Loretta Zderad and Josephine Paterson. Humanism is found as a thread in other nursing models, including Neuman's Health Care Systems Model, and is a basis for the views of Hildegarde Peplau, Dorothy Johnson, Martha Rogers, and Dorothy Orem.

Existential phenomenological theorists include Rollo May and R. D. Laing.

The Humanistic Perspective

Maslow: Theory of Motivation and Hierarchy of Needs

Abraham Maslow originated the term *Third Force* to show the perspectives of creativity and potential for freedom in the person, aspects that he felt were neglected in psychoanalytic and learning theories. Maslow studied normal people and sought to understand mental illness through a study of mental health, the opposite of analytic theorists (48). One of his most important concepts is *self-actualization, the tendency to develop potentialities and become a better person,* and the need to help the person achieve the sense of self-direction that is implicit in self-actualization. Implicit in this concept is the idea that people are not static but are always in the process of becoming something different and better (48, 86, 87, 88, 123).

The needs that motivate self-actualization can be represented in a hierarchy of relative order and predominance. The basic needs, in their order, are as follows (48, 86, 87).

1. *Physiological needs* include the needs for oxygen, water, food, temperature control, elimination, shelter, exercise, sleep, sensory stimulation, and sexual activity. These needs cease to exist as active means of determining behavior when satisfied, reemerging only if they are blocked or frustrated.

2. *Safety needs* include the needs for security, dependency, consistency, stability, fairness, structure, order, and limits; protection from immediate or future danger; freedom from fear, anxiety, and chaos; and a certain amount of routine.

3. *Love and belonging needs* derive from societal factors and include needs for identification with significant others, affection from and affiliation with others, recognition and approval, companionship, and group interactions. Love is not synonymous with sexual needs, but sexual needs may be motivated by a need for love and affection.

4. *Self-esteem and esteem for others* are concerned with the concept of self as a worthwhile person and an awareness of individuality. Included are needs for self-respect; respect from others; a sense of confidence, dignity, competence, independence, prestige, status, and success; and recognition from others for accomplishments.

5. *Self-actualization needs* include needs for self-fulfillment, ongoing emotional and spiritual development, reaching individual potentialities, using talents, being productive and having peak experiences. Self-actualization involves experiencing something fully, vividly, with full concentration and without self-consciousness.

6. *Knowledge and understanding* needs involve curiosity; a desire to know as much as possible; attraction to the mysterious, unknown, and unexplained; a desire to understand, systematize, organize, analyze, to look for relations and meanings; and a desire to construct a value system. The person who cannot meet these needs feels bored, apathetic, self-hate, depressed, and loses interest in life, self, and others.

7. *Aesthetic needs* include needs for beauty, harmony, and order, and are expressed in efforts to make the surroundings as attractive as possible, as well as in art, music, literature, dance, or other creative forms.

The self-actualized person also has a high need for knowledge and aesthetic experiences. This person views self and others objectively, clearly, and realistically. Hopes, wishes, fears, and defensive mechanisms do not distort observations. Because of superior perception and ability to make judgments, the person has a clearer notion of reality and right and wrong than most people. Yet the person has humility, listens carefully, admits what is not known, and learns from others. This person is dedicated to some work, task, duty, or vocation that is considered important. Work is exciting and pleasurable: the distinction between work and play blurs. Apparently commitment to an important job, hard work, discipline, and ability to do or to achieve are major requirements for growth, self-actualization, and happiness. The self-actualized person is creative; flexible; spontaneous in thinking, feeling, and behavior; and open and willing to make mistakes in an attempt to accomplish something. Courage, the ability to risk, to take a stand, to give criticism and ridicule, to take on a challenge, and to resist the influences of culture is combined with a sense of humility. Most people have far more creativity than is used; creativity rests on hard work, extreme self-discipline and perseverance, and training or in-depth study (48, 86, 87, 88, 139).

The self-actualized person has an integrated personality, a high degree of autonomy, and few conscious or unconscious conflicts. He/she is not afraid of personal desires or impulses but feels a sense of self-control and can manage them. This person finds pleasure in helping others, following a moral code, acting responsibly as a citizen, and being involved in work to improve society. Although this person is independent, can rely on self, and enjoys privacy and being alone, he/she also enjoys the company of others. The person is both individualistic and social, friendly, and loving. The self-actualizer depends less on others and therefore feels less ambivalence, hostility, and anxiety in relationships with others. The person does not seek prestige, honors, or rewards, although he/she may receive them (48).

The self-actualizing person feels a sense of kinship with all people, regardless of color, race, creed, class, education, political beliefs, or national boundaries. He/she is not threatened by differences; yet the person tends to have only a few deep, close, personal friendships, and the friends will be very similar to the individual. Outward appearance is less important than personality characteristics in friends. The person is very tolerant of another's shortcomings but very intolerant and righteously indignant about immoral, illegal, or unethical behavior in others. This person develops warm and deep relationships and is not exploitative, whether with friends, spouse, children, or work colleagues. Maslow's data contradict the stereotype of basic hostility between the sexes; this does not exist between two mature and self-actualizing persons. Rather, relationships between opposite sexes or with the same sex becomes stronger over time. Yet this person may be constructively and honestly critical when necessary (48).

The self-actualizer, superior in maturity and emotional health, is part of a small percentage of people. He/she has pains and problems but also gets more out of life and is bothered less by boredom, anxiety, fear, shame, or lack of purpose. The person has many interests, the ability to enjoy the simple things in life, and a sense of humor that does not ridicule others. There is disciplined ability to work through problems, less vulnerability to external threats, a deep commitment to democracy and ethical and moral behavior, and attraction to learning and the unknown. Self-acceptance and acceptance of others are basic to relationships. He/she is sufficiently philosophical to be patient and seek or accept slow, orderly change, rather than sudden changes, and to be both practical and theoretical (48).

Maslow's study of self-actualizing people refutes Freudian Theory that the human unconscious or id is only bad or dangerous. In self-actualizing people, the unconscious is creative, loving, and positive (48).

Maslow ranked these basic human needs from lowest to highest. They do not necessarily occur in a fixed order. But the physiological and safety needs, (deficiency needs) are dominant and must be met before higher needs can be achieved. Personal growth needs are those for love and belonging, self-esteem and recognition, and self-actualization. The highest needs of self-actualization, knowledge, and aesthetic expression may never be as fully gratified as those at lower levels. Individual growth and self-fulfillment are a continuing, lifelong process of developing, emerging, and becoming. Self-actualization involves risk (48, 87).

Maslow recognized the inadequacy of his motivational theory in explaining why, if the human is growth-oriented, so many fail to develop their potential. He theorized that the person has simultaneously a tendency toward inertia and growth, toward rest and activity. The difference in the direction of the tendency is in the environmental conditions. Certain environmental and social conditions are necessary for meeting basic needs, especially the growth needs. For the person to be motivated toward self-actualization, there must be freedom to speak, to pursue creative potential, and to inquire; an atmosphere of justice, honesty, fairness, and order; and environmental stimulation and challenge (48). Many people have trouble moving toward self-actualization because of the environment in which they live. For example, socialization practices may hinder women in utilizing their intellectual abilities to the greatest extent. Or men may be inhibited from expressing emotions of tenderness, love, or need of others by cultural norms. Deprivation of growth needs results in feelings of despair and depression, and a sense that life is meaningless (48, 56, 87, 88, 119).

Maslow thought that the neurotic is a person who is prevented from, or is preventing the self from, attaining basic needs. Thus, the person feels threatened, insecure, and unfulfilled. The therapist must show the client love and respect. The client must be encouraged to express affection to the therapist. When this reciprocal relationship is established, the client can begin movement toward meeting higher-level basic needs and maturity (48, 56, 119).

Rogers: Theory on Self-Concept and Client-Centered Therapy

Carl Rogers is, along with Maslow, one of the leaders of Humanistic Psychology. He has questioned several traditional concepts of science and has developed a perspective on personality with a focus on self-concept. Self-actualization is also a key concept in his theory. Rogers assumed that the person sees self as the center of a continually changing world and that he/she responds to the world as it is perceived. The person responds as a whole in the direction of self-actualization. The ability to achieve self-understanding, self-actualization, self-regard, and perception of social acceptance by others is based on experience and interaction with other people. The person who, as a child, felt wanted and highly valued is likely to have a positive self-image, be thought well of by others, and have the capacity to achieve self-actualization. Optimal adjustment results in what Rogers calls the fully functioning person. The fully functioning person accepts self, avoids a personality facade, is genuine and honest, is increasingly self-directive and autonomous, is open to new experiences, avoids being driven by other people's expectations or the cultural norms, and has a low level of anxiety (112, 115).

The person also has an ideal self, an idea of what he/she wishes to be, which may or may not be congruent with the "real" self. When a discrepancy develops between the "ideal" self and "real" self, a state of tension and confusion results. For example, interactions with the environment may present an unfavorable picture of the self, which will result in internal conflict. Feelings of unworthiness may produce anxiety and defensive psychological reactions (112).

Although the ways in which they have talked about behavior contrast sharply, both Rogers and Freud have developed their theoretical positions on the basis of similar observational data: the behavior of clients and therapists in psychotherapy. However, Rogers rejects the psychoanalytic notion that the individual is by nature irrational and unsocialized. He asserts, on the contrary, that each person is basically rational, socialized, and constructive (116). Behavior is goal-directed and motivated by needs. Unlike the intrapsychic and interpersonal theorists, Rogers states that current needs are the only ones the person endeavors to satisfy (111, 112).

Rogers identifies neurotic and psychotic people as those whose self-concepts and experiences do not match up. They are afraid to accept their own experiences as valid, so they distort them, either to protect themselves or to win approval from others. A therapist can help them give up the false self that has been formulated (111).

Rogers's technique of client-centered therapy brings about behavioral change by conveying complete acceptance, respect, and empathy for the client. The therapist neither provides interpretations nor gives advice. Providing this high degree of acceptance allows the person to meet basic needs that should have been met in childhood by significant people, to incorporate into the self-structure threatening feelings that were previously excluded, and to become aware of unconscious material that is controlling life. Perceptions and behavior change. The person may then continue the self-actualizing process. Recently Rogers has given the therapist a more active role that includes the therapist sharing emotions and feelings in an interchange with the client (111). Chapter 6 discusses use of Rogers's technique as it can be applied to the nurse-client relationship.

May and Laing: The Existential-Phenomenological Perspective

Existentialism, a theory of individual meaning, began with the nineteenth-century writings of the Danish philosopher Soren Kierkegaard. He introduced the idea of relational truth, that the subject (the human being) can never be separated from the object (what is observed), coupled with a phenomenological approach. He was interested in individual rather than group responses and in reaction to the immediate experience. The existentialist is not interested in explaining why things occur but rather in understanding a person's subjective experience (92, 119).

A person's only reality exists in his/her inner awareness and in the personal manner in which he/she experiences the world. This experiencing of reality is a freeing experience in that the person is not bound by the rules of others, yet it is oppressive in that the person can only derive in life what he/she makes for and of self. The person makes choices that change meaning and existence but is not free to avoid choice. Making choices is being alive, and the person must accept responsibility for the choices and their consequences. To establish personal goals is living authentically; to let others determine personal goals is behaving inauthentically (92, 119).

There are similarities as well as differences between Psychoanalytic and Existential theories. Both are interested in the basic question of human existence and an alleviation of suffering, and both blame society for interfering with people's healthful development. An important difference is the phenomenological viewpoint of the existentialists and their rejection of causality of behavior. The emphasis on "becoming" also contrasts with Freud's more pessimistic view. Becoming means that a situation is never static; change is always possible. The goal is to become completely human, and the person is always free to work toward that goal. Existentialists ask such questions as, "Who am I?" "Is there a meaning to life?" "How do I become an individual?" The denial of determinism, the basis of modern science, is probably the aspect of Existential Psychology most frequently criticized by other psychologists (119).

Existential and Humanist views are similar in the focus on the individual and the perception and meaning of events held by the person. Both Rogers and Maslow presented very hopeful, optimistic schemes for personal growth and development of the full human potential. In contrast, the framework of Existentialism is rather gloomy and pessimistic and focuses on internal conflicts of a crisis nature. The crises that are considered most important are those having to do with such issues as despair, anxiety, dread, aloneness, death, and meaninglessness. Existential Theory holds that internal conflicts result when people feel too separate from the world in which they exist (56).

If, as the existentialists maintain, most people are free to choose, why are so many people unhappy and dissatisfied? Why does maladaptive behavior exist? Not everyone chooses wisely; some choose to live authentically, others unauthentically. Also, for each person there are certain factors that limit what he/she may become: innate characteristics, such as learning ability or physical appearance, presence of a disabling disease, or environmental factors, including influence of the parental and later environments. Other unavoidable factors are guilt, which comes from a person's failure to fulfill all possibilities, and a dread of nothingness, not only of death but of alienation from the world (119).

May

Rollo May is one of the most prominent American existential theorists; he was originally a psychoanalyst. Two areas where he has made original contributions to Existential Psychology are his concept of anxiety and his ideas about dependency feelings as a central conflict in human development.

Since we live in a transitional age, values and goals are continually changing. This causes the person to question beliefs and to feel lost and helpless. Because of disintegration of values, the person feels isolated from other humans and empty inside. Emptiness comes from the feeling of powerlessness over events. With emptiness comes a feeling of loneliness. When values are in an upheaval, people turn to other people. The more they reach out, the more lonely they become because, according to May, the one way to over-come loneliness in the long run is to develop inner resources and values. Instead, people react to loneliness by doing things like going to boring parties to prove they are acceptable, clinging to loveless relationships, and seeking companionship to avoid anxiety that comes with loneliness and emptiness (90, 119).

Anxiety is created when a person is faced with the fundamental choice to move either forward or backward. Anxiety is not just an unpleasant feeling; it is the threat of imminent nonbeing. The person who has been rejected may question others and use the anxiety to change behavior constructively. Or he/she may avoid questions because of embarrassment, thus blocking further development. If anxiety is not used constructively, it causes guilt. Freud thought of guilt as a result of ignoring cultural prohibitions. May thinks of it as the response of a person who can choose but fails to do so (89, 119).

May thinks the person goes through definite stages of development. The pattern that carries through all these stages is the dependency struggle. Children are physically dependent on parents or others for a number of years. Even after this physical dependence ceases, psychological dependence remains. The Oedipal conflict described by Freud is seen by May not as a sexual conflict but as a dependency struggle. He describes it as occurring at age two and again in adolescence. This rebellion involves defiance of parents and rejection of societal rules. Although necessary in development, it is a rigid response and should not be confused with freedom.

May thinks of neurosis and psychosis as attempts to adjust to the threat of nonbeing by repressing or distorting experience so that some aspect of being can be preserved while accepting nonbeing in the rest of life (89, 90, 91).

The primary task of the therapist is to help the empty, lonely person expand experiences, fulfill personal uniqueness, and make constructive choices (56, 89, 90, 119). May would agree with Rogers's description of what he has learned as a therapist. The following statements describe the existential therapist (89, 90, 91).

> The therapist must be genuinely him/herself and not act with a facade.
> The therapist must listen with acceptance, and allow the other person to feel and be him/herself.
> The therapist, by being genuine and letting the client be, does not feel a need to rush in and fix things, to use a technique, to give assistance.
> The therapist is supportive to the client searching for personal awareness and meaning.

Perhaps neither May nor Rogers would ascribe to the view of Joan Middleton, who believes that, as an existentialist, the therapist is not able to help any other person except to offer a unique personality and respect to the other (92).

Laing

R. D. Laing, an English existential psychiatrist, has directed attention to deviant types of con-scious experience and has intensively studied and worked with schizophrenics. He believes that the anxious, insecure person feels unreal and dead rather than alive; questions his/her identity and autonomy; feels unauthentic, bad, and worthless; and may feel the self divorced from the body. This person experiences the outer world differently than others and must find ways to prove that he/she is real and has an identity (75, 76, 77).

Laing is interested in three modes of human experience: perception, memory, and imagination. He believes that if a disturbed person's perceptions, memories, and fantasies were known and understood, that person's behavior would make sense (54).

Laing's view of the person includes the general environment and family. Experiences are perceived through rules taught in the family and imposed by culture. The experience then becomes an image or memory. Behavior is a reflection of the images or memories of earlier experiences. Self-identity comes from what other people (and the individual) says he/she is (76).

Laing believes that although an unusual state of mind may be "different," it does not necessarily imply madness. The problem of schizophrenia is one of a split between the false facade a person represents to the world and the true inner reality or identity that goes unexpressed. The bizarre behavior of the schizophrenic results from stripping away of the false facade and the direct expression of inner preoccupations, distortions, and fears. The problem might not be the madness of the schizophrenic, but the falseness of interpersonal relations in modern life. The schizophrenic consciously experiences thoughts that people usually manage to hide. Laing has described schizophrenia as a growth experience, an attempt to solve an existential crisis, because from the psychotic turmoil may emerge a truer outer-self, the facade we present to others. Laing, like Rogers and others, believes false facades are created when great pressure is put on individuals to please other people, including parents. Schizophrenia may result from an abnormal socialization process that reinforces conventionality rather than genuine and spontaneous behavior (54, 75, 76, 77).

The client's abnormal behavior or symptoms are seen as a healing reaction to the problems being experienced, and in keeping with the medical model, Laing suggests that these symptoms must be allowed to run their course. Laing deviates from the Freudian approach, however, by not only insisting that we should not treat the symptoms, but also that we must not treat even the underlying disorder. Regression is seen as expected and acceptable behavior, and the client is allowed to live through the regression without interference so that the person can learn or acquire a genuine identity. The therapist describes the underlying images and fantasies to expose them and confirms the client's experiences (56, 75, 76, 77).

You may wish to examine your philosophical base carefully before adhering to existentialism in nursing practice. Yet, knowledge of the beliefs and approaches of May and Laing may help you better understand your client.

CURRENT ECOLOGICAL THEORIES ABOUT HUMAN DEVELOPMENT AND BEHAVIOR

Basic Principles

Ecology is an emerging science that is concerned with the community and the total setting in which life and behavior occur, and has contributed to the formulation of community psychology. The most basic ecological principle is that the continuity and survival of any ecological system (ecosystem) depend on a deliberate balance of factors influencing the interactions between the organism or person and the environment. For example, in a closed-top terrarium with plants and small animals, there is a steady exchange of oxygen and carbon dioxide between the plants and animals and sufficient moisture to maintain plant growth. If there is a sudden change in the ecosystem, the entire environment can be destroyed. The human community may not seem that fragile, but again the ecosystem is evident. A small town may be in a steady state until a minority family moves in, causing everyone to be hypervigilant about the family and the behavior of its members. Certain townspeople may refuse to associate with or give service to the minority family. This causes disruption in the life of the community. Another example might be a large city, which is able to provide adequate social services for its needy until a political change causes industries to move from the city, taking population and needed funds with them, so that there are fewer social or welfare services for poor families. The equilibrium of the city (ecosystem) has been disrupted (26).

The ecological approach can be quite helpful in examining how the community contributes to and manages mental health problems. The ecological approach raises several important issues:

1. *The interdependence or interrelation of social or organizational systems in the community.* Ecological analysis assumes that the operation of all community services are indirectly related. If a service does not exist, certain needs are not met or people must find other resources.

2. *The interdependence or relation between the physical environment and individual behavior.* Studies of overcrowding illustrate that the social environment affects behavior and may contribute to abnormal behavior.

3. *The interdependence or relation of the individual to the immediate social environment.* It has been found that group size has definite effects on individual behavior.

4. *The adaptation of every person in order to survive and prosper* within the natural environment.

5. *The change of systems.* No form of life remains static (56, 67, 68, 69).

Social Causation Versus Social Selection

Surveys in any urban or geographic area show that abnormal behavior and diagnosed emotional illness have a higher frequency in some areas than others. The high frequency areas tend to have substandard housing, high crime rate, and a high successful suicide rate. There are two conflicting explanations for the results:

1. *Social Causation Theory* believes that the poverty, poor schools, crime, poor housing, and prejudice often found in low income, deteriorating neighborhoods may increase the stress felt by already vulnerable people. Negative or unpleasant life events such as job loss, divorce, death in the family, or financial troubles are related to an increased chance of maladaptive behavior or physical illness (56).

2. *Social Selection Theory*, in contrast, states that the lower socioeconomic group has a greater incidence of maladaptive behavior

because people who do not function well show downward mobility from their original social status, increasing the proportion of people in the lower socioeconomic group who show maladaptive behavior. A number of studies support the Social Selection Theory, at least for disorders such as schizophrenia and alcoholism (30).

Those who believe in the community perspective support the Social Causation Theory. Although social selection may be a factor, the Social Causation Theory believes that stress-producing situations may aggravate existing disorders for people in the lower economic level. These people have less power to control their environment and fewer resources to deal with stress. There is also some evidence that lower economic-level families transmit a rigid set of behaviors and values to their children, which makes it harder for them to cope in a complex world (74).

Community Factors That Affect Behavior

Sociological Variables

Sociological variables, including socioeconomic level, position in the community and prestige related to birth, race, cultural ties, and power roles all affect behavior and adaptation of the person and family. Statistics show that abnormal behavior is found more frequently and intensely in: (1) poor families, (2) persons without meaningful social ties or roles (which may include the poor), and (3) persons who have suffered intense stress, loss of significant relationships, or severe crises (26, 56).

The findings by A. B. Hollingshead and F. C. Redlich in 1958 appear to still be applicable (61). Although presenting symptoms may be the same for people from all socioeconomic levels, those who are higher on the social economic ladder may be given different diagnostic labels than poorer people. Further, the more affluent people can obtain treatment earlier and more intensively, so that they are likely to exhibit fewer long-term abnormal symptoms than those who are lower in social status. Persons with abnormal behavior or who are eventually admitted to a psychiatric setting are more likely to be seen first in a court or welfare agency if they are poor, and by a physician or therapist if they are in middle or upper economic levels. In turn, treatment is more likely to consist of pharmaceuticals, shock treatments, or custodial care for the poor, in contrast to counseling for the more privileged. Length of treatment or hospitalization also varies with ability to pay. The poor and minorities are more likely to be labeled "deviant," receive negative responses from society and health professionals, and have difficulty returning to society (122). Urbanization, rapid social changes, social stressers, discrimination, unemployment, poor housing, inadequate diet and health care, feelings of *anomie* (*not being a part of society*), and negative self-image also contribute to stress and behavioral dysfunction in the vulnerable, immature person or in one without a support system. Persons whose social system is disrupted, for example, by loss of employment, or who do not find the opportunities to meet their achievement needs, appear susceptible to abnormal behavior (56, 103, 119).

Cultures

Cultures vary in their definitions of normal and abnormal behavior, which makes cross-cultural comparisons of mental health difficult. Variations in symptom content are also culturally related. For example, the schizophrenic African native may have delusions of being bewitched or poisoned, or his delusions of grandeur may consist of being a chief or medicine man (56). What is depression in our culture may be defined as physical illness in the Oriental culture. Or the person who is diagnosed as schizophrenic in our mainstream culture may be regarded as just being eccentric or different in some isolated rural areas of Appalachia, as being special in the Hutterite culture, or as being divine in some preliterate cultures. Senile psychosis appears rare in cultures that revere their elderly or where people live only 20 or 30 years. What is labeled homosexuality in our culture, such as men embracing, is considered normal man-to-man behavior in the Arab culture. Also the diagnosed mentally ill person behaves differently in different cultures; for example, the Japanese schizophrenic or manic is less aggressive than his counterpart from America. The black man who believes that the policeman might shoot first and then ask questions later *may not* be paranoid (17). Suicide incidence also varies considerably from culture to culture.

W. H. Grier and P. M. Cobbs agree that Blacks and other minorities must be evaluated by different psychological criteria than those used for Caucasions. They cite a number of important adaptive personality traits that Blacks have adopted in order to survive in white society, including "cultural paranoia." Although white observers might classify these traits as "abnormal," Grier and Cobbs believe that these patterns are not only normal but essential for black Americans in coping with the problems stemming from racism (52). Many Blacks have had identity conflicts in adapting to white society.

In this sense, the adaptive behavior of the individual may be viewed as healthy depending on the cultural context of such behavior. Soldiers are rewarded for killing people during wartime. Yet, when the war is over, such behavior is considered homicide. The behavior is not fundamentally different, but the cultural context of the behavior has changed.

Mental health problems of black Americans and other minorities must also be considered in the context of the social problems of their communities —high unemployment, inadequate housing, poor nutrition, and inferior educational programs. There can be no simple psychological remedies for problems that are, at the same time, economic and political. These individuals with behavior problems must be given adequate mental health assistance (56).

Thus the *social subcommunity* of which the individual is a part is a critical reference point in all evaluations of behavior in that values and behavior are usually intimately related to the values of the familiar and respected group (the subcommunity). For example, a teenage boy in a tough, working-class neighborhood may be proud of his fighting skills and receive respect and admiration from peers. Should this youth later become a clergyman, he may come to see his former qualities as deviant and distasteful (56).

Geographical Moves

Geographical moves from one location to another, or from one subculture to another, create many adjustments for the person as he/she attempts to meet norms of the new community. Such individuals are a high-risk group because of the difficulty of these transactions. Dysfunctional behavior may be a problem among those who migrate (56).

Status and Role Factors

Status and role factors also influence an individual's behavior. Certain types of behaviors may be expected from a person because of age, sex, race, religion, or occupation. The individual may experience role conflicts when there are discrepancies between norms and values and the demands of occupation, sex, religion, or age. If the person occupies two or more roles or social strata, he/she may manifest dysfunctional behavior (122).

Labeling

Labeling occurs whenever people are categorized on some basis, such as their roles, life styles, residence, age, or behavior. The label, whether or not it is accurate or fair, affects other people's responses to the person. For example, the role of the mental patient is deeply ingrained as socially unacceptable, and labeling someone as mentally ill is often permanently damaging. The damage takes many forms, including discrimination by others and personal feelings of self-doubt and inadequacy (28). Various studies confirm the negative effects of negative labeling (117). Labels attached to the so-called deviant person, whether those labels refer to the emotionally ill according to the *Diagnostic and Statistical Manual III* published by the American Psychiatric Association and used by the medical profession (see Appendix at end of book) or to someone from a specific racial or minority group, may result in failure to see other characteristics of the person, rejection from others, a negative self-concept, and eventually general incompetence in the labeled person. Labels, even when true, imply deviance and tend to exaggerate differences between people; they isolate the labeled person and interfere with objectivity in the professional (28, 56).

Some professionals, as well as some lay people, think abnormal behavior results from individual failure. In this view, an individual's psychological problems are the result of some personal circumstance, such as deficient achievement of developmental tasks, immaturity, character defect, or maladjustment. In some cases, this ideology extends so far as to blame the victims for their own problems and failures. Typically, such stereotypes are applied in judging lower socioeconomic group and minorities: "It's their own fault." "They really don't want to work." (56)

An alternate view is to see the individual problems as stemming from social causes. The broad economic, political, cultural, and social patterns of the nation and particular subcultures can be viewed as determinants of individual responses. One result of this broader social context viewpoint is the growing feeling that the community is the place to begin making changes if individual dysfunction is to be decreased (56).

A Systems Perspective: General Systems Theory Applied to Behavior

General Systems Theory, first proposed by Ludwig von Bertalanffy, presents a comprehensive, holistic, and interdisciplinary view. This theory does not represent a separate discipline but advocates that nothing is determined by a single cause or explained by a single factor (133). Nothing can be studied as a lone entity: the environment; various sociocultural components; political-legal, religious, educational, and other social institutions or organizations; the person, family, group, or community; or the health care delivery organization. All have interrelating parts, and all components interact with each other (100). Further, any entity is more than the sum of its parts. A general systems perspective presents a humanistic view of the person as a holistic, goal-directed, self-maintaining, creative individual of intrinsic worth, capable of self-reflection upon his/her uniqueness (123).

A system is a combination of two or more interdependent parts, persons, or objects that are united by some form or order into a recognizable unit and are in equilibrium (13, 23, 100, 133).

People satisfy their needs within social systems. The *social system is groups of people joined cooperatively to achieve certain common goals, using an organized set of practices to regulate behavior* (9). The person occupies various positions and has defined roles in the social system. The person and his/her health are shaped by the system; in turn, people create and change social systems (100).

Characteristics of any system include the following elements or components (3, 13, 85, 100):

1. *Parts are the basic components and are the interdependent units*. None can operate

without the other. Change in one part affects the entire unit. For example, the person as a whole system is made up of physical, emotional, mental, spiritual, and social aspects. Physically, he/she is made up of body systems: neurological, cardiovascular, etc. The health agency is one part of the health care system, and it in turn is made up of parts: physical plant, employees, clients, and departments that give services.

2. *Attributes are characteristics of the parts*, such as temperament or health of the person, or the roles, education, or age of health agency employees. These are variables that affect interactions.

3. *Information or communication is the sending of messages and getting feedback*, or exchange of energy or matter that is essential for growth, development, and life maintenance.

4. *Boundary is a barrier or area of demarcation that limits or keeps a system distinct from its environment*; prevents entrance of undesirable or extraneous matter, energy, or information; and aids information exchange. The person's skin, family, home, or health agency building are boundaries. Yet the boundary is not always rigid and must be permeable in open systems. Relatives outside the home are part of the family. The boundary may also be an imaginary line, such as the feeling that comes from belonging to a certain racial or ethnic group.

5. *Organization is the formal or informal arrangement of parts to form a whole and complex entity* so that the organism or institution has a working order that results in established hierarchy, rules, or customs. The person can be organized or categorized according to physical structure, basic needs, cognitive and developmental stages, and achievement of developmental tasks. In the family or health agency, the hierarchy provides organization that is based on power (ability to control others) and responsibility. Nursing care may be organized into primary or team nursing. Specialization in medical practice is also a way of organizing care. Organization in an institution is also maintained by norms, roles, and customs that each member must learn.

6. *Goals are the purposes of or reasons for the system to exist.* The system must be able to determine its work, adapt, and accomplish what is necessary to maintain life.

7. *Environment refers to the social and physical world outside the system, boundaries or community in which the system exists.* A constant exchange of energy and information must exist with the surrounding specified environment if the system is to be useful, creative, and open. If this information or energy exchange does not occur, the system becomes ineffective and closed.

8. *Evolutionary processes, changes within the person and the environment, proceeding from simple to complex, occur in all systems.* The interaction between the person and environment results in a more complex person and environment. The person undergoes changes in physical, psychological, and social growth throughout the life span, within certain parameters.

Von Bertalanffy identified two types of systems. (1) The **closed system** is *an entity or complex of components that is isolated from its environment.* Once the components are in the system, no new components are added (133). (2) All living organisms, such as the human or various social systems, are classified as **open systems** because they are *characterized by the ability to exchange energy, matter, and information with the environment in order to evolve into higher levels of heterogeneity, organization, and order.* Because of this dynamic interaction of the system with the environment and the ability for self-direction and monitoring, the final products tend to resemble each other (equifinality) even though they began with different initial components. The environment will influence, but will not determine, the final state (100). Every person is an open social system. Physically there is a hierarchy of components such as cells and organ systems. Emotionally there are levels of needs and feelings. Cognitively a person has memories, knowledge, and intellectual strategies. Socially the person is in a relative rank in a hierarchy of prestige roles, such as boss, worker, adult, or child. Although internal stimuli are at work, such as those governed by the nervous and endocrine systems, outer stimuli also affect the person. The boundaries or environment—such as one's skin, the limits set by others, one's status, home, and community—influence the person's needs and goal achievement. To remain healthy, the person must have feedback: the condition of the skin tells about temperature control; an emotional reaction signifies a sense of security, a job well done, or a failure; a pain signifies malfunction or injury. In turn, the person influences the world through his/her behavior (100).

The state of health of a system can be identified by determining: (1) how well it adapts to environmental constraints, (2) how closely output meets goals, (3) how efficiently internal and external resources are used for meeting goals, and (4) the degree of differentiation among component parts and their ability to function cooperatively to meet system goals.

When the system finds that its usual adaptation mechanisms or responses fail, then it can: (1) alter itself, (2) alter the environment, (3) withdraw from the environment, or (4) alter its purpose, goal, or concept of desirable state.

Von Bertalanffy was concerned with explaining the behavior of the human system as a whole and did not concern himself with pathological behavior and its treatment. His theories indicate that pathological behavior must be viewed in light of current culture and time. Many variables contribute to the formation of current behavior; there is no one cause (133).

Martha Rogers in her Theory of Man views the person holistically and as an open system in constant interchange with the environment with life processes evolving in one direction along the space-time continuum (116). The person is characterized by sensation, emotion, pattern, organization, and ability to use abstraction, imagery, language and thought. Life processes are homeodynamic.

A HUMANISTIC, INTERACTIONAL VIEW OF NURSING PRACTICE

The theories that are discussed in this chapter can be utilized in developing a conceptual framework for nursing, since theories from another discipline can be combined with nursing theory that has already been formulated as a result of nursing research. Table 2-10 summarizes the nursing implications of many of the theories described in this chapter.

We have attempted to describe the most valuable contributions of the major theoretical perspectives concerning development and behavior. A certain viewpoint may contribute to understanding one set of conditions. Under a different set, another viewpoint may be more helpful. Such an approach is called an *eclectic or interactional approach* to behavior. How a situation influences behavior depends on the particular vulnerabilities,

capabilities, preoccupations, and adaptations of the person experiencing the particular set of conditions. Additionally, the variables emphasized by different theoretical perspectives interact or exert combined effects. Dysfunctional or abnormal behavior, or emotional illness, can result from any, or perhaps all, of a large number of factors.

Throughout this book, the authors will be presenting many viewpoints, including First, Second, and Third Force theories and biological, psychological, and ecological (community) perspectives for any condition or emotional illness. However, the Third Force theorists, especially the humanists, will provide the basis for our discussions of the nursing process. We consider the humanistic approach to be essential in a caring, professional person.

TABLE 2-10.   Nursing Implications of Selected Theories

THEORIST/THEORY	NURSING IMPLICATIONS OF THEORY
Skinner's Operant Conditioning Theory	1. In teaching or therapy, follow the guidelines previously described for a behavior modification program. 2. The general procedure for behavior modification is to: a. Plan what behavior is to be established; plan what is to be taught and at what specific time. Objectives are specific. Follow the teaching or treatment plan explicitly.

TABLE 2-10. Continued

THEORIST/THEORY	NURSING IMPLICATIONS OF THEORY
	b. Determine available reinforcers. Feedback from physical sensations, excelling over others, or the teacher's affection—all may reinforce. The only way to determine whether a consequence is rewarding is to observe its effect on the behavior associated with it. c. Identify the responses that can be made by the person. d. Plan how reinforcements can be efficiently scheduled so the behavior will be repeated. Reinforcements must immediately follow the desired behavior.
Freud's Psychoanalytic Theory	1. Insight into own behavior can add to personal maturity and understanding of others. 2. Constructs of id, ego, superego, conscious-unconscious continuum, manifestations of anxiety and defense mechanisms, and psychosexual development are useful in assessment and therapy. 3. All behavior meaningful; outer behavior may hide inner need or conflict. 4. Use knowledge of psychosexual development to teach parents about norms and meaning of child's behavior. 5. Transference and resistance must be worked through in therapy.
Erikson's Epigenetic Theory	1. Assessment of and insight into own stage of development. 2. Use knowledge of eight stages and psychosexual tasks in assessment, therapy, and teaching parents about child development. 3. Help clients and staff realize that emotional development is lifelong process and that society influences health and behavior.
Sullivan's Interpersonal Theory	1. One Genus Postulate basic to nursing practice with clients from all settings and backgrounds. 2. Assess developmental stage and task; teach family about normal development and development of self-system. 3. Promote syntaxic rather than parataxic mode of experiencing through intervention. 4. Promote positive experiences for client so that "good-me" or positive self-concept can develop.
Berne's Transactional Analysis	1. Analyze own dominant ego stage, psychological position, type of transactions engaged in, and kind of strokes (reinforcement) sought. 2. Assess feeling state as most accurate way to determine ego state. 3. Assess posture, nonverbal behavior, and language of client to determine ego state. 4. Assess how person gets along with others to determine ego state, transaction styles, and psychological position of client.

TABLE 2-10.   Continued

THEORIST/THEORY	NURSING IMPLICATIONS OF THEORY
	5. Use knowledge of games, types of transactions, and strokes in therapy. Help client gain feeling of "I'm OK—you're OK," and behaviors to attain positive strokes from others.
	6. Theory useful in personal and professional life, with family, friends, and colleagues as well as clients.
Bandura's Social Learning Theory	1. Your appearance and behavior are a model for client.
	2. Determine who significant adults were in the person's life and who role models were.
	3. In teaching, demonstrate desired self-care behavior.
	4. Recovered person visiting an ill client can serve as model for rehabilitation and a normal life, e.g., person with mastectomy, colostomy, amputation, alcoholism.
	5. Demonstrate nurturing approaches or discipline methods to child client so that parents can learn effective child-rearing methods.
	6. Nurse-client relationship is a behavioral model of trust and interpersonal relations for the client.
Rotter's Cognitive Social Learning Theory	1. Client's feeling about the amount of control in situation affects his decision making about life event, pursuit of health practices, various goals, or self-actualization; following medical orders; initiation of preventive measures.
	2. Intervention involves helping person gain realistic expectations of own abilities and the situation.
Piaget's Theory of Cognitive Development	1. Teach parents about process of child's cognitive development and the implications for education, purchase of toys, and interactions.
	2. Assess cognitive stage of client as basis for planning content and presentation in teaching sessions.
	3. Assess cognitive development to determine language and abstraction level to use in therapy.
	4. Use knowledge of cognitive development in play therapy.
	5. Use knowledge of Preoperational and Concrete Phases to understand and work with many adult clients, including those diagnosed as schizophrenic.
Bruner's Cognitive Construct Theory	1. Assess person's major mode of managing reality; intervene to facilitate client's use of symbolic mode. Whether person talks, forms images, or acts out problems depends on cultural background, past experiences, degree of curiosity, and exploration abilities.
	2. See self as facilitator, providing opportunities for client to learn and mature, rather than in control of client.
	3. Nursing intervention and therapy should foster: a. Positive self-image. b. Attitude of curiosity. c. Self-confidence in solving problems. d. Knowledge base for self-care.

TABLE 2-10. Continued

THEORIST/THEORY	NURSING IMPLICATIONS OF THEORY
	e. Reflectiveness about self and environment.
	f. Ability to explore alternatives; opportunity for intuitive thinking.
	g. Intellectual and affective honesty.
	h. Willingness to live in harmony and participate honestly in community affairs.
	4. Teaching should foster independence and discovery. Utilize Bruner's four features of a theory of instruction:
	a. *Predisposition to learn.* Be concerned with the experiences and contexts that will tend to make the person willing and able to learn.
	b. *Structure of knowledge.* Know how to organize or structure a body of knowledge so that it can be most readily grasped by the learner.
	c. *Sequence.* Present the materials in the most effective sequence.
	d. *Reinforcement.* Specify the nature and pacing of rewards, moving from extrinsic rewards to intrinsic ones in your reinforcement of the learner.
	5. Emphasize intrinsic motivation with individual, family, group, or community. Emotional health comes from inner motivation and process; it cannot be forced by outer demands. Self-care practices result from inner motivation.
Lewin's Gestalt Field Psychology	1. Examine your life space; enlarge it to become more empathic nurse.
	2. Focus on the total person and environment rather than on pathology and treatment.
	3. Knowledge of laws of perception enhances assessment and therapy.
	4. Assessment of client enhanced by understanding of concept of life space, psychological environment, nonpsychological foreign hull, and the inner and outer areas of the psychological person, and forces that motivate behavior. Determine psychological position of client in reference to various goals, ideas, and activities.
	5. Recognize in therapy that person occupies a series of overlapping life spaces that are continuous and similar but not identical, which can account for the lack of response or misunderstandings.
	6. Determine vectors of valences (attracting and repelling powers) of various objects, events, ideas, and regions of life space to ascertain ability to change behavior.
	7. In teaching or therapy, life space of person must be expanded in order to increase client's awareness of personal and other behavior, to try new behavior, and to move into new situations.

TABLE 2-10. Continued

THEORIST/THEORY	NURSING IMPLICATIONS OF THEORY
	8. In teaching or counseling, there must be an intersection of your life space with life space of the client.
Kohlberg's Theory of Moral Development	1. Assess own level of moral development. 2. Assess client's level of moral development when working with children, adolescents, or adults. 3. Through your modeling, clarification, explanation, and validation, contribute to client's moral development.
Maslow's Theory of Motivation and Hierarchy of Needs	1. Assessment can be done around hierarchy of needs. Planning and intervention must consider need hierarchy and priorities in care. 2. Person is a unified whole, not divided into components of needs. 3. Higher level needs can be met simultaneously with some lower-level needs. 4. Concepts of needs and motivation can be used in teaching and therapy. By meeting needs of client on one level, you can help client mature and feel motivated to meet growth needs.
Roger's Theory of Self- and Client-Centered Therapy	1. Assess own self-concept and self-actualization needs prior to counseling clients. 2. Assess client's self-concept; promote positive experiences and contribute to development of positive self-concept. 3. In therapy, assume as much as possible client's frame of reference to perceive world as he/she does. 4. Be accepting, warm, genuine, and empathic to help client discover self and mature.
General Systems Theory	1. Consider self as an individual system as well as part of other systems. 2. Consider client (individual, family, group, or community) as part of a system in implementing nursing process. 3. Consider client in totality and the relationships and interactions between parts: physiological, psychological, spiritual, and sociocultural. Dysfunction in one part affects all parts. 4. Client, as a system, has definite range for absorption, processing, and retention of stimuli. Avoid overstimulation or deprivation of stimuli. Assess needs and intervene accordingly. 5. Help client determine resources and supportive systems that will maintain or return function and wellness.

REFERENCES

1. Adler, Alfred, *The Practice and Theory of Individual Psychology*. London: Routledge & Kegan Paul Ltd., 1923.

2. Almy, M., E. Chittenden, and P. Miller, *Young Children's Thinking: Studies of Some Aspects of Piaget's Theory*. New York: Teachers College Press, 1967.

3. Anderson, Ralph, and I. Carter, *Human Behavior in the Social Environment*. Chicago: Aldine Publishing Company, 1974.

4. Babcock, Dorothy, "Transactional Analysis," *American Journal of Nursing*, 76, no. 7 (1976), 1152-55.

5. Baldwin, Alfred, *Theories of Child Development*. New York: John Wiley & Sons, Inc., 1967.

6. Baltes, Margaret, and Melissa Zerbe, "Re-establishing Self-Feeding in a Nursing Home Resident," *Nursing Research*, 25, no. 1 (1976), 24-26.

7. Bandura, Albert, *Social Learning Theory*. Morristown, N.J.: General Learning Press, 1971.

8. Barr, Norman, "The Responsible World of Reality Therapy," *Psychology Today*, 7, no. 2 (1974), 64-68.

9. Bell, Earl, *Social Foundations of Human Behavior*. New York: Harper & Row, Publishers, Inc., 1961.

10. Berne, Eric, *Transactional Analysis in Psychotherapy*. New York: Grove Press, Inc., 1961.

11. ——, *Games People Play*. New York: Grove Press, Inc., 1964.

12. Bernie, Rosemarian, and Wilbert Fordyce, *Behavior Modification and the Nursing Process*. St. Louis: The C. V. Mosby Company, 1973.

13. Berrien, Kenneth, *General and Social Systems*. New Brunswick, N.J.: Rutgers University Press, 1968.

14. Bigge, Morris, *Learning Theories for Teachers*, 3rd ed. New York: Harper & Row, Publishers, Inc., 1976.

15. Binswanger, L., *Being-in-the-World*. New York: Basic Books, Inc., 1963.

16. Bower, Fay Louise, *The Process of Planning Nursing Care: A Theoretical Model*. St. Louis: The C. V. Mosby Company, 1972.

17. Brody, E. B., "Color and Identity Conflict in Young Boys," *Psychiatry*, 26 (1963), 188-201.

18. Bruner, Jerome, *The Process of Education*. Cambridge, Mass.: Harvard University Press, 1960.

19. ——, *Toward a Theory of Instruction*. Cambridge, Mass.: Harvard University Press, 1966.

20. Bruner, Jerome, ed., *Learning about Learning: A Conference Report*. Monograph No. 15. Washington, D.C.: U.S. Department of Health, Education and Welfare, 1966.

21. Bruner, Jerome, and Jeremy Anglin, *Beyond the Information Given: Studies in the Psychology of Knowing*. New York: W. W. Norton & Co., Inc., 1973.

22. Bugelski, B. R., *The Psychology of Learning Applied to Teaching*. Indianapolis: The Bobbs-Merrill Co., Inc., 1964.

23. Buckley, Walter, *Sociology and Modern Systems Theory*. Englewood Cliffs, N.J.: Prentice-Hall, Inc., 1967.

24. Carruth, Beatrice, "Modifying Behavior through Social Learning," *American Journal of Nursing*, 76, no. 11 (1976), 1084-6.

25. Carter, Susan, "The Nurse Educator: Humanist or Behaviorist?" *Nursing Outlook*, 26, no. 9 (1978), 554-57.

26. Clausen, J. A., "Sociology and Psychiatry," in *Comprehensive Textbook of Psychiatry II*, Vol. 1, 2nd ed., eds. A. M. Fredman, H. I. Kaplan, and B. J. Sadock. Baltimore: The Williams & Wilkins Company, 1975.

27. Combs, Arthur, and Donald Snygg: *Individual Behavior: A Perceptual Approach to Behavior*. New York: Harper & Row, Publishers, Inc., 1959.

28. Cullen, Agnes, "Labeling Theory and Social Science," *Perspectives in Psychiatric Care*, 12, no. 3 (1974), 123-25.

29. Dollard, J., and Neal Miller, *Personality and Psychotherapy*. New York: McGraw-Hill Book Company, 1950.

30. Dunham, H. W., "Social Class and Schizophrenia," *American Journal of Orthopsychiatry*, 34 (1964), 634-42.

31. Eissler, Ruth et al., eds., *The Psychoanalytic Study of the Child*, Vol. 25. New York: International Universities Press, 1970.

32. Erikson, Erik, *Childhood and Society*, 2nd ed. New York: W. W. Norton & Co., Inc., 1963.

33. Erickson, Marilyn, *Child Psychopathology: Assessment, Etiology, and Treatment*. Englewood Cliffs, N.J.: Prentice-Hall, Inc., 1978.

34. Fagan, J., and L. Shepard, eds., *Gestalt Therapy Now*. New York: Harper Colophon Books, 1970.

35. ——, *What Is Gestalt Therapy?* New York: Perennial Library: Harper & Row, Publishers, Inc., 1970.

36. Freud, Anna, *The Ego and the Mechanisms of Defense*. London: Hogarth Press, Ltd., 1937.

37. Freud, Sigmund, *New Introductory Lectures in Psychoanalysis*. New York: W. W. Norton & Co., Inc., 1933.

38. ——, *A General Introduction to Psychoanalysis*. New York: Simon & Schuster, 1935.

39. ——, *The Problem of Anxiety*. New York: W. W. Norton & Co., Inc., 1936.

40. ——, *Ego and the Id*. London: Hogarth Press, 1947.

41. ——, *Inhibitions, Symptoms, and Anxiety*. London: Hogarth Press, 1948.

42. ——, *Outline of Psychoanalysis*. New York: W. W. Norton & Co., Inc., 1949.

43. Fromm, Eric, *The Art of Loving*. New York: Harper & Row, Publishers, Inc., 1963.

44. Gagne, Robert, *The Conditions of Learning*, 3rd ed. New York: Holt, Rinehart and Winston, 1977.

45. Gershon, E. et al., "Genetic Studies and Biologic Strategies in the Affective Disorders," in *Progress in Medical Genetics*, Vol. II, eds. A. Steinberg, A. Bearn, A. Motulsky, and B. Childs. Philadelphia: W. B. Saunders Company, 1977.

46. Glaser, William, *Reality Therapy: A New Approach to Psychiatry*. New York: Harper & Row, Publishers, Inc., 1965.

47. ——, *Mental Health or Mental Illness*. New York: Harper & Row, Publishers, Inc., 1961.

48. Goble Frank, *The Third Force: The Psychology of Abraham Maslow*. New York: Grossman Publisher, 1970.

49. Goldiamond, Israel, "A Diary of Self-Modification," *Psychology Today*, 3, no. 11 (1973), 95–100.

50. Gordon, J. W., "Who Is Mad? Who Is Insane? R. D. Laing: In Search of a New Psychiatry," *Atlantic*, 227 (1971), 50–66.

51. Graves, Joy, "Psychoanalytic Theory. A Critique," *Perspectives in Psychiatric Care*, 11, no. 3 (1973), 114–20.

52. Grier, W. H., and P. M. Cobbs, *Black Rage*. New York: Basic Books, Inc., 1968.

53. Grubbs, Judy, "An Interpretation of the Johnson Behavioral System Model for Nursing Practice," in *Conceptual Models for Nursing Practice*, 2nd ed., eds. Joan P. Riehl and Callista Roy. New York: Appleton-Century-Crofts, 1980.

54. Haber, Judith et al., *Comprehensive Psychiatric Nursing*. New York: McGraw-Hill Book Company, 1978.

55. Hamden-Turner, Charles, and Phillip Whitter, "Morals: Left and Right," *Psychology Today*, 4, no. 11 (1971).

56. Hermatz, Morton, *Abnormal Psychology*. Englewood Cliffs, N.J.: Prentice-Hall, Inc., 1978.

57. Harris, Thomas A., *I'm OK — You're OK*. New York: Harper & Row, Publishers, Inc., 1967.

58. Hartmann, Heinz, *Essays on Ego Psychology*. New York: International Universities Press, 1964.

59. Heidbreder, Edna, *Seven Psychologies*. Englewood Cliffs, N.J.: Prentice-Hall, Inc., 1961.

60. Hilgard, Ernest, and Gordon Bower, *Theories of Learning*, 4th ed. Englewood Cliffs, N.J.: Prentice-Hall, Inc., 1975.

61. Hollingshead, A. B., and F. C. Redlich, *Social Class and Mental Illness: A Community Study*. New York: John Wiley & Sons, Inc., 1958.

62. Horney, Karen, *The Neurotic Personality in Our Time*. New York: W. W. Norton & Co., Inc., 1937.

63. Jourard, Sidney, *Disclosing Man to Himself*. New York: D. Van Nostrand Company, 1968.

64. Jung, Carl, *The Psychology of the Unconscious*, B. M. Hinkle, trans. New York: Dodd, Mead & Company, 1927.

65. ——, *Man and His Symbols*. New York: Doubleday & Co., Inc., 1964.

66. ——, "Psychological Types," in *Collected Works of Carl G. Jung*, Vol. 6, ed. G. Adler et al. Princeton, N.J.: Princeton University Press, 1971.

67. Kelly, J. G., "Ecological Constraints on Mental Health Services," *American Psychologist*, 21 (1966), 535–39.

68. ——, "Towards an Ecological Conception of Preventive Intervention," in *Research Contributions from Psychology to Community Mental Health*. ed. J. W. Carter. New York: Behavioral Publications, 1968.

69. ——, "Naturalistic Observations in Contrasting Social Environments," in *Naturalistic Viewpoints in Psychological Research*, eds. E. P. Williams and H. L. Raush. New York: Holt, Rinehart and Winston, 1969.

70. Kohlberg, L. "Moral Education in Schools," *School Review*, 74 (1966), 7.

71. ——, "A Cognitive Developmental Approach to Moral Education," *The Humanist*, 1 (November-December, 1972), 15 ff.

72. ——, *Recent Research in Moral Development*. New York: Holt, Rinehart and Winston, 1977.

73. Kohlberg, Lawrence, and Elliot Turiel, "Moral Development and Moral Education," in *Psychology and Education Practice*, ed. G. S. Lesser. Chicago: Scott, Foreman & Company, 1971.

74. Kohn, M. L., "Social Class and Schizophrenia: A Critical Review and Reformulation," *Schizophrenia Bulletin*, 7 (1973), 60–79.

75. Laing, R. D., *The Divided Self: An Existential Study in Sanity and Madness*. Baltimore: Penguin Books, 1965.

76. ——, *The Politics of Experience*. New York: Pantheon Books, Inc., 1967.

77. ——, *Self and Others*. Baltimore: Penguin Books, 1975.

78. Landis, Dylan, "A Scan for Mental Illness," *Discovery* (1980), pp. 26–28.

79. Latner, J., *The Gestalt Therapy Book*. New York: Julian Press, Inc., 1973.

80. LeBow, Michael, *Behavior Modification*. Englewood Cliffs, N.J.: Prentice-Hall, Inc., 1973.

81. Levinthal, Charles, *The Physiological Approach in Psychology*. Englewood Cliffs, N.J.: Prentice-Hall, Inc., 1979.

82. Lewin, Kurt, *A Dynamic Theory of Personality: Selected Papers*. New York: McGraw-Hill Book Company, 1935.

83. ——, *Theory in Social Science*. New York: Harper & Row, Publishers, Inc., 1951.

84. Lewin, Pamela, and Eric Berne, "Games Nurses Play," *American Journal of Nursing*, 72, no. 3 (1972), 483–87.

85. Loomis, C. P., *Social Systems*. New York: D. Van Nostrand Company, 1960.

86. Maslow, Abraham, *Towards a Psychology of Being*, 2nd ed. New York: D. Van Nostrand Company, 1968.

87. ——, *Motivation and Personality*, 2nd ed. New York: Harper & Row, Publishers, Inc., 1970.

88. ——, *The Farther Reaches of Human Nature*. New York: The Viking Press, 1971.

89. May, Rollo, *Existential Psychology*. New York: Random House, Inc., 1960.

90. ——, *Psychology and the Human Dilemma*. New York: D. Van Nostrand Company, 1967.

91. May, Rollo, E. Angel, and H. Ellenberg, *Existence: A New Dimension in Psychiatry and Psychology*. New York: Basic Books, Inc., 1958.

92. Middleton, Joan, "Existentialist as Helper?" *Canadian Psychiatric Nursing*, 20, no. 3 (1979), 7–8.

93. Miller, Neal, "Learnable Drives and Rewards," in *Handbook of Experimental Psychology*, ed. S. S. Stevens. New York: John Wiley & Sons, Inc., 1951.

94. ——, "Central Stimulation and Other New Approaches to Motivation and Reward," *American Psychologist*, 13 (1958), 100–108.

95. ——, "Chemical Coding of Behavior in the Brain," *Science*, 148 (1965), 328–38.

96. ——, "Learning of Visceral and Glandular Responses," *Science*, 163 (1969), 434–45.

97. ——, "Interaction between Learned and Physical Factors in Mental Illness," in *Annual Review of Behavior Therapy*, eds. C. P. Frank and G. Wilson. New York: Brunner & Mazel, Inc., 1973.

98. Mowrer, O. H., *Learning Theory and Personality Dynamics*. New York: The Ronald Press Company, 1960.

99. Munroe, Ruth, *Schools of Psychoanalytic Thought*. New York: Holt, Rinehart and Winston, 1955.

100. Murray, Ruth, and Judith Zentner, *Nursing Concepts for Health Promotion*, 2nd ed. Englewood Cliffs, N.J.: Prentice-Hall, Inc., 1979.

101. Neuman, Betty, "The Betty Neuman Health-Care Systems Model: A Total Person Approach to Patient Problems," in *Conceptual Models for Nursing Practice*, 2nd ed., eds. Joan P. Riehl and Callista Roy. New York: Appleton-Century-Crofts, 1980.

102. Orem, Dorothy, *Nursing: Concepts of Practice*. New York: McGraw-Hill Book Company, 1971.

103. Parloff, Morris, "Shopping for the Right Therapy," *Saturday Review*, February 21, 1976, pp. 14–20.

104. Patterson Josephine, and Loretta Zderad, *Humanistic Nursing*. New York: John Wiley & Sons, Inc., 1976.

105. Peplau, Hildegarde, *Interpersonal Relations in Nursing*. New York: G. P. Putnam's Sons, 1952.

106. Perls, F. S., *Gestalt Therapy Verbatim*. Lafayette, Calif.: Real People Press, 1969.

107. Piaget, Jean, *Six Psychological Studies*. New York: Random House, Inc., 1967.

108. Pugh, Elizabeth, "Dynamics of Teaching-Learning Interaction," *Nursing Forum*, 15, no. 1 (1976), 47–58.

109. Redmond, Gertrude, "A Study of Modification of Socially Acceptable Eating Behavior," *Perspectives of Psychiatric Care*, 11, no. 3 (1973), 126–28.

110. Riehl, Joan, and Sister Callista Roy, "Theory and Models," in *Conceptual Models for Nursing Practice*, 2nd ed., eds. Joan Riehl and Callista Roy. New York: Appleton-Century-Crofts, 1980.

111. Rogers, Carl, *Client-Centered Therapy*. Boston: Houghton Mifflin Company, 1951.

112. ——, *On Becoming a Person*. Boston: Houghton Mifflin Company, 1961.

113. ——, *Freedom to Learn*. Columbus, Ohio: Charles E. Merrill Publishing Company, 1969.

114. ——, *On Encounter Groups*. New York: Harper & Row, Publishers, Inc., 1970.

115. ——, "A Theory of Personality," in *Theories of Psychopathology*, ed. T. Millan. Philadelphia: W. B. Saunders Company, 1973.

116. Rogers, Martha, *An Introduction to the Theoretical Basis of Nursing*. Philadelphia: F. A. Davis Company, 1970.

117. Rosenhan, D., "On Being Sane in Insane Places," *Science*, 179 (1973), 250–58.

118. Rottkamp, Barbara, "A Behavior Modification Approach to Nursing Therapeutics in Body-Positioning of Spinal Cord Injured Patients," *Nursing Research*, 25, no. 3 (1976), 181–86.

119. Saranson, Irwin, and Barbara Saranson, *Abnormal Psychology: The Problem of Adaptive Behavior*, 3rd ed. Englewood Cliffs, N.J.: Prentice-Hall, Inc., 1980.

120. "Scanning the Human Mind," *Newsweek*, September 30, 1980, p. 63.

121. Schacter, S., and J. Singer, "Cognitive, Social, and Physiological Determinants of Emotional State," *Physiological Review*, 69 (1962), 379–99.

122. Scheff, T. T., "The Role of the Mentally Ill and the Dynamics of Mental Disorder," *Sociometry*, 26 (1963), 436–53.

123. Schuster, Clara, and Shirley Ashburn, *The Process of Human Development*. Boston: Little, Brown & Company, 1980.

124. Skinner, B. F., *Walden Two*. New York: Macmillan Publishing Co., Inc., 1948.

125. ——, *Beyond Freedom and Dignity*. New York: Alfred A. Knopf, Inc., 1971.

126. ——, *Cumulative Record,* 3rd ed. New York: Appleton-Century-Crofts, 1972.

127. Snow, Richard, "Theory Construction for Research on Teaching," in *Second Handbook of Research on Teaching*, ed. Robert Travers, pp. 77–112. Chicago: Rand McNally College Publishing Company, 1973.

128. Staub, Erwin, *Personality: Basic Aspects and Current Research*. Englewood Cliffs, N.J.: Prentice-Hall, Inc., 1980.

129. Sullivan, Harry Stack, *The Interpersonal Theory of Psychiatry*. New York: W. W. Norton & Co., Inc., 1953.

130. Swanson, Mary, and A. M. Woolson, "A New Approach to the Use of Learning Theory with Psychiatric Patients," *Perspectives in Psychiatric Care*, 10, no. 2 (1972), 55–68.

131. Thompson, Clara, "The Different Schools of Psycho-analysis," *American Journal of Nursing*, 57, no. 10 (1957), 1304–7.

132. Tudor, Mary, *Child Development*. New York: McGraw-Hill Book Company, 1981.

133. Von Bertalanffy, Ludwig, *General System Theory*. New York: George Braziller, Inc., 1968.

134. Wadsworth, Barry, *Piaget's Theory of Cognitive Development*, 2nd ed. New York: Longman, Inc., 1979.

135. Whitman, Helen, and Shelby Lukes, "Behavior Modification for Terminally Ill Patients," *American Journal of Nursing*, 75, no. 1 (1975), 98–101.

136. Winick, M., *Malnutrition and Brain Development*. New York: Oxford University Press, 1976.

137. Wolpe, Joseph, *The Practice of Behavior Therapy*, 2nd ed. New York: Pergamon Press, Inc., 1973.

138. Zubek, J., ed., *Sensory Deprivation: Fifteen Years of Research*. New York: Appleton-Century-Crofts, 1969.

CLASSROOM DISCUSSIONS

139. Combs, Charles, Ph.D., Professor, Educ. 602 Theories of Learning and Development, Southern Illinois University, Edwardsville, Illinois.

140. Russell, Ivan, Ph.D., Professor, Educ. 602 Theories of Learning and Development, Southern Illinois University, Edwardsville, Illinois.

3

Basic Concepts about the Individual

Study of this chapter will assist you to:

1. Integrate theories presented in Chapter 2 into a holistic view of the person.

2. Assess your client's behavior with consideration for biological, cultural, family, social-system, environmental, and psychodynamic influences.

3. Describe psychodynamic aspects of the person: his/her drives, needs, conflicts, perceptions, emotions, values, attitudes, and beliefs.

4. Explore effects of the psychodynamic aspects on the person's behavior.

5. Formulate your own view of the person as a whole, unique, interrelating individual.

6. Examine yourself as a whole person.

This chapter contributed by M. Marilyn Huelskoetter, R.N., M.S.N., with additions by Ruth Murray, R.N., M.S.N.

As a nurse working with people who are striving for emotional health, as well as those struggling with emotional illness, you need the deepest possible knowledge and understanding of the human being and of behaviors and their meaning. You must also understand how to communicate and build relationships as well as how to use the nursing process as it is described throughout this book.

This chapter presents concepts and principles related to the characteristics, needs, perceptions, feelings, values, attitudes, beliefs, and other facets of human life, as well as some influences exerted on the person throughout his/her years of development. This chapter will help you to better understand the human condition and the uniqueness of each person from a *humanistic and holistic viewpoint* and to synthesize the theories presented in Chapter 2. When we speak of the person, we speak of *any* person—the client you work with, as well as yourself.

INTRODUCTION TO THE WHOLE PERSON

There is order and organization in nature and the world. The human, included in this universal whole, coexists within it. When you ask yourself, "Who is the person?" you should first see the human as a member of the greater system of the universe. Each person, as part of the larger whole, is influenced by and exerts influence on other forms of life. Each person comprises a discrete system composed of atoms, cells, tissues, and organ systems, which function as an organized, dynamic whole (17, 48). At the same time each person grows in a circle of human experiences. In turn this experiental world is composed of emotional, cognitive, spiritual, and sociocultural aspects. Thus the human stands between and is comprised of two worlds—the biological and the experiential.

Biological Characteristics

Every person born into this universe possesses a genetically determined biological system of characteristics common to all mankind. These characteristics are brought to the person upon conception and are carried on 46 chromosomes (23 pairs from the mother and father, each) in the nuclei of the somatic cell. With this fusion the individual will have, for any given trait, two genes that will come together in patterns of either recessiveness or dominance. These traits will combine uniquely in each individual. The *totality of this genetic endowment is called the person's* **genotype**. The *overtly manifested characteristics of the individual are called the* **phenotype**. The study of genetics is rapidly progressing and is useful to help you gain further knowledge of the person. Your study of human anatomy and physiology will assist you in understanding the human body as well as the manner in which it develops and functions.

Human endowment is also presented through the family genetic heritage. The child will not only have eyes with organ characteristics, but will have *blue* eyes because of parental lineage (26). A pedigree chart or family tree can help you trace patterns of specific traits.

The growth of the person, an extremely complex process, proceeds from birth through maturity. The sequence, timing, and direction of this growth take place in a predictable manner. This unfolding process involves the interaction of genetic traits, predispositions, and potentialities (45).

Growth is an increase in body size, or a change in function, structure, and complexity of cells and processes (37). These changes occur in four ways: (1) *incremental growth* (*maintaining excess over normal daily losses, as in urine and perspiration*), (2) *replacement growth* (*maintaining normal refills as in the life cycle of red blood cells*), (3) *hypertrophy* (*increase in cellular structure size*), and (4) *hyperplasia* (*increase in number of cells*) (37). As the person grows, both physical and emotional changes occur. In order to exist, the entire human body constantly changes in at least some small way. All the components of the body exist in a dynamic relationship, influencing each other; this provides adaptation to stimuli and stressors and the ability to maintain a uniformity of function. The capacity to adapt is inherent in every individual. Throughout all these processes, energy is in a continual state of change—in growth, regulation of activity, and the mediation of stress.

Experiential Influences

Embryonic and fetal experiences begin the process of individuation; the person's genetic endowment interacts with the intrauterine environment. This combination molds the emerging person in a unique way and comes into fruition after birth (25, 57). Notice the observable behavioral differences in newborns. Although all neonates have similar physical characteristics, researchers have found significant individual differences between babies in behavioral responses during the first few days of life (17, 20). At birth every individual is truly unique, similar and yet not identical, to any other person that has ever lived (57).

The person's continuing experiences are dependent on a variety of variables, including family, culture, social systems, and environmental stimuli. Although we separate these four variables to aid understanding, in real life they cannot be separated, and they influence the child in a way that is unique or specific, even though the experience may be similar to that of others. Think of the difference in the life experiences of a youngster growing up in a medium-size North American city, within a one-parent family, and those of a youngster of the same age in a communal family in Equatorial Africa. Even after physical maturity, the experiences of the adult are important and unique, although similar. For example, the aging process can progress differently for a Hopi Indian grandfather living and working among his people and family than for an elderly man of the same generation living alone in an American inner city.

Development is the dynamic process that occurs in structure, behavior, and personality over time and that evolves as a result of changing physical and mental capacity, life experiences, and learning. Thus the person constantly moves toward a new level of maturity and integration (37). These developmental processes involve interplay of biological characteristics; of experiential, family, social, cultural, and environmental influences that act upon the person; and of psychological mechanisms that mediate between them (37).

The person develops in a dynamic manner. As the individual is confronted by the constantly changing world, adaptive responses occur that are at the highest possible level for that specific time. All circumstances considered, the person's behavior and physiological responses are the best of which he/she is capable at any given point in time. There is inherent in every person a potential for growth, change, and movement toward health, but each response of the individual continues to develop the very unique differences in that person.

Cultural Influences

Culture is the sum total of learned patterns of living. Every group of people has learned over time to adapt its life style in order to continue survival. Such ways of adaptation become a body of knowledge and custom and are passed on to each new generation. A child born into a family group quickly begins to assimilate these ways as the family shapes the young life. Throughout life, including the first year, culture has a tremendous impact on the maturing person's experiences, life style, health habits, values, attitudes, and ways of thinking and doing. As parents and others communicate and live with the child, these family ways are taught.

Diversity of customs depends on a variety of cultural influences, such as economic level, ethnic or racial background, regional factors, occupation and religion of family members, and even historical placement. Life in the 1750s was very different from life in the 1980s. If you desire to understand another person, you must study the relevant culture in depth. Refer to Chapter 9 for further information.

Cultural variables bring about differences that are paramount. We are, however, more alike than we are different (56). Even though two people from different cultures may show strikingly different overt behaviors, experiences, and preferences, they have the same basic needs. People from different cultures may search for the same ideals in life, hold the same values, and express similar emotions. These similarities have to do with commonalities in the human experience and can be understood and experienced by every person. Such similar human experiences include hunger, pain, death, anxiety, loneliness, alienation, illness, loss, compassion, and joy (59), although outward manifestations of these inner experiences and feelings may differ from culture to culture.

Family Influences

The *family is a basic social system, a primary reference group made up of two or more persons living together over time* (37). In our society the family is given the task of raising the young; sharing goals and identity; and providing for, supporting, and promoting the adaptive capacities of one another. The family works toward achieving basic developmental tasks. These include:

1. Allocation of resources, including space, shelter, time, social interaction, and finances.
2. Provision of physical and emotional maintenance by meeting basic needs.
3. Division of labor between the sexes and members of various ages.
4. Socialization of family members so that they behave in a culturally approved way.
5. Reproduction, recruitment through marriage of offspring, and release of family members.
6. Maintenance of order among family members through rituals, customs, traditions, mores, and discipline.
7. Placement of members in larger society as productive citizens.
8. Maintenance of motivation and morale of the family unit (12).

To what extent the individual accomplishes these tasks will largely depend on family influences. Family influence is present from birth to later maturity, but the greatest influence is exerted during childhood. Early family experiences are the foundation of the child's future development and personality.

The human at birth is completely dependent and helpless and must be totally cared for by a nurturing person. The infant must *be* cared for, *feel* cared for, and *learn to trust* that he/she will continue to be cared for. The mother forms a bond, a kind of merging of personalities, as she holds the baby securely in a close extrauterine relationship (31). The mother's sensitivity to the child's needs fosters the child's sense of security (56). This relationship will have marked influence on the infant's future identity, ego capacities, and interpersonal relationships. If the infant's experiences are safe and nurturing, the child moves ahead and out of the bonded mother-child unit into a still close family membership.

The situation is unique and different for each child and family member within the family circle, depending on ordinal position, current stressors, changing environments, and previously mentioned variables, all of which interplay to form a network of influences that are similar but different. Children, parents, and the family unit as a whole form different constellations at different points of development; each parent and child will differ at various stages of development. Relationships change as a result. Thus, each child emerges from the family with similarities but also true uniqueness. Nurses are increasingly recognizing the importance of the family in the development and personality of the individual. Chapter 10 treats this subject in greater depth.

Social-System Influences

As a result of the interplay of family influences, the sphere of the child's life will continually widen, resulting in ever-increasing self-autonomy and variety of personal options. Just as you might note a widening circle after throwing a pebble in a pond, so does the social circle widen into varying groups and influences for this child (see Figure 3-1).

Although the primary relationship with the mother continues throughout childhood, it changes in complexion through the years. The first symbiotic relationship nurtures, satisfies, and develops a sense of self in the child, encouraging development of trust. Gradually the mother assists the infant's movement beyond the first bond; the child's horizons expand into deeper relationships with others—a father figure, grandparents, siblings, or other relatives. Through developing motor, cognitive, and language skills and handling of routines and activities, the young child develops greater self-confidence, autonomy, and social contacts. Home, the center of the child's first existence, broadens out to new experiences. The mother assists the child to diminish the intense attachment to her and supports the growing independence. Parents participate in the socialization process as they respond to the child's behavior. The child learns to master and gain satisfaction from social skills.

Roles begin to be structured to help the child

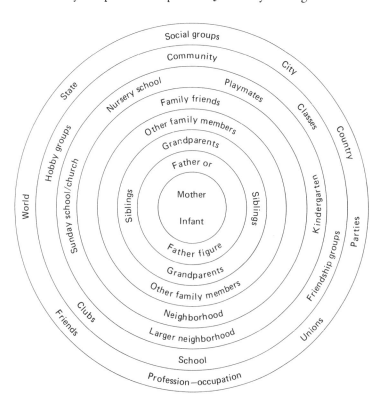

FIGURE 3-1   Social systems and interactions of the individual.

avoid anxiety and gain mastery. A *role is what a person does in relation to others:* first, in response to parents, then, as a male or female, and later, in response to a variety of situations. There is an increased opportunity to socialize and learn roles within schools, clubs, and social groups. This process continues to finally include membership in occupations, professions, and extended groups, as well as an awareness of the neighborhood, community, and society at large.

Social adaptation means adjusting self to a group. The person acts and reacts to other people in a variety of groups. The person establishes a **status** (*a position in relation to others*) and maintains a **position** (*the place a person holds in a group*). A **social system** *consists of a plurality of individuals acting toward and reacting with each other.* As the person moves within a social system, he/she experiences a changing sense of self-identity and satisfaction with relationships (37). Any social situation, whether making friends in the community, moving to another community, death of a loved one, or occupational choice, may have a lasting effect on the person's life, resulting in

significant influence on behavior. Throughout life and until death, group and social experiences will continue to influence the person.

Environmental Influences

An intimate relationship exists between the person and his/her total environment. The types of food and shelter, sense of safety and life space, and total life style of the individual—all are related to geographic, climatic, and spatial surroundings. The environment is constantly changing and must be considered in all of its complexity in its relationship to the person. The physical environment contains a wide variety of potential stimuli: gravity; light and sound waves; meteorological stimuli such as temperature variation; wind velocity; atmospheric pressure; humidity; solar radiation; air pollutants; ozone, oxygen, carbon dioxide, and carbon monoxide levels; electromagnetic fields; day–night and seasonal periodicity; and infectious microorganisms. The physical environment affects both physical and emotional health (37).

PSYCHODYNAMIC ASPECTS OF THE WHOLE PERSON

To understand the whole person, we must look at the interaction, manifestation, and consequences of forces of psychic energy moving within the individual. The term **psychodynamics** *refers to the science and explanation of the movement of directing, restraining, or inhibiting forces that arise from motivational needs and drives and that affect intrapersonal and interpersonal behavior.*

Motivation

Motivation is a force propelling a person into activity. It can be termed the *"why" of behavior.* Motivation exists on the three levels of behavior: (1) conscious, (2) preconscious, and (3) unconscious (11). *Needs, requirements for life,* and *drives, a hereditary, transmitted force,* are related to the biological, physiological, emotional, cognitive, spiritual, sociocultural, and family components of the person and are motivating forces (25).

Human Needs

Need is a necessary requirement for the continu-

ation of life, a condition characterized by tension or discomfort. The word *need* describes a single aspect or a part of the person, yet the concept of need is far too complicated to be reduced to a simple definition. We do this to illustrate and understand, but any need is actually a total bodily phenomenon and involves the whole person with a total response. Basic needs, and the behavior to meet these needs, are influenced by the brain and cognitive processes, biochemical responses, anatomical and muscular activity, physiological and neurological activity, and psychological and sociological responses. Since the person also interacts with the environment, the interchange with environmental forces and interpersonal relationships will also affect these needs.

Maslow described needs according to a hierarchy (see Chapter 2). In this text, needs will be divided into three broad categories: physiological, libidinal (sensual and affectional), and ego developmental. *Physiological needs are cyclic, perpetual, and imperative for survival.* They include need for oxygen, water, food, elimination, sleep, temperature control or shelter, safety, and movement (37).

Libidinal needs refer to both sensual-sexual and affectional-emotional needs. Sensual-sexual needs are not uniformly rhythmic in humans, although menstrual cycle hormonal rhythms are correlated with emotional and behavioral changes in some women. The basis of sensual-sexual needs is organic, but these needs take on psychologic meanings. Affectional-emotional needs are constant and are at the core of normal psychic dependence. The person must be given love, security, respect, support, care, and protection for proper emotional and physical development (37).

Ego developmental needs refer to the need for cognitive, perceptual, and memory development, training, and education. The person must have opportunity for and help with mastery of age-adequate behaviors, including: (1) motor coordination, (2) emotional autonomy, independence, and self-identity, as these behaviors relate to self and culture, (3) social skills, (4) communication skills (speech, reading, writing, nonverbal), (5) adaptive mechanisms, (6) moral development, (7) control of drives, (8) problem solving, and (9) work skills, as well as (10) opportunity for the development of creative and self-actualization behavior (37).

Libidinal and ego developmental needs emerge together; they influence each other, and they are equally significant for psychic and physical well-being. Ego development proceeds from mastery of simple to complex tasks (37).

Humans are very adaptable in meeting their needs, but adaptive potentials are not unlimited. In prehistoric evolution, humans met many stressors, but their genetic constitutions could adapt over time. Now humans face threats created by modern technology that have no precedent in the evolutionary past. The rate of biologic evolution is too slow to keep up with the effects of technological and social changes. Thus, certain needs may not be met, and other needs may be created. These unmet needs affect health status (37).

A number of theorists have postulated a framework for explaining basic needs in relation to development. Refer to Chapter 2 for further explanation.

Conflicting Needs

Human beings have many needs, some of which may be in conflict with others. *Conflict is a struggle between two or more strong opposing forces at any level in the hierarchy of needs.* These forces may vary in direction, degree, nature, and consequences (5). Conflicts are influenced by the person's experiences, cultural norms, values, and standards. For example, an adolescent boy may be attracted to a young woman and he may want to meet her. If his past experiences with girlfriends have been hurtful ones, he may experience a conflict situation, simultaneously wanting to approach and avoid the girl.

There are four kinds of conflict situations in which there are both conscious and unconscious components (23). At times, a conflict may be totally unconscious.

1. *Approach-approach*, where *both goals have positive attraction.* For example, Mary wants to be a nurse and an artist.
2. *Approach-avoidance*, where *one goal is attractive and the other has more disadvantages than advantages.* For example, Mary wants to drive the car to Florida but is afraid of having an accident.
3. *Avoidance-avoidance*, where *both goals or situations have disadvantages, but one must be chosen.* For example, Jack knows he will fail the course if he takes it, and he doesn't want to fail, but the course is required.
4. *Double-avoidance approach*, where *two alternative goals have advantages and disadvantages relative to each other.* For example, John wants to go to a party and also to stay home and work. If he goes to the party he cannot complete his work; if he stays home, he cannot see his friends.

All people experience many conflict situations. Some are conscious. In such cases, the person is very aware of the situation, but may have difficulty choosing what step to take. Some conflicts are unconscious, causing the person to suffer from symptoms of neurosis.

Needs can be satisfied, producing personal satisfaction. Or needs may be blocked or frustrated, producing stress, anxiety, and symptoms, as shown in Figure 3-2 and as described in this chapter.

Conflict can occur at any level, including within the person, group, social situation, or in a local, regional, national, or world community. Conflict develops as untrustworthy behavior of one person brings about tension in another. The other person then responds with untrustworthy behavior himself, creating a spiral. Negotiation and efforts at communication may decrease tension, increasing the options or moves available to each person. Conflictual feelings may then diminish (40).

Conflict is not necessarily destructive. Two or more opposing forces may stimulate change. Differences in motivation, attitudes, values, feelings, and opinions among people are healthy and inevitable (38). Expression of these differences can result in learning, new appreciation of people, and behavioral changes.

Behavior

Behavior may be defined as all the activity involved in living. This includes actions, feelings, thinking, and conscious as well as unconscious activity. Behavior is *activity directed toward satisfaction of needs—personal, group, and community* (1). Behavior is modified by many variables, but the person tries to function as an integrated whole. All behavior has significance and can be understood from the person's dynamic intrapsychic and interpersonal experiences (21). *Overt behavior can be observed and is discernible to others. Covert behavior is not obvious and must be inferred.* A person does not always recognize his/her own behavior or the reasons for it (42). Much behavior is outside awareness, is repressed, and cannot be recalled. There is potential within each person to change and to develop or strive toward psychological health. Whatever the behavior, it is the best the individual can do at the time.

Assumptions about behavior, based on Second and Third Force theories, include the following (9):

1. Behavior is relevant, meaningful, purposeful, and has a cause, either past or present.
2. Behavior has more than one cause and serves more than one purpose.
3. Behavior is learned, for the most part, in relations with others.
4. Behavior is determined by (and pertinent to) the individual's perception, rather than by external events. Perception is the reality.
5. Behavior changes when perceptions change and needs or goals are met.
6. Behavior is determined by the context of the situation, which is affected by past and present experiences and future anticipations.

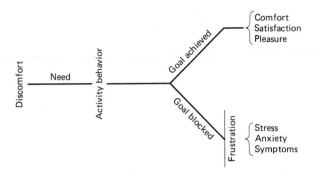

FIGURE 3-2   Need achievement and frustration.

7. Variables that influence perception, and thus behavior, include:
   a. The person's needs, including maintaining a sense of security and adequacy.
   b. Biological, physical, emotional, and social status; the limits and capabilities of the person.
   c. Length of time of exposure to an event and the opportunity to be in contact with the stimuli or event.
   d. Goals and values, and the techniques, strategies, or roles to reach these goals and to maintain values.
   e. Development of the phenomenal self, based on self-perception, personal abilities, and perceptions of the situation, which give continuity and consistency to the personality.
   f. Self-concept, the basic frame of reference from which all perceptions gain their meaning.
   g. Availability of perceptions and level and character of differentiations made by the person.

Perception

Perception is the basis for personal reality; it is basic to behavior and influences emotions and feelings, attitudes, values, and beliefs. Sensations occur within a context of other stimuli; thus figure-ground relationships are basic to perception (see Chapter 2). Cognitive processes within the person, including innate and developed sensory abilities, acuity, and attention paid to stimuli, also will influence the context of perception (2, 42).

Many factors, in addition to neurophysiological structures and functions, influence the ability to perceive and interpret stimuli. These factors include (2, 9, 18, 42):

1. Past experience, pleasant or unpleasant, with the same or similar stimuli, or familiarity with a situation, object, or event.
2. Size, shape, and intensity (brightness) of an object.
3. Duration or repetition of an event or object.
4. Variations or changes of stimuli, so that all or part of an object or event does not remain the same in color, sound, position, movement, or tempo.
5. Presence of additional stimuli, objects, or events.
6. Perceptual set, in that the person takes in information about a situation, object, or another human that meets his/her needs, expectations, wishes, needs, fantasies, or values.
7. Ability to focus on stimuli by forcing self to be vigilant; giving self a break in routine, a reward, or feedback; seeking interesting aspects in the stimuli and using techniques to maintain concentration.

Behavior is influenced by perceptions and interpretations. Based on individual interpretation, two people experiencing the same situation may react quite differently, just as two people may view the same person quite differently. Interactions may be helped or hindered, depending on individual interpretations and the resulting reactions and activity.

Attributes and characteristics similar to those previously encountered help distinguish people, objects, and events from the background or environment. People are taught within the culture and family to assign a specific *label* to similar people or situations, and these labels help the person to feel that he/she knows a great deal about someone or something, although such knowledge is based on limited information. Thus, a few signs and symptoms can help you quickly to make a diagnosis and intervene. But labeling may hinder relationships because labels are the basis of stereotypes, generalizations, and preconceptions about people, all of which prevent observation of the person's uniqueness. Labels also contribute to a feeling that something is not important, is already known, or is present when it actually is not (9, 18).

Perceptual errors frequently occur. Perception of others may be influenced by *judgment errors* or *perceptual distortions.* You observe the behavior of another and make an inference about the behavior. This inference about the reasons for such behavior, or your interpretation of the behavior, may be incorrect or inappropriate. Frequently such behavioral interpretations about another are made after an initial impression instead of after longer contact, so they may be incorrect. The impressions, inferences, and judgment errors form a frame of reference for continuing perceptions, which in turn guide behavior with another. You may also use a frame of reference in working with people that is habitual, superficial, or even outside of your awareness. Therefore relationships may be hindered as a result of distorted perceptions and judgment errors because you cannot appreciate and communicate with the person as he/she really is (18).

Logical error occurs when you assume that certain personality traits go together and that all of these traits exist in one person, even though only one of the traits is observed. If the person has a characteristic you do not appreciate, your interaction can be hindered before you learn of the many distinct characteristics that make up that person. The *halo effect* may cause a distortion in either direction since you evaluate someone on a number of characteristics based on an overall positive or negative impression.

Leniency error is a reaction opposite to logical error. You may make many positive judgments about another, avoiding identification of negative or undesirable characteristics. Giving a person the benefit of doubt may help a relationship. However, **objectivity** *(seeing as many aspects of the person as possible)* and honesty are needed if a relationship is to endure and if you are to help another to mature (18).

Emotions and Feelings

Affect may be identified as a feeling state, a signal of pleasant or unpleasant feeling that accompanies mental ideas. Affect and feeling can be used synonymously. **Mood** *is a sustained feeling state.* **Emotion** *is the biochemical, somatic expression of feeling tone. It is a transitory, physical, subjective reaction.*

Every person is an emotional being and has

feelings at some level. Feelings are uniquely sensed by each person. Situations that arouse feelings in one person may not create a reaction in another. Also the reasons for two persons feeling similarly in the same situation may be quite different. What triggers a feeling response one time may not at another time, depending on the interpretation of events. Some people ignore or cover up feelings. Sometimes feelings are so frightening that they must be covered by other feelings. Defenses may be used to disguise such feelings. (Refer to Table 2-3.) Many people use anger, a powerful feeling with which they are comfortable, to cover up uncomfortable feelings from a close or intimate situation. Some feelings become unbearable over a period of time and are redirected into a psychotic symptom; for example, an anxious person may hallucinate.

Feeling states vary in intensity and may be expressed openly or subtly. The following adjectives describe only a few of the many feelings that can be experienced:

I feel intimate — close — hopeful — delighted.
I feel loving — joyful — happy — cheerful.
I feel alienated — suspicious — lonely — isolated.
I feel angry — hostile — resentful — disgusted.
I feel ugly — dejected — sad — helpless.
I feel anxious — inadequate — cautious — afraid.

The relationship between mind and body is widely recognized. Feelings are experienced in physical terms. We say, "Pain in the neck," "Grit your teeth," "I'm turned on," and "Keep a stiff upper lip." You can name others. Feelings touch off physical reactions, as described in Chapter 12. An angry word can result in tension, diarrhea, or shortness of breath. An organ can manifest feeling states, such as a bleeding ulcer, an inflamed colon, a skin rash, or a tension headache. Certainly emotions are more difficult to define and measure than physical states. A blush, increased blood pressure and pulse, change in the strength of grip, galvanic skin response, and the polygraph are among the ways to measure feeling states. Although emotions and their effects are difficult to measure, this does not mean that emotions are not present. Emotions have an impact on the person and on interpersonal relationships.

That the unborn child experiences feeling states has been inferred from research when anxiety and stress in the mother precipitate overactivity in the child (7). Before and during birth, it is believed that the infant feels discomfort, anxiety, pain, and periods of relief from discomfort (5). Phyllis Greenacre felt that the anxiety pattern began at birth, and Freud and Rank believed that the entire birth process was the prototype of anxiety (19). The reactions to the loss of the warm, protected environment during birth has been referred to as *separation anxiety*.

The basic needs of the newborn are security and love. The infant is thought to have two emotional states — pleasure and discomfort. The infant is unable to give love but needs to receive much in the form of talking, touching, cuddling, and holding. René Spitz, in his classic studies with infants in foundling homes, found a high mortality rate due to the lack of love (53). Harlow showed that infant monkeys had to have a loving attachment to the mothering monkey in order to progress in their ability to relate to peer monkeys and to grow to have a parental attachment (23). If the emotional environment is safe and loving, the young child will grow in trust and the ability to feel love. As attachments of the child continue throughout childhood, he/she experiences a greater variety of feelings and a deepening emotional life. Confidence, ability to be more spontaneous, and greater freedom with self ensue. As Carl Rogers states, feelings can "bubble up," bringing about a greater authenticity of person (49).

Further, the child learns to censor feelings from interactions with parents, family, and culture. Everyone learns this to some degree. The child learns early to, "Be a good girl," "Don't cry," "Be seen and not heard," or "Keep feelings to yourself." The child's behavior may reflect the thought that, to get along with parents, he/she must not be angry (or warm or open or reserved). A value judgment begins to be placed on feeling, and *should have* and *should not have* feelings eventuate. Notice the different ways in which people in some cultures respond to their own feelings. For example, people with a Jewish, Southern European, or Spanish-speaking background are usually more emotionally expressive than people from some other cultural groups. This trait is also usually true with women, in contrast to men, in our culture. Notice how certain individuals have greater difficulty with some kinds of feelings, such as feelings of anger, love, intimacy, or sexuality. What the child learns about feelings, and consequent behaviors, is carried over into adult life. The behavioral responses to feelings may become a lifetime pattern or personality trait.

A child may also learn to respond to certain feelings with other feelings. If the person feels it is *bad* to feel angry, then the self-concept, self-esteem, and confidence are affected when anger is present. Guilt may arise. The person may also act out feelings that are feared. The adolescent may steal tires; the young girl may become pregnant; or the nurse may delay answering a call light for a given patient as a way to express unconscious anger. The person who restricts his feelings may experience physiological symptoms of pain or distress. There may also be changes within tissues if intense feelings are prolonged. Certainly the more the individual restricts and censors his/her feelings, the less healthy he/she will be, the less satisfying will be the human relationships, and the less self-awareness will exist.

Values

Values involve priorities—preferring one object, person, or way of life over another. They are conceptions of what is important, prized, held dear, or thought of as desirable to the person and to his/her group, family, or community. Values set a standard for determining action; they are criteria for choosing alternatives and a basis for recognizing self and others. Values represent what is good, what one ought to do, what should be, and that to which the person gives time, energy, and money. Values affect communication, thinking, and learning, and they color our perceptions. They are complex and have strong motivational, cognitive, affective, and behavioral components (48). Values become internalized as the person makes the belief system part of the self. Yet this may be difficult to identify since values may function both consciously and unconsciously (60, 61, 62, 63).

As you live each day, you will constantly be choosing. What will you do? Whom will you be with? What patient will you care for first? You will have goals—momentary and unconscious ones, as well as long-term, life-directed, and conscious ones. Your values will affect your choices of behavior.

Values are made up of a set, or cluster, of attitudes. When they become organized into a group, they are called a value system. You have more attitudes than values, and more beliefs than

attitudes. A value may be seen as an attitude at a higher level of abstraction (65).

Values have their roots in the development of conscience. In early childhood years, the child introjects the parents's value system and learns what to do and what not to do. The child learns rules and regulations of the family in order to please and gain love of the family and others, even when such rules are restrictive or cause discomfort. Later, new standards and values are learned, as school, other children and adults, and social influences impinge on the child. The child begins to realize that at times there must be choices, and that these must be made between what he/she wants to do and what feels right. Piaget discusses how children go through a period of professing reverence for rules but only in terms of the rules being external to the mind (43, 64). Judgments of the child are only in terms of the letter of the law, without true understanding of them. The child of three or four plays games, imitating rules, and perhaps bending them to win. The child of seven or eight learns rules and considers them immutable, and a child of twelve considers rules as a contract that may be changed (33). The child's peers not only influence the child but also the family. The peers increasingly become the arbitrator of values and standards. As the young person moves toward independence from the family, he/she should demonstrate a personal set of standards, based on a developed conscience, rather than using standards imposed by someone else. However, family values will remain influential, even though peer values are also influential.

As the person develops intellectually and socially, rules will be understood in the context of overall community life. Fairness will be perceived in terms of equality, and justice in terms of weighing all relationships and circumstances to reach a decision. The child moves from the stage of imposed rules and authority to adulthood, with free choice based on internalized rules and principles. Thus development of a value system is related to moral development. See Kohlberg's Theory, Chapter 2.

All of us live in multiple communities and become subject to a variety of value systems. As we play and work with various groups, the value systems of these groups will influence us. There may be an internal struggle as a result of competing values; confusion and inability to identify personal choices may result. Some early values may be rejected, and some will be accepted. Thus a relatively unchanging base for standards or values will have come together for a mature or older adult, influenced by many situations and experiences of growth and change.

Attitudes

An *attitude is a state of mind, a feeling state ingrained in the personality and organized through experience, causing readiness to respond in a certain manner.* The person learns a tendency to think, feel, or act in a certain way. Experiences with parents and family are essential influences in molding attitudes. Peers, friends, and other groups later become influential. Culture sets the broad limits (1). Feelings largely determine attitudes. Studies have shown that when the emotional component of attitudes is changed, cognitive components fall in line and are changed without any additional information (65). In turn, the individual will react in a characteristic pattern in a certain situation.

Attitudes have many attributes: they are complex, differ in content, and have varying intensities. Jeanine Auger characterized them by five primary dimensions (1):

1. *Extremeness*—relative degree of positive or negative value attached to object.
2. *Content*—precise meaning in which attitude is directed.
3. *Clarity or structure*—highly differentiated or lacking in structure.
4. *Degree of integration*—how isolated the attitude is or how it is related to other attitudes.
5. *Strength of belief*—resistance to attitudinal change based on belief in cognitive content.

Attitudes have three components: (1) affect, emotion, or feeling involved—such as good or bad, like or dislike; (2) cognition and statement of thinking and level of belief; and (3) behavior—how the attitude is carried out in activity.

Attitudes may be in conflict, vary in motive, and serve a variety of functions. Attitudes help people understand the world because they tend to organize and simplify the world in the minds of the people involved. Attitudes protect self-esteem, allow for expression of fundamental values, and cause the person to react in such a way as to maximize rewards from others and the environment (58). Content or meaning of an event toward which the attitude is directed will depend on individual perception of the event. How a person perceives anything will be influenced by the individual's self-concept, past experiences, and relationships with people who are considered important.

Beliefs

A *belief is an idea, set of attitudes, or opinion that is held with personal conviction or confidence, based upon faith rather than fact.* This belief can center around a person, an object, a plan of action, a fantasy, or an impression. The emotional attitude, not cognitive component, gives strength to making an idea a belief. *Rational belief is supported by available evidence.* *Blind belief is not supported by evidence,* and *irrational belief is held despite available evidence.* Research shows that people usually know more about statements they believe than about statements they do not believe (67). People tend to seek additional information to support an idea they already hold, rather than direct themselves toward a new or challenging idea.

A child begins to develop beliefs into a system early in life as he/she learns from parents. This belief system contributes to the child's development of values. As values and beliefs develop, there is an interchange of the two. The belief will sharpen the values, and a value system can further develop beliefs.

The person has many beliefs. Beliefs can be changed more easily than attitudes and values. Beliefs tend to reinforce the cognitive elements of attitudes as well as values. To embrace a belief, one must take a risk, square it with existing values, and then let it expand into a system.

In this section, we have presented concepts and facts about the person—you and your client—and have touched on some areas that make the person unique. Values, attitudes, and beliefs all influence behavior and emotional health. But the essence of the person lies in the mystery of the spirit, which is difficult to define or identify. The person is not just so many cells or a number of traits but a multitude of qualities, experiences, and characteristics, each in itself and in the combination, a different whole. A mystery—this person! At the very core of psychiatric nursing is listening and hearing. If you can bring yourself to each client with an earnestness to discover the mystery of the person, with an attentive listening to what is said, and a hearing of what is not said, you may find the true spirit of the person.

AWARENESS OF SELF AS A WHOLE PERSON

You, too, are a unique person, and you bring *yourself* to this psychiatric/mental health experience. In giving emotional care, you are important since you are the tool you use. Socrates said, "Know thyself." Lidz said, "One cannot come to know very much about others, without learning to know oneself, how one's life fits together, and how one defends against experiencing insecurities and anxieties" (33). The knowledge of who you are, with all of your complexities, will be one of your goals in psychiatric/mental health nursing. This is not an intellectual finding, nor does it happen overnight. Knowledge of self as a whole person can become a reality only with a gradual awakening to yourself, which involves an attitude of emotional openness, a searching attitude, a wanting to know, an honest evaluation of your own behavior, and a willingness to take chances. To reveal yourself openly and honestly takes the rawest kind of courage (44).

You arrive at the experience of psychiatric/mental health nursing with a background of experiences, feelings, values, attitudes, and beliefs. You may believe in nursing and the importance of healthful living. You may have a positive attitude toward people and helping others. You may value health. At the same time, you may have learned a negative attitude toward psychiatry and mental illness from societal attitudes. You may believe that:

> Mental health is earned by hard work and positive thinking.
> Good people are mentally healthy.
> Sin brings on mental illness.
> Hard work and activity will keep a mind healthy.
> Mentally ill people are dangerous.
> All mentally ill people should be in institutions.
> All mentally ill individuals hurt other people.

These beliefs may cause you to respond negatively toward your client. But even if you have grown into adulthood without such preconceptions concerning the mentally ill, the elderly, the alcoholic, or the delinquent, you may find people within the profession negatively judging these people. Or you may value cleanliness, beauty, youth, intelligence, power, and competition. These values also can cause you difficulty in building a relationship with your client.

Although you may be unaware of your feelings, beliefs, attitudes, and values, they may be expressed in your relationships, method of communication, ability to be empathic, and understanding of others. Few people realize how frequently they communicate nonverbally their values, attitudes, and feelings to others, and how these affect behavior. You may say to a patient, "I care about you," while, by inflection, expression, gesture, and deeds of omission, you say, "I do not." It is important, inasmuch as possible, to be aware of your feelings. The more you are aware of them, the less frequently you will act them out. Know your beliefs. Examine your attitudes. Clarify your values. What are some qualities about yourself that make you feel good and proud? What matters to you? About what do you become indignant or self-righteous? Ask yourself these questions to get clues to your values. Look at your parents and siblings. Check with them on some of the proverbs you were taught as a child. For example, the motto "The early bird catches the worm" taught you to value promptness. You may be able to identify only what is important to you.

You may also be able to express affective reactions and feelings concerning these values. You may be able to identify pleasure felt when achievement is experienced. You may be able to acknowledge what causes pain, frustration, and a sense of loss. The highest level of awareness comes when you are able to identify the extent to which you would sacrifice for these values. How much effort would be spent in their service? How much conflict or stress endured? How much sacrifice?

For how long? Look for your values. Look to them on all levels. Is there consistency? Consistent patterns of behavior over a period of time will indicate your enduring values. Core values will be consistent, enduring, and worthy of high risk.

Self-awareness also involves feelings: a curiosity, a wanting to know what makes you act as you do, and a willingness to work at the process of self-awareness or introspection. Self-awareness is not an easy task. It is difficult, personal, and private. You cannot completely understand every aspect of yourself and your behavior. Some people avoid understanding; they work at keeping themselves hidden, not only to others but also to themselves. Self-awareness allows for personal improvement.

Your authors encourage you to try to understand yourself. Perhaps asking yourself the questions in Table 3-1 will help you explore areas for further thought and observation.

Think about the assessment. Think about your values, feelings, attitudes, and beliefs. Can you make connections or conclusions? Try to

TABLE 3-1. Self-Assessment Tool

1. *Assessing my environment:*

   How do I respond to the world around me?

   What is my world like? Do I seek out similar environments?

   How do I respond to the people I am with: my classmates, teachers, landlord?

   Can I discuss problems with others? Who are these others?

   Do I have close relationships? With whom?

   What do I do when I disagree with others? Fight or withdraw? Talk or cry?

   How do others respond to me?

   How do I feel about others in my situation?

   How do I handle stress? Are my stressful situations similar over a period of time?

   Do I consider others around me? Do I usually think of myself? Do I always think of others?

   How do I respond to the people with whom I work?

   What type of space am I most comfortable in?

2. *Assessing my own person and inner processes:*

   How do I explain problems to myself?

   What do I do when I become threatened and scared?

   Do I become defensive? Most people do, but how do I react?

   Do I recognize when I am anxious? What type of physiological and psychological signs are shown?

   What type of adaptive mechanisms do I use? Are they used frequently or occasionally?

   How do I respond when others are anxious?

   How do I respond to a withdrawn person, or to an angry or sexually aggressive person?

   Do I use displacement, taking my feelings out on others?

   Do I use projection, attributing my feeling of inadequacy to others?

   Do I use intellectualization, i.e., knowledge and intellectual verbage, to cover up when I am afraid?

3. *Assessing my thinking processes and thoughts of fantasy:*

   What do I think about, or what is on my mind?

   What percentage of my thoughts center on myself?

   What is on my mind when I am caring for my clients?

   What is my greatest mind investment?

   What do I daydream about?

   What are my dreams like?

   What type of feelings do I have when I dream?

describe some of your thoughts. Get feedback from colleagues and friends. Talk it over with a close friend or your instructor. Make a contract with yourself that this will be an ongoing process. Do not drop it. Seek out more knowledge in courses, experiences, and interactions with others. This can mean growth and change for you. Occasionally stop and evaluate where you are in the process.

Learning about self can be one of the more important tasks in nursing and in life. Some feel that self-understanding comes only through under-standing others (4). When you focus on the other person, you transcend yourself and become more involved in how the other person sees the world. This, then, is the I-thou relationship described by Buber. Perhaps this is what nursing is all about and why we use this chapter to set the stage for understanding the other person, your client. As A. Schutz stated, "I experience myself through you, and you experience yourself through me." (50). In this experience you may begin to really discover who you are.

REFERENCES

1. Auger, Jeanine, *Behavioral Systems and Nursing,* pp. 132–36. Englewood Cliffs, N.J.: Prentice-Hall, Inc., 1976.

2. Bigge, Morris, *Learning Theories for Teachers,* 3rd ed. New York: Harper & Row, Publishers, Inc., 1976.

3. Boyer, Barbara, "Valuing: Teaching the Process of Values Clarification," in *Current Perspectives in Psychiatric Nursing, Issues and Trends,* eds. Carol Kneisl and Holly Wilson. St. Louis: The C. V. Mosby Company, 1978.

4. Brennan, James, "Self-Understanding and Social Feeling," *Psychology in the World Today,* ed. Robert Guthrie. Reading, Mass.: Addison-Wesley Publishing Co., Inc., 1968.

5. Brown, Martha, and Grace Fowler, *Psychodynamic Nursing,* 3rd ed. Philadelphia: W. B. Saunders Company, 1967.

6. Burgess, Ann, and Aaron Lazare, "Nursing Management of Feelings, Thoughts, and Behavior," *Journal of Psychiatric Nursing and Mental Health Services,* 10, no. 6 (1972), 7–11.

7. Caplan, Gerald, *Theory and Practice of Mental Health Consultation.* New York: Basic Books, Inc., 1970.

8. Cohn, L., "Barriers and Values in the Nurse-Client Relationship," *O. R. Nursing Journal,* 3, no. 6 (1978), 3–8.

9. Combs, Arthur, and Donald Snygg, *Individual Behavior: A Perceptual Approach to Behavior.* New York: Harper & Row, Publishers, Inc., 1959.

10. Curran, C. L., "Construction of a Reliable Instrument to Measure Attitudes," *Nurse Educator,* 3, no. 6 (1978), 6–8.

11. Dixon, Samuel L., *Working with People in Crisis, Theory and Practice.* St. Louis: The C. V. Mosby Company, 1979.

12. Duvall, Evelyn, *Family Development,* 4th ed. Philadelphia: J. B. Lippincott Company, 1971.

13. Fischer, Valentina, and Arlene Connolly, *Promotion of Physical Comfort and Safety.* Dubuque, Iowa: Wm. C. Brown Company, Publishers, 1970.

14. Fish, Sharon, and J. A. Shelly, *Spiritual Care: The Nurse's Role.* Downers Grove, Ill.: Inter-Varsity Press, 1978.

15. Flaskerud, J. H., "Use of Vignettes to Elicit Responses Toward Broad Concepts. . .The Measurement of Attitudes, Beliefs, Values and Perceptions," *Nursing Research,* 28, no. 4 (1978), 210–12.

16. Francis, Gloria, and Barbara Munjas, *Promoting Psychological Comfort.* Dubuque, Iowa: Wm. C. Brown Company, Publishers, 1968.

17. Frank, L. K., "Human Development: An Emerging Scientific Discipline," in *Modern Perspectives in Child Development,* eds. A. J. Solnit and S. A. Province, pp. 10–36. New York: International Universities Press, 1963.

18. Grasha, Anthony, *Practical Applications of Psychology.* Cambridge, Mass.: Winthrop Publishers, Inc., 1978.

19. Greenacre, Phyllis, *Trauma, Growth, and Personality.* New York: W. W. Norton & Co., Inc., 1952.

20. Guthrie, Robert, *Psychology in the World Today, An Interdisciplinary Approach,* pp. 100–102. Reading, Mass.: Addison-Wesley Publishing Company, 1968.

21. Haber, Judith et al., *Comprehensive Psychiatric Nursing,* pp. 4–8. New York: McGraw-Hill Book Company, 1978.

22. Hager, R., "Evaluation of Group Psychotherapy, a Question of Values," *Journal of Psychiatric Nursing,* 16, no. 6 (1978), 26–28.

23. Harwatz, Morton, *Abnormal Psychology.* Englewood Cliffs, N.J.: Prentice-Hall, Inc., 1978.

24. Hayman, Howard, "Models of Human Nature and Their Impact on Health Education," *Nursing Digest,* 3, no. 5 (1975), 37–40.

25. Hofling, Charles, and Madeleine Leininger, *Basic Psychiatric Concepts in Nursing.* Philadelphia: J. B. Lippincott Company, 1967.

26. Jensen, Margaret, Ralph Benson, and Irene Babok, *Maternity Care, the Nurse and the Family.* St Louis: The C. V. Mosby Company, 1977.

27. Johnson, Mae M., Mary Lou David, and Mary Jo Belitch, *Problem Solving in Nursing Practice.* Dubuque, Iowa: Wm. C. Brown Company, Publishers, 1970.

28. Jourard, S. M., *Transparent Self.* New York: D. Van Nostrand Company, 1964.

29. Kirschenbaum, H., *Advanced Value Clarification.* LaJolla, Calif.: University Associates, Inc., 1977.

30. Kirschenbaum, H., and S. B. Simon, *Readings in Values Clarification.* Minneapolis: Winston Press, 1973.

31. Klaus, M., and J. Kennell, *Maternal-Infant Bonding.* St. Louis: The C. V. Mosby Company, 1976.

32. La Rocco, S. A., "An Introduction to Role Theory for Nurses," *Supervisor Nurse,* 9, no. 12 (1978), 41–45.

33. Lidz, Theodore, *The Person.* New York: Basic Books, Inc., 1968.

34. Maslow, Abraham, and Bela Mittelmann, *Principles of Abnormal Psychology.* New York: Harper & Row, Publishers, Inc., 1951.

35. Masserman, Jules, "Psychoanalysis and Human Values." *Science and Psychoanalysis, Vol. III.* New York: Grune & Stratton, Inc., 1960.

36. Menninger, Karl, *The Human Mind,* 3rd ed. New York: Alfred A. Knopf, Inc., 1945.

37. Murray, Ruth, and Judith Zentner, *Nursing Concepts for Health Promotion,* 2nd ed. Englewood Cliffs, N.J.: Prentice-Hall, Inc., 1979.

38. Nichols, Barbara, "Dealing with Conflict," *Journal of Continuing Education in Nursing,* 10, no. 6 (1979), 24–27.

39. Nunokowa, Walter, *Human Values and Abnormal Behavior.* Glenview, Ill.: Scott, Foresman & Company, 1965.

40. Osgood, C. E., *An Alternative to War or Surrender.* Urbana, Ill.: University of Illinois Press, 1962.

41. Payne, Dorris, and Patricia Clunn, *Psychiatric—Mental Health Nursing,* 2nd ed. Vienna: Hans Huber Publishers, 1977.

42. Perls, Fritz, *Gestalt Therapy Verbatum.* Lafayette, Calif.: Real People Press, 1969.

43. Piaget, Jean, *The Moral Judgment of the Child.* New York: Harcourt Brace Jovanovich, Inc., 1932.

44. Powell, John, *Why Am I Afraid to Tell You Who I Am?* Niles, Ill.: Argus Communications, 1969.

45. *Psychology Encyclopedia.* Guilford, Conn.: The Rushkin Publishing Group Inc., 1973.

46. Raths, L. E. et al., *Values and Teaching.* Columbus, Ohio: Charles E. Merrill Publishing Company, 1966.

47. Robb, S. S., "Attitudes and Intentions of Baccalaureate Nursing Students toward the Elderly," *Nursing Research,* 28, no. 1 (1979), 43–50.

48. Roberts, Sharon, *Behavioral Concepts and Nursing throughout the Life Span.* Englewood Cliffs, N.J.: Prentice-Hall, Inc., 1978.

49. Rogers, Carl, *On Becoming a Person.* Boston: Houghton Mifflin Company, 1961.

50. Schutz, A., *Collected Papers,* Vol. 2. The Hague: Martinus Nyhoff, 1964.

51. Simon, B. S. et al., *Values Clarification: A Handbook of Practical Strategies and Students.* New York: Hart Publishing Company, 1972.

52. Smith, J. M., "The Psychology of Changing Attitudes," *Occupational Health Nursing,* 30, no. 10 (1978), 468–73.

53. Spitz, René, *The First Year of Life.* New York: International Universities Press, 1965.

54. Steele, Shirley, and Vera Harmon, *Values Clarification in Nursing.* New York: Appleton-Century-Crofts, 1979.

55. Stillman, M. J., "Territoriality and Personal Space," *American Journal of Nursing,* 78, no. 10 (1978), 1670–72.

56. Sullivan, Harry S., *The Interpersonal Theory of Psychiatry.* New York: W. W. Norton & Co., Inc., 1953.

57. Sutterley, Doris, and Gloria Donnelly, *Perspectives in Human Development,* p. 63. Philadelphia: J. B. Lippincott Company, 1973.

58. Travelbee, Joyce, *Interpersonal Aspects of Nursing,* pp. 25–30. Philadelphia: F. A. Davis Company, 1971.

59. Triandis, Harry, *Attitude and Attitude Change.* New York: John Wiley & Sons, Inc., 1971.

60. Uustal, Diane, "Searching for Values," *Image,* 9, no. 2 (1977), 15–17.

61. ——, "The Use of Values in Nursing Practice," *Journal of Continuing Education in Nursing,* 8, no. 3 (1977), 8–13.

62. ——, *Values and Ethics: Considerations in Nursing Practice.* North Scituate, Mass.: Duxbury Press, 1978.

63. ——, "Values Clarification in Nursing: Application to Practice," *American Journal of Nursing,* 78, no. 12 (1978), 2058–63.

64. Wadsworth, Barry, *Piaget's Theory of Cognitive Devel-*

opment, 2nd ed. New York: David McKay Co., Inc., 1978.

65. Walman, Benjamin, *Handbook of General Psychology.* Englewood Cliffs, N.J.: Prentice-Hall, Inc., 1973.

66. Wiley, L., "Finding and Using Your Patient's Strengths," *Nursing '79,* 9, no. 3 (1979), 40–45.

67. Wilson, Holly, and Carol Kneisl, *Psychiatric Nursing.* Reading, Mass.: Addison-Wesley Publishing Co., Inc., 1979.

II

Nursing Behaviors in the Psychiatric/Mental Health Setting

4

The Nursing Process and Emotional Care

Study of this chapter will assist you to:

1. Define nursing utilizing models from various nursing leaders.

2. Identify client as person, family, group, or community.

3. Describe why and how to assess the client who needs emotional care.

4. Formulate an assessment tool, based on information presented in this chapter, for use with clients.

5. Determine a nursing diagnosis that is based on assessment and related to actions that you can take to overcome client problems.

6. Write short-term and long-term client-care goals and an individualized plan of care.

7. Discuss interventions pertinent to psychiatric/mental health nursing.

8. Implement appropriate interventions for the client.

9. Evaluate effectiveness of your nursing approach and care measures, using information presented in this chapter.

10. Discuss the importance of standards of practice for psychiatric nursing.

11. Discuss your philosophy of nursing.

12. Relate information about the nursing process from this chapter to the content in the remaining chapters.

This chapter contributed by Ruth Murray, R.N., M.S.N.

In this chapter five steps in the nursing process will be explored in relation to care of the emotionally ill client. The five steps are: (1) assessment, (2) statement of nursing diagnosis, (3) formulation of client-care goals and plan of care, (4) intervention, and (5) evaluation, which involves ongoing assessment. Application of the nursing process to the emotionally ill person, the dysfunctional family, and the group seeking a new level of health will also be discussed in following chapters.

DEFINITIONS OF NURSING

Many leaders in nursing have defined nursing. You may want to read various references at the end of this chapter to help you formulate your own definition of nursing.

The authors define **nursing** *as an art and science in which verbal, nonverbal, tangible, and intangible health-related activities are systematically performed by a specially educated and licensed compassionate person to promote or maintain biopsychosocial health of the person/family/group, as well as to comfort, protect, or stabilize the same during life or in the face of death, and to aid in their recovery. These activities, legally defined, involve use of self and may be performed independently or collaboratively with other health team members, but always with the person/family/group or community as actively involved as possible in the process* (88).

Psychiatric/mental health nursing *is a specialized area of practice, utilizing theories of human behavior for its scientific basis and employing the purposeful use of self in a therapeutic relationship with one or more people as its art, in order to provide emotional care to the client and to facilitate the process of learning more positive or effective behaviors and of achieving increasing emotional maturity. In this interpersonal process with the client, the nurse works with the client so that present needs are met and more mature needs and motivations emerge and can be met* (103, 123). Although psychiatric/mental health nursing is a specialty area, its principles are applicable to all areas of nursing. This emotional care of the person is directed at any one of the three levels of prevention—primary, secondary, or tertiary—to be discussed in Chapter 25. Thus, psychiatric/mental health nursing has as its ultimate goal the promotion of optimum emotional health for the person, family, group, community, and society (102). Essential to the psychodynamic processes involved in giving emotional care are the abilities to understand personal behavior as well as the behaviors of others, to identify feelings and thoughts and the problem areas, and to apply principles of human relations to the situation.

Throughout this book we refer to *emotional care* when discussing psychiatric/mental health problems or nursing care. The term **emotional** more specifically *defines the affective part of the person, the feelings and attitudes, which are expressed in behavioral responses*. The term **mental** more specifically *refers to the cognitive or intellectual function of the person*. Certainly intellectual function may be impaired in emotional illness, but this is not consistently true. Additionally, cognitively impaired persons may be cared for by psychiatric services in an institution. Often the words are used interchangeably without any clarification as to which sphere of the person is impaired. The word **psychological** *covers both intellectual/mental and emotional components;* this term is rather new in usage and often is not used by professionals who adhere to the medical model, which uses the term *psychiatric*.

Because generally our society uses the word *mental* to denote *emotional* when referring to health and illness, the last chapter will use that term also when discussing the three levels of preventive care.

The term **client** *is used to mean the person, family, group, or community system that you will work with as a nurse*. The person, family, group, or population in a community, as client, may be *cared for in any setting,* including the hospital, emergency service, clinic, doctor's office, outpatient department, neighborhood health center, health department service, home, storefront, or long-term care institution.

HISTORY OF PSYCHIATRIC NURSING

Nursing is an emerging profession based on the criteria that describe a "profession" (119). The multiple entry levels into nursing continue to confuse the public and cause other professional groups to see nurses as technicians. However, the baccalaureate and master's prepared psychiatric nurse is considered a professional person, at least by nurses. Certainly nursing meets a social need and is based on socially acceptable scientific principles. The professional nurse demonstrates unique skills, critical thinking, and systematic inquiry, and uses discretion and judgment in practice. The psychiatric nurse, perhaps more so than some others, makes decisions that cannot be standardized to time, manner of performance, or habit, nor regularly subjected to the direction of another person. Nurses, including psychiatric/mental health nurses, have a group consciousness and a special language, and they recognize societal obligations by adhering to a code of ethics. The professional nurse is drawn to nursing, recognizes her/his unique knowledge and skill, and does not aspire to join another profession.

Nursing is rapidly gaining professional status and is developing a body of knowledge based on nursing research. The nursing profession is continuing its efforts to gain autonomy for individual practitioners, to control professional activity, and to participate in the formulation of public policy. Psychiatric nurses have been in the forefront of these efforts.

Although the history of psychiatric nursing followed that of psychiatry and medical management for many decades, in the past three decades, psychiatric/mental health nursing has progressed considerably under the leadership of many forward-looking and committed psychiatric nurses in education and service. Table 4-1 summarizes some of the nurse leaders and their major contribution(s) along with some events that have affected the history of psychiatric nursing. This table cannot mention all of the nurses who have made a significant contribution in psychiatric nursing, nor can it do justice to either the leaders or their contributions, but the summary does indicate that committed, caring, educated people can indeed make a difference in nursing care.

TABLE 4-1. Summary of Historical Contributions to Psychiatric/Mental Health Nursing

HISTORICAL ERA	PSYCHIATRIC NURSING LEADER	CONTRIBUTION
Pre-1860		Nursing care for the young, ill, and helpless historically has existed as long as the human race. Care was given by family members, relatives, servants, neighbors, members of religious orders or humanitarian societies, or by convalescing patients or prisoners.
1782–1815		Nursing school established by Dr. Franz May in Germany. Believed that quality of nursing care could not be improved unless nurses were well treated by their superiors.
1860	Florence Nightingale	Established Nightingale School at St. Thomas Hospital, London, after Crimean War and worked with untrained women caring for soldiers. Founder of modern-day nursing.
1860–1880		Emphasized maintaining healthful environment, personal hygiene, cleanliness, and healthful living habits such as adequate nutrition, exercise, and sleep so that nature could heal. Emphasized kindness toward patients along with custodial care.
	Linda Richards	First graduate nurse and first psychiatric nurse in the United States. After study under Miss Nightingale, organized nursing services and educational programs in Boston City Hospital and in several state mental hospitals in Illinois.
	Dorothea Lynde Dix	Worked to reform psychiatric care in mental hospitals and to correct overcrowding and the insufficient number of of overworked physicians and attendants.
1882		First school to prepare nurses to care for acutely and chronically mentally ill opened at McLean Hospital, Waverly, Massachusetts, through collaboration of Linda Richards and Dr. Edward Cowles.
1890–1930		Nurses recognized by some administrative psychiatrists in state and private hospitals for their preparation. Nurses relieved of menial housekeeping chores to engage in physical, custodial care of patients. Role primarily to assist physician or carry out procedures for physical care. Few psychological nursing skills. Psychologically concerned with maintaining kind, tolerant attitude and humane treatment.
1920	Harriet Bailey	First nurse educator to write a psychiatric nursing text, *Nursing Mental Diseases,* 1920, published by Macmillan. When Assistant Superintendent of Nurses at the Henry Phipps Clinic, Johns Hopkins Hospital, she wrote of the importance of a nurse knowing dynamics of mental ill-

TABLE 4-1. Continued

HISTORICAL ERA	PSYCHIATRIC NURSING LEADER	CONTRIBUTION
		ness and of teaching mental nursing, and worked for student experiences in psychiatry. She argued for more holistic care of patients. Also was advisor to New York State Board of Regents pertaining to nurses' education and laws governing nurses.
1930–1960		Medical profession emphasized somatic treatment. Nurse's role to care for physical needs and assist with somatic therapies.
1937		Psychiatric nursing a requirement by National League for Nursing in basic nursing curriculum.
1946		National Mental Health Act passed, authorizing establishment of National Institute of Mental Health, with funds and programs to train professional psychiatric personnel, conduct psychiatric research, and aid development of mental health programs at the state level. Provided impetus for psychiatric nursing as a specialty.
1950–1960		Nurse's role included physical care and medications and maintenance of therapeutic milieu. Less emphasis on physical restraints. Nurses gradually realized that somatic therapy alone is not adequate to treat mental disease.
1952	Hildegarde Peplau	Formulated first systematic theoretical framework in psychiatric nursing; presented in *Interpersonal Relationships in Nursing,* 1952, published by Putnam's. Emphasized that nursing is an interpersonal process and that psychological techniques and theoretical concepts are essential to nursing practice. Psychoanalytic, interpersonal, and communication theories utilized by nurses.
	Francis Sleeper	Addressed American Psychiatric Association in 1952; advocated use of psychiatric nurse as a psychotherapist rather than a caretaker.
	Gwen Tudor Will	Presented in 1952 a sociopsychologic nursing approach to schizophrenic patients. Approach became classic. Showed powerful effect of nursing relationship. Described effects of institutionalization, dynamics of mutual withdrawal and behavior in the relationship, and theoretical principles as basis for intervention.
1953		"The Therapeutic Community" by Maxwell Jones, in Great Britian, laid basis for movement in United States toward therapeutic milieu and nurse's role in this therapy.
1956		National Conference on Graduate Education in Psychiatric Nursing introduced concept of psychiatric clinical nurse

TABLE 4-1. Continued

HISTORICAL ERA	PSYCHIATRIC NURSING LEADER	CONTRIBUTION
		specialist. Theoreticians begin to differentiate functions based on Master's level of preparation in nursing.
1957	June Mellow	Introduced second theoretical approach to psychiatric nursing; utilized psychoanalytic theory in one-to-one approach to schizophrenic. Emphasized providing corrective emotional experience rather than investigating pathological processes or interpersonal developmental processes.
	Garland Lewis	Developed psychiatric aide education project nationwide.
1958		American Nurses Association established Conference Group on Psychiatric Nursing.
1959		Accredited schools of nursing had to have own psychiatric nursing curriculum and instructor, per National League for Nursing. Could no longer buy services of hospitals to supply education.
1960–1970	Hildegrade Peplau Gertrud Ujhely Joyce Travelbee Shirley Burd Loretta Bermosk Joyce Hays Catherine Norris Gertrude Stokes W. Hargreaves Dorothy Gregg Sheila Rouslin	Nursing leaders emphasized importance of self-awareness and use of self, nurse-patient relationships therapy, therapeutic communication, and psychosocial aspects of general nursing.
1960	Ida Orlando	Initiated term *nursing process* and began to delineate its components. Presented general theoretical framework for all nurse-patient relationships with focus on client ascertaining meaning of behavior and explaining help needed. Emphasized deliberative actions by nurse in interpersonal process. Wrote classic book, *The Dynamic Nurse-Patient Relationship,* 1961, published by Putnam's. Framework used by some practitioners in psychiatric settings.
		Comprehensive Community Mental Health Act passed, 1960; provided impetus for nurses moving from hospital to community setting.
1961		Joint Congressional Commission Report, 1961, *Action for Mental Health, Final Report of the Joint Commission on Mental Illness and Mental Health,* published by Basic

TABLE 4-1. Continued

HISTORICAL ERA	PSYCHIATRIC NURSING LEADER	CONTRIBUTION
		Books, Inc., gave historical overview of attitudes and behavior toward mentally ill, changed public attitudes to mentally ill being treated in the community and reduced state mental hospital populations, promoted establishment of community mental health centers, and championed mental health. Encouraged nurse to develop therapeutic effectiveness in group and milieu therapies as well as individual therapy.
		Legislation and publication for improvement of mental health services and preventive services created new roles and positions for psychiatric nurses and emphasized need for more graduate education in psychiatric nursing.
		Role of nurse expanded to that of consultant, case-finder, therapist, and cotherapist.
		Nurse functioned more as member of health team on collegial level in community mental health centers. Role blurring between health professionals evident. Nurses evolved roles in various settings other than hospitals, including outpatient programs, day hospitals, halfway houses, and aftercare programs.
	Anne Burgess Donna Aguilera	Engaged in crisis work and short-term therapy as well as in long-term therapy.
	Hildegarde Peplau	Promoted primary role of nurse as psychotherapist or counselor rather than as mother surrogate, socializer, or manager.
1967		American Nurses Association presented Position Paper on Psychiatric Nursing, endorsing role of clinical specialist as therapist in individual, group, family, and milieu therapies.
1969	M. Meldman	Nurse psychotherapist moved into private practice.
	Luther Christman	Emphasized importance of joint position in education and service for graduate-prepared nurses.
1970–1980		Psychiatric nurse clinical specialist role created increasingly in hospitals and other agencies to work with nonpsychiatric as well as psychiatric clients. Consultation and liaison roles in nonpsychiatric agencies increased.
	Sheila Rouslin	Certification of clinical specialists in psychiatric nursing begun by Division of Psychiatric Mental Health Nursing, New Jersey State Nurses Association because of her leadership. Later, certification developed by American Nurses Association.
	Shirley Smoyak	Client defined as individual, group, family, or community.

TABLE 4-1.   Continued

HISTORICAL ERA	PSYCHIATRIC NURSING LEADER	CONTRIBUTION
	Gwen Marram Irene Burnside	Group and family psychotherapy by graduate-prepared nurses emphasized by nursing leaders.
	Carolyn Clark	Systems framework was used increasingly by psychiatric nurses.
		Change agent, health maintenance, and research roles emphasized in latter half of decade.
	Bonnie Bullough	Legal and ethical aspects of psychiatric care emphasized.
	Madeleine Leininger	Care of whole person reemphasized.
	Audra Pambram Ildaura Murillo- Rhode Hector Gonzales Doris Mosley Paulette D'Angi	Implications of cultural diversity for mental health services and psychiatric treatment emphasized. Alternate methods of treatment increasingly utilized.
		Practice as autonomous member of team and in independent or private practice increased in latter half of decade. Work with citizens, consumer groups, and consumer organizations increased toward end of decade.
1978		President's Commission Report of 1978 describes stigma as primary barrier to providing mental health services and offered possible interventions. Concluded that effects of deinstitutionalization and discharge of patients to community facilities have not worked as expected because of lack of financial, social, medical, and nursing resources and lack of coordination of services with clients and families.

MODELS FOR NURSING

There are a number of conceptual models for nursing. These **conceptual models** *are a matrix of concepts that direct or describe the focus of inquiry or a network in which theories, concepts, principles, and data patterns are merged.* Joan Riehl and Sister C. Roy classify models as developmental, as a system, or as interactional (109). You may gain in-depth knowledge of these models by reading their text *Conceptual Models for Nursing Practice* (109) and other references at the end of this chapter. All of the models described present a systematic study of problems related to practice and link theory and facts to the real world.

Table 4-2 briefly outlines some of the major nursing theories and theorists.

The basis for the nursing model utilized by

the authors is the Humanistic Nursing Model formulated by Josephine Paterson and Loretta Zderad. In this model, **nursing** *is an existential experience lived between the nurse and client, whereby each nursing situation reciprocally evokes and affects expression and manifestations of people's capacity for existence.* Thus, the nurse has responsibility for realistic self-awareness as well as awareness of others. Humanistic nursing means more than a benevolent, technically competent subject-object, one-way interaction, with the nurse "doing" for the client. Instead, nursing is a responsible, searching, nurturing, transactional relation-ship between a nurse and client. The nurse's self-awareness, self-acceptance, being in touch with others, and self-actualization enable her/him to share with others in a relationship. The nurse recognizes the complexity of the person and the human experience, is concerned with the person's perception of experience, and is willing to share that experience. Nursing practice involves ability to struggle with the person through peak experiences, such as birth, death, grief, and illness, in an "I-Thou" relationship, doing and being with the person. Nursing is an art-science, lived by the nurse (100).

TABLE 4-2. Summary of Major Nursing Theories (Models) and Theorists

THEORIST	THEORY/MODEL
Florence Nightingale	Emphasized interrelationship between person's environment and state of health.
Hildegarde Peplau	Developmental–Interpersonal Relationship Theory (see description in text).
Joyce Travelbee	Interpersonal Theory; an elaboration of Peplau's theory.
Sister Madeleine Clemence (utilizing Gabriel Marcel)	Existentialism: Study of the person in his/her real existence. Emphasis on being and becoming. Responsibility of person to shape his/her own self. Human existence goal-directed. Person's courageous choices result in personal growth, fuller human stature, greater participation in being. Nurse must be committed and have full, willing, and open-eyed acceptance of full share of life, love given and received, and joys and sorrows that are common lot of humanity. Nurse must be willing to take risks and take responsibility for actions. Nurse enables client to exercise full freedom, to become authentic, to use the illness situation for maturing. Nurse establishes I-Thou relationship by sharing human experience and emotions; thus uses self therapeutically.
Josephine Patterson Loretta Zderad	Humanistic Nursing Model (see description in text).
Dagmar Brodt	Synergistic Theory: Simultaneous combination of separate agencies, physical and emotional comfort measures, produces greater effect than either independent action when nurse providing care, cure, and coordination through use of nursing process.
Martha Rogers	Theoretical Basis of Nursing: Science of Unitarian Man. Emphasis on wholeness of the person. Perceives person through principles of homeodynamics. Concepts of energy fields, openness, pattern and organization, and four-dimensionality explain person. Unified concept of human function includes mutual and simultaneous interaction between person and the environment, coherence and integrity of human process, and promotion of human and environmental patterns for maximum health potential.

TABLE 4-2. Continued

THEORIST	THEORY/MODEL
Dorothy Johnson	Behavioral System Model: Person a collection of behavioral subsystems that interrelate to whole person or system and have specific tasks; these are achievement, affiliative, aggressive/protective, dependency, eliminative, ingestive, restorative, and sexual. Each subsystem has structure and function; is open and linked. Subsystems and system as a whole are self-maintaining and self-perpetuating as long as internal and external environmental conditions remain orderly and predictable, conditions and resources necessary for function are met, and subsystem interrelations are harmonious. Otherwise, malfunction and illness result, and nursing problems identified. Nursing an external regulatory force to preserve organization and integration of person's behavior at optimal level when health threatened.
Dorothea Orem	Self-Care Concept of Nursing: Person is a biopsychosocial being, a self-care agent, who has universal self-care requirements, occupies a dynamic position on wellness-illness continuum, and can engage in decisions and actions for health. Self-care agency defined as voluntary set of actions or potential for action that person initiates and performs for maintenance of health or well-being. Therapeutic self-care demand defined as complex of requirements that assist person with maintenance of present health or movement to desirable state. Self-care deficit defined as inadequacy in self-care agent to meet actual or potential demands. Nursing system a complex set of actions combined to assist self-care agent achieve health and overcome self-care deficits, or to foster self-care abilities, with specific roles and responsibilities for person and nurse. Nursing needed when therapeutic self-care demand exceeds assets of self-care agency of an individual or group. Basic goals of nursing action to accomplish client's self-care demand and to move client toward responsible action in matters of self-care. Intervention deals with nursing agency—the partly compensatory, wholly compensatory, and supportive–educative system that nurse can use. Nursing modified and eventually eliminated when progressive favorable change in health state of person or when person becomes self-directing in care to prevent illness and maintain or improve health.
Betty Neuman	Betty Neuman Health-Care Systems Model: Model derived from Gestalt, Field, Systems, and Selye's Stress-Adaptation theories. Study of person, group, or community and the response of the open system to stress. Person unique but also composite of normal characteristics that are interrelated. Stressors are intra-, inter-, and extrapersonal forces. Variables or stressors affecting person are physiological, psychological, sociocultural, and developmental. When line of defense or resistance inadequate, malfunction or illness occurs. Nursing can be initiated at primary, secondary, or tertiary levels of

TABLE 4-2.   Continued

THEORIST	THEORY/MODEL
	prevention to assist person to maintain balance between internal and external environment.
Marilyn Chrisman Marsha Fowler	Systems—In-Change Model: Emphasizes structure and process. Refers to interdependent biologic, social, and personal systems, in continual process of change, which interact with environment along developmental continuum. Feedback among the systems and with environment is crucial. Changes produce stress, which disturbs equilibrium. Nurse must assess for and intervene with compensatory or regulatory mechanisms that help person achieve, restore, or maintain integrity. Utilizes stress and adaptation theories in nursing practice.
Sister Callista Roy	Roy Adaptation Model: Systems model with interactionist levels of analysis. Client has four interrelated subsystems or modes of adaptation to meet needs: physiologic needs, self-concept, role function, and interdependence. The person, a dynamic, integrated being, strives to maintain a balance in response to internal or external environmental changes, forces, or stimuli; this is called *adaptation.* Adaptation results from response to stimuli: focal (immediate), contextual (environmental), and residual (subjective, resulting from past background). Adaptation constantly occurring. Maladaptive response not promoting person's equilibrium or integrity is disruptive. Adaptation ability depends on degree of change and coping abilities and time. Person and interaction with environment are units for nursing assessment; nursing intervention involves manipulation of system environment. The nurse is concerned with promoting health by assisting person to adapt in subsystems.
Joan Riehl	Riehl Interaction Model: Based on Symbolic Interactionism and Self-Concept Theory. Person lives in symbolic and physical stimuli. Person learns meanings, values, and actions through communication of symbols. Self-concept is key element between behavior and social organization to which the individual belongs. Self-concept (responding to self as object) is essential to behave as a human. Symbolic interaction occurs between people who interpret or define each other's actions instead of just reacting to them. Responses based on meanings attached to such actions. Role-taking is a cognitive activity; person takes into self another's attitude or perceptual field—symbolic process by which person puts self in another's place to gain insight, anticipate another's behavior, and act accordingly.

Another important nursing model utilized by the authors is the Interpersonal Model developed by H. Peplau (102) and expanded by J. Travelbee (123). Probably the most specific model for psychiatric nursing is the Developmental-Interpersonal Relationship Framework developed by Hildegarde Peplau. She defines *nursing as a significant therapeutic interpersonal process that functions cooperatively with other human processes and focuses on support processes, self-repair, and self-renewal to foster health and growth for the person.* She has *four assumptions* in the model (15, 102):

1. The person is an organism, living in an unstable equilibrium, with the ability to learn skills for solving problems and adapting to tensions created by basic needs. *The learning of more positive behaviors is called **growth**.*

2. The kind of person each nurse becomes makes a substantial difference in what each client learns while being nursed through illness. In the interpersonal process, both nurse and client respond to, stimulate each other, and experience growth.

3. A function of nursing is to foster personality maturity for productive living, using principles and methods to guide the process of grappling with everyday interpersonal difficulties.

4. The nursing profession has legal responsibility for effective use of nursing and consequences to clients.

The goal of nursing action is the forward movement of personality in the direction of creative, constructive, productive behavior for personal and community life. To accomplish this goal, the nurse meets the person's needs and assists psychological and interpersonal conditions of self-repair and self-renewal. The main factors inhibiting personality development are unmet needs, frustration, or conflict of goals. The setting of nursing is anywhere that people are in need and occurs at all three levels: primary, secondary, and tertiary. Primary prevention is the preferred focus. The main mode of intervention is the interpersonal process between the client and nurse, which is divided into the four phases of orientation, identification, exploitation, and resolution. These phases are described more fully in Chapter 6 (15, 102).

Joyce Travelbee elaborated on the interpersonal process in nursing and described the **therapeutic use of self** as *the ability to use one's person consciously and in full awareness in an attempt to establish relatedness and structure nursing interventions* (123).

The authors realize that readers of this text may be using any one of the various models summarized in Table 4-2. We consider the information in this text to be essential and basic to the understanding and care of people who hurt emotionally, who have a negative self-concept, and whose behavior interferes with their interpersonal relationships and social role functions. Thus the holistic approach to the Humanistic-Interpersonal Model, synthesizing the frameworks of Paterson and Zderad, Peplau, Travelbee, and major Second and Third Force theorists, is used throughout the text since that framework is basic to the personalized care spoken to by every conceptual model in nursing. The basic ideas presented here can also be reworked into the terminology of any of the major models.

THE NURSING PROCESS

As a nurse, you do more than can be overtly seen by others, especially when you are engaged in emotional care. You use the **nursing process,** *a dynamic method through which nursing is practiced.* The nursing process is *an ongoing, systematic series of actions, interactions, and transactions with a person(s) in need of health care, using the problem-solving method, so that empathic and intellectual processes and scientific knowledge form the basis for outward actions observable to others.* The problem-solving process in nursing is analogous to the problem-solving process used by other professionals, as shown in Table 4-3.

The nursing process provides a foundation for humanistic, knowledgeable, organized, holistic, and individualized nursing care. The process can be used with any theoretical framework, any type of client, and in any setting. The nursing process also provides the framework for nursing research, as well as for the nurse's accountability to society.

TABLE 4-3.   Comparison of Problem-Solving Method and Nursing Process

PROBLEM-SOLVING METHOD	STEP OF NURSING PROCESS
1. Preparation: Problem identi-fication	1. Assessment Statement of nursing diagnosis
2. Production: Potential solution sought Alternate solutions are tried to solve problem	2. Identification of client-care goals Formulation of plan of care Intervention
3. Judgment: Evaluation of effec-tiveness of selected solution	3. Evaluation of the effectiveness of plan of care and intervention

Assessment

In *assessment, data about the person, family, group, or situation are obtained by means of astute observation, listening, and examination; by purposeful communication; and by the use of special skills and techniques, through application of a theory and scientific knowledge about the person, family, group, or community, and behavior.* Information from other health team members can be utilized to gain a broader perspective. The information about the objective and subjective status of the client(s) is analyzed, interrelated, and interpreted through using inferences, knowledge, personal or health team experience, records, and a variety of other sources as indicated. Nursing judgments are based on this information (1, 12, 16).

First-level assessment is done on initial contact with the client of any age or situation to determine the feelings, perceived threat to self, ability to adapt to the threat, and immediate necessary actions. Second-level assessment continues throughout the time of contact with the client; it adds depth and breadth to the understanding of physical, emotional, mental, spiritual, family, social, and cultural characteristics and needs. This more comprehensive view enables you to plan and give care better suited to the whole individual or situation (12, 16, 58).

Data are collected and analyzed to help you determine patterns of behavior that are adaptive and functional and can be maintained or reinforced;

that are functional but must be temporarily modified because of the constraints of the illness, hospitalization, or institutionalization; and that are dysfunctional and require nursing intervention (6). The data become part of the health history. The articles by E. Baer, M. McGowan, and D. McGivern (8), E. T. Eggland (38), and G. K. McFarland and F. E. Apostopes (80) give additional information on obtaining a health history.

Assessment Tools

An *assessment tool is an organized means of recording information obtained in first- and second-level assessments.* It is distinct from a medical history in that it focuses on the client's own feelings, perceptions, and reactions, that is, on the perceived illness and health care needs, instead of primarily on pathology and diagnostic labels. The form serves as a guide to obtain information that does not repeat data collected by other health team members, although it may include aspects of the medical or social history that are pertinent to nursing care. The nursing assessment provides a composite picture of the client; other health team members may also use it as an introduction to the client.

Although the form used and the kind of information collected must be adapted to your individual work setting and clientele, there are certain components that should be included in any assessment. Some factors are more pertinent for children and youth; others are more pertinent to adults. Refer to Chapter 5 for interviewing guidelines.

Assessment of the normal or emotionally ill child or adolescent can be done initially by watching the person when he/she is alone and quiet, at play, and in interaction with others. Observe appearance, apparent affect or mood, sensorimotor development, use of language, capacity for play and fantasy, and manner of relating to peers or adults.

Assessment of the psychological status of the child client is a challenge because of developmental stage and related abstraction ability, level of language development, and limitations of formal psychometric tests. The child's cultural and environmental background also can influence test skills and results. Or the child may be unable to cooperate with testing because of fear, anxiety, fatigue, or emotional status. Thus the assessment data gained from observation, listening, and play, as well as data obtained from parents or other adults, are usually not sufficient (3). Tests must also be used.

The Denver Developmental Screening Test is simple and reliable for assessing developmental status from birth to six and one-half years of age. A thorough description of the test is available in several books (43, 54).

The Goodenough Draw-A-Man Test is easily administered to children ages four to six (31). The test is scored by counting the number of parts of the body the child draws. Test results are abnormal when the total number of points for the child's drawing is less than the standard number for that age. The test gives a gross estimate of the child's mental age and feelings about self but must be used in conjunction with other tests. A variation of this test is the Draw-A-Person (DAP) Test, in which the subject draws a person and then another of the opposite sex for assessment of body image. This is also used with subjects of any age.

The Peabody Picture Vocabulary Test assesses verbal intellectual capacity (54). The child is asked to pick from among four pictures, the one that best describes each word the examiner uses. The child with speech impairment or who is very shy can be assessed with this test because it only involves pointing to pictures.

The child who demonstrates developmental lags, school failure, or emotional problems should be referred to a child psychologist or child psychiatrist for formal psychometric and IQ evaluation (31, 34, 43, 127). Chapter 21 further discusses assessment of the child and adolescent.

The older child and adolescent typically have better language and abstraction skills but may be equally as challenging to assess and test because of their feelings and ability to withhold or distort information, in addition to illness factors. Diane Critchley describes a method for organizing content of the mental status examination of the adolescent, suggests verbal and nonverbal activity for involving the youth and observations that should be made, and concludes with a developmental clinical formulation (34). Tests that are used with the adults are also used with the adolescent, especially after age sixteen.

The nursing models listed in Table 4-2 also propose an assessment format that can be used if you are utilizing one of those models in your education and practice. Most of the models would have to be adjusted somewhat for use with the child; none are specific for children or adolescents or for psychological examinations.

Adult assessment which is also applicable to the adolescent, is described by many authors. Joyce Snyder and Margo Wilson describe the following factors to be included in the psychological assessment: (1) response to stress, and coping and defense mechanisms, (2) interpersonal relationships, (3) motivation and life style, (4) thought processes and verbal behavior, (5) nonverbal behavior, (6) awareness and handling of feelings, (7) support systems, (8) talents, strengths, and assets, (9) physical health, and (10) nurse's impression of the interview and interaction (121). Janis Reynolds and Jann Logsdon describe a tool for assessing mental status that includes information about identifying data; responses based on the nurse's judgment, such as appearance, motor movement, and level of consciousness; and responses based on the person's self-description about illness, family, living arrangements, and life patterns (107). Other authors also give information about psychological assessment (5, 53). Sometimes initial assessment is done by telephone. Read the section on telephone crisis work in Chapter 8 and an article by Donna Murphy and Eleanor Chronopoulous for more information on special points to consider in telephone assessment (87). You may wish to read any of the above references for additional information on assessment.

In the Appendix at the end of this chapter you will find sociocultural and psychological assessment tools that can help you formulate your own tool. *The guide is extensive in order to assist you in formulating your own tools. You may also choose to use only a portion of a tool. Suggested techniques for phrasing the questions are also given.* However, *it is unlikely that you would ever ask the client all of the questions in one or two interviews or in the exact order or phraseology given in the tool. The tool must be adapted to the uniqueness of both you and the client and to the situation.*

You will find a family assessment tool in Chapter 10, and information on group assessment in Chapter 11. Assessment in crisis situations is covered in Chapter 8. Guidelines for assessment basic to specific nursing diagnosis are then presented in the chapters in Unit IV.

Tests that are widely used by psychologists and psychiatrists include:

1. Weschsler Adult Intelligence Scale (WAIS). (There is also a form for children ages 6–16.)
2. Stanford-Binet Intelligence Scale (also used with children).
3. Vineland Social Maturity Scale to determine social competence in mentally retarded persons.
4. Shipley-Hartford Scale to compare vocabulary and abstract ability to detect intellectual impairment.
5. Rorschach Inkblot Test—a projective test of ten standardized inkblots used to elicit associations, which are then interpreted.
6. Thematic Apperception Technique (TAT)—a projective test of twenty pictures, some of which are selected and the client is asked to tell a story in response to the picture. The story is then interpreted. (The Children's Apperception Test (CAT) is a similar technique.)
7. Bender (Visual-Motor) Gestalt Test, which involves the client in copying geometric figures to determine presence of brain damage and a projective technique with associations about the figures to interpret personality makeup.
8. Minnesota Multiphasic Personality Inventory (MMPI)—a pencil-and-paper test to measure personality traits and psychopathology.

More information about these tests can be obtained from any psychological testing text.

Use of Assessment Tools

You may think that obtaining a lengthy assessment is too time-consuming and impractical. But it is a necessary activity for humanizing and individualizing care. A nurse-client relationship is begun during assessment. Assessment conveys interest and concern and establishes a sense of mutual trust. Nursing diagnoses and realistic care objectives cannot be formulated without the information obtained in an assessment or without the client's involvement. Nor can the last step, evaluation of the process, be done effectively unless there are baseline data. Every nursing unit should have a guide for assessment, and all of the nurses should be involved in its development, trial usage, and revision so that the tool can be useful in daily practice.

Communication skills will help you obtain assessment and nursing history data. *Use open-ended statements.* Observe and respond to the person's feelings; convey understanding of implied communication. Remain silent so that the person can elaborate on answers. Be attentive to the nonverbal behavior and its meaning that accompanies verbal behavior. Asking a barrage of direct questions will stifle the person's expression, resulting in superficial, brief, or no answers. The interviewer who is too active obtains less pertinent data. *An assessment tool is not meant to be used as a probe. Ask questions related to what the person is saying to fill in the needed information.* In that way you may get information that was not anticipated but which is important. Information about certain aspects, such as the person's interpretation of reality or ability to abstract, can best be obtained by observation, attentive listening, or indirect questions.

Do not feel compelled to fill in all the spaces on the assessment tool the first time you meet the person/family. You will get more accurate information if you use the assessment tool for both first- and second-level assessment. Determine *patterns* of behavior instead of making conclusions based on one observation or interview. The more skillful you are as a communicator, the better your data will be as the basis for continued care.

Part of your skill in communication will be to know when the client is too ill or too anxious for a lengthy assessment. Recognize when your persistent assessment causes the mute, withdrawn, agitated, or suspicious person to feel worse and to demonstrate more behaviors of illness.

Observation skills are essential in assessment. Use of eyes, ears, perception and interpretation, and touch are all means through which you observe. A seldom discussed vehicle for observation is your own affect, emotion, or sense of self. Use your emotional response to observe your client. Ask yourself: What is my response to the person? What do I perceive? Do I feel a sense of coldness and detachment, or warmth and friendliness? How did the person respond to me in the interview? Did I feel the client's high level of anxiety? Depression? Suspicion? Dependency? If you have not experienced the emotion of another, you are missing a sense that you could be sharpening for more astute assessment.

Regardless of the tool's format, the tool will enable you to (88):

1. Assemble information systematically.
2. Determine the need for more information.
3. Select and organize information.
4. Recall knowledge and theory that apply to the client.
5. Locate other sources of information, such as past records, the family, or other health team members.
6. Continue to appraise the client/situation over time in order to validate prior information for use in emotional care.

Avoid the following obstacles when using an assessment tool: (1) having a partial or stereotyped view of the client, (2) perceiving client as an object or thing instead of as a person, (3) viewing the person in terms of potential to meet your needs instead of in terms of how you can better meet his/her needs, and (4) using the tool as a task in itself instead of as a basis for humanistic, individualized care.

Statement of Nursing Diagnosis

Once a sufficient amount of information has been collected about the client and situation, the infor-

mation can be analyzed and interpreted so that an explicit statement can be made about human responses, presenting problems, or unmet needs related to health that require nursing care.

Nursing diagnosis is a concise term or phrase, based on assessment data, that describes any of the following client situations as they are amenable to nursing intervention: (1) actual or potential behavior at variance with the desired state, (2) adaptive response or effort directed to an actual or potential stressor or crisis, (3) a commonly recurring condition or unmet needs that interfere with health and adaptation, or (4) a present or anticipated difficulty. According to researchers working with classification of nursing diagnoses, the diagnostic statement or label should be validated with the client and should provide: (1) a definition of the *client's strengths and deficiencies,* the concern, the actual or potential problem, or unhealthy behavior, (2) reference to *etiology* or factors that relate to, contribute to, are associated with, or maintain the unhealthy response or prevent desired change, (3) guidelines for *intervention,* and (4) indication of *prognosis,* the potential or desired outcome (20, 50, 73, 86). Most statements of nursing diagnoses do not include all four components because of lack of specific nursing research.

Nursing diagnoses do not label medical entities or the pathological or disease process. They refer to conditions that can be helped by nursing action. Diagnoses that have been accepted by the Third National Conference on Classification of Nursing Diagnosis, which are being tested and may be revised, and which refer to clients needing psychiatric/mental health nursing, are as follows (47):

Anxiety
Consciousness, Altered Levels of
Comfort, Alterations in
Coping Patterns, Maladapted Individual
Coping, Ineffective Family
Family Process, Inadequate
Grieving
Injury, Potential for
Knowledge, Lack of
Manipulation
Mobility, Impairment of
Parenting, Alterations in
Role Disturbances

Self-Care Activities, Alterations in
Self-Concept, Alterations in
Sensory-Perceptual Alterations
Sexuality, Alterations in Patterns of
Spirituality, Matters of
Social Isolation
Thought Processes, Impaired
Verbal Communication, Impairment of

Many of the above nursing diagnoses will be discussed in this text, but the above list is not comprehensive. Other diagnoses will be included, based on the author's knowledge and experience. Perhaps in the future there will be a generally accepted list and classification of nursing diagnoses.

Generally, the nursing diagnosis is written so that the first part of the phrase states the behavior assessed by the nurse that is amenable to nursing care, and the second part of the phrase gives direction to nursing action.

In this text, the authors will also refer to medical diagnoses since you must know these terms, and the signs and symptoms associated with the diagnoses, in order to work collaboratively with the other health care professionals who use the medically based diagnoses. Further, medical problems generate nursing diagnoses pertinent to the physical and psychological status, and nursing implications of medical diagnoses will be your responsibility in meeting client needs.

A dynamic diagnosis is also important for understanding of and intervention with the client. The nurse should use knowledge of the ego, id, superego, conscious, unconscious, defense mechanisms, and the person's developmental history, all of which contribute to the illness. The dynamic diagnosis will help you better determine and work with the person's strengths, limits, needs, feelings, self-concept, and potential for maturity. Reference will be made to the dynamics of behavior throughout the text to enhance understanding of the person and interpersonal processes.

Formulation of Client-Care Goals and Plan of Care

After assessment and statement of nursing diagnosis, various nursing actions, approaches, or solutions are considered in view of the nature and probable source of the person's unmet needs. At this point

client-care goals, statements about a predicted or desired client outcome, can be formulated in collaboration with the person/family/group. Your judgment, insights, and initiative are crucial so that the direction of goal setting is toward health restoration, maintenance, and promotion, to avoid conflicting goals, and to avoid interfering with other therapies. If conditions are such that the individual cannot be involved in goal setting and planning, the family or significant group should be involved if possible. *Short-term goals are individualized to the client, related to assessment of current overt needs, derived from the diagnosis, and can be accomplished in a short span of time, perhaps in one-to-ten days. Long-term goals are based on assessment of continuing needs, are future-oriented, and state in general terms the ultimate desired result of nursing intervention.*

Priority of goals is affected by the following criteria (16):

1. Priority of nursing diagnoses, identified in collaboration with the person, family, group, or community when possible.
2. Severity of health problem or life situation and actual or potential problems.
3. Resources (and their availability) that are needed by client or nurse.
4. Receptivity to nursing care by client.
5. Cost in terms of money or energy to client, nurse, agency, and society.
6. Demands of external constraints, such as agency policies or legal factors.

Short-term goals for the hospitalized client might include relief from stressful preoccupations or from depressed response to surgery. Long-term goals might include decreased social isolation or increased self-esteem. Short-term goals for the person who comes to a mental health clinic might include management of stresses related to work and financial obligations. Long-term goals might include resolution of the crisis of death of a loved one. Goals reflect the psychomotor, physiological, cognitive, affective, spiritual, or social needs or concerns of the client.

The nursing care plan is written when goals are formulated, priorities are set, and the ways to meeting goals are determined. The *nursing care plan is a brief introduction to the client, a record summarizing information obtained from assessment that is required to implement appropriate nursing care and to meet specific goals for the person, family, group, or community at a given time.* The written plan includes: (1) the client's needs, problems, values, attitudes, and feelings, (2) client-care goals and priority in reaching them, (3) *nursing orders, or the approaches of action that have been selected from the available alternatives,* (4) care measures prescribed by the physician, (5) general measures determined by the person's situation or agency policy, (6) expected behavioral outcomes, and (7) evaluative criteria to measure actions. The plan is a blueprint for action (41).

Purposes of the care plan include: to carry information; to establish care priorities that incorporate the client's perception of personal needs; to promote care that is individualized, comprehensive, coordinated, and shows continuity; and to facilitate ongoing and accurate evaluation of care (16).

The care plan is begun when the client comes for help; it must be updated as more information is obtained or as the health status or situation changes. The nurse who first contacts the person is usually responsible for beginning a care plan. Thereafter, all nursing personnel should be encouraged to write observations and care suggestions on the plan (16).

The nursing care plan may be used for a long period of time in the mental health clinic, residential center, or extended care facility. In hospital stays, which are frequently limited in duration, the nursing care plan is used for short-term care intervals and should become a permanent part of the client's record so that it is available for understanding the person on future admissions and for further care planning. Additionally, a copy of the care plan should be sent with the client upon transfer or referral to another agency.

Intervention

Intervention refers to all of the actions that you engage in, as well as the therapeutic approach you use, to promote the client's well-being (86). According to the definition of nursing given earlier, intervention includes verbal and nonverbal communication, visible actions, and your approach and reactions to the person as you promote or maintain biopsychosocial health and comfort, protect and enhance the client's stability, or aid recovery of the person. Intervention occurs when you prevent harm or further dysfunction or assist the client to function as effectively as possible. Many tasks done unwittingly are nursing interventions and should be defined as such to the client. The scientific rationale for doing nursing activity should also be explained to the client when pertinent.

Fay Bower classifies intervention into three nursing actions: supportive, generative, and protective (16). *Supportive nursing actions provide comfort, treatment, and restoration. These measures augment or maximize present strengths and adaptive capacity, enhance coping with stress, prevent additional health problems, and provide guidance, encouragement, or relief to enable the person to regain health. Generative nursing actions are innovative and rehabilitative. They encourage development of different approaches to coping with stress or crisis* and are especially used when assisting another with struggles involved in role changes or identity crisis. *Protective nursing actions are measures that promote health and prevent disease, improve or correct situations, or prevent complications and disease sequelae.* Examples include health teaching about drug therapy, anticipatory guidance, or reminiscence group therapy.

Since the nursing process is a problem-solving method, your nursing actions should be considered as hypotheses to be tested in practice. When the actions are demonstrated to be effective and can be validated as the best way to meet needs, they become part of the ongoing individualized nursing care plan.

Interdependent and Independent Interventions

Nursing care can be divided into interdependent and independent functions (74). The *interdependent area* of psychiatric-mental health nursing *refers to nursing care associated with a physician's prescriptions (orders for patient care):* administering medications and treatments and performing related care. These tasks comprise nursing responsibilities that are expected for patient safety and comfort and will not be specifically ordered. For example, observation of drug side effects and toxicity and prevention of their results (such as falls because of postural hypotension) are implicit in the medication order (74).

Independent areas of psychiatric-mental health nursing *are generally covered under the nursing process* (74).

Independent interventions that do not need a doctor's order and foster humanistic care include the following:

1. Reducing stressors, if possible, and reducing anxiety by being supportive and available, while recognizing that some stress and anxiety are necessary for survival, learning, emotional development, and self-actualization.

2. Establishing, maintaining, and terminating a therapeutic relationship with a person, family, or group.

3. Listening and maintaining communication. For example, help client work through feelings of anger, depression, suspicion, denial, and overcome the resulting behaviors; help client gain a sense of control and understanding over a situation, engage in problem solving, and move to appropriate goals; or foster reminiscing in the elderly.

4. Maintaining sensory stimulation to avoid withdrawal, social isolation, or retreat into fantasy or unreality; or reducing excessive stimulation.

5. Establishing and maintaining a therapeutic milieu. For example, a safe, predictable, warm, caring, open emotional and spiritual climate; attractive and comfortable physical arrangements; constructive policies; flexible visiting hours and procedures for operating the unit; and harmonious staff relations all enhance self-concept and optimal behavioral function and contribute to the client's care and treatment plan.

6. Promoting reality by working with the clients on current problems of living.

7. Encouraging the person to participate in his/her own care to foster a sense of progress and accomplishment; attending to grooming and basic life functions when the person is unable to care for self.

8. Accepting and using the surrogate parent role, which may include helping the person with decisions or self-care activities and assuming certain responsibilities when the person has an energy or adaptive deficit.

9. Teaching about mental health practices in personal and family life, effects of feelings, effective coping skills, and adaptive, independent, effective behavioral functioning.

10. Encouraging the person to behave in a way that will elicit positive responses and reinforcement from others.

11. Assuming role of socializing agent concerned with improvement and promotion of the client's social, recreational, and occupational competence.

12. Assisting with desensitization to or avoidance of factors that threaten security or adaptation.

13. Coordinating care of the client to avoid fragmentation and depersonalization and promoting continuity of care, including use of referrals.

14. Collaborating with the client in preparation for discharge and reintegration into community life.

15. Working with client and family to make changes in life style or home environment so that needs can be better met and frictions reduced.

16. Participating with other health workers and professionals in cooperative, collaborative efforts for joint planning and consistency of care.

17. Being an advocate for the client by helping other team members to understand the client's perspective about his life situation.

18. Collaborating with consumer groups and other health professionals, the community political structure, and community agencies and resources to develop the best possible mental health and psychiatric services and to bring about necessary changes in the health care system.

Spiritual needs of clients are often ignored because staff wish to avoid adding to delusions or neurotic behavior. Nurses become so involved in trying to meet psychological and socialization needs of patients that the importance of spiritual care is overlooked. A chaplain or the client's clergyman should be considered part of the treatment team. Nurses may also assume direct responsibility for spiritual care. The article by Verna Carsen describes the method and effectiveness of group prayer meetings (21).

Independent nursing functions are fostered in a setting that uses primary nursing care as the organizational plan for delivering nursing care (28, 40) but can also be seen in team nursing.

Direct and Indirect Interventions

Nursing functions can also be divided into direct and indirect measures (74). *Direct nursing care includes individual psychotherapy, group therapy, family therapy, and sociotherapy. Therapy* in the broadest sense *refers to any behavior or planned activity that promotes growth and well-being.* Individual psychotherapy is done within the context of the nurse-client relationship. Group therapy may be done along or with a nurse or another professional as cotherapist. Group therapy may involve any of the levels of activity or kinds of therapy described in Chapter 11 and may be carried out either as a dependent or independent function. Sociotherapy is usually done in collaboration with others and may include responsibilities related to milieu therapy and socializing of the client, through teaching of basic living and social skills, recreation, drama, dance, or other art forms. Sociotherapy may also include participation with the client in prevention or rehabilitation measures in the home, community, church, school, job, or the long-term residential or corrective institution.

Working with the family is essential for maintaining mental health of the individual, as well as the family unit. You may or may not do formal therapy with the family, but your support and teaching will be important. Family members often have basic needs that are overlooked. Even though the family members may sometimes seem to contribute to the person's illness, they deserve the same consideration as the individual client. They should not be treated as infants, as incompetent, or with disdain. Family members also need to be comforted emotionally, and sometimes physically, when they are feeling anxious, guilty, or worried. They need to be informed as fully as possible about the situation and expected results of the treatment and care. Family members also need encouragement and support as they encounter the stress of illness in the loved one and work to restore and maintain his/her well-being and prevent further complications in the person (52). Your work with the family will sometimes consist of being firm and of being an advocate for the client as you help the family recognize how they contribute to the client's illness. For example, the client may maintain an identity and emotional health only if he/she is able to live independently from the rest of the family. Chapter 10 gives additional information about working with the family.

Indirect nursing roles refer to the administrative/leadership roles and functions; clinical teaching of other personnel, students, or various community groups; consultation with other services, agencies, or professionals; and participation in research. You may be involved in direct nursing care while in any of these indirect roles and may serve as a role model to others.

Roles in Nursing Intervention

Nursing roles have changed with the emerging and expanding nature of the profession. Bonnie Bullough (18) and Marion Kalkman and Ann Davis (63) give a history of role expansion and describe a number of factors that have been influential in these emerging roles. As a psychiatric/mental health nurse, you may carry out any of the following roles:

1. General practitioner, with a number of clients, in a variety of settings.
2. Clinical specialist (nurse clinician).
3. Primary therapist.
4. Client educator.
5. Manager or coordinator of care, including maintaining a therapeutic milieu.
6. Collaborator with, leader of, or referral source to health team.
7. Role model for client and health team.
8. Change agent.
9. Client advocate.
10. Researcher.
11. Consultant to or liaison nurse with nurses and health team members from other specialty areas.
12. Health planner.

However, in your assumption of nursing role, do not become so objective, specialized or set in a role that you lose your ability to be flexible and to give humanistic care (103).

As a *practicing nurse,* you may work with hospitalized or nonhospitalized clients in a variety of settings. You will implement the direct and dependent nursing interventions as well as some of the indirect and independent interventions. How you will practice may be dictated by the agency, unless you are an active spokesman for carrying out any of the roles that are discussed here. However, the practitioner must always strive to carry out the nursing process, to provide humanistic, individualized care. You will be responsible for predicting the client's behavior, often based on subtle clues, and preventing destructive behavior. You will be expected to do more than just react to behavior. In your nursing practice, you may use a contract with your client (64, 132).

A *contract is an explicit mutual agreement between you and the client that defines the nature of your relationship, your mutual expectations, the different but equal responsibilities toward a common goal(s), and accountability for the outcome.* The contract can be verbal or written, but it should be part of the approach to all clients. Terms in the contract include appointment time and place, or the specific care activities and their timing that are involved for the hospitalized person. Tentative duration of treatment, specific contributions of other professionals, and fees, if any, are included in the contract. The contract should be evaluated periodically by nurse and client to be sure each is meeting the contract terms and goals, and the terms should be changed when alterations are necessary. If an aspect of a contract is broken by the client, do not become judgmental. Renegotiate the terms.

Implicit in the contract is that the client is essentially in charge of his/her personal life and usually able to make decisions, that both parties have rights and responsibilities, and that they will work together toward a goal. If the contract is written, both client and counselor sign it and retain a copy. Receiving help on a contractual basis has the following effects:

1. Clarifies short-term and long-term goals.
2. Avoids rescuer-victim or superordinate-subordinate roles and promotes collaboration between nurse and client.
3. Enhances self-mastery and social skills of client.
4. Facilitates emotional development of client.
5. Decreases chance of failure in helping client.
6. Prepares the client better for discharge.

A contract should not be used to manipulate a client, even if you feel your idea is best.

Some psychiatric nurses feel a contract with a client is similar to a business arrangement and is not appropriate to an affective relationship. Others feel a contract should be used with certain clients and not others. For example, you would not use a contract to structure a highly organized routine with an obsessive, rigid person who is striving for flexibility, but you would use a contract with an immature, disorganized person to assist with goal setting. A contract cannot be negotiated if the person is psychotic, highly anxious, in panic, or cognitively impaired. However, when you work with any of these people, you can perceive the situation as contractual on your part. Then a verbal, or written, contract can be developed when the person is able to understand, since such a client would need care for some time. For further information on contracting, refer to the article by Mary-Eve Zangarie and Patricia Duffy (132).

Clinical Specialist

The clinical specialist is a nurse with a master's degree in psychiatric/mental health nursing, is expert in providing client care, and demonstrates authoritative nursing on the basis of knowledge and expert skills. This nurse selects a caseload, works with managers and staff, and functions as an educator and role model for the staff. The clinical specialist is the key to moving nursing from intuitive, traditional, and authority-based practice to one that can be supported by theory and research. This role calls for skill in teaching, in supervision, and in research, as well as an ability to deal with organizational politics (13, 69, 78). Beverly Benfer gives some practical suggestions for fulfilling the clinical specialist role and working with other professionals in the health care agency (13).

Nurse Therapist

The nurse therapist has at least graduate preparation in psychiatric/mental health nursing and has developed skills, under supervision, in individual, group and/or family therapy. The nurse therapist will practice in the manner described in Chapters 2, 5, 6, and 8, as well as implement measures described in the other chapters. Being a therapist in an agency is analogous to primary nursing in other settings (27). The nurse therapist may also be in private practice (2, 82).

Client Education

Client education is an important part of nursing care. Often nurses in hospitals cite various reasons for not doing client education, including lack of time to teach, uncertainty about specifics to teach, and difficulty teaching at the person's level of understanding (72). Frequently psychiatric clients are considered more difficult to teach than medical, surgical, or obstetrical clients. Yet psychiatric clients also have a right to know what is being done to them and why; they have a right to be taught about emotional or physical illness, effective behavior, and self-care on a level they can understand. Often teaching is neglected because teaching materials are not available in the agency or are not organized to be easily used by the nurse or client (72). There may also be a lack of an organized system for family and client teaching and discharge planning on the psychiatric unit. Standardized printed material or audiovisual media may be useful for the psychiatric client, but because of individual perceptions or confusions, the more humanistic way to teach will probably be through personal contact and face-to-face sessions (84). Further, the person may not be able to read. An interpersonal relationship is also a better way than printed material to teach about improving interpersonal skills. You can use printed materials and audiovisual materials in teaching, but do so in conjunction with the interpersonal relationship.

Some other guidelines are useful for teaching the client and family and are presented in Table 4-4. Refer also to the theorists in Chapter 2.

TABLE 4-4.   Principles of Teaching in Emotional Care

GENERAL APPROACH

1. Convey respect; be genuine.
2. Reduce social distance between self and other as much as possible.
3. Promote sense of trust and an open interaction; a trusting relationship fosters self-understanding and motivation to follow a teaching plan.
4. Elicit description of feelings from the client about the subject matter or situation in order to relieve tension.
5. Be organized in presentation.
6. Use a comfortable setting and audiovisual aids as indicated.
7. Encourage questions, disagreement, and comments to ensure that your presentation stays focused on client needs.
8. Encourage, support, and reinforce as you present content.

TEACHING SPECIFIC CONTENT

1. Begin at knowledge level of client.
2. Determine what client wants to know and already knows.
3. Answer the client's questions first; the client will then be more receptive to the information presented.
4. Build on what the client knows. Gently refute myths or misunderstandings.
5. Relate information to behavior patterns, life style, and sociocultural background to increase likelihood of being followed by the client.
6. Assist client in reworking your ideas to fit cultural, religious, or family values and customs to ensure that the material to be learned will be practiced.
7. Be logical in sequence of content.
8. Present more basic or simpler content prior to more advanced or complex information.
9. Present one idea, or a group of related ideas, at a time, rather than many diverse ideas together.

TABLE 4-4.   Continued

TEACHING SPECIFIC CONTENT

---

10. Demonstrate as you describe directions, suggestions, or ideas, if possible.
11. Break content into units and a series of sessions, if necessary. Do not present too many ideas at one time.
12. Teach the family as thoroughly as the client to ensure that suggestions on interpersonal relationships and other concerns will be followed.
13. Present the same information to friends, employer, occupational health nurse, school-teacher, clergyman, or significant community leader, if possible.

EVALUATION OF TEACHING

---

1. Check frequently to determine if content is of interest or being understood.
2. Have client repeat content or give examples of application of content.
3. Have client review previously covered content, and its application, at each teaching session.
4. Determine the amount of learning that has occurred.

As a teacher, be aware of the importance of your behavior as a model for the client (9, 49). Often the client is in an unfamiliar situation or is unsure of what to do. Watching and imitating others are done to define the situation and determine what is normal and expected. Because modeling effects are strongest in ambiguous situations where people do not know what to expect, (9) your response to a client upon admission to the hospital or initial contact in the home or clinic will have a more powerful impact than your later behavior. Opportunities to teach about self-care or effective behavior will be greatest when the client feels uncertain about solutions. Sometimes you will teach best when you think out loud while helping a client solve problems. Then the client learns how to arrive at an answer, how to think things through. One of the most helpful things you can teach another is how to develop effective problem-solving strategies (49).

You will also be a model in how to cope with stress as you interact with a difficult team member, handle an emergency situation, or handle broken equipment. Do not underestimate how much you are watched by the client. Your nonverbal behavior in a situation or your verbal response to colleagues may undermine all of your previous excellent suggestions to a client.

Socialization also occurs through modeling (9). Often the psychiatric client lacks basic social interaction skills. Your interactions with him/her show how to converse socially, how to treat others respectfully and kindly, how to listen, how to follow rules and maintain inner control, and how to express feelings in an acceptable way. Your socially appropriate behavior can be a norm for the client to follow, whether or not you want it to be. Just as the child follows the parent and must see ideal behavior patterns in order to develop them, so the client must see some credible, ideal and healthy behavior in the nurse to use as a guide. Your verbal and nonverbal behavior are models for the client, and they must be consistent with each other to avoid confusion or frustration. What you say about and to others in front of your client can either build or interfere with the client's sense of trust and his/her respect and positive feelings toward self, you and others. Modeling and reinforcing sociable behavior can help the client enhance interpersonal skills.

Manager or Coordinator

The manager or coordinator of care may work less directly with clients, but he or she is responsible for maintaining an environment that is accepting, calm, facilitative of a positive self-concept and movement toward self-actualization, and conducive to self-discovery—for both clients and staff. One study showed that maintaining a therapeutic milieu was valued by patients often more than other nursing interventions, and that the psychologic climate of the agency has a predictable effect on the person (71). The nursing milieu can have a healing effect. The nurse is the expert in the constructive use of environment for the client, from admission through the postdischarge period. *In the therapeutic milieu or community, the nurse has the responsibility to:*

Represent cultural norms.

Set limits constructively.

Prevent antisocial or destructive elements from affecting clients or staff.

Offer friendliness, security, stability, and individual attention to each client.

Act as clarifier and interpreter when the client experiences difficulty.

Collaborate with other team members to promote policies and procedures that help each client achieve his/her maximum potential.

As manager of the milieu, the nurse should be represented on all agency committees, including planning committees for building or remodeling a unit.

Bernard Kutner describes factors to consider in the therapeutic milieu for a disabled person (68). Although the physically disabled person may have to learn some new physical skills for home and job, milieu therapy for both emotionally and physically disabled people involves helping the person gain new roles and skills, readapt old ones, and develop social skills necessary to enter and manage the roles. Managing care also involves working closely with staff to ensure that all nursing care, and diagnostic and treatment measures are accomplished. The nurse is typically responsible for coordinating the multitude of activities associated with the client's total treatment plan.

Collaborator, Leader, and Referral Source

Collaborator, leader, and referral source are interrelated aspects of working with the health team. Most psychiatric, as well as other health-care settings, use a multidisciplinary team approach; you must be an expert in clinical nursing as well as in coordinating care and collaborating with others. You will have opportunity to work with occupational, music, recreational, art, and psychodrama therapists. Collaboration is enhanced when you understand the contributions of these therapists. The role of the occupational therapist is described by Wilma West (128). Music therapy for clients is described by Stacie Beavers (11), E. T. Gasten (45), and Sylvia Parriott (98). Recreational therapy is discussed by E. Aveden (7), Thomas Collingwood (33), Valerie Hunt (55), and G. O'Morrow (93). Art as therapy is described by Sadie Dreikurs (37). The use of psychodrama is explained by M. Goldberg (48). Role blurring or diffusion occurs between the psychiatric nurse specialist, social worker, psychologist, psychiatrist, and mental health technician since all of these team members claim to engage in counseling and in establishing a relationship with the client. However, as a nurse, you maintain a holistic view of the patient, over the 24-hour day, and a flexibility in approach that is often not seen in the other team members. Therefore, in this role, you must have a clear concept of psychodynamics, a firm understanding of your unique contribution to client care, and be able to assertively interpret your role and its interface with other professionals' roles to other workers as well as to the client. Often the nurse is seen by other professionals only in the dependent role, primarily in medication administration and related responsibilities. Unless you can clearly explain other nursing roles and responsibilities, there is a danger that the client will not receive the benefits of the full realm of nursing care—because other professionals tend to exclude the nurse from the independent areas of function. Thus, the nurse must cooperate and collaborate with other team members. Sometimes the nurse's suggestions will be followed or adapted, and the committed professional nurse is a model for holistic, humane, individualized care.

The nurse must also know how and when to make a *referral*. The following guidelines will be useful:

1. Know the available community resources and the services offered.
2. Recognize when you are unable to further assist or work with the client; be honest about your own limits and your perceived need for a referral. Avoid implying rejection of the client.
3. Explore client readiness for referral. The client may also have ideas about referrals and sources of help.
4. Determine what other professionals had contact with the client and confer with them about the possibility of referral.
5. Discuss the possibility of referral with a specific person at the selected agency prior to referral.
6. If the client is a minor, inform parents of your recommendations and obtain their consent and cooperation.
7. Be honest in explaining services of the referral agency. Do not make false promises about another agency's services or roles.
8. Describe specifics about location, how to get to the referral place/person, where to park and enter, and what to expect upon arrival.
9. Have the client (or parent) make the initial appointment for the new service, but tell the person that you have called the agency and that he/she is expected.
10. Do not release information to the referral agency or person without written permission from the client (or parent).
11. Request the client to give you feedback about the referral agency/person to help you evaluate your decision and to help you make a satisfactory referral selection if needed for future needy individuals or families.

Change Agent

The change agent is another important nursing role. Chapter 7 discusses the change process and what must be considered when you initiate change. Be assertive in getting your ideas put into action.

Client Advocate

Client advocate is one of the newer roles in nursing. This role is complex and often incorporates the roles of consultant and health planner. Chapter 24 discusses advocacy and its meaning for nursing, nurse, and client.

Investigation or Research

The investigative or research role of the nurse is also quite new. Research is the method of inquiry characteristic of science. In nursing, the emergence of nursing theory, nursing as a profession, and nursing research go hand in hand. Essential characteristics of a researcher are to keep an open mind to the inconsistencies of practice, be willing to ask questions that others ignore, and look at the usual situation in a creative way. Without these characteristics, even expert knowledge of the research process will result in little nursing research (42). The ethical and legal aspects of research must also be considered (75).

Consultant

The role of consultant (1, 83) is often combined with those of clinical specialist, nurse therapist, client educator, change agent, and researcher. Chapter 26 discusses important considerations in the consultant role.

Health Planner

The role of health planner (81) is not seen as part of nursing by some nurses, but if we are to make lasting improvements in health care services, the nurse must be among the people who help to establish and implement broad policies. The holistic view of the client, commitment to the unique individual, and the caring attitude that are an integral part of nursing may be foreign to the politician, legislator, and administrator. Without the persistent voice of the nurse, the values that we hold dear in nursing care will be legislated out of existence as efficiency, economy, and bureaucracy take over.

Evaluation

Evaluation is the purposeful examination and use of measurement data, devices, and methods to determine effectiveness of nursing actions and your approach toward achieving short-term and long-term client-care goals, as well as to determine the problems that have been resolved, those that are still unresolved, and any new ones that have arisen. It is the last step of the nursing process, but it cannot be separated from assessment, formulating a nurs-

ing diagnosis, determining objectives and planning care, and intervention (88). Evaluation and reassessment go together.

Evaluation first includes predicting outcomes through long-term and short-term goals. These outcomes are expressed in terms of anticipated responses—responses that result from nursing intervention and that indicate progress in achieving emotional health. Statements of goals help you not only to determine specific interventions to use but also to predict the specific client behaviors that would indicate that these goals have been achieved. When a predicted outcome is reached, a new goal corresponding to progress in status is written.

Goals are based on priorities of care, establish the criteria for evaluation, and must be observable either to the client or to the nurse, so that the cause of unexpected outcomes can be determined and further negative effects can be avoided.

Evaluation should be continuous during care so that insights gained can be used to reassess the person, modify plans, and improve care throughout the nursing process. Evaluation benefits both client and nurse at the end of the nursing process because it provides a final statement about progress that was made by the client and is a critical examination of nursing practice. Areas to scrutinize before or at discharge include: The use of knowledge in practice, accuracy of assessment and diagnosis, effectiveness of intervention on client outcome, consistency of approach, success of communication, and cooperation of other health team members (92).

Evaluation of care is directly related to **accountability,** *the state of being responsible for your actions and being able to explain, define, or measure the results of your decision making.* Accountability involves measuring your effectiveness against a set of criteria—the agency's policies, the unit's general care standards, the Standards of Nursing Practice, and the client's care objectives. Accountability involves validating intangibles, such as attitudes and subtle nuances, as well as overt care measures. You are accountable to the person/family/group, agency, doctor, other health team members, and the community. Your accountability assures optimum health care delivery (122).

STANDARDS OF PRACTICE FOR PSYCHIATRIC/MENTAL HEALTH NURSING

The Standards of Psychiatric Nursing Practice were developed by the American Nurses Association to provide guidelines for the nurse, to improve nursing practice, and to provide a means of evaluating quality of client care. The Standards expand on the nursing process and are summarized in the following list (4):

1. Collect data through observations based on knowledge, analyze and interpret data, and make inferences from the data to be used in care planning and treatment.

2. Involve client in the nursing process to the fullest extent possible.

3. Develop the nursing care plan, using the problem-solving approach.

4. Do health teaching to individuals, families, and groups to promote satisfying and productive living patterns.

5. Utilize activities of daily living as a basis for intervention to: provide comfort and care, reinforce client strengths, encourage constructive behavioral changes, engage in health teaching, and ensure consistency and continuity of care.

6. Carry out somatic treatments, as ordered, and related nursing responsibilities.

7. Establish and maintain a therapeutic milieu to serve the best interests of the client in the treatment setting.

8. Participate with interdisciplinary teams to provide the best possible care.

9. Utilize psychotherapeutic interventions to assist clients to achieve their maximum development.

10. Be adequately prepared and accountable for the practice of psychotherapy with an individual, family, or group.

11. Consult, cooperate, and collaborate with community groups and agencies, including legislative bodies and regional and state planning groups, to promote mental health, prevent mental illness, and provide treatment and rehabilitation services in a broad sense and throughout the community.

12. Provide learning experiences for other nursing personnel by being a role model, leader, teacher, and supervisor.

13. Assume responsibility for personal continued educational and professional development and for the professional development of others.

14. Contribute to nursing and mental health through innovative practice and development of theory through research.

A copy of the Standards can be obtained from the American Nurses' Association, 2420 Pershing Road, Kansas City, Missouri, 64108.

A PHILOSOPHY OF NURSING

As a nurse, you are in a special position to think about the meaning and sequence of life as you care for the person/family/group—ill or well. Your philosophy of nursing should be the foundation for your use of nursing theory and knowledge and skill in nursing practice. Often nurses prefer to avoid thinking about philosophy. Now that you have a general perspective on the nursing process as the method for giving care, consideration of the guiding principles about people and health care is essential. You may want to return to a study of various philosophers, such as Sidney Jourard (61) or Rollo May (77), or review Table 4-2 in this chapter in order to help you clarify your own philosophy of care. You may also want to read what other nursing authors have written about their philosophy. Authors who will provide helpful insights include Lynn Bernstein (14), Sister Madeleine Clemence (30), Donna Diers and David Evans (36), Sarah Fuller (44), and Elaine LaMonica (70).

The following paragraphs reflect the basic beliefs of the authors of this text about nursing and emotional care for the person/family/group and community population. We adhere principally to ideas presented by the Third Force theorists.

Life is a movement, a changing and growing process. You, the nurse, as a living being, constantly undergo change. The health care system in which you work is changing, and your roles are affected by these changes. The people you care for are also changing; they are maturing as unique individuals. They are not just a conglomerate mass isolated by an age bracket or a kind of illness. Each person has unique potential, abilities, needs, desires, and feelings. Each has the potential to make decisions pertinent to the self. The emotionally ill person with his/her individual perceptions and potential for change and further development is intrinsically valuable. Each person is unique and different, yet similar to yourself in basic needs. The client continues to adapt to a changing self and changing life situation. He/she maintains a faith in something or someone greater than self and uses inner strengths as well as relationships with others to maximize potential. Behavior falls on a continuum from wellness to illness to dying, and the client attempts to remain responsible to self, others, and the environment as long as possible.

You, the nurse, functioning as an individual citizen and as a professional health worker, can add much to the dimension of the client's life through humanistic nursing. You see the human aspect of each person and that the person has the capacity to give meaning to experience. You look at the situation from the person's viewpoint as well as from your own. You are significant to the well-being and ongoing development and maturity of the client by demonstrating a humanistic concern for the whole person; by being nurturing, compassionate, empathic, courteous, authentic, and nonpossessive in your behavior; and by treating the person with dignity. What you are and what you do are significant to those in your care. You enter into a partnership with the client, a partnership that is based on trust and mutual respect. You assure the person that his/her rights will be honored, that appropriate information will be shared, that choices will be encouraged, and that he/she can contribute to the individualized, not standardized, care plan. You are responsible for the overall welfare of the person to whom you give service, and in this commitment, the client's needs have priority over your own needs, and over institutional traditions or the doctor's standard orders. You are responsible for personalizing care while you work with the client to gain more positive feelings about self and others and to move toward health through goal-directed care. Your caring fosters a sense of self-worth and release from emotional pain. Your expressions of concern, support, caring, empathy, and love can provide a transfer of energy from one person to another. Accepting, caring, and loving cannot be expressed in behavioristic objectives or efficient outcomes, or be easily measured or quantified, but we cannot deny the existence of their qualities or their impact on lives. (Perhaps we can measure their effects with a thoughtfully designed research method.)

Nursing is a human and humane service that

encourages the person to meet his/her potential, not just a service directed toward humans who are considered as little more than machines. Nursing is *being* with another, *not* just *doing* for another. Nursing should keep the nurse human and humane, as well as enhance the humanity of others.

Giving the kind of high-level care just described is possible if you are aware of your own values, biases, and beliefs, and if you base your nursing practice on a belief system. Thus, your knowledge of the nursing process, your methods of practice, and your awareness of the philosophy underlying your actions must be combined with knowledge of the client. Then your nursing will be a practice of excellence, with a sense of humility, caring, discipline, perseverance, responsibility, and commitment toward the client along with appropriate enthusiasm and skepticism about the profession (36).

REFERENCES

1. Adamson, Frances, "A Mental Health Consultant At Work," *American Journal of Nursing,* 70, no. 10 (1970), 2164–66.

2. Alford, Dolores, and Janet Jansen, "Reflections on Private Practice," *American Journal of Nursing,* 76, no. 12 (1976), 1966–68.

3. Allmond, B. W., "Psychological Testing of Children: Review and Commentary," *Pediatric Clinics of North America,* 21 (1974), 187–94.

4. *American Nurses Association Standards of Psychiatric and Mental Health Nursing Practice.* Kansas City, Mo: American Nurses Association, 1973.

5. Anderson, Marcia, "A Psychosocial Screening Tool for Ambulatory Health Care Clients," *Nursing Research,* 29, no. 6 (1980), 347–51.

6. Auger, J., *Behavioral Systems and Nursing.* Englewood Cliffs, N.J.: Prentice-Hall, Inc., 1976.

7. Aveden, E., "The Function of Recreation Service in the Rehabilitation Process," *Rehabilitation Literature,* 27, no. 8 (1966), 226–29.

8. Baer, E., McGowan, M., and McGivern, D., "How to Take a Health History," *American Journal of Nursing,* 77, no. 7 (1977), 1190–93.

9. Bandura, Albert, *Social Learning Theory.* Morristown, N.J.: General Learning Press, 1971.

10. Bates, Barbara, *A Guide to Physical Examination.* Philadelphia: J. B. Lippincott Company, 1974.

11. Beavers, Stacie, "Music Therapy," *American Journal of Nursing,* 69, no. 1 (1969), 89–92.

12. Beland, Irene, and Joyce Passos, *Clinical Nursing: Pathophysiological and Psychosocial Approaches,* 3rd ed. New York: Macmillan Publishing Co., Inc., 1975.

13. Benfer, Beverly, "Defining the Role and Function of the Psychiatric Nurse as a Member of the Team," *Perspectives in Psychiatric Care,* 18, no. 4 (1980), 166–77.

14. Bernstein, Lynn, "The Psychiatric Patient as a Human Being: A Philosophy of Care," *Free Association,* 5, no. 4 (1978), 3.

15. Blake, Mary, "The Peplau Developmental Model for Nursing Practice," in *Conceptual Models for Nursing Practice*, 2nd ed., eds. Joan Riehl and Sister Callista Roy, pp. 53–59. New York: Appleton-Century-Crofts, 1980.

16. Bower, Fay, *The Process of Planning Nursing Care: A Theoretical Model.* St. Louis: The C. V. Mosby Company, 1972.

17. Brodt, Dagmar, "The Synergistic Theory of Nursing," *American Journal of Nursing,* 69, no. 8 (1969), 1674–76.

18. Bullough, Bonnie, "Influences in Role Expansion," *American Journal of Nursing,* 76, no. 9 (1976), 1476–81.

19. Burgess, Ann, *Nursing: Levels of Health Intervention.* Englewood Cliffs, N.J.: Prentice-Hall, Inc., 1978.

20. Campbell, Claire, *Nursing Diagnosis and Intervention in Nursing Practice.* New York: John Wiley & Sons, Inc., 1978.

21. Carsen, Verna, "Meeting the Spiritual Needs of Hospitalized Psychiatric Patients," *Perspectives in Psychiatric Care,* 18, no. 1 (1980), 17–20.

22. Carter, Susan, "The Nurse Educator: Humanist or Behaviorist?" *Nursing Outlook,* 26, no. 9 (1978), 554–57.

23. Chrisman, Marilyn, and Marsha Fowler, "The Systems in Change Model for Nursing Practice," in *Conceptual Models for Nursing Practice,* 2nd ed., eds. Joan Riehl and Sister Callista Roy, pp. 74–102. New York: Appleton-Century-Crofts, 1980.

24. Christman, Luther, "Accountability and Autonomy Are More than Rhetoric," *Nurse Educator,* 3, no. 4 (1978), 3–6.

25. Church, Olga, and Kathleen Buckwalter, "Harriet

Bailey: A Psychiatric Nurse Pioneer," *Perspectives in Psychiatric Care,* 18, no. 2 (1980), 62–66.

26. Ciske, Karen, "Primary Nursing: An Organization That Promotes Professional Practice," *Journal of Nursing Administration,* 4, no. 1 (1974), 28–31.

27. —, "Accountability—The Essence of Primary Nursing," *American Journal of Nursing,* 79, no. 5 (1979), 890–94.

28. Ciske, Karen, and Gloria Mayer, eds., *Primary Nursing.* Wakefield, Mass.: Nursing Resources/Concept Development, Inc., 1980.

29. Clark, Deborah, and Kathleen Long, "Nurses as Health Educators with Emotionally Disturbed Children," *Perspectives in Psychiatric Care,* 17, no. 4 (1979), 167–73.

30. Clemence, Sister Madeleine, "Existentialism: A Philosophy of Commitment," *American Journal of Nursing,* 66, no. 3 (1966), 500–505.

31. Coleman, J. M., "The Draw-a-Man Test as a Predictor of School Readiness and as an Index of Emotional and Physical Maturity," *Pediatrics,* 24 (1959), 275–81.

32. Coleman, Leatrice, "Orem's Self-Care Concept of Nursing," in *Conceptual Models for Nursing Practice,* 2nd ed., eds. Joan Riehl and Sister Callista Roy, pp. 315–28. New York: Appleton-Century-Crofts, 1980.

33. Collingwood, Thomas, "The Effects of Physical Training upon Self-Concept and Body Attitude," *Journal of Clinical Psychology,* 27, no. 3 (1971), 411–12.

34. Critchley, Diane, "Mental Status Examinations with Children and Adolescents," *Nursing Clinics of North America,* 14, no. 3 (1979), 429–41.

35. Curtis, Joy, Marilyn Rothbert, and Bernice Christian, "A Practical Evaluation of Nursing Care as Part of the Nursing Process," *Nursing Digest,* 3, no. 3 (1975), 20–21.

36. Diers, Donna, and David Evans, "Excellence in Nursing," *Image,* 12, no. 2 (1980), 27–30.

37. Dreikurs, Sadie, "Art Therapy for Psychiatric Patients," *Perspectives in Psychiatric Care,* 7, no. 3 (1969), 102–3, 134–43.

38. Eggland, E. T., "How to Take a Meaningful Nursing History," *Nursing '77,* 7, no. 7 (1977), 22–30.

39. Evans, Frances Monet Carter, *The Role of the Nurse in Community Mental Health.* New York: Macmillan Publishing Co., Inc., 1968.

40. Felton, G., "Increasing the Quality of Nursing Care by Introducing the Concept of Primary Nursing: A Model Project," *Nursing Research,* 24, no. 1 (1975), 27–32.

41. Forman, Mary, "Building a Better Nursing Care Plan," *American Journal of Nursing,* 79, no. 6 (1979), 1086–87

42. Fox, David, and Ilse Lesser, *Readings on the Research Process in Nursing.* New York: Appleton-Century-Crofts, 1981.

43. Frankenberg, W., A. Goldstein, and B. Camp, "The Revised Denver Developmental Screening Test: Its Accuracy as a Screening Instrument," *Journal of Pediatrics,* 79 (1971), 988–95.

44. Fuller, Sarah, "Holistic Man and the Science and Practice of Nursing," *Nursing Outlook,* 26, no. 11 (1978), 700–704.

45. Gasten, E. Thayer, *Music in Therapy.* New York: Macmillan Publishing Co., Inc., 1968.

46. Gebbie, Kristine, ed., *Proceedings of the Third National Conference on the Classification of Nursing Diagnosis.* Wakefield, Mass.: Contemporary Publishing, 1980.

47. Gebbie, Kristine, and Mary Lavin, eds., *Classification of Nursing Diagnosis.* St. Louis: The C. V. Mosby Company, 1975.

48. Goldberg, Merle, "The Theory and Practice of Psychodrama," *Canada's Mental Health,* 22, nos. 1-2 (1974), 13–16.

49. Good, Thomas, and Jeri Brophy, *Looking in Classrooms,* pp. 119–45. New York: Harper & Row, Publishers, Inc., 1973.

50. Gordon, M., "Nursing Diagnosis and the Diagnostic Process," *American Journal of Nursing,* 76, no. 8 (1976), 1298–1300.

51. Grubbs, Judy, "The Johnson Behavioral System Model for Nursing Practice," in *Conceptual Models for Nursing Practice,* 2nd ed., eds. Joan Riehl and Sister Callista Roy, pp. 217–54. New York: Appleton-Century-Crofts, 1980.

52. Guralnik, David, ed., *Webster's New World Dictionary of the American Language,* 2nd College Ed. New York: William Collins and World Publishing Co., Inc., 1972.

53. Heagarty, J. R., "Psychological Assessment of the Mentally Handicapped: Part V. The Psychologist, His Tests, and the Nurse," *Nursing Mirror,* 143, no. 25 (December 16, 1976), 59–60.

54. Heagarty, Margaret et al., *Child Health: Basics for Primary Care.* New York: Appleton-Century-Crofts, 1980.

55. Hunt, Valerie, *Recreation for the Handicapped.* Englewood Cliffs, N.J.: Prentice-Hall, Inc., 1955.

56. Jacobs, Charles, Tom Christoffel, and Nancy Dixon,

Measuring the Quality of Patient Care: The Rationale for Outcome Audit. Cambridge, Mass.: Ballinger Publishing Co., 1976.

57. Johnson, Donald, *Psychology: A Problem-Solving Approach.* New York: Harper & Row, Publishers, Inc., 1961.

58. Johnson, Dorothy, "The Behavioral System Model for Nursing," in *Conceptual Models for Nursing Practice,* 2nd ed., eds. Joan Riehl and Sister Callista Roy, pp. 207-16. New York: Appleton-Century-Crofts, 1980.

59. Joint Commission on Mental Illness and Health, *Action for Mental Health, Final Report of the Joint Commission on Mental Illness and Health.* New York: Basic Books, Inc., 1961.

60. Joseph, Lynda, "Self-Care and the Nursing Process," *Nursing Clinics of North America,* 15, no. 1 (1980), 131-43.

61. Jourard, Sidney, *Disclosing Man to Himself.* New York: D. Van Nostrand Company, 1968.

62. Kalisch, P. A., and B. J. Kalisch, *The Advance of American Nursing.* Boston: Little, Brown & Company, 1978.

63. Kalkman, Marion, and Anne Davis, *New Dimensions in Mental Health—Psychiatric Nursing,* 4th ed. New York: McGraw-Hill Book Company, 1974.

64. Kavchak, Mary et al., "Motivating the Unmotivated Patient," *Nursing '74,* 4, no. 2 (1974), 31-36.

65. King, Imogene, "A Conceptual Frame of Reference for Nursing," *Nursing Research,* 17, no. 1 (1968), 27-31.

66. Kinlein, M. Lucille, "The Self-Care Concept," *American Journal of Nursing,* 77, no. 4 (1977), 598-601.

67. Kuntz, Sandra, Joan Stehle, and Ruth Marshall, "The Psychiatric Clinical Specialist: The Progression of a Specialty," *Perspectives in Psychiatric Care,* 18, no. 2 (1980), 90-92.

68. Kutner, Bernard, "Milieu Therapy," in *The Psychological and Social Impact of Physical Disability,* eds. Robert Marinelli and Arthur Dell Orto, pp. 334-41. New York: Springer Publishing Co., Inc., 1977.

69. Lamberton, Martha, "Adult Nurse Clinician on a Psychiatric Unit," *American Journal of Nursing,* 76, no. 12 (1976), 1961-63.

70. LaMonica, Elaine, *The Nursing Process: A Humanistic Approach.* Reading, Mass.: Addison-Wesley Publishing Co., Inc., 1979.

71. Leonard, Callista, "Patient Attitudes toward Nursing Interventions," *Nursing Research,* 24, no. 5 (1975), 335-39.

72. Letterman, Anita, and Joanne Gordon, "Improving Patient Education in a Small Community Hospital: A Packet System for Patient Teaching," *Missouri Nurse,* 49, no. 3 (1980), 4-6.

73. Little, D., and D. Carnevali, *Nursing Care Planning,* 2nd ed. Philadelphia: J. B. Lippincott Company, 1976.

74. Longo, Dianne, and Reg Arthur Williams, eds., *Clinical Practice in Psychosocial Nursing: Assessment and Intervention,* pp. 357-58. New York: Appleton-Century-Crofts, 1978.

75. MacKay, Ruth, and John Soule, "Nurses as Investigators: Some Ethical and Legal Issues," *Nursing Digest,* 5, no. 1 (1977), 7-9.

76. Marram, Gwen, Margaret Barrett, and Em Bevis, *Primary Nursing: A Model for Individualized Care,* 2nd ed. St. Louis: The C. V. Mosby Company, Inc., 1979.

77. May, Rollo, *Existential Psychology.* New York: Random House, Inc., 1960.

78. McCain, R. Faye, "Nursing by Assessment—Not Intuition," *American Journal of Nursing,* 65, no. 4 (1965), 82-84.

79. McDinagh, Mary Jo, Virginia Tribles, and Ann Crism, "Nurse Therapists in a State Psychiatric Hospital," *American Journal of Nursing,* 80, no. 1 (1980), 103-4.

80. McFarland, G. K., and F. E. Apostoles, "The Nursing History in a Psychiatric Setting: Adaptations for a Variety of Nursing Care Patterns and Patient Populations," *Journal of Psychiatric Nursing,* 13, no. 4 (1975), 12-17.

81. McLemore, Melinda, "Nurses as Health Planners: Our New Legal Status," *Nursing Digest,* 5, no. 1 (1977), 59-60.

82. McShane, Nancy, and Elizabeth Smith, "Starting a Private Practice in Mental Health Nursing," *American Journal of Nursing,* 78, no. 12 (1978), 2068-70.

83. Moore, Jean, "Community Mental Health Consultation in Police Court," *Perspectives in Psychiatric Care,* 18, no. 5 (1980), 204-9.

84. Moore, S. H. et al., "Effect of a Self-Care Book on Physician Visits: A Randomized Trial," *Journal of American Medical Association,* 243 (June 13, 1980), 2317-20.

85. Morgan, Arthur, and Judith Moreno, *The Practice of Mental Health Nursing: A Community Approach.* Philadelphia: J. B. Lippincott Company, 1973.

86. Mundinger, Mary, and Grace Jauron, "Developing a

Nursing Diagnosis," *Nursing Outlook,* 23, no. 2 (1975), 94–98.

87. Murphy, Donna, and Eleanor Chronopoulous, "What Is the Problem? How Long Have You Been Ill?" *American Journal of Nursing,* 79, no. 3 (1979), 505–6.

88. Murray, Ruth, Marilyn Huelskoetter, and Dorothy O'Driscoll, *The Nursing Process in Later Maturity.* Englewood Cliffs, N.J.: Prentice-Hall, Inc., 1980.

89. Murray, Ruth, and Judith Zentner, *Nursing Concepts for Health Promotion* 2nd ed. Englewood Cliffs, N.J.: Prentice-Hall, Inc., 1979.

90. Nelson, Jill, and Dianne Schilke, "The Evolution of Psychiatric Liaison Nursing," *Perspectives in Psychiatric Care,* 14, no. 2 (1976), 60–65.

91. Neuman, Betty, "The Betty Neuman Health-Care Systems Model: A Total Person Approach to Patient Problems," in *Conceptual Models for Nursing Practice,* 2nd ed., eds. Joan Riehl and Sister Callista Roy, pp. 119–34. New York: Appleton-Century-Crofts, 1980.

92. O'Driscoll, Dorothy, "The Nursing Process and Long-Term Care," *Journal of Gerontology Nursing,* 2, no. 3 (1976), 34–37.

93. O'Morrow, G., "Recreation Counseling: A Challenge to Rehabilitation," *Rehabilitation Literature,* 31, no. 8 (1970), 226–33.

94. Orem, Dorothea, *Nursing: Concepts of Practice.* New York: McGraw-Hill Book Company, 1971.

95. Orlando, Ida, *The Dynamic Nurse-Patient Relationship.* New York: McGraw-Hill Book Company, 1961.

96. ——, *The Discipline and Teaching of Nursing Process.* New York: G. P. Putnam's Sons, 1972.

97. Palmer, Irene, "Florence Nightingale: Reformer, Reactionary, Researcher," *Nursing Research,* 26, no. 2 (1977), 84–89.

98. Parriott, Sylvia, "Music as Therapy," *American Journal of Nursing,* 69, no. 8 (1969), 1723–26.

99. Partridge, Kay, "Nursing Values in a Changing Society," *Nursing Outlook,* 26, no. 6 (1978), 356–60.

100. Paterson, Josephine, and Loretta Zderad, *Humanistic Nursing.* New York: John Wiley & Sons, Inc., 1976.

101. Payne, Dorris, *Psychiatric Mental Health Nursing: Nursing Outline Series.* Flushing, N.Y.: Medical Examination Publishing Company, 1974.

102. Peplau, Hildegarde, *Interpersonal Relations in Nursing.* New York: G. P. Putnam's Sons, 1952.

103. Pilette, Patricia, "Caution: Objectivity and Specializa-

tion May Be Hazardous to Your Humanity," *American Journal of Nursing,* 80, no. 9 (1980), 1588–90.

104. President's Commission on Mental Health, *Task Panel Reports, Vol. II.* Washington, D.C.: U.S. Government Printing Office, 1978.

105. Price, Mary, "Nursing Diagnosis: Making a Concept Come Alive," *American Journal of Nursing,* 80, no. 4 (1980), 668–69.

106. Read, Donald, "The Search for the Person in the Teacher," *Health Values: Achieving High Level of Wellness,* 1, no. 4 (1977), 149–54.

107. Reynolds, Janis, and Jann Logsdon, "Assessing Your Patient's Mental Status," *Nursing '79,* 9, no. 8 (1979), 26–33.

108. Riehl, Joan, "The Riehl Interaction Model," in *Conceptual Models for Nursing Practice,* 2nd ed., eds. Joan Riehl and Sister Callister Roy, pp. 350–56. New York: Appleton-Century-Crofts, 1980.

109. Riehl, Joan, and Sister Callista Roy, eds., *Conceptual Models for Nursing Practice,* 2nd ed. New York: Appleton-Century-Crofts, 1980.

110. Roberts, Sharon, *Behavioral Concepts and Nursing Throughout the Life Span.* Englewood Cliffs, N.J.: Prentice-Hall, Inc., 1978.

111. Rogers, Martha, *The Theoretical Basis for Nursing.* Philadelphia: F. A. Davis Company, 1970.

112. Roy, Sister Callista, "A Diagnostic Classification System for Nursing," *Nursing Outlook,* 23, no. 2 (1975), 90–94.

113. ——, *Introduction to Nursing: An Adaptation Model.* Englewood Cliffs, N.J.: Prentice-Hall, Inc., 1976.

114. ——, "Relating Nursing Theory to Education: A New Era," *Nurse Educator,* 4, no. 2 (1979), 16–18.

115. ——, "A Case Study Viewed According to Different Models," in *Conceptual Models for Nursing Practice,* 2nd ed., eds. Joan Riehl and Sister Callista Roy, pp. 381–92. New York: Appleton-Century-Crofts, 1980.

116. ——, "The Roy Adaptation Model," in *Conceptual Models for Nursing Practice,* 2nd ed., eds. Joan Riehl and Sister Callista Roy, pp. 179–88. New York: Appleton-Century-Crofts, 1980.

117. Ruell, Virginia, "Nurse-Managed Care for Psychiatric Patients," *American Journal of Nursing,* 75, no. 7 (1975), 1156–57.

118. Saxton, Dolores, and Patricia Hyland, *Planning and Implementing Nursing Intervention.* St. Louis: The C. V. Mosby Company, 1975.

119. Shepard, William, "The Professionalization of Public

Health," *American Journal of Public Health,* 38, no. 1 (1948), 146.

120. Slavinsky, Ann, and Judith Krauss, "Mutual Withdrawal or Gwen Tudor Revisited," *Perspectives in Psychiatric Nursing,* 18, no. 5 (1980), 194–203.

121. Snyder, Joyce, and Margo Wilson, "Elements of a Psychological Assessment," *American Journal of Nursing,* 77, no. 2 (1977), 235–39.

122. Stevens, Barbara, "Accountability of the Clinical Specialist: The Administrator's View," *Nursing Digest,* 5, no. 1 (1977), 77–79.

123. Travelbee, Joyce, *Interpersonal Aspects of Nursing.* Philadelphia: F. A. Davis Company, 1971.

124. Wandelt, Mabel, and Joel Ager, *Quality Patient Care Scale.* New York: Appleton-Century-Crofts, 1974.

125. Wandelt, Mabel, and Doris Slater Stewart, *Slater Nursing Competencies Rating Scale.* New York: Appleton-Century-Crofts, 1975.

126. Weindenbach, Ernestine, "Nurses' Wisdom in Nursing Theory," *American Journal of Nursing,* 70, no. 5 (1970), 1057–62.

127. Weiner, I., and R. Goldberg, "Psychologic Testing of Children," *Pediatric Clinics of North America,* 21 (1974), 175–86.

128. West, Wilma, "Occupational Therapy Philosophy and Perspective," *American Journal of Nursing,* 68, no. 8 (1968), 1708–11.

129. White, Marjorie, "Inside Family Life: An Arena for Health Education," *Nursing Forum,* 18, no. 3 (1979), 246–52.

130. Wilson, Holly, and Carol Kneisl, *Psychiatric Nursing.* Reading, Mass.: Addison-Wesley Publishing Co., Inc., 1979.

131. Yura, Helen, and Mary Walsh, *The Nursing Process,* 2nd ed. New York: Appleton-Century-Crofts, 1973.

132. Zangari, Mary-Eve, and Patricia Duffy, "Contracting with Patients in Day-to-Day Practice," *American Journal of Nursing,* 80, no. 3 (1980), 451–55.

Appendix A

Assessment of Psychological/Sociological Status

I. IDENTIFYING DATA

Name:

Age:

Marital status:

Children:

Other members of household:

Occupation (past or present):

Where employed:

Ever employed in different occupation?

If yes, why did you change?

Date of admission/First contract?

Sex:

Race/Ethnicity:

How long?

When?

Referral source:

II. HEALTH HISTORY

General Appearance:

Observe height-weight ratio, facies, posture, general body movement and apparent energy level, gait, eye contact, gestures, mannerisms, stereotypy in movement, hygiene, dress.

Listen for statements about body functions and apparent mood, content of thoughts, and process of thinking.

This assessment tool contributed by Ruth Murray, R.N., M.S.N. and M. Marilyn Huelskoetter, R.N., M.S.N.

Questions for Client:

Describe siginificant aspects of your health history.

Have you had previous admissions to a hospital, clinic or other health care agency? Counseling or other psychological intervention?

What does it mean for you to be in the hospital/clinic?

How difficult is it to get to health services? Available transportation? Hours of service? Do you have some form of health insurance?

What medication are you using?

Describe any drug allergies or reactions.

Describe your major present problem or area of concern. What does this illness/problem/concern mean to you? How does it affect you?

When did the problem begin? Was the onset sudden or gradual?

If physical illness is present, what factors contribute to it? (emotional, family, work, food, activity, others)

What do you consider as the stressful event that triggered your problem?

What physical symptoms do you have? Describe major body functions: sleep, appetite, digestion, elimination, sexual functions. Has there been a recent weight gain or loss? Any skin problems?

Describe any problems with managing personal hygiene and self-care activities.

Have you ever experienced a similar problem(s)? If you have, what was the problem and how did you handle it? Did you feel your coping patterns were successful?

III. LIFE STYLE AND FAMILY PATTERNS

Describe where you live. (geographic area, neighborhood, residence) Describe any threats or hazards to yourself.

Who lives with you? What is their relationship to you?

How does your family (or those living with you) affect you? Describe your position (place) in the family. What does the family depend on you for? (What is your role?)

Tell me how you usually spend your day. Are you able to care for yourself? Your family? Your home? What time of the day do you feel most energetic and alert?

What special practices (religious or other rituals)

or foods do you consider essential to your life style?

Describe family events or rituals that are important to you. How do these affect your health?

Describe your work and where you work. Describe any threats or hazards to yourself. How does your work affect your health?

What changes have occurred in your life because of your illness/admission to hospital or clinic?

Describe what you consider as your economic level. (or) Are you worried about money or do you feel comfortably fixed? Will this illness/hospitalization create a financial strain? Do you have concerns about the fees for service?

IV. COMMUNITY PATTERNS

What do you consider your place in the community?

Describe the groups you belong to and your role/

responsibility in these groups. How much satisfaction do you get from group activities?

V. PERCEPTUAL ABILITY

Describe your sensory ability or any impairment related to:

Vision
Hearing

Smell
Taste
Touch
Balance
Pain or unusual body perceptions

Do bright lights or loud noises bother you?

If you are more sensitive to light or noise now, is it related to your illness or to conditions existing in the hospital/residence?

Describe any special visions and when and where they occur? (hallucinations)

Do you ever see something different from what is really present? (illusions)

Do you hear voices? If so, what do they say and are you able to converse with them?

What are your food preferences? What foods are distasteful and what foods are enjoyable to you?

Describe any feelings you have in various body parts? Are you especially aware of any body part or function?

What situations require assistance for you to maintain balance/mobility? What kind of assistance do you need?

VI. EMOTIONAL STATUS

Self-Concept/Body Image:

(It may be helpful at times to have the client draw a picture of him/herself. Not only might you be able to see how the client views him/herself, but you might discover conflict areas, stage of development, as well as intellectual achievement and ability.)

How would you describe yourself? Assets? Limits? Satisfaction with yourself?

What do you like best about yourself? Like least?

How do you refer to yourself?

If it were possible, what is the primary aspect of yourself that you would like to change?

In what stage of life do you consider yourself?

How do you feel you handle yourself and your life? Have you a sense of independence/self-control/autonomy?

Describe your attitude toward life.

What are your interests?

Feelings:

Describe your feelings. (tension, anger, sadness, depression, suspiciousness, confusion, aloneness, being different, being overwhelmed, hopelessness, helplessness)

Ego Ideal:

Tell me the goals or aspirations you presently have.

Do you feel you have managed to achieve your goals in life? How do you plan to achieve them?

Superego:

Which of the following comes first for you: pleasure, your goals, or essential tasks? (sense of responsibility)

How do you respond to situations that require you to do something you are reluctant to do:

Do you ignore the task?
Do you plunge in and complete it as soon as possible?
Do you delay the task as long as possible?

What rules or customs are difficult for you to follow?

Describe what you consider the most important teachings that were given to you by your parents or family—the ones that you live by.

What causes you to feel guilty? To feel angry with yourself?

Sense of Autonomy:

What does the term *fate* mean to you?

What do you feel has control over what is happening to you?

How much control do you exert over others? In any situation?

How has this illness/situation affected your feelings of control or lack of control?

VII. ADAPTIVE ABILITY

What situations or persons make you feel calm, secure, happy?

What situations or persons cause you to feel upset, embarrassed, anxious, or angry? How do you handle these situations or persons?

What is your usual pattern of relating to those close to you? To strangers? To a group situation?

How much does another's reaction or behavior influence how you will act?

How important is another person's behavior or feelings to you?

What is your reaction to frustration? To success?

Have others told you that you have good judgment or can cope in a situation?

Which of the following are you likely to do:

Go along with the person or situation to keep peace?

Blame others if something goes wrong for you?

Consider yourself the cause if something goes wrong?

Feel more angry than is warranted by the situation?

Let others know abruptly of your feelings?

Say little about your feelings, hoping the other person will guess how you are feeling?

Feel reluctant to act in an unfamiliar situation without permission or encouragement from someone?

Feel confident in unfamiliar situations and take charge of things if it is indicated?

Encourage others to do their best work possible?

Consider that others are unlikely to do the job as well as yourself?

What do you find best relieves your tension? (eating, smoking, drinking, drugs, sleep, activity, sexual activity, physical activity, etc.)

What results do you usually get from your behavior?

How have you managed past crises? Describe your feelings as you tried to cope.

VIII. VALUES

Tell me your ideas about the following:

The importance of the environment around you. (man-environment relationship)

Which do you prefer? (being alone or with others/ with a group; privacy vs. group interaction)

How important are your possessions? Do you like your own or are you willing to share material goods/furnishings/clothes, etc? (possessions: personal vs. shared)

How important is lots of room/space? Do you prefer small or large living areas? Do you mind being crowded? (value on space)

Do you like to have things done promptly? How do you feel if you know that you or someone else is going to be late to an event? (time orientation)

Do you tend to rely on past experiences, think mostly about the present, or frequently plan ahead into the future? (past-present-future orientation)

Would you rather be busy or be able to sit and think, read, or relax? (work/activity—leisure values)

How much time do you spend in work tasks daily?

How do you feel when you hear the word *change*? (attitude to change)

How often do you make or have you made changes in your life? (value on change)

What changes would you like to make in yourself? Others? Your environment?

How much schooling do you have? How important is education to you? (value of education)

What do you consider necessary to get ahead in life? (value on achievement)

What customs, special practices, or rituals do you

and your family engage in to keep healthy? Do you and your family have any specific beliefs or observe any specific traditions concerning health? (health illness values/definitions)

When do you consider yourself or members of your family healthy? Ill? What do you do when you or members of your family become ill?

IX. RELATIONS TO OTHERS

Tell me how you prefer doing activities—alone or with others?

With whom do you share your feelings? Is talking to another about feelings easy or difficult?

Who can you trust to help you in time of need? (immediate family, other relatives, friends, acquaintances, strangers)

Whom or what do you care about most in your life?

Who do you think cares most about you?

How do you see your life fitting into the lives of others?

How dependent on/independent of your family/friends are you?

How have your usual interactions and family responsibilities been disrupted by your illness?

Has there been a change in your sexual pattern?

X. RELIGIOUS PRACTICES

Are you active in a church or religious denomination?

If you do not subscribe to a particular religious creed, have you any basic beliefs/philosophy/values that are important? How do these affect your health?

Describe any special beliefs/religious practices that you adhere to? How do these affect your health?

How do you see your relationship to God during this period of time? What effect does God have on your health/illness?

What can the nurse do to assist you in practicing religious rituals/beliefs during your illness/hospitalization?

XI. USE OF LEISURE

What activities do you enjoy for recreation or relaxation?

How often do you engage in these activities? With whom? Where?

How do these activities affect your health?

XII. LANGUAGE AND COMMUNICATION PATTERNS
(Observe and listen for)

Ability to express thoughts and feelings. (Talks freely or hesitantly, writes, draws, uses nonverbal behavior primarily.)

Describe vocabulary. (Note variety of words used, repetition of words, slang, or correct grammar.)

Enunciation of words, voice tone, inflection, volume.

Expression of speech. (how quick to answer, rapidity in flow of speech, hesitations, smooth vs. uneven rate, urgency of speech, distortions, excesses or deficiency in speech)

Ability to express ideas. (coherent, logical, confused, circumstantial, tangential, poverty of ideation, excessive detail)

XIII. COGNITIVE STATUS (observe and listen for)

Level of consciousness. (alert, lethargic, confused, stuporous, comatose)

Orientation to time, place, person.

Emotional level.

Ability to recall far past, immediate past, and present events. (What brought you here? Tell me about the events that led to your illness/hospitalization/admission. Tell me some major things about yourself and your past life.)

Attention span. (Does person respond to immediate stimuli? Estimate length of concentration or attention span; whether distracted by extraneous stimuli; how capable of following train of thought; what stimuli distract; how long interview proceeded before person showed fatigue; whether preoccupied with self or some event.)

Speed of response to verbal stimuli. (Answers immediately, quickly, or slowly; hesitates; ignores certain statements.)

Preoccupation, obsessions, ideas of reference.

Remains in reverie state or in primary process.

(Daydreams, fantasizes, talks about material that seems nonsensical or is difficult to follow.)

Ability to do logical thinking or problem solving. (Or unable to do cause-effect associations; states loose, magical, or nonsensical logic.)

Ability to grasp ideas, follow directions, or carry trend of thought.

Ability to abstract and deal with symbols. (Answers questions literally, is able to elaborate or explain, can give meanings for behavior situations, can explain proverbial statements.)

Presence of delusions or degree of reality in belief system.

Apparent insight into problem/situation. (What have you been told about your illness? What do you think is the cause of your problem? Why do you think you have been admitted to the hospital? Can you tell me about your current situation?)

Aware of need for more knowledge about illness situation. (What questions or concerns do you have about your illness, hospital stay, admission?)

XIV. EGO FUNCTIONS

Interviewer should note the following during the interview:

What was the primary emotion? Was it appropriate to the situation?

During the interview, what nonverbal behavior accompanied statements?

What questions elicited behavioral manifestations of discomfort or anxiety?

Was there accentuated use of any one pattern of behavior during the interview?

Did the person use "they" instead of "I" when responding to questions? Was he/she aware of body parts and functions without excessive preoccupation with himself/herself?

Was the person realistic or did he/she show disturbed reality testing? For example, is the person adapting to reality? Does he/she show poor judgment? Does he/she understand the consequences of behavior? Does reality interfere with creative behavior? Presence of delusions? Hallucinations?

Has the person learned the socially acceptable method of dealing with drives and feelings?

What defense mechanisms are apparently commonly used? What defense mechanisms were used during the interview?

Does behavior appear overcontrolled, undercontrolled, or without control? Describe.

Does the person appear able to have the various aspects of the personality integrated? What aspects of behavior appear fragmented or lacking in unity of autonomy?

XV. SUICIDAL RISK (See also Chapter 8.)

Have there been past suicidal attempts? Describe what triggered the attempt and the outcome.

What recent stresses or losses have been endured?

Has there been a recent change in mood or attitude? Is a sense of depression, agitation, and hopelessness present? Describe.

Have you thought about death, wanting to die, or life after death? (Does the person talk about wanting to die, either initiating the topic or after you introduce the topic?)

Does the person have a plan for suicide that is logical, organized, detailed, and refers to highly lethal methods?

SUMMARY OF IMPRESSIONS

Note any discrepancies between the patient's/client's perception and that of the interviewer/caregiver.

Impression of your feelings about the client and your feelings during the interview. (What was the progression of rapport, trust, relationship?)

Intrapersonal Factors:

Physical. (appearance, posture, facies, dress, hygiene, range of body functions, physical findings that evidence anxiety)

Psychological. (cognitive and perceptual abilities, thought processes, emotional status, ego functions, adaptive/defensive mechanisms used, feelings about self and body image, values, attitudes, needs, expectations, aspirations, behavior patterns, creative expressions, needs, strengths, limits)

Developmental. (degree of apparent normalcy, apparent stage of behavior and coping/defensive mechanisms, past learning history, perception of environment and family values, goals and ideas and the influence of these, how current level of functioning and life style relate to culture/ethnicity, age, and sex of person)

Social. (superego functions, behavior/socialization patterns, use of language and communication skills, activities of daily living, perception of relations to others, value system, customs, taboos or superstitions, understanding of own roles and roles of others)

Interpersonal Factors. (family structures; relationship with family, friends, and others; communication ability; socialization level; expectations of family, friends, care-givers, and others in present situation; ability to anticipate consequences of behavior; resources)

Extrapersonal Factors. (cultural factors; social class level; occupation; work-related resources; environmental or work-related stresses; residence and geographical location; financial resources; relationship to community; community resources; effect of time of day, temperature, and weather on behavior; use of space and privacy)

The special uniquenesses of this person:

Factors that may enhance and inhibit working with health care providers, response to nursing care, and progress in treatment:

Nursing diagnosis:

Recommendations for short-term and long-term goals:

Client goals:

Nursing goals:

Appendix B

Assessment of the Child/Adolescent

Some of the previously listed elements in the socio-cultural and psychological assessment tool are applicable. Information may be gained from the young client or parents/guardians. The following data may be obtained in conjunction with parental interview, during a physical examination, or during play activities.

I. GENERAL OBSERVATIONS

Growth norms—height, weight, body build:

Appearance—facial expression; hygiene and dress of the child:

General behavior—loud, quiet, active, withdrawn; movements:

Use of toys:

Play with other children, if present:

Other responses:

II. DEVELOPMENTAL STATUS

Review prenatal, perinatal, and neonatal history; note any problem areas.

Learn a developmental history since birth, including age of walking, talking, toilet training, motor control, and other major tasks.

III. HEALTH HISTORY

Describe past illnesses or behavioral/developmental concerns or problems.

Describe current problem/illness and characteristics of symptoms/behavior.

Describe general physical condition, including sensory status; medication use; substance abuse.

IV. FAMILY STATUS

Distance or closeness to parents:

Position in family—siblings, primary caregiver:

Interaction pattern and relations with parents and others in family:

Effect of behavior on family:

Family's perception of child:

Parent's communication with child:

V. SCHOOL HISTORY (if applicable)

Kind of schooling and age of entry:

Perceptions about school:

Success or failure in school:

Peer and teacher relations:

VI. PSYCHOLOGICAL STATUS (observe and note)

Speech. (vocabulary, verbal patterns, word pronunciation)

Nonverbal behavior. (mannerisms, posture, stereotyped or ritualistic movements)

Cognitive ability. (apparent intellectual level; memory ability; ability to concentrate, attend to questions, and comprehend; preoccupations with own thoughts, obsessions)

Fantasy. (content in keeping with development level)

Emotional status. (appropriate affect for the situation; capacity to experience range of emotions; ability to cope with stressful situation; orientation to person, time, and place; sense of reality; usual temperament or mood)

VII. SUMMARY

Is child's behavior abnormal in relation to age, developmental level, sex, type and persistence of pattern, life circumstances, sociocultural setting, family perception?

Strengths and limitations:

Special uniquenesses:

5

Therapeutic Communication for Emotional Care

Study of this chapter will assist you to:

1. Define communication and describe the elements in the communication process.

2. Identify the levels of communication and use this knowledge during the nursing process.

3. List and describe the tools used in communication.

4. Discuss ways to effectively use language of size, time, space, and color, as well as words.

5. Observe various clients and situations and determine whether your observations meet the criteria and what factors influenced your observations and perceptions.

6. Describe the different types of nonverbal behavior and how each affects communication.

7. Analyze silent periods to determine the type of silence and its effect on communication.

8. Practice attentive listening and explore its impact on the other person.

9. State the definition of an interview and list its purposes.

10. Discuss interviewing methods and the rationale for steps in the method.

11. Interview a person, well or ill, using the correct methods, and analyze the effectiveness of the interview.

12. List and describe methods of therapeutic communication and the rationale for each method.

13. Relate effective use of tools of communication to therapeutic communication with the client.

14. Practice therapeutic communication with a client and analyze the pattern of communication, using knowledge of rationale.

15. Describe modifications in communication ap-

This chapter contributed by Ruth Murray, R.N., M.S.N.

proach that will be effective with a client or adolescent.

16. Discuss ways to modify a communication approach to be effective with clients who have communication disorders or specific behaviors that hinder communication.

17. Practice therapeutic communication with persons of different ages and with varying behavioral patterns.

18. Discuss barriers to and ineffective methods of communication, identify personal use of these, and analyze why they are ineffective.

19. Explore how use of effective communication methods is basic to humanistic nursing care in any setting and contributes to health and the functioning of any system.

Communication is the matrix for all thought and relationships between people. Early sensory experiences shape subsequent learning abilities in speech, cognition, and symbol recognition, and in the capacity for maturing communication. Perception of self, the world, and one's place in it results from communication. Both verbal and nonveral communication are learned in a cultural setting, and if the person does not communicate in the way prescribed by the culture, many difficulties arise, for he/she cannot conform to social expectations. Disordered thinking, feeling, and actions result, along with mental anguish, and perhaps emotional and physical illness (97).

Communication is basic to the nursing process and to the care of emotionally ill clients. It is used in assessing and understanding the client, in setting goals and a care plan, and in nursing intervention. Communication helps people express thoughts and feelings, clarify problems, receive information, consider alternate ways of coping or adapting, and remain realistic through feedback from the environment. Essentially you and the client learn something about yourselves, how to identify health needs, and if and how to meet them.

DEFINITIONS

The word *communication* comes from the Latin verb *communicare,* "to make common, share, participate, or impart" (48). *Communication establishes a sense of commonness with another and permits the sharing of information, signals, or messages in the form of ideas and feelings.* A series of messages exchanged between persons forms an interchange or communication. Communication is a continuous dynamic process by which one mind may affect another through written or oral language, gestures, facial expressions, music, painting, sculpture, drama, dance, or other signs.

Communication pattern refers to the relatively consistent network of messages sent and received in short- or long-term exchanges, the habitual way of interacting with others. Part of this pattern is the *social amenities pattern, the interaction that uses socially prescribed rules, ceremonies, or cus-*

toms according to the situation and usually results in superficial communication. The social pattern includes *small talk, social chitchat that encompasses mundane topics* and is used to kill time, to test the reactions of others, to avoid involvement, or to serve as a bridge to significant conversation. The *information pattern* differs in that it *involves a request for or giving of information or orders,* but it is not likely to establish intimate understandings because there is little disclosure of self. Neither the social nor the informational pattern is adequate by itself in the nursing process. The communication pattern in the nurse-patient-family relationship should be a *dialogue,* involving *purposeful, reciprocal, close expression between the participants* and focusing on the problems of the one seeking help rather than on the helper. Yet there should be an openness that contributes to the growth of all participants involved (109).

THE COMMUNICATION PROCESS

Every communication process includes a sender, a transmitting device, signals, a receiver, and feedback, as shown in Figure 5-1. The sender attempts to convey a message, idea, or information through appropriate use of symbols or signals directed to another specific person or group. That the message is sent does not guarantee that it will be received, let alone by the person for whom it is intended.

Many factors influence how the message is sent and whether, how, and by whom it will be received, including: the needs and condition of both the sender and receiver, emotionally, physically, and intellectually; the occasion or setting; and the sender's knowledge about and relationship with the receiver. Other factors include the content of the message or vocabulary to be decoded, the mood or attitude present in the situation, and the communication experience already in operation.

The receiver in turn perceives, interprets, and responds to the message. Through some process, he gives feedback to the sender, confirming that the message has been sent. The receiver at that point becomes the sender of a message. If the original message sent does not result in a response or feedback, there is no official interchange.

Communication and related behavior can be studied only in their proper context. Studying only the information, the command, the question—the words—is not enough. Behavior and the way of communicating are not static; they vary with the specific situation. In certain situations, seemingly inappropriate responses may be highly appropriate behavior. For example, the apparently senseless talk of an emotionally ill person may be the only feasible reaction in an untenable family situation—the only way of achieving family equilibrium. Or a child's aggressive behavior may be the only way of maintaining initiative and self-respect when the

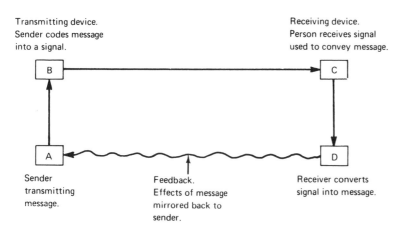

FIGURE 5-1   Elements in the communication process. [From R. Murray and J. Zentner, *Nursing Concepts for Health Promotion*, 2nd ed. ©1979, p. 64. Reprinted by permission of Prentice-Hall, Inc., Englewood Cliffs, N.J.]

mother communicates overprotection or "smothering" nonverbally. Thus communication is influenced by the family and social systems in which the person lives.

In the strictest sense, all behavior in the presence of others is communication, and all communication affects behavior (115). How you gesture, posture, dress, move, speak, behave, or fail to carry out certain behaviors will provide an understandable signal for someone. For example, two persons sitting side by side in an emergency room may neither speak nor look at one another. Yet there is a communication process present, for each behaviorally conveys to the other that he/she does not wish to engage in an interchange of words, for whatever reason. Contrast this with two persons sitting side by side who do not speak but occasionally look at one another and smile. Then a few words are exchanged. The initial nonverbal expressions encourage the eventual verbal exchange. Thus anything perceptibly present or absent can serve as a signal of communication, one that need only be decoded to be meaningful.

LEVELS OF COMMUNICATION

Communication occurs on several levels because of the perceptions of each person involved in the communication, and each level becomes increasingly abstract, as demonstrated in Figure 5-2. When two persons are communicating, the following levels may occur (115):

1. This is how I perceive me.
2. This is how I perceive you.
3. This is how I perceive you seeing and hearing me.
4. This is how I think you see me seeing you.

In a nurse-client dialogue, on *Level 1,* you are thinking only of the yourself while talking to the client. Self-awareness is important, but awareness must include more than that. Level 1 communication is not helpful to another. On *Level 2,* you are thinking of yourself by also observing the patient's behavior and hearing what is said. This level is more appropriate for communication of the client's needs.

On *Level 3,* you are aware of how the client might be perceiving you in addition to being aware of what both you and the client are saying, doing, and feeling. Thus you can better consider the effect of yourself on the other and the behavioral cues from the person and respond to them. In addition, you may ask for validation of personal perceptions— whether or not the person is actually perceiving you as you believe. For *Level 4* communication to occur, you must be very alert, feeling energetic and attuned to the situation. Now, in addition to the above, you consider how the client thinks you are perceiving him/her—your feelings and attitudes toward the other as he/she perceives them. Level 4 takes considerable empathy, but it will allow you to be most helpful in communicating with the emotionally ill person. These levels increase in complexity with increasing numbers of people. If you understand the levels of communication, you can anticipate the communication process, hear "hidden meanings," and recognize your impact upon the process (88, 115).

TOOLS OF COMMUNICATION

The tools of communication—language, observation and perception, nonverbal behavior, silence, listening, and watching—are closely interrelated and are used simultaneously, although they are discussed separately in the following pages. Knowledge of these tools is essential when using the nursing process (as discussed in Chapter 4), as well as for effective functioning in any system.

Basic to the use of any tool of communication is acknowledgment of and working with your own feelings. Chapters 1 and 3 refer to your self-assessment, as do other chapters. The reference by Lynne Jungman, Thora Kron, and Mary Paynich are also pertinent (62, 68, 87).

Language

Language is basic to communication. Without language, the higher-order cognitive processes of

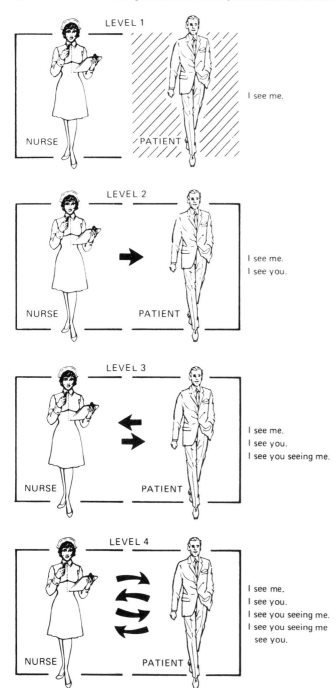

FIGURE 5-2 Levels of communication. [From R. Murray and J. Zentner, *Nursing Concepts for Health Promotion*, 2nd ed. ©1979, p. 66. Reprinted by permission of Prentice-Hall, Inc., Englewood Cliffs, N.J.]

thinking, reasoning, and generalizing cannot be attained. ***Words*** *are tools or symbols* used to express ideas and feelings or to indicate objects; *they are not the same as the experience*, although words shape experience, and they influence cultural per-

ceptions, communicate facts, convey interpretations, and affect relationships (84, 92).

The functions of language can be divided into three classifications: expressive, arousing, and descriptive. A speech act is *expressive* if it informs us of a speaker's state of mind or emotions; it is also likely to serve the function of *arousal*, triggering an emotional response in the receiver of the message. The *descriptive* function serves to inform another person, to convey observations, memories, ideas, or inferences (115).

Visual images are more likely to serve the function of arousal than is language. Viewing a picture can arouse strong emotion, for much of the self can be projected into the image. Yet the visual image is unable to show the many contexts of description or tense of which verbal language is capable, for in listening, the personality of the speaker more easily strikes us (43).

The same words may have different meaning for different people, and you must constantly be prepared to define the meaning of a word or phrase. Also, word meanings change over time and in different situations. Consciously or unconsciously, the person selects the part of the world that is experienced at any time. No two people are in exactly the same spot at exactly the same time; therefore, all our experiences are to some extent different. Many problems in communication arise because we fail to remember that individual experiences are never identical. When two persons talk with one another, communication is established by determining mutual experiences. If the experience being discussed is new to a person, he/she may have difficulty making sense out of it. Much difficulty in introducing new ideas and much resistance to change arise from the fact that we have to learn *what* to experience in events as we live through them.

Words may be used both to express feelings and to avoid expressing them. When a person says he feels "fine," he may be functioning at optimum level, or he may be physically ill but wish to stop further inquiry by responding with the word "fine." Words may also be used in deliberately obscure ways in order to convey hidden meanings, to test your interest in finding out such meanings, to judge the degree of your concern for the person, or to express hostility without fear of retaliation. There is always **latent** or *hidden content* in the person's message. Latent content can be heard as you listen for underlying ***themes*** (*repetition of key words,* *feelings, or ideas)*, for verbal nuances or cues, the double or omitted message, or "the slip of the tongue." Latent content also becomes apparent when you observe incongruency between words and nonverbal behavior, or between the words and their context of use (3, 95).

Nonlinguistic aspects of speech, such as silence, how much of the time the person talks, rate of speech, how soon the other person stops talking, interruptions, rate of speech errors, hesitations, pauses such as "ers" and "ahs," and repetitions also give important signals. Many of these signals indicate anxiety or other feelings, as do loudness, high pitch, rapidity of speech, and breathiness. A depressed person talks slowly and at a low pitch and tolerates longer silences. An aggressive, dominating person talks loudly and rapidly, enunciates precisely, interrupts others more often, and may include ridicule, teasing, joking, or direct insult in speech (5).

Language of Size

In addition to the language of words, there is the language of size, time, space, and color. The language of physical and psychological size is related to the impact, influence, or potential for helping that one person has in regard to another person. Large physical size conveys dominance, power, authority, and control. Large psychological size is perceived when someone is highly knowledgeable, extrovertive, aggressive, loud, rapid-speaking, or moving; also when someone is stern, distant, holds the body rigidly, or keeps others at a distance by physical, verbal, or emotional maneuvers. The psychologically large person may be expected by others to solve problems, to see that all goes well, and to take care of them. Alternately, the psychologically large person may also be seen as someone to avoid, who stifles development and creativity, or who must have the final word. Regardless of the perception, size may interfere with communication (45). Examples of large psychological size include the business executive, teacher, doctor, or nurse as they relate with others in their environment.

The person who is large (psychologically and/or physically) will have to develop insight about and a feeling for others' perceptions and then develop methods to convey accessibility to and acceptance of others. Although changes in interpersonal communication take time and no one principle changes everything, using the principles of thera-peutic communication described later in this chapter when interacting with others will be a positive move. Changing nonverbal behavior, including various mannerisms, facial expressions, gestures, movement patterns, or even style of dress, may help the person seem more empathic and approachable. Asking questions to initiate conversation, clarifying points, and trying to elicit feedback through use of words and silence can decrease negative effects of large physical or psychological size. Actively working to learn another's name, being attentive and concerned, and avoiding jargon, ridicule, sarcasm, and emphasis on status and titles will also reduce the negative effects of psychological size (45). Take a personal inventory. Do others consider you physically or psychologically large or small? How do you consider yourself? Does your size enhance or inhibit communication with others?

Language of Time

The language of time conveys feelings not expressed by words and may depend on the culture and concept of time. If you frequently look at your watch, or walk too fast for the client to stay abreast, or keep a person waiting past the hour of an appointment, you may be conveying rejection, neglect, or lack of concern. Be mindful of how you use time with others.

Language of Space

The language of space—the distance between you and another—helps determine the nature of the communication. ***Proxemics* *is the term for the study of human use and perception of social and personal space*** (51). Physical distancing varies with the setting and is culturally learned, as well as individually determined, based on personal comfort with and need for space. Placing a person near the center of a group is one way of saying that he/she is important. The amount of space given a person—the size of desk or office, hospital room or ward cubicle—conveys differential importance or status.

Also the distance maintained between the client and yourself must be taken into consideration in regard to the particular situation and the client's needs because distance may convey feelings varying from concern to rejection (50, 103). For example, when we meet someone, we stand at a slight angle to the person, ready for conversation, but we still maintain contact with the outside world. More direct facing and more eye contact, along with a side-by-side position, occur when two people are interested in each other or are emotionally close and wish to exclude others. Rejection of another is shown by moving at a right angle to that person (98).

You can also use physical space to foster communication. For example, place chairs in a circular arrangement to foster face-to-face contact. Avoid talking to someone with a desk or table between you. Sit rather than stand when possible, and sit in the same type of chair as the client. Sit face to face rather than side by side. Thus you can use space and furnishings to bring people together rather than to keep them apart.

Territoriality or *personal space refers to an area with invisible boundaries surrounding the person's body.* According to studies in proxemics by Edward Hall (50), four distinct zones of interpersonal space exist, primarily in front of us. The intimate zone ranges from 0 to 18 inches; the personal zone from 18 inches to 4 feet; the social consultative zone from 4 to 12 feet; and the public zone from 12 feet and beyond. Different zones are appropriate for different interactions and relationships. For example, the couple, or the parent and child, or the nurse and client may interact in the *intimate* zone, which entails a close, personal relationship, such as comforting, lovemaking, protection, and sometimes psychotherapy, depending on who is involved. Some details of the person's appearance are observable only in this zone, although visual perception of the other may be slightly distorted. Persons talk softly or whisper; body heat and odors are transmitted. The nurse and doctor may work together on a procedure with a client in the *personal* zone, but later remain in the *social consultative* zone as they discuss the client's progress. The personal zone is the amount of space usually maintained between family members and between friends, or between counselor and counselee. In the personal zone, touch is possible, and visual perception and loudness of voice are normal. The social zone is used when impersonal business is conducted, or by people who are working together or in casual social gatherings. In group therapy, you may be in the personal zone with some people and the social zone with others. Sensory involvement and communication are often less intense. As you teach a class of expectant parents, you would tend to maintain the *public* zone. Distance of the public zone is outside of the sphere of personal involvement. Others are perceived as somewhat smaller than life size, and verbal com-

munication is stylized and formal. Attraction is also indicated by the zone. People who are attracted to each other at a business meeting stand farther apart than they would at a party. Everyone is expected to be closer at a party than at a meeting. The intimate zone is reserved for someone who is highly attractive or to whom we feel close (50, 51, 52).

Language of Color

The language of color elicits fairly specific responses. In American culture, warm colors such as yellow, red, and orange stimulate creative, happy responses. Cool colors such as blue, green, and gray tend to encourage meditation and deliberation and have a dampening effect on equality of communication. Color in the environment can be planned to be therapeutic and to enhance communication in nursing if you are aware of what is being conveyed through colors in the surroundings (9). Be aware of what the color of your uniform (or other dress) and hair means to the client. For example, white clothing may arouse fear in children with past illness experiences. Or the male patient may perceive any redheaded nurse as quick-tempered or "sexy" until he can learn otherwise.

Observation and Perception

The second tool of communication is observation and perception. *Observation is the act of noting and recording facts and events. Perception is the personal interpretation of observations* (48). Rarely do observations exist alone. Meanings or judgments about observed events are based on knowledge, experience, and/or bias. The observer is part of the observed. What you communicate depends on the quality of your observations and your interpretation of them. Observations are made because of curiosity, a desire to understand others, a need for security or self-preservation, or any combination of these. In nursing, each client's needs vary and constantly change. Since you are the one health team member who has continuous contact with the client, and since the diagnosis, treatment, and prognosis frequently are determined by your observations, your keen perception will help guide the other team workers in their services.

Factors influencing observation and perception are similar to those influencing the communication process generally and include the following (2, 4, 5, 6, 45):

1. Physical, mental, and emotional states, feelings, and needs.
2. Cultural, social, and philosophical values and background.
3. The senses that are involved and their functional ability.
4. Past experiences associated with the present situation and its context.
5. Meaning of the observed event.
6. Interests, preoccupations, preconceptions, and motivational level.
7. Tendency to make judgments on the basis of first impressions and then avoiding changing that impression.
8. Tendency to view others' opinions or ideas as more like or unlike your own than they really are.
9. Tendency to judge others on the basis of possession of central traits that are considered important to you personally, such as cleanliness.
10. Tendency to assume that a person has traits you value positively if you are impressed favorably with the person, or has traits you dislike if you are unfavorably impressed.
11. Tendency to assign certain traits to a specific group and assume that all members of the group have these traits.
12. Knowledge of or familiarity with the situation being observed.
13. Practice in purposeful observation.
14. Environmental conditions and distractions.
15. Availability of technical devices.
16. Presence, attitudes, and reactions of others—even if your observations and perceptions are accurate, if they do not agree with group consensus, you are likely to conform to group opinion.

You perceive best what you are prepared to perceive and that to which you direct your attention unless other stimuli are exceedingly unusual, intense, or compelling. Some stimuli are admitted to the nervous system in whole, some in part, and some are not received at all. Thus you must consciously attend to sensory stimuli—visual, auditory, tactile, olfactory—and identify, sort, separate, and combine those entering the mind in order to communicate significant observations.

One aspect of communication to remember in client care is that when two sounds are presented simultaneously to both ears, any verbal signals such as words, nonsense syllables, and separate speech sound are more readily heard and identified by the right ear; whereas music and environmental noises are better recognized by the left ear—if the person hears equally well with both ears (60).

In nursing, observations must fulfill certain criteria. They must be purposeful, planned, objective, accurate, complete, and orderly. In *purposeful* observation, you decide what to observe and why the observation is important. *Planned* observation considers timing, duration, interval between observations, and kind and location of observations. An observation is *objective* when it can be validated directly, indirectly, or through replication by others and is not based on personal bias. *Accuracy* involves use of knowledge, concentration, memory, and problem solving. A *complete* observation meets the purposes for which it is made. *Orderly* or systematic observation permits relating parts of data gathered, observing the commonplace and general data, and then focusing on minute details (88). Whenever you make an *interpretation*, it should be stated as such.

Perception of the same event varies from person to person and within the same person at different times, depending on personal feelings, what he/she is prepared for or wishes to see, as well as the total context. In addition, an individual often simplifies things not understood, leaving out important facts or substituting others, even if distortion results. Recognize this tendency in relation to yourself, the client, family, and your coworkers because perception of the event determines action. Refer also to Chapters 2 and 3 for discussion of perception.

Hildegarde Peplau describes four types of relationships between the observer and the observed in nursing (88):

1. *The spectator relationship:* The person is not aware of being observed; the nurse is outside the focus of attention. This could occur when you observe the sleeping or critically ill person.
2. *The interviewer relationship:* The person is more or less aware of being studied and that you are noting statements or responses to a situation or question. This could occur during the admission procedure or during nursing rounds.
3. *The collector relationship:* You use records or

reports prepared by other health care workers to learn what has happened to the client. This occurs in the change-of-shift conference, team conferences, or when reading the chart to assist in planning care.

4. *The participant-observer relationship:* You engage in ordinary acts connected with nursing, such as morning care, teaching, or counseling, and at the same time observe the relationship between the client and yourself. The client is aware that he/she is getting care but is not necessarily aware that his/her responses to a situation are being observed and studied.

Body Action or Nonverbal Behavior

Movement or action is the third tool of communication—for example: finger pointing, head nodding, and other specific gestures; eye behavior, gaze, a wink, eyebrow movement, pupil dilation; mouth movements, smile, and other facial expressions; a touch or a slap on the back, general posture, and head and general body movements; and body sounds such as belching, knuckle cracking, and laughing. These nonverbal behaviors are described in various references at the end of the chapter.

Nonverbal communication is powerful and honest, but its meaning varies from culture to culture and even within a culture. Many signals are sent without a person's being aware of it. Research shows that nonverbal behavior conveys 65 percent of the message. Nonverbal behavior relates to verbal behavior in that it repeats, clarifies, contradicts, modifies, emphasizes, and regulates the flow of communication. The significance of nonverbal behavior comes not from looking at an isolated movement but from examining the total composite of the person's nonverbal behavior. One person may consistently use eye contact to communicate closeness; another may use touch; a third may use body position and distance (11, 24, 31, 37, 54). Other helpful references include Ray Birdwhistel (15), Flora Davis (26), Randall Harrison (55), Mark Knapp (65), and Ted Polhemus (93).

You must be aware of your own as well as the client's nonverbal behavior. Nonverbal behavior many times will state what a person is unable to say verbally. Listen for clues. For example, the skin flush, the tiny tremor around the eyes or corners of the mouth, the brief hesitations in speech may indicate stress or agitation in the person. In the United States, certain preening behavior has sexual overtones: stroking the hair, adjusting clothing, or changing position to accentuate maleness or femaleness (98).

Eye contact in the United States indicates positive self-concept, interest in the person, and attentiveness to what is being said. In social conversation or teaching, the speaker glances away from the listener at intervals as an indication of collecting thoughts, planning what is to be said. During close, intimate care, such as during nursing procedures, you will use intermittent eye contact to show interest but also respect for privacy. In the counseling situation, you will keep eye contact with the counselee throughout the session unless he/she looks away. Be aware of the importance of eye behavior. Our pupils dilate in response to fear, anxiety, and arousal, and also when we see an attractive person or pleasing object or are being presented with an attractive idea or positive line of reasoning. Our pupils constrict whenever something unattractive is encountered (57, 58).

Several taboos related to nonverbal behavior exist in the United States. For example, touching, standing close to, or looking directly at a stranger, a person of the same sex, or someone we are not attracted to may be considered impolite and intrusive. As a relationship grows closer, the area open to touch increases, the amount of direct eye contact increases, and the distance between the two people decreases (51, 103, 104).

Body Language

Through **body language,** *moving or positioning the body or some portion of it, (kinesic behavior) a person conveys what cannot or will not be verbalized.* This body language may be used simultaneously with verbal activity (15). The many kinds of body motions or kinesic behavior can be categorized as follows (65):

1. **Emblems:** *Nonverbal actions that have a direct verbal translation or dictionary definition, usually consisting of a word, phrase; or symbol.* Sign language of the deaf, signals used in television production or in the operating room, or the gesture of thumb and forefinger touching to form a circle, to say "A-OK" ("Everything is all right") are examples.
2. **Illustrators:** *Nonverbal acts directly tied to*

or accompanying speech. Pointing a finger to indicate direction or an object, or pounding the fist in the opposite hand to emphasize phrases are examples.

3. *Affect displays: Facial contortions that display emotional states,* such as a smile, frown, down-turned lips.

4. *Regulators: Movements that maintain and regulate the back-and-forth nature of speaking and listening between people.* Head nods or turning your gaze toward another indicates its his/her turn to talk; an intermittent head nod and eye contact indicate listening.

5. *Adaptors: Nonverbal behaviors that are learned as a way to meet needs, manage emotions, develop social contacts, or convey feelings, including aggression and sexual interest.* Arms across the chest or hands on hips, leg swinging, finger tapping, or a friendly wave are examples.

Expression of self through movement is learned before speech, so that under stress, the person often reverts to such preverbal communication (4, 17). For example, an individual may overtly manifest the expression he/she feels is expected in the existing situation—the smile that is only a facade—rather than show what is really felt. Thus nonverbal behavior is likely to express hidden meanings, although these must be interpreted with extreme care. Laughter is not always a sign of humor or happiness; it may be a device to cover anxiety, to show ridicule, or to seek attention.

Certain facial expressions and eye behavior can give clues to a person's feelings. Research shows that generally in this country you will observe the following expressions. A constant stare with immobile facial muscles indicates coldness. During fear, eyes open wide, eyebrows raise, and the mouth opens with lips tense and drawn back. In anger, eyes fix in a hard stare with the upper lids lowered and eyebrows drawn down, and the lips are tightly compressed. With feelings of disgust, eyes narrow, the upper lip curls upward, and the nose moves. During sadness, the eyes look down, the inner corners of the eyebrows raise, the lips turn down, and the lower lip may tremble. With embarrassment, modesty, or self-consciousness, the eyes look down and away, the face is contorted and flushed, and the person pretends a smile, rubs the eyes, nose, or face, or twitches his hair or beard/mustache. Surprise is shown by raised eyebrows and direct gaze.

The eyes rolled upward may be associated with fatigue, or a suggestion that another's behavior is inappropriate, or an effort at organizing one's thoughts (32, 65, 93).

Aggressive, controlling, and manipulative actions include threatening gestures, such as a direct look, a sharp movement of the head toward the other person, a frown, and hand raising. Flight behaviors include retreat, closed eyes, withdrawing chin into chest, and crouching. These defensive behaviors often occur when a dominant person sits too close to a subordinate. Notice these behaviors, along with other signs of tension, such as rocking, leg swinging, or foot tapping, so that you do not push yourself onto a client (31, 65, 103).

Personality characteristics may also be associated with gaze patterns, although the statistical relationship is weak. People who gaze at another person about 15 percent of the time are seen as cold, pessimistic, cautious, immature, evasive, submissive, indifferent, and sensitive. Persons who gaze at someone about 80 percent of the time are seen as friendly, self-confident, natural, mature, sincere, involved, and dominant. Dependent individuals use eye behavior not only to communicate more positive attitudes but also to elicit such attitudes when they are not forthcoming. Extroverts seem to gaze more frequently than introverts and for longer periods of time, especially while talking. Eye behavior, especially direct gaze, is also a good predictor of aggressiveness or competitiveness. An unaggressive person is three times more likely than an aggressive person to be deterred to a considerable degree when stared at (65). There have been research studies that suggest special gazing patterns (usually less gaze time) for autistic, schizophrenic, depressed, and neurotic persons, and for persons with low self-concept. Finally, it seems that males and females can be expected to differ in the amount of gaze time shown. Females seem to look more than males when measured for gaze frequency, duration, and reciprocity, and such differences have been observed in early elementary school. Although women tend to look at others more, they also tend to avert their eyes more than men, especially in response to being stared at by a man. Only one male from the thirty observed performed this behavior, whereas it was seen in twelve of the thirty females (65).

Posture also may indicate feeling. A slightly relaxed, leaning forward position can indicate a closeness, interest in, or attraction to a person, object, or event. The male indicates attraction by the closed posture: arms in front of body with legs closed. The female indicates attraction with a more open posture: arms down at the side (50). Rigid muscles, flexed body, and caution in moving a body part communicate physical pain.

Thus body language is often a reliable index of the real meaning of what is being said or communicated because the person is generally unable to exert as much conscious control over this aspect of behavior as over the words used. But knowledge of the person's sociocultural heritage is essential since various body parts are used differently in different cultures to enhance conversation. For example, in India and Greece the use of the eyes is all-important, whereas in Africa the torso is frequently moved. And in America, head nodding is common. The amount of movement also varies culturally (31).

Furthermore, normal distance for conversation is much closer in Latin countries than in the United States; you may feel uncomfortable when the South American male client stands in the intimate zone while he is describing his symptoms to you. More physical contact occurs between people in many cultures, for example, Italian, Greek, Jewish, Mexican, and Puerto Rican, than between people in the United States. Touching between same-sexed pairs, including male pairs, rather than between opposite-sexed pairs, is more common among Arabs or South Vietnamese than it is among Americans. This may be misinterpreted as a homosexual "pass" in the United States. These subtle cultural variations in the use of nonverbal signals often lead to serious misunderstandings and resentments. Misinterpretations of nonverbal signals can sometimes be avoided only by verbal validation of their meaning, but speaking of the nonverbal signal may often cause embarrassment because many of these signals are sent without much, or any, thought (31, 50, 52, 65).

Other cultural differences should be noted. For example, more than brief eye contact is generally initially avoided by the American Indian, rural Appalachian, the Vietnamese, and Black American. Although eye contact is taboo in Far Eastern countries, prolonged avoidance of eye contact in the United States is interpreted as lack of attention, rudeness, or mental illness. Gestures are used by Americans and the English to denote activity and by the Italian or Jewish persons to emphaaize words. The use of facial expression varies with the culture. Italian, Jewish, Black, and Spanish-speaking persons smile readily or use facial movements, along with gestures and words, to express feelings—happy, unhappy, or physical pain. Oriental, American Indian, English, Irish, and Northern European persons show less facial expression, and verbalize less, in response to feelings, particularly with strangers. Sometimes facial expression is deliberately used to convey the opposite meaning; in Oriental countries it is customary to conceal emotions and bad news with a smile.

Even verbal techniques vary between cultures. Americans put commands in the form of queries or suggestions. The English talk with considerable understatement so that they will not be considered boastful. Arab speech contains much emphasis and exaggeration. The Japanese kiss to show deference to superiors, a signal that would be interpreted as an insult and would be rejected by many in the United States (5, 31, 51). Length of sentences and speech forms also vary with social class of a country. The working class typically uses short, simple sentences and are more direct than the more educated class of people (5).

Observe the nonverbal behavior of the whole person in order to interpret communication correctly because an isolated gesture or expression may require a completely different interpretation in the proper context. In addition, validate your impressions with other health team members who have observed the person, as well as the person, for the *same nonverbal behavior can be interpreted differently by different people.* Also look for inconsistencies between nonverbal and verbal behavior. For example, a person's eyes may be cold even though his words are affectionate. And the meaning of words may be altered or even contradicted by the way the words are said.

Touch or tactile sensation is an important nonverbal tool in communication, for touching another with some part of the body or an extension of it is an outside event that stimulates a response. Touch, like movement, begins in utero and precedes speech as a form of communication; thus the relationship between touch and communication begins in infancy and remains throughout life as a means of returning to direct experience. Without tactile stimulation that is gentle and nurturing, the child may not live, or he/she may have seriously impaired development. Touching stimulates an infant's chemistry for mental and physical growth (8, 44, 61, 80, 116).

Once the child reaches school age, he or she is

touched less and less, even by the parents. Americans teach their children not to touch themselves unnecessarily and to keep their hands off grown-ups' objects and others' possessions in general, thereby dampening the child's natural curiosity and desire to explore (80).

Americans tend to connect touch or physical contact with sexual connotations. Other cultures also consider touching taboo; the English and Germans carry untouchability further than Americans do. On the other hand, highly tactile cultures exist—the Spanish, Italians, French, Jews, and South Americans (26).

Within our culture, differences also exist among socioeconomic classes in the use of and response to touch as a form of nonverbal communication. People in the upper and middle socioeconomic levels use touch less in communicating and are generally less responsive to this type of behavior as a positive reinforcement tool than are people in the lower socioeconomic level (80).

In some cultures, touch is considered magical and healing. In the United States, however, there is still a considerable taboo on casual touching, in part the result of residual Victorian sexual prudery (27). However, certain health care workers are beginning to combine laying on of hands (touch) and prayer and therapeutic touch with other forms of scientific treatment (16, 19, 66, 67).

Touch has many meanings. Touch may convey (20, 38, 110):

1. An active striving to connect with another, a commitment of availability.

2. A purposeful means of communication and expression.

3. A feeling state, such as warmth, rapport, love, excitement, happiness, and approval; or frustration, anger, aggression, and punishment.

4. A quality of behavior, such as empathy, interest, encouragement, nurturance, caring, trust, concern, gentleness, protection, and competence; or aggression and physical or psychological assault or intrusion.

5. A means of integrating body boundaries and image into the self-concept.

6. A means of defining oneself to and differentiating oneself from another person.

7. An establishment or invasion of territory or of personal space and privacy.

8. A relationship with another, a giving to or taking from, or being taken advantage of.

9. A mode of sensation, perception, and experience.

10. A direction or suggestion to be followed.

Certainly touch must be used judiciously and not forced on anyone. But a great deal of communication, closeness, mutual encouragement, reality contact, comforting, and caring can be conveyed between two people when they touch. The message conveyed through touch depends on the attitude of the people involved and the meaning of touch both to the person touching and to the person touched. In general, the need for intimacy and touch is so strong that the satisfaction of that need is a greater influence on behavior than is the fear of closeness or of possible rejection (28, 61, 113).

When another human being reaches out to you, hopefully you will be there as a fellow, caring human being. Between people who care about one another, touch can communicate feelings where words would fail. In the healing professions, affective use of touch is indispensable. Thus touch is an important tool in the nurse-patient relationship and in the healing art of communication. The back rub, the hand on the shoulder, the squeeze of a hand—each encourages closeness and communication between you and your client (24, 44, 67). More information about the use of touch can be found in various references at the end of the chapter. Marie Boguslawski (16), Dolores Krieger (66), and Lynn Miller (79) give additional information on therapeutic touch as a method of healing.

Silence

Silence is the fourth tool of communication, even though silence may also interfere with communication. Since one of your essential tasks is to encourage verbal description, you need to intervene effectively when your client is silent. However, do not cut off silence prematurely because of your own anxiety. Much can be learned from the silence by examining the data preceding the silence and observing the person during the silence. Table 5-1 summarizes the kinds of silence, their characteristics, and interventions.

TABLE 5-1.   Types of Silence and Interventions

TYPE OF SILENCE	CHARACTERISTICS	INTERVENTIONS
Blank, Empty, Blocked	Client says nothing; states, "I have nothing to say." Nonverbal behavior shows anxiety or tension.	Initiate conversation, perhaps of social nature. Reflect feeling, "It is hard for you to talk now."
Stubborn, Resistive	Client feels angry; tries to gain control over another; sets up power struggle.	Avoid reciprocal anger or impatience. Sit in silence; show interest in person. Reflect, "I wonder what is going on within you," or "Tell me your feelings." (See p. 200 and Chapter 15 for more detail.)
Fearful	Client previously intimidated by people when tried to talk; currently intimidated by hallucinations, thoughts, or people.	Stay with person; recognize efforts to talk. Be kind and positive. Accept whatever is said. State, "It's OK; you can tell me." Reflect, "It's scary for you to talk," or "You feel afraid?"
Thoughtful	Client resolving difficulties, doing problem solving.	Avoid interrupting thoughts. Suggest, "Share your thoughts with me." Show acceptance.

Listening

Listening is the fifth tool of communication. We have two ears and one mouth, which should give us a clue! Everyone loves a listener, but few people are skilled listeners.

Because listening gives no chance for self-assertion, instruction, or giving opinion, most people think listening is a passive act requiring no special talent. The evidence is to the contrary. You have to learn to listen attentively and to curb the desire to speak.

The act of listening consists of more than just hearing. Listening occurs only when the mind is purposefully attentive to what is being said or communicated. The mind is a selective organizer and responder to experience. On the average, we receive thousands of exteroceptive and proprioceptive impressions every second. Thus a drastic selective process is necessary to prevent the brain's higher centers from being overwhelmed by irrelevant data. Decisions concerning what is relevant and essential and what is irrelevant vary from person to person and are largely determined by processes and criteria outside the person's awareness. A person may say something that another does not hear because of the latter's selective response, his selective inattention. Selective hearing and listening are influenced considerably by past experience and associations as well as by the need to decrease anxiety over what is being said in the present situation (23, 33, 49, 118).

Listening is a faster process than speaking. No matter how fast the speaker's mind is racing, he/she cannot articulate more than about 200 words per minute, but the listener can take in words as quickly as he/she can think. The endings of most sentences can be guessed before they are completed. In fact, a person may hear the end of the sentence inaccurately because of the false sense of security and selective inattention caused by this phenomenon. In the nursing situation you should listen attentively throughout the length of each sentence, rather than guess or assume what will be said (33).

Listening manners are vital and may have a subtle but powerful impact on the other person. Elements of good listening include the following points (25, 34, 39, 71):

1. Show the person that you are listening by looking at him/her; avoid extraneous or distracting movements, handling various objects in the setting, or carrying out other procedures. Some clients need continuous eye contact as an indication of your attentiveness; others feel uncomfortable and may prefer that you occasionally shift your gaze.

2. Change facial expression in accordance with the topic and personal reactions. A client benefits from nonverbal expressions of face and body that are congruent with your words and feelings. Much message sending, acceptance, and empathy are shown nonverbally.

3. Put aside personal filters—values, biases, ideas, attitudes, and experiences—to the extent possible to avoid missing what the other is saying. Personal filters contribute to moralistic judgments, making assumptions before the other has finished speaking, or formulating an answer or interpreting too soon. Personal filters prevent hearing the subtle message, the meanings and values that are being discussed. Filters prevent real understanding of the client's perspective.

4. Be patient—willing to wait until the person has spoken. Then formulate your response. Silence during the dialogue promotes thoughtfulness.

5. Use multidimensional listening. Try to understand not only the content but also the intent, feelings, inconsistencies, and nonverbal behavior. Attend to all aspects of the communication, not just the obvious words.

6. Use validation. Restate what you heard and ask, "Did I hear and understand you correctly?"

A message is not a spear of thought thrust into the listener's mind by a speaker or writer. Meaning is transferred only when the listener rearranges his mind in accordance with the speaker's voice or printed word signals. Your attitude while listening to another person is an important form of feedback. Learn to adapt and to control your own behavior in order to listen attentively and to stimulate the communication of others.

INTERVIEWING AS PART OF THE COMMUNICATION PROCESS

All activities in nursing involve communication, and verbal communication with clients often involves interviewing.

Definition and Factors Involved in Interviewing

An **interview** is an interchange between two persons in which one seeks information from another without gaining personal advantage, and the other gives information about self without suffering disadvantage (89). The interview is a conversation directed to a definite purpose other than satisfaction in the meeting itself. Interviewing in the nursing situation involves the following five factors (12, 88):

1. The interview is usually conducted in connection with other nursing activities in which you do something for the client so that he/she can see and feel the immediate effect of nursing efforts; or you use interviewing to determine how best to give care or to evaluate the effectiveness of care given.

2. Either you or the other person may initiate the interview.

3. The situation of the interview is flexible in regard to the setting, interruptions, and availability of time for client and nurse. The setting may be the waiting room, home, office, factory, or bedside. Interruptions may occur from other health team members, other clients, or visitors. Time limits may be beyond your control because of intervening demands, so that you may have to return several times to the person to achieve the purpose of the interview.

4. The person is usually physically and emotionally confined or restricted and is relatively dependent on you and the climate created by you.

5. There is a continuum of people who represent "the nurse" over a 24-hour period. Each nurse, in the process of continuity of care, participates within the framework of the total plan of care. Thus each nurse may achieve a portion of the purposes of the interview, for example, teaching or gathering information, and the entire nursing team should work together toward the total purpose.

Purposes of the Interview

In nursing, the following purposes can be achieved through an interview (12, 14, 35, 46):

Establishing rapport to convey to the person that he/she is important, that someone cares; developing or maintaining feelings of self-esteem; diminishing feelings of isolation.

Establishing and maintaining the nurse-client relationship.

Listening in order to provide release of tension or to allow expression of feelings.

Obtaining information; identifying and clarifying needs.

Giving information or teaching.

Counseling to clarify a problem; encouraging self-understanding and constructive problem solving in the person.

Referring the person to other resources of help as necessary.

Your Role as Interviewer

Your self—your personality—is the principal tool of the therapeutic interview or communication. Your character structure, values, and sensitivity to the feelings of others will influence your attitude and helpfulness toward people.

As a beginner you are more likely to have certain problems in interviewing and therapeutic communication than your more experienced colleagues. Often there is a strong fear that you will do something wrong or be criticized by others. Defense mechanisms used to control your anxiety may reduce your sensitivity to the emotional responses of others. Fear of being inadequate can be projected onto the client or onto other health workers. You may feel competitive toward professional peers and wish to perform better than they.

You may feel guilty about "using" or "practicing on" the client. With experience, you will learn to work through these feelings; you will become increasingly aware of relationships and subtleties and will recognize your contributions to a relationship (18).

At first you may bombard the patient with questions. Later you will learn when a person has completed the answer to your question or when slight encouragement to go on is needed. As competence grows with experience, you will be able to hear the content of words and simultaneously consider feelings, deduce what he/she is inferring or omitting, and gauge your emotional response. In addition, you will be able to actively intervene when necessary, rather than sit and passively listen.

In order to gain this competence, take careful notes during or after each interview. Also regular sessions should be held with a teacher or supervisor who can guide you and promote self-understanding.

Techniques of Interviewing

Prepare for the interview as much as possible, by the use of records, by application of general knowledge to the specific situation, and by being alert and observant to the situation. Know or define what information is needed to achieve the purpose of the interview. What you ask or say is dependent on the purpose of the interview. Avoid, however, the "self-fulfilling prophecy," that is, setting up the interview situation in such a way that the person tells you (or seems to tell you) only what you have predetermined he/she will or can tell you. If selective inattention causes you to see or hear only what you wish to, much information will be missed or misinterpreted, and you will not be fully helpful to the person.

As mentioned previously, the personality and attitude of the interviewer can influence the interviewee's responses. The emotional climate and immediate conditions surrounding the interview also affect both you and the other person. The following techniques will help promote productive interviews (12, 46, 56, 63, 74, 90):

Establish rapport. Create a warm, accepting climate and a feeling of security and confidentiality so that the person feels free to talk about what is important to him/her.

Arrange comfortable positions for both yourself and the person so that full attention can be given to the interview.

Control the external environment as much as possible. This is sometimes difficult or impossible to do, but try to minimize external distractions or noise, regulate ventilation and lighting, and arrange the setting to reduce physical distance.

Wear clothing that conveys the image of a professional and is appropriate for the situation. Consider wearing casual clothing without excessive adornment instead of a uniform when working in the school, home, or occupational setting. Consider what expectations the interviewee may have of you. In some cases he/she will respond more readily to your casual dress; at other times the person may need your professional dress as part of the image to help him/her talk confidentially.

Begin by stating and validating with the client the purpose of the interview. Either you or the interviewee may introduce the theme. You may start the session by briefly expressing friendly interest in the everyday affairs of the person, but avoid continuing trivial conversation. Maintain the proposed structure.

Use a vocabulary on the level of awareness or understanding of the person. Avoid professional jargon or words too abstract for the interviewee's level of understanding or health condition.

Avoid preconceived ideas, prejudices, or biases. Avoid imposing personal values on others.

Be precise in what you say, so the meaning is understood. Say as little as possible to keep the interview moving. Ask questions that are well-timed, open-ended, and pertinent to the situation. This pattern allows the person to stamp his/her own style, organization, and personality on the answers and on the interview. Getting unanticipated data can be as useful in an interview as in giving care. Meaningless questions get meaningless answers. Questions that bombard the person produce unreliable information. Open-ended sentences usually keep the person talking at his/her own pace. Careful timing of your messages, verbal and nonverbal, as well as allowing time for the interviewee to understand and respond, is essential in nursing.

Avoid asking questions in ways that get socially acceptable answers. The interviewee often reponds to questions with what he/she thinks the interviewer wants to hear, either to be well thought of, to gain status, or to show that he/she knows what other people do and what is considered socially acceptable.

Be gentle and tactful when asking questions about home life or personal matters. What you consider common information may be considered very private by some. Matters about which it would be tactless to inquire directly can often be arrived at indirectly by peripheral questions. If a subject meets resistance, change the topic; when the anxiety is reduced, return to the matter for further discussion. Remember, what the person does not say is as important as what is said.

Be an attentive listener. Show interest by nodding, responding with, "I see," etc. Remain silent and control your responses when another's comments evoke a personal meaning and thus trigger an emotional response in you. While the person is talking, find the nonverbal answers to the following: What does this experience mean for him/her? Why is this content being told at this time? What is the meaning of the choice of words, the repetition of key words, the inflection of voice, the hesitant or aggressive expression of words, the topic chosen? Listen for feelings, needs, and goals. Recognize the levels of meaning in communication previously discussed, and listen for what is not discussed. Do not answer too fast or ask a question too soon. If necessary, learn if the words mean the same to you as to the interviewee. Explore each clue as you let the person tell his/her story.

Carefully observe nonverbal messages for signs of anxiety, frustration, anger, loneliness, or guilt. Look for feelings of pressure hidden by the person's attempts to be calm. Encourage the free expression of feelings, for feelings often bring facts with them. Focus on emotionally-charged topics. Ventilation of feeling is the key resolution of many emotional difficulties and opens the door to new data as well as increased understanding and insight in the client.

Encourage spontaneity. Provide movement in the interview by picking up verbal leads, clues, bits of seemingly unrelated information, and nonverbal signals from the client. If the person asks you a personal question, redirect it to him/her; it may be the topic he/she unconsciously (or even consciously), wishes to speak about. Only occasionally will it be pertinent for you to answer personal questions. Sometimes brief self-disclosure will help the interviewee feel comfortable and elicit additional data. Be sure to disclose such information for the benefit of the client, not yourself.

Ask questions beginning with "What . . . ?" "Where . . . ?" "Who . . . ?" and "When . . . ?" to gain factual information. Words connoting moral judgments should be avoided; they are not conducive to a feeling of neutrality, acceptance, or freedom of expression. The "How" question may be difficult for the person to answer because it asks, "In what manner . . . ?" or "For what reason . . . ?" and the individual may lack sufficient knowledge to answer. The "Why" question should also be avoided, for this asks for insights that the person should not be expected to give.

Indicate when the interview is terminated, and terminate it graciously if the interviewee does not do so first. Make a transition in interviewing or use a natural stopping point if the problem has been resolved, if the information has been obtained or given, or if the person changes the topic. You may say, "There is one more question I'd like to ask . . .," or "Just two more points I want to clarify . . .," or "Before I leave, do you have any other questions, comments, or ideas to share?"

Keep data obtained in the interview confidential and share this information only with the appropriate and necessary health team members, leaving out personal assumptions. If you are sharing an opinion or interpretation, state it as such, rather than have it appear to be what the other person said or did. The person should be told what information will be shared and with whom.

Evaluate the interview. Were the purposes accomplished? Recognize that not everyone can successfully interview everyone. Others may see you differently from the way you see yourself. Evaluate yourself in each situation.

You must be sincere, knowledgeable about the purpose of the interview, and skillful in using tools of communication during the interview as well as in establishing and maintaining a climate conducive to successful data collection. The effective interview takes a great deal of energy and attention.

In summary, move the interview through the following cycle to get maximum information and make accurate interpretations (35, 76, 89, 109):

1. Begin with low use of authority and completely open-ended questions.
2. Ask related and more direct questions as necessary to explore the problem with the client.
3. Use increasingly, but gradually, more authority and more direct questions to get additional necessary information.
4. Note and explore with the client any incongruity between what the person says at different points of the interview, and between what the person says and your observation of his/her nonverbal behavior.
5. Be aware of your own feelings and behavior through the progression of the interview.

Remember, you are the interviewer, but you do not control or own the interview. The leads, the expression, and the direction should be a participatory endeavor for both the client and you.

Whenever you communicate with a client, you will be facing the feelings of both yourself and the client. Guidelines for conceptualizing about and dealing with personal and client feelings include the following (71, 83, 117):

1. Own your thoughts and feelings. Say "I think," and "I feel." Avoid the nebulous "They . . ." or "My mother always said . . . ." As you speak in the first person, and take responsibility for your thoughts and feelings, you will help the client to also take responsibility for personal thoughts and feelings. The more distressed the person, the more likely that he/she cannot identify or accept personal thoughts or feelings, which in turn interferes with being responsible for personal behavior. Projection is a frequently used mechanism and interferes with honest communication and development.
2. Avoid judging or evaluating the rightness or

wrongness of another's thoughts or feelings. The person is a judge of his/her own thoughts and feelings and can be helped to explore and understand these evaluations, and in the process, to mature.

3. Avoid projecting your feelings, desires, aspirations, or ideas upon the client. Do not assume how the client feels. Allow the person to be authentic, to struggle, to determine his/her life course. Do not lay blame or anger on the client, nor hopes, aspirations, or ideals for his/her life. Do not try to make the client into an image of you, or what you think you want to be.

4. The client may project or attribute personal feelings to you. Identify your feelings and help the client to clarify which feelings belong to you and which belong to him/her. Help the client to see you as you are, not as he/she assumes or wishes you to be.

THERAPEUTIC COMMUNICATION

Analysis of your communication pattern will help you improve your methods. Realize that you cannot become skilled in therapeutic communication without supervised and thoughtful practice. However, as you talk with another, don't get so busy thinking about a list of methods that you forget to focus on the person. Your keen interest in the other person and your use of personal style are essential if you are to be truly effective (107, 111).

To be effective while communicating with the patient or family, use simple, clear words geared to the person's intelligence and experience. Develop a well-modulated tone of voice, especially with the sick person, since auditory sensitivity is increased during illness. Principles, attitudes, and methods essential in therapeutic communication have been discussed by J. Hays and K. Larson (56), R. MacKinnon and R. Michels (72), H. Peplau (88, 89, 90), J. Ruesch and G. Bateson (97), and J. Travelbee (109).

Effective Methods

Basic methods for conducting purposeful, helpful communication with a person, well or ill, along with their rationale, are given in Table 5-2. Some of these methods elaborate on earlier suggestions for interviewing.

The quality of any response depends on the degree of mutual trust in the relationship. Techniques can be highly successful, or they can misfire or be abused, depending on how they are used, on your attitude at the time, and on the other person's interpretation. Techniques are stepping stones to better understanding, an understanding that nurtures the trust, relationship, and expression of feeling. There must be a feeling of caring, or safety and security in your company, and a feeling that you want to help the person help him/herself. The more important or highly personal a feeling or idea is, the more difficult it is to say. This situation causes hesitancy in revealing thoughts, feelings, or intimate needs. By using therapeutic principles such as those previously listed you will help the person and family identify you as someone to whom ideas and feelings can be safely and productively revealed (42).

Communication with the Child and Adolescent

Perceive the child or adolescent as the unique person he/she is—*not* as a miniature adult, an infantile being, an extension of the parents, or a nonentity as you focus on the parents. Be respectful. Consider the developmental level of the child in your approach. Take time to establish rapport with this young person, as well as with family members if they are present. Acknowledge if you have cared for the child or parents before or acknowledge some special event, such as birthday, school entry, club membership for the child, or progress with health care. The child tends to mirror the parents' feelings and attitudes, so it is essential to establish a sense of rapport and trust with parents to help the child become more calm and reassured.

Plan to talk with the child/adolescent alone at some point in the assessment or intervention, but do not force a separation if either party protests greatly. If parents are with the offspring, at some point you will want to ask them to wait in a separate

TABLE 5-2. Effective Communication Methods and Their Rationale

COMMUNICATION METHOD	RATIONALE
Be accepting in nonverbal and verbal behavior. (Does not mean agreement with person's words or behavior).	All behavior is motivated and purposeful. Promotes climate in which person feels safe and respected. Indicates that you are following the person's trend of thought and encourages further talking while you remain nonjudgmental.
Use thoughtful silence at intervals, while continuing to look at and focus on person.	Indicates accessibility to mute, withdrawn, or depressed person. Encourages person to talk and set own pace. Gives both you and client time to organize thoughts. Aids consideration of alternate courses of action; provides opportunity for explanation of feelings; gives time for contemplation. Conserves energy and promotes relaxation in physically ill person.
Use "I" and "We" in proper content; call person by name and title, as preferred.	Strengthens identity of person in relation to others.
State open-ended, general, leading statements or questions: "Tell me about it." "What are you feeling?"	Encourages person to take the initiative in introducing topics and to think through problems. May gain pertinent information that you would not think to ask about because client has freedom to pursue feelings and ideas important to him/her.
Ask related or peripheral questions when indicated: "And what else happened?" "You have four children. What are their ages?"	Explores or clarifies pertinent topic. Adds to data base. Encourages person to work through larger or related issues and to engage in problem solving. Explores subject in depth without appearing to pry. Helps person see implications, relationships, or consequences. Helps keep communication flowing and person talking.
Encourage description of feelings: "Tell what you feel."	Helps person identify, face, and resolve own feelings. Validates your observation Deepens your empathy and insight.
Place described events in time sequence: "What happened then?" "What did you do after that?" "And then what?"	Clarifies how event occurred or explains relationships associated with given event. Places event in context or manageable perspective. Helps identify recurrent patterns or difficulties or significant cause-effect relationships.
State your observations about the person: "You appear . . ." "I sense that you . . ." "I notice that you . . ."	Acknowledges client's feelings, needs, behavior, or efforts at a task. Offers content to which person can respond. Encourages comparisons or mutual

TABLE 5-2.   Continued

COMMUNICATION METHOD	RATIONALE
	understanding of client's behavior. Validates your impressions. Helps person notice own behavior and its effects; encourages self-awareness. Reinforces behavior. Adds to person's self-esteem.
State the implied, what client has hinted, or a feeling that may be a consequence of an event.	Expresses acceptability of feeling or idea. Clarifies information. Conveys your attention, interest, and empathy. May be used as subtle form of suggestion for action.
Paraphrase; translate into your own words the feelings, questions, ideas, key words of other person: "I hear you saying . . ." "You feel . . ."	Indicates careful listening and focus on client. Encourages further talking. Validates and summarizes what you think client has said. Conveys empathy and understanding. Indicates that person's words, ideas, feelings, opinions, or decisions are important. Promotes integration of feelings with content being discussed.
Restate or repeat main idea expressed by client.	Conveys interest and careful listening or desire to clarify a vague point. Helps to reformulate certain statements or to emphasize key words to help client recognize less obvious meanings or associations.
Clarify: "Could you explain that further?" "Explain that to me again."	Indicates interest and desire to understand. Helps the person become clearer to him/herself. Encourages exploration of subject in depth or of meaning behind what is being said.
Make reflective statement, integrating feelings and content.	Indicates active listening and empathy. Synthesizes your perceptions and provides feedback to client. Shares your perception of congruity between person's statements and other behavior. Provides client with new ways of considering ideas, behavior, or a situation. Identifies and encourages understanding of latent meanings.
Suggest collaboration and a cooperative relationship.	Offers to do activities *with*, not *for* or *to* person. Encourages person to participate in identifying and appraising problems. Involves person as active partner in care. Tells person you are available and interested. Provides reassurance.
Offer information; self-disclose by sharing	Makes facts available whenever client

TABLE 5-2.   Continued

COMMUNICATION METHOD	RATIONALE
own thoughts and feelings briefly, if appropriate.	needs or asks for them. Builds trust; orients; enables decision making. Reduces client's anxiety, frustration, or other distressing feelings that hinder comfort, recovery, or realistic action. Helps client focus on deeper concerns.
Encourage evaluation of situation.	Helps client appraise quality of his/her experience and consider people and events in relation to own and others' experience and values. Assists person in determining how others affect him/her, and personal affect on others. Promotes understanding of own situation and avoidance of uncritically adopting opinions, values, or behavior of others.
Encourage formulation of plan of action.	Conveys that person is expected to be active participant in own care. Helps person consider alternate courses of action. Helps person plan how to handle future problems.
Voice doubt; present own perceptions or facts; suggest alternate line of reasoning: "What gives you that impression?" "Isn't that unusual?" "I find that hard to believe." Respond to underlying feeling.	Promotes realistic thinking. Helps person consider that others do not perceive events as he does nor draw the same conclusions. May reinforce doubts person already has about an idea or course of action. Avoids argument. May help to gradually reduce delusion. Conveys acceptance that delusion is the client's reality; acknowledges the communication; and attempts to establish common ground.
Seek consensual validation of words; give definition or meaning when indicated.	Ensures that words being used mean the same to both you and client. Clarifies ideas for you and client as client defines meaning for self. Avoids misunderstanding. May help to gradually reduce autistic thinking.
Summarize; condense what speaker said, using speaker's own words.	Synthesizes and emphasizes important points of dialogue. Helps both you and client leave session with same ideas in mind. Emphasizes progress made toward self-awareness, problem solving, and personal development. Provides sense of closure.

area so you can speak more privately with the child. Confidentiality may be important; the child/adolescent may share secrets with you that will not be shared with parents. You may need to clarify the confidentiality issue by saying, "Unless there is a chance of harm to you, I will keep the secrets you tell me." Or, "If I feel that your health and safety depends on it, I'll tell your parents what you told me, but I'll tell you first that I'm going to do so" (35).

If at all possible, conduct interviews or teaching/counseling sessions when the child is comfortable, and in an environment free of distracting machines, fear-producing instruments, or uncomfortable procedures (35).

Combine the following guidelines with ideas presented in the assessment tool for the child at the end of Chapter 4 when you are doing an assessment. Combine the following guidelines with the suggestions for effective teaching given in Chapter 4 when you are doing health education with the young person. The principles of therapeutic communication described earlier are useful to combine with the following guidelines when giving emotional care to the child/adolescent.

Preschool or School-age Child

The *preschool or school-age child* has a relatively short attention span, especially when ill. Simple words and direct statements or questions about concrete or tangible topics or experiences are more effective than abstractions. Since all adults are viewed as omnipotent by the young child, avoid stimulating fantasies, if possible, by what you say. Speak softly and gently, but with confidence. Use of toys can be helpful to promote relaxation, emphasize a point, encourage expression of feelings, and engage the client in an interchange. A playful attitude is helpful with the young child, for example, talking on a play telephone may enable you to elicit information from a very shy child (35), as well as help the child express fears, anxiety, anger, concerns, or fantasies about self, parents, and death itself.

Preadolescent and Adolescent

The *preadolescent and adolescent* will appreciate an adultlike approach, sentence structure and words appropriate to the understanding level, focus on him/her rather than the parents, and a private environment. Talk to this person first if you are obtaining assessment information; if you talk first to the parents you may get no further response from the youth. Be observant of nonverbal behavior that indicates anxiety, embarrassment, or rebellion: body position, seating placement, eye contact or avoidance, shrug of shoulders, clenched fists. Note manner of speaking as well as interaction with parents (35). Modify your approach, using principles discussed earlier in the chapter, to reduce the sense of threat as much as possible. If you are teaching, give information directly to the youth while including the parents. If you observe that the family is very parent-centered, then you will need to re-emphasize your teaching points with the parents to ensure compliance.

Parents

The parent(s) accompanying the child should be acknowledged for their ability to add information, make decisions about the care of the child, and their ability to carry out necessary care measures. Further, determine how the parent feels about the child's health problem and what has been done, and the effectiveness of the intervention to date. Take time to learn what else the parent feels should be done; this can give you clues both for assessment and intervention. Convey that it is normal to feel angry or frustrated with one's child. For example, instead of saying, "Do you ever get angry at the child?", (which may connote disapproval) you might ask, "What do you do when you feel angry at the child?" (35) Be able to move from your informal, though respectful approach to the child or adolescent to a more formal one with the parents, as indicated by their behavior and manner or response. Do not continue with the child-directed manner of conversation when speaking to the mother, or speak in a simple, childlike way to mother and in a professional, adult manner to the father.

Communicating with the Client Who Has Communication Difficulties

You will need to gather data from clients with sensory impairments. When you interview a person with a communication disorder, caused by hearing impairment, aphasia, inability to speak the language, or visual impairment, the basic principles still apply although the specific condition will necessitate some adaptations. However, the guidelines presented in Tables 5-3, 5-4, and 5-5 will be helpful. For anyone with a communication disorder, develop rapport and a trust relationship slowly to overcome the reticence of suspicion that might be present. Intro-duce yourself and your purpose. Use appropriate nonverbal behavior to convey ideas. Use an inter-mediary, such as a family member or interpreter, if available and necessary, but *not* to the exclusion of talking with the client.

Guidelines for interviewing or communicating with clients who have specific nursing diagnoses are discussed in Part IV.

TABLE 5-3. Communication with the Hearing Impaired Client

1. When you meet a person who seems inattentive or slow to understand you, consider that hearing, rather than manners or intellect, may be the reason. Some hard-of-hearing persons refuse to wear a hearing aid. Others wear aids so inconspicuous that you may not see them at first glance. Others cannot be helped by a hearing aid.

2. Be sure the person's hearing aid is in place, turned on, and in working order. Batteries need frequent replacement.

3. The hard-of-hearing may depend to a considerable extent on reading your lips to un-derstand what you are saying, even if they are wearing a hearing aid. No hearing aid can completely restore hearing. Always speak in a *good light,* face the person and the light as you speak, and do not have objects in or covering your mouth (gum, cigarettes, hand).

4. When you are in a group which includes a hard-of-hearing person, try to carry on your conversation with others in such a way that he/she can watch your lips. Never take advantage of the disability by carrying on a private conversation in his/her pre-sence in low tones that cannot be heard.

5. Speak distinctly but naturally. Shouting does not clarify speech sounds, and mouthing or exaggerating your words, or speaking too slowly, makes you harder to understand. On the other hand, try not to speak too rapidly.

6. Avoid excessive environmental noise, which, when magnified by a hearing aid, is dis-tracting and distressing and overrides normal conversational tones.

7. Do not start to speak to a hard-of-hearing person abruptly. Attract attention first by facing him/her and looking straight into the person's eyes. If necessary, touch the hand or shoulder lightly. Promote understanding by starting with a key word or phrase, e.g., "Let's plan our week-end now," "Speaking of teen-agers . . ." *If he/she does not understand you, don't repeat the same words.* Substitute synonyms: "It's time to make plans for Saturday."

8. If the person you are speaking to has one "good" ear, always stand or sit on that side when you address him/her. Do not be afraid to ask a person with an obvious hearing loss whether he/she has a good ear and, if so, which one it is. The person will be grate-ful that you care enough to find out.

9. *Facial expressions and gestures are important clues to meaning.* Remember that an affectionate or amused tone of voice may be lost on a hard-of-hearing person.

10. In conversation with a person who is especially hard-of-hearing, or having difficulty understanding, occasionally jot down key words on paper. The person will be grate-ful for the courtesy.

11. Many hard-of-hearing persons, especially teen-agers, who dislike being different, are unduly sensitive about their handicap and pretend to understand when they do not.

TABLE 5-3.   Continued

When you detect this situation, tactfully repeat your meaning in different words until it gets across.

12. The speech of a person who has been hard-of-hearing for years may be difficult to understand, since natural pitch and inflection are the result of imitating the speech of others. To catch such a person's meaning more easily, watch the face while he/she talks.

13. If you do not understand the person, ask for a repeat rather than ignoring the person.

14. Use common sense and tact in determining which of these suggestions apply to the particular hard-of-hearing person you meet. Some persons with only a slight loss might feel embarrassed by any special attention you pay them. Others, whose loss is greater, will be profoundly grateful for it.

TABLE 5-4.   Communication with the Visually Impaired Client

1. Talk to the person in a normal tone of voice. Being visually impaired is no indication that he/she cannot hear well.

2. Accept the normal things which a blind person might do, such as consulting a watch for the correct time, dialing a telephone, or writing name in longhand, without calling attention to them.

3. When you offer assistance, do so directly. Ask, "May I be of help?" Speak in a normal, friendly tone.

4. Be explicit in giving verbal directions.

5. Advise the person when you are leaving so that he/she will not be embarrassed by talking when no one is listening.

6. There is no need to avoid the use of the word "see" when talking with a blind person.

7. In guiding the person, permit him/her to take your arm. Never grab the visually impaired person's arm for he/she cannot anticipate your movements. Proceed at a normal pace. Hesitate slightly before stepping up or down.

8. When assisting the person to a chair, simply place his/her hand on the back or arm of the chair. This is enough to give location.

9. Never leave the person without a way to secure help. Have a call signal available.

10. Never leave a blind person in an open area. Instead, lead him/her to the side of a room, to a chair, or some landmark from which direction can be realized.

11. A half-open door, low stools, or loose cords or rugs are dangerous obstacles for the visually impaired person.

12. When serving food to a visually impaired person who is eating without a sighted companion, offer to read the menu. As you place each item on the table call attention to it. Food locations should be described on a plate according to the face of the clock. If the person wants you to cut food, he/she will tell you.

13. Be sure to tell who else is present in the environment.

TABLE 5-4.   Continued

---

14. Encourage use of a magnifying glass if it is helpful.

15. Read mail to the person and assist him/her with business matters, if necessary.

16. Describe the environment, people, and events surrounding the person to enrich his/her experience and understanding.

TABLE 5-5.   Communication with the Aphasic or Mute Client

---

1. Be aware of the cause, type, and manifestations of aphasia.

2. Use nonverbal behavior, including facial set, eye and facial expression, body posture, gestures, and voice tone to convey messages congruent with your spoken word.

3. Stand nearby, within the person's line of vision, to enable better listening and response.

4. Speak slowly, with a normal tone of voice.

5. Use simple short sentences; ask direct questions but do not bombard with questions.

6. Be prepared to use mimicking of speech, if person is capable.

7. Use visual aids, concrete objects, or pantomine with your words, if appropriate.

8. Give the person adequate time to respond to each question; do not supply words for the person.

9. Maintain a calm, quiet, accepting environment to enhance concentration and listening, to encourage attempts at communication and speech, and to reduce person's frustration.

10. Rephrase or repeat the question if the person did not understand or remember what you said.

11. Give the person a pad and pencil, or flash cards with pictures or words on them, if appropriate, to answer your questions.

12. Realize that an answer may indicate automatic speech and not real understanding.

13. Continue to converse even though person does not appear to understand.

14. Discuss topics pertinent to person's adaptation in the setting.

15. Assist family members to converse with the person.

Communication Approaches for Specific Behaviors

Overtalkativeness

Interviewing the overtalkative person can be a special challenge. You may feel irritated because the person is describing trivial details, repeating unnecessarily, or because you cannot get relevant information within a reasonable time period. Further, you may feel defensive because of the aggressive tone of voice or dominating manner. Realize that behavior is meaningful. Try to determine what is behind the overtalkativeness—anxiety, desire to keep pertinent information from you, fear of closeness, low self-esteem or inferiority covered by this compensatory behavior, habit, or psychopathology. Be respectful, firm, and supportive. Your own behavior can help to manage the interview.

Ask specific questions that cover only one idea at a time. Do not encourage further talking with nods of approval, a smile, or "um hum." Show limited interest by facial expression or averted eyes when the person is speaking repetitively or of truly trivial details or extraneous topics. Keep the interview focused by courteously interrupting; you may need to lean forward and touch the person's arm as you interrupt to clarify a point or ask another specific question. Do not show hurry or impatience; your anxiety will trigger off more anxiety in the person, and more talking will result. There are times when all you can do is sit back, relax, and accept the situation gracefully, since your efforts at focusing on time limitation will go unheeded (35). During this time, *listen carefully.* The apparent trivia may not be unnecessary detail, but rather truly pertinent information that adds considerably to your insights about the person.

Fear of Helplessness

The person who fears helplessness needs overt and active show of concern, competence, and trustworthiness. Give an adequate, but not overwhelming, explanation about what you are doing or whatever is happening so that the person feels an increasing sense of worth, support, and mastery (35).

Fear of Dependency

The person who fears dependency may act strong and independent, avoiding essential care. Reinforce a sense of strength by saying that to seek help is a sign of strength and independence. Reinforce other behavior that shows initiative. Some people cannot accept or express warmth or tenderness and become brusque, distant, irritable, embarrassed, or angry when you are warm and friendly.

Do not be overly solicitous. You will be perceived as less threatening if you are warm but passively friendly (35).

Anger

The person who is angry may feel very helpless, dependent, sensitive to failure, or fear expression of angry or sexual feelings. Anger may be a response to anxiety, against closeness and warmth, or be habitual. Be prepared for indirect expressions of anger, for example, joking, fantasies, or overly sweet or solicitous behavior. The person will benefit from your acceptance, warmth, recognition of anger, and encouragement to express anger directly, even if at first the person protests. Do not take the anger personally or return anger to the person. Acknowledge it and talk with the person about his/her feelings and behavior. If the person is trying to maintain distance with angry expressions, your reserved but warm and consistent response will be better tolerated than if you are too demonstrative. Do not push too hard for information. Explore gently or delay exploring areas that get an angry response (35).

Denial

The person who minimizes or denies symptoms or a situation may consciously or unconsciously mislead you during an interview. Denial may be an adaptive mechanism in response to anxiety, fear, shame, or guilt, or it may be a character trait. The person who denies may present disparities between the condition and self-reports, may overstate feelings of health and well-being, or may be vehement about absent or minimal symptoms. Pursue the person's behavior, symptoms, or life situation cautiously but steadily. Reflect back self-reported cue words like "only" or "a little," and use questions to point out the disparities between verbal and nonverbal behavior. You will usually need to get essential data from others who know the client, or at least to verify the information you obtain (35).

BARRIERS TO EFFECTIVE COMMUNICATION

Various authors have written about communication patterns to be avoided by persons in the helping professions and the rationale for their avoidance. For additional information, refer to G. Bingham

(13), S. Eldred (34), G. Flynn (38), M. Hardiman (53), J. Hays and K. Larson (56), H. Hewitt and B. Pesznecker (59), L. Jungmen (62), D. Little (70), L. Meadow and G. Gass (76), M. Paynich (87), and R. Veninga (112). The following approaches and techniques will interfere with helpful communication with the client and family, whether you are conducting an interview or communicating in any other nursing situation. Continually study your personal pattern of communication, verbal and nonverbal, to make sure that you avoid these practices.

Conveying your feelings of anxiety, anger, judgment, ambivalence, condescension, denial, isolation, lack of control, or lack of physical or emotional health will negatively influence your initial and continued response to another. Such feelings also interfere with your ability to listen and will certainly cause the other person to withdraw, since rapport cannot be established. Accept and work through your feelings with a supervisor. Refer to Chapter 6, pp. 198–199 and 201–203, for further discussion.

The appearance of being too busy, of not having time to listen, of not giving sufficient time for an answer, or apparently not really wanting to hear is equally forceful in "cutting off" another. Establishing contact on a social rather than on a therapeutic basis also limits communication to superficial issues.

Using the wrong vocabulary — vocabulary that is abstract or intangible, or full of jargon, slang, or implied status; talking too much; or using unnecessarily long sentences or words out of context can be interpreted by the person as your unwillingness to communicate. But words alone do not block. Perhaps even more crucial can be your attitudes and prejudices resulting from your personal and cultural background and your failure to understand the receiver's background. Think about what the message will mean to the person, depending on age, sex, personality, socioeconomic status, cultural background, occupation, religion, and degree and nature of illness.

Failing to understand the reason for the person's reluctance to make a message clear (resulting from the feeling that what he/she needs to express is socially unacceptable or inappropriate) can prevent therapeutic communication. Questions may not be asked for fear of getting an obscure answer or for fear of being reprimanded for such questioning. This fearful silence can cause a sense of futility and a closure of communication. Lack of dialogue prohibits evaluating the effectiveness of any message and blocks further attempts at communication. Also avoid interpreting cooperation or passivity as understanding. Sometimes the person answers yes to please you but really does not understand you at all.

Making inappropriate use of facts, introducing unrelated information, offering premature interpretation, wrong timing, saying something important when the person is upset or not feeling well and thus unable to hear what is really said — all these provoke anxiety and prohibit problem solving on the part of the person.

Making glib statements, offering false reassurance by saying, "Everything is OK," or unfairly indicating that there is no cause for anxiety — these are dishonest ways of evaluating the client's personal feelings and communicate a lack of understanding and empathy. You cannot foretell the future accurately; therefore you cannot honestly say that there is nothing to worry about. Such verbal behavior belittles the person who feels he/she has legitimate problems, and it discourages further expression of feelings and trust, although it may relieve your own anxieties.

Using cliches, stereotyped responses, trite expressions, and empty or patronizing verbalisms stated without thought, such as, "It's always worse at night," "I know," "You'll be OK," or "Who is to say?" makes the person uncomfortable and prohibits you from maintaining objectivity. Such statements, unfortunately common, do not allow for any expression of feelings or show of understanding. You cannot understand a person as he/she really is if you respond automatically. Also, do not jump to conclusions based on initial impressions.

Being too strongly opinionated in any aspect of your conversation with another presents a barrier since you do not allow for a different response. Neither should you be totally neutral; recognition should be given for accomplishments. However, approval or agreement and disapproval or disagreement carry overtones of judgment about the person.

Expressing unnecessary approval, stating that something the person does or feels is particularly good, implies that the opposite is bad and limits freedom of the client to think, speak, or act in ways that may displease you. Excess praise arouses undue ambition, competition, and a sense of superiority, closing off possible learning experiences because the person may continue to speak and act only in ways that will bring approval. This approach does not allow the person to live up to his/her potential. Similarly, *excessive agreement*, indicating the person is right, can be equally inhibiting, for you leave little opportunity to modify a point of view later without admitting error. Do not take sides with the person, but use the time to help him/her gather data so that personal opinions and conclusions can be drawn.

Expressing undue disapproval, denouncing another's behavior or ideas, implies that you have the right to pass judgment on the person's thoughts and feelings and that he/she must please you. This moralistic attitude diverts your attention away from the other's needs and directs attention to your own. Also *excessive disagreement*, opposition to another's beliefs or values, implies that he/she is wrong and you are right, and it raises defensiveness. Disagreement usually results in resistance to change and shows lack of respect. Similarly, *rejection*, refusing to consider, or showing comtempt for, the person's idea and behavior, closes off the topic from exploration and also rejects the individual. Every person has no doubt experienced some degree of disapproval, disagreement, and rejection in the past; but such responses from others reinforce loneliness, hopelessness, and alienation and may even contribute to illness. This person may then avoid help rather than risk further disapproval, disagreement, or rejection.

Giving advice; stating personal experiences, opinion, or value judgments; giving pep talks; telling another what should be done—such behavior emphasizes yourself, elevates your self-esteem, and relieves your anxiety; it implies that you know what is best and that the person is incapable of self-direction. Such behavior inhibits spontaneity, prevents struggling with and thinking problems through, and may unnecessarily keep the person in a state of prolonged dependency. Occasional self-disclosure can be useful if brief and pertinent. But talking about yourself is usually of little interest or relevance to the person or family in need of help. Remember that when a person asks for your advice, opinion, or judgment, a decision has often already been made; the person is actually seeking a sounding board or validation for an idea. (Instead, such queries should be met with questions like: "What

have you been told to do?" "What would you like to do?" "What do you plan to do?" Then you can facilitate the person's problem solving by using the effective methods of communication previously described.)

Probing, persistent, pointed, or yes-no questioning or misuse of confrontation places the person on the defensive and makes him/her feel manipulated and valued only for what is being said. Often data obtained will not be accurate because the person gives answers he/she feels you want to hear or, to protect him/herself, will give no answers.

Requiring explanations, demanding proof, challenging or asking "Why . . . ?"—when the person cannot provide a reason for thoughts, feelings, and behavior and for events—this forces an invention of reasons, partial answers, expanded delusions, or rationalization since he/she feels "on the spot." Emotionally-charged topics will be avoided. If the "whys," the reasons, were known, the person could handle the situation.

Belittling the person's feelings (equating intense and overwhelming feelings expressed by the client with those felt by everyone or yourself) implies that such feelings are not valid; that he/she is bad; or that the discomfort is mild, temporary, unimportant, or self-limiting. Such statements indicate a lack of understanding, and no constructive assistance is offered. When someone is concerned with his/her personal misery, he/she is not concerned about nor interested in the misery of others; the client expects you to be concerned and interested in his/her feelings and problems. Don't say, "Everyone feels that way."

Making only literal responses or asking questions related only to practical matters cuts off the exploration of feelings. Individuals often cannot state feelings directly or in conventional phrasing but must use symbolism or statements with hidden meanings. If you respond to symbolism on its literal level, you may be showing a lack of understanding. For example, if the client says, "I'm a real doll," the meaning may be that he/she is, "feeling likable," "less than human," or "conspicuous." Similarly, a statement such as "It's a gray day" may have no reference to the weather.

Interpreting the person's behavior or confronting him/her with analytical meanings of behavior may cause great anxiety, denial, or withdrawal and indicates your limited confidence in his/her capacity to cope with, work through, or understand personal problems. Self-understanding does not come directly from someone else but from assistance from another.

Interrupting or abruptly changing the subject takes control of the conversation, often to escape from something anxiety-provoking. However, the new topic may be of no interest or relevance to the client. Such verbal behavior is rude, shows a lack of empathy, and indicates your anxiety and egocentrism. The other's thoughts and spontaneity are interrupted, the flow of ideas is cut off or becomes confused, and you will get inadequate information or be unable to do effective counseling or teaching. The relevance of what is being said may not be immediately apparent, but you should remain hopeful for later understanding.

Defending or protecting someone or something (nurses, doctors, hospital) from verbal attack by the client is unnecessary and implies that he/she has no right to express impressions, opinions, or feelings. Stating that the criticism is unjust or unfounded doesn't change feelings because such feelings are valid to the client. Moreover, what he/she says may be true. Genuine acceptance, understanding, and competent care of the person can make such defense unnecessary.

Examples of nontherapeutic communication are seen daily and are given in a number of references at the end of the chapter. The effects of nontherapeutic communication on the acutely ill patient in the intensive care unit is described by Mary Anne Noble (85). Nontherapeutic communication is the antithesis of emotional care.

IMPLICATIONS FOR HEALTH PROMOTION

Application to Nursing

Therapeutic communication is basic to humanistic nursing in any setting, with any client. You must recognize, own, and cope with personal feelings in the nurse-client-family relationship. Since the main barrier to communication is emotions, you must develop skill in building bridges over these barriers. The basic bridge to effective communication is feeling. Everyone seeks *warmth, security, assurance,* and *appreciation.* When these qualities are present, tough problems can be taken in stride, especially when commitment is combined with skillful use of the methods described in this chapter.

Study yourself to discover those points at which you could be responsible for blocking communication through your own shortcomings. Know your likes and dislikes. Recognize them for what they are and keep them under control. For you to accept another person, you must first accept yourself. You must be aware of your own needs in order to help another meet his/her needs.

Cultivate an understanding of the part played by body language in human interactions and be as aware of what you are saying with your body movements as you are of what others say with theirs. Feelings are frequently expressed by gestures, attitudes, gait and body posture, and facial expressions. For more information on the science of body language, refer to J. Benthall and T. Polhemus (11), R. Birdwhistell (15), C. Christophers (22), I. Eibl-Eibesfeldt (31), P. Ekiman and W. Friesen (32), J. Faust (37), E. Hall (50, 51, 52), R. Harper, et al. (54), R. Harrison (55), M. Knapp (65), A. Scheflen (98), R. Sommer (103), and J. Spiegel and P. Machotka (104).

For the person to make full use of therapeutic communication, he/she must feel safe with you and feel respected by and trusting of you. Revealing one's innermost thoughts and feelings to someone one scarcely knows is difficult for any individual, even when help is needed and expected. Your use of communication techniques in counseling should make no attempt to influence the speed or direction of the person's problem-solving efforts; be a facilitator instead of a doer or a teller.

You are in a key position to apply an understanding of the communication process and to carry out therapeutic communication methods in all kinds of nursing—while conducting routine procedures, teaching, counseling, giving support, or establishing a therapeutic milieu and working with other staff members. Thus you can enable the person and family to achieve optimum wellness and to prevent future health problems. In addition, through communication, you will learn of the effectiveness of the care you have given.

Application to Daily Living

Although this chapter has centered around nurse-client interaction, the discussions of the communication process, of interviewing, and of techniques and blocks to communication could apply equally well to associations with your colleagues and other health team members. In fact, application of all information in this chapter to your everyday relationships with family and friends can promote an increasingly appropriate, harmonious living pattern. The smoother the communication system, the smoother all other systems will function.

Appropriate, realistic, constructive communication between persons is a basic step toward mental, emotional, and, indirectly (but no less significantly), physical health. Communication patterns that block or resist the other person reduce feelings of autonomy and equality and increase feelings of being misunderstood. The resultant emotions —frustration, anger, depression, and the like—will eventually affect the relationship between the persons involved as well as the physiological functioning of the body.

As a nurse you will find yourself refining your personal pattern of communication, practicing therapeutic communication with others, and teaching others patterns of communication that promote health individually, within the family, within the group, and within the community.

REFERENCES

1. Aasterud, Margaret, "Explanation to the Patient," *Nursing Forum,* 2, no. 4 (1963), 36–44.

2. Allport, Floyd, *Theories of Perception and the Concept of Structure.* New York: John Wiley & Sons, Inc., 1955.

3. Almore, Mary, "Dyadic Communication," *American Journal of Nursing,* 79, no. 6 (1979), 1076–77.

4. "Anxiety: Recognition and Intervention—A Programmed Instruction," *American Journal of Nursing,* 65, no. 9 (1965), 130–52.

5. Argyle, Michael, *The Psychology of Interpersonal Behavior.* Baltimore: Penguin Books, 1967.

6. Asch, S. E., "Effects of Group Pressure on the Modification and Distortion of Judgments," in *Groups, Leadership, and Men,* ed. H. Geutzkow. Pittsburgh: Carnegie Institute, 1951.

7. Ball, Geraldine, "Speaking without Words," *American Journal of Nursing,* 60, no. 5 (1960), 692–93.

8. Barnett, Kathryn, "A Theoretical Construct of the Concepts of Touch as They Relate to Nursing," *Nursing Research,* 21, no. 2 (1972), 102–10.

9. Bartholet, M., "Effects of Color on Dynamics of Patient Care," *Nursing Outlook,* 6, no. 10 (1968), 51–53.

10. Bender, R. E., "Communicating with the Deaf," *American Journal of Nursing,* 66, no. 4 (1966), 757–60.

11. Benthall, Jonathan, and Ted Polhemus, eds., *The Body as a Medium of Expression.* New York: E. P. Dutton & Co., Inc., 1975.

12. Bermosk, Loretta, "Interviewing: A Key to Therapeutic Communication in Nursing Practice," *Nursing Clinics of North America,* 1, no. 2 (1966), 205–14.

13. Bigham, Gloria, "To Communicate with Negro Patients," *American Journal of Nursing,* 64, no. 9 (1964), 113–15.

14. Bird, Brian, *Talking with Patients.* Philadelphia: J.B. Lippincott Company, 1965.

15. Birdwhistell, Ray, *Kinesics and Context.* Philadelphia: University of Pennsylvania Press, 1970.

16. Boguslawski, Marie, "The Use of Therapeutic Touch," *Journal of Continuing Education in Nursing,* 10, no. 4 (1979), 9–15.

17. Burkhardt, M., "Response to Anxiety," *American Journal of Nursing,* 69, no. 10 (1969), 2153–54.

18. Burton, Genevieve, *Personal, Impersonal, and Interpersonal Relations,* 3rd ed. New York: Springer Publishing Co., Inc., 1970.

19. Cashar, Leah, and Barbara Dixson, "The Therapeutic Use of Touch," *Journal of Psychiatric Nursing,* 5, no. 5 (1967), 442–51.

20. Coad-Denton, Alice, "Therapeutic Superficiality and Intimacy," in *Clinical Practice in Psychosocial Nursing,* eds. Diane Longo and Rex Williams, pp. 28–40. New York: Appleton-Century-Crofts, 1978.

21. Christo, S., "A Nursing Approach to Adult Aphasia," *Canadian Nurse,* 74, no. 8 (1978), 34–39.

22. Christoffers, Carol, "Movigenic Intervention: An Expanded Dimension," *Journal of Psychiatric Nursing and Mental Health Services,* 6, no. 6 (1968), 349–60.

23. Cohen, M., "Easy to Listen To," *American Journal of Nursing,* 66, no. 9 (1966), 1999–2001.

24. Cooper, Jeffrey, "Actions Really Do Speak Louder Than Words," *Nursing '79,* 9, no. 4 (1979), 113–18.

25. Davis, Anne J., "The Skills of Communication," *American Journal of Nursing,* 63, no. 1 (1963), 66–70.

26. Davis, Flora, *Inside Intuition: What We Know about Nonverbal Communication.* New York: McGraw-Hill Book Company, 1973.

27. DeThomaso, Marita, "Touch Power and the Screen of Loneliness," *Perspectives in Psychiatric Care,* 9, no. 3 (1971), 112–17.

28. Durr, Carol, "Hands That Help—But How?" *Nursing Forum,* 10 (1971), 392–400.

29. Dye, Mary C., "Clarifying Patients' Communication," *American Journal of Nursing,* 63, no. 8 (1963), 56–59.

30. Egolf, Donald, and S. Chester, "Speechless Messages," *Hearing and Speech Action,* 43, no. 4 (1975), 12–15.

31. Eibl-Eibesfeldt, I., "Similarities and Differences between Cultures in Expressive Movements," *Nonverbal Communication,* ed. R. A. Hinde, pp. 297–312. Cambridge, England: Cambridge University Press, 1972.

32. Ekiman, Paul, and Wallace Friesen, *Unmasking the Face.* Englewood Cliffs, N.J.: Prentice-Hall, Inc., 1975.

33. Elder, R., "What Is the Patient Saying?" *Nursing Forum,* 2, no. 1 (1963), 25–37.

34. Eldred, S., "Improving Nurse-Patient Communication," *American Journal of Nursing,* 60, no. 11 (1960), 1600–1602.

35. Enelow, Allen, and Scott Swisher, *Interviewing and Patient Care,* 2nd ed. New York: Oxford University Press, 1979.

36. Evans, Frances, *Psychosocial Nursing: Theory and Practice in Hospital and Community Mental Health,* pp. 103–41. New York: Macmillan Publishing Co., Inc., 1971.

37. Faust, Julius, *Body Language.* New York: M. Evans and Co., Inc., 1970.

38. Flynn, G., "The Nurse's Role: Interference or Intervention?" *Perspectives in Psychiatric Care,* 7, no. 4 (1969), 170–76.

39. Freund, H., "Listening with Any Ear at All," *American Journal of Nursing,* 69, no. 8 (1969), 1650–53.

40. Gibran, Kahlil, *The Prophet,* p. 21. New York: Alfred A. Knopf, Inc., 1963.

41. Goffman, Irving, *Relations in Public Places.* New York: Basic Books, Inc., 1971.

42. Goldin, P., and B. Russell, "Therapeutic Communication," *American Journal of Nursing,* 69, no. 9 (1969), 1928–30.

43. Gombrich, E. H., "The Visual Images," *Scientific American,* 227, no. 3 (1972), 82–96.

44. Goodykoontz, Lynne, "Touch: Attitudes and Practice," *Nursing Forum,* 18, no. 1 (1979), 4–17.

45. Grasha, Anthony, *Practical Application of Psychology.* Cambridge, Mass.: Winthrop Publishers, Inc., 1978.

46. Greenhill, Maurice H., "Interviewing with a Purpose," *American Journal of Nursing,* 56, no. 10 (1956), 1259–62.

47. Gunther, Bernard, *Sense Relaxation.* New York: Crowell-Collier Books, 1968.

48. Guralnik, David, ed., *Webster's New World Dictionary,* 2nd College Ed. New York: William Collins & World Publishing Co., Inc., 1972.

49. Haggerty, Virginia, "Listening: An Experiment in Nursing," *Nursing Forum,* 10, no. 4 (1971), 382–91.

50. Hall, Edward, *Hidden Dimension.* New York: Doubleday & Co., Inc., 1966.

51. ——, "Proxemics," in *Nonverbal Communication,* ed. Shirley Weitz, pp. 205–29. New York: Oxford University Press, 1974.

52. ——, *The Silent Language.* New York: Doubleday & Co., Inc., 1959.

53. Hardiman, M., "Interviewing or Social Chit-Chat?" *American Journal of Nursing,* 71, no. 7 (1971), 1379–81.

54. Harper, Robert, Arthur Wiens, and Joseph Matarazzo, *Nonverbal Communication: The State of the Art.* New York: John Wiley & Sons, Inc., 1978.

55. Harrison, Randall, *Beyond Words.* Englewood Cliffs, N.J.: Prentice-Hall, Inc., 1974.

56. Hays, J., and K. Larson, *Interacting with Patients.* New York: Macmillan Publishing Co., Inc., 1963.

57. Hess, E. H., "Attitude and Pupil Size," *Scientific American,* 212 (April 1965), 46–54.

58. ——, "The Role of Pupil Size in Communication," *Scientific American,* 233, no. 5 (1975), 110–19.

59. Hewitt, H., and B. Pesznecker, "Blocks to Communicating with Patients," *American Journal of Nursing,* 64, no. 7 (1964), 101–3.

60. Jakobson, Roman, "Verbal Communication," *Scientific American,* 227, no. 3 (1972), 73–80.

61. Johnson, B., "The Meaning of Touch in Nursing," *Nursing Outlook,* 13, no. 2 (1965), 59–60.

62. Jungman, Lynne, "When Your Feelings Get in the Way," *American Journal of Nursing,* 79, no. 6 (1979), 1074–75.

63. Juzwiak, M., "How Skilled Interviewing Helps Patients and Nurses," *R.N.,* 29, no. 8 (1966), 33 ff.

64. King, Imogene, *Towards a Theory for Nursing.* New York: John Wiley & Sons, Inc., 1971.

65. Knapp, Mark, *Nonverbal Communication in Human Interaction,* 2nd ed. New York: Holt, Rinehart and Winston.

66. Krieger, Dolores, "Therapeutic Touch: The Imprimatur of Nursing," *American Journal of Nursing,* 75, no. 5 (1975), 784-87.

67. Krieger, Dolores, Erik Pepper, and Sonia Ancoli, "Therapeutic Touch: Searching for Evidence of Physiological Change," *American Journal of Nursing,* 79, no. 4 (1979), 660-65.

68. Kron, Thora, *Communication in Nursing.* Philadelphia: W. B. Saunders Company, 1967.

69. LaMeri, Russell, *Dance Composition: The Basic Elements.* Lee, Mass.: Jacobs Pillow Dance Festival, Inc., 1965.

70. Little, D. E., "The Say-Something-Tell-Nothing Concept of Nursing," *Nursing Forum,* 2, no. 1 (1963), 38-45.

71. Litwack, Lawrence, Janice Litwack, and Mary Ballou, *Health Counseling.* New York: Appleton-Century-Crofts, 1980.

72. MacKinnon, Roger, and Robert Michels, *The Psychiatric Interview in Clinical Practice,* pp. 1-64. Philadelphia: W. B. Saunders Company, 1971.

73. Mahl, George, *Gestures and Body Movements in Interviews.* Paper prepared for the Third Research in Psychotherapy Conference, Chicago, June 1-4, 1966.

74. Manthey, M., "A Guide for Interviewing," *American Journal of Nursing,* 67, no. 10 (1967), 2088-90.

75. Mattes, Norman, "Are You Listening? *American Journal of Nursing,* 58, no. 6 (1958), 827-28.

76. Meadow, Lloyd, and Gertrude Gass, "Problems of the Novice Interviewer," *American Journal of Nursing,* 63, no. 2 (1963), 97-99.

77. Meyers, M., "The Effect of Types of Communication on Patients' Reactions to Stress," *Nursing Research,* 13, no. 2 (1964), 126-31.

78. Mickens, Patricia, "The Influence of the Therapist on Resistive Silence," *Perspectives in Psychiatric Care,* 9, no. 4 (1971), 161-66.

79. Miller, Lynn, "An Explanation of Therapeutic Touch," *Nursing Forum,* 18, no. 3 (1979), 278-87.

80. Montagu, Ashley, *Touching: The Human Significance of Skin.* New York: Columbia University Press, 1971.

81. Muencke, M., "Overcoming the Language Barrier," *Nursing Outlook,* 18, no. 4 (1970), 53-54.

82. Muller, Theresa, "Dynamics of Communication in Nursing," *American Journal of Nursing,* 63, no. 1 (1963), 9-16.

83. Murray, Jeanne, "Self-Knowledge and the Nursing Interview," *Nursing Forum,* 2, no. 1 (1963), 69-79.

84. Murray, Ruth, and Judith Zentner, *Nursing Concepts for Health Promotion,* 2nd ed. Englewood Cliffs, N.J.: Prentice-Hall, Inc., 1979.

85. Noble, Mary Anne, "Communication in the ICU: Therapeutic or Disturbing?" *Nursing Outlook,* 27, no. 3 (1979), 195-98.

86. O'Sullivan, Ann, "Privileged Communication," *American Journal of Nursing,* 80, no. 5 (1980), 947-50.

87. Paynich, Mary, "Cultural Barriers to Nurse Communication," *American Journal of Nursing,* 64, no. 2 (1964), 87-90.

88. Peplau, Hildegarde, *Interpersonal Relations in Nursing.* New York: G. P. Putnam's Sons, 1952.

89. ____, *Basic Principles of Patient Counseling,* 2nd ed. Philadelphia: Smith, Kline and French Laboratories, 1969.

90. ____, "Talking with Patients," *American Journal of Nursing,* 70, no. 7 (1970), 964-66.

91. Piotrowski, M., "Aphasia: Providing Better Nursing Care," *Nursing Clinics of North America,* 13, no. 3 (1978), 543-54.

92. Pirandello, L., "Language and Thought," *Perspectives in Psychiatric Care,* 8, no. 5 (1970), 230 ff.

93. Polhemus, Ted, ed., *The Body Reader: Social Aspects of the Human Body.* New York: Pantheon Books, Inc., 1978.

94. Prange, A., and H. Martin, "Aids to Understanding Patients, *American Journal of Nursing,* 62, no. 7 (1962), 98-100.

95. Ramaekers, Sister Mary James, "Communication Blocks Revisited," *American Journal of Nursing,* 79, no. 6 (1979), 1079-81.

96. Rodger, B., "Therapeutic Communication and Post-hypnotic Suggestion," *American Journal of Nursing,* 72, no. 4 (1972), 714-17.

97. Ruesch, Jurgen, and Gregory Bateson, *Communication.* New York: W. W. Norton & Co., Inc., 1951.

98. Scheflen, Albert, *Body Language and Social Order.* Englewood Cliffs, N.J.: Prentice-Hall, Inc., 1972.

99. ____, "Quasi-Courtship Behavior in Psychotherapy,"

in *Nonverbal Communication,* ed. Shirley Weitz, pp. 182–98. New York: Oxford University Press, 1974.

100. "Simple Courtesy and the Hard of Hearing," St. Louis Hearing and Speech Center, St. Louis, Missouri, 1977.

101. Skipper, James, "Communication and the Hospitalized Patient," in *Social Interaction and Patient Care,* eds. James Skipper and Robert Leonard, pp. 61–82. Philadelphia: J. B. Lippincott Company, 1965.

102. Skipper, James, D. Tagliacozzo, and H. Mauksch, "What Communication Means to Patients," *American Journal of Nursing,* 64, no. 4 (1964), 101–3.

103. Sommer, Robert, *Personal Space.* Englewood Cliffs, N.J.: Prentice-Hall, Inc., 1969.

104. Speigel, John, and Pavel Machotka, *Messages of the Body.* New York: The Free Press, 1974.

105. Suhrie, Eleanor Brady, "The Importance of Listening," *Nursing Outlook,* 8, no. 12 (1960), 687.

106. Tarasuk, M., J. Rhymes, and R. Leonard, "An Experimental Test of the Importance of Communication Skills for Effective Nursing," in *Social Interaction and Patient Care,* eds. James Skipper and Robert Leonard, pp. 110–20. Philadelphia: J. B. Lippincott Company, 1965.

107. Taylor, M., "The Process Recording: Aid to Interviewing," *Canadian Nurse,* 64, no. 10 (1968), 49.

108. Thomas, M., J. Baker, and N. Estes, "Anger: A Tool for Developing Self-Awareness," *American Journal of Nursing,* 70, no. 12 (1970), 2586–90.

109. Travelbee, Joyce, *Intervention in Psychiatric Nursing.* Philadelphia: F. A. Davis Company, 1969.

110. Ujhely, Gertrud, "Touch: Reflections and Perceptions," *Nursing Forum,* 18, no. 1 (1979), 18–32.

111. Underwood, P., "Communication through Role Playing," *American Journal of Nursing,* 71, no. 6 (1971), 1184–86.

112. Veninga, Robert, "Communications: A Patient's Eye View," *American Journal of Nursing,* 73, no. 2 (1973), 320–22.

113. Waddell, Elizabeth, "Quality Touching to Communicate Caring," *Nursing Forum,* 18, no. 3 (1979), 288–92.

114. Ward, Anita, "My Silent Patient," *Perspectives in Psychiatric Care,* 7, no. 2 (1969), 87–91.

115. Watzlawich, P., J. Beavin, and D. Jackson, *Pragmatics of Human Communication.* New York: W. W. Norton & Co., Inc., 1967.

116. Weiss, S. J., "The Language of Touch," *Nursing Research,* 28, no. 2 (1979), 76–80.

117. Wicks, Robert, *Counseling Strategies and Intervention Techniques for the Human Services.* Philadelphia: J. B. Lippincott Company, 1979.

118. Wilson, L., "Listening," in *Behavioral Concepts and Nursing Intervention*, coord, C. Carlson, pp. 153–70. Philadelphia: J. B. Lippincott Company, 1970.

INTERVIEW

119. Leighninger, R. D., Director, St. Louis Society for the Blind, St. Louis Missouri.

6

The Helping Relationship

Study of this chapter will assist you to:

1. Discuss your nursing role with the emotionally ill person and his/her family.

2. Differentiate between the social interchange and the helping relationship.

3. Describe characteristics of a helping person and explore how these apply to yourself.

4. Define characteristics of the helping relationship and explore behaviors that indicate these characteristics to the client.

5. Discuss principles of human behavior and give examples of how they apply to a client.

6. Review guidelines for your behavior in a helping relationship and relate them to principles of human behavior and characteristics of a helping relationship.

7. Discuss constraints in a helping relationship and how these behaviors can be avoided.

8. Explore examples of nontherapeutic behaviors that could arise while you are working with a client.

9. Describe the phases of the nurse-client relationship and the characteristic behaviors of nurse and client in each phase.

10. Explore how to adapt behavior in order to establish a therapeutic relationship with a verbally or sensory-impaired person.

11. Work with a client to establish and maintain a relationship.

12. Analyze your behavior in a relationship with a client and evaluate your effectiveness.

This chapter contributed by Ruth Murray, R.N., M.S.N.

THE NURSE AS COUNSELOR AND THERAPIST

As you use the nursing process daily with a client, you will function in a variety of nursing roles, including that of counselor or nurse therapist. (See Chapter 4). There are many areas in which counseling is indicated. Counseling does not necessarily require major problems; it can be useful in any of the following ways (38).

1. Identifying, stating, and reducing or resolving troublesome feelings, anxiety, and stress.
2. Clarifying conflict; ordering of needs and goals.
3. Formulating a decision; sorting out alternatives and variables; gaining different perspectives; setting either short- or long-term goals.
4. Clarifying and reinforcing values; determining implications or consequences of values, decisions, and actions.
5. Adjusting to developmental or situational crises. (Refer to Chapter 8.)
6. Changing behavior from problem producing to problem solving.
7. Achieving new insights or self-understanding and new levels of maturity.

8. Reducing psychopathology and emotional illness.

Thus, you may do most of your counseling outside of the psychiatric setting. You may be a counselor to a school child or adolescent, a neighbor or friend, new parents, an employee, or a family member, as well as the identified patient. You may counsel in your home, the school or church, the clinic or doctor's office, the senior citizens' center or child day-care center, the hospital or nursing home. You may counsel medical, surgical, or obstetrical clients as well as psychiatric clients.

How the person reacts to you, your attitudes, appearance, and behavior will be influenced at least initially by his/her past experiences with people. If these experiences have been pleasant, he/she will respond more quickly to your caring. If primarily anxiety and tension have been felt in contacts with others, he/she is likely to be distant, to respond slowly, or even to tell you to go away. Your intentions may be tested with overtly obnoxious behavior, but under this apparent rejection of you there will be strong interpersonal needs. Knowing this should stimulate you to continue to reach out, to care.

Essential in the emotional care of the person/ family/group is the establishment and maintenance of a relationship. Your goals may be limited because you cannot always change the person's pathology and you cannot reverse past negative influences, but you can help the person accept self, find meaning in life, accept others, interact with you, and grow from the experience. This total care involves not only physical care but also genuine concern for the client's self-worth as a human, regardless of his/her social value or capacity for achievement (14). *Central to nursing is caring behavior* (37). All of us need loving contact with other people in order to stay human in the fullest sense. Neither the infant nor the emotionally ill person can survive, emotionally or physically, unless someone cares.

This chapter will discuss the helping relationship as it is applicable to any person you care for, not only the emotionally ill client. Specific aspects of the nurse-client relationship will also be discussed in other chapters.

WHAT IS A RELATIONSHIP?

Definitions

Relationship refers to connectedness in interaction, where each person has an effect upon the other. There are different types of relationships: parent-child, husband-wife, teacher-student, friend-friend, and nurse-client. A *helping relationship can be defined as an interpersonal process in which one person facilitates the personal development or growth of another over time by assisting that person to mature; to become more adaptive, integrated, and open to personal experience; and to find meaning in the present situation.*

The *nurse-client relationship results from a series of interactions between a nurse and client over a period of time, with the nurse focusing on the needs and problems of the person/family/group while using the scientific knowledge and specific skills of the nursing profession.* The helping relationship develops through interest in, encounter with, and commitment to the person.

The Social Exchange (as Contrasted to the Nurse-Client Relationship)

The social exchange or interaction consists of the following characteristics, in contrast to the nurse-client relationship.

1. The contact is primarily for pleasure and companionship.
2. Neither person is in a position of responsibility for helping the other.
3. No specific skill or knowledge is required.
4. The interaction is between peers, often of the same social status.
5. The people involved can, and often do, pursue an encounter for the satisfaction of personal or selfish interests.
6. There is no explicit formulation of goals.
7. There is no sense of accountability for the other person.
8. Evaluation of interactions does not concern personal effectiveness in the interaction.

The following pages describe characteristics of the helping person, the helping relationship, and the nurse-client relationship.

CHARACTERISTICS OF THE HELPING PERSON

The capacity to be a helping person is strengthened by a genuine desire to be responsible and sensitive to another person. In addition, experience with a variety of people will increase your awareness of others' reactions and feelings, and the feedback you receive from others will teach you a great deal on both the emotional and cognitive levels.

Characteristics of a helping person in a humanistic approach with a client include being (59):

Respectful—Feeling and communicating an attitude of seeing the client as a unique human being, filled with dignity, worth, and strengths, regardless of outward appearance or behavior; being willing to *work* at communicating with and understanding the client because he/she is in need of emotional care.

Genuine—Communicating spontaneously, yet tactfully, what is felt and thought, with proper timing and without disturbing the client, rather than using professional jargon, facade, or rigid counselor or nurse role behaviors.

Attentive—Conveying an active listening to verbal and nonverbal messages and an attitude of working with the person.

Accepting—Conveying that the person does not have to put on a facade and that the person will not shock you with his/her statements; enabling the client to change at his/her own pace; acknowledging personal and client's feelings aroused in the encounter; to "be for" the client in a nonsentimental, caring way.

Positive—Showing warmth, caring, respect, and agape love; being able to reinforce the client for what he/she does well.

Strong—Maintaining separate identity from the client; withstanding the testing.

Secure—Permitting the client to remain separate and unique; respecting his/her needs and your own; feeling safe as the client moves emotionally close; feeling no need to exploit the other person.

Knowledgeable—Having an expertise based on study, experience, and supervision.

Sensitive—Being perceptive to feelings; avoiding threatening behavior, responding to cultural values, customs, norms as they affect behavior; using knowledge that is pertinent to the client's situation.

Empathic—Looking at the client's world from his/her viewpoint; being open to his/her values, feelings, beliefs, and verbal statements; stating your understanding of his/her verbal or nonverbal expressions of feelings and experiences.

Nonjudgmental—Refraining from evaluating the client moralistically, or telling the client what to do.

Congruent—Being natural, relaxed, trustworthy, and dependable, and demonstrating consistency in behavior and between verbal and nonverbal messages.

Unambiguous—Avoiding contradictory messages.

Creative—Viewing the client as a person in the process of becoming, not being bound by the past, and viewing yourself in the process of becoming or maturing as well.

Other characteristics that correlate highly with being effective in a helping relationship are being open instead of closed in interaction with others, perceiving others as friendly and capable instead of unfriendly and incapable, and perceiving a relationship as freeing instead of controlling another (6).

Establishing and maintaining a relationship or counseling another does not involve putting on a facade of behavior to match a list of characteristics. Rather, both you and the client will change and continue to mature. As the helper, you are present as a total person, blending potentials, talents, and skills while assisting the client to come to grips with his needs, conflicts, and self (47).

Working with another in a helping relationship is challenging and rewarding. You will not always have all the characteristics just described; at times you will be handling personal stresses that will lower your energy and sense of involvement. You may become irritated and impatient while working with the client. Accept the fact that you are not perfect and that you are always in the process of becoming. Analyzing your behavior in relation to the person/family/group can help you to determine your effect on them and can help you to be more effective. Just as you help the person to develop, you will also continue to expand your personality to better gain the above characteristics. As you open a panorama of possibilities to another, your own potential unfolds. Remember that the most important thing you can share with a client is your own uniqueness as a person. As you give of yourself to the client, you will in return be given to—rewarded with warmth and sharing from the client.

The nursing experience in itself can bring about a cool efficiency, an overt indifference, and an impersonal attitude and environment for the client. The distant behavior that may result when a nurse is not rewarded by the work system for demonstrating helping characteristics seems to be an occupational hazard of nursing. Yet, in an increasingly mechanical world we have to remain human and treat our clients as human (18).

CHARACTERISTICS OF THE HELPING RELATIONSHIP

The nurse-client relationship depends primarily on your experience, your attitudes toward self and client, and the nature of your involvement. The relationship develops out of what you and the other person are. Set techniques or rules do not exist to ensure a relationship, but the following discussion may help you understand the components that enhance its achievement.

Rapport

A relationship begins with the ability to establish *rapport, creating a sense of harmony between individuals* (22). To establish rapport quickly, you must have the following social skills and feelings (1):

1. A warm, friendly manner, appropriate smile, and comfortable eye contact.
2. Ability to perceive and treat the other as an equal, to eliminate social barriers, to convey acceptance, and to promote a sense of trust.
3. Ability to establish a smooth, easy pattern of conversation, or silence, when indicated.
4. Ability to find a common interest or experience.
5. Ability to show a keen, empathetic interest in the other, to give full attention, to listen carefully, and to indicate there is plenty of time.
6. Ability to accurately adopt another's terminology and conventions to make the person feel at home.

Trust

Trust is the firm belief in the honesty, integrity, reliability, and justice of another person without fear of outcome, the inner certainty that the other person's behavior is predictable under a given set of circumstances (22, 59).

The capacity to develop a trusting relationship is built upon your attitude toward people, your flexibility in responding, and what you are personally. Techniques and knowledge are not enough. You will learn through experience which aspects of your personality are most effective with and helpful to others. Trust is based on consistency rather than on compatibility. The person cannot reveal him/herself nor share important information unless he/she can rely on you and believes that you will react with the same behavioral characteristics at each session, and that you will keep the content from the interview confidential, as mutually agreed upon. You may have to delay obtaining certain information until a sense of trust is established because the client may feel at first very threatened by an interview or examination (6, 59). In addition, you must feel that you can predict the person's behavior because you have an understanding of that person. If you show fear of the person, he/she will probably lack trust in you and in him/herself.

The emotionally ill person is often slow to respond to your trustworthiness or to feel trust in you. Often this person has a history of being rejected, unloved, exploited, or misused. The person may continue to wait for you to make a wrong move, or to say the wrong thing because of feelings of mistrust toward people from the past. As one client said to this author, "I never met anyone like you. I've never had anybody stay when I act like this. For the first two months I kept thinking you'd tell me not to come back. Instead, when I missed appointments, you'd call me!"

Unconditional Positive Regard and Acceptance

Two qualities often described as essential to a relationship are positive, warm feelings and acceptance (59). Is it possible to give expert and truly professional care and not feel positively toward your client? Most texts and most clients would say no. The human spirit loses its sense of vitality and sometimes even the will to live when surrounded by hostile persons.

Realistically, it is not possible to like everyone, just as it is not possible to establish and maintain a relationship with everyone. But you will find some clients you will be genuinely interested in and can feel affection for; other nurses will respond that way to other clients, although there are a few people whom no one seems to feel any rapport with or interest in. Your willingness to reach out, to stimulate more likable behavior in a client, to learn more about his/her uniqueness will be the result of your *unconditional positive regard, your belief in the dignity, worth, and importance of the person, regardless of his/her behavior* (59).

Every person, when the outer mask is removed, has some likable and interesting characteristic. The rewards of your efforts to become involved with the difficult client will be to learn about the person and his/her life style, and in the process, learn something about yourself, your persistence, your beliefs about people, your commitment to nursing, and your interactional skills. Anyone can respond to someone who is attractive and gracious. The challenge (and the measure of the nurse) lies in the ability to relate to the person everyone else has given up on—such as the hostile or withdrawn person, the person who is readmitted frequently without apparent change in behavior, the grotesque alcoholic, and the wobbly old lady who bites and spits.

Some people are hard to accept. *Acceptance means interest in, concern for, and patience with another because he/she is a human being with dignity; it means avoidance of moralistic judgment; it means the feeling that this person is worth all of your attention, skill, understanding, and energy* (57). Acceptance means to relate to the inner core of the person, understanding but not agreeing with, nor necessarily permitting, inappropriate behavior. Acceptance means not to show your feelings of shock or disapproval aroused by the person's behavior and not to feel a need to control that behavior (55). Acceptance means to acknowledge that the cultural practices about healing are crucial to helping the client feel better or change behavior. Acceptance means recognizing the right of another to have beliefs, values, and standards that contradict your own. You do not condemn the person's behavior; you do not zealously insist that he/she change behavior just because it displeases you. Instead, you assist the person, if possible, to change behavior to become more acceptable to others. The person feels accepted if he feels neither above you nor below you, neither dominated by you nor alone without needed guidance. He/she senses you are not bored by the interaction. If the person feels your acceptance, he/she feels free to disclose private information about him/herself and to call for your assistance without fear or embarrassment. He/she feels at ease with you. He/she feels good about him/herself in your presence. The client may describe feelings of acceptance by saying, "Maybe I shouldn't say this, and to other people, I wouldn't, but you're O.K. You'll hear me out."

Empathy

Unconditional positive regard and acceptance are easier to achieve if you have developed empathic understanding of people. *Empathy is feeling with the person and simultaneously understanding the dynamics of behavior* (59). As you and the client feel and think together, your feelings for him/her impel you to act.

Empathy is the ability to sense the client's private world as if it were your own, without ever losing the "as if" quality; to sense the client's anger, fear, or confusion as if it were your own, without your own feelings getting bound up in the interaction. You may sense what the client is thinking or feeling before such thoughts or feelings are described. The client may say, "You pick up my vibes," or "You *really* do know what I'm talking about!" Empathy involves using your feelings to help the person identify and then understand his/her feelings, problems, and behavior objectively and from a broader frame of reference, from the viewpoint of others. As you help the client understand the factors and feelings underlying his/her behavior, the themes in verbal messages, and the implied feelings behind the behavior, the person can then begin to resolve his/her feelings and to change such behavior.

You are empathic to the degree that you stay open to your environment and to others' behavior and feelings, and to the degree that you are able to abstract from your own life experience, by way of recall or generalizations, common factors that are applicable to the client's problems.

Certain qualities enhance empathic skills. The ability to empathize varies with the client, time, and nurse. Certainly a general interest in people, basic knowledge of human behavior and cultural customs, and a warm, flexible personality will encourage empathy. Other characteristics that enable you to be more empathic are (74):

1. Similarity with the client in values, experiences, social class, culture, occupational and economic level, religion, age, personality traits, or sameness of sex.
2. Ability to be alert, to listen with the "third ear," to become involved in another, to abandon self-consciousness.
3. Ability to cope with egocentricity, anxiety, fears, or other feelings or stresses that might interfere with listening to and feeling with another.
4. Variety of life experiences that help you to acquire a broad understanding of people, flexibility, and spontaneity.
5. Ability to maintain an adequate health and energy level.
6. Ability to interpret correctly and to avoid distorting perceptions.

Empathy involves the following dimensions (8):

1. *Tone*—Expressing warmth and spontaneity nonverbally and verbally.
2. *Pace*—Timing remarks or behavior appropriate to the client's feelings and needs.
3. *Perception*—Abstracting the core or essential meaning of the client's feelings and concerns and discussing them in acceptable terms.
4. *Leading*—Being resourceful in formulating questions or statements that move the interview in the direction of the client's feelings and concerns.
5. *Vocabulary*—Being able to use a variety of words, phrases, or statements that are expressive of emotion.

Empathy is not the same as sympathy or pity. The sympathetic person becomes stricken with emotion because he/she projects self into the other person's place. The sympathizer may be secretly happy that a certain situation has not occurred, or may feel guilty in his/her luck. In contrast, the empathic person shares the experience but maintains objectivity (34). Empathy can be found in any situation, in grief and joy.

Pity is contrary to helping. To cause another to feel like a victim debases the person and conveys that he/she will remain debased and helpless. Pity conveys that the other person receives help because you are obligated and pseudoaltruistic. Spontaneous and genuine helping is done by one human being for another simply because you are both human (6).

How do you communicate empathy? Face the person and maintain eye contact. Adopt an open, relaxed posture. Lean toward the client. Use verbal and nonverbal communication so that the person experiences a feeling of being understood. *Your* statements serve as an emotional mirror or as a reflection of feelings without distorting ideas or giving advice. For example, you may say:

"You feel *caught.*" (using a single word)
"You feel *down in the dumps.*" (using a descriptive or idiomatic phrase)
"You feel like *dancing in the streets.*" (using a behavioral statement)
"You feel *unwanted* because you think *she does not love you.*" (stating primary emotional state and experience underlying the feeling)
"You feel *reluctant to talk* about your problems with me because past experiences with people cause you to *feel uncertain about me too.*" (stating primary feeling and related behavior based on prior experience)

Avoid a response like, "I know how you feel," or "Everyone feels like that." Such a response makes the person unsure about your truly understanding him/her. It is a rote response and is not based on genuine understanding of current feelings.

Talk on the person's level of understanding and adjust your pace of speech and tone of voice to that set by the client. For example, if you use a declarative, harsh tone of voice, it will seem as if you are telling the client what he/she thinks and feels, rather than *reflecting* his/her feelings. Using language that is not understood will convey a lack of respect, regardless of the accuracy of your interpretation.

Evaluate the person's true feelings. Sometimes he/she is not aware of nor ready to admit certain feelings and needs time to be allowed to deny them.

Reflect the person's feelings frequently and tentatively for correction, clarification, elaboration, and validation, and remain open to the response. A client who feels free to correct you moves on to a higher level of self-understanding. If he/she cannot refute your reflection or feels accused by the way you respond, he/she builds up defenses and then withdraws, thereby defeating the primary purpose of the relationship. Some examples of how to begin your reflections are: "If I understand you correctly, you feel . . .," or "Is this right?"

Respond actively and frequently enough to the client without interrupting, to indicate that you are focusing on his/her speech and feelings (43).

Focus on feelings rather than on the content or intellectual ideas or opinions. Refer to the content or the basis for the feelings only *after* you speak to the feelings. For example, you may paraphrase a client's description of the husband's behavior when she tries to talk to him: "You feel angry and hurt because you can't talk about your feelings to your husband and because he doesn't understand your real needs." "You feel belittled because no matter what you say to your husband, he responds with jokes about your feelings rather than saying he cares."

At times you may use self-disclosure to briefly refer to having experienced what the client is describing, in order to help the client realize he/she is not alone in this situation, that you really do understand, and that there is a need for behavioral change. However, self-disclosure must *never*: (a) place the focus on you instead of on the client; (b) distract the client from his/her work; (c) add to the problems of the client or trigger feelings of concern for you; (d) be overly dramatic or ill-timed.

Be concrete as you reflect and paraphrase the client's message. Speak to *specific* feelings, experiences, and behaviors rather than in vague generalities. Use precise words to describe or clarify. For example, avoid statements like, "Things are bad for you." Instead, be precise, and say, "Today your classmates ridiculed you for being overweight and you feel belittled and angry." Help the client to avoid storytelling but rather to describe relevant content.

Use immediacy; talk about what is happening between yourself and the client in the here and now of the relationship as a way to help the client explore his/her interpersonal style and view self from another frame of reference. Do not dwell on the past, although you may use an understanding of the past to help the person gain new insights and change behavior. Bring in the past as it relates to the present situation or the person's needs.

The ultimate purpose of the empathic response is to convey to the person a depth of understanding about him/her and the situation so that he/she can expand and clarify understanding of self and others (10); thus the client receives relief from loneliness and overcomes feelings of isolation and being alone with problems. Your willingness to understand how the person feels about him/herself and his/her world implies that the viewpoint is valuable. Also, the focus of evaluation is within the client, so that he/she becomes less dependent on the opinions of others and grows to value self. Empathetic understanding is not a passive process, and it will not happen without effort. You must concentrate intensely on the person and listen to your feelings and the client simultaneously. Since intense concentration allows you little time to reflect on personal needs, values, and ideals, it prevents judgmental thoughts or behavior (34).

Improvement of patients is correlated with empathic response, regardless of their diagnoses. Not only are high empathic levels correlated with improvement, but low levels of empathy can contribute to increased disturbance in patients. A lack of empathy displayed by nurses could therefore actually hinder a patient's recovery (32).

Purposeful Communication

A helping relationship involves *careful listening to the client's total message* rather than selective listening to the parts that are most enjoyable or easy. There are times when you will have to ignore your own needs and the clock. You will have to listen to ideas, values, or attitudes contradictory to your own; or listen to offensive language; or observe behavior that makes you uncomfortable. If you cannot see past these factors, you will not be able to be helpful. Be prepared for such communication. At some point in the relationship, work through your own feelings, and respond to the person so that underlying feelings and needs can be handled. Refer to Chapter 5 for in-depth discussion of therapeutic communication.

Confidentiality in the relationship can be a concern. Tell the client that what he/she shares with you is shared generally with your instructor/supervisor to promote your own learning and to enhance your ability to give appropriate care. Although most of what the client tells you will remain between you, the client, and the instructor, there are times that you may have to tell the client that the "secret" will have to be shared with the therapy team. For example, the client who describes a suicidal or homicidal plan should know that you will share this information with the agency staff. Thus he/she will not feel deceived, and the necessary therapy can be initiated by the team with the client and family (40). Honesty with your client has ethical as well as legal implications. (See Chapter 23.) Help the client to realize also that when you chart information told to you, the remarks in the chart include only the content that is significant to the team members. If the client asks to read the chart, obtain information pertinent to your agency about permission.

Goal Formulation

A helping relationship differs from a social relationship in that in the helping relationship there is explicit formulation of goals. There are certain goals that you hope to accomplish, and the client can participate with you in setting these goals. As the relationship progresses, new problems or concerns will be identified, and new goals will have to be set. The relationship is structured in that you share with the client what he/she can expect and you listen to what the client expects of you. Together you determine the course of the relationship; intentions and expectations are verbally and nonverbally conveyed to each other, and the expectations change as the relationship progresses (6).

General goals of the nurse-client relationship include (66):

1. Increasing the person's self-esteem and promoting a positive self-concept and sense of security.
2. Decreasing the person's anxiety to a level that promotes behavioral change in a positive direction.
3. Providing a gratifying, positive experience.
4. Assisting the person in improving communication skills and in participating comfortably with others.

5. Providing the opportunity for the person to grow emotionally.
6. Helping the person find meaning in the life situation.
7. Maintaining and stimulating the person biologically, mentally, emotionally, and socially.
8. Gathering data in order to gain in-depth assessment and provide individualized care.

Humor

Intense interaction between two or more people cannot endure unless a sense of humor surfaces at times. *Humor is the ability to see the ludicrous or the incongruities of a situation, to be amused by one's own imperfections or the whimsical aspects of life, to see the funny side of an otherwise serious situation* (22). Humor does not necessarily mean joking and teasing. It does not involve the put-down of another, and it does not always evoke laughter. Humor may be expressed as a tiny smile that lingers, or the mental chuckle that occurs when you are sober-faced.

The purposes of humor include releasing tension, anxiety, or hostility; cautiously distracting from sadness, crying, or guilt; decreasing social distance; conveying a sense of empathy to another; expressing warmth and affection; encouraging learning or task accomplishment; and denying painful feelings or a threatening situation.

The client may have an experienced use of humor beneath his/her signs of emotional illness or cognitive impairment. He/she may test you with a few dry statements to see if you are really alert and if you can make the cognitive connections that are insinuated. Too often these dry statements receive only a grunt in reply, or worse, they are ignored because the person is labeled senile, confused, or crazy. If you do not respond to rational humor, the person loses emotional and social input and self-esteem. You lose when you cannot expand your mind with humor. You dry up emotionally, and you have lost an opportunity to learn, to mature, and to enjoy.

UNDERSTANDING BEHAVIOR IN THE RELATIONSHIP

Principles of Human Behavior

Basic elements of human behavior to consider in any nurse-client relationship include the following

ideas. Refer also to assumptions about behavior in Chapter 3.

The person is an open system and maintains the self through exchanges with other people and with various environmental stimuli. Input and output are required for life maintenance and reproduction. Since the person is not self-sufficient, he/she must remain open to the ministrations of others in order to have certain needs met (58). The emotionally ill person may be less open to environmental stimuli and other people, and needs encouragement to become more open.

Change in one part of a system produces change(s) in all parts. Helping another produces effects not always anticipated by the helper or by the person receiving help because of the resultant changes in that person. Helping another, that is, forming and maintaining a relationship, does not provide total freedom from discomfort, but it often changes the discomforts or the individual's ability to cope with them. The essence of life is change, not bliss. Helping—relating—affirms and stimulates a person's power to change, to overcome helplessness in adversity (58), to cope with stressors, and to affiliate with people.

Human behavior has purpose or is goal-directed. Therefore, the behavior is commonly preceded by imagining the desired result. The person visualizes the future and tries to bring it about. The helper tries to understand the client by understanding his/her needs, goals, or purposes in order to encourage the client to pursue them, if realistic. Behavior may seem purposeless, but it is directed to meeting needs and goals, even if these are not apparent at first. The goals or satisfactions sought are based on recall of earlier satisfactions and how these were obtained. Because of the tendency to regress under stress, the person who needs help will be hoping to have things done for him/her. Yet, receiving help from a stranger or impersonal caretaker is difficult. On the one hand, if you do not have a good relationship with your client, you may not be aware of the deep-felt need for help. On the other hand, when you do have a helping, trusting relationship, you can expect the person to make extra demands on you when he/she feels great need, indicating feelings of security with you. In response, you may feel impatient or irritable. Your goals and the client's goals may differ, and these differences need to be resolved (55, 56, 58, 59).

When one need or goal is met, the person has energy to pursue another need, interest, or goal (58). Behavior changes direction, but it does not come to an end. You can help the client use time constructively so that he/she can meet priority goals.

Human behavior is learned or unconsciously motivated and is based on past experience. Behavior that had a satisfactory outcome is likely to be repeated; behavior that brought pain is likely to be extinguished. However, people go through different developmental levels, and the conditions under which they have to apply learning will change over time. Human learning can become obsolete; the person may behave in a situation in a way that was appropriate in the past but is inappropriate in the present situation. Thus, he/she needs your help to understand how to change behavior. Whether or not he can unlearn behavior is questionable. Can something once learned ever be extinguished? If what was learned in the past seemed good or brought gratification, it might interfere with learning something new and supposedly better. Additionally, people seem to seek gratification in times of stress by reverting to earlier, more comfortable kinds of behavior. Thus, as a helper, you enable the person to acquire additional learning so that he/she has alternatives in coping. A feeling of being able to choose among alternatives improves the self-image because the person feels less helpless (58). Sometimes behavior occurs without apparent reason and in spite of the client's protestations that he/she doesn't mean to do such acts. This is because unmet needs or tensions are often unconscious motivations. And although anticipations of the future can be a powerful motivator, past experiences often set the stage for current behavior. Thus the unconscious factors and past experiences contribute to the behavior of the emotionally ill person.

If behavior is unsuccessful, tension increases, and self-esteem fails. The unsuccessful person creates a new need, a need for psychological repair. Because the emotionally ill person often feels unsuccessful and worthless, you can foster a positive self-concept and help him/her to a higher level of maturity or to find new coping patterns that improve self-evaluation.

Loneliness is a very basic and common feeling in people, especially in the emotionally ill person. People in distress may have many acquaintances, but they seldom have anyone who has the time, interest, understanding, or skill to help alleviate their suffering. The distressed person feels lonely. You can help to offset the loneliness through an individual relationship. Involvement in a group, as described in the Chapter 11, also offsets loneliness.

Human development is on a spiral of increasing maturity, alternating with periods of status quo or decline. The person grows from helplessness into strength, but periodically returns to some degree of helplessness or earlier form of behavior. The person throughout life needs some experiences of being strong and adequate. You can help the person to combat the helpless or inadequacy feelings and to feel emotionally energetic enough to move forward with developmental tasks. The emotionally ill person needs much support to begin to move up the spiral of emotional health and maturity. There will be times when he/she seems to hold on to feelings of helplessness, dependency, passivity, or immature behavior. An infant never completely has all its dependency needs met. In times of stress this form of dependency is again sought. You, the helper, with your own personal stresses, may also develop regressive tendencies and unconsciously and defensively become an ally of the client's regression. Dependency and helplessness in the client may be used vicariously by the helper to increase feelings of omnipotence and satisfaction or to enhance self-evaluation (58). Such behavior should be guarded against.

Humans have an innate drive toward health, but prolonged and/or severe anxiety may result in personality disorganization and emotional illness (55, 65). Peplau's view of the person is optimistic. Clients are thought to know what they need, although they may need help in becoming aware of their needs (55).

Guidelines for Your Behavior

When you relate to and work with any client, consider the following guidelines and approaches that build on the principles discussed in Chapter 5.

The total complement of nonverbal clues should be observed; facial expression alone is not a good indicator of feelings. For example, the client's smile can be a mask for anxiety, fear, uncertainty, anger, or suspicion. Also be aware that your facial expression may not convey what you intend or actually feel. When you counsel, be conscious of your facial expression and body posture. Sit comfortably, feet on floor, arms in an open position, hands relaxed, in order to convey an open and calm feeling. What is your facial expression? It is relaxed and welcoming with a pleasant smile? Or do you smile excessively, frown, look worried or stern? Look at the person; hold eye contact without being aggressive or intrusive. Are your eyes warm or cold? How do you move your eyes? When you look at

the person, you indicate interest, attention, listening, caring. When you look away from the person, you temporarily lose track of what is being said; you may be focusing on what you plan to say rather than on the feelings between you and the client. Your eyes tend to dart upward when you focus on facts or content of the dialogue, or when you state clichés, or when you feel superior or judgmental. Eyes glancing down may convey a barrier, feelings of uninvolvement, or inferiority. Sideward glances may indicate evasiveness or suspicion to the client. What is the position of your head? Try to keep your head level and square on your shoulders. A tilted head may convey doubt, disinterest, disapproval, lack of genuineness. How do you use your hands? Palms or hands held upward indicate that you want the client to continue talking. Hands held down and passively do not invite information. Hands held up and vertically say "Stop." Such a hand position may help you interrupt unobtrusively in order to respond to what the client is saying. Where do you place your feet? The sole of the foot directed toward the client as you cross or stretch your legs may nonverbally say you are kicking the client. If you lean back in the chair, you may be conveying lack of interest in, or superiority toward, the client. Arms crossed over the chest may convey an air of authority or judgmental attitudes.

The *quiet, cooperative, or depressed person has as great a need to talk and to receive attention as does the outgoing, uncooperative, or demanding person.* The quiet client is popular, but cooperation may be a way of bargaining for security and attention. Refer to Chapter 5 and Unit IV for suggestions on how to talk with clients with different kinds of behavior.

Some clients will be hard to accept and will cause you anxiety because they are demanding, regressed, uninhibited in action or speech, stubborn, hallucinating, suspicious, or, because of their illness, generally unpleasant to be with. *Such behavior may be the best that the individual can demonstrate at that point;* behavior is the result of trying to handle feelings and maintain identity and integrity. Often such behavior is difficult to tolerate because it reminds you of characteristics you do not like within your own personality, or it reminds you that you could also behave like that when you are under stress, ill, or old. The person may be embarrassed by his/her behavior even though he/she cannot control it. Without belittling or punishing the person, you can convey that the nature of the behavior is temporary, that the person is accepted even though the behavior is unacceptable, that you trust his/her capacity to grow and evolve more appropriate behavior as emotional health returns.

If tears make you uncomfortable, consider that the crying client is paying you a great compliment; that is, he/she feels secure enough with you to cry in your presence. The person senses your acceptance and caring. Most clients know the social sanctions against crying and will feel embarrassed when tears come spontaneously. Although mood is more unstable in the emotionally ill, and the person may cry more easily—this does not necessarily mean he/she will cry in front of just anyone. Convey that it is all right to cry, that you do not consider the person a baby or less of a man or woman. Give the person time to regain composure before continuing the conversation or activity.

Clients of different ethnic or racial backgrounds may react differently with you because of their past experiences with people. First, realize the meaning of Sullivan's One Genus Postulate: All people are more similar than different (65). Acknowledge similarities as well as differences. If the person has suffered much rejection or persecution during life, he/she may be suspicious of your intentions and behavior as you try to establish a relationship. Social conditions and related life stressors can contribute to negative self-concept in people from a minority culture. The Black, Oriental, Spanish-speaking or American Indian living in the United States will be keenly mindful of the history of abuse their people have suffered. Thus their way to avoid continued rejection and hurt is to remain unresponsive to contacts from others. Yet the person has a need for care, attention, respect, and security. Do not be rebuffed by apathy, withdrawal, or mute behavior. Acknowledge verbally that you know that life can be difficult.

Consistent availability combined with intervals of deeper exploration of feelings will be accepted over time. Sometimes it takes months before the rejecting person senses and responds to your interest and is able to establish trust. The person from a minority culture may perceive counseling or psychiatric service as a privilege only for middle-class whites and may be reluctant to become involved in something so unfamiliar that also involves closeness with another. The apparently passive attitude may be related to a fatalistic outlook about improving life conditions as well as to lack of trust in you and what you are attempting to do. Over time you can help the client avoid using color or cultural background as a defense and instead use a problem-solving approach to identifying alternatives for behavior.

You may become attached to, or possessive of, a client and be unwilling to relinquish him/her to the family when the discharge date arrives. This frequently happens in the case of children, but it can happen with clients of any age. There is nothing wrong with liking a client. In fact, it helps. But your emotional involvement with that person will be different from that with a friend or relative. Except in the nursing home or long-term residence for the aged, your relationship is not permanent; you begin as strangers and you are in a service role to the person. The best way to show that you like someone is to accept the person as he/she is, meet his/her needs promptly, and help expand his/her relationships to others. Termination means that you have achieved a goal. Further, the most significant people to the client are usually his family. Thus helping the client and family to relate more comfortably to each other is usually necessary.

The Superficiality-Intimacy Continuum in Relationships

Both social and therapeutic relationships have levels of superficiality and intimacy, but the manifestation of these levels differs (13). In a social relationship, *superficiality is characterized by limited self-disclosure, discussion of general topics, and minimum knowledge of the other participant.* Rarely are personal goals, perceptions, and needs shared. Such interactions occur in large social gatherings, in time-limited interactions, and in initial social contacts. In such a social relationship, *intimacy is shared interpersonal closeness in an interaction where there is awareness of psychologic interdependence, mutual acceptance of each other, feelings of safety and security, a nonevaluative exchange, and mutual disclosure of perceptions, needs, desires, behavior, and feelings.* An atmosphere of closeness, satisfaction, general support, acceptance, and trust results because actions occur among close friends, family, and housemates (13).

In a therapeutic relationship, the progression from superficiality to intimacy emerges differently. There is not the same kind of mutual sharing. Although you may share some feelings briefly, primarily the client shares feelings and thoughts *with you.* You facilitate the client's explanation of needs, taking risks, problem solving, and developing coping skills. The client is not asked to respond to your

needs. Thus there is not the interdependence that exists in social relations (13).

Table 6-1 compares how a helping relationship moves from the superficial to the intimate.

TABLE 6-1.   Superficial to Intimate Continuum in Therapeutic Relationships

CHANGES THAT OCCUR	STEPS IN DIRECTION OF CHANGE FROM SUPERFICIAL TO INTIMATE
Focus of interaction	1. Topics about unknown events or people, or about people and events that are understood by therapist. 2. Topics are mutually known and are of concern to the client. Therapist does not share concerns or problems of personal life.
Pertinence of topic	1. Conversation is like a social exchange until trust is established. 2. Topics are increasingly pertinent to client's needs and feelings.
Time orientation	1. Conversation is future-oriented; avoids present and past concerns. 2. Focuses on present feelings and concerns; explores past issues and future anticipations in relation to present problem.
Relationship of experiences to topics	1. Lack of involvement or interest in topic at hand; events or feelings vaguely or abstractly described. 2. Specific experiences, feelings, and perceptions explored in depth, clearly and concretely, with sense of involvement by client and nurse. Distortion reduced.
Use and expression of feelings	1. Discussion of feelings avoided or brief. 2. Discussion of feelings in increasing depth, at client's pace.
Recognition of individual worth and autonomy	1. Respect for, but superficial involvement between client and therapist. 2. Integrity, worth, autonomy, and uniqueness of client are understood and respected. Therapist values own autonomy and uniqueness. Mutual consensus in adopting rules for interaction. No competition between client and therapist. Both develop emotionally.

Ethics in the Relationship: Four Models

Consider the ethical aspects of your relationship with the client. There are four models for looking at ethical relationships (2, 68).

Priestly Model

The health professional is paternalistic to the patient who comes for treatment, comfort, and counsel. The patient cannot expect to collaborate with the professional in goal setting or planning.

The professional makes all the necessary decisions without considering the patient's values. Often the emotionally ill person is treated in this way.

Engineering Model

The health professional is viewed as an applied scientist without values related to health care. The professional presents the facts to the client, who is expected to make the decision related to treatment and care. The professional then carries out the client's wish, even if it is contrary to the professional's moral code. Or the professional sets aside personal values and carries out requests of another professional, the agency, or system. The professional under this model acts, or is treated as, a means to an end. For example, the nurse whose only role is to give medications and assist with electroshock treatments, wait for physician's orders for everything, and direct patients in the hospital from one activity to another operates under this ethic.

Contractual Model or Covenant

The health professional and client collaborate to identify obligations, responsibilities, and benefits for both parties during the treatment period. Clients are viewed as having control over significant decisions affecting their lives and bodies. The professional takes no action without consulting the client, or the family if the client is unable to respond. However, the client realizes that the professional has both the knowledge and expertise necessary to make some decisions, as well as the skills to carry out certain tasks, which the client cannot do. Thus, the client does not expect to be consulted on all details. Under this model, the professional has the right not to make a contract if the client is requesting services that are against the professional's moral code or value system. This model values both professional and client and allows each to articulate personal values prior to decision making. The limits in this model refer to: (1) the agency setting in which the nurse is employed and where she/he is expected to carry out duties, regardless of personal values and feelings, and (2) the person or family who cannot or will not identify goals and needs or make decisions when a life-threatening situation or crisis is present. This ethic is pertinent when the client presents self for treatment, but there are times that the client is so ill that the family is the contractual party.

Collegial Model

The client is treated as a colleague or peer. This model is probably unrealistic in most situations and at times could be detrimental to either the professional or the client, especially if the professional lost objectivity about the treatment or care that was essential or actions that should be avoided for the client's well-being.

Constraints in the Helping Relationship

Certain limits exist for both you, the helper, and the client. Relationship means involvement and commitment; it takes time. The client's dependency may create demands for extra time or responsibility. You will have to consider feelings and needs, meet important demands, and set limits whenever necessary (5). An honest response about your limitations of time and energy is most helpful. The person usually accepts the fact that you have other demands placed upon you—if they are explained objectively. Such honesty often stimulates the person to try to do all possible for him/herself. If you can respond without anger or without a sense of excessive obligation, the person will not feel rejected. Thus, undue dependency will be avoided.

Differences between you, the helper, and the client can be an obstacle to a satisfactory exchange. Perceiving each other as different will prevent two people from coming closer. Helping is an overcoming of distance and difference between helper and client. You cannot empathize or engage in sharing if the real differences of two unique persons, such as age, sex, educational level, or sociocultural background, are not worked through (56).

Inequity in a relationship, in which the client's needs are sufficiently met but there is insufficient gratification for the helper, may cause the ending of a relationship. If you feel depleted and cannot feel a sense of doing good, being worthwhile, learning about people and life, developing professional skills, or maturing, you can no longer meet the dependency needs of the other. Much of this sense of depletion or inequity can be prevented if you have other relationships—with friends and colleagues—to support you. You should not expect to have personal needs, other than those just listed, met by the client. Instead, focus on his/her needs. There is not much tangible payoff. You must have considerable ego strength if you are to interact in a therapeutic way with a number of clients. You cannot live out your problems and find answers by listening to the client. This may be one reason why some nurses never form relationships with clients.

Yet, you may have certain needs, as a helper, met through client relationships. Loneliness in the client is relieved by the security of being attended to, and your loneliness may be relieved by people seeking your help. The client's sense of helplessness needs hope that things will get better, that there are other ways of handling the situation, and that it won't cost too much in time and money. And you may have a need to convey hope, optimism, and confidence and to use your imagination and skills to meet the challenge of stimulating another to handle a situation. You may need to convey to the client what you have learned by overcoming obstacles in your life (58). While encouraging a client, you must control your ambitions for his/her improvement.

The client may not be willing to change sufficiently to resolve the problem. The person may not be able to give up his/her discomforts because these may be a core part of his/her identity (58). Review the steps in the change process, Chapter 7, to understand why the client may be unable to change.

As a helper, you may use the professional role to resolve your own developmental difficulties that remain from earlier life. The risk is that as the client talks, you will relive your own conflicts and fears of past developmental eras. In that case, the client's problems may not be resolved; they are likely to be maintained unconsciously by you as you work out your own problems through the person. You must be aware of any inappropriate feelings and overreactions. Keep your personal life out of the reaction to and concern with the client. You will also need a change in your professional and personal life at times so that you will be able to remain helpful and feel revitalized. Continuing education and seeking help from a friend or counselor by talking through your reactions and the possible causes can serve this purpose (56, 58).

As a helper, you may treat the client or his/her problems as trivial. It is important for anyone in distress to feel that his/her existence has meaning. If the client does not have a philosophical, religious, or political affiliation that permits transcending personal destiny, the helping existence can be the only chance to gain such meaning. Treating the client as insignificant in the formative states of the relationship increases the burden of loneliness and helplessness, and it decreases the chance of a working relationship (58).

Your inability to recognize or handle the transference phenomenon will hinder progress in a relationship. Arising most likely during the identification phase of the relationship, **transference is the process whereby the client inappropriately, unrealistically, but unconsciously displaces onto you or invests in you, the helper, the patterns of behavior and emotional reactions that originated with authority figures in childhood, usually with parents.** Transference may be positive; that is, all the attitudes, emotions, or responses to you are loving or happy because the client sees in you his/her parents who fostered such responses. Positive transference also includes expression of unmet needs or desires, or delegated omnipotence; that is, the person repeatedly states how wonderful you are and how he/she wishes to be like you. Negative transference occurs when the client responds to you with anger or hate, such as he/she felt toward his/her parents earlier (40). Either negative or positive transference can be threatening to you. The client who has positive feelings may tell you, "You are perfect," "You are an angel," "You are the Great Spirit (or God) moving in me." This may be seen as manipulating or delusional. Yet the client may be talking about your importance to him/her. The negative or rebellious statements may be interpreted as "acting out" rather than a behavior that is developmentally based and must be worked through.

Transference is not simply positive or negative, and it is not age- or sex-related. It is a re-creation of the various stages of the emotional development or a reflection of complex attitudes toward others who were important earlier in life. Transference is triggered because the client is developing a closeness to you. Realistic characteristics about you can trigger transference: your appearance, age, sex, personal manner, social, and ethnic background. The desire for affection, respect, and gratification of dependency needs may also trigger transference. The client seeks evidence that you can or will love him/her, often through making demands upon you. Legitimate or realistic requests should be met early in the relationship. Later, refusals to meet requests that are unnecessary or that the person can meet, along with discussion and interpretation of the significance of this behavior, are warranted (40).

Questions about your personal life may involve

a different kind of transference. Most often these questions are concerned about your status or ability to understand the person. Occasionally a direct answer to the question is appropriate, but usually it is more appropriate to inquire, "What leads to your question?" or "What did you have in mind?" It may be helpful to interpret, for example, "You ask about my age because you are unsure of me?" (40).

Competitive feelings resulting from earlier relationships with siblings or parents may be expressed toward you in transference. Such a client clearly strives to be one jump ahead of you; he/she makes belittling and disparaging remarks about you, challenges your statements or abilities, or constantly interrupts you. When the person is obviously competitive, it is helpful to make a remark about it, for example, "I didn't know we were having a race," or "You feel that you are competing with me?" Or you may wish to explore earlier or current relationships with siblings or parents. At times, it is best to ignore competitive behavior; often such behavior is motivated by feelings of inferiority (40).

Because of transference male patients may show interest in the power, status, or economic success of a male nurse, whereas they may be concerned about the motherly, seductive, or domineering behavior of the female nurse. Female clients are frequently concerned about the male nurse's attitude toward the role of women, whether he can be seduced, what his wife is like, and what sort of father he is. The female client may feel competitive toward the female nurse and be interested in her career and adequacy as a woman and mother (40).

Or clients may treat you as a child, for example, by bringing food or other gifts, cautioning you about health or hard work, or reprimanding you. Elderly male clients may offer fatherly advice about financial matters, home, or cars; elderly females may give maternal advice (40).

As the helper, you may experience the phenomenon of **countertransference**—*inappropriate, emotional response to the client as if he/she were an important figure in your life.* The helpful measure in this situation would be to respond to the client realistically, as he/she really is. Countertransference works in much the same ways as transference does for the client. You may become dependent on the client's praise or affection; unconsciously invite gifts or favors; offer excessive reassurance or help that is not really necessary; suppress a need to show anger; or display knowledge, social, or professional

status in order to solicit affection or admiration. Persons in the healing professions may have a desire to be all-knowing and all-powerful, but if you assume such a role, the person cannot overcome feelings of inferiority and helplessness. Countertransference includes overidentification with the client; you exert pressure on him/her to improve, and you attempt to make the person over in your own image. The countertransference response of wishing to be the client's child, grandchild, or younger sibling may occur with older people, especially if they actually resemble your parents, grandparents, or siblings (40).

If you are experiencing countertransference, you may have any of the following reactions (53):

1. Thoughts wander from the client, or the client's words trigger unrelated thoughts.
2. Inattention to the client's verbal and nonverbal behavior.
3. Feelings of impatience with the client's progress, insensitivity to or lack of empathy for his/her needs, or feelings of being unable to help.
4. Conflicting feelings of intense affection, dislike, defensiveness, indifference, or angry sympathy with the person.
5. Overconcern about the person between sessions or overemotional reaction to the client's troubles.

Countertransference can be overcome through guidance from a supervisor and a willingness to examine your personal behavior and comments. C. Vidoni provides further insights into the feelings and effects of countertransference in the therapist (70).

The client may be physically attractive and sexually arousing to you. Such feelings can be disturbing. Feelings of attraction can be especially threatening to you if they are aroused by a client of the same sex. You may sense that to be therapeutic, you must be objective and neuter. Accept that both you and the client are sexual beings, and that you may be attracted, often only briefly, to various persons you encounter. Sexually-aroused feelings do not mean you are a homosexual (if attracted to the same sex) or promiscuous (if attracted to the opposite sex). Feelings of affection, physical attraction, and biological sexual response are often intermingled, but they can be recognized as such and be consciously controlled and sublimated so that a warm relationship can develop.

The client may also feel sexually attracted to you and may invite you to become intimate. Acknowledge the underlying feelings of the client without belittling or rejecting. Usually the person is really talking about a need for love, attention, and caring rather than a need for the physical act of intercourse. Clearly define that the therapeutic relationship does not include dating, intercourse, or physically acting out affection. Rather, a therapeutic relationship means to emotionally accept, care for, and extend affection to help another gain a positive self-concept and confidence and skills to establish a close bond with others.

Feelings of sexual attraction between you and the client can be important. Those feelings may help to initiate a warm bond and relationship between you. Talk about these feelings with an instructor or supervisor. You may feel embarrassed and hesitant in admitting sexual or attraction feelings; yet anyone who has worked intimately with other people and who has also been self-aware, will acknowledge having had such feelings at sometime in his/her professional life. Usually admitting the feelings to yourself and talking with your supervisor about your response, as well as exploring ways to direct these feelings, can defuse the feelings and the anxiety associated with them. Then you can continue to face the client and be in close proximity without fear of losing self-control. Further, if the client suggests intimate behavior, you can explain briefly that such activity is not a part of your relationship but that you can explore together such underlying feelings and needs and appropriate ways to meet them.

Resistance is likely to occur at some time during a relationship. Your inability to recognize or handle it is the main obstacle. **Resistance** *is an attitude on the part of the client that avoids exploring symptoms, refusing to change behavior, and thereby avoiding the feeling of anxiety in the relationship.* Resistance is the client's way of protecting him/herself when you are touching painful areas of his/her life. Content that is basic to the problem and that is kept out of awareness or is repressed prevents development of understanding and also wards off threatening impulses. Resistance may occur when the person is unwilling to give up the secondary benefits that the illness or behavior provides (40).

Either positive or negative transference can cause resistance (40). If the client expresses only affection for you, you may reply, "You spend so much time talking about your feelings for me that you haven't talked about yourself." If a client becomes silent after initial talkative sessions, you may remark, "Perhaps you're not talking much because of some feelings concerning me?" The client may expect to have the life situation improved by identifying with you or telling you information that he/she thinks would please you.

Resistance is commonly expressed by silence. The client may say, "I have nothing to say." Although this may be uncomfortable, sit quietly and wait for him/her to talk, unless this is early in the relationship. The person may be testing your sincerity. You may not be trusted. Or the ill or elderly person may think more slowly than a well or younger person. Initially, after waiting in silence, it may be helpful to use open-ended, explorative questions to promote a fuller assessment (40). It can be helpful to state interest in why he/she is silent, saying, "Perhaps there is something that is difficult for you to discuss," or "You seem to be holding back."

Silence can be provoked in the client if you are too active—asking too many questions that can be answered with yes or no or always providing the answers. This discourages spontaneity, constricts the flow of ideas, and may encourage a negative transference (40).

Intellectualization, when the person talks as if he/she understands self and the problems but then cannot go on to act on that supposed understanding, may be a form of resistance. Usually there is an absence of appropriate emotion with the intellectual constructs. Intellectualization may include learning and using your professional jargon. You can discourage the resistance that comes with intellectualizing in several ways. Avoid "why" questions. Ask instead for elaboration and details. Avoid questions that seem to seek an answer that pleases you or that you specifically want. Avoid using technical terms or professional psychological jargon (40). As the person feels safe in the relationship, he/she may be able to drop this defense with you.

Preoccupation, persistently focusing on certain symptoms, problems, one phase of life, or trivial details, is another form of resistance. You can demonstrate to the person that such behavior is not helpful and that it prohibits finding solutions (40). You may say, "You seem to have difficulty talking about anything except . . . ," or "Tell me first about . . . , and then you can tell me the other details."

Emotional displays as well as apathy, stoicism, or apparent boredom may be forms of resistance. One emotion may be used to defend against deeper, more painful ones. Frequently, "happy sessions" indicate that the client obtains sufficient emotional gratification during the session to ward off anxiety, but this can reduce his/her motivation to change behavior (40). Therefore it is important to explore the process with the person.

Frequent requests to change the time or date of the interview, arriving late, or using minor physical illness to avoid the interview may be forms of resistance (6, 40). Explore the client's feelings about your interactions and the meaning of the behavior, and avoid giving undue attention to it.

Several problems arise in handling resistance. As a helper, you may feel hurt, impatient, angry, inadequate, or unaccepting to the client when he/she is resistant. Working through these feelings with another professional and with the client will avoid a crescendo of feelings that may be damaging to the relationship. You may also think that the resistance results from your lack of expertise or misperception. Remember that the client may talk about irrelevant matters or may not fully trust you, not because of what you are doing, but because of earlier experiences with other people. Again, an open, honest discussion with the client will be useful. Security and concern will be transferred to the client in the closeness of the relationship, which in turn will help him become more secure and confident.

If the above constraints are ignored, the helper-client relationship is likely to deteriorate (6).

Characteristics of a Nontherapeutic Relationship

There may be people with whom you cannot form a helpful relationship. There may be situations in which it would be best for the client if someone else were to work with him/her. You need to be aware of your own feelings of discomfort with a client, and you should be able to accept the fact that you cannot work with a certain person. Often the reasons will be obscure; you may want to work through the reasons with an instructor or supervisor for your own personal growth.

How can you or other colleagues know if an interaction is detrimental to the client? The following is a list of nontherapeutic characteristics that will help you analyze your effect upon the client.

You may increase the client's anxiety or feel increased anxiety with him/her. Often anxiety is manifested by anger, inappropriate laughing or humor, or withdrawal. Anxiety is always present when two strangers first begin to interact, but the anxiety should not be overwhelming. With time, the support of colleagues, and continued contact with the person, your anxiety should diminish. The more comfortable you become, the more comfortable the client will become. If this does not happen, unconscious forces may be operating. If neither you nor the client can cope with the discomfort, you must analyze the situation instead of pushing ahead blindly. Often the situation is resolved by the client's withdrawing from you—physically and emotionally. If such withdrawal persists, you should talk over the situation with an experienced colleague, so that the final outcome will be best for both the client and you. Every helper who works with dependent or helpless people has the responsibility to stop when unable to function effectively, whether in physical or emotional care.

You may feel anger toward the client. Your anger may be a reaction to his/her overt behavior and your fear of acting that way. Your anger may be a counterreaction to the client's anger that is related to something else but is directed toward you. You can stop the cycle by recognizing your own feelings as well as the helplessness felt by the client, by talking with him/her to determine possible sources of anger, and by avoiding either a hostile or too sweet response. Do not joke about anger in yourself or the client and do not reject or punish the client for anger. Make sure that you are not the cause of anger because of actions that demean, aggravate, or neglect him/her. If the person arouses anger in you, seek help from a skilled colleague to work through possible reasons for your anger, to talk about how you demonstrate anger in your behavior, and to work out how to handle such feelings. Anger prevents understanding the person and seeing him/her as a unique person of worth. If your anger overpowers the client, he/she will either withdraw or attempt to defend him/herself in other ways. A barrage of anger keeps the client from maturing.

You may think you are the only person who can care for the client or that you can solve all the problems. Such a feeling of omnipotence is usually unfounded. Although nursing can meet some of your own needs for approval, gratification, security, esteem, and achievement, do not rely only on the job and your client to meet your needs. *Also* you cannot meet all of your client's needs, even when you are very important to him/her. In a relationship that encourages growth, you can help the person reach out to others, and vice versa. Work with the health care team to promote consistent goal setting and for the client's health. Avoid disagreeing with other health care workers in front of the client or neglecting to keep other health team members informed.

You may have difficulty with dependency and independency within a relationship. You may want to have others depend on you. Therefore, you do things for the client that he/she can do for him/herself. Such smothering discourages independent behavior. On the other hand, you may not be able to tolerate the person's dependency, clinging, helplessness, or need for total assistance. Seek help to work through your own feelings. Accept the client as he/she is. Recall the behavioral principle that the person cannot become independent emotionally or physically unless dependency needs are first met. Also remember that the person values whatever independency he/she is capable of, fears dependency, and hates being infantilized.

You may want to treat the client as a social friend or look for companionship in him/her. The result is that you usually meet your personal needs, but at the client's expense. Avoid using the client as a confidante to solve your own problems or as an audience for talks about your personal life or to get attention or praise. Avoid using the client to promote your own political, religious, or philosophical views, even when he/she uses you as a sounding board for such views. Talk about yourself and your activities with friends, family, or colleagues, not with the client.

Sometimes the client may ask you questions about yourself and show an interest in you as a person. Some information may be important so that he/she has a feeling of knowing you and a sense of personal contact. However, experience has proven that a brief answer about yourself generally is sufficient for his/her curiosity or it takes care of the person's idea of the social graces, that is, showing an interest in the other. If fact, after your brief answer, the person frequently interrupts and begins talking about him/herself. Your reply may have

stimulated his/her thoughts, and the person usually enjoys sharing ideas with someone who will listen.

You may place the client in a me-you pattern, perceiving and interacting with him/her as grandparent, parent, aunt, uncle, or someone else whom you know. Although you may feel affection for and interest in the client because he/she reminds you of someone you like (or feel dislike or repulsion for the opposite reason), the person deserves to be seen as a unique being. If you talk to him/her the way you would to someone you know personally, or have unrealistic expectations, the client will not perceive your affection or interest. Instead, he/she will sense that you talking to someone else, feel used, and may withdraw. At best, a distorted relationship results from interacting with someone as if he/she were someone else. You are likely to miss important cues and may intervene in a way that does not meet his/her needs.

You may consciously or unconsciously use intimidation to control the client. Intimidation is making another afraid, forcing or deterring behavior with threats or violence, or overpowering another with awe (22). Rituals and policies can also intimidate. A common practice that is sometimes used as part of a behavior modification program is isolation: the nurses stop going to the client's room, they answer the lights slowly or not at all, and they generally withhold services from someone whom they consider a nuisance (52). The client conforms; he/she does not ring the bell or ask for services. Any sense of self-worth is lost because the client realizes that others think that his/her personal needs are unimportant. Furthermore, the fears of neglect are verified. And the staff may (incorrectly) evaluate their behavior modification program as effective!

If you always have to win in an interaction, you set up the other person to lose. Competition in a nurse-client relationship is destructive; the client ends up losing, and so do you. If the client senses that you must come out on top and be the authority in every conversation, he/she will feel intimidated and will run emotionally, if not physically. You also lose an opportunity to be helpful, to learn something from another person, and to learn about yourself.

If you joke or tease in a harsh or belittling manner, if you use jestful sarcasm, if you laugh at the client's appearance or behavior, if you play childish games to get him/her to cooperate or be pleasant, or if you use him/her as a scapegoat, you will be the cause of the client's anger, hate, despair, hopelessness, and finally complete withdrawal and regression.

You may also use nontherapeutic communication techniques that will reduce the chance of forming or maintaining a relationship. To probe, challenge, offhandedly ask questions about very private matters, or ask "why" is threatening. Interrupting, speaking too rapidly or in a condescending way, or talking too loudly to the person who hears well or too softly to the hearing-impaired conveys a lack of interest or knowledge of the person. Controlling the conversational topic according to your needs or interests is rude, egotistical, and unprofessional, and it is frustrating to the client. If you control the conversation, you will never learn what is really most important to the person. Asking a barrage of direct questions will get a nod, a yes or no answer, or a blank stare. Direct questions are appropriate at times, but too often health profes-

sionals think they know what information is needed and ask questions accordingly. The result is assumptions, not data. Using jargon, standing at a distance, or conveying by your posture that you are in a hurry will cause the client to say very little or nothing at all. Falsely reassuring or using glib clichés when he/she knows all is not well may cause withdrawal. The feelings he/she was trying to express will remain inside, drain energy, cause anger or irritability, or even cause confusion and disorientation as a means of avoiding the reality he/she faces. Never tell the person to be cheerful when he/she doesn't feel cheery. In trying to cheer him/her, you may create a new problem when the person feels guilt feelings because he/she is not living up to your expectations. Review Chapter 5 for other communication approaches that are a deterrent to a therapeutic relationship.

PHASES OF THE NURSE-CLIENT RELATIONSHIP

Working with the emotionally ill to establish and maintain a relationship is similar to working with any other client. The differences are that at first the client's symptoms or pathology may be challenging for you, the person's response to therapy may be slower than that seen in acute care settings, and the length of stay may be longer. If you work in a nursing home, an extended care facility, or a residence for severely emotionally ill or the elderly, the person's stay may extend for years—until he/she dies. In such cases, because you usually have an opportunity to know this client in greater depth, you can form a more meaningful relationship. This is one of the rewards of psychiatric nursing.

The nurse-client relationship is goal-directed and usually is divided into four phases: (1) orientation or establishment, (2) identification, (3) working or therapeutic phase, and (4) termination (28, 55). Because of the long-term contact that is typical with the aged, chronically ill, or institutionalized emotionally ill, another phase has been identified and inserted, that of maintenance, which differs from and follows the working phase and will also be explained.

Throughout the relationship you will feel and demonstrate the characteristics of a helping relationship described earlier in this chapter. Then you will be a humanistic therapist. As a humanistic nurse,

you will see yourself serving the client or facilitating his/her emotional growth as more important than the system, rules, or institution. You will help the client navigate through the system, and this assistance begins in the orientation phase. You will be concerned about the whole person and his/her family unit. You will not see yourself or the client as a machine or as a thing. You will not use a standardized care plan; you will apply nursing principles and knowledge in an individualized way. You will help the person grow in a self-determined direction and will facilitate effective interpersonal and communication skills.

Orientation, Initial, or Establishment Phase

The orientation, or initial, phase of the relationship begins when you first meet the client, when he/she seeks assistance or is brought for care. In this phase, the nurse explains the nature and purpose of the relationship, the role of the nurse, and the client's responsibilities. You may carry out essential interventions simultaneously, or shortly thereafter, as indicated. However, your main tasks are to introduce yourself; learn who he/she is; and become oriented to his/her expectations, health needs, and goals through assessment. Orient the client to your role, the admission procedures, the general aspects of the agency, your health care goals, and his/her role in the health care system. Formulate a tentative care plan and determine whether or not it matches the client's impression of the problem. Explore how long you will be caring for him/her and how you will work together (28, 55).

Early in this phase you can make a written or informal verbal contract with the person who seeks counseling or who is hospitalized. The contract includes a commitment to see the client through the problem or refer him/her to appropriate assistance. The contract explicitly defines the relationship, roles, and mutual explanations. Refer to Chapter 4 for further information.

You begin as strangers to each other. The client is anxious about his/her problems, the treatment and/or hospitalization, and your reaction. Your anxiety centers on the client's reaction to you and your ability to help. Establishing rapport and showing unconditional positive regard and acceptance are vital for assessing and orientating the person and for beginning a relationship. The client should begin to sense that you are trustworthy. He/she may test you with various behaviors or questions in order to learn if you can be trusted, if you are congruent or consistent. While you are assessing and getting acquainted with the person, you are also examining your own thoughts, feelings, actions, and expectations. During this time the client may be assessing you as carefully as you are assessing him/her: the client observes and listens for your voice tone, the words you say and how you say them, your facial expressions, mannerisms, posture, and dress. The person watches carefully for your response: Do you act bored, inattentive, hurried, or rejecting? Such behavior may slow or prevent a relationship (28, 55).

This phase has been likened developmentally to that of infancy because the client depends on you. If you demonstrate that you are a caring, nurturing, safe person, the client will begin to feel more secure. During the days or weeks that follow, he/she will disclose more of self, so that you get to know new facets of the client as a person. Answers to questions on the nursing history or assessment form may change as the client learns to trust you enough to give you the true answers or as you help him/her to better know him/herself. Throughout this period you are also giving more information about his/her situation, yourself, and the health care system (28, 54, 55).

Identification Phase

The identification phase has been compared developmentally to the childhood phase. During this period the client responds selectively to the person (nurse) who seems to offer the needed help. If you have been perceived as accepting, congruent, trustworthy, and empathetic, you become the identification figure, a surrogate parent. The client then chooses to actively enter the relationship (28, 55).

This is the time when the client and you become better acquainted as you mutually explore deeper feelings, needs, and goals. He/she trusts your decisions and actions, works closely with you, follows your suggestions, and claims you as "the nurse who has all the answers." Because of the time you spend with the client and your response, you may become an ego-ideal for the client. This is a positive transference in which he/she imitates your speech, mannerisms, dress, or ideas. The person may make admiring statements about you. It may be helpful to explore with the client why he/she wants to emulate you, for in the process you can help him/her better understand him/herself and further establish self-identity (28, 55).

If earlier experiences with people were traumatic, the client will take longer to feel trust and to move into this phase. He/she may become isolated, withdraw, act independent, or not accept needed help. If you wish to form a relationship, you will have to remain available and carry out the behaviors of the orientation phase for a longer period of time, that is, until you see a response from the client (28, 55).

You may feel uncomfortable during this phase because the client is compliant, dependent on you, and moving emotionally close. Accept this dependency without fostering it unnecessarily. This is a time when you can teach a great deal, a time when you can guide learning about self and better coping with the situation. Because he/she feels close to you, your responsiveness and empathy can help him/her mature emotionally. You continue the steps of the nursing process throughout this phase, guiding, but also providing opportunities for self-care and increasing emotional security and independence (28, 55).

Working or Therapeutic Phase

During the working phase the problem and underlying needs are explored in the relationship. Developmentally this phase is similar to adolescence. During this phase the client becomes more independent and uses all of the services and resources offered by the health team that meet his/her needs. The person becomes more assertive and self-reliant as he/she tries out self-care measures, insists on doing things a personal way, or tries new ways of behaving with others. By now, he/she is usually regaining physical and emotional health and functioning optimally. Therefore, the client's behavior may change as he/she becomes more involved in making decisions about certain aspects of the situation. Although the client seems more independent, explorative, manipulative, and even self-centered and demanding, you can now work as partners in meeting his/her health care goals. You are active as a counselor, support, and resource person. If you enjoy the dependent client, you may feel uncomfortable during this phase. If so, you should explore why you feel uncomfortable (28, 55).

During this phase you gain an even better understanding of the client and the meaning of illness and the life situation to him/her. You help him/her work through problems at a personal pace; you offer support, and you help him/her gain insight to the greatest degree possible (28, 55).

You will be a factor in mobilizing clients to change dysfunctional behavior when you engage in the helping relationship. In attempting to motivate behavioral change and emotional development, you may assign therapeutic tasks or homework assignments to be done between counseling sessions. These tasks can be valuable, when the client agrees to them, for the following reasons:

1. The client continues to be emotionally close to you, strengthening the relationship.
2. The client perceives that you feel change is possible, which instills hope and initiative in the client.
3. When tasks are accomplished, you can acknowledge the achievement, reinforce positive behavioral changes, and enhance the client's self-esteem.
4. Tasks can teach problem-solving skills; help restructure a personal, family, or job system;

help overcome resistance to change; and test the flexibility and maturing of the client.

5. The client experiences that what is discussed in sessions can be applied to life situations (20).

Connie Goldberg describes tasks that can be assigned in conjunction with therapy sessions (20).

During interviews in this phase, the main responsibility for speaking rests with the client, who exercises options on what he wants to talk about. You listen carefully and are silent more of the time than he/she is. Feedback about what you see and hear, intent behind speech, and observations about inconsistency between verbal and nonverbal behavior are given. You point out to the client unused strengths and resources. You invite the client to examine how he/she and you are relating to each other. You challenge, without being judgmental, discrepancies in the client's communication and life and invite him/her to explore and resolve these discrepancies. Interpretation is indicated. Ultimately interpretation will be considered and the meaning integrated, which will convey a feeling of self-control and self-worth to the client when he/she discovers the connection between thoughts, feelings, and resultant behavior, with your validation, of course (28, 55, 58).

You point out options of behavior and experiences to the client that he/she does not see for him/herself. You convey hope that something can be done, inject optimism into the situation, and provide an element of confidence that the required changes will not be too expensive in pain, money, or time. You stimulate the client to change, to lessen feelings of helplessness, and to increase ability to cope. You enable the person to develop behavioral change strategies and action plans, or to acquire additional learning so that he/she has alternatives in coping and can solve problems, which in turn will improve self-image. You encourage expression of feelings, recognizing the importance of each person experiencing, understanding, and sharing his/her feelings with a confidant (24, 45, 48).

At the same time, you do not make decisions about life style for the client. You are accepting and nonpunitive if the person does not aspire to your every suggestion or does not use your help the way you anticipated. Your self-image should not depend on how the client uses your help. You recognize the client is not a carbon copy of you (28, 55, 58).

The helping process does not always proceed smoothly. Sometimes all you can do is relieve the client's loneliness until conditions change and coping seems possible. This method of helping requires patience, a defense against becoming irritated by an apparent lack of success, humility regarding one's own powers of invention, and at best, being satisfied with contributing to the client's survival (58).

If the client was admitted to an acute care setting or to a home health agency, he/she may now be preparing for convalescence and discharge from your services. The person has made the most of the services offered and is ready to resume his/her former life style to the greatest degree possible. This would be the beginning of the termination phase. However, if the client was admitted to a long-term care setting or geriatric residence, or if you work with elderly clients in the community through an independent practice, your relationship is not terminated, although the nature of the relationship does change after a while. *Instead* you are entering the maintenance phase with the client.

Maintenance Phase

Often the nurse who works in an acute-care setting does not really experience the rewards of a relationship with the patient. The short stay typical of hospitalization or even the few visits given by a home health nurse allow nothing more than establishing rapport, if that. Nurses may talk glibly about nurse-client relationships, but in many settings this relationship may never exist for the client. Although we have instant coffee, instant tea, and instant potatoes, you can't have instant relationships. You cannot measure out a portion of yourself to another, stir once, and be friends.

Relationships are only possible in the setting in which a client is followed by the same nurse over a period of time, for example, in a rehabilitation center, nursing home, senior residence, or psychiatric/mental health agency. Primary nursing, in an acute care setting, can allow for relationship formation because the same nurse cares for the patient during the hospitalization. Some home health agencies will provide care over a long period of time; they do not insist on a rapid turnover of cases. Also the nurse in independent practice or in an ambulatory care clinic may see the same clients over a period of years.

The relationship that pertains to total health care and that extends over years is different from the nurse-patient relationship that is usually described in books. There is no termination, or at least not for a long time. Often termination only comes with the death of the person. The active, working, therapeutic stage goes on until the person has reached his/her potential. In this situation, the client has reached a plateau where support and maintenance are essential for daily living. The client may live at home, following your directions for health promotion measures, and may call on you for assistance only when chronic illness becomes uncontrolled or when he/she suffers a new condition of pathology or of aging. Or the client may be in an institution and need maximal or minimal assistance with daily physical care. What characterizes this phase is that you must actively pursue interventions in order to maintain emotional and social well-being. The kinds of activities that you may implement are described further in another article by this author (49). The reward will be the gratification of seeing a person reassert his/her will to live, to become creative in coping with problems or making "ends meet," and to remain independent.

This author has carried out the maintenance stage for years with elderly people who wanted to remain living in their own apartments but who could not manage without a helpful relationship because they were alone, without family, and with few resources. Thus, a number of elderly clients have remained as physically intact as possible, emotionally well, mentally alert, socially aware, and independent because this author does not define nursing in a narrow sense. Jo Carr and Imogene Sorley have aptly described this phase (11):

> Depth relationships have a mutual history of shared joy and anguish, a mellowed blend of caring and being cared for, of listening and removing masks, of openness and honesty . . . . All of this takes time, effort, and expenditure of self. [P. 31]

Termination Phase

The termination phase is marked by the client's becoming as healthy and independent as possible. Events in the relationship and the growth that has occurred are summarized by client and nurse. Old needs have been adequately met; goals have been accomplished, and he/she is ready to be discharged from your services or from the health care system.

This is a time of impending separation as you plan together how the person will continue to interact and manage life's patterns and stresses. This phase is likened developmentally to adulthood; the client is freeing him/herself from your help and is generating strength and ability to stand alone. The illness and any changes in behavior and body are integrated into the total self-concept (28, 55). As the crisis of illness is resolved, you and the client work collaboratively on an adult-to-adult basis.

Termination is an important phase; plan for it. In the acute care setting the client may be discharged so abruptly that neither thought nor time is given to how he/she will manage at home, in the community, or on the job.

During this phase you and the client must work through feelings about separation—sometimes past separations as well as the present termination. Mutual attachment has developed between you and someone you care for over a period of time. Each of you has invested something of the self in the other. Either one or both of you may feel uncertain about the other person's ability to manage without you. Tell the client your confidence in his/her ability to manage. Avoid increasing dependency on you just to meet your own needs. The client may feel very insecure and stressed about termination of the relationship. When the client leaves the health care system, both you and the person should feel no regret about discharge, since follow-up care, either physically or emotionally, should be planned for if it is necessary (28, 67).

Sometimes the client gives a gift to the nurse in an effort to convey feelings of appreciation, warmth, caring, and to leave an object that ensures being remembered. Usually the gift is not expensive, but it may be significant to the client. Unless it is an item essential to the client, accept the gift graciously and explore feelings behind the gift. Share appropriate feelings about the client with him/her. Discuss the importance of this relationship to you.

At times the client may either consciously or unconsciously try to delay discharge and termina-tion with a variety of reasons to delay discharge, such as inability to manage, or the development of new symptoms, either as a result of anxiety or in the form of malingering. The symptoms and excuses tell you of inner feelings—lack of trust in self, loneliness and helplessness, or the need for a continued relationship (55).

These feelings will be magnified if you do not prepare the person for termination or if you try to discontinue being with the person when you feel that he/she is improving and no longer needs you. The person needs an opportunity to resolve the feelings he/she is experiencing, or rejection and abandonment will be felt. The person needs to go through a mourning process in relation to this separation, so that when future separations and losses occur, he/she will be better able to cope with them.

Other feelings the client may experience during the termination phase include ambivalence or anger about the loss of relationship and care, a sense of rejection by you, grief and depression, or guilt about having done something wrong or about not having met your expectations. The client may perceive the discharge and termination as being pushed out. He/she may feel that you no longer like or care for him/her and may deny that termination is near by not entering into discharge plans, decision making, and self-care, or by talking about how your relationship will continue.

Preparation for termination should begin early in the relationship when you tell the client about how long you expect to care for him/her and how long he/she is expected to remain in the health care agency. As the time for discharge approaches, talk about feelings—yours and the other person's—as well as about realistic discharge and teaching plans. Let the person know that caring for him/her has been a meaningful experience for you. Help him/her to see the gains made during the relationship. Talk about separation, loss, and termination as part of the life cycle, about the worth of past relationships, and about the anticipation of future relationships. This talk can involve valuable reminiscing for the client and renewed hope for the future (55).

RELATIONSHIP WITH THE VERBALLY OR SENSORY-IMPAIRED CLIENT

The psychiatric client may be aphasic because of organic pathology, mute because of emotional illness, too physically ill to talk, deaf, or regressed to the point that he cannot carry on a logical conversation. Nevertheless, you can have a relationship with such a client. All that has been discussed so far would also be applicable to some extent to this client.

The most essential aspect of a relationship with the verbally or sensory-impaired person is your attitude or approach. You can convey that you are trustworthy, dependable, interested in, accepting of, empathic, and respectful by your posture, tone of voice, use of touch, and thoroughness of physical care. If you are repulsed by the client, you convey this feeling both nonverbally and vocally. The verbally and sensory-impaired person is very vulnerable to the hostility, aggression, or sadism of his/her caretakers; often he/she cannot defend him/herself physically and cannot call for help because of immobility.

The principles of communication discussed in Chapter 5 and throughout this chapter would apply to a considerable extent here. You may also use more direct questions, for the client may only be able to nod yes or no. And the attitude that your communication techniques convey would be equally important with a person who could not reply. You should talk to the person as if he/she could reply. Countless cases exist in which the mute patient finally talked because therapeutic communication techniques were used. If the aphasia is reversible, the person will be better motivated to try to talk. If the person is regressed, he/she will sense your caring and respect and, as a result, his/her behavior may change in a positive direction. If the person is deaf, he/she will see your caring; if blind, he/she will hear your caring voice.

In relating to the mute person, utilize the following guidelines in addition to those in Chapter 5 (29):

1. The person has a basic need for a comfortable, relatively anxiety-free nonverbal or verbal experience with another human.
2. The person cannot remain completely isolated from other humans; there is either a negative or positive response, however minimal, to the presence of others.
3. You cannot know the thought content of the mute person; psychotherapeutic intervention with pathology awaits verbalization.
4. Your presence and nonverbal therapeutic approach act as a stimulus to the client's perceptual powers.
5. Your use of a caring approach, expectation of speech, and concise statements stimulate

auditory experience, verbal images, and desire to speak, and become the basis on which verbal behavior can be modeled.
6. You should focus on events and people in the immediate environment to promote reorganization of spatial and time perception and related speech in the client.
7. Your ability to reduce anxiety and touch the client emotionally promotes communication, and over time, speech.

When stimulating verbal communication in the mute client, sit nearby, tell the person your name and that you will be coming at a regular time each day to speak with him/her. State time of day and how long you will be there, and keep the appointment. Acknowledge any nonverbal behavior on the part of the client and repeat that you are there to listen to what he/she has to say. You may need to repeat this approach for many days or weeks as you slowly help the client feel safe with you. After a few days, you may bring an object with you, placing it in the client's line of vision, to stimulate verbal response or description. Perhaps a bouquet of flowers; or a picture of flowers, a pet, a sports activity, or of the client or one of his/her family members; or a fishbowl; or a craft article made in occupational therapy—any of these may be of interest to the client. Try to elicit a brief description or response about the object without increasing the person's discomfort. Reinforce nonverbal or unintelligible responses. Later you can focus on eliciting more precise speech. Sometimes the use of a book or magazine is helpful; you may take turns reading sentences (29). Eventually the client will realize that this interpersonal situation is different from those he previously experienced. Your caring, your wanting to listen and talk with him/her, and your creating of a safe and trusting feeling will contribute to his/her desire to speak— perhaps at first about objects and events in the immediate environment, and finally about personal ideas, feelings, and life experiences.

The nurse-client relationship is an integral part of the nursing process. You will need to assess the client in order to determine which needs can be met through a helping relationship. Your therapeutic approach is a nursing intervention and is important in combination with any other nursing interventions. Understanding the phases of the relationship will help you understand the person's changing behavior.

The authors emphasize use of the Humanistic framework for nursing practice; and this author emphasizes a Rogerian model for counseling. However, you may utilize information from other theorists when you counsel, and apply knowledge from First and Second Force theorists through a Humanistic approach. An example of an eclectic use of theory is given by G. P. Ney (53). L. Loesch and N. Loesch discuss that the Rogerian model may not be effective for all clients, and emphasize eclecticism in the use of theory as they describe how other theorists can be used in a counseling approach (39).

EVALUATION

Evaluation of the nursing process must include evaluation of the approach you use and its effectiveness in promoting wellness. You may be very skillful in relating to people generally, and those skills may be useful in the professional helping relationship. However, you will want to evaluate your helpful characteristics and whether or not you use constraining or nontherapeutic approaches.

You may also use the following list to gain self-awareness about why you involve yourself in a client relationship. You must achieve sufficient satisfaction from the interpersonal exchange, or your dissatisfaction may defeat the client. Helping others regain function and health is satisfying, but there may be other returns as well. To enter into the therapeutic process may result in some personal therapeutic release, including some of the following factors (71):

The pleasure of being able to give love, have it received and reciprocated.

The release of being able to reveal and examine yourself and to be open.

A feeling of power and control that another human being depends on you.

A sense of security, or relative safety from the ills and troubles of the client. Someone else is climbing the mountain and facing the danger while you observe.

Intellectual intrigue with the puzzle to be worked through.

Enhancement of your personal life by the vicarious experience of many other circumstances.

Feelings of worth and responsibility because of involvement in the success of a human being.

Messianic feelings of being the possible savior of a human life and having the power to relieve pain and suffering.

Confirmation of competence by the client's gratitude.

Wise investment of efforts; precious time was not wasted when the client shows gains.

Feelings of alliance and commonality with the human condition.

Practice with the disrupting elements of life that strengthens self and develops skill in personal solutions.

Enjoyment of the competition for insightful discoveries and their validation when the client achieves accordingly.

As the client gains, you have a feeling of the appropriateness of the chosen field.

REFERENCES

1. Argyle, Michael, *The Psychology of Interpersonal Behavior.* Baltimore: Penguin Books, 1967.

2. Aroskar, Mila, "Ethics of Nurse-Patient Relationships," *Nurse Educator,* 5, no. 2 (1980), 18-20.

3. Baumgartner, M., "Empathy," *Behavioral Concepts and Nursing Intervention,* ed. C. Carlson, pp. 29-39. Philadelphia: J. B. Lippincott Company, 1970.

4. Bender, R. E., "Communicating with the Deaf," *American Journal of Nursing,* 66, no. 4 (1966), 757-60.

5. Benjamin, Alfred, *The Helping Interview.* Boston: Houghton Mifflin Company, 1969.

6. Blocker, Donald, *Developmental Counseling.* New York: The Ronald Press Company, 1966.

7. Brammer, Lawrence, *The Helping Relationship: Pro-

cess and Skills, 2nd ed. Englewood Cliffs, N.J.: Prentice-Hall, Inc., 1979.

8. Buckheimer, A., "The Development of Ideas about Empathy," *Journal of Counseling Psychology,* 10, no. 1 (1963), 61–71.

9. Burkhardt, M., "Response to Anxiety," *American Journal of Nursing,* 69, no. 10 (1969), 2153–54.

10. Carkhuff, Robert R., *Helping and Human Relations.* New York: Holt, Rinehart and Winston, 1969.

11. Carr, Jo, and Imogene Sorley, *Mockingbirds and Angel Songs and Other Prayers.* Nashville, Tenn.: Abingdon Press, 1975.

12. Cashar, Leah, and Barbara Dixon, "The Therapeutic Use of Touch," *Journal of Psychiatric Nursing and Mental Health Services,* 5, no. 5 (1967), 442–51.

13. Coad-Denton, Alice, "Therapeutic Superficiality and Intimacy," in *Clinical Practice in Psychosocial Nursing,* eds. Diane Longo and Rex Williams, pp. 28–40. New York: Appleton-Century-Crofts, 1978.

14. Cowley, Michele, "No Cure, Just Care," *American Journal of Nursing,* 74, no. 11 (1974), 2010–12.

15. Dejean, Sherrilyn, "Empathy: A Necessary Ingredient of Care," *American Journal of Nursing,* 68, no. 3 (1968), 559–60.

16. Durr, Carol, "Hands That Help—But How?" *Nursing Forum,* 4, no. 4 (1971), 393–400.

17. Ehmann, Virginia E., "Empathy: Its Origin, Characteristics, and Process," *Perspectives in Psychiatric Care,* 9, no. 2 (1971), 72–80.

18. Garant, Carol, "Stalls in the Therapeutic Process," *American Journal of Nursing,* 80, no. 12 (1980), 2166–69.

19. "Gentle Be Present," *American Journal of Nursing,* 74, no. 9 (1974), 1611.

20. Goldberg, Connie, "Therapeutic Tasks: Strategies for Change," *Perspectives in Psychiatric Care,* 18, no. 4 (1980), 156–62.

21. Greenhill, Maurice, "Interviewing with a Purpose," *American Journal of Nursing,* 56, no. 10 (1956), 1259–62.

22. Guralnik, David, ed., *Webster's New World Dictionary,* 2nd College Ed. New York: William Collins and World Publishing Co., Inc., 1972.

23. Hale, S., and J. Richardson, "Terminating the Nurse-Patient Relationship," *American Journal of Nursing,* 63, no. 9 (1963), 116–19.

24. Hardiman, M., "Interviewing or Social Chit-Chat," *American Journal of Nursing,* 71, no. 7 (1971), 1379–81.

25. Hardy, Jean, "The Importance of Touch for Patient and Nurse," *Journal of Practical Nursing,* 25, no. 6 (1975), 26–27.

26. Hays, J., and K. Larson, *Interacting with Patients.* New York: Macmillan Publishing Co., Inc., 1963.

27. Hewitt, H., and B. Pesznecker, "Blocks to Communicating with Patients," *American Journal of Nursing,* 64, no. 7 (1964), 101–3.

28. Hofling, Charles, Madeleine Leininger, and Elizabeth Gregg, *Basic Psychiatric Concepts in Nursing,* 2nd ed. Philadelphia: J. B. Lippincott Company, 1967.

29. Hurtean, Phyllis, "The Psychiatric Nurse and the Mute Patient," *American Journal of Nursing,* 62, no. 6 (1962), 55–60.

30. Ingles, Thelma, "Understanding the Nurse-Patient Relationship," in *Issues in Nursing,* eds. Bonnie Bullough and Vern Bullough. New York: Springer Publishing Co., Inc., 1966.

31. Johnson, Betty, "The Meaning of Touch in Nursing," *Nursing Outlook,* 13, no. 2 (1965), 59–60.

32. Kalisch, Beatrice J., "Strategies for Developing Nurse Empathy," *Nursing Outlook,* 19, no. 11 (1971), 714–18.

33. ——, "An Experiment in the Development of Empathy in Nursing Students," *Nursing Research,* 20, no. 3 (1971), 202–11.

34. ——, "What Is Empathy?" *American Journal of Nursing,* 73, no. 9 (1973), 1548–52.

35. Kimball, C. P., "Psychotherapeutic Intervention in Acute Medical Situations," *General Hospital Psychiatry,* 1, no. 2 (1979), 150–55.

36. Kreiger, Dolores, "Therapeutic Touch: The Imprimatur of Nursing," *American Journal of Nursing,* 75, no. 5 (1975), 784–87.

37. Leininger, Madeleine, "The Phenomenon of Caring," *Nursing Research Report,* 12, no. 1 (1977), 2, 14.

38. Litwick, L., J. Litwick, and M. Ballou, *Health Counseling.* New York: Appleton-Century-Crofts, 1980.

39. Loesch, Larry, and Nancy Loesch, "What Do You Say After You Say Mm-hmm?" *American Journal of Nursing,* 75, no. 5 (1975), 807–9.

40. Mackinnon, Robert, and Robert Michaels, *The Psychiatric Interview in Clinical Practice.* Philadelphia: W. B. Saunders Company, 1971.

41. Manaser, Janice, and Anita Werner, *Instruments for Study of Nurse-Patient Interaction.* New York: Macmillan Publishing Co., Inc., 1964.

42. Mansfield, Elaine, "Empathy: Concept and Identified Psychiatric Behavior," *Nursing Research,* 22, no. 6 (1973), 525–30.

43. McCorkle, Ruth, "Effects of Touch on Seriously Ill Patients," *Nursing Research,* 23, no. 2 (1974), 125–32.

44. Meadow, Lloyd, and Gertrude Gass, "Problems of the Novice Interviewer," *American Journal of Nursing,* 63, no. 2 (1963), 97–99.

45. Mitchell, Ann, "Barriers to Therapeutic Communication with Black Clients," *Nursing Outlook,* 26, no. 2 (1978), 109–12.

46. Montagu, M., *Touching: The Human Significance of the Skin.* New York: Columbia University Press, 1971.

47. Moustakas, Clark, *Creativity and Conformity.* New York: Van Nostrand Reinhold Company, 1967.

48. Murray, Jeanne, "Self-Knowledge and the Nursing Interview," *Nursing Forum,* 2, no. 1 (1963), 69–79.

49. Murray, Ruth, "Caring," *American Journal of Nursing,* 72, no. 7 (1972), 1286–87.

50. Murray, Ruth, Marilyn Huelskoetter, and Dorothy O'Driscoll, *The Nursing Process in Later Maturity,* pp. 51–81. Englewood Cliffs, N.J.: Prentice-Hall, Inc., 1980.

51. Murray, Ruth, and Judith Zentner, *Nursing Concepts for Health Promotion,* 2nd ed. Englewood Cliffs, N.J.: Prentice-Hall, Inc., 1979.

52. Nehring, Virginia, and Barbara Geach, "Patients' Evaluation of Their Care: Why They Don't Complain," *Nursing Outlook,* 21, no. 5 (1973), 322–24.

53. Ney, G. Phillip, "Combined Approaches in the Treatment of Conflicted Children and Their Families," *Canada's Mental Health,* 24, no. 2 (1976), 2–8.

54. Orlando, Ida, *The Dynamic Nurse-Patient Relationship.* New York: G. P. Putnam's Sons, 1961.

55. Peplau, Hildegarde, *Interpersonal Relations in Nursing.* New York: G. P. Putnam's Sons, 1952.

56. ____, *Basic Principles of Patient Counseling,* 2nd ed. Philadelphia: Smith, Kline, and French Laboratories, 1969.

57. ____, "Professional Closeness," *Nursing Forum,* 8, no. 4 (1969), 346.

58. Pollak, Otto, *Human Behavior and the Helping Professions.* Jamaica, N.Y.: Spectrum Publications, Inc., 1976.

59. Rogers, Carl, *Client-Centered Therapy.* Boston: Houghton Mifflin Company, 1951.

60. Rosendahl, P., "Effectiveness of Empathy, Non-Possessive Warmth, and Genuineness of Nursing Students," *Nursing Research,* 22, no. 3 (1973), 253–57.

61. Ruesch, J., and Gregory Bateson, *Communication.* New York: W. W. Norton & Co., Inc., 1951.

62. Ryden, M., "An Approach to Ethical Decision-Making," *Nursing Outlook,* 26, no. 11 (1978), 705–6.

63. Scheideman, Jean, "Problem Patients Do Not Exist," *American Journal of Nursing,* 79, no. 6 (1979), 1082–83.

64. Speroff, B. J., "Empathy Is Important in Nursing," *Nursing Outlook,* 4, no. 6 (1956), 326–28.

65. Sullivan, Harry, *The Interpersonal Theory of Psychiatry.* New York: W. W. Norton & Co., Inc., 1953.

66. Travelbee, Joyce, *Intervention in Psychiatric Nursing.* Philadelphia: F. A. Davis Company, 1969.

67. Triplett, June L., "Empathy Is . . . ," *Nursing Clinics of North America,* 4, no. 4 (1969), 673–82.

68. Veatch, Robert, "Models for Ethical Medicine in a Revolutionary Age," *Hastings Center Report,* 2, no. 6 (1972), 5–6.

69. Veninga, Robert, "Communications: A Patient's Eye View," *American Journal of Nursing,* 73, no. 2 (1973), 320–22.

70. Vidoni, C., "The Development of Intense Counter-transference Feelings in the Therapist Toward a Patient," *American Journal of Nursing,* 75, no. 3 (1975), 407–9.

71. Whitehouse, Frederick, "The Concept of Therapy: A Review of Some Essentials," in *The Psychological and Social Impact of Physical Disability,* eds. Robert Marnelli and Arthur Dell Orto, pp. 299–318. New York: Springer Publishing Co., 1972.

72. Wicks, Robert, *Counseling Strategies and Intervention Techniques for the Human Services.* Philadelphia: J. B. Lippincott Company, 1977.

73. Wiedenbach, Ernestine, "The Helping Art of Nursing," *American Journal of Nursing,* 63, no. 11 (1963), 54–57.

74. Zderad, Loretta, "Empathetic Realization of a Human Capacity," *Nursing Clinics of North America,* 4, no. 4 (1969), 655–62.

7

The Change Process

Study of this chapter will assist you to:

1. Define and describe the change process and consequent reactions.

2. Analyze the dynamics generally involved in planned change.

3. Compare and contrast the change process as it occurs in the individual, group, organizational, and community systems.

4. Describe risks and the underlying dynamics that are involved in the change process.

5. Explore predisposing factors and common manifestations of resistance toward change.

6. Assess personal reactions to change as a prerequisite for being a change agent.

7. Assess a system's need for and response to change.

8. Formulate nursing diagnosis(es) that relate to inability to cope with change.

9. Formulate a plan with the client for coping with change.

10. Utilize principles described in this and other chapters in your role as change agent.

11. Evaluate your effectiveness in working through change with clients.

This chapter contributed by M. Marilyn Huelskoetter, R.N., M.S.N. and Evelyn Romano, R.N., M.S.N., with additions by Ruth Murray, R.N., M.S.N.

Change is a natural, inevitable, constant, and dynamic process. In Western society we value change and see it as positive because to us it means progress. You probably see yourself as a person wanting to keep up with the changing times and as a nurse wanting to become a change agent, to use planned change theory, and to implement new ideas and growth for your client—individual, group, organization, or community. This chapter will give you a general understanding of change, how it comes about, progresses, and is maintained, and how it affects you as a person and a nurse. Knowledge of the change process is essential in psychiatric/mental health nursing. Often emotional distress occurs because of the person's inability to cope with the stress of change. Further, you will always be functioning in the capacity of change agent as you work with people.

A MODEL OF THE CHANGE PROCESS

In this chapter, the Change Model, incorporating elements of Systems Theory and the Development Model of Change, will be discussed (42). According to Systems Theory, an individual, group, or community is a functioning dynamic whole and is considered an open system, attempting to maintain a state of equilibrium as it maintains life. Within the boundaries of a system there is movement or a continuously changing state to maintain life. When the forces operating within and upon the system are in a balanced relationship to one another, the system is in a steady state. Groups, or the departments of an organization, when operating together with harmony between members as they work on group goals, are in a steady state. In the environment, systems in the form of plants or animals are constantly changing and modifying themselves for survival. Forms for survival may change, but life itself is sustained in a steady state as the interrelated parts function together in a process where there is energy flow and movement in spurts and increments. As this process continues there are times when tension occurs because of a lack of integration of the parts. This tension, in the broadest sense, creates conflict, stress, or strain, with resulting movement of the system to reduce the tension (10). Thus the tension motivates the system toward action or change. The change process is the process of tension reduction, and the change agent's role is to diagnose and initiate action (42).

Underlying the Developmental Model of Change is the assumption of constant change and development in any organism. Change is seen as natural, end-related, and purposeful. Difficulties arise when there is a discrepancy between potential growth and actual growth, development, or change.

THE PROCESS OF CHANGE

What Is Change?

Change is a dynamic process. We all experience it. It can be external to us, coming from forces around us—the wind, air, and temperature. Or it can be the internal personal change we experience as we grow, mature, and develop our own personalities. The developmental change process is complex, continuous, orderly, and unique to the person (53). As the person develops from the cell to the fully grown person and until death, change is occurring.

Change *can be spontaneous, or it can be planned.* Theories of change had their beginning in the work of Kurt Lewin, who saw the concept of change having three basic stages: (1) unfreezing (motivation to change, disturbing the equilibrium, or breaking habit by introducing new behaviors while retaining old patterns), (2) moving (change itself, creating new habits and modifying attitudes), and (3) refreezing (integration of change into a steady state of behavior) (37). W. Bennis and his colleagues developed the concept of planned change (6, 7). They believed *change should be a conscious, deliberate, and collaborative effort to solve problems, which can be applied to any system. Planned change is a goal-directed activity that involves problem solving or decision making.* Planned change is change with a purpose; it begins as an idea or plan of one person or group and may spread to a larger group or community.

Change as a process that is either spontaneous or planned includes the following responses: (1) feelings of tension, anxiety, or even fear, (2) a sense of need, (3) feelings of hope, (4) a search, (5) decision and goal setting, (6) commitment to goals and change, (7) creative behavior, and (8) change in behavior. These responses occur

The change agent's role is to diagnose problems, remove obstacles, and encourage new patterns of behavior (50).

The Change Model looks at the forces producing and resisting change and emphasizes study of ways to arrive at planned change through unfreezing of behavior and collaborative processes. The parts of the system and the developmental processes of the individual, group, and organization are involved in the change process (42).

in a pattern and will be discussed in the following pages.

Change Causes Anxiety and Fear

People feel uneasy about change that occurs within the self, job, or environment. Consider how you feel about change in your own life. Quickly write your answers to the questions in Table 7-1. As you think of changes you have experienced, you may be more aware of the anxiety and fear, as well as the anticipation and challenge, associated with change. In growing up you may have felt fear and anxiety as you started a new school, moved to a new neighborhood, or joined a new club. As a schoolchild and adolescent, you may have had many fears as you developed and moved into new experiences and opportunities. As an adult, you may have felt anxiety associated with a new role as wife and husband, mother or father. Certainly happiness, challenge, and excitement exist with change, but also an apprehension of the unknown. With just the thought of change, people may express feelings of confusion, anger, threat, and bewilderment. As environmental changes occur, many people become less changeable. In remembering how you felt, you may understand how others feel. Shakespeare was speaking of death, but his statement also applies to change:

> And makes us rather bear those ills we have, than fly
> to others we know not of. [Hamlet]

The result of anxiety and fear is a reluctance to change; *any real change comes slowly.* The pace will be an individual matter; some people will change more quickly than others. Many times the more successful, orderly, and precise the person, the more slowly he/she will be able to change attitudes, behaviors, values, beliefs, or life style. You may understand how difficult it is to change ingrained life patterns but not understand how equally difficult it may be for a person to change a daily habit or routine. As a nurse working with change, you should expect change to be frightening for the client and to come slowly.

TABLE 7-1.   Change Experience Sheet

Answer all questions as quickly and spontaneously as possible.

1. When I think of change I think of_____
2. A change of style of life makes me feel _____
3. When I am asked to be orderly and systematic I_____
4. When I perceive a difficult situation and become dissatisfied I_____
5. When I am given a new task to try I_____
6. When another person disagrees with me I_____
7. When I am asked to take a job risk I feel_____
8. To be "open" means to be _____
9. Identify a personal characteristic in yourself that you would like others to perceive.

_____

10. Identify a personal characteristic in yourself which you wish to modify.

_____

11. What restrains you from making changes you desire?_____

Recognition of Need Produces Motivation

A sense of need may arise with a crisis, conflict, disorganization, or dissatisfaction, any of which can produce tension. The tension brings about unorganized energy, energy that is available either for nonproductive activity or for productive activity and for problem solving. Energy may be felt in the form of anxiety, tension, and discomfort; it propels the person into some form of activity, including aggressive, withdrawn, or neurotic behavior; somatic symptoms; or a cognitive-intellectual process of goal formation with problem solving, learning, and resolution (2). The cognitive-intellectual process is the more productive means of resolution and becomes a step in the change process. Defenses and nonproductive behavior bring about blocking and resistance.

Hope: Basis for Belief in a Solution

Hope is the eternal light in the distance that motivates a search for knowledge, ideas, and actions that contribute to a solution. It is the sense of possibility that keeps the prisoner alive and the dying person strengthened throughout the last stages. Hope is the energizer that motivates the person to continue to move on, the organization to continue to strive, and the community to work together. Sharon Roberts describes hope as the best resource of humanity; it brings transcendence to any situation (41). It is a necessary concept in the process of change.

You may be able to strengthen hope by looking for, evaluating, and confronting the client with his/her strengths, weaknesses, and potential for change. The better you know the client, the more impact you will have upon nurturing and fostering hope.

The Search Process: Seeking Possible Alternatives

Searching for a solution may take a variety of forms. Change may come to the individual as he/she consciously works out thoughts and fantasies; unconsciously processes ideas, thoughts, dreams, or daydreams; and intellectually and psychologically searches for insight. As a nurse and crisis worker, you are a change agent as you assist the person to problem solve and search for insight and options from which to choose. An organization or community may over time informally search, by trial and error, for a solution to a need or problem, as well as formally search through the use of standard procedures and administrative skills. Search for a plan or an idea occurs in the system by observation, data collection, task analysis, and the exchange of ideas through established channels and at various levels of meetings.

Decision Brings About Goal Setting and Action

A decision includes a plan of action, implementation of the plan, and feedback. The plan must include some type of goal setting. This may involve a formal operation whereby a work group within an organization establishes goals, sets target dates with time plans, and creates guidelines for participants. The process might include task groups, follow-through, and evaluation. Sometimes a decision comes through an informal process whereby the decision results from a gradual process of growth and maturation.

You need to consider several areas in setting goals for change: yourself, the client, and the system where the change is to occur. This knowledge should include understanding the dynamics of both yourself and the client, the strengths and weaknesses of people within the system and of the overall system itself, and the communication channels and abilities. Set priorities and determine which change is important and needed. Avoid changing just for change's sake. Look at the goals and envision the stresses that might be encountered. If the potential for change is not carried within the client or system, then failure will occur. Consideration of these areas and realistic appraisal of and commitment to goals will assist the client or system to move into the next phase and achieve change.

Commitment to the Goals and the Process

To have change continue there must be an involvement in the continuation of the process. To climb a mountain you must want to, be willing to expend the energy, and be interested in going all the way to the top. This involves dedication, willingness to take chances, compromise, evaluation, feedback, and perhaps taking another path. *Commitment means energy involvement.* This is true of the individual, group, organization, or community. When more than one individual is involved, the commitment must be the total response, even though the reaction is made up of individual feelings and responses.

The Creative Act of Change

E. O. Bevis stated that creativity in change is the act of change (7). To *create implies to bring about the new: in thought, attitude, behavior, idea, or product.* The new is the end result of the change process. The system (person, organization, or community) integrates the change, and it becomes stabilized and productive again.

Change is followed by periods of stability and consolidation. If change is too rapid, a movement backward occurs, and the system must regain equilibrium before moving ahead again. The system must stabilize a rapid gain and use resources and energies for production and maintenance rather than for internal change. If the system cannot produce a sufficient output, it cannot maintain an adequate level of exchange with its environment. These internal reorganization changes may consume a major amount of the energy, but another period of productivity and stability will follow. Forward movement and stability alternate. You might think of climbing stairs. Picture yourself taking two up and one back in order to gain your breath, then going forward again. Such is the process of change.

After any change there will be feedback. You may have noticed this from other people, perhaps in the form of comments or facial reaction, when you changed your hair style, habit of dress, or behavioral pattern. You should understand the meaning of feedback. It may be positive or negative, involve approval or disapproval. Feedback in response to change may bring about other modifications and additional change. Feedback brings further ideas, needs, and renewal of the process. This is the full process of creative change.

As you work with clients in crisis, stress, and

emotional pain, you will want to help them bring about change in their lives so that they can move toward a more secure, stabilized state of mental health. First approach your own attitudes and feelings about change itself. Evaluate how you handle change and, as much as possible, observe your own behavior. Be open to yourself. Ask your friends

and trusted persons for feedback on the way you handle changes. The more you can resolve and deal with your own feelings, the more you will be able to assist others. Study the change process. Get to know your client. Only in the environment of trust will the newest change be allowed freedom to stabilize and be integrated.

TYPES AND DYNAMICS OF CHANGE

Developmental or Situational Change

There are two types of change that any client undergoes—developmental and situational. *Developmental changes have to do with psychosocial change in the person's experiences and the normal life cycle stages* and can therefore be a part of planned change. Some family examples are the arrival of a new baby, when children reach puberty, or when retirement occurs. In organizations, these individual life cycle stages in the members can create problems, conflicts, and a need for action. Developmental changes in an organization would include an expansion or decline in the company in response to economic and consumer pressures. *Situational changes are those that are external or accidental (unplanned) to the client.* Examples of situational changes include when a child dies, a family member is seriously injured by a tragic accident, or economic decline for a person or a group. A natural disaster causing property damage could be a situational change for an individual, family, group, or community. Further information about developmental and situational crises that result in change can be found in Chapter 8.

Our society is characterized by rapid change, which is one of the most common psychosocial stressors. Throughout the entire life span, individuals experience separation from others, which changes their interpersonal relationships and life styles. Even pleasant and positive changes are potential stressors. For example, a job promotion that is considered positive can carry with it increased responsibilities and the need to develop new ways of behaving and interacting. Change interferes with the existing adaptive patterns for fulfilling needs of love, self-esteem, and self-actualization. With each change, interpersonal relationships are affected, which in turn necessitates further individual and group change.

General Dynamics of Change

The characteristics that are essential for change and evolvement of maturity in the therapeutic one-to-one relationship are equally applicable to other categories of interactions in which the purpose of the interaction is to promote change. The relationship between group member and group leader, organizational groups to management leader, and community groups to community leader may also fall into this category of interactions when the goal is to promote a change in functioning. In other words, the dynamics of the change process are generally the same in any type of change; the major differences lie in the complexities surrounding the change. The degree of successful change will depend on the ability of the change agent to facilitate a helping relationship with the client—whether it be one-to-one, individual-group, groups-organization, or groups-community.

Basic to effective change is the understanding that in any client or system there is a synthesis of subparts or subsystems. Regardless of size, there are certain similarities in terms of the relationship between subparts or subsystems that make for health, growth and collaboration, or for dysfunction and conflict. The degree of change-growth potential depends on how well the parts of the system are put together. For it is along the interfaces between parts of the system that human organization, whether within a person, group, organization, or community, is either sealed and bonded or stressed and broken (6). These counterforces produce either security or anxiety in man and either collaboration or competition in groups or the community. Therefore, in order for change to become effective, you must assist the client or system to look at the relationships between subparts and subsystems.

Conditions for individual, group, organization, or community change are basically the same. The process will be analogous for each type of system. Change in each type of system will be discussed in the following pages.

Change in the Person

The mind and body are inextricably related. If either is at odds over the satisfaction of any need in the human system, there is a problem. There are innumerable possibilities for subsystem conflicts within each individual. If a client is to maintain a reasonably stable health state, there must be compatible relationships between all parts within and between his/her own subsystems.

Thus the person is constantly confronted by the need to change and make choices between goals, values, and ideas. When an individual consults a counselor for help in making appropriate decisions regarding his/her life, the counselor's role is to assist in illuminating alternatives or options, to help the person make responsible choices between them, and to promote emotional harmony and stability in the client. The following conditions in the psychotherapeutic process, further described in Chapter 6, seem to be present when the phenomenon of change occurs in the person.

Facing the problem comes first. The person is in a situation that he/she perceives as being a serious and meaningful problem and with which he/she has unsuccessfully attempted to cope. The problem may be difficulty at work, unhappiness about personal behavior, or feelings of being overwhelmed by confusion and conflicts. Therefore, the person wants to change, yet feels ambivalence, anxiety, and fear before discovering what is wrong and attempting change.

If meaningful change is to take place in the relationship, it is necessary that the therapist (change agent) be a genuine, unified, integrated person, with characteristics like those of the helper described in Chapter 6. The extent to which the therapist provides a climate of acceptance, empathy, warmth, and nonjudgmental caring will influence the extent of constructive change in the client. The therapist opens the way for the client to broaden self-understanding and to change.

Change in the Small Group

All groups have differentiated parts or subgroups in the form of group members, each with differing goals, values, or procedures. Sometimes subgrouping and divisions are unchanging and sometimes fluid. Probably the most important factor for understanding the group is to understand the relationship among and between the subgroups. An example of a small group might be the family. The subgroupings are caused by differences of sex, age, and role. The management of a family might be thought of, in large part, as the management of relationships between these subgroups.

In many significant ways the individual and the group change processes are very similar. They are also distinctly different. They are similar in that they both arise from a common purpose and from a shared conception of the human potential for change. The differences arise primarily from the number of people involved. In the individual therapeutic process there are several people involved. The additional number of people involves more than just the extension of the individual therapeutic process to six or seven persons at one time; it provides a qualitatively different experience with distinctly different therapeutic outcomes. Chapter 11 discusses the group process in greater depth.

Similarities between Individual and Group Therapies in the Change Process

As in the individual therapeutic process, if the person is to grow (change) from the group experience, he/she must feel genuinely accepted by the therapist (change agent). As in the individual therapeutic process, there must be freedom to look at self in a climate in which the therapist seeks to understand the client's life from his/her viewpoint. It is necessary that the individual, as well as the group as a whole, feel respected at every step of the way. It is also advantageous, and probably necessary, for the individual in the group, and the group as a whole, to feel confidence in ability to make choices, no matter what the direction, and to have responsibility for behavioral change. In essence, the attitudes of confidence and respect that are so important for the therapist (change agent) to nurture in the individual client relationship are equally as important in the group relationship.

Another similarity is the unity of content and feeling found in the group. Actually, this concept may be hard to understand since individual problems of the group member could understandably serve to exert a centrifugal effect on the group. In actuality, this has not been found to occur. Invariably, there are really only a few kinds of problems that people can have. Most of these involve a breakdown in interpersonal relationships, resulting in lowered self-esteem. However, this similarity of content in group discussions is probably secondary to the feelings of unity that develop from the sharing of feelings. As in the individual therapeutic process, the goal of the process is to gain from the experience itself.

Differences between Individual and Group Therapies in the Change Process

Although there are significant similarities between the individual and group therapeutic process, there are also some distinctive differences. One of the most important of these differences has to do with the fact that the group situation brings into focus the problem with interpersonal relationships and provides an immediate opportunity for finding new and more meaningful ways of relating. It is, after all, a negative experience with other significant persons that created the discrepancies in the client's self-perception and that brings him/her into the therapeutic process. When these experiences have been hurtful, the person reacts by adapting a coping pattern that is rigid and controlled and that is not too effective, even if it does prevent total personality disintegration. The person is desperately in need of some experience that will help him/her change behavior and feel closer to others. The group therapeutic process, in which the expectation is that people will come closer together, offers such an experience. The group experience also offers a diversity of values that the individual may use as he/she perceives this material to be meaningful. Another opportunity that the group therapeutic process offers for change, which is not present in the individual therapeutic process, is that in the group the individual may be simultaneously giving and receiving help. Perhaps the most significant aspect of the group experience is that it is a considerably more meaningful experience to be understood and accepted by several people who are honestly sharing their feelings rather than only by the therapist (change agent).

A group's adaptive behavior will be most appropriate and effective when each member is maximally involved in making creative contributions. Although groups usually do not operate at this ideal level where members are given this opportunity, given the appropriate conditions, the group can develop so that is does approach the maximum utilization of potential and engage in change.

Change in the Organization

An organization, no matter what size, is made up of many subgroups (6). This is especially true in modern-day society where specialization is a predominant occupational characteristic. Specialized subgroups are utilized to carry out many of the required assignments.

A hospital, for example, will need many different groups for clinical services: nursing, maintenance, administration, purchasing, education, public relations, and others. A government facility may need military, civilian, and computer operations personnel; research and development groups; division; branches; sections; and so on.

The organization may be viewed as a matrix of specialized services, talents, and resources overlaid on centralized functions. For example, a nurse working on a ward is dependent on the laundry department for linens. Or a teacher must communicate with the audiovisual department for a film to show to the class.

The total organization really represents a composite of its various groups. Each group may be seen as a human subsystem, one that can further be divided into even smaller human subsystems. For example, a hospital nursing service department consists of various levels of nursing personnel. The nurses in one typical group identify themselves as supervisors assigned to particular services throughout the hospital. Within each service, head nurses are differentiated from staff nurses, and they in turn are differentiated into various specialized subgroups, such as psychiatric, obstetrical, medical, surgical, or pediatric.

Organizational change requires alterations in the behavior of individuals and groups. A certain degree of upset always accompanies organizational change. Some people welcome the upset because they found prior conditions restrictive. Others, who had no complaints about the previous conditions, may look forward to the change because they can see potential personal gains. However, change in the status quo is likely to be looked at suspiciously by those who are uncertain of just what the new change might bring. This is especially true of older individuals who have been with the organization for a long time and who view another change as requiring a costly expenditure of energy to which they have little or no desire to commit themselves.

Because organizational change necessitates an alteration in the behavior of individuals and groups, attention must be given to the psychological factors involved. These factors may work either to facilitate or retard the change. The psychological factors usually operative in organizational change are: (1) leadership attitudes, (2) identification of individuals with the organization, (3) influence of the immediate work group, (4) a sense of involvement and participation, and (5) release and acceptance of authority (25).

Top leadership support for new proposals is the first important factor that acts to facilitate change. For the most part, workers will respond to what their leaders want. Because of this, there should be no doubt about the position of the leadership toward the change. If the leadership presents an unsure position toward the change, then it is very likely that the members further down the line will also feel unsure. They, in fact, may openly oppose the change or take what to them is a safe path of passive resistance (25).

Most individuals in the organization view their own future as being internally linked with the fortunes of the organization, which is another powerful force in favor of effecting change. The more the organization grows and the more stable it becomes, the better and more stable the jobs will be. This kind of pervasive identification is of great help to a leadership seeking acceptance of its proposal for change (25).

A person's behavior is greatly affected by the responses he/she receives from the group to which he/she belongs. This kind of group influence can be a useful management tool in facilitating the acceptance of change. If the dominant members of the group have positive attitudes toward the new proposal, then it is likely that the other group members will become accepting of the proposal also. On the other hand, if the leaders within the group show serious disagreement, mem-

bers may be encouraged to doubt benefits of the proposed change (25).

In general, *people are more likely to accept and facilitate change if they have had an opportunity to share in the formulation of the proposals.* However, it is extremely important that the desire of leadership for input be genuine. If the leadership planners just go through the motion of inviting input from others after the change has already been determined, then the members will feel belittled or manipulated. Not only will they question the integrity of the leadership, but they also may respond negatively to the proposals for change (25).

People do not relinquish authority easily. It is not easy to relinquish the power and prestige that are concomitant to authority; rather *a large number of people seek to increase authority* (25). This conflict is significant in some large psychiatric facilities that are changing from a centralized organizational structure to one of decentralization. Such a change is frequently met with resistance from those in top positions since they are the ones who will be giving up their direct authority over services, whereas the proposal will receive much support from the newly appointed unit directors since they will secure a great increase in authority.

Sometimes a person may feel that the proposal for change is so pervasive that he/she either must accept the change or resign. Another person might be thoroughly opposed to the plan but pretend a show of absolute compliance, sit back, and wait for errors to show up in the implementation of the new proposal.

Although there are various emotional factors that determine a person's response to major changes in the organization, the new proposals, if they make sense, will carry themselves. The success of management in effecting major changes with the least amount of difficulty will be dependent on the skill it exercises in promoting growth-oriented responses in favor of change. The same process used to promote change in the individual can be utilized to promote change in the organization. An organization, just as a person, has an emotional life. In fact, feelings of individuals within the organization are often critical elements in determining the emotional life of the organization. Reduction of anxiety and open communication are major psychological mechanisms that must be dealt with by management if the proposed change is to be significantly effective.

Change in the Community

Conditions similar to the organization may be observed if one takes the community as the unit of analysis. The community consists of human systems that are easily distinguished by language, geographic location, and association of interests. Each group in a community is a human subsystem that in turn is divisible into smaller subsystems. It is important for these groups or subsystems, whether formal or informal, to perceive their goals as being the same as the overall goals of the community, or if different, to see their own goals being satisfied as a direct result of working for the goals of the community. It is the management of the interrelationships between each group and the smaller subsystems that will determine the effective function of a particular community.

The community can be referred to as a "unified field (37)." Change in one segment will create change in other segments of the community in one way or another. The response of each segment can be quite varied, depending on the way the change is experienced and perceived. But whatever the response, the idea of the dynamic community would lead one to believe that these are overall responses rather than haphazard responses based on individual idiosyncrasies. Since groups within the community act to maintain stability, and other forces or changes cause instability and disequilibrium. Changes in any one group in the community will produce changes in the community as a whole. When group behavior is such that it serves to reduce group instability and disequilibrium, it may be referred to as *adaptive behavior.* The degree to which the group's behavior is adaptive depends on the appropriateness of methods used by the group as it relates to the internal imbalance of stability and disequilibrium.

On occasion, groups or units of a community come into conflict. This conflict between groups can affect the overall goals of the community. The problem is said to exist because as groups become more committed to their own goals, they are apt to compete with each other and seek to undermine the activities of rival groups. When this occurs, they become a liability to the community as a whole. The problem then becomes how to establish collaborative intergroup relations.

RISKS INVOLVED IN THE CHANGE PROCESS

Any change brings about a reaction. Change may evoke restlessness, discomfort, and anxiety, as well as feelings of joy, excitement, and involvement. Two people may be in the same situation, but they respond differently based on their personal uniqueness, life experiences, support systems, and environment. We can say, however, that in most circumstances a person will react to major change as if it were a risk—with a sense of tension, anxiety, or fear.

The greatest risk involved in change is the risk of losing the wholeness or identity that makes up the person, organization, group, or community. The person may have so many changes that *psychosis, breakdown of the organization of the personality,* occurs. The individual (or group, organization, or community) may become so disorganized with change that he/she is unable to function effectively or meet goals or tasks.

Through personality development, the individual lays down a foundation that is either stable or unstable and that provides the essence of self—the spirit, values, beliefs, standards, sense of purpose, direction, and basic principles. In the organization this function includes the charter, philosophy, staff, job descriptions, board members, community support, ground rules, and informal and formal organizational structure. To prepare or to evaluate change in ourselves, others, and the organization, we must first look to the foundation and the principles that do not change, to see if there is security. We know from the principle of leverage that in order to pick something up, there must be a solid base upon which to move. A solid base gives more freedom for the movement that occurs during change.

In assessing a person's risk potential, ask the following questions: If there is not perceived security or a solid base, can successful change be planned? If change does occur, what is needed to create greater security? The individual can work to develop self through various ways, such as self-awareness exercises and realistic appraisal of self, feedback from support systems, a group or personal experience with a helping professional person, or other personal growth experiences.

The change agent must also assess the organization or community to know that changes can occur and what support systems are needed so that change can occur as smoothly and productively as possible. We want to rule change and not have it rule us. The wise change agent will ask how the system will react to the change and whether the risk can be handled. If not wisely considered, the system may end up with a goal that had not been chosen originally. If the equilibrium does not accommodate for the envisioned change, the result may nullify the efforts at progress.

A second risk involved in the change process is the stress response involved, a response that is normal, expected, and needs to be considered. Frequently when we feel anxious and uncomfortable, we look for some hidden meaning and overlook the stressors involved in the situation. Certainly stress is present when trying out new behaviors or confronting conflict situations or dissatisfactions. However, frequently the discomfort is associated with the stress of change itself. Review Chapter 12 to get a broader perspective of the effects of stress.

A third risk that always occurs with change is loss. Whether perceived as positive or negative, change involves a sense of loss for the familiar— for the way it used to be. Sometimes a yearning for the "tried and true" causes us to slip back into old behavior patterns or recreate a familiar situation, in spite of overt goals for change. The feelings of hurt, pain, and suffering arising from the loss experience are also uncomfortable. The more we understand the experience of loss, and how best to deal with it, the more successful will be the

progress during change. Review Chapter 8 on loss and grief reactions.

A risk of change is also psychological or physiological illness. Two researchers, T. Holmes and R. Rahe, have correlated life changes with illness susceptibility in their Social Readjustment Scale (30). When enough life changes occur within one year, illness frequently occurs. See Chapters 8 and 12 for further description.

Risk of change also brings up other unfamiliar and frightening feelings. Change can bring about feelings of detachment or vulnerability. As growth and change takes place, you are more vulnerable until you have become comfortable with the new way. Also, you may react to these experiences in ways previously unfamiliar to you. Hidden in the cleavage lines of each personality are responses that come forth in times of least resistance. In one instance, you may feel attacked when in reality no one is attacking you. Or you may momentarily fear that you are exercising too much initiative or creativity. You may not feel free with new demands, or you may feel closed in with either too much intimacy or too much isolation. These feelings may be fleeting and will submerge with time and as progress is made.

Change does involve risk. At the same time there is within each human being the need to progress and move ahead. The desire for development and the hope that life will improve spur us on for greater changes and risks. Risks are diminished with greater knowledge of self, others, the involved social system, the change process, and the available support systems. Risks decrease when: (1) the system and change agent are sufficiently organized and knowledgeable; (2) the planned change is not too great, and it is not implemented with too much speed; (3) freedom of movement is based on flexibility and security; and (4) a personal commitment is given to the specific change.

RESISTANCE TO CHANGE

A common reaction to change is resistance. **Resistance** *is any behavior that will oppose, obstruct, or block movement in the change process.* Resistance can be an **active process** *whereby the person directly confronts the environment by refusing to comply, openly opposing new ideas, blaming the change agent when something goes wrong, actively disagreeing with a new activity, or attacking the change*

agent. Resistance can also be a **passive process** *whereby the person avoids or delays change indirectly* through conscious strategies, apathy, silence, detachment, expressions of hopelessness, or unconscious use of defense mechanisms, such as projection, displacement, or denial (39).

In an organization, resistance can be manifested by absenteeism, resignations, requests for transfers, reduction in performance, drifting back into old patterns of behavior, postponing deadlines for action, communication breakdowns, or uncooperative, aggressive, and defensive behaviors. The more threatening the situation, the more intense will be the resistance. Individuals resist change in themselves because of disturbed equilibrium, vested interests, or poor timing, or because of fear and anxiety concerning emotional, social, or financial security, and stability, prestige, and social status position.

In the organization, resistance increases when: (1) notification of a change is not clearly communicated, (2) norms and customs of the organization are ignored, (3) excessive work pressure is involved, (4) little consideration is given to possible problem areas, and (5) management is poorly organized (39). The more pressure or forces operating to move individuals, the more resistance can be expected (6). In some instances, resistance occurs because the person is satisfied with the status quo and does not wish to expend the energy demanded by any change (42).

Whether you are working for personal growth with a client, or as a change agent in a organization or community agency, it is important to be aware of resistance and to search for ways to prevent an undue amount, as well as to overcome it.

Know as much as possible about the client and the system, the reasons for the resistance, and what measures might be used for eliminating difficulty. Perhaps the major problem is lack of trust. Almost any situation will be a threatening one if trust is not present either between client and nurse or within the group or organization. Active and open communication needs to be encouraged with continued protection of the relationship between nurse and client. Sometimes answers to questions or information to alleviate fears will help. Participation and decision making frequently will encourage involvement. Supportive persons may be helpful to the individual confronting change. Support may also come from the maturity within the person, from members within the small group, or from allies within or outside of the organization. Give the client time to readjust and change. The change process takes time.

A paradoxical form of resistance may also occur—resistance to stability and order. Some people are so attracted to the ever-changing, accelerated pace of life that they feel bored, tense, or depressed when the system is stable. They want action, without regard for its outcome. The goal is excitement, not constructive, thoughtful change. Because of the reaction they evoke in others, these people may in the long run be the greatest obstacle to planned change. Their impatience with studies, surveys, pilot projects, consultants, and colleagues may ensure failure of a plan for change (42).

ROLE OF CHANGE AGENT IN THE NURSING PROCESS

In order for you to be a change agent using a Humanistic Framework to effect positive change, you must be aware of your own reactions to change and be able to change your behavior. Then you can develop a collaborative relationship between yourself and the client system—whether individual, group, organization, or community. You must use yourself as a "helper" in releasing energy that moves toward alteration and then stability in human systems of any size. As a change agent, you will facilitate a process that, in essence, comes from the members themselves. Perhaps the most important skill that the change agent possesses is interpersonal competence.

The components of the nursing process—assessment, problem identification (nursing diagnosis), goal establishment, intervention, and evaluation—can be utilized by the change agent to facilitate change in the client system.

Assessment

As a change agent, collect as much information as possible about the client system by listening and observing. Take note of how people relate to one another and how various groups of individuals work together. Listen and observe for signs of stress that might be harmful to the client during the process of the proposed change. In addition, listen and observe for indications of trust, respect, confidence, openness, and other signs of health. Determine centers of resistance. Listen closely to others' feelings and suggestions.

Problem Identification or Nursing Diagnosis

The second step is identification of problems that emerge from the data assessment. Often the biggest problem at issue is that the problems are not clear — people are not getting along and do not know why they are not getting along. It is not easy to formulate a clear definition of a problem. Often it takes several attempts before interpersonal issues can be clearly stated. The competent change agent works back and forth between initial assessment information, tentatively stated problems, and newly gathered information in an effort to formulate statements of the problem that are mutually understood and agreed to by all involved parties.

Goal Formulation and Planning

Once the relevant data have been collected and the initial nursing diagnosis of need for change is formulated, appropriate goals to be achieved from the change should be outlined. Goals should be stated as desired outcomes. Formulate goals and the plan of action by getting input from all people who are involved in the change so that the goals are mutually understood and shared. Be patient with resistive people; involve them gradually in goal setting, if possible.

Intervention

The principles described for an individual therapist (Chapter 6) or for the group leader (Chapter 11) are applicable in intervention for change. When you work with an organizational or community system, the following approach is useful. Using insights gained from discussion of Second and Third Force theorists in Chapter 2 and the developing person in Chapter 3 will help you use a humanistic approach as you assist others with making change.

Acknowledge feelings of the people involved. Include suggestions from the average worker in the system if possible. Do not rush to give all of the solutions. Plan specific interventions, through collaboration with others, that are designed to make the change seem inviting and thus facilitate the change. Promote psychological bonding by helping to create a therapeutic climate in which knowledge, opinions, and feelings can be discussed and mutual endeavors can be shared. Serve as a linking agent between individuals and groups. Listen for conflict between individuals and groups, and use effective interpersonal skills to collaborate with and bring individuals and groups together that need to be brought together in order to effect the proposed change. If there are negative feelings involving relationships, lift the issues to a level in which they can be vented and worked through. As a change agent, seek to establish, through a collaborative relationship with the client system, a psychological climate of respect, warmth, trust, openness, and understanding. In fact, the degree to which a collaborative relationship is established with the client system will determine the durability and genuine significance of the change. The conditions necessary for the establishment of a collaborative relationship have been discussed earlier in the chapter as conditions necessary for therapeutic growth (change) to take place. These questions for growth (change) apply whether the client system is individual, group, organization, or community.

Utilize the following principles of change when you are a change agent with any system (14):

1. The person takes part in change to the extent he/she has participated in planning.
2. The person accepts change better when the new message or expected behavior is not too different from that already in practice.
3. The person may respond better to gradual shaping of behavior, and the consequent change is likely to be more effective and long-lasting than the response to rapid change strategies.
4. The person changes to the extent that the reward or benefit is greater than the pain or disruption.
5. The person changes to the extent that others are also seen as changing.
6. The person maintains changed behavior to the extent that it is rewarded, supported, and satisfying.
7. The person needs time to detach from old behavior patterns while exploring and acclimating to new patterns.
8. The person who is highly anxious or mourning a loss created by the change learns or applies little about desired changes.

Evaluation

At some point during the change, your efforts to assist the client system toward change will cease and the client will have learned to adapt comfortably to the change. In the evaluative process, analyze both the positive and negative elements that the change has produced and the effectiveness of methods used to accomplish the change. Evaluate also your effectiveness as a model for creating and accepting change. Did the change consider the unique perceptions and needs of the client, whether individual, family, group, organization, or community? Were the principles of change adhered to?

The change agent might be compared to a gardener tending a flower garden. The gardener watches and helps the plants grow in their own direction, and feeds, waters, and weeds the garden. Although at times the gardener modifies and intervenes in the growth process by cutting off excess foliage or picking off excess buds, generally the gardener allows nature to take its course and encourages the desired outcome of beautiful flowers through nurturing of the roots and the stalk of the plant. So be it with the change agent.

REFERENCES

1. Anderson, Ralph, and Irl Carter, *Human Behavior in the Social Environment*, pp. 18–19. Chicago: Aldine Publishing Company, 1974.

2. Argyris, Chris, *Intervention Theory and Method: A Behavioral Science View*. Reading, Mass.: Addison-Wesley Publishing Co., Inc., 1973.

3. Aspree, Elsie, "The Process of Change," *Supervisor Nurse,* 6, no. 10 (1975), 15–24.

4. Auger, Jeanine, *Behavioral Systems and Nursing,* pp. 98–99. Englewood Cliffs, N.J.: Prentice-Hall, Inc., 1976.

5. Barron, Frank, and William Dement, *New Directions in Psychology.* New York: Holt, Rinehart and Winston, 1965.

6. Bennis, Warren, Kenneth D. Benne, and Robert Chin, eds., *The Planning of Change,* 2nd ed. New York: Holt, Rinehart and Winston, 1969.

7. Bevis, Em Olivia, *Curriculum Building in Nursing, A Process.* St. Louis: The C. V. Mosby Company, 1973.

8. Bluhn, John, "Planning for Social Change: Dilemmas for Health Planning," *Contemporary Community Nursing,* ed. John Bluhn, pp. 450–59. Boston: Little, Brown & Company, 1975.

9. Bocker, B., P. Duhent, and E. Eiserman, *Psychiatric/ Mental Health Nursing: Contemporary Readings.* New York: Van Nostrand Reinhold Company, 1978.

10. Brown, Esther Lucille, *Nursing Reconsidered: A Study of Change.* Philadelphia: J. B. Lippincott Company, 1970.

11. Brownlee, Ann, *Community, Culture and Care,* pp. 212–13. St. Louis: The C. V. Mosby Company, 1978.

12. Bullard, Dexter, ed., *Psychoanalysis and Psychotherapy: Selected Papers of Frieda Fromm-Reichman.* Chicago: University of Chicago Press, 1959.

13. Burd, Shirley, and Margaret Marshall, *Some Clinical Approaches to Psychiatric Nursing,* pp. 328–29. New York: Macmillan Publishing Co., Inc., 1963.

14. Bushnell, Marilyn, "Institutions in Transition," *Perspectives of Psychiatric Care,* 17, no. 6 (1979), 260–65.

15. Cannon, W., *The Wisdom of the Body.* New York: W. W. Norton & Co., Inc., 1939.

16. Craig, Anne, and Barbara Hyatt, "Chronicity in Mental Illness: A Theory on the Role of Change," *Perspectives in Psychiatric Care,* 16, no. 3 (1978), 139–54.

17. Crum, M. R., et al., "Open-Mindedness, Rigidity, and the Tendency to Change Inferences among Psychiatric Nursing Staff: A Pilot Study," *Nursing Research,* 27, no. 1 (1978), 42–47.

18. Delaughery, Grace, Kristine Gebbie, and Betty Neuman, *Community Mental Health Nursing.* Baltimore: The Williams & Wilkins Company, 1971, pp. 130–40.

19. Denner, Bruce, and Richard Price, *Community Mental Health,* pp. 200–202. New York: Holt, Rinehart, and Winston, 1973.

20. Epstein, R. B., *Coping with Change through Assessment and Evaluation: Theory and Process of Change,* pp. 1–12. New York: National League for Nursing, 1976.

21. Foster, J., "The Group Solution to Isolation," *Nursing Mirror,* 147 (October 12, 1978), 28–29.

22. Friedman, Alfred, et al., eds. *Comprehensive Textbook of Psychiatry—II.* Baltimore: The Williams Wilkins Company, 1975.

23. Gassett, Hester, "Participative Planned Change," *Supervisor Nurse,* 7, no. 3 (1976), 34–40.

24. Ginzberg, E. and Reilly, R., *Effecting Change in Large Organizations.* New York: Columbia University Press, 1957.

25. Gordon, Marjory, "The Clinical Specialist as a Change Agent," *Nursing Outlook,* 17, no. 3 (1969), 14–20.

26. Haiman, Theodore, *Supervisory Management for Health Care Institutions.* St. Louis: The Catholic Hospital Association, 1974.

27. Hensey, Paul, and Kenneth Blanchard, *Management of Organizational Behavior: Utilizing Human Resources,* 2nd ed. Englewood Cliffs, N.J.: Prentice-Hall, Inc., 1972.

28. Hirschowitz, Ralph, O. "The Development of the Staff for Institutional Change," *Adult Leadership* (January 1975), pp. 211-13.

29. Hoffer, Eric, *The Ordeal of Change.* New York: Harper & Row, Publishers, Inc., 1963.

30. Holmes, T., and R. Rahe, "The Social Readjustment Rating Scale," *Journal of Psychosomatic Research,* 11, no. 8 (1967), 213-17.

31. Jacobs, B. P., "Loneliness When Age Brings a Crisis: The Nurse Can Restore Hope," *Nursing Mirror,* 147 (1978), 25-27.

32. Jensen, Diane, "Crisis Resolved: Impact through Planned Change," *Nursing Clinics of North America,* 8, no. 4 (1973), 735-42.

33. Joel, Lucille, and Doris Collins, *Psychiatric Nursing: Theory and Application,* pp. 386-93. New York: McGraw-Hill Book Company, 1978.

34. Johnson, Mae, et al., *Problem Solving in Nursing Practice.* Dubuque, Iowa: Wm. C. Brown Company Publishers, 1974.

35. Kenney, M., et al., "Planned Change in the Critical Care Unit," *Heart-Lung,* 7, no. 1 (1978), 85-89.

36. Kravetz, Diane, and Alice Sargent, "Consciousness-Raising Groups: A Resocialization Process for Personal and Social Change," *Supervisor Nurse,* 6, no. 10 (1975), 26-35.

37. Lewin, Kurt, *Field Therapy in Social Science.* New York: Harper & Row, Publishers, Inc., Brothers, 1951.

38. Lippitt, Ronald, Jeanne Watson, and Bruce Westley, *The Dynamics of Planned Change,* pp. 145-82. New York: Harcourt Brace and Jovanovich, Inc., 1958.

39. Olson, Elizabeth, "Strategies and Techniques for the Nurse Change Agent," *The Nursing Clinics of North America,* 14, no. 2 (1979), 323-37.

40. Riehl, Joan, and Sister Callista Roy, *Conceptual Models for Nursing Practice,* pp. 60–63. New York: Appleton-Century-Crofts, 1974.

41. Roberts, Sharon, *Behavioral Concepts and Nursing throughout the Life Span.* Englewood Cliffs, N.J.: Prentice-Hall, Inc., 1978.

42. Rodgers, Janet, "Change Process," in *Management for Nurses: A Multidisciplinary Approach,* eds. S. Stone, et al., pp. 174-83. St. Louis: The C. V. Mosby Company, 1980.

43. Rogers, Carl, *Client Centered Therapy.* Boston: Houghton Mifflin Company, 1951.

44. ——, "The Necessary and Sufficient Conditions of Therapeutic Personality Change," *Journal of Consulting Psychology,* Vol. 21: no. 2 (1957).

45. Schuler, Sandra, and Lenore Campbell, "The Theme Is Change," *Journal of Psychiatric Nursing and Mental Health Services,* 12, no. 4 (1974), 15-21.

46. Spradley, Barbara, ed., *Contemporary Community Nursing.* Boston: Little, Brown Company, 1975.

47. Stevens, Barbara, "Effecting Change," *Journal of Nursing Administration,* 5, no. 2 (1975), 23-26.

48. Stotland, Ezra, *The Psychology of Hope,* pp. 1-28. San Francisco: Jossey-Bass, Inc., 1969.

49. Strochan, J., "The Change-Loss Connection in Counselling," *Canadian Journal of Psychiatric Nursing,* 20 (January-February 1979), 6-8.

50. Sullivan, Harry Stack, *The Interpersonal Theory of Psychiatry.* New York: W. W. Norton & Co., Inc., 1953.

51. Sullivan, M. E., "Processes of Change in an Expanded Role in Nursing in a Mental Health Setting," *Journal of Psychiatric Nursing and Mental Health Services,* 15, no. 2 (1977), 18-24.

52. Sutterley, Doris Cook, and Gloria Ferraro Donnelly, *Perspectives in Human Development.* Philadelphia: J. B. Lippincott Company, 1973.

53. Sweeney, Anita, et al., "Courage to Change," *Journal of Psychiatric Nursing and Mental Health Services,* no. 2 (1969), 73-76.

54. Tofler, Alvin, *Future Shock.* New York: Random House, Inc., 1970.

55. Welch, Lynne, "Planned Change in Nursing: The Theory," *The Nursing Clinics of North America,* 14, no. 2 (1979), 307-22.

56. Wolff, K. C., "Change: Implementation of Primary Nursing through Advocacy," *Journal of Nursing Administration,* 7, no. 12 (1977), 24-27.

8

Crisis Intervention to Promote Psychological Adaptation

Study of this chapter will assist you to:

1. Differentiate between crisis and stress.

2. Identify the types of crises and list examples of each.

3. Relate the crisis of separation and loss, and the concomitant grief and mourning, to both developmental and situational crises.

4. Describe factors that influence coping with, and the outcome of, a crisis.

5. List the phases of crisis and describe the normal behavioral responses in each phase.

6. Define grief and mourning, and explain how the mourning process relates to the acknowledgment phase of crisis.

7. Compare and contrast reactions of family unit, group, and community to those of an individual during a crisis.

8. Examine behavioral manifestations of ineffective crisis resolution.

9. Relate the steps of the nursing process to crisis therapy.

10. Explore the necessity of integrating crisis theory into your philosophy of care.

11. Describe assessment parameters for the client in crisis.

12. Utilize assessment data for formulating a plan of care.

13. Demonstrate principles of crisis intervention with the client.

14. Relate levels of prevention to crisis intervention.

15. Modify application of principles of crisis intervention for use in telephone counseling.

This chapter contributed by Ruth Murray, R.N., M.S.N. and Virginia Luetje, R.N., M.S.N.

16. Assess and counsel the person in a suicidal crisis.

17. Apply principles of crisis therapy with persons throughout the life span, and with a family unit or group.

18. Modify principles of crisis assessment, planning, and intervention with persons who have verbal, hearing, or cognitive impairments.

19. Describe the crisis of illness, injury, hospitalization, and death for the person and family.

20. Utilize principles of crisis therapy with the person who has psychiatric or nonpsychiatric illness and with his/her family.

21. Demonstrate principles of crisis therapy with the client who has experienced loss or death of a significant person.

22. Apply principles of crisis therapy during care of the victim of sexual assault.

23. Prepare for crisis work with survivors of a disaster in the community.

24. Examine ways to maintain personal physical and emotional health in the face of ongoing crisis work that is a part of nursing.

Crisis theory provides nursing with a theoretical model of the adaptive processes that follow certain kinds of stressful, unmanageable events in life. The theory organizes events that appear haphazard and unpredictable, and it guides your intervention when working with persons in crisis.

DEFINITIONS AND CHARACTERISTICS

Crisis is any temporary situation that threatens the person's self-concept, necessitates reorganization of the psychological structure and behavior, causes a sudden alteration in the person's expectation of self, and cannot be handled with the person's usual coping mechanisms (19, 36). Crises always involve change and loss. Either the changes or losses that occur result in the person's inability to cope, or as a result of the crisis the person is no longer the same. He/she will have to change behavior in order to remain adaptive and functional, and in the process, loss will be felt. Resolution of the crisis and growth mean that something is lost even while something else is gained.

During crisis, the person's ordinary behavior is no longer successful—emotionally, intellectually,

The basic premise is that the person, family, group, and/or community in crisis are all essentially normal, capable of self-help, and capable of greater maturity with minimal help. In nursing, the emotionally ill and their families can be considered to be in crisis as discussed in this chapter.

or physically. Old habits are disturbed, and the person feels motivated to try new responses in order to cope with the new situation. Although behavior is inadequate or inappropriate to the present situation and may be different from normal; it should not be considered pathological. For example, rage or bitter prolonged crying by a usually jovial person may be an emotional release that paves the way for problem solving.

The crisis may also reactivate old, unresolved crises or conflicts, which can impose an additional burden to be handled at the present time. However, the crisis is a turning point, and with its resultant mobilization of energy, it operates as a second chance for resolving earlier crises or for correcting faulty problem solving. The time of crisis serves as a catalyst or opportunity for growth emotionally. Readjustment of behavior occurs; if all goes well, a state of equilibrium or behavior that is more mature than the previous status results. On the other hand, because of the stress involved and the felt threat to the equilibrium, the person is also more vulnerable to regression and emotional or physical illness. The outcome—either increased, the same level of, or decreased maturity, or illness—depends on how the person handles the situation and on the help others give. Encountering and resolving crisis is a normal process that each person or family faces many times during a lifetime.

Stress must be differentiated from crisis. *Stress is the everyday wear and tear on the body, the effects of the pace of life at any moment, positive and negative, physical, emotional, or mental* (101). All living things are constantly under stress; and anything, pleasant or unpleasant, that speeds up the intensity of life causes a temporary increase in stress or in the wear and tear upon the body. For example, a day of vacation or one of challenging work can be equally stressful. Stress does not consist merely of damage, but also of the adaptation to stress, and can be positive and life-promoting. During a stressful period, the person may use normal coping mechanisms. The temporary upsets in equilibrium are solved by previously learned coping techniques and various mechanisms of tension discharge, such as talking or physical activity. Nonetheless, stress, especially if persistent and intense, has a potential for reducing the person's level of emotional health, whereas crisis has a potential for raising the level of emotional health. Yet both may have either a positive or negative outcome (87, 94, 101). The effects of stress are further discussed in Chapter 12.

Not all persons facing the same hazardous event will be in a state of crisis. But some events or situations are viewed as a crisis by all persons, of any age, in that some behavioral adjustment must be made by anyone facing that situation. Research by T. Holmes and R. Rahe has shown that the number and seriousness of certain kinds of life changes or crises, ranging from death of a loved one to receiving a parking ticket, that are encountered within a year will increase the person's chance of facing other crises, including illness or accidental injury. (See Table 8-1.) Crises also vary in degree; a situation may be perceived as major, moderate, or minimal in the degree of discomfort caused and in the amount of behavioral change demanded.

TABLE 8-1. Social Readjustment Rating Scale
—Based on Life Change Unit (LCU) Scale

LIFE EVENT	MEAN VALUE
1. Death of spouse	100
2. Divorce	73
3. Marital separation	65
4. Jail term	63
5. Death of close family member	63
6. Personal injury or illness	53
7. Marriage	50
8. Fired at work	47
9. Marital reconciliation	45
10. Retirement	45
11. Change in health of family member	44
12. Pregnancy	40
13. Sex difficulties	39
14. Gain of new family member	39
15. Business readjustment	39
16. Change in financial state	38
17. Death of close friend	37

TABLE 8-1.   Continued

LIFE EVENT	MEAN VALUE
18. Change to different line of work	36
19. Change in number of arguments with spouse	35
20. Mortgage over $10,000	31
21. Foreclosure of mortgage or loan	30
22. Change in responsibilities at work	29
23. Son or daughter leaving home	29
24. Trouble with in-laws	29
25. Outstanding personal achievement	28
26. Wife begins or stops work	26
27. Beginning or end of school	26
28. Change in living conditions	25
29. Change in personal habits	24
30. Trouble with boss	23
31. Change in work hours or conditions	20
32. Change in residence	20
33. Change in schools	20
34. Change in recreation	19
35. Change in church activities	19
36. Change in social activities	18
37. Mortgage or loan less than $10,000	17
38. Change in sleeping habits	16
39. Change in number of family get-togethers	15
40. Change in eating habits	15
41. Vacation	13
42. Christmas	12
43. Minor violations of the law	11

LIFE CRISIS CATEGORIES AND LCU SCORES (FOR ONE YEAR)

CATEGORY OF LIFE CRISIS	LCU SCORE
No life crisis	0–49
Mild life crisis	150–199
Moderate life crisis	200–299
Major life crisis	300 or more

TYPES OF CRISES

Crises are divided into two categories: (1) developmental, maturational, or normative, and (2) situational or accidental (19).

Developmental Crises

Developmental crises occur during transition points,

those periods that every person and family experience in the process of biopsychosocial maturation. These are times in development when new relationships are formed and old relationships take on new aspects. There are new expectations of the person, and certain emotional tasks must be accomplished in order to move on to the next phase of development. The onset of the developmental or maturational crisis is gradual because it occurs as the person moves from one stage of development to another. The crisis resolves when the individual succeeds in new age-level behaviors; disruption does not last for the entire developmental phase.

Role theory is helpful for understanding why normal development leaves the person vulnerable to crisis (106). *Role is a goal-directed pattern of behavior learned within the cultural setting and carried out by the person in the social group or situation because both the person and group expect this behavior.* No role exists in isolation. It is always patterned to dovetail with or complement the role of another. When one person changes a role, the role partners—other persons in the system—undergo reciprocal role or behavioral changes. The times of developmental crisis are mainly periods of many role changes, although they may be slow and gradual and vary from one culture or social class to another. A maturational crisis occurs when the person is unable to make role changes appropriate to the new level of maturity. The stressful events are the social and biological pressures on the individual to see him/herself in a new and different role and act accordingly (106).

There are three main reasons why someone may be unable to make role changes necessary to prevent a maturational crisis:

1. The person may be unable to picture him/herself in a new role. Roles are learned, and adequate role models may not exist.
2. The person may be unable to make role changes because of a lack of intrapersonal resources—for example, inadequate communication skills; the realization that with life passing, certain goals will not be achieved; or the lack of past opportunities to learn how to cope with crises because of overprotection.
3. Others in the social system may refuse to see the person in a different role. For example, when the adolescent tries to move from childhood to the adult role, the parent may persist in keeping him in the child role (106).

The main developmental crises are entry into school, puberty, leaving home, graduation from school, marriage, pregnancy, childbirth, middle age, menopause, retirement and facing death of others and of the self.

However, certain turning points in life may not be crises, based on the person's ability to anticipate the next stage, to prepare, and to learn expected behaviors. The more clear cut the cultural definitions, the less frightening is the future situation because the person has models of behavior and can prepare in advance for change. The person's capacity to imagine the future is an important aspect of this process. For example, it is quite common to live out, in fantasy, what the future will hold; to identify potential problems; or to make some decisions in advance. However, in a fast-changing society, few turning points are clearly defined; thus the person may have difficulty in adjusting and will experience crises (2).

Several factors help the person adjust to a new life era: (1) desire for a change and boredom with present experiences, (2) agenda for a life course; present versus future plans, (3) accomplishments in the present era, (4) past success in coping with turning points, (5) group support in meeting turning points, and (6) examples of how peers have coped with similar situations (2).

Situational Crises

The *situational crisis is an external event or situation, not necessarily a part of normal living, often sudden, unexpected, and unfortunate, that looms larger than the person's immediate resources or ability to cope and thereby demands a change in behavior.* Life goals are threatened; tension and anxiety are evoked; unresolved problems and crises from the past are reawakened. The amount of time taken for healthy or unhealthy adaptation to occur is usually from one to six weeks, although resolution may take longer. A situational crisis may occur at the same time as a developmental crisis.

Situational crises include natural disasters, such as a hurricane, tornado, earthquake, or flood; loss through separation, divorce, or death of a loved one; losing one's job, money, or valued possessions; or a job change. Additions in the family, such as unwanted pregnancy, the return of a prisoner of war or deserter, adoption of a child, or remarriage resulting in a stepparent and step-siblings, also can cause a change in life style and are potential crises. Illness, hospitalization, or institutionalization; a power struggle on the job; a sudden change in role responsibilities; or a forced geographical relocation are other examples. Rape, suicide, homicide, or imprisonment can also be classified as this type of crisis (26).

The Crisis of Separation and Loss

Life is a series of losses. The crisis of separation and loss can be either developmental or situational in origin, and both kinds of losses may occur simultaneously. Loss and the universal reaction to loss— grief and mourning—are experienced by everyone at some time in life.

Loss is giving up external or internal supports required by the person to satisfy basic needs. In regard to loss, the term *object may mean a person, thing, relationship, or situation.*

Grief is a sequence of subjective states, a special intense form of sorrow caused by loss, either through separation or death of a loved person or loss of an object that is felt to be a part of the self or that provides psychological gratification. Grief is the emotion involved in the work of mourning. Absence of that which is lost is felt as a gap in one's sense of continuity and self-concept.

Mourning is a psychological process involving a range of reactions whereby the person suffers through the grief following either loss of a significant or valued object or person or realization that such a loss could occur. It is the process whereby disengagement occurs from an emotionally demanding relationship so that the person is able to reinvest emotionally in a new and productive relationship (88).

As a person's interdependence with others grows, the likelihood increases that separation, loss of something valuable, or death of a loved one will induce a crisis. The capacity to have warm and loving relationships also leaves the person vulnerable to sadness, despair, and grief. The more that was emotionally invested in that which is lost, the greater the threat is felt.

Every person is also subjected to separations or losses that are subtle and may not be recognized. Any crisis, developmental or situational, involves some degree of loss. If nothing else, there is a loss through change in old behavior patterns and the addition of different coping mechanisms. The process of achieving independence in psychosocial development in the course of normal upbringing involves a whole series of separations. The way these early separations are dealt with affects how later separations and loss, including death, will be resolved. Examples of loss situations, either partial or total, temporary or permanent, throughout the life span include the following:

1. Period of weaning in infancy; learning to wait.
2. First haircut, even when it involves pride and anticipation.
3. Period of increasing locomotion, exploration, and bowel and bladder control and resultant loss of dependency.
4. Loss of baby teeth, baby possessions, toys, clothes, or pets.
5. Change in the body, body image, and self-attitude with ongoing growth and development.
6. Change in body size and shape and in feelings accompanying pregnancy and childbirth; loss of body part or function, external or internal, through accident, illness, or aging.
7. Departure of children from the home when they go to school or marry.
8. Menopause and loss of childbearing functions.
9. Loss of hearing, vision, memory, strength, and other changes and losses associated with old age.
10. Changes and losses in relationships with others as the person moves from childhood to adulthood—loss of friends and lovers; separation from or death of family members; changes in residence, occupation, or place of business; promotions and graduations.
11. Losses with symbolic meanings, such as the loss of a symptom that attracted others' attention; a loss or change that necessitates a change in body image; or "loss of face," honor or prestige.
12. Loss of home due to natural disaster or relocation projects; loss of possessions or money.
13. Loss experienced with divorce or incapacitation of a loved one.

Thus the person brings to any major crisis a backlog of experience that predisposes him/her either to successfully integrate a personal tragedy or to fail to absorb another loss or change. The significance of the present reaction may become clear only when you understand the person's earlier separations and losses.

FACTORS INFLUENCING THE OUTCOME OF CRISIS

Many factors influence how the person, family, group, or community will react to and cope with crises situations (1, 19, 36).

1. *Perception of the event.* If the event (or the consequences of it) threatens the self-concept; conflicts with the value system, self-expectations, or wishes for the future; or is demoralizing or damaging, the situation is defined as *hazardous.* The perception of the event is reality for the person, regardless of how others might define reality. How the person perceives an event depends in large measure on past experience. For example, two persons live through the disaster of a tornado. One loses house and all possessions; the other has house damage but everything is intact. The latter may react with greater shock, denial, anger, or depression than the person who loses home and possessions because of each one's different perceptions— the meaning of the loss to each individual. Degree of perceived dependency on a lost object is also crucial; the greater the dependency, the more difficult the resolution of loss.

2. *Physical and emotional status,* including degree of health, amount of energy present, age, genetic endowment, and biological rhythms of the person, or the general well-being of the community.

3. *Coping techniques or mechanisms and level of personal maturity.* If adaptive capacities are already strained, or if the stress is overwhelming, the person will cling to old habits, and behavior will very likely be inappropriate to the task at hand. The person and family who have met developmental tasks all along and who perceive themselves as able to cope will adapt more easily in any crisis.

4. *Previous experiences with similar situations.* The person, family, or group needs to learn to cope with stress, change, and loss. If past crises were handled by distorting reality or by withdrawing, when similar crises arise, burdens of the prior failure will be added to the problem of coping with the new situation. Unresolved crises are cumulative in effect. The most recent crisis revives the denial, depression, anger, or maladaptation that was left unsettled from past crises. If the person successfully deals with crises, self-confidence and self-esteem will thereby be increased, and future crises will be handled more effectively. Success brings more success. If the community evolved an effective disaster plan after a previous crisis, the next disaster crisis will generally cause less disruption.

5. *Realistic aspects of the current situation,* such as personal or material losses, the extent to which community services are interrupted, or changes in living pattern necessitated by the loss.

6. *Cultural influences.* How the person is trained and socialized in the home to solve problems and meet crisis situations; the use of religious, cultural, or legal ceremonies or rituals to handle separation or loss and facilitate mourning; expectations of how the social group will support the person or family during crisis; and the method established by the community to provide help—all influence present behavior.

7. *The availability and response of family and close friends, community groups, or other helping resources,* including professional persons. The less available the environmental or emotional support systems are to decrease stress or buttress the coping response, the more hazardous the event will be. The family system, by its influence on development of self-concept and maturity, can increase or decrease the person's vulnerability to crisis. If prior to loss, the person derived satisfaction from a variety of objects, people, interests, and roles, he/she now has more bases of support and can more readily form new relationships. When involvement with others is concentrated on only a few family members— as, for example, in the nuclear versus the extended family support system—vulnerability

is increased. The reaction to crisis is increased in today's mobile, urbanized society because traditional support systems of long-term family and friends have been disrupted to varying degrees. Thus the professional person is more likely to be needed and sought. Even a small amount of influence exerted by a significant person can be enough to decide the outcome for emotional health and against emotional illness. Sustained emotional health is in large measure a result of a life history of successfully resolving crises.

The crisis-prone person or family often demonstrates the following characteristics: (1) rapid encountering of one stressful situation after another, with inadequate time to adjust to or cope with any one situation; (2) a history of inadequate coping skills; (3) lack of communication skills or inability to ask for help because of emotional isolation from others; (4) feelings locked into solving problems alone because of loss of persons or things that were viewed as supportive or because of feelings of racial or ethnic prejudice, demoralization, or alienation; and (5) inadequate family, social, religious, economic, or employment supportive resources. Frequent illness or accidents, legal problems, or abuse of alcohol or other drugs also may increase the risk of other crises (50).

Crisis effects are reduced by: (1) anticipating and preparing for the so-called unpredictable events, such as change of developmental stages, natural disasters, or death, (2) redefining or changing goals when something seems insurmountable, (3) developing communication skills and a support system, and (4) seeking help to work through each crisis and unresolved past crises (50).

PHASES OF CRISIS

All crises require a sudden and then a later restructuring of biopsychosocial integration before normal function can be restored. The phases involved are: shock, followed closely by general realization of the crisis; the defensive retreat; acknowledgment and mourning; and finally, adaptation or resolution (36, 66, 71).

Individual Reactions

Table 8-2 presents the feelings and behaviors that may be experienced by the person during the phases of crisis.

Stages of the Mourning Process

Stages of the mourning process occur in the third phase, Acknowledgment of Reality. Resolving loss, whether the death of a loved one or the loss of a significant object, status, or job, involves a number of steps.

The loss is first felt as a defect in the psychic self as the mourner becomes aware of innumerable ways in which he/she was dependent on the lost object as a source of gratification, for a feeling of well-being, for effective functioning, and for sense of self. The mourner is not ready to accept a new object in place of the old one, although passively and transiently a more dependent relationship may be accepted with remaining objects, roles, or persons.

Increased preoccupation with the loss, a heightened desire to talk about the loss, a search for evidence of failure "to do right," verbal self-accusation and ambivalence toward that which is lost become manifested with increasing acknowledgment.

With any love relationship, the person will also at times feel anger or dislike toward, or desire to be rid of, the relationship, along with the love feelings. The greater the ambivalence felt toward the lost object, person, or status, the greater the feelings of guilt and shame. In addition, the grieving person may feel angry at the lost (deceased, divorced, or separated) person for leaving. Guilt and angry feelings, a normal but often unacceptable part of grieving, are frequently displaced onto others: the doctor, nurse, employer, family member, or God. These feelings may also be handled through projection or reaction formation. If guilt is not resolved, then self-blame for the loss and preoccupation with it, with future losses, or with personal death, will occur.

The person continues to want to talk about the lost object or person, the pleasant memories, the meaning of the loss, and the events associated with it. Unfortunately, talking about the loss several weeks or months after it has happened is

TABLE 8-2. Individual Reactions in the Crisis Phases

PHASE AND DURATION	FEELINGS	COGNITIVE MANIFESTATIONS	PHYSICAL SYMPTOMS	INTERPERSONAL/SOCIAL BEHAVIOR
Initial Impact; Shock (duration of 1 to 24–48 hours)	Anxiety. Helplessness. Chaos. Overwhelmed. Hopeless. Incomplete. Detached. Despair. Depersonalized. Panic. Self-concept threatened. Self-esteem low. Anguish may be expressed by silent, audible, or uncontrollable crying.	Altered sensorium. Disorganized thinking. Unable to plan, reason logically, or understand situation. Impaired judgment. Preoccupation with image or hallucination of lost object/person.	Somatic distress. May suffer physical illness or injury and ignore symptoms. Shortness of breath. Choking. Sighing. Hyperventilation. Weakness. Fatigue. Tremors. Anorexia. Lump in throat or abdomen.	Disorganized behavior, Habitual or automatic behaviors used unsuccessfully. Withdrawn. Docile. Hyperactive. May appear overtly as if nothing happened or may be unable to carry out routine behavior. Lacks initiative for daily tasks. May need assistance meeting basic needs.
	In *Developmental Crisis*, the response more gradual. Feelings less intense. May feel anxiety, frustration, lack of confidence, discouragement, imperfection, unfamiliarity with self, loss of self-control as realizes new responsibilities. Cannot move emotionally into next stage or change life perception.			*Developmental Crisis* May try to do more than is biologically or emotionally realistic. Unable to achieve behavior appropriate to role or to change inappropriate behavior in relationships.
Defensive Retreat (duration of hours to weeks)	May feel tense and inadequate, but usually feels as if nothing is wrong because of use of repression and defense mechanisms. Apathetic or euphoric. Feelings displaced onto other objects.	Tries habitual coping mechanisms unsuccessfully. May try to redefine problem unrealistically. Fantasizes about what could be done, how well past problems handled. Avoids thinking about event. May be disori-	Denies symptoms unless presence of physical illness.	Tries habitual behaviors and defense mechanisms unsuccessfully. Usually withdraws from others indirectly. Superficial response. May avoid reality with overactivity. Resistant to change suggested by others. Unwilling to initiate new behavior. Ineffective, disorgan-

238

TABLE 8-2. Continued

PHASE AND DURATION	FEELINGS	COGNITIVE MANIFESTATIONS	PHYSICAL SYMPTOMS	INTERPERSONAL/SOCIAL BEHAVIOR
		ented. Maintains rigid thinking. States same ideas over and over. May be unable to devise alternate courses of action or predict effects of behavior. Denies through rationalization about cause for situation.		ized behavior. May be unable to maintain daily activities, work performance, or social roles. Denies through demands, complaints, or projections of inadequacy.

(Note: Temporary retreat emotionally, mentally, and socially is adaptive and protective from perceived stress and loss and overwhelming anxiety. Allows time to gradually realize what has happened; avoids debilitating effects of high anxiety or panic. Initially person fluctuates between the phases of Defensive Retreat and Acknowledgment of Reality.)

PHASE AND DURATION	FEELINGS	COGNITIVE MANIFESTATIONS	PHYSICAL SYMPTOMS	INTERPERSONAL/SOCIAL BEHAVIOR
Acknowledgment of Reality (duration varies)	Tension and anxiety rise. Loneliness. Irritable. Depressed. Agitated. Apathetic. Self-hate. Low self-esteem. Gradually self-satisfaction increased; self-concept becomes more positive. Gains self-confidence in ability to cope.	Becomes aware of facts about change, loss, event. Asks questions. Slowly redefines situation. Attempts problem solving. May be disorganized in thinking. Trial-and-error approach to problems. Gradually makes appropriate plans. Gives up unattainable goals. Validates personal experiences and feelings. Coping skills improved.	Symptoms may reappear or intensify. New symptoms may occur. May somatize feelings. Gradually regains physical health.	Gradually demonstrates appropriate behaviors and resumes roles. Utilizes suggestions. Tries new approaches. Greater maturity demonstrated.
Resolution; Adaption; Change (duration of mourning	Painful feelings integrated into self-concept and sense of maturity. New sense of worth. Firm identity. Gradual increase in self-	Perceives crisis situation in positive way. Integrates crisis event into self. Problem solving successful. Discusses	Functions at optimum level.	Discovers new resources. Uses support systems and resources appropriately. Resumes status and roles. Strengthens relations with others. Adaptive

239

TABLE 8-2. Continued

PHASE AND DURATION	FEELINGS	COGNITIVE MANIFESTATIONS	PHYSICAL SYMPTOMS	INTERPERSONAL/SOCIAL BEHAVIOR
and crisis work may be 6 to 12 months)	satisfaction about mastery of situation. Gradual lowering of anxiety. Does not feel bitter.	feelings about event. Organizes thinking and planning. Redefines priorities. Does not blame self or others. Remembers comfortably and realistically pleasures and disappointments of lost relationship.		in relationships. Life style may be changed.

often discouraged by family or friends, yet talking about the loss is one way of reinforcing reality as well as of expiating guilt through repeated self-assurance that all possible action was taken to prevent the loss. This repetitious talking about the loss is adaptive and continues until the person forms a memory, almost completely devoid of negative characteristics of the lost object, to replace the object that no longer exists. This process of idealization follows the difficult and painful experience of alternating guilt, remorse, fear, and regret for real or fantasied past acts of hostility, neglect, and lack of appreciation, or even for personal responsibility for the loss or death.

If the loss was a loved person, identification follows idealization. The mourner consciously adopts some of the behavior and admired qualities of the dead person. He/she changes interests in the direction of activities formerly enjoyed by the lost loved one, adopts the person's goals and ideals, or even takes on certain mannerisms of the deceased. In addition to developing symptoms that are a normal part of mourning, the person may develop symptoms similar to those suffered by the deceased loved person. This identification process maintains a tie with the deceased loved one and appeases some of the guilt felt for harboring earlier aggressive or angry feelings toward the dead person. How such symptoms are expressed depends on the person's constitutional factors as well as on past learning about which symptoms are most likely to get attention or to be defined as illness by the self and others. As this final identification is accomplished, preoccupation with the deceased, ambivalence, guilt, and sadness decrease, and thoughts return to life. If strong guilt is present, the person is more likely to take on undesirable characteristics, including the last disease symptoms, of the deceased. This negative identity may lead to quickly seeking a substitute relationship or object, absorbing oneself in work, overindulging in alcohol or drugs, literally fleeing from the situation, or psychopathology, especially depression.

Feelings are then gradually withdrawn from the lost object. A yearning to be with the lost person is replaced by a wish to renew life. The person gradually unlearns old ways of living and learns new life patterns. The lost object becomes detached from the person and is enshrined in the form of a memory, memorial, or monument. At first, the person's renewed concern for others may be directed toward other mourners or other persons in crisis since it is easier to feel closeness with someone who has experienced a similar loss.

Finally, the person becomes interested in new objects and relationships and allows himself new pleasures and enjoyments. At first the replacements must be very much like the former object, but eventually new relationships are formed and objects are acquired that are equally or even more satisfying than before.

Difficulty in achieving resolution is compounded by the negative influences discussed earlier and by additional hardships or complications caused by the crisis itself, such as deteriorating illness of self or family member. Ineffective mastery or problem solving or lack of expression of feelings associated with the crisis may cause a restricted level of functioning in one or all spheres of the personality. The problem may be repressed and permanently denied and unresolved, or major disorganization such as neurosis, psychosis, socially maladjusted behavior, or chronic physical disability may occur in a small percentage of people. Resolution of mourning is delayed whenever the person confronts a chronic situation, such as birth of a defective child. Acute grief is manifested at the birth of the child (or onset of the situation), but mourning is drawn out as long as the child lives (or the situation continues) (55).

Table 8-2 has outlined the predictable phases of crisis; however, each stage is not sharply demarcated. One stage may merge into another, or certain behaviors may not appear at all, particularly in developmental crises in which the person's functioning may be appropriate in one sphere but less so in another aspect of personality. In addition, the person may be at the beginning of one phase but then return to the previous phase behaviorally. Thus the person may demonstrate some behaviors indicative of one phase—such as defensive retreat—and simultaneously demonstrate a few behaviors of shock or of acknowledgment (82).

Although the adolescent may manifest some reactions to crisis in the same way as the adult, there is considerably more angry acting-out behavior and emotional lability. The child usually manifests behavior related to a sense of loss. In some cases, however, he/she may overtly appear untouched by the crisis, although play, questions, or conversation with a fantasy friend may reveal that he/she does not really understand what is happening, blames self for the event, or fears further catastrophe. The child often has more difficulty resolving crises because of lack of experience, of verbal skills, and of abstract thinking ability (50).

Family Reactions

The family unit undergoes essentially the same phases of crisis and manifests similar reactions as the designated client, although the intensity and timing may be different.

All families have problems, and all families have ways of managing them, successfully or otherwise. Success in coping depends on: (1) the family's perception of the disruptive event, (2) the family values, (3) sociocultural background, (4) external resources and support system available to the family, and (5) the ability of individual family members to come to the aid of the family unit (50).

If the source of trouble is from within the family, it is usually perceived as more distressing than an external source of trouble since internal problems reflect lack of harmony and inadequacy in the members. Shock and defensive retreat reactions may be more pronounced during times of internal trouble. As acknowledgment of reality occurs, there is a strong tendency to scapegoat family members to restore family balance. Crisis events for the family include the developmental and situational crisis previously discussed, which could also be categorized as follows (86):

1. *Dismemberment:* Loss of family member through death, divorce, separation, marriage, or geographic mobility.
2. *Accession:* Addition of family member through birth, adoption, marriage, or foster placement, or older relative moving into the home.
3. *Demoralization:* Loss of morale in the family unit through delinquency, legal problems, or events that cause alienation from the community or carry a social stigma.
4. *A combination of the above.*

Group or Community Reactions

A social group or entire neighborhood may feel the impact of an individual or family in crisis.

Various factors influence the crisis proneness of a group or community, as listed below (50, 67):

1. Personal strengths, characteristics, and level of need satisfaction of its members.
2. Social and economic stability of family units or groups versus social and economic inequities among ethnic, racial, or socioeconomic groups.
3. Adherence versus rebellion against social norms by families and groups.
4. Adequacy of community resources to meet social, economic, health, welfare, and recreational needs of individuals and families.
5. Geographic, environmental, and climatic resources and characteristics that surround the group or community.

The community is also affected by natural disasters, such as a flood, tornado, hurricane, or blizzard; by disasters resulting from advances in our civilization, such as chemical or radiation spills and electrical blackouts; and by disasters for which man is responsible, such as fire or war.

Reactions of a community to any of these disasters will be influenced by the following factors (25, 46, 50, 67, 69):

1. Element of surprise versus preparedness. If warnings are not given about an impending crisis — or if warnings are given without an action plan — panic, shock, denial, and defensive retreat are more likely to occur.
2. Separation of family members. Children are especially affected by separation; the family should be evacuated from a disaster area as a unit.
3. Availability of outside help.
4. Leadership. Someone must make decisions and give directions. Usually the police, Red Cross and Civil Defense workers, National Guard, military, or professionals in a community are seen as authoritative persons. Coordination of the activities of all of these groups is essential to deliver services and avoid chaos.
5. Communication. Public information centers have to be established to avoid rumor, provide

reassurance and direction, and ensure that all citizens get information about coping measures, evacuation, reconstruction, rehabilitation, and available financial aid. Otherwise citizens will later be bitter and suspicious when some learn that others benefited more than they did.

6. Measures taken to help reorientation. Communication networks lay the foundation for re-identification of individuals into family and social groups and for registration of survivors.

7. Presence of plans for individuals and social institutions to cope with disaster, including evacuation of a population from a stricken area if necessary. Emergency plans focus on the following concerns:

   a. Preservation of life and health through rescue, triage, inoculation, and treatment of the injured.

   b. Conservation and distribution of resources, such as shelter, water, food, and blankets.

   c. Conservation of public order by police surveillance to prevent looting and further accidents or injuries.

   d. Maintenance of morale through dispatching health and welfare workers to the disaster scene.

   e. Administration of health services.

Communities in crisis have characteristics in common with individuals in crisis. The most immediate social consequences of a disaster is disruption of normal social patterns and services; the community is socially paralyzed.

In a major disaster, about 75 to 90 percent of the victims will be in shock, followed by the phase of defensive retreat, in response to warnings of disaster, orders of evacuation, destruction of homes, and disruption of water, electricity, heat, food supplies, communication, traffic, and transportation. Further, there is potential inability of the health agencies to care for the injured and ill because of manpower and supply shortages or damage. In addition to individual reactions, an atmosphere of tension, fear, confusion, and suspicion exists; facts are distorted and rumors are rampant. Normal functioning is reduced as businesses, vital services, schools, and recreational areas may be closed. Although some people are

in shock or denial, there will be a few who take advantage of the chaos to loot and steal, and a few businesses may profiteer (25, 46, 50, 67).

Response to external emergencies is often quicker than the response to internal stresses or crises. About 10 to 25 percent of the victims remain reality-oriented, calm, and able to develop and implement a plan of action; these people often are those with advance training. But these crisis workers may react with at least brief periods of shock and defensive retreat after most of the immediate work is done (46, 50).

When reality is acknowledged, people in the community at first become more cohesive as they help each other; then individual problems become the focus. People find shelter, look for someone to be with, want to be cared for, express a sense of loss through crying and talking, and share with others how they managed to survive. During this time, depending on the amount of damage, anger and frustration are keenly felt as the person evaluates the damage and feels robbed of possessions that have been worked for throughout life. The older, dependent, or incapacitated person may become seriously ill or die because he/she feels unable to start all over again. If loved ones were killed, grief and mourning for them as well as for lost possessions occur. Guilt reactions as a result of being unable to save the loved one, of being spared death, and of relief at being alive are common. Reactive depression, anxiety reactions, regression, dreams, suicidal thoughts, physical illness, psychotic episodes, and neurotic reactions occur and may last for several months or a year after the disaster. The more severe the disaster, the longer these reactions last. Some people's psyches may be permanently damaged. Older people who suffer a disaster are statistically more likely to die within the year following the disaster. Also psychological effects are more severe and slower to resolve when survivors perceive the disaster as a result of human callousness or error rather than as an act of God or nature (25, 46, 50, 67, 120).

Resolution occurs in individuals as previously described and is related to the individual's psychological health before the crisis as well as to the kind of help given to the family unit during the disaster, the kind of crisis and extent of damage, and the ability of the community to repair damage and return to normal function. Perhaps the best sign of community resolution is a well-developed disaster plan of action, one that can be implemented in the event of another crisis, and community-wide education for individual and family preparedness for disaster (46, 50).

INEFFECTIVE RESOLUTION OF CRISIS

If there is no adaptive resolution or change in behavior to cope with the crisis, dysfunctional or ineffective reactions occur as an attempt to lower tension and to resolve the situation.

There may be a delayed reaction in that the crisis event and its consequences are denied and repressed. At times, denial may be manifested as hope. *Hope is the confident assumption or faith that a certain outcome must occur or that a dread event or its consequences will not occur.* Hope is a way of coping with stressful or crisis situations and differs from wishing for a certain outcome. Although sustained hope has occasionally facilitated recovery from a declared incurable disease, hope may also contribute to ineffective resolution of crises when the person fails to acknowledge the inevitable, maintains that an impossible outcome will occur, avoids reality, or escapes responsibility (9).

Denial may also be manifested as prolonged euphoria. Denial is more likely in cases of marginal disability than in severe disability because reality is less avoidable over a period of time when the person has multiple or severe disabilities (29, 102, 122).

After loss of a loved one, the person using extreme denial may continue to act as though the lost person is still alive and present. For example, the survivor may continue to set a place at the table for the deceased or keep all the possessions of the lost one. Or the person may acknowledge the death but deny the significance of the loss emotionally or intellectually. He/she may not take care of business matters because the deceased person was the person who previously did this.

A dysfunctional reaction will eventually be precipitated when a crisis occurs that recalls buried feelings which then renders the person ineffective in functioning. A crisis may produce various other reactions of distorted or inappropriate behavior, although neurosis, psychosis, or socially ineffective behavior occurs only in a small percentage of people.

As mentioned above, in the crisis of death of a loved one, the person may prolong identification with the deceased by developing symptoms like those in the last illness of the deceased. And eventually organic pathological changes specific to the disease can occur (22, 49, 89). Sometimes such illness occurs on the anniversary of the loss. Or the grieving person may develop a different disease, caused by the mind-body relationship, in which physiological changes occur because of the effects of the emotional state on body parts, which eventually causes organ damage (49). Illness resulting from the effects of the emotional state is also called *psychosomatic illness.* Such reactions are further described in Chapter 12.

Studies have shown a definite relationship between loss and crisis and symptom formation and illness. Both morbidity and mortality are related to the damaging effects of emotions on the body when crisis cannot be adequately resolved. See references at the end of this chapter by A. Carr and B. Schoenberg (22), G. Engel (35), L. Hinkle, et al. (49), T. Holmes and R. Rahe (51), E. Shontz (102), and B. Wright (122).

Dysfunctional reactions may include expressing hostility for an excessively prolonged time against authority figures such as doctors, nurses, policemen, parents, or teachers. Prolonged sadness, apathy, lack of initiative, irritability, suspicion, and withdrawing from others because of internalized anger or shock can be equally detrimental to relationships with others and to the person's overall conduct. Feelings of isolation, worthlessness, hopelessness, and guilt may become magnified to the point of inducing suicide attempts. Or the person may suppress his/her own personality, taking on traits of the lost person.

The person who stays compulsively busy or is ritualistic may become ineffective in his/her attempts to cope. Alcohol, drugs, or excessive eating may become a crutch or escape when activity no longer provides adequate tension release. Or the person may engage in action detrimental to the self economically or socially through excessive generosity or foolish financial dealings (which represent self-punishment) or through delinquency. The latter situation invites apprehension, punishment, and, at times, someone else making decisions for him/her.

THE NURSING PROCESS AND CRISIS INTERVENTION

You will see people in crisis in a variety of settings: in the emergency room, clinic, recovery room, coronary-care unit, surgical intensive-care unit, industrial or school dispensary, and in the medical, surgical, obstetrical, pediatric, and psychiatric units. In most of these settings, you will collaborate with the physician and other health team members. In the mental or neighborhood health center, you may function as primary therapist within agency policy or with other health team members. In telephone crisis work, you may be the sole therapist.

Your philosophy of care must include the concept of crisis. The person in crisis is at a turning point. He/she is ready for great changes in a relatively short period of time because of the felt tension, pain, and disequilibrium associated with crisis. These feelings motivate efforts to try to alter the situation. Distress creates an openness to assistance and change. Expert help is expected, and the nurse is perceived as an expert. Even a minimal amount of support and help can influence the outcome of a crisis to a significant degree.

Crisis therapy is based on the theory that immediate aid during crisis will help the person to adapt in a healthy manner. The minimal goal of therapy is psychological resolution of the immediate crisis and restoration of coping mechanisms to at least the level of functioning that existed before the crisis event. The maximal goal is to bring about a change in behavior that is more mature than that of the precrisis level. Crisis work involves reinstating earlier stress-reducing behavior or developing new adaptive techniques. Underlying these goals is the assumption that the person seeking help has unused resources that, with minimum assistance, can be called upon to function effectively in everyday living.

Factors influencing the successful course of crisis therapy include the following:

1. The ability of the therapist to establish rapport and convey warmth and caring quickly, often to a stranger.
2. A positive attitude on the part of the therapist, including emphasis on the value of crisis work.
3. Constructive use of time, in that assessment is done as quickly as possible: to accurately define the nature of the crisis, to identify the person's response to the event, to devise a course of action for resolving the crisis, and to relieve the most distressing symptoms.
4. Use of nontraditional treatment practices where needed. Appointment time and place must be determined by the extent of stress response and impaired functioning that the person is experiencing, as well as by the skill of the therapist, the number and kind of resources in the community to assist the person, and the type of crisis.
5. Understanding of the differences between the value systems of the therapist and the person or family. The therapist must be open to what constitutes a problem for another. The life style and values of the person may be foreign to or in conflict with those of the therapist, but the person needs acceptance in order to maintain his/her basic life style and value system.

The following description of use of the nursing process emphasizes nursing behaviors that utilize the Humanistic Framework.

Assessment

Collecting data must be systematic, yet flexible, and rapid enough to interrupt the crisis but thorough enough to define the problem and phase of crisis and to identify and achieve the desired outcomes.

The following should be assessed: the anxiety level and feelings of the person, ego functioning (perception, judgment, memory, problem solving), presence of emotional and physical symptoms, whether the person is suicidal or homicidal, usual living patterns and work arrangements, interpersonal and social situation, and crisis event and its onset. Nonverbal behavior and the consistency between verbal and nonverbal behavior must be noted. The person does not always mean what he/she says and will not always act in a way that directly expresses true feelings. If the person cannot identify the problem because of disorganized thinking, focus attention on what was occurring just prior to the situation and onset of symptoms. Constructing a sequence of events helps reorientation.

After determining the extent of the problem, focus the person's perception on the event—for example, the illness or loss. What does this situation mean? How does he/she see its effect on the future? Is the event seen realistically? What hardships have been created by the crisis—for example, job loss due to depression or mental illness, which in turn causes financial and family problems and loss of self-esteem?

Ascertain if the person plans to kill self or another person. If so, ask how and when. If the intention is carefully planned and details are specific, hospitalization and psychiatric evaluation must be arranged to protect the person and others.

Your next questions should be directed to the availability of help and supportive others versus the extent of isolation from significant relationships. What is the person's relationship with supportive others? Crisis intervention is sharply limited in time. The more persons who are in some way helping the person, the better. Then, too, when crisis therapy is terminated, if helpful others are involved, they can continue to give support to the person. Assess the adaptive capacities of the others involved in the situation who have not sought help but who might also be experiencing crises. If no helpful resources are available, you become a temporary support system while helping the person to establish a relationship with a person or group in the community or work setting.

Ascertain what the person usually does when encountering a problem. What are the coping skills? Has anything like this happened before? What was done to decrease tension? If he/she is trying the same method now and it is not working, what does the person think would decrease his/her stress symptoms? Activity that has been done in the far past to cope successfully could be tried again. Determine strengths and not just problems and limitations. Asking the individual what he/she sees as an *ideal* solution for the current situation will give you an indication of what type of solutions will be acceptable.

Through assessment you can determine why this situation is a crisis to this person, why he/she is unable to alter the life style to cope with the situation, and what in the life style can be altered so that the crisis can be resolved.

Throughout assessment, use a straightforward but empathic approach. Use simple questions that are open and nonthreatening but directive enough to give structure to the interview and to gain optimum information.

Such an assessment would also be done with a family unit in that you would assess the status of individual members as well as the perceptions, emotional status, and resources of the family as a whole.

When assessing the person, family, or group after a community disaster, you would again seek information related to the above points. Assessment would also include questions about damage to home and possessions, effects of disruption of services, and need for community, state, or federal aid during the recovery period.

Planning Intervention

Based on your assessment, your *nursing diagnosis* will be *crisis state*, _____ *phase*, related to (*situation or developmental era*). As you study data collected in the manner described in the preceding section, the person should also be actively involved in seeking a potential solution. You cannot solve the problem for the client; you can only help the person to help him/herself.

The following criteria are useful for planning crisis intervention (50):

1. Collaborate *with* the client (person or family) to the extent possible, in establishing goals and planning action. Encourage the person or family to make decisions; avoid assuming control. If the client is in shock, highly anxious, dependent, or in defensive retreat, you will have to be more directive, as the person or family may not be able to formulate even short-term goals or plans. However, you should convey during planning that you believe the person or family will be able to get in control of the situation.

2. Consider the uniqueness of the client's values, feelings, thoughts, behavior, perceptions, needs, and sociocultural and religious background.

3. Consider the precrisis adaptive capacity of the client, to the extent that you can assess previous coping styles and life styles. Understanding the person's past and current status and environmental resources enables you to facilitate coping behaviors.

4. Be problem-oriented; deal with the immediate situation and problems contributing to the crisis. Underlying psychological, marital, or social problems should be handled after the crisis is resolved.

5. Formulate a plan that is realistic, time-limited, clearly stated, concrete, and flexible. Provide evidence that something will happen to change the present state of discomfort and that the chaos can be handled in terms familiar to the client.

6. Explore and provide for alternative solutions so that if one plan does not work, the person will not experience failure. Positive guidelines for action should be given to the person when he/she leaves each session (including the first session), so that alternate solutions can be tested. This permits evaluation of coping behavior at each successive session so that additional solutions can be sought if necessary. Further, having specific tasks to do helps the person feel more in control of self and the situation.

The plan for intervention is determined by assessing the nature of the crisis (whether it is acute or chronically recurring), the reactions of others significant to the person, and the strengths and resources of all persons involved. The plan for intervention must extend beyond the person to others involved less directly in the crisis.

Intervention: Principles and Techniques

Principles of intervention, which follow, can be accomplished by using your knowledge of crisis theory, therapeutic communication (discussed in Chapter 5), establishment of a nurse-client relationship (discussed in Chapter 6), and general principles of intervention and use of roles discussed under the nursing process (Chapter 4).

1. *Begin with comfort strategies.* Through verbal and nonverbal behavior, establish rapport, show acceptance of the person, and establish a positive, concerned relationship so that he/she feels a sense of hope, self-worth, lessened anxiety, and an expectation of management. Let the person or family know that coming for help is a sign of strength and good judgment and that you and the client will work together. This intervention begins simultaneously with assessment.

2. *Work first with feelings; then you will be able to get the facts.* Encourage expression of feeling by acknowledging the validity of the

tension and concern the person feels and that the feelings being experienced are normal.

3. *Help the person confront the crisis by talking about present feelings* of denial, anger, guilt, or grief. Catharsis lowers tension, clarifies the problem, promotes comprehension of the reality and of the consequences of the situation, and mobilizes energy for constructive action.

4. *Encourage the person to talk about the losses and changes involved* in the crisis and to reminisce about the lost person, relationship, or object. Help the person to work through the stages of mourning previously described.

5. *Clarify the person's perception of current difficulties.* Effective problem solving depends on appropriate perception.

6. *Explain to the person the relationship between the crisis situation and his/her present behavior and feelings.* The person feels less overwhelmed and better able to manage when he/she understands that such emotions are normal in the context of crisis and that symptoms will disappear.

7. *Recognize denial as a normal reaction during defensive retreat from the crisis.* Cope with personal feelings about the person's behavior and situation; observe behavior objectively. Avoid reinforcing denial. Gently represent reality. State your awareness of how appalling the events seem to the person. Work with other resource persons for information, collaboration, maintenance of support, and representation of reality.

8. *Help him/her find facts,* since facts are less awesome than speculations or fantasies about the situation or the unknown.

9. *Give the person time to experience the feelings and to fully express them.* Frequently we are so concerned about reality, problem solving, and fast solutions that we try to hurry the person through the crisis. The crisis phases and stages of mourning previously discussed take time to work through, and the client needs the release of feelings and the feeling of contact with the therapist before any real crisis work can be done.

10. *Avoid giving false reassurance.* Acknowledge the validity of fears and other feelings. Show faith in the person's ability to manage; you

should not reduce motivation to cope and adapt by saying that everything will be fine.

11. *Do not encourage the person to blame or shove responsibility on others for the crisis event,* since this process avoids the truth, reduces motivation to take responsibility for personal behavior, and discourages adaptation. Listen initially to rationalizations; then raise doubt about such statements through questioning.

12. *Help the person confront the crisis in amounts or "doses" that can be managed,* being cautious not to overly soften the impact of the event. The reality of the situation must be kept in the foreground, although periods of relief from facing the whole situation are needed. Help him/her first gain an intellectual understanding of the crisis; then encourage an emotional understanding and adjustment. In this way, the person can more objectively handle the real situation.

13. *Encourage the person to do what he/she can for self; explore coping mechanisms to assist the person in examining alternate ways of coping* and in seeking and using new behaviors or alternate ways of satisfying needs. Help him/her to learn or relearn basic social skills as necessary and to fit behavior to the demands presented by the crisis.

14. *Strengthen or reinforce previously learned behavior patterns that can be effective but are not presently being used.* You should only explore past life occurrences in relation to the existing crisis, particularly if feelings aroused in past crises have been unresolved and are influencing the present behavior. The present experience can bring forth defensive behaviors used in the past that are no longer useful. If indicated, establish a new contract to do long-term therapy with the person in relation to the unresolved crisis, or discuss your observations with the client and refer him/her to another professional.

15. *Involve the client in decision making and working on specific tasks.* Search for boundaries to the problem and appraise the meaning of the crisis event. Help the person or family to determine what problem to work on initially, if there appear to be several. Set priorities, and help the client answer the questions

of how, when, where, and by whom in relation to carrying out an action plan.

16. *Reinforce useful suggestions.* Look for realistic strengths to focus on and reinforce. Do whatever you can to help the client reestablish a positive self-concept, a sense of wholeness, and confidence in his/her ability to manage this crisis and ongoing stresses.

17. *Help the person establish necessary social relationships and effective personal behavior.* If he/she has lost or is otherwise removed from all significant persons, as might be true for the elderly or new immigrants, introduce him/her to new people to help fill the void and to obtain support and gratification. Also help the person find appropriate outlets for tension, such as leisure activities, hobbies, or physical exercise. Sometimes these activities can be shared with others.

18. *Assist the person in seeking and accepting help.* By acknowledging that trouble exists, he/she is more likely to use personal resources and to accept the help offered by others. If necessary, encourage acceptance of help with the everyday tasks of living, and encourage mobilization of inner strengths as well as help from concerned others in the environment.

19. *You must be familiar with community resources to which the person or family can be referred for additional service.* Community services in a metropolitan area are often described in a special directory, including address, phone number, key personnel, and available services. Referral agencies may include Family and Children's Services, Catholic or Lutheran Charities, Salvation Army, Traveler's Aid Society, Red Cross, International Institute, Housing and Urban Development, Retired Senior Volunteer Programs, Parents-without-Partners, widows' groups, meals-on-wheels, home health agencies, crisis phone lines, telephone and transportation services, health department, and special housing for youth or the elderly. If you do refer the client, follow the guidelines described in Chapter 4.

Often during crisis you may be confronted by an angry, bitter, or accusatory person or family who berates you; or even by other health team members or the agency who accuse you of negligence. Keep two things in mind: (1) Their statements may be accurate and justified, or (2) such statements may serve as the only way that these individuals (clients or helpers) can cope with their own aggression, helplessness, or guilt at the time. Provide the best care possible and show genuine concern, but do not become verbally involved in the dispute. Also do not take the behavior personally if it does not apply to you.

Anticipate that people facing loss may behave ineffectively and will need to be treated with tact, patience, warmth, and empathy, as well as be encouraged to express feelings without feeling guilty about doing so. However, you should set limits on behavior that would be destructive to the person or to others.

Clarify and reemphasize the person's responsibility for his/her behavior, decisions, and way of life. For example, the person in crisis from illness and hospitalization should be assisted in learning the expected role. Then uncertainty about expectations for self and others can be replaced with the feeling that he/she is a participating member of the treatment team. Therefore, orientation to the hospital division's policies and routines, to the room (and roommate, if any), to other personnel, to diagnostic procedures, and to preoperative and postoperative care is needed. When the patient is conversant about the possible outcomes of the illness, he/she can participate in decisions about present care goals and future health needs. When he/she knows what to expect from the health team members, behavior can be adaptive.

Group work for six to ten sessions is sometimes indicated in crisis work to (50, 108):

1. Assess coping mechanisms that are revealed through group interaction; certain group behavior may have contributed to the person's crisis situation.
2. Help the person realize the impact of his/her behavior on others.
3. Relieve the sense of isolation, facilitate establishing a social network, and utilize the group as a resource for the person.

In most cases however, crisis work with the individual is usually preferred to group work since precipitating events and preceptions of the events are often quite individual. Further, individuals move through the phases of crisis at their own unique pace, which may be out of step with others in the group.

Helping the person or family resolve a crisis constructively involves a process of reestablishment with self, significant others, and the community. The client's isolation is reduced as ties are reestablished to the world of work or school, and to community organizations or church. Resolution is best facilitated by confronting reality at the person's pace; medications should be used only in cases of extreme anxiety or when there is fear of losing control. Tranquilizers and sedatives can decrease motivation to solve problems and to engage in psychic growth.

To facilitate crisis resolution, you may have to use multiple support strategies, including your counseling and relationship, intense support over a number of consecutive hours, environmental manipulation and support, work with the family unit, group sessions, and referral to community resources.

When you do crisis work, keep in mind the model of primary, secondary, and tertiary prevention (19). Refer to Chapter 25 for additional discussion of the three levels of prevention.

Levels of Prevention
Primary prevention

Primary prevention, or *preventing a crisis,* can be achieved by helping the person work through developmental periods or anticipated situations (19). The anticipation of life crises is an important concept in health promotion and therefore has broad implications in nursing. If the person can prepare for what may happen with the "work of worry" or anticipatory grieving, he/she will be less vulnerable to physical or mental illness (56). The more thorough the thinking, planning, or "work of worry" before a crisis, the more adequate the subsequent adjustment and the less severe the impact felt. However, persons with either excessively high or excessively low levels of fear or worry are less able to prepare for crisis. A high-level worrier feels such fear that something bad will happen that he cannot effectively plan ahead. A low-level worrier does not adequately contemplate impending stress and crisis and feels overwhelmed when it comes. A moderately worrisome person can express tension, physically, emotionally, and verbally, but maintains self-control and thus can rationally plan and adjust personal behavior to the situation (63).

You can help the person do the "work of worry" or anticipatory grieving in many different situations by: (1) premarital counseling to increase the chance of healthy resolution of stressful marital events and the achievement of appropriate developmental tasks; (2) teaching and counseling in prenatal classes to prepare for childbirth and child care; (3) talking with a mother whose child will soon enter school or be married; (4) preretirement counseling to help the person plan ahead to meet the problems and developmental tasks associated with retirement; (5) counseling the family of a terminally ill patient; and (6) talking preoperatively with the person who is undergoing major surgery and body-image changes (19). Primary prevention also includes job or school counseling, disaster planning, maintaining health practices, taking prescribed medicines, developing leisure activities to promote relaxation, planning for changes that may occur in life, and deliberately thinking about ways to effectively cope with stresses at home or on the job.

Preventive intervention is not designed to bring about major changes in the maturity or personality structure of the person, but rather to maintain the usual level of functioning of equilibrium.

Secondary prevention

Secondary prevention involves early identification of the crisis so the person can avoid maladaptive behavior. The person is helped to adapt to the crisis, thereby reducing the intensity and duration of reaction. He/she is quickly given support, is encouraged to use personal energies and available resources constructively, and is helped to understand that the manifested feelings and behavior are a normal response to the situation (19).

Examples of secondary prevention in crisis therapy are counseling the school dropout; working with women who have not resolved the crisis of motherhood, menopause, or widowhood; working through feelings with the person who is mourning the birth of a child with a congenital anomaly, or the loss of a significant body part after surgery or injury, or loss of a significant person, object, or role; and counseling the psychiatric patient who has a reactive depression or the man who is drinking excessively because of job problems.

Tertiary prevention

Tertiary prevention is aimed at preventing further decompensation or impairment after the person has partially resolved a crisis, so that he/she can live a useful role in the community. The person's behavior may initially interfere with rehabilitation. When the meaning or implications of the crisis and feelings about it can be resolved, the person will be able to become involved in rehabilitation related to physical or emotional illness. Progress depends strongly on the nurse's counseling role and on continuity in the nurse-client relationship. Through this kind of intervention, the person may eventually rework the crisis and become behaviorally more effective. Examples of tertiary prevention are group therapy with chronically ill or disabled persons to help them cope with their health problems, counseling to help a person work through delayed mourning, counseling the alcoholic or drug-abusing person, and use of remotivation techniques to prevent further disengagement in the aged (19).

Crisis Therapy

Crisis therapy is basically brief and specific to the present situation and involves placing attainable goals directly before the person. Thus principles of crisis intervention are relevant to all persons, including people who are concerned primarily with the here and now; who prefer brief, concrete intervention; and who seek assistance for specific problems.

The person or family in crisis becomes especially susceptible to the influence of significant others. A little help directed purposefully and with the right timing is more effective than more help given at a period of less emotional accessibility. View yourself as intervening in a social system, always cognizant of the individual and family as well as of the larger network of relationships. You may not be the only resource to the person. You can also use skills of other health team members—the doctor, social worker, chaplain, psychologist, and occupational therapist—either directly for consultation or for referral (75).

Evaluation

However, crisis intervention is not a panacea for all social, emotional, or physical problems. It is not synonymous with brief psychotherapy or psychoanalysis. But effective crisis intervention can be an important link to in-depth psychotherapy, for during a crisis the person is more likely to consider getting help for recurring conflict areas and continued personal growth.

Crisis resolution and anticipatory planning complete the process of crisis intervention. Crisis work is then reviewed, and the accomplishments of the person in working through the predicament should be emphasized. Adaptive coping mechanisms and appropriate behavior that the person has successfully used should be reinforced. Positive changes in behavior should be summarized to allow reexperiencing and reconfirming the progress made. Give assistance as needed in making realistic plans for the future, and discuss with the person ways in which the present experience may help coping with future crises. The person should leave with self-confidence in managing his/her life and with the awareness that assistance will be available in the future if necessary.

In order to continue to do effective crisis intervention, the step of evaluation in the nursing process must be carried out as discussed in Chapter 4.

CRISIS COUNSELING BY TELEPHONE

The ringing clinic telephone is answered. A tremulous young female voice asks, "Do you do pregnancy tests without informing parents?"

In the emergency department the nurse is called to the phone because a panicky male voice has inquired, "If ya' hit up Thorazine, will it break down in the bloodstream?"

The voice at the other end of the line of a nursing division phone is saying, "You were so nice to me there. You were the only ones who cared. Thanks for trying, but it's no use." The speech of the caller is heavily slurred.

Situations such as the above emphasize the need for telephone counseling skills in nurses who have been taught to rely primarily on face-to-face encounter (41, 64, 68, 90).

Telephone Crisis Centers

In the last decade, telephone crisis centers have proliferated. There are hot lines for concerns including, but not limited to: child, adult, or substance abuse; divorce counseling; gay life difficulties; loneliness; rape; runaway youths or crisis situations; sexual information and counsel; middle-age crises; and outreach to the desperate, depressed, and suicidal. Experience and research both indicate that the telephone is a valuable tool of preventive psychotherapy.

Typically, a telephone crisis center operates with a small salaried professional and clerical staff aided by a much larger group of volunteers trained and supervised in doing telephone crisis work. Nurses are often well represented in telephone crisis centers (90).

Telephone crisis centers usually provide training specific to their own particular goals and related to their own particular problem calls. You may want to gain the training and experience a specific telephone counseling center can offer. You will also want to be informed about other telephone crisis lines that are locally accessible. Learn about their services and skills, the training and supervision provided for the crisis workers, and their biases. Is their service prompt, responsive, and reliable? What information and referral services can they provide you as a practitioner? Become well acquainted with the strengths and limitations of crisis lines that your clients may use (90).

Characteristics of Telephone Therapy

Unique qualities of telephone therapy are: (1) client in control, (2) client anonymity, (3) geographic and personal barriers between client and therapist, (4) anonymity of the therapist, and (5) client's incentive to call.

The above variables can create in you considerable anxiety, anger, and a sense of helplessness. The caller can hang up at any point when he/she feels too threatened. You are also without your institutional supports and cannot physically do anything to control an impulsive or hysterical client. You are operating on reduced cues—only those that you can hear. Ironically, these feelings and factors are a basis for identification with the caller's needs.

The caller, too, may feel anxious, angry, and helpless. He/she has to depend on you not to terminate the call without having been helpful. The usual support systems are lacking. The person needs to trust you in spite of having reduced cues as to whether or not you are trustworthy.

The therapist's anonymity in most crisis phone calls can enhance crisis work (119). The caller may decide that you are older and parental or that you are young and romantic. This projection of traits may enable him/her to confide in you. The caller's illusions need not be shattered unless they lead to unrealistic expectations, which you then can gently but honestly clarify.

Assessment by Telephone

If the caller has just swallowed an overdose of pills, offer immediate concern and interest so that the caller can trust you enough to reveal name and location. *Trust is the key goal.* Listen to the slurred speech and tolerate a wavering level of consciousness. It is self-restraining, difficult, but essential to initially say, "Tell me what has happened that you feel you want to stop living," rather than, "Tell me who you are and where you are." An open phone line dropped to the floor when the unconsciousness comes can still be traced. A hung-up phone cannot! Thus, your overriding concern is to keep the person on the phone until someone has personally arrived to help the caller. The highly ambivalent caller will usually provide some means for you to help once he/she senses your concern. You might then say, "I can feel the wish of some part of you to give life another chance. That part of you is fighting hard for your life. I want to get help to you. Tell me how to find you."

When you hear overt panic and hysteria in the caller who has attempted suicide, you can be more direct and say, "I'm sending someone over to take you to an emergency room. Tell me the address where you are now." You can work out arrangements to send a relative, ambulance, or police, depending on the situation. You do all the decision making that the caller cannot do, but none that he/she can do.

As you try to discover who the person is, you might say, "My name is Jane Watson, but people usually call me Janie. What is your name?" (You may want to use a professional name or alias to keep from being reached via a listed home phone number.) With a caller still reluctant to give a name, you may want to suggest, "We'd find it easier to talk if we used names. Since our conversation is confidential, you can give me a name to call you."

The caller is often choosing the phone as a means of self-revelation because he/she feels the problem is embarrassing or even contemptible. Thus your restraint from conveying judgment is essential. If the person can lay out the difficulties to you and find acceptance via phone, the next step of accepting a referral for face-to-face therapy or emergency treatment may be taken.

Suicidal Crisis

In one crisis situation, the caller described to the nurse how earlier in the day she had rented a certain motel room while she could be sure there was a vacancy. Later in the evening the caller returned to the motel room and swallowed an indeterminate number of barbiturate sleeping capsules. Some 30 minutes later as her suicidal ambivalance increased, she left the motel room and went to a phone booth to place her call. Her speech became thicker as she talked. She was upset over the loss of a boyfriend she hoped to marry and thereby regain custody of her two children who had been placed in foster care. As the nurse helped her consider alternative mechanisms for regaining custody, the caller agreed to go to an emergency room but insisted vehemently that she drive herself there! "My car's got a dented front fender already. I just won't go off and leave it here." The nurse was able to determine the make and year of the car. When she could not persuade the caller to accept other arrangements, the nurse planned with the caller the best route to an emergency room. As soon as the call was terminated, the nurse telephoned the local police to tell them of the situation, describing the car and its anticipated route, although the exact model was unknown. The police intervened and succeeded in getting the caller and her car to the emergency room. The caller was admitted to the hospital.

In assessing the caller who is depressed, bitter, or overwhelmed by crisis, determine the degree of suicide risk by asking direct questions. Ask questions that determine the extent of clinical depression, extent of drug and alcohol use, family history of suicide or depression, history of previous suicidal thoughts or attempts, and information about any current suicidal plan, such as details of the suicidal plan, the lethality potential of the plan, and available means for carrying through with the plan. Contrary to a common fear that asking about suicide will give the client the idea of suicide, your questions about suicide may provide a helpful catharsis (32).

If you learn of a specific, potentially lethal plan, you need to take immediate preventive action. The variables of depression, current suicide plan, previous suicide attempts, and abusive use of alcohol are all highly significant in determining suicidal risk (96, 97, 98). In such situations you must help the caller to obtain an emergency psychiatric evaluation. Take steps to ensure that the caller is not alone, and inform caring friends or relatives of the caller's suicidal intent and its seriousness.

Sometimes professionals who have been too well trained in defeating the manipulative behaviors of clients are dangerously reluctant to respond to telephoned threats or attempts of suicide. They feel it is wrong to risk getting themselves manipulated. The authors believe that it is more helpful to follow the philosophy that a client is functioning in the best way he/she knows at that moment. Thus, your short-term goal is to respond with caring

to the client's cry for help. You will carry out the interventions given in Table 8-3. Essential long-term goals include modifying self-defeating, manipulative patterns and teaching the client that reliance on dramatic suicidal rescues can be a fatal mistake that he/she doesn't really want to make.

Some professionals may argue that the client has the "right" to suicide; however, the client also has the right to make informed choices. Persons in crisis are often psychologically blocked in their ability to make informed choices. Most nurses will at some point see the barely surviving, suicidal attempter, who stares coldly and says, "Why didn't you let me die?" In fact, you may see many such attemptors. However, you may also see a crisis successfully resolved with a client saying, "Thank you for your help. My crisis is over."

How do you define successful resolution? We suggest that successful resolution of a suicidal crisis involves the capacity to live meaningfully until forces beyond anyone's control pull the client irreversibly away from meaningful living. The nurse's role is to help the client see alternatives, regain hope, and feel the respect of human worth until such time when the client can again find life to be meaningful.

TABLE 8-3.   Response to Telephone Reports of Overdose Suicide Attempts

1. Convey concern and interest.
2. Keep communication (and phone line) open.
3. Encourage the caller's trust in your desire to help.
4. Remind the caller that:
   a. There is a life-force struggling to exert itself even in the midst of the attempt.
   b. Other choices more meaningful than suicide can still be explored.
   c. He/she owes self the right to nonsuicidal solutions.
5. Ask:
   a. What the caller has ingested. How much the caller has ingested.
   b. Age, height, weight.
   c. What the caller expects will happen.
   d. Who is nearby to help.
   e. Address and phone number of caller's location.
6. Work out with the caller a plan for emergency evaluation, using nearby persons and/or ambulance or police.
7. Arrange for overdose containers to be taken along to emergency department.
8. Keep in touch with the caller, at least until emergency department assistance has been received.
9. Tell the caller that you will contact the emergency department involved to give pertinent information.

Intervention by Telephone

The call makes progress as you help the caller consider personal strengths and resources, develop a plan of problem resolution, and take steps toward adaptation. You help the caller convert a problem statement into a process of effective problem solving.

Telephone intervention may involve only a single call in which you are a reflective sounding board, while the caller reaches an appropriate plan of action. Or the intervention may involve a succession of five or six phone calls in which the caller increasingly moves toward effective action.

The principles of crisis intervention do not change because you are talking by phone instead of sitting face-to-face. The therapeutic communication methods identified in Chapter 5 remain the same. Silence may still be either thoughtful, expectant, anxious, or resistive. But the silence may feel much longer when you cannot look at the silent person for cues. Do you hear even a sigh? Do you hear sound of movement, such as a creak of a chair when someone shifts weight in it? Do you hear the inhale and pushed exhale of a tense drag on a cigarette?

In response to silence you can state your aural observations: "I heard your sigh. I wonder what you are thinking?" "It sounds as though you are shifting your weight. Was my last question uncomfortable to consider?" "You're quiet. It feels to me as though you may be thinking about something important and trying to decide whether or not to tell me."

Even into a dead silence that is becoming uncomfortably long, you can offer, "I'm still here. I'm interested in knowing what's troubling you." You need to verbally clarify your own silences, feelings, and reactions. Since the caller cannot see your thoughtful, furrowed brow, you need to say, "I'm thinking about what you've told me and wondering what alternatives you've already considered." The person can hear if your vocal cords tighten in mounting frustration and he/she needs you to tell him the source of the frustration.

On occasion a telephone caller will find that he cannot deal with even the amount of exposure he has created by dialing the phone. You may hear the click of the phone being hung up and fear that you have failed. Maybe you have not failed.

You may have succeeded. The caller may have reached a caring, empathetic voice when disinterest and rejection were expected. Now that the person found the opposite, he/she may hang up to reflect on whether or not to expose him/herself further. The first contact with you will enhance the chance of calling back for further help.

In many situations the telephone contact cannot provide sufficient therapy. Plan instead to be a bridge between the person in crisis and the appropriate referral source. You might say, "You have family concerns that are very frustrating to you. You deserve an intense effort on someone's part to help you work out solutions. I can't do that in this call. I believe you can get this help at. . . " (name, address, phone, hours of service, and fee range of referral resources nearby). Referrals are most likely to be accepted if they are located nearby and are within the economic reach of the caller.

Avoid doing an oversell of referrals. Be optimistic when you give a referral but also add that you would like to hear from the caller again if this referral isn't helpful once he/she gives it a fair try.

Very often the caller is not seeking information for self but for a loved one. Then you will indirectly provide health information, assessment guidelines, and information on available treatment resources to the person in crisis (87). In an emergency situation, however, you should make every attempt to talk directly with the subject whom the caller has in mind.

Evaluation

In phone counseling you often must base evaluation of your intervention on a single phone encounter. Only occasionally will you ever know whether or not your intervention was the turning point toward effective resolution. Yet by examining and practicing the skills used in telephone crisis work you can develop confidence. Role playing done sitting back to back with your peers can help you develop skills of telephone therapy as they react and analyze your verbal statements and tone of voice (90).

Once, a "holler" to a neighbor and a "back fence conference" provided emergency crisis intervention. Today, the telephone can do the same. You can use it as one more tool in expanded nursing care.

ADAPTATIONS IN CRISIS INTERVENTION

With the Child and Adolescent

Specific guidelines for assessing, communicating, and working with the child and adolescent who are demonstrating specific behaviors are discussed throughout the book and in Chapter 21; these guidelines are applicable in crisis work. Although the level of maturity may be a constraint, the child and adolescent can resolve a crisis on their own developmental level. But the adult must help them face and accept their feelings, answer questions realistically, and give them time and support to go through the mourning process that is part of acknowledgment. The best assistance is an adult who is a role model in facing loss and change and who can share feelings that are a part of grief and mourning. In turn, you must give support and assistance to the grieving adult so that he/she can remain supportive to the grieving child. Loss and crisis can be resolved by a child, and the rest of the family, when memories of the loss are retained and the person can take action directed at substituting for or replacing the loss (44, 50).

With the Elderly Person

Utilize the principles of crisis intervention previously described. Focus on the present event; the elderly person may tend to bring many associations from earlier life into assessment and during exploration in intervention. Have the person repeat the story as often as necessary; reminiscence is adaptive. Recounting the crisis event lowers tension; reduces anger, guilt, resentment, or fear; clarifies the problem; promotes comprehension of reality and consequences of the situation; and mobilizes energy for constructive action. The senior citizen will need reinforcement about personal strengths, past effective crisis management, and present effective suggestions and behavior. Support and assistance may need to be continued longer than for a younger person. The older person may be more cautious about trying new behavior, taking risks, or changing behavioral patterns. Work closely with the spouse or significant other as you plan and intervene with the elderly; interdependence is usually great in elderly families. Be cognizant as you do crisis work with the elderly person that an intensely traumatic event may never really be resolved in the sense that the phases of crisis have been dis-cussed here. Often the loss is mourned well over a year, and the person may die still suffering the anguish of loss. However, your ongoing acceptance, support, relationship, and assistance will be appreciated and may make the difference between mere existence and at least some enjoyment from life for the client.

With the Family or Group

The family or group undergo the same phases of crisis and manifest similar reactions as the individual client, although the intensity and timing may be different. Thus the same nursing approach previously discussed is needed. Guidelines for assessing and working with the family and group that are discussed in Chapters 10 and 11 will also be useful.

With the Verbally or Hearing-Impaired Person

The guidelines for communication discussed in Chapter 5 are useful here. Learning the individual's perception of the event, helping the person express feelings, and working through solutions will take patience and empathy. Other helpful techniques include the use of sign language, nonverbal methods, possibly an interpreter, and information from significant others. However, be cognizant that others may not always accurately or adequately reflect the verbally impaired person's feelings or thoughts. Sometimes a speech or occupational therapist or counselor who works regularly with such clients can be helpful to you.

With the Cognitively Impaired Person

The mentally retarded or other persons who suffer cognitive impairment, for whatever reasons, will be quite aware that a crisis event, change, or loss surrounds them, even if they cannot coherently talk about it. Often you can assess that the cognitively impaired person, evenly the profoundly retarded, is in crisis because of a behavioral change, such as becoming more irritable, crying, withdrawing from others, regressing from his/her accomplishments, or manifesting physical symptoms. Adults who are caring for and managing the environment for such a person need to examine and work through their own feelings and behavior in response to the crisis. Further, the following interventions will be helpful:

1. Tell the person what has happened.
2. Demonstrate additional nurturing and touching.
3. Talk soothingly to the person about feelings and concerns that he/she might be experiencing and how everything possible will be done to ensure the person's comfort and safety.
4. Remove the person from disruptive others.
5. Remove distractions or upsetting stimuli from the person's environment.
6. Reinforce all behavior that shows response to others and is appropriate to the setting.
7. Utilize play therapy if the person is capable of this.
8. Bring in stimuli (persons, pets, objects, music, etc.) that are a substitute for the loss or change and that provide comfort to the distressed person.

The person with borderline retardation may also have unique difficulties in a crisis situation. The self-image may have long-ago incorporated the feeling, "I'm almost as good as everybody else—yet not quite." Thus, in crisis, he/she may feel easily defeated in spite of supportive efforts on your part. Help by: (1) stating sincere admiration of the person's efforts, (2) pointing out that he/she is doing well and working hard, (3) being specific and tangible in explaining the events without conveying that the person is unduly limited, (4) encouraging the person to consider and reflect on the power and control he/she can exert in a given situation, and (5) conveying to the entire health team that this individual's abilities need to be assessed very carefully to avoid stereotyping or under- or overestimation.

Remember, the person who is cognitively imparied should be seen as important because he/she is a human being, not because of present abilities. Respond to the person as someone with dignity. That initial contact will help you to further work with the person.

With the Ill or Injured Person

Physical and emotional illness and the resultant hospitalization are viewed as crises by most people,

as discussed in Chapter 12. Utilize the principles of communication written in Chapter 5 and the principles of crisis intervention previously discussed in this chapter to help the person and family work through reactions to the stages of illness and to plan for discharge and the degree of wellness possible.

Often the emotionally ill person's physical or emotional illness is related to past unresolved conflicts and crises triggered off by present crisis. This adds an additional burden to the emotional overload carried by the person experiencing the crisis. As the person improves in feeling, thinking, and behavior, and begins to function autonomously, explore the crisis of emotional illness, hospitalization, and eventual discharge with him/her. Since admission of a family member to a psychiatric unit or hospital carries at least some stigma, the family will also need crisis intervention to help it work through feelings related to the stigma as well as other problems related to a hospitalized family member.

The chronically ill psychiatric patient who resides in the community also experiences acute episodes or crises periodically and will need special assistance. Crises may be related to work problems, loss of a loved one, geographical move, financial strains, instability of others in the environment, or mismanagement of medications and resultant behavioral problems. The institutionalized person can experience crises when staff members or ward routines change, when discontinuance of disability pay is threatened, when staff expects the person to begin vocational or educational rehabilitation because of apparent behavioral improvement, or when discharge is planned. Various group activities, as discussed in Chapter 11, as well as crisis intervention, may be indicated to help adjustment.

With a Person Experiencing Loss of a Loved One

Your role with the person experiencing any kind of significant loss is essentially the same as with the person and family experiencing the greatest loss—death. A thorough account of these nursing measures can be found in a text by Mary Castles and Ruth Murray (23).

Reactions to loss are not always obvious. In assessing the patient who is admitted for a medical or surgical illness following a serious loss, direct your assessment and intervention to the mourning process as well as to the illness. Recognize the necessity of grief work for this patient if he/she is to achieve an optimum level of wellness. Illness may be a reaction to grief; help him/her make the connection.

The principles of crisis intervention described earlier in this chapter and the concepts of primary, secondary, and tertiary prevention are applicable to the person experiencing loss.

You can help the person finish the mourning process by giving support during disengagement from the significant object and the search for new and rewarding relationships and patterns of living. *The person cannot be hurried through mourning to crisis resolution.* Encouragement as well as a time and place to talk, weep, and resolve grief is needed. Help the person develop a philosophy about life to the point where he/she can again tolerate stress and change behavior to meet the situation, rather than using excess behavioral mechanisms, such as denial or aggression, to protect him/herself from reality. Encourage the person to do what he/she can for the self. Explore experimentation with new modes of living and behaving and with new relationships. Encourage change and growth with your sharing of ideas and support, but do not try to rush the person through mourning.

The person who has been in mourning for some time demonstrates denial, feelings of emptiness, self-depreciation, anger at self and others, self-pity, somatic complaints, hopelessness, and helplessness. Although such behavior may be disturbing, it is to be expected. The person needs respect and acceptance from you and others before self-respect and acceptance of the life situation are possible.

In addition to dealing with the kinds of death-losses that today's prevailing culture may accept and respond to effectively, some individuals have to deal with unusual and "questionable death" losses. Perhaps there is no clear-cut death, but the family will mourn a person who becomes "missing." Sometimes a family is chronically faced with the limbo of hope versus despair for a missing member. You may find such individuals on any unit of any hospital or walking into a clinic with unexplained hypertension or other physical symptoms. Try to be ready to look beyond the obvious and into despair or mourning as explanation for their symptoms. Analogous to the grief for a missing person is the grief over a family member's personality deterioration, which is like a slow

dying. Do not overlook the feelings and needs of the family.

Some families and friends have to cope with the suicide event of someone important to them. They are "entitled" to all mourning behaviors. Help them know this. They may need an opportunity to intellectually separate normal mourning of sudden death events from their feelings regarding the suicide. Perhaps they need someone who can understand the "relief" that a distressed family or friend feels when they no longer have to be perpetually concerned with how to aid the individual who has now committed suicide. They may be angry at the suicidally deceased. Or they may be preoccupied with feeling they should have somehow prevented the suicide (18, 50). Maybe they need a caring, objective listener who will attend empathically to tales not only of insensitive neighbors and friends but of probing law officers who had to ascertain whether the death was homicide or suicide. Often surviving parents and relatives need guidance in ways of giving honest, yet appropriate age-level explanations to children who are involved. Refer when you reach your limits!

Your peers and other health professionals may also be in crisis. They (as well as yourself) may have to face the loss of a client or patient who was very significant to their (or your) experience of caring. Be gentle and sensitive. When you cannot be helpful to your colleagues, explain that you care but are limited by your own pain. Suggest another person who can be helpful. Be kind to yourself by seeking out a trusted friend, another colleague, or a counselor at the first available moment in order to sort out your own feelings and gain support through the experience. Then you may be able, in turn, to be helpful to colleagues—if not this time, then at a later crisis point.

With the Person Experiencing Delayed Resolution

You have an opportunity to help prevent delayed or ineffective resolution through appropriate crisis intervention. When assessing the patient in any illness situation, determine if the problems and needs could be the result of an earlier crisis or unresolved conflicts, which are now causing symptoms of emotional illness or inappropriate behavior.

Working with a person who has maladaptive

behavior can be a slow process. You should not expect too much of yourself or of the person, for in your disappointment and frustration you may withdraw, thus preventing crisis resolution. Recognize your strengths and limitations and decide whether or not the patient can use help beyond what you can offer. Accept the fact that because this person is unique, or because of the complexity and severity of the problem, available knowledge and techniques may not be sufficient to help him/her. On the other hand, knowing that there is a possibility of failure should not preclude trying to help. Your help may be the stepping stone to later resolution and deeper maturity.

Provide an environment in which the person can experience the phases of recovery from ineffective behavior or emotional or physical illness. Encourage reminiscence about what he/she used to do, the expression of feelings, optimistic but realistic anticipations of the future, and using appropriate rehabilitative measures.

With the Victim of Physical Assault

To be helpful to the assaulted victim, you must understand that the significant event is that the victim *perceives self* as having been violated (48). A sense of control of the body and destiny becomes part of our psyches once we successfully master the independence strivings of early childhood. Few events can so overwhelmingly and suddenly undermine that essential sense of body integrity as being the victim of bodily or sexual assault. For example, D. K. Ipema identifies loss of choice as a central issue facing rape and other assault victims (53).

Reports of clinical studies of rape victims seemingly date back only a decade or so to that of S. Sutherland and S. Scherl in 1970 (109). There is an even greater lack of clinical information in considering male victims of sexual abuse. Yet a young male approached this author during a break from a class on rape. He had this to say: "You know, I thought I wouldn't be able to relate to this topic at all. But a few years ago a buddy of mine was dragged into a carload of five guys. They all used him sexually. He went through a lot of these things you are describing. He was only fifteen at the time."

Although you are going to find this discussion primarily confined to the area where the data exist,

i.e., female rape victim of unknown or barely known attacker, you are encouraged to think much more broadly. Any of the following persons may feel like violated victims: the wife forced into sexual submission by her husband, the youngster intimidated into "sexual play" by older children or into an incestuous act, or the adolescent (male or female) psychologically coerced by another into sexual activity not freely willed. Their needs may be similar if not identical to those of rape victims, and the following intervention principles will apply (1):

> (1) emotional catharsis, (2) exploring self-blame, (3) active support and encouragement on a short-term basis, and (4) assistance in identifying the situational supports available.

In counseling the sexually assaulted victim, try to hear what that individual's experience was for her/him. Put aside your beliefs, such as the victim's role in inviting or encouraging the assault. Avoid vicariously fabricating in your own mind what the experience must have been like. The client will need you to provide opportunities for sorting through her/his own conflicting reactions, whether they are vengeful rage, guilt regarding some element of satisfaction, crippling anxiety in the face of such vulnerability, or some combination of all of these and more.

Emergency Care

Emergency care of rape victims involves four kinds of assistance: (1) emergency medical treatment, (2) prevention of pregnancy and venereal disease, (3) psychological support, and (4) correct collection and preservation of legal evidence (107).

The staff in the emergency department must be familiar with local law enforcement practices as far as the evidence to be obtained for legal purposes. Clearly defined hospital regulations must be carried out for obtaining treatment consent as well as for gathering and handling clothing and specimens so that a chain of evidence is maintained.

The sexual assault victim should be provided with a private area for examination and treatment immediately upon arrival. You must act as the victim's advocate throughout the entire examination and treatment (8). D. Silverman points out some common difficulties as well as opportunities for support when the health worker involved is male (103). Decisions have to be made about the order of attending to injuries, doing examinations, and obtaining historical data. These decisions may vary with circumstances. However, the way in which staff proceed in the emergency room will make a difference in whether the victim is further traumatized or whether healing begins.

A number of actions can reduce trauma (116):

1. Rapid registration procedure with minimal questioning.
2. Continuous presence of a sympathetic, knowledgeable advocate.
3. Caution in words used in victim's earshot. ("Alleged rape" may be an objective term for a staff member but will communicate skeptical disbelief to an overhearing victim.)
4. Privacy.
5. Not asking the victim to undress or climb into stirrups until immediately before the exam.
6. Explaining why questions and procedures are necessary as well as inviting the victim's questions.
7. Avoiding "why" questions.
8. Softening the effect of certain questions by explaining that they must be asked.
9. Restoring to the victim a sense of control over events that are happening.

You may find yourself caring for a victim trying to make an extremely stressful decision, i.e., what to do about reporting to police or pressing charges. Assisting in this situation will necessitate your familiarity with local law enforcement and legal options. However, there are some general guidelines. The victim does have the right to request only medical attention and to refuse legal examination (8). Be aware that a victim experiencing shock and fear in the immediate aftermath of assault may reject legal options; yet in a later stage of integration, the victim may wish that legal evidence had been gathered and preserved in order to pursue civil court processes. Some police officers wish to talk to victims whether or not prosecution is likely to follow, so that they can obtain significant data about the *modus operandi* of a repeat rapist. Consider your own desire of seeing society become safer. The choice may also be affected by what costs for various procedures are going to be billed to the victim. Often the victim has to bear the entire cost of related medical care! All legal decisions rest with the client, but a victim should be informed that choosing to have evidence legally collected and/or to report the event to law officers does not compel him/her to prosecute. The prosecution decision can be postponed until some of the shock of the event has diminished.

A victim or legal guardian trying to decide about consent for legal evidence collection should know that many procedures are involved. The attack must have happened in at least the past 72 hours for most of the evidence to have any validity. However a police report can still be made even if several days have gone by. Evidence is destroyed by baths, showers, clothing changes, douches, and hygienic actions that victims have often taken immediately after the attack in order to feel "clean" again. Evidence collection generally involves the following: an appropriately taken history and physical exam, photography of clothing and wounds, collection of clothing, fingernail scrapings, pubic hair trimmings, pubic hair combing, collection of any dried seminal materials from skin, Wood's light check of pelvic area, vaginal aspiration, swabs, washings, cultures, smears, anal-rectal examinations, rectal cultures and washing, pharyngeal cultures, specimens of saliva, urine, seminal ejaculate, and blood samples (8). As these extensive exams and intrusive procedures can easily be perceived as further violations of sexual integrity, you can readily see how indispensable the support of emergency personnel is to successful crisis resolution.

The victim's need to feel protected from venereal disease can be met by tests done immediately, by a gonococcal swab repeated five to six days later, and by blood tests for syphilis six weeks later (107). Many clients will want to have a prophylactic antibiotic regimen to avoid possible venereal disease.

Respond to pregnancy concerns by inquiring about current birth control practices and the date of the last menstrual period. A pregnancy test may be indicated if there is a possibility that the client was pregnant at the time of the rape. The raped client often fears getting pregnant as a result of the rape. What will be done in a given emergency room depends on the religious affiliation and stance of the specific hospital. The client may choose to handle fears of pregnancy by taking a drug, such as diethylstilbestrol to remove a fertilized ovum; with the procedure of dilation and curettage; or by waiting to see what the future holds. The guiding principle lies in enabling the client to make a counseled and informed choice, to know the risks and side effects involved, and to feel that she has at this point exerted choice and control over her future.

Psychological Care

Psychological care of rape victims has traditionally been done poorly, yet it is essential to the person's resolution of the crisis. Sutherland and Scherl brought long-avoided attention to the crisis-dimensions of rape with their description of a three-phased adjustment response to rape: (1) acute reaction, (2) outward adjustment, and (3) integration and resolution (109). A. Burgess and L. Holmstrom, interviewing a much larger group of subjects, classified reactions into a two-phased response: (1) an acute phase of disorganization, and (2) a long-term process of reorganization (14). The contributions of both author-pairs have been summarized in Table 8-4 in order to suggest intervention guidelines for each phase of crisis-response. The use of the crisis model seems to make a clear and positive difference in the future health of rape victims (17, 53, 109).

TABLE 8-4.   Feelings of Rape Victims and Principles for Counseling

REACTIONS TO RAPE	NURSING INTERVENTION
A. IMMEDIATE IMPACT OR SHOCK PHASE	**A. IMMEDIATE INTERVENTION**
1. Acute emotional reactions, ranging from panic and hysterical emoting to overly subdued self-control.	1. Provide for continuous presence of an empathic , supportive other.
2. Fear of further harm from the attacker.	2. Assist in planning actions to alleviate rational fears, i.e., going to a friend's house instead of home.
3. Feelings may include self-blame, guilt, shame, embarrassment, humiliation, anger, and vengefulness.	3. Provide opportunities for emotional release. Do not minimize. Offer validation of feelings. Explain that the feelings have been experienced by other victims.
4. Concerns about whom to tell and how to tell them.	4. Offer "rehearsal discussion." Offer to talk mutually with significant others.
5. Difficulty with lack of confidence in decision making.	5. Provide clear information on medical and legal procedures and options. Comment on client's survival strengths and capacities. Inform client regarding community resources, such as rape crisis centers, that are available to victims and family. Suggest victim consult a trusted other before making any sudden or impulsive changes in usual life patterns.
6. Episodes of extreme anxiety, insomnia, nightmares, anorexia, nausea, and symptoms related to injuries suffered or treatment given.	6. Help client anticipate and plan a response to physical symptoms that may occur later.

TABLE 8-4.   Continued

REACTIONS TO RAPE	NURSING INTERVENTION
B. OUTWARD ADJUSTMENT (DEFENSIVE RETREAT)	**B. SUPPORTIVE INTERVENTION**
1. Appears outwardly to be managing extremely well. May be puzzled about why there is not more reaction.	1. Initiate follow-up contact and offer continuing interest that is nonintrusive and nonthreatening. State that you are interested in knowing how things are going for the client, but don't push if the client seems reluctant to talk.
2. Shows inclination to make drastic lifestyle changes: moving, changing jobs, dropping out of school, avoiding former friends and interests.	2. Repeat information about available resources, if available, such as rape crisis center, crisis telephone service, and counseling services.
C. INTEGRATION (ACKNOWLEDGEMENT AND REORGANIZATION)	**C. RESTORATIVE INTERVENTION***
1. Depression, possibly including suicidal feelings.	1. Assess depressive, suicidal, phobic status. Respond as indicated by severity of symptoms.
2. Nightmares.	2-5. Deliver or arrange for skilled counseling so victim can successfully rebuild an assaulted self-image; make final decisions related to legal options; and healthfully resolve issues related to self and sexual relationships, fears of sex, men, strangers, touch, and being alone.
3. Fears and phobias related to sensory experiences and situations emotionally associated with the rape event.	
4. Reliving a preoccupation with the rape event.	
5. Rage toward attacker, police, legal or health care system, and health care personnel.	

Special considerations

Special considerations are needed for certain victims of rape and those associated with the victim. Burgess and Holmstrom alert clinicians to a Silent Rape Reaction (14). Victims who did not tell anyone about a rape at the time it happened may experience another crisis years later when events unlock the blocked emotions associated with that long-ago assault. Being aware of this will help you to explore the possibility of an ages-past sexual assault when you are puzzled about the basis for apparently unexplained current reactions a client is having to an event.

M. T. Notman and C. C. Nadelson help us consider some special factors that are relevant when the sexual assault victims are children or adolescents (84). Rape as the first sexual experience may leave a victim quite confused about the relationship between sexuality, violence, and humiliation. To be sexually assaulted during the years of independence strivings can leave a victim anxious that desired independence is not a safe pursuit. Adolescents have to deal with peer group issues. School phobia and truancy may be a result.

Parents may feel guilt that they did not somehow protect the child or adolescent. They have a need to blame someone, whether it be attacker, child, or themselves. Sexual assault may be the proverbial straw in a family where members are already crippled by a general inability to discuss sexuality. Acute family crisis may result. Parents anxious about sexuality may react defensively to a fear that their child provoked the assault.

Consider indications for concurrent counseling of any male(s) significant to the rape victim (1, 38). At a time when appropriate support to the victim is so indispensable, you may first have to help the significant male(s) deal with feelings of rage, impotence, or doubts related to cultural myths, as well as individual defenses. The following example illustrates this point.

> The rape crisis counselor for M. V. was initially puzzled by what was occurring between M. V. and J. T., her fiancé. M. V. had described J. T. as a very supportive potential mate. J. T. had first been very distressed and grief-stricken on hearing of his fiancee's rape. He tearfully clung to M. V. and repeatedly declared his love and support. Yet 24 hours later, M. V. was numbly wondering if the rape meant all was destroyed in her relationship with J. T. She could not believe how accusatory he had become toward her. The counselor offered to talk with J. T., wondering if he was reacting primarily to cultural stereotypes that victims cannot be raped unwillingly. When the counselor used a nonpresumptive approach of exploratory and active listening, a quite different context of events emerged. When the rape occurred, M. V. had been moving from one apartment to another. She had asked J. T. to help her and he had agreed. On the evening that they planned to transport several carloads of small items, J. T. decided he needed to work overtime. He told this to M. V. Anxious to get the move accomplished, M. V. said she would go ahead and get started on her own. It was in the hallway of the apartment being vacated that M. V. was accosted. J. T. had pushed away the guilt he was feeling about the decision to work overtime and instead projected onto M. V. the responsibility for the rape by accusing her of foolhardy independence. The guilt issues were explored and resolved. This

might not have been accomplished without the intervention of an astute counselor.

Rape Prevention

Rape prevention is often not possible. Victims may only have a choice between submission or survival. They may react with paralyzing fear, especially when weapons or physical brutality are involved. The victim is usually at a disadvantage in terms of physical strength. "Fighting back" requires not only physical self-defense skills but a psychological overcoming of cultural inhibitions (12).

D. Aguilera and J. Messick's review of the patterns of the stranger-to-stranger rape reinforce the admonitions that women have heard since childhood (1). Pattern rapists are opportunists and generally preselect a victim, or type of victim, and an environment conducive to their success. For example, a nursing colleague was raped by a man who upon entering through an insecure bedroom window threw a sack of just-purchased hamburgers on the floor for the victim's growling dog. That, in addition to the rapist's knife, made submission seem the only viable choice.

Some women increase their odds of avoiding rape by massive security arrangements for their apartments or homes. Some feel safer by remaining aloof, unfriendly, and doing nothing that may draw attention to themselves. Some refuse to give or accept help from strangers. Some potential victims avoid actual rape by not showing intimidation or submissive behavior. By striving for a cool, problem-solving mentality, the person may sometimes realize possibilities for escape. It is important to be prudent, discrete, and self-directed. When all that fails, most of us would endure physical abuse to preserve our mind and spirit for life. Hopes rest on a future world that provides no encouragement or reinforcement for those meeting sick needs through pathological aggression. See also Chapter 19.

With the Person, Family, or Group after a Disaster

Basic principles of intervention already discussed apply to victims of disaster (or any crime). At times you may have to screen, assess, triage, and work with groups of people or families because the number of counselors is limited, or because everyone is encountering the same crisis. For example, you may work with a group in crisis related to housing, financial problems, employment, specific physical problems, or military service, or having been prisoners of war.

When working with groups of people in disaster events, remove the panic-stricken persons from the main group and place them with someone who will be nurturing. After providing for safety, catharsis, and a sense of security, you may assign small, supervised tasks, since physical activity helps to occupy the mind, work off emotional tension, and increase a sense of worth (25, 45, 50, 104).

Remember that any action that helps the survivor feel valued as a person and safe is important. Provide for basic physical needs. Listen with concern; be nonjudgmental and matter-of-fact; encourage catharsis of feelings of fear, panic, despair, loss, and grief; promote awareness of what has happened; and avoid isolation of the person during shock and defensive retreat. Later, you can give the person specific tasks to do. You should accompany the person or family in the return to the scene of tragedy or damaged homesite. As reality is acknowledged, you can help the person explore how he/she will reconstruct the life style. Help the person make contact with relatives or friends. Give information about social, financial, health, and other resources (46, 50, 67).

You can also call on those victims who are calm, in control, and realistic to assist you in needed tasks, such as movement of people through an interview line, talking with moderately distressed persons, playing with children, working together to keep the group within a shelter entertained, monitoring housekeeping tasks in a shelter, or as a last resort, staying with and restraining a troublesome, overactive victim.

Crisis workers need special consideration also, since they may give much of themselves physically and emotionally during a mass disaster. Insist on at least brief rest periods and privacy and adequate meals for each worker, to avoid later ineffective behavior or illness. After the disaster work is over, the worker should take time to get in touch with his/her personal feelings related to the disaster, to talk about the experience, to resolve any guilt or anger that remains, and to work through the meaning of this crisis for him/herself. Only then can the worker be effective in the next disaster.

Read literature published by the Red Cross and Civil Defense to gain indepth information on evacuation, triage, and the specific responsibilities related to all aspects of survival and care in the event of a large-scale natural disaster, a man-made disaster, or thermonuclear warfare. Several articles give specific information on the following: (1) how a community reacted and coped with a potential disaster (67, 104); (2) how a hospital, nursing department, and health team coped with a natural disaster that stopped community function (46); (3) how an agency and health workers coped with smaller-sized, contained disasters (25, 69).

REFERENCES

1. Aguilera, D., and J. Messick, *Crisis Intervention: Theory and Methodology,* 3rd ed. St. Louis: The C. V. Mosby Company, 1978.

2. Atchley, Robert, "The Life Course, Age Grading, and Age-Linked Demands for Decision Making," in *Life Span Developmental Psychology,* eds. Nancy Datan and Leon Ginsberg, pp. 261–78. New York: Academic Press, Inc., 1975.

3. Barker, R., "Social Psychology of Acute Illness," in *Adjustment to Physical Handicap and Illness: A Survey of the Social Psychology of Physique and Disability,* eds. R. Barker et al., pp. 309–45. New York: Social Science Research Council (Bull. 55, rev.), 1953.

4. Beck, Aaron, "Etiologies of Depression," in *The Medical Management of Depression,* eds. Denis Hill and Leo Hollister, pp. 17-20. New York: Lakeside Laboratories, 1970.

5. Benoliel, Jeanne, "Assessment of Loss and Grief," *Journal of Thanatology,* 1, no. 3 (1971), 182–93.

6. Berlinger, Beverly, "Nursing a Patient in Crisis," *American Journal of Nursing,* 70, no. 10 (1970), 2154-57.

7. Blackwell, B., "Stigma," in *Behavioral Concepts and Nursing Intervention,* coord. C. Carlson, pp. 317-30. Philadelphia: J. B. Lippincott Company, 1970.

8. Braen, G. Richard, *The Rape Examination.* Chicago: Abbott Laboratories, 1976.

9. Brammer, Lawrence, *The Helping Relationship: Process and Skills,* 2nd ed. Englewood Cliffs, N.J.: Prentice-Hall, Inc., 1979.

10. Broden, Alexander, "Reaction to Loss in the Aged," in *Loss and Grief: Psychological Management in Medical Practice*, eds. B. Schoenberg et al., pp. 199-217. New York: Columbia University Press, 1970.

11. Brown, H. F., V. Burdett, and C. Liddell, "The Crisis of Relocation," in *Crisis Intervention: Selected Readings*, ed. H. Parad, pp. 248-60. New York: Family Service Association of America, 1965.

12. Brownmiller, Susan, *Against Our Will: Men, Women, and Rape*. New York: Simon and Schuster, Inc., 1975.

13. Bunn, T. A., and A. M. Clarke, "Crisis Intervention: An Experimental Study of the Effects of a Brief Period of Counseling on the Anxiety of Relatives of Seriously Injured or Ill Hospital Patients," *British Journal of Medical Psychology*, 52, no. 2 (1979), 191-95.

14. Burgess, Ann, and Lynda Holmstrom, "The Rape Victim in the Emergency Ward," *American Journal of Nursing*, 73, no. 10 (1973), 1740-45.

15. ____, "Rape Trauma Syndrome," *American Journal of Psychiatry*, 131, no. 9 (1974), 981-86.

16. ____, *Rape: Victims of Crisis*. Bowie, Md.: Robert J. Brady Company, 1974.

17. ____, *Rape: Crisis and Recovery*. Bowie, Md.: Robert J. Brady Company, 1979.

18. Cain, Albert C., ed., *Survivors of Suicide*. Springfield, Ill.: Charles C Thomas, Publisher, 1972.

19. Caplan, Gerald, *Principles of Preventive Psychiatry*. New York: Basic Books, Inc., 1964.

20. Carlson, C., "Grief and Mourning," in *Behavioral Concepts and Nursing Intervention*, coord. C. Carlson, pp. 95-116. Philadelphia: J. B. Lippincott Company, 1970.

21. Carnevali, Doris, "Preoperative Anxiety," *American Journal of Nursing*, 66, no. 7 (1966), 1536-38.

22. Carr, A., and B. Schoenberg, "Object Loss and Somatic Symptom Formation," in *Loss and Grief: Psychological Management in Medical Practice*, eds. B. Schoenberg et al., pp. 36-48. New York: Columbia University Press, 1970.

23. Castles, Mary, and Ruth Murray, *Dying in an Institution*. New York: Appleton-Century-Crofts, 1980.

24. Chiles, John, "A Practical Therapeutic Use of the Telephone," *American Journal of Psychiatry*, 131, no. 9 (1974), 1030-31.

25. Ciuca, R., C. Downie, and M. Morris, "When a Disaster Strikes, How Do you Meet Emotional Needs?" *American Journal of Nursing*, 77, no. 3 (1977), 454-56.

26. Clark, Terri, "Counseling Victims of Rape," *American Journal of Nursing*, 76, no. 12 (1976), 1964-66.

27. Cline, David, and J. Chosy, "A Prospective Study of Life Changes and Subsequent Health Changes," *Archives General Psychiatry*, 29, no. 7 (1972), 51-53.

28. Cohen, Racquel, and Frederick Ahearn, *Handbook for Mental Health Care of Disaster Victims*. Baltimore: Johns Hopkins University Press, 1980.

29. Cowen, E., and P. Bob, "Marginality of Disability and Adjustment," *Perceptual and Motor Skills*, 23 (1966), 869-70.

30. Datan, Nancy, and Leon Ginsberg, eds., *Life Span Developmental Psychology*. New York: Academic Press, Inc., 1975.

31. DeMott, Benjamin, "The Pro-Incest Lobby," *Psychology Today* (March 1980), pp. 11-18.

32. Diran, Margaret, "You Can Prevent Suicide," *Nursing '76*, 6, no. 1 (1976), 60-64.

33. Dixon, Samuel, *Working with People in Crisis: Theory and Practice*. St. Louis: The C. V. Mosby Company, 1979.

34. Donner, Gail, "Parenthood as Crisis: A Role for the Psychiatric Nurse," *Perspectives in Psychiatric Care*, 10, no. 2 (1972), 84-87.

35. Engel, George, *Psychological Development in Health and Disease*. Philadelphia: W. B. Saunders Company, 1962.

36. Fink, Stephen, "Crisis and Motivation: A Theoretical Model," *Archives of Physical Medicine and Rehabilitation*, 48, no. 11 (1967), 592-97.

37. Gebbie, K., "Treatment Dropouts and the Role of the Crisis Therapist," *Journal of Psychiatric Nursing and Mental Health Services*, 6, no. 6 (1968), 328-33.

38. Ginnetti, John, Jr., "Counseling the Man in the Rape Victim's Life," *Nursing '79*, 9, no. 7 (1979), 43.

39. Gordon, Gerald, *Role Therapy and Illness*. New Haven: College and University Press, 1966.

40. Grace, Helen, "Symposium on Crisis Intervention," *Nursing Clinics of North America*, 9, no. 1 (1974), 1-96.

41. Greene, Robert, and Frank Mullen, "A Crisis Telephone Service in a Nonmetropolitan Area," *Hospital and Community Psychiatry*, 24, no. 2 (1973), 94-97.

42. Grier, Anne, and C. Knight Aldrich, "The Growth of a Crisis Intervention Unit under the Direction of a Clinical Specialist in Psychiatric Nursing," *Perspectives in Psychiatric Care*, 10, no. 2 (1972), 72-83.

43. Hackett, T., N. Cassem, and J. Raker, "Patient Delay in Cancer," *New England Journal of Medicine*, 289 (July 5, 1973), 14-20.

44. Hall, Joanne, and Barbara Weaver, *Nursing of Families*

in Crisis. Philadelphia: J. B. Lippincott Company, 1974.

45. Hargreaves, Anne, "Coping with Disaster," *American Journal of Nursing,* 80, no. 4 (1980), 683.

46. Hargreaves, Anne, et al., "Blizzard '78: Dealing with Disaster," *American Journal of Nursing,* 79, no. 2 (1979), 268–71.

47. Herman, Sonya, "Divorce: A Grief Process," *Perspectives in Psychiatric Care,* 2, no. 3 (1974), 108–12.

48. Hilberman, Elaine, *The Rape Victim.* New York: Basic Books, Inc., 1976.

49. Hinkle, Lawrence, et al., "An Investigation of the Relation between Life Experience, Personality Characteristics and General Susceptibility to Illness," *Psychosomatic Medicine,* 20, no. 4 (1958), 278–95.

50. Hoff, Lee Ann, *People in Crisis: Understanding and Helping.* Reading, Mass.: Addison-Wesley Publishing Co., Inc., 1978.

51. Holmes, T., and R. Rahe, "The Social Readjustment Rating Scale," *Journal of Psychosomatic Research,* 11, no. 8 (1967), 213–17.

52. Holstrom, Lynda, and Ann Burgess, "Assessing Trauma in the Rape Victim," *American Journal of Nursing,* 75, no. 8 (1975), 1288–91.

53. Ipema, Donna K., "Rape: The Process of Recovery," *Nursing Research,* 28, no. 5 (1979), 272–75.

54. Jackson, Edgar, *Understanding Grief.* Nashville: Abington Press, 1967.

55. Jackson, Pat, "Chronic Grief," *American Journal of Nursing,* 74, no. 7 (1974), 1288–91.

56. Janis, Irving, *Psychological Stress.* New York: John Wiley & Sons, Inc., 1958.

57. ——, "Vigilance and Decision Making in Personal Crisis," in *Coping and Adaptation,* eds. George Coelho, David Hamburg, and John Adams, pp. 134–75. New York: Basic Books, Inc., 1974.

58. Johnson, Dorothy, "Powerlessness: A Significant Determinant in Patient Behavior," *Journal of Nursing Education,* 6, no. 2 (1967), 39–44.

59. Johnson, Jean, "Effects of Restructuring Patients' Expectations on Their Reactions to Threatening Events," *Nursing Research,* 21, no. 6 (1972), 499–504.

60. Joselson, Maurice, and Ruth Joselson, "Do Perceptual Changes Occur in Crisis? A Case Study," *Journal of Psychiatric Nursing and Mental Health Services,* 10, no. 5 (1972), 6–10.

61. Keining, Sr. Mary Martha, "Denial of Illness," in *Behavioral Concepts and Nursing Intervention,* coord.

C. Carlson, pp. 9–28. Philadelphia: J. B. Lippincott Company, 1970.

62. King, Glen, "How to Handle Hotline Calls," *MH* (formerly *Mental Hygiene*), 58, no. 4 (1974), 10–13.

63. King, Joan, "The Initial Interview: Basis for Assessment in Crisis Intervention," *Perspectives in Psychiatric Care,* 9, no. 6 (1971), 247–56.

64. Larson, Virginia, "What Hospitalization Means to Patients," *American Journal of Nursing,* 61, no. 5 (1961), 44.

65. Lederer, Henry, "How the Sick View Their World," *Journal of Social Issues,* 8 (1952), 4–15.

66. Lee, J., "Emotional Reactions to Trauma," *Nursing Clinics of North America,* 5, no. 4 (1970), 577–87.

67. Lesher, Dolores, and Audrey Bomberger, "Experience at Three-Mile Island," *American Journal of Nursing,* 79, no. 8 (August 1979), 1403–8.

68. Lester, David, and Gene Brockopp, eds., *Crisis Intervention and Counseling by Telephone.* Springfield, Ill.: Charles C Thomas, Publisher, 1973.

69. Lewis, Edith, "Fire on the Ninth Floor," *American Journal of Nursing,* 62, no. 2 (1962), 50–55.

70. Lewis, Garland, "Communications: A Factor in Meeting Emotional Crisis," *Nursing Outlook,* 13, no. 3 (1965), 36–39.

71. Lindemann, Eric, "Symptomology and Management of Acute Grief," *American Journal of Psychiatry,* 101 (1944), 141–48.

72. Maloney, Elizabeth, "The Subjective and Objective Definition of Crisis," *Perspectives in Psychiatric Care,* 9, no. 6 (1971), 257–68.

73. McCormick, Glen, and Margaret Williams, "Stroke: The Double Crisis," *American Journal of Nursing,* 79, no. 8 (1979), 1410–11.

74. McDaniels, James, *Physical Disability and Human Behavior.* New York: Pergamon Press, Inc., 1969.

75. McDonald, J. M., *Rape: Offenders and Their Victims.* Springfield, Ill.: Charles C Thomas, Publisher, 1971.

76. Mechanic, D., "The Concept of Illness Behavior," *Journal of Chronic Diseases,* 15 (1962), 184–94.

77. Messick, Janice, "Crisis Intervention Concepts: Implications for Nursing Practices," *Journal of Psychiatric Nursing and Mental Health Services,* 10, no. 5 (1972), 3–5.

78. Miles, Margaret, "SIDS: Parents Are the Patients," *Journal of Emergency Nursing* (March-April 1977), pp. 29–32.

79. Morley, W., "Crisis: Paradigm of Intervention," *Journal of Psychiatric Nursing,* 5, no. 6 (1967), 531–44.

80. Muhlenkamp, Ann, Lucille Gress, and Mary Flood, "Perception of Life Change Events by the Elderly," *Nursing Research,* 24, no. 12 (1975), 109–13.

81. Murray, Ruth, and Judith Zentner, *Nursing Assessment and Health Promotion through the Life Span,* 2nd ed. Englewood Cliffs, N.J.: Prentice-Hall, Inc., 1979.

82. ——, *Nursing Concepts for Health Promotion,* 2nd ed. Englewood Cliffs, N.J.: Prentice-Hall, Inc., 1979.

83. Murray, Ruth, M. Marilyn Huelskoetter, and Dorothy O'Driscoll, *The Nursing Process in Later Maturity.* Englewood Cliffs, N.J.: Prentice-Hall, Inc., 1980.

84. Notman, M. T., and C. C. Nadelson, "The Rape Victim: Psychodynamic Considerations," *American Journal of Psychiatry,* 133, no. 4 (1976), 408–13.

85. Palmer, Ellen, "Student Reactions to Disaster," *American Journal of Nursing,* 80, no. 4 (1980), 680–82.

86. Parad, H., ed., *Crisis Intervention: Selected Readings.* New York: Family Service Association of America, 1965.

87. Pederson, Andreas, and Haroutun Babigian, "Providing Mental Health Information through a 24-Hour Telephone Service," *Hospital and Community Psychiatry,* 23, no. 5 (1972), 139–41.

88. Peretz, David, "Development, Object-Relationships, and Loss," in *Loss and Grief: Psychological Management in Medical Practice,* eds. B. Schoenberg et al., pp. 3–19. New York: Columbia University Press, 1970.

89. ——, "Reaction to Loss," in *Loss and Grief: Psychological Management in Medical Practice,* eds. B. Schoenberg et al., pp. 20–35. New York: Columbia University Press, 1970.

90. "Personal Experience and Communication with Staff and Training Committee (1967-1977)," Life Crisis Services, Inc., Gwen Harvey, Director, St. Louis, Mo.: 1977.

91. Polak, Paul, "The Crisis of Admission," *Social Psychiatry,* 2, no. 4 (1967), 150–57.

92. Rahe, Richard, "Life Change Events and Mental Illness: An Overview," *Journal of Human Stress,* 5, no. 9 (1979), 2–10.

93. Rahe, R., and A. Arthur, "Life-Change Patterns Surrounding Illness Perception," *Journal of Psychosomatic Research,* 11, no. 3 (1968), 341–45.

94. Rapaport, Lydia, "The State of Crisis: Some Theoretical Considerations," in *Crisis Intervention: Selected Readings,* ed. Howard Parad. New York: Family Service Association of America, 1965.

95. Reeves, Robert, "The Hospital Chaplain Looks at Grief," in *Loss and Grief: Psychological Management in Medical Practice,* eds. B. Schoenberg et al., pp. 362–72. New York: Columbia University Press, 1970.

96. Resnik, H. L. P., Joseph Sweeney, and Audrey Resnik, "Telephone: A Lifeline for Potential Suicides," *RN,* 37, no. 10 (1974), 1–2.

97. Robins, Eli, et al., "The Communication of Suicidal Intent: A Study of 134 Consecutive Cases of Successful (Completed) Suicide," *The American Journal of Psychiatry,* 115, no. 8 (1959), 724–33.

98. ——, "Some Clinical Considerations in the Prevention of Suicide Based on a Study of 134 Successful Suicides," *The American Journal of Public Health,* 49, no. 7 (1959), 888–89.

99. Robischon, Paulette, "The Challenge of Crisis Theory for Nursing," *Nursing Outlook,* 15, no. 7 (1967), 28–32.

100. Schutz, William, *FIRO: A Three-Dimensional Theory of Interpersonal Behavior.* New York: Holt, Rinehart and Winston, 1960.

101. Selye, Hans, "The Stress Syndrome," *American Journal of Nursing,* 65, no. 3 (1965), 97–99.

102. Shontz, F., *The Psychological Aspects of Physical Illness and Disability.* New York: Macmillan Publishing Co., Inc., 1975.

103. Silverman, Daniel, "First Do No More Harm: Female Rape Victims and the Male Counselor," *American Journal of Orthopsychiatry,* 47, no. 1 (1977), 91–96.

104. Slater, Reda, "Triage Nurse in the Emergency Department," *American Journal of Nursing,* 70, no. 1 (1970), 127–29.

105. Smith, Dorothy, "Survivors of Serious Illness," *American Journal of Nursing,* 79, no. 3 (1979), 441–46.

106. Spiegel, John, "The Resolution of Role Conflict within the Family," in *A Modern Introduction to the Family,* eds. Norman Bell and Ezra Vogel. New York: The Free Press, 1963.

107. Sredl, Darlene, Catherine Klenke, and Mario Rojkind, "Offering the Rape Victim Real Help," *Nursing '79,* 9, no. 7 (July, 1979), 38–43.

108. Steiner, Jerome, "Group Function within the Mourning Process," *Archives of the Foundation of Thanatology,* 2, no. 2 (1970), 80–82.

109. Sutherland, S., and D. Scherl, "Patterns of Response among Victims of Rape," *American Journal of Orthopsychiatry,* 40, no. 3 (1970), 503–11.

110. Thomas, Edwin, "Problems of Disability from the Perspective of Role Theory," *Journal of Health and Human Behavior,* 7, no. 1 (1966), 2-14.

111. Toth, Susan, and André Toth, "Empathic Intervention with the Widow," *American Journal of Nursing,* 80, no. 9 (1980), 1652-53.

112. Turner, Ralph, "Role Taking: Process Versus Conformity," in *Human Behavior and Social Process,* ed. Arnold Rose, pp. 20-38. Boston: Houghton Mifflin Company, 1962.

113. Ujhely, Gertrude, "What Is Realistic Emotional Support?" *American Journal of Nursing,* 63, no. 7 (1963), 758-62.

114. ____, "Grief and Depression: Implications for Preventive and Therapeutic Care," *Nursing Forum,* 5, no. 2 (1966), 23-25.

115. Venokur, A., and M. Seiger, "Desirable Versus Undesirable Life Events: Their Relationship to Stress and Mental Distress," *Journal of Personal and Social Psychology,* 32, no. 8 (1975), 329-37.

116. Welch, Mary Scott, "Rape and the Trauma of Inadequate Care," *Nursing Digest,* 5, no. 1 (Spring, 1977), pp. 50-52.

117. Williams, Florence, "Intervention in Maturational Crisis," *Perspectives in Psychiatric Care,* 9, no. 6 (1971), 240-46.

118. Williams, Reg Arthur, "Crisis Intervention," in *Clinical Practice in Psychosocial Nursing: Assessment and Intervention,* eds. Dianne Longo and Reg Arthur Williams, pp. 191-209. New York: Appleton-Century-Crofts, 1978.

119. Williams, Tim, and John Douds, *Crisis Intervention and Counseling by Telephone,* eds. David Lester and Gene Brockopp. Springfield, Ill.: Charles C Thomas, Publisher, 1973.

120. Willis, Wayne, "Bereavement Management in the Emergency Department," *Journal of Emergency Nursing* (March-April, 1977), pp. 35-39.

121. Wise, Doreen, "Crisis Intervention before Cardiac Surgery," *American Journal of Nursing,* 76, no. 8 (1976), 1316-18.

122. Wright, Beatrice, *Physical Disability: A Psychological Approach.* New York: Harper & Row, Publishers, Inc., 1960.

The Nursing Process with Special Systems in Psychiatric/Mental Health Nursing

9

The Contribution of Culture: Implications for the Nursing Process

Study of this chapter will assist you to:

1. Identify basic assumptions of cultural diversity that relate to the implementation of the nursing process.

2. Identify cultural factors that influence the mental health status of individuals and groups.

3. Discuss common stereotypes that may have negative effects on the delivery of mental health services to people of various cultural backgrounds.

4. Develop skills in cultural assessment of clients.

5. Initiate appropriate nursing interventions with persons from a different culture.

6. Analyze the relationship of the individual's sociocultural background to his/her response to nursing interventions.

7. Discuss how knowledge of culture can influence the effective delivery of mental health care.

This chapter contributed by Wayne Hooker, R.N., Ph.D., and Doris Edwards, R.N., M.S.N.

Harry Stack Sullivan, in the following quote, stated that the individual, regardless of the cultural background, is more similar to, than different from, persons from another background.

> Everyone is much more simply human than otherwise .... Man—however undistinguished biologically—as long as he is entitled to the term human personality, will be very much more like every other instance of human personality than he is like anything else in the world. [70, pp. 32–33]

In other words, basic human needs are similar from one cultural group to the next. And any differences that are apparent probably relate to the manner in which people of a particular culture make their needs known and the manner in which these needs are satisfied. Thus the nurse in offering quality care must do so by reviewing the client in his/her totality.

Providing effective mental health care to clients based on viewing the individual as a whole person with individual needs has for years received emphasis in the nursing literature. Therefore, if quality care is indeed the right of every human being—regardless of status, values, and cultural background—then concerted action by nurses is required, rather than the rhetoric that has been so evident up to now, so that all people will receive effective care.

During the last decade, attention has been focused more and more on culturally diverse populations and on the relationship of cultural diversity to the different mental health needs of individuals. Studies are currently being conducted, and similarities and differences are being delimited. The nurse must learn this information and adjust to social changes that affect the delivery of mental health services to the culturally diverse groups.

As a nurse, you must become involved with the collective society if you are to understand those to be served. The overall goal is to understand the uniqueness of the client as fully as possible, based on a consideration of how the person's culture has contributed to his/her uniqueness. Then you can avoid stereotypes and can provide sensitive care to individuals from a variety of cultural backgrounds.

BASIC GUIDELINES CONCERNING CULTURAL DIVERSITY AND THE NURSING PROCESS

In implementing the nursing process for culturally diverse people, the following guidelines may help you to assess, plan care, and provide effective intervention.

1. Increased awareness of your personal beliefs will assist you to be open to the discovery of the values of persons who differ from you.
2. Sensitivity to the uniqueness of each person is required to work effectively with everyone, and certainly with clients from different cultures.
3. Any care provided clients should be relevant to the life style and unique needs of these people, and you must determine the order of priority that will be most helpful to them.
4. Some specific knowledge about culturally diverse groups and the individuals within these groups is required in order to provide sensitive, quality health care.
5. Knowledge and skills can be gained from a variety of sources, including the literature and experiential learning.
6. Consider yourself not only a teacher but also a learner—with members of the various cultural groups as teachers.
7. Clients should be worked with at their level of functioning, with their strengths receiving major focus.

When you utilize the above guidelines for working with persons who are different from you, your role as a helping person will be strengthened.

DEFINITIONS OF CULTURE

In the consideration of culture as an important aspect of assessment and implementation of care, you should formulate a definition that has meaning for you. Madeleine Leininger states that there are more than 250 definitions of culture that have been recorded, although in its broadest sense, *culture refers to a way of life practiced by a group of people* (43).

Culture can further be defined as *the sum total of the learned ways of doing, feeling, and thinking, past and present, of a social group at a given period in time.* These learned ways are transmitted from one generation to the next, as well as to individuals who join the group. Culture is the group's design for living and includes every facet that surrounds the person: the physical and social world values, attitudes, roles, goals in life, knowledge, beliefs, customs, morals, laws, skills, acquired habits, and capabilities that help the group to survive and live together (58).

A *subculture is defined as a social group within a larger culture made up of persons of the same or similar socioeconomic level, racial, or ethnic origin, religion, occupation, education, geographic background, or age who have an identity of their own and similar values and goals but who also relate to the total culture in certain ways* (58).

All people from any cultural group are surrounded by the components of a culture. When you provide care for someone, be aware that the following cultural components influence how the person looks at self and attains and maintains his/her health. These components may also influence the client's expectations of you and of the care to be received.

A communication system.
Knowledge, methods, and objects for providing for basic needs.
Family and sexual patterns of behavior and roles.
Other human patterns of social exchange such as competition or collaboration.
Goals and direction for life.
Customs and mores.
Artistic expressions.
Religious or magical ideas and practices.
Recreational and leisure-time interests and activities.

These components, along with societal and governmental controls, forms of property, and means of transportation and exchange of goods, affect each person, often in ways that are not obvious to the casual observer (58, 60).

Margaret Mead differentiates culture into three different kinds. *Postfigurative refers to a culture in which change is slow and the behavior of the new generation is much like the behavior of the former generation because children learn primarily from the generations that preceded them.* There are no expectations for opportunities of change in the ways of life, and a sense of continuity pervades from the past, through the present, and on to the future. In a postfigurative culture, you see a linear relationship or hierarchy of age groups in which there is an emphasis on the extended family with biological and cultural relationships through time (53).

Cofigurative refers to a culture in which both children and adults learn from their peers, which provides some opportunities for change. The adults model for the younger generation and must approve change. In the cofigurative culture, there is a collateral or more or less equal relationship between the various age groups. Collateral relations imply that the person is part of a family and social system, with certain responsibilities to the cultural group (53).

Prefigurative refers to a culture in which adults are able to learn from their children. In this culture, there is increased opportunity for individuality in behavior, and the person maintains autonomy in that he does not have to completely submit to authority. Personal goals may take precedence over group goals (53).

These variations set the stage for human behavior in terms of how the person sees his/her relation to nature, the sense of time dimension, the type of valued dominant personality, and the patterns of relationships with others. Overall, these variations can affect mental health as well as definitions of mental health and illness. If culture is a sum total of learning, and therefore, a product of where the learning took place, ethnicity is a very important consideration in assessment and planning of nursing care. Does your client behave differently because his/her behavior was learned in a setting entirely different from the dominant culture in which he/she is now attempting to interact? Anthropologists report that there are more than 2,000 subcultures; thus it would be impossible to know everything about every subculture. However, concepts of culture and subculture must be used in assessing clients, in evaluating individual needs, and in lessening the possibility of stereotyping.

CULTURAL PATTERNING

Many observations support the theme that survival of life, in all forms, is maintained through groups and grouping. This can be seen as a permanent pattern or as an occurrence due to specific stress situations. For the human, groups have greater meaning and significance than for other forms of biological life. The person achieves optimum development and fulfillment only through groups. The foundation for group interaction is laid in the earliest relationship with another individual (the mother). However, this first relationship has to be extended beyond the family if mental health and intellectual development are to be achieved. In this process, groups are of primary importance. Growth of personality cannot be gained only from interaction with other individuals; rather, group experiences are necessary because the person has to deal with and interact with a variety of persons. The survival of the human race has depended on the ability of individuals to merge into a system of relationships over a period of time. This enduring system of relationships leads to the formation of cultural patterning. And it is through cultural patterning that social systems, family interaction, and technology are preserved. In the person's attempt to cope with an ever-changing environment, stressors are somewhat lessened through cultural patterning and through the perpetuation of beliefs, values, and customs that remain constant within the group.

The history of a cultural group is basic to the maintenance of it's customs, rituals, beliefs, and values. Beliefs and values aid the preservation of customs, and rituals strengthen family unity and give direction to child-rearing patterns. A historical heritage with established beliefs and rituals helps the group to relate to and understand individual role status changes and special events, such as birth, maturity, marriage, illness, and death.

Some groups have been less successful than others at maintaining their historical cultures. For example, the history of black Americans began when they were first introduced into this country in the early 1600s. Black people were not brought to America by their own choice but were forcefully separated from their primarily African cultural heritage. They were separated from their own tribes and families upon their arrival and were obliged to express racial identity and culture according to the perceptions and expectations of the dominant white culture. The native African languages were lost because of restrictions on their use, and the English or French tongue was superimposed on the many languages spoken by the African slaves (58).

Mexican-Americans in the Southwest also found themselves unwilling immigrants through annexation or conquest. These people, however, were able to maintain their language, cultural heritage, and identification with a specific historical past.

The American Indians' historical harmony with nature has shaped their particular view of life, health practices, and social interaction. The American Indian is historically more aware of the earth, and life is coordinated with the seasons. This is in contrast to the average middle-class white American (Caucasian) who has a sense of control over his/her life because of a history of attempting to dominate nature. The Caucasian's historical view of self as overcoming nature when it is an obstacle also influences the philosophy of life, health care practices, and social interactions.

Poor people have a cultural history and patterning also. A stereotypic view of poor persons from ethnic groups is that they seem reluctant to give up certain ways of life. This is especially true if these people have had the disadvantage of a poor education, which limits them to few new life experiences. There are generational differences too. For example, ethnic persons newly arrived in the country may also have an added language barrier, which inhibits communications and experiences with the dominant culture. Yet, if certain ways have worked historically for a group of people, they will be hesitant to give them up, at least until better ways are proven. Holding onto customs also depends on whether the person came by choice, was brought to the country, or was indigenous.

In the past few years, there seems to be a new wave of pride in ethnic identity. You may see Blacks who attempt to maintain the African identity in simulating African dress. Mexican-Americans, Polish-Americans, Italian-Americans, Oriental-Americans, and other national groups celebrate their ethnic holidays and follow some of their historical customs. These kinds of behavior are not necessarily an attempt to cling to old ways. Rather, following ethnic traditions is a statement to the dominant culture that through the assimilation process it is not necessary to lose the historical and cultural heritage of the group.

THE IMPACT OF ETHNICITY ON MENTAL ILLNESS AND PSYCHIATRIC TREATMENT

There are many conceptual and measurement problems in researching mental health in different cultures because each culture defines health from a different perspective. C. Gaitz and J. Scott report that cultural factors may influence the scores in research studies, but such scores do not indicate whether one ethnic group has more or less incidences of mental illness than another (28). Added to this is the problem of the many different definitions of *mental health*; such as: *a balance in a person's internal life and adaptation to reality; an orderly progression through life's developmental stages without upsets; a growth toward maturity in which the individual is able to achieve the capacity to love rather than remain in a state of helplessness with the need for love.* Normal behavior is relative to the specific culture, and different personality characteristics

are promoted by each culture. Thus results of studies are difficult to compare because each study tends to place emphasis on different cultural factors.

Most such studies have shown that cultural factors, such as family relationships, child rearing practices, language, and attitudes toward illness, as well as social and economic status, do exert an important influence on mental health statistics. However, it is also true that these differences in statistics may reflect largely different ethnic modes of expression rather than actual differences in the incidence of mental disorders. Further, economic factors affect mental health as shown in a study by C. Gaitz and J. Scott (28) on Mexican-Americans who experience low socioeconomic status in terms of substandard housing, little education, poor physical health, little political influence, communication problems, and social exclusion. Both ethnicity and economic factors must be considered in mental health assessments, and low economic status may override ethnic differences.

Take the example of the traditional Mexican-American family where the wife is somewhat isolated. Her contacts with others are usually limited to female relatives who live close by. The Mexican-American husband is said to rule his home, and the wife and children are expected to show him respect and accept his decisions without question. Moreover, it is considered unbecoming for a wife to show anger or withhold affection from her husband. This denial of freedom and suppression of emotions in the Mexican-American wife are said to give rise to hysterical behavior, behavior that gains some attention and concern from the husband and family. The consequence of this is that certain illnesses are found among Mexican-Americans, especially among Mexican-American women, that are considered to be superstitious by Anglo-Americans. One such illness is *susto,* or fright, caused by something that is natural but unexpected, such as a sudden loud noise. This fright is said to be responsible for insomnia, restlessness, and loss of appetite. This contrasts with *espanto,* which is fright from an unnatural source, such as spirits, and causes some of the same symptoms as *susto. Coraje* is a rage in which the individual becomes hyperactive and may scream and cry.

That members of any one culture, regardless of education, may define mental health and treatment differently from members of another culture was demonstrated in a study of J. Flaskerud (24). Mental health professionals and lay people from the dominant Caucasian culture in the United States used similar definitions of mental illness, but a group of lay people from the Appalachian culture (also Caucasian) defined mental illness behavior quite differently. For example, behaviors defined as mental illness by the dominant Caucasian culture were labeled as lazy, mean, immoral, psychic, or criminal by the Appalachians. The Appalachians recommended that these behaviors be tolerated or punished by the social group or legal system, in contrast to recommendations for some type of psychiatric management by non-Appalachian groups.

As another example, Bonnie and Vern Bullough report that admission rates to mental hospitals are higher and the hospital stay is longer for black Americans than for white Americans (7). But when socioeconomic status is carefully controlled, psy-

chosis rates among the two populations appeared similar. On the other hand, in a comparison of studies concerning psychological disorders, Bruce and Barbara Dohrenwend found conflicting reports of incidence of mental disorders among black and white populations in the United States (19).

Many studies demonstrate an underrepresentation of Mexican-American clients in community mental health centers, particularly as compared to Caucasian clients. A view expressed by G. Jaco (36) and W. Madsen (50) is that underrepresentation of the Mexican-American in mental health centers is the result of less mental disorders among Mexican-Americans than among Anglos. Madsen felt that the Caucasian experiences stressors to a greater degree because he/she experiences them in an individual way, whereas the stressors experienced by the Mexican-American are shared and to some extent lessened by family support. Madsen's research was conducted in Hidalgo County in Texas and covered the four-year period from 1957 to 1961.

A study by M. Karno and R. Edgerton came to a different conclusion (39). Although Mexican-Americans are underrepresented in mental health clinics in Los Angelos, interview responses indicated that they do not perceive and define mental illness in significantly different ways from white Americans. Furthermore, the underrepresentation does not indicate a lower incidence of mental illness than that found in other ethnic groups in the United States. Rather, these authors propose that the underrepresentation is caused by the language barrier, by the use of family physicians for emotional problems rather than established mental health agencies, and by the lack of psychiatric facilities that can meet the specific need of the Mexican-American.

E. F. Torrey reports that traditional mental health services are irrelevant for most urban Mexican-Americans. His observations were made of mental health centers in San Jose and Santa Clara Counties in California. Torrey points out the following six areas of irrelevancy (73):

1. Services are inaccessible to Mexican-Americans.
2. Language considerations make the services irrelevant because of the low ratio of Spanish-speaking therapists.
3. Services are class-bound; traditional mental health services are structured for the middle class and are not relevant to the needs of the poor Mexican-American.

4. Services are culture-bound; studies from cognitive anthropology suggest that psychotherapy may also be culture-bound.

5. The community mental health center is perceived by Mexican-Americans to be an Anglo instrument to perpetuate the Anglo's dominance.

6. Mexican-Americans have their own systems of mental health services, i.e., *curanderos,* or folk healers, and mental health "ombudsmen."

Therefore, the limited number of Mexican-Americans in community mental health centers may not be the result of a decreased incidence of mental disorders. Rather, the decreased use of clinics reflects that these clinics do not meet a perceived need.

The conclusion from available evidence is that there is at present no correlation between ethnic identity and type or amount of mental disorder within a given population.

J. J. Yamamato, C. Quinton, and N. Pally discuss therapist-client attitudes in a study that was performed in California (79). The group studied consisted of outpatients of which 65 percent were Caucasian, 25 percent were Black, 9 percent were Mexican-American, and 1 percent were Oriental. The purpose of the study was to find out what happened to a minority group patient after he/she applied for treatment and was initially seen by a therapist. The paper explores the relationship between patients and their Caucasian therapists. The conclusions of the study revealed some problems in the therapist-patient situation, such as felt prejudice and dislike. Yet, the non-Caucasian patient seldom criticized his/her therapist. One conclusion of the study, in spite of relatively few complaints from minority patients, was that the minority group patient received the least intensive therapy, and many dropped from the program before therapy had been completed.

H. Gonzales states that the Mexican-American client who has emotional problems should seek the help of a psychiatrist who is versed in the relevant cultural beliefs about disease, health, and life, so that the psychiatrist will avoid mistaking a cultural belief for a mental disorder (30). Thus, increasing evidence suggests that all mental health practitioners must be sensitive to the life experiences and unique characteristics of persons from different ethnic backgrounds.

THE CULTURE OF POVERTY

It is not the purpose of this chapter to debate the various theories of the culture of poverty. You should, however, be aware that not everyone perceives these theories in the same manner. Some proponents of the idea of a culture of poverty even negate the ethnic consideration altogether. The phrase, *culture of poverty, refers, in part, to the ready-made set of behavioral solutions for everyday problems, the life style, way of thinking, attitudes, and beliefs that emerge and remain when a person is forced to get along in his/her everyday activities without money* (14).

Some studies of cultural and minority groups have been limited to the poor segment of the cultural and minority populations, ignoring the values and life styles of the middle and upper classes of the cultural groups. For example, in studies by Oscar Lewis, information about a few *atypical* families was applied to all people, from which Lewis developed his theory on the culture of poverty. Lewis stated that the culture of poverty tends to perpetuate itself. He claimed that by the time children living in a slum area are ages six or seven, they have usually absorbed the basic attitudes and values of their subculture; and he concludes that they are psychologically unready to take full advantage of changing conditions or improving opportunities that may develop later in their lifetime (14).

E. Casavantes also contributes to the idea that ethnicity and poverty are synonymous. In an article concerning Mexican-Americans, he uses several attributes that are said to characterize Mexican-Americans, but these are really characteristics of people living in poverty, not just of Mexican-Americans. He has not considered the characteristics of Mexican-Americans of higher economic levels (12).

Such studies perpetuate stereotypes about poverty and ethnicity and interfere with understanding the problems of being poor, as well as overlooking the unique characteristics of people of various ethnic and racial backgrounds. In the *Culture of Poverty Revisited,* a critique by the Mental Health Committee against Racism, another perspective is presented. The committee maintains that culture of poverty theories by Lewis and others are racist and erroneous in many ways and may also be politically dangerous (14).

THE PROBLEM OF STEREOTYPING

Because culture is a way of life practiced by a group of people, and this way of life is learned along with a set of beliefs and values, it is easy to understand that a person can learn to become closed to the values and beliefs of others. *The belief that your own ways of doing things and your values and beliefs are the only right ones is called ethnocentricity.* You can surmount ethnocentricity and cultural biases by studying your own and other people's cultures and by interacting with people from other racial, ethnic, or religious groups and cultures. Do you identify with mainstream America or with a specific cultural or subcultural group? You have to analyze your own value systems as well as your attitudes toward, and biases about, people. Are your beliefs the remains of stereotypes and prejudices from your past learning experiences? We often tend to combine various racial or ethnic groups together. For instance, there are about 200 American Indian tribes with differing languages and customs, and you cannot assign the same beliefs, values, and behavior to all of them.

Furthermore, visual and linguistic cues are not always valid guidelines for assessment of persons. These cues alone, without other varifying data, can lead you to stereotype. Every person must be considered as an individual, whose behavior is the product of where learning took place. That a person has dark skin, blue eyes, a large nose, or other prominent features does not indicate that his/her values, beliefs, and behavior will fit neatly into a prescribed pattern. Also a person who speaks with an accent will not necessarily demonstrate a set pattern of values, beliefs, and behavior that are thought to be representative of a particular cultural group. For example, Spanish-speaking persons are immigrants from more than twenty countries—each with different histories, geographic locations, cultures, and subcultures. The Puerto Rican-American and Mexican-American share some of the same values, but they differ in the way they use folk healers, in their food preference, and in their adaptation to the dominant culture.

Stereotypes may be perpetuated by research studies or other literature. The problem of making accurate conclusions concerning the Mexican-American family has been discussed in a study by M. Montiel (55). He maintains that studies often emphasize pathology rather than the diversity and strengths of the Mexican-American family. It has been referred to as "paternalistic," "traditional," "male-dominated," "familistic," "automistic," and "authoritarian." Montiel claims that this variety of descriptions inhibits a meaningful understanding of the Mexican-American family. He asserts that social scientists have assumed that the Mexican-American family is male-dominated and that the mother assumes an inferior position in the family; yet these assumptions have not been documented. His paper discusses the concept of *machismo* in terms of the assumption that the Mexican-American family is male-dominated. According to Montiel, the numerous studies of the Mexican-American family, although based on empirical evidence, are open to serious question.

Stereotypes about middle-class and wealthy people also exist and may be as inaccurate and damaging as are stereotypes about poor or ethnic people. Stereotypes about any group come about because someone has had only limited experience with one member, or a few members, or a certain group. This minimal experience is then applied to all members of the group. Stereotyping also arises from personal feelings of fear, inadequacy, and conflict, whereby the individual projects these feelings upon a group of people. In this case, the subculture will then be defined by a variety of inappropriate or disparaging adjectives having personal significance and meaning only to the person who is doing the projecting.

The important thing is never to base your opinions about people, or any group of people, on just one or a few experiences. Stay open to the unique values, beliefs, and life styles of each person, regardless of that person's color, religion, property, or appearance. Then you will know that all Jehovah's Witnesses, all Catholics, all black people, all white people, all poor people, all wealthy people, all thin people, or all obese people are *not* alike. Their similar needs are manifested differently, even though there may be some similarities in appearance, values, statements, or behavior. You must see the uniquenesses as well as the similarities.

M. T. Busch and K. S. Babich deal candidly with some of the reasons that have inhibited our ability to provide effective care to all clients. Not only do nurses lack awareness about cultural groups, but there is also denial by some that differences, uniquenesses, and similarities even exist (8). In addition, although information is increasing and studies are being undertaken, much of the information on various ethnic or economic groups may be inaccurate, and therefore it tends to perpetuate the stereotypes regarding ethnicity and mental illness. Furthermore, the groups being studied frequently have little input into the studies being done about them, so misconceptions and generalizations continue to persist based on this inaccurate data.

INTERACTION PATTERNS RELATED TO CULTURAL GROUPS

The Extended Family

The statement is often made that family relationships are stronger among certain ethnic groups than among the dominant Caucasian groups. Casavantes maintains that this pattern of strong family relationships is true particularly of poor people, who have few resources and need to rely on the support of the extended family to meet their physical and emotional needs (12). Middle-class or wealthy persons have resources outside of the extended family and are able to avail themselves of physical and emotional supports within the community. If persons do not have money and other resources to engage in outside the recreational and social activities, they tend to spend more time together, and they depend on the integrated family group for recreational and social outlets. Yet, in some religious, family, and cultural groups, such as Jewish, Mormon, Appalachian, black American, American Indian, Islamic, Buddhist or Hindu cultures, the extended family is considered important regardless of the economic level of the person. The relatives are sought for validation, advice, and support during health and illness (14, 42).

Social Interaction

Persons of minority cultural groups and poor persons are frequently viewed as nonjoiners in social, church, and civic organizations. However, this is not usually true of black people, especially the women, who are frequently staunch and active supporters/members of a church or fraternal organization. The church and other fraternal organizations provide the black person with emotional, spiritual, and interpersonal support and camaraderie. Actually, there are many reasons other than race and low economic status as to why minorities and poor people are found to be nonjoiners, for example: (1) lack of leisure time in which to participate in group activities, (2) lack of transportation, (3) lack of money for appropriate clothes or dress, or (4) feelings of being unwelcome and/or excluded from certain social and civic groups. Minorities and poor persons may have feelings of helplessness and hopelessness; they perceive that joining groups does not change anything in the long run (14). Therefore, this sense of powerlessness can lead to the immobilization of disadvantaged persons, resulting in a feeling of not being in control of their destiny—even in matters such as illness and death.

Mexican-Americans are said not to be joiners because of their concept that the family itself is sufficient. To join other groups is considered disloyal to the family. This is contrasted to white Americans who are often viewed as compulsive joiners (50).

Some groups purposefully remain aloof from the dominant society. For example the Amish, Hutterites, some reservation Indians, and some Appalachians do not wish to have their lives or their children influenced by mainstream America. As people in various ethnic groups become better educated, have better jobs, and have access to more political power within a community, the amount of participation in social and civic groups often becomes greater. This, however, usually occurs as the subordinate group becomes more assimilated into the dominant culture. Perhaps as assimilation increases, the cultural identity becomes diminished. This raises two questions:

1. Does a person's ethnic group identity, other group identity, or economic status determine

his/her pattern of joining or not joining community groups?

2. Is assimilation (and decrease in a person's cultural identity) necessary to gain power and acceptance within a dominant culture?

As indicated in this section, the amount of participation in the larger society can influence whether the person seeks health or medical care from the institutions or agencies in the community. Thus isolation in the community may well contribute to illness as well as to inadequate care.

The Concept of Machismo

The term *machismo* refers to a controversial aspect of the male's self-concept in the Mexican-American culture, as well as in most traditional cultures. *Machismo* comes from the word *macho*, which simply means "male." The expectations of the Mexican-American male is that he must demonstrate *machismo* rather than behavior indicative of nurturing or of intellectual or artistic interests. A part of the *macho* image is to brag about various conquests and masculine behavior and to refuse to do anything considered to be feminine, such as housekeeping or caring for infants and children. According to Casavantes, this demonstration of *machismo* may be an overcompensation (12). For example, a man is considered *macho* when he is working and providing for his family, since he is able to maintain his identity if he has a job. Therefore, the man who has no job or a job of which he is not proud, will have a problem of lowered self-esteem when he is unable to protect, provide for, and give care to his family. He then compensates for his lack of self-esteem by a demonstration of excessive *machismo*. This is probably what leads to his refusal to have anything to do with things that are womanly.

In this consideration of *machismo*, there has been neglect of the identity component of self-concept in broader terms; rather, the literature has concentrated on a cluster of values and traits associated with the concept of *machismo* as a prominent aspect of the male's self-concept in Mexican-American culture and has ignored other aspects.

The concept of *machismo* has far-reaching consequences in terms of unfair treatment of women, the aggressive behavior seen in society, harsh child-rearing patterns, social attitudes toward educational pursuits, and possibly in regard to emo-

tional health as well. Male alcohol use and abuse in the Mexican-American culture are also purported to be influenced by the *macho* image. A "man" should be able to drink heavily and tolerate it well; not to do so is perceived as being unmanly. Therefore, it is reported that the Mexican-American male is reluctant to recognize and seek treatment for problems with alcohol. And if there is a problem of alcoholism in these men, it is tolerated, and the alcoholic is protected within the structure of the extended family.

The use of physical force among poor persons and minorities in the form of fighting to solve interpersonal differences and to punish children is supposedly part of the *macho* image. However, this idea is controversial and not supported by adequate research findings. Fighting may be the result of frustration from lack of employment and achievement opportunities and from the social limitations placed on persons in lower socioeconomic and some ethnic groups.

Other Ethnic Misconceptions

Studies of black family patterns of behavior and interaction have been criticized from both a political and scientific point of view, but nevertheless, many such findings have been incorporated into our current assumptions about black families. These studies depict the patterns of interaction in the black family as being pathological and unstable, with any stability depending on the presence of a controlling, domineering mother. This pathologic family interaction is said to affect the male, so that in later life he is unable to adjust to the role of husband and father and is unable to form mature lasting relationships with others (14).

Contrary to the implications of some research, white people are not always in the middle economic level and therefore stable, and black people are not always in the lower economic level and therefore unstable.

The Need for Immediate Gratification

A common sociological stereotype of poor people, and particularly of black people, is that they are unable to delay gratification for material possessions, in contrast to the middle-class value that you must carefully plan for the future and delay or deny small gratifications along the way for some future payoff. The fact is that it is difficult for the poor person to plan economically for the future because he/she often does not have the financial resources that provide for more than a day-to-day existence. Also, reality for poor people and minorities may well be that the outside environment cannot be depended upon. Thus for poor persons and minorities, promises made for future gain are often not kept (14).

In psychiatric nursing, the phrase, *unable to delay gratification* has a connotation quite different from the economic or sociological meaning. We speak of a personality trait, the **inability to delay gratification,** when *referring to someone who is infantile, narcissistic, egocentric, immature, or even sociopathic.* Do not impart this meaning to poor people or minorities as you read about their being unable to delay gratification. Being poor or of a

minority group does not imply immaturity. Emotional maturity is not correlated to economic level or cultural group.

There is actually no substantial evidence to support the idea that poor people and minorities are unable to delay gratification. This stereotype, however, is posited as influencing the kind and amount of mental health services that the poor receive. Some professionals believe that poor people are only receptive to and interested in crisis treatment, or that they are not good candidates for psychotherapy because they need to see rapid change. Therapists who view their clients in this way do not provide them with opportunities to experience long-range planning because they do not perceive the client as being able to comply with such a plan of care.

THE NURSING PROCESS

Assessment

An important aspect of the nursing process is the collection of valid data for client assessments. This implies the need to gain knowledge regarding cultural variations. The assessment tool, Appendix A, in Chapter 4 can serve as a guide.

Although the possession of sound knowledge regarding cultural variations does not guarantee the provision of the most effective care to meet a client's needs, it does provide you with basic foundations upon which to implement the nursing process. However, when you possess such knowledge, do not assume that knowledge by itself presupposes that you can relate to all people within this group. The temptation to be avoided is the categorization of people into groups, and for the sake of expediency, to label or type them. Since the nursing process focuses on the individual, it is imperative that you take into consideration the diversity among individuals within the designated group.

Realize, too, that the culture of poverty theories are probably more useful for sociologists or other disciplines than for nurses. Therefore, remember that when you care for persons who are poor, you should also attend to the person's cultural heritage. In assessing and planning nursing care, always consider beliefs, values, and ways of living that may be different from your own. This is especially important so that you care for the person

from a culture different than your own as an unique individual.

Communication is an important step in assessment and serves as a basis for interaction between persons. Communication is also the means by which culture is transmitted and preserved. Verbal communication requires a vocabulary, or repertoire of words, and a grammatical structure. Along with the vocabulary and grammatical structure, you can perceive significant cues from the client's voice qualities, intonation, rhythm, and speed, as well as from the pronounciation in verbal communication. Along with the verbal cues, you can also perceive nonverbal communication by way of gestures, facial expressions, and body posture. Furthermore, there are many variations of verbal and nonverbal communications among families and groups within and specific to a culture. These variations give rise to specific meanings for a designated group. Variations in communication may be as simple as the currently popular language of a family group, or they may be complicated and widespread. The border version of Spanish spoken in the Southwest, referred to as "Tex-Mex," and "black English" are examples of extremes.

The *interview* is one way to communicate with clients from all cultures. Proceed with the interview unhurriedly and adhere to acceptable social or cultural amenities. Start with statements that refer to general social topics. When gathering information, begin with general questions and give time for response or unrelated conversation. Do not be too efficient and begin the interview for specific data immediately. Such an approach may appear rude and uncaring. Persons of European background and Spanish-speaking, rural, and elderly clients expect and value a bit of "small talk" before getting down to the business of the interview. Then, once the interview has begun, the Spanish-speaking client, as well as these other clients, will talk freely. Many ethnic clients respond better to a nondirective approach and the use of open-ended questions rather than to a direct question-and-answer approach. The nondirective approach is especially useful with Spanish-speaking clients, who tend to be passive with Caucasians, and also with Oriental clients, who may tend to be rather nonexpressive.

Spanish-speaking clients and American Indians are said to be more reluctant to talk about matters concerning sex than many young Americans or Oriental clients, who may discuss these matters rather freely. If this subject is necessary, the reticent client will probably respond more openly to sexual questions with an interviewer of the same sex. Usually any sexual matter regarding a male child should be discussed with the father rather than with the mother in Spanish-speaking, Pakistani, or Arabian families. The principles of communication discussed in Chapter 5 are applicable to people from any cultural background.

Many sources describe American Indians as being private persons who do not readily discuss personal affairs. With the American Indian, interpersonal relationships are developed slowly, and trust is attained only over a period of time. Once trust is established, the American Indian usually talks freely about self and culture. This poses a dilemma for the interviewer because you frequently do not have the opportunity to interact with a person over the period of time necessary to establish trust. Be aware that the Navajo Indian is ethically unable to speak for another person—even a close relative. This ethic, of course, makes it difficult for the interviewer in his/her attempt to obtain a personal history from any person other than the client. Some cooperation, however, will usually be given in an emergency situation. In interacting with American Indians, it is important to listen carefully and to give your full attention to the interview. It is also to your advantage when interviewing an American Indian to avoid situations in which the client will feel hurried.

Eye contact is an important tool in assessment, both for observation and to initiate interaction. The dominant American culture values eye contact as symbolic of positive self-concept, openness, interest in the other person, attentiveness to events and feedback, honesty, and "above board" behavior. Lack of eye contact from another person is interpreted as a sign of shyness, lack of interest, subordination, humility, guilt, embarrassment, low self-esteem, rudeness, or dishonesty. The value of the establishment of eye contact in nurse-client relationships is usually taught to beginning nursing students as an integral component of the repertoire of skills used in the interview and helping interaction with clients. Review Chapter 5 for information about cultural differences in use of eye contact, as well as in facial expression, gestures, posture, and body contact.

Most black and Mexican-American clients are comfortable with eye contact and even may interpret lack of eye contact from the professional helper as disinterest in them. J. McKenzie and H. Chrisman report that eye contact is important with some Filipino-Americans because they may believe that a witch will turn away from your gaze. Therefore, it is important to establish eye contact or face the possibility of being considered a witch (52)!

Other groups find eye contact difficult. Some Oriental people and many American Indians consider eye contact an impolite act and an invasion of privacy, which accounts for their hesitancy to make eye contact with persons of the opposite sex or persons who are perceived to be superiors. You can understand that if the helping professional is considered to be a superior, which is often the case, the client would not be expected to make direct eye contact with the helper and probably would be embarrassed if direct eye contact were initiated by the helper. Also, some subcultures in the United States, such as some Appalachians, consider immediate direct eye contact impolite because of the interpretation of eye contact as aggressive or hostile behavior. The elderly Orthodox Jewish male avoids eye contact with all females except his wife so that his behavior will not be interpreted as seductive.

Equally as important as the cultural implications of eye contact are the personal expressions of the individual. Feelings are expressed in the eyes, and you can assess much as the person talks to you.

The fearful person may not be able to look at you, whereas the suspicious, guarded person may intently hold eye contact without apparent difficulty.

Intervention

Cultural variations among clients appear in a variety of ways, all of which have implications for you as a nurse. Some examples include: (1) the manner in which illness behaviors are manifested, (2) the way interactions with others are established, and (3) the way mental health services are utilized. It is your responsibility to develop increased knowledge of and sensitivity to the cultural aspects of client behaviors.

Unless these cultural components of behavior are considered, the nurse may label the client's behavior as abnormal. Also stereotypic beliefs may continue to be perpetuated, and the patient is not likely to receive the quality of care required.

Thus you must recognize the client as a total functioning individual with special needs that only can be met through providing comprehensive care, which takes into consideration the specific cultural aspects of the client's behavior as well as the physical and psychological aspects. Within the cultural context, you should modify intervention in response to particular ethnic patterns of behavior. Respond to those patterns that affect the client's state of illness, health-seeking behaviors, and responses to therapeutic modalities. With this information, you are better able to plan nursing interventions specific to an individual's needs.

When you intervene with a client from a cultural background different than your own, your knowledge of the major values, usual customs and norms, and preferred life-style practices is important, but remember that not all members of that culture will follow these same practices. Table 9-1 summarizes some beliefs, religious practices, and life-style implications of some religious cultures/subcultures. (The summary is not meant to be comprehensive.) The impact of these beliefs and practices upon the care needed during hospitalization or home care is also summarized as a part of the nurse's responsibility. The table is not meant to stereotype clients but rather should be used as a guide in working with them. In addition, you should always check with a client or family member about any individual beliefs, preferences, and needs. Then your modifications in nursing care will be appropriate.

Touching may be considered a part of nursing intervention, but touch must be used appropriately for it to convey caring or to be effective. Touching, or lack of touch, has cultural significance and symbolism and is a learned behavior. You know that in the dominant culture, a person learns to offer his hand on various interpersonal encounters. The firm, hearty handshake is symbolic of good character and a sign of strength. The mainstream culture also tolerates hugs and embraces among intimates and a pat on the shoulder as a gesture of camaraderie.

In most American Indian groups, the hand is offered in some interpersonal interactions, but the expectation in this touch situation is different. Rather than a firm handshake, there will be a light touch or grasp or even just a passing of hands. Some American Indians interpret vigorous handshaking as an aggressive action and are offended by a firm lengthy handshake.

Touching in Mexican culture can be symbolic of an "undoing" or prevention of harm ritual, especially with infants and small children, because of the concept of *mal ojo,* the evil eye. Some persons in the Mexican culture believe that *mal ojo* can unintentionally be "put on" a child by the admiring look from a stranger. The manifestation of *mal ojo* in a child is said to be seen as lethargy, not eating well, and crying excessively. The threat of *mal ojo* is not present if the admiring person touches the child while looking at him/her. You will often see Mexican children being patted on the face when adults talk to them; this touching is reassuring to the parents that *mal ojo* has not been "put on" the child.

All groups have rules, often unspoken, about who touches who, when, and where. Be mindful of the person's reaction to your touch during care so that you are not perceived as unnecessarily intrusive.

Everyone has a main culture and probably belongs to a subculture as well. At this point in time, mental health care providers are predominantly from the dominant culture of the United States, which is white and middle class. Thus there is a need for additional professional care providers representative of the various other cultural groups. This need has been emphasized in the American Nurses Association's efforts to encourage the recruitment of ethnic persons as well as men for the profession of nursing. This glaring deficit, at this

TABLE 9-1. Summary of Major Beliefs and Health Care Implications of Selected Religious Cultures/Subcultures

RELIGION	DEITY	BELIEF	WORSHIP PRACTICES	EFFECT OF RELIGION ON LIFE STYLE	FOOD PREFERENCE	NURSE'S RESPONSIBILITY RELATED TO CLIENT BELIEF/NEED
Buddhism Zen, sect of Buddhism Shintoism, Japan's state religion	Guatama, Buddha, and Kwannon, the Goddess of compassion.	Strive to reach Nirvana, divine state of release, ultimate reality, and perfect knowledge, in order to remove ignorance and maintain equilibrium in life. Reach Nirvana by eight rights: knowledge, intentions, speech, conduct, livelihood, effort, mindfulness, and concentration. Values of happiness: goodness, beauty, and profit. Zen: seek absolute truth in honesty and simple acts.	Meditation/books. Two godshelves in home: One has wooden tablet with name of the household's patron deity, symbolic form of goddess of rice, texts, and prized objects. The second is a Buddha shelf. Different Buddhist sects emphasize different values and rituals of worship. Believe in reincarnation, which is either immediate or after 49 days. Zen: Meditation and word puzzles. Shintoism: Worship of emperor, ancestor, or heroes.	Moral code of life comes from religion. Lying or killing is not condoned. Emphasize beauty and cleanliness. Discourage use of tobacco. Zen: Simple acts are emphasized. Shintoism: Intense loyalty to every aspect of nature; ancestral spirits are in nature.	Vegetarian. No intoxicants. Moderation in eating and and drinking.	Family help care for ill member and give emotional support. Religion discourages use of drugs; assess carefully for pain. Cleanliness important. Question about feelings regarding medical or surgical treatment on holy days. Prepare for death; help patient remain alert, resist confusion or distraction, and remain calm. Last rite chanting is often practiced at bedside soon after death. Contact the deceased's Buddhist priest or have the family make contact.
Christianity	All worship Jesus; God.	Christ's crucifixion, resurrection, and ascension to redeem mankind and rule with God.	Sunday is day of worship unless specified otherwise.	All, or most, will feel religion is important support and that it guides life style. Knowledge is gained from reading Bible.	All will wish to see spiritual advisor when ill and to read Bible or other religious literature and follow usual practices.	
Roman Catholic	Venerate Virgin Mary and Saints.	Jesus Christ established Church; appointed apostles. Authority of Church in the Scriptures, Pope, and Bishop. Believe in heaven, hell, purgatory, resurrection, and Second coming of Christ.	Mass and Holy Communion may be celebrated daily. Sacraments of Confession, Holy Communion, and Sacrament of Sick may be received more than once. Baptism, Confirmation, and Matrimony are sacraments received only once. Ritual and tradition are important in worship.	Infant baptism or adult baptism when join church. Oppose abortion.	Nothing special, except fasting or abstaining from meat on Ash Wednesday and Good Friday. Some Catholics may fast every Friday and other holy days.	Client finds comfort in having rosary, Bible, prayer book, crucifix, medals. Infant baptism mandatory, especially urgent if prognosis is poor. Baptism demanded if aborted fetus may not be clinically dead. For baptismal purposes, death a certainty only if obvious evidence of tissue necrosis. Tell priest if you baptize baby; done only once. Inquire about dietary preferences, and fasting. May want information on natural family planning. The Rite for Anointing of the Sick is mandatory. If the prognosis is poor, the patient or his family may request it. In sudden death, priest is called to anoint and administer Viaticum, if possible, or special prayers are said. Amputated limb may be buried in consecrated ground. No blanket mandate for this but may be required within a given diocese. Donation or transplantation of organs is approved providing the recipient's potential benefit is proportionate to the donor's potential harm.

TABLE 9-1. Continued

RELIGION	DEITY	BELIEF	WORSHIP PRACTICES	EFFECT OF RELIGION ON LIFE STYLE	FOOD PREFERENCE	NURSE'S RESPONSIBILITY RELATED TO CLIENT BELIEF/NEED
Orthodox						
Eastern (Turkey, Egypt, Syria, Cyprus, Bulgaria, Rumania, Albania, Poland, Czeckoslovakia.		Similar to Roman Catholic; no Pope.	Divine Liturgy, Eucharistic Service, in native language and possibly also in English.	Infant baptism by immersion, followed by Confirmation. Feel inspiration and insight directly from God.	Fasting each Wednesday, each Friday, and 40 days before Christmas and Easter. Avoid meat, dairy products, and olive oil.	Prayer book and icons important. Infant baptism if death imminent. Check consequences of fast days on health; fasting not necessary when ill. Blessing for the sick (unction) is not last rite but a form of healing by prayer. Last rites obligatory if death impending; cremation discouraged.
Greek				Infant baptism significant; to be done within 40 days after birth. Oppose abortion.	Fasting periods on Wednesday, Friday, and during Lent; avoid meat and dairy products.	Prayer book and icons important. Infant baptism if death imminent. Patient prepares by fasting for Holy Communion and Sacrament of Holy Unction. Fasting not mandatory during illness. Opposes euthanasia. Every reasonable effort should be made to preserve life until terminated by God. Cremation or autopsies that may cause dismemberment are discouraged. Last rites administered for the dying.
Russian				Baptism by priest only, on certain days.	Fasting on Wednesday, Friday, and during Lent. No meat or dairy products.	Prayer book and icons important. No baptism of infant. Check consequences of fasting on health. Cross necklace important; should be replaced immediately when patient returns from surgery. Do not shave male patients except in preparation for surgery. Patients do not believe in autopsies, embalming, or cremation. Traditionally, after death, arms crossed, fingers set in a cross. Clothing at death must be of natural fiber so that the body will change to ashes sooner.
Protestantism (Many denominations and sects)	Jesus Christ; God.	Bible ultimate authority. God has not given any one person or group sole authority to interpret His truths. Freedom of spiritual searching and reinterpretation. Finding God's will is ultimate goal. Some groups, including some American Indian, Appalachian, Black, and rural people, may combine culture and denominational beliefs and magic into their religion.	Read Bible for knowledge and spiritual guidance. Practices vary with denomination or sect.	Some denominations hold liberal precepts, so their belief affects life style less directly; others hold fundamental precepts and place constraints on life style—religion is part of daily living.		
Baptist		Oppose infant baptism; only believers are baptized by immersion.	Liturgically free; some groups very fundamental.	Some fundamentalist groups resist modern scientific treatment that might be related to "false teachings."	Some groups condemn coffee and tea. Most condemn alcoholic beverages. Some groups may fast on Sundays or other special days, especially in Black Baptist Churches.	No infant baptism. Client may be fatalistic: believes illness is punishment from God; passive about care. Inquire about effect of fasting if client is on special diet, a diabetic, or has disease dependent on dietary regulation.

	Beliefs	Organization / Liturgy	Social practices	Diet	Birth, death, and medical practices
Brethren (Grace) (Plymouth)		Liturgically free; fundamental.	Some are pacifists and conscientious objectors in wartime.	Most abstain from alcohol, tobacco, and illicit drugs.	No infant baptism. Anointing with oil for physical healing and spiritual uplift. No last rites.
Church of Christ, Scientist (Christian Scientist)	Deny existence of illness and pain. God is Divine Mind. Spirit is real and eternal; matter is unreal illusion.		Avoid most medical treatment unless family force it or if not fully practicing Christian Science. Avoid use of tobacco. Because of beliefs, do not seek physical examinations, immunizations (unless required by law), biopsies, psychotherapy, or hypnotism.	Avoid coffee and alcohol.	No infant baptism. If hospitalized or receiving medical treatment, guilt feelings may be intense. Be supportive. Allow practitioner or reader to visit freely as desired. Use nursing measures to alleviate pain. Patient may refuse blood transfusions as well as intravenous fluids and medication. No last rites or autopsy, unless sudden death.
Church of Christ	Church is body of Christ, with Christ as head.		Believe humans limited in understanding; Christ omniscient.	Avoid alcoholic beverages.	No infant baptism. Anointing with oil and laying on of hands for healing. No last rites.
Church of God		Identified by geographical headquarters; about 200 independent church groups in the U.S. use this name in their title.		Most avoid alcoholic beverages.	No infant baptism.
Church of Jesus Christ of Latter-Day Saints (Mormon)	Inspiration from Book of Mormon, which supplements Bible. Body is "temple of God." Believe dead can hear Gospel.	No official congregational leader, but a group called seventy and high priest are in authority.	Each Mormon is an official missionary. Marriage in temple seals relationship for eternity. Church attends to all needs of members, including education, recreation, and financial aid. Health and prevention highly valued; disease results from failure to obey laws of health and God. Faith keeps one well.	Eat in moderation; limit meat. Avoid coffee and tea. No alcoholic beverages. Avoids use of tobacco.	No infant baptism, but baptism of dead essential; living person serves as proxy. Laying on of hands for healing. White undergarment with special marks at navel and right knee is to remain on; considered a safeguard against danger.
Episcopalian		Liturgically formal.	Some believe in spiritual healing.	May fast from meat on Friday.	Infant baptism mandatory, but not for aborted fetus or stillbirth. Patient fasts in preparation for Holy Communion, which may be daily, thus check effects on disease. Rite for Anointing Sick (last rites) not mandatory.
Friends (Quakers)	God is in every person and is approached directly. Authority resides in self.	No minister, no religious symbols, no formal creed. Follow inner light to share inspiration.	Pacifist; conscientious objector in wartime; obeys inner light in daily living. Simplicity, honesty, physical and mental health, and harmonious living with family and others valued. Relates to all people as equals.	Moderation in eating. Most avoid alcoholic beverages and drugs.	No infant baptism. Health teaching important. Give explanations about medical technology used in care. Share information about condition as indicated.
Jehovah's Witnesses	Levitical Commandment given by God to Moses that no one in House of David should eat blood or he would be cut off from people; reference in Acts, *New Testament*, prohibits tasting of blood.	Liturgically free. Use of literature.	Pacifist; conscientious objector in wartime. Individual does not take oath or participate in national holidays or ceremonies.	Avoid food to which blood is added, e.g., certain sausages and lunch meats.	No infant baptism. Opposed to blood transfusion. (Hospital administrator or doctor may seek court order to be appointed guardian of child in times of emergency need for blood.) No last rites.

TABLE 9-1. Continued

RELIGION	DEITY	BELIEF	WORSHIP PRACTICES	EFFECT OF RELIGION ON LIFE STYLE	FOOD PREFERENCE	NURSE'S RESPONSIBILITY RELATED TO CLIENT BELIEF/NEED
Mennonite			No sacraments.	Deep concern for individual dignity and self-determination.	Most avoid alcoholic beverages.	No infant baptism. Shock therapy, psychotherapy, and hypnotism conflict with individual will and personality.
Nazarene			Liturgically free.	Avoid use of tobacco. Believe in divine healing.	Avoid alcohol.	No need to baptize infant. Stillborn is buried. Laying on of hands for healing. No last rites.
Pentecostal		Many different groups, which have specific beliefs.	Liturgically free.	Believe in divine healing through prayer.		No infant baptism. Prayer, anointing with oil, laying on of hands, speaking in tongues, shouting, and singing important for healing of patient.
Unitarian/ Universalist			No official sacrament.	Reason and practicality are emphasized. Individual responsibility important.		Infant baptism not necessary. Cremation preferred to burial. Check before calling clergy to visit.
Seventh-Day Adventists		Rely more on Old Testament law than do other Christian Churches. Following commandments is key to salvation. Believe in man's choice and God's sovereignty. Dead are asleep until return of Jesus Christ, when rewards and punishments will be given.	Spiritual literature important.	Body is temple of Holy Spirit and should be protected. Values health and healthy living. Religion strongly affects values, behavior, and life style. Following Commandments is important. Duty to prepare mankind for Second Coming of Christ. Avoid use of tobacco.	Vegetarian (no meat) or lacto-ovo-vegetarian (may eat milk and eggs but no meat). Pork and fish without fins and scales prohibited. Avoid coffee and tea. Avoid alcoholic beverages.	No infant baptism. Health measures, prevention, and health education important. Some believe in divine healing and anointing with oil. Avoid administering narcotics and stimulants. Use nursing measures for pain; medication last resort. Check on food preferences. Sabbath is Friday sundown until Saturday sundown for most groups. Client may refuse medical treatment and use of secular items, such as television, on Sabbath.
Hindu	Trinity: Brahma (Creator) Vishnu (Preserver) (God of love), and Shiva (Destroyer.)	Concept of Brahman, Divine Intelligence and Supreme Reality, part of all physical being. To unite real and inner self (atman) with Brahman is greatest desire. Desire freedom and touching the infinite. Reincarnation depends on knowledge, past deeds, past experience. Every birth a rebirth.	Read literature. Meditate by Shrine in home with pictures of incarnations and burning incense. Prayer for freedom is best. Prayer for bodily cure is low form of prayer.	Live in moderation. Death is accepted, a rebirth; the atman (basic self) remains the same. Yoga is the training course to reach God. Strive for self-discipline, self-control, cleanliness, contentment. Avoid injury, deceit, stealing. Religion pervades life style.	Vegetarian. No alcoholic beverages. Other restrictions conform to sect doctrine. Fasting is important part of religious practice. Yoga is important for person on special diet or with diabetes or other diseases regulated by food.	Medical care last resort; client considers help will come from own inner resources. Nurse should treat client with respect and convey sense of dignity. Reinforce need for medical care and explain care measures. Client may reject help; stoic. Assess carefully for pain. Provide privacy. Assist to maintain religious practices. Cleanliness and dietary preferences important. Certain prescribed rites are followed after death: The priest may tie a thread around the neck or wrist to signify blessing; the thread should not be removed. Immediately after death, the priest will pour water into the mouth of the corpse; the family will wash the body. They are particular about who touches their dead. Bodies are cremated. Loss of limb considered sign of wrongdoing in previous life.

Religion	Name of Supreme Being	Beliefs	Scriptures/Practices	Religious Practices	Dietary	Health/Death Practices
Islam	Allah; Mohammed is the prophet.	Direct relationship with Allah. Believe in heaven and hell and eternal soul. Necessary to live good life.	Use Quran (Koran), (scriptures), and the Hadith (traditions) for guidelines in devotional life, thinking, and social obligations. Pray five times daily, need water for ritual washing before prayer and a prayer rug. Face Mecca or east when praying. No worship of images.	Daily prayers and affirmation of Allah. Emphasize good life, responsibility to society. Ramadan is month of fasting; no eating from sunrise to sundown. Moderation in eating and drinking. Submission to Allah is important. Moderation in all activities.	Avoid pork and products with pork in them. No intoxicants.	Excused from religious practices when ill but may still want to pray to Allah and face Mecca. No spiritual advisor to call. Family visits are important. Cleanliness important. After 130 days, fetus treated as fully developed human. Fatalistic view about illness; resigned to death, but encourage prolonging life. Patient must confess sins and beg forgiveness before death, and family should be present. The family washes and prepares the body, folds hands, turns the body to face Mecca. Only relatives or friends may touch the body. Unless required by law, no postmortem or no body part should be removed.
Black Muslim (Nation of Islam)				Moderation in all activities.		No baptism. Carefully prescribed procedure for washing and shrouding dead and performing funeral rites. Cleanliness important.
Judaism	God	Orthodox—literal interpretation; Conservative in between; Reform—Old Testament is written by inspired men but can be interpreted. Belief about resurrection is individual. Believes soul lives on in memory of others, memorials, good works.	Use Torah, first five books of Bible, and its enlargement, and Talmud. Sabbath and morning prayer—use prayer book and phylacteries, leather strips with boxes containing scriptures. Holy days: Rosh Hashanah (new year); Yom Kippur (day of atonement); Passover (celebrates deliverance from Egyptian bondage).	Sabbath is from Friday sundown to Saturday sundown. Orthodox males wear yarmulka (skullcap) continuously. Value family, education, and sense of community. Value enjoyment of life now and share with God; no value to suffering. Emphasize social concern and each person contributes according to ability. Year of mourning after death, with intensity of mourning decreasing with time—3 days, 7 days, 30 days, and anniversary memorials.	Orthodox eat only kosher (ritually prepared) foods. Milk consumed before meat, or meat eaten six hours before milk consumed. Does not eat pig, horse, shrimp, lobster, crab, oyster, birds of prey if Orthodox; others may restrict diet. Special utensils and dishes for Orthodox. Fasts on Yom Kippur and Tisha Bab; may fast other times but excluded if ill.	No infant baptism. Circumcision of baby on eighth day if Orthodox. Preventive measures, avoiding illness, are important. Concerned about future consequences of illness and medications. Preoccupied with health; will convey that pain is present and want relief. Nursing measures for pain important. On Sabbath, Orthodox Jews may refuse freshly cooked foods, medicine, treatment, surgery, and use of radio or television. Orthodox male may not shave. Nurse should avoid loss of yarmulka, prayer books, or phylacteries. Nurse must arrange for kosher or preferred food; food may be served on paper plates. Check consequences of fasting on person's condition. Visits from family members important. If patient without family, notify synagogue so other people may visit. Family or friends to be with dying person. No artificial means to prolong life if patient vegetative. Confession by dying person like a rite of passage. Human remains ritually washed following death by members of the Ritual Burial Society. Burial should take place as soon as possible. Cremation not permitted. All Orthodox Jews and some Conservatives opposed to autopsy. Organs or other tissues available to the family for burial. Parts of the body are not donated to medical science or removed, even during autopsy. Donation or transplantation of organs requires rabbinical consultation. A fetus is to be buried, not discarded.

time, creates the necessity for increased knowledge of cultural diversities in order to adequately meet the needs of your clients, whoever they are and wherever they may be.

Some nurse educators believe, and rightly so, that you would not really have to be concerned about cultural diversities in nursing interventions if it were possible to be truly empathic with clients. Of course, this requires a large measure of self-awareness, self-understanding, and maturity, as well as a healthy level of self-esteem. You will find that in the attainment of these attributes, you never reach the ultimate level. Rather, growth toward empathy at the highest level is a lifelong process of observation, assessment, analysis, intervention, and evaluation. You will find, however, that in each succeeding situation with a client from a different culture—in which you have successfully intervened—you will have gained a valuable growth-enhancing experience.

Any intervention provided to the client should be relevant to the client's particular needs. For example, long-term psychotherapy/supportive services may be appropriate for one client, whereas quick crisis intervention may be appropriate for another. Different intervention needs may be present even though both clients are from the same cultural background and may present the same pathology.

The use of intervention by someone who has common life experiences with the client would be ideal, and if this were possible, it would be a positive move toward getting the client the appropriate care. However, this should not be construed to mean that only a client and therapist with the same cultural background would be appropriate. Rather, you must always consider the unique needs of every individual, and all interventions should be tailored to the life experiences of the client regardless of his/her background. Remember that many modes of intervention are aimed primarily at the treatment of the white middle class and therefore may not be appropriate for your client.

The goal of intervention, above all else, is to decrease the negative effects of emotional illness and help patients achieve improved social roles regardless of the cultural background.

The interventions described throughout this text are applicable to people from any background. However, be mindful of the need to modify your approach for specific cultural, subcultural, or ethnic values, norms, or customs. Ability to apply principles but modify specific measures with the client is the mark of individualized, humanistic nursing care.

Evaluation

The final phase of the nursing process is evaluation of the interaction between the nurse and the client. It is at this time that you look at the client's behavioral changes that have resulted from your planned interventions. You should rethink your interaction with the client to identify changes in the client's behavior. If there are changes, what factors in your approach brought about these changes? If there are no changes, what factors influenced or inhibited planned-for changes from occurring? For example, your evaluation could consider some of the following points:

1. Has the client kept appointments for services? If not, why not? What could you have done differently? Could agency policies or procedures be changed to give better care?
2. What is your feeling when you are with the client? How does the client feel about self? Do you perceive the client's feelings toward you? Does your interaction indicate that you perceive the client's feelings accurately and with empathy?
3. What is the client's response to your verbal and nonverbal behavior? What is his/her response to other health care workers? Is the response to others different? In what way?
4. Has the client been able to change in the direction of increased self-esteem, improved coping with problems, and improved communication with and acceptance by others?

In rethinking the nursing process, pinpoint areas where problems have been solved as well as areas where problems remain unsolved. It is not always possible to solve a problem, but an area of unsolved problems does not necessarily mean that you have been unsuccessful or that your assessment and interventions were inadequate. However, reassessment may be necessary, and other approaches may need to be considered. This is a part of the evaluation process since evaluation often leads to discovery of some ineffective approaches and serves as a guide for further assessment and interventions that may prove to be more effective in the future.

REFERENCES

1. Ailinger, Rita, *Incorporating Cultural Dimensions into the Baccalaureate Nursing Curriculum*, pp. 69–73. National League for Nursing Publication No. 15-1622. New York: National League for Nursing, 1977.

2. Baker, Frank, "From Community Mental Health Service to Human Service Ideology," *American Journal of Public Health*, 64, no. 6 (1974), 576–81.

3. Barry, Herbert, "Cultural Variations in the Development of Mental Illness," in R. B. Edgerton and S. C. Plog, eds., *Changing Perspectives in Mental Illness*. New York: Holt, Rinehart and Winston, 1964.

4. Branch, Marie, "Models for Introducing Cultural Diversity in Nursing Curricula," *Journal of Nursing Education*, 15, no. 2 (1976), 7–13.

5. Branch, Marie, and Phyllis Paxton, *Providing Safe Nursing Care for Ethnic People of Color*. New York: Appleton-Century-Crofts, 1976.

6. Brink, Pamela, ed., *Transcultural Nursing*. Englewood Cliffs, N.J.: Prentice-Hall, Inc., 1976.

7. Bullough, Bonnie, and Vern Bullough, *Poverty, Ethnic Identity and Health Care*. New York: Appleton-Century-Crofts, 1972.

8. Busch, M. T., and K. S. Babich, "Cultural Variation," in D. C. Longo and R. A. Williams, eds., *Clinical Practice in Psychosocial Nursing: Assessment and Intervention*. New York: Appleton-Century-Crofts, 1978.

9. Bush, Mary, Jean Ullom, and Oliver Osborne, "The Meaning of Mental Health: A Report of Two Ethnoscientific Studies," *Nursing Research*, 24, no. 2 (1975), 130–38.

10. Byerly, Elizabeth, *Cultural Components in the Baccalaureate Nursing Curriculum, Philosophy, Goals and Processes*, pp. 74–84. National League for Nursing Publication No. 15-1622. New York: National League for Nursing, 1977.

11. Caplan, Gerald, *The Theory and Practice of Mental Health Consultation*. New York: Basic Books, Inc., 1970.

12. Casavantes, Edward, "Pride and Prejudice: A Mexican-American Dilemma," *Chicanos: Social and Psychological Perspectives*, 2nd ed., p. 914. St. Louis: The C. V. Mosby Company, 1976.

13. Cole, Robert, "Eskimos, Chicanos, Indians," *Children of Crisis*, vol. 4, pp. 231–392. Boston: Little, Brown & Company, 1977.

14. *Culture of Poverty Revisited*. A critique by the Mental Health Committee against Racism. New York: Mental Health Committee against Racism, n.d.

15. Damon, Albert, "Race, Ethnic Group, and Disease," *Social Biology*, 16, no. 2 (1969), 69–79.

16. Delgado, Melvin, "Therapy Latino Style: Implications for Psychiatric Care," *Perspectives in Psychiatric Care*, 13, no. 3 (1979), 107–13.

17. Di Angi, Paulette, "Barriers to the Black and White Therapeutic Relationship," *Perspectives in Psychiatric Care*, 14, no. 4 (1976), 180–83.

18. ____, "Erikson's Theory of Personality Development as Applied to the Black Child," *Perspectives in Psychiatric Care*, 14, no. 4 (1976), 184–85.

19. Dohrenwend, Bruce, and Barbara Dohrenwend, *Social Status and Psychological Disorder*, pp. 24, 131. New York: John Wiley & Sons, Inc., 1969.

20. Evans, Frances Monet Carter, *The Role of the Nurse in Community Mental Health*. New York: Macmillan Publishing Co., Inc., 1968.

21. Fabrega, Horacio, and Carole Wallace, "Value Identification and Psychiatric Disability: An Analysis Involving Americans of Mexican Descent," in C. A. Hernandez, M. J. Haug, and N. N. Wagner, eds., *Chicanos: Social and Psychological Perspectives*, 2nd ed., pp. 253–61. St. Louis: The C. V. Mosby Company, 1976.

22. Feldman, Saul, and Gerald Thielbar, *Lifestyles: Diversity in American Society*, 2nd ed. Boston: Little, Brown & Company, 1975.

23. Finney, Joseph, ed., *Culture Change, Mental Health, and Poverty*. New York: Simon & Schuster, 1970.

24. Flaskerud, Jacquelyn, "Perceptions of Problematic Behaviors by Appalachians, Mental Health Professionals, and Lay Non-Appalachians," *Nursing Research*, 29, no. 3 (1980), 140–49.

25. Freeman, Howard, Sol Levine, and S. Reeder, *Handbook of Medical Sociology*, 2nd ed. Englewood Cliffs, N.J.: Prentice-Hall, Inc., 1972.

26. Freeman, Howard, and Clarence Sherwood, *Social Research and Social Policy*. Englewood Cliffs, N.J.: Prentice-Hall, Inc., 1972.

27. Fuentes, José Angel, "The Need for Effective and Comprehensive Planning for Migrant Workers," *American Journal of Public Health*, 64, no. 1 (1974), 2–9.

28. Gaitz, Charles, and Judith Scott, "Mental Health of Mexican-Americans: Do Ethnic Factors Make a Difference?" *Geriatrics* (November 1974), pp. 103–10.

29. Goldman, Elaine, ed., *Community Mental Health Nursing*. New York: Appleton-Century-Crofts, 1972.

30. Gonzales, Hector, *Health Care Needs of the Mexican-*

American, pp. 21–28. National League for Nursing Publication No. 14-1625. New York: National League for Nursing, 1976.

31. Gresser, Linda, "Healing Hands: A New Mexico Herbalist, *The Herbalist,* 5, nos. 4–5 (1980), 7.

32. Henry, Beverly, and Elizabeth DiGiacomo-Geffers, "The Hospitalized Rich and Famous," *American Journal of Nursing,* 80, no. 8 (1980), 1426–29.

33. Hollingshead, August, and Frederick Redlich, *Social Class and Mental Illness.* New York: John Wiley & Sons, Inc., 1958.

34. Hooker, Wayne D., "Mental Health Care in the Lower Rio Grande Valley," *The Missouri Nurse,* 48, no. 4 (1979), 12–15.

35. Hutchinson, Sarah, "The American Indian Senior Citizens View of Women," *Bulletin of American Association of Social Psychiatry,* 1, no. 3 (1980), 13–15.

36. Jaco, Gartly, "Mental Health of Spanish-Americans in Texas," in M. K. Opler ed., *Culture and Mental Health,* p. 467. New York: Macmillan Publishing Co., Inc., 1959.

37. Kagan, Spencer, and Philip Ender, "Maternal Response to Success and Failure of Anglo-American, Mexican-American, and Mexican Children," *Child Development,* 46 (1975), 452–58.

38. Karno, Marvin, and Robert Edgerton, "Perception of Mental Illness in a Mexican-American Community," *Archives of General Psychiatry,* 20 (1969), 233–38.

39. Karno, Marvin, and Armando Morales, "A Community Mental Health Service for Mexican-Americans in Metropolis," in C. A. Hernandez, M. J. Haug, and N. N. Wagner, eds., *Chicanos: Social and Psychological Perspectives,* 2nd ed., pp. 237–41. St. Louis: The C. V. Mosby Company, 1976.

40. Kiev, Ari, "Transcultural Psychiatry; Research Problems and Perspectives," in R. B. Edgerton and S. C. Plog, eds., *Changing Perspectives in Mental Illness.* New York: Holt, Rinehart and Winston, 1964.

41. Koshi, Peter, "Cultural Diversity in the Nursing Curriculum," *Journal of Nursing Education,* 15, no. 2 (1976), 14–21.

42. LaFargue, Jane, "A Survival Strategy: Kinship Networks," *American Journal of Nursing,* 80, no. 9 (1980), 1636–40.

43. Leininger, Madeleine, *Nursing and Anthropology: Two Worlds to Blend.* New York: John Wiley & Sons, Inc., 1970.

44. ——, *Contemporary Issues in Mental Health Nursing.* Boston: Little, Brown & Company, 1973.

45. ——, *Cultural and Transcultural Nursing: Meaning and Significance for Nurses,* pp. 85–103. National League for Nursing Publication No. 15-1622. New York: National League for Nursing, 1977.

46. ——, "Cultural Diversities of Health and Nursing Care," *Nursing Clinics of North America,* 12, no. 1 (1977), 5–18.

47. ——, *Transcultural Nursing.* New York: John Wiley & Sons, Inc., 1978.

48. Lewis, Edith, and Mary Browning, eds., *The Nurse in Community Mental Health.* New York: The American Journal of Nursing Company, 1972.

49. Longo, Dianne, and Reg Arthur Williams, *Clinical Practice in Psychosocial Nursing: Assessment and Intervention.* New York: Appleton-Century-Crofts, 1978.

50. Madsen, William, "Mexican-Americans and Anglo-Americans: A Comparative Study of Mental Illness in Texas," in R. B. Edgerton and S. C. Plog, eds., *Changing Perspectives in Mental Illness.* New York: Holt, Rinehart and Winston, 1964.

51. Martinez, Richard Argijo, *Hispanic Culture and Health Care.* St. Louis: The C. V. Mosby Company, 1978.

52. McKenzie, Joan, and Noel Chrisman, "Health Herbs, Gods, and Magic: Folk Health Beliefs among Filipino-Americans," *Nursing Outlook,* 25, no. 5 (1977), 326–39.

53. Mead, Margaret, *Culture and Commitment: A Study of the Generation Gap,* p. 1. New York: Natural History Press/Doubleday & Co., Inc., 1970.

54. Mechanic, David, *Mental Health and Social Policy.* Englewood Cliffs, N.J.: Prentice-Hall, Inc., 1969.

55. Montiel, Miguel, "The Chicano Family: A Review of Research," *Social Work* (March 1973), pp. 22–31.

56. Moseley, Jewell, and Virgil Clift, *Cultural Characteristics of Minority Groups of Color,* pp. 18–34. National League for Nursing Publication No. 15-1622. New York: National League for Nursing, 1977.

57. Murphy, Jane, and Alexander Leighton, *Approaches to Cross-Cultural Psychiatry.* New York: Atherton Press, 1967.

58. Murray, Ruth, and Judith Zentner, *Concepts for Health Promotion,* 2nd ed., pp. 382–436. Englewood Cliffs, N.J.: Prentice-Hall, Inc., 1979.

59. Newman, William M., *American Pluralism—A Study of Minority Groups and Social Theory.* New York: Harper & Row, Publishers, Inc., 1973.

60. Opler, Marvin, *Cultural and Social Psychiatry.* New York: Atherton Press, 1967.

61. Ozbum, William, and M. Nimkoff, *Sociology,* 2nd ed. Boston: Houghton Mifflin Company, 1950.

62. Ramey, Craig, and Frances Campbell, "Parental Attitudes and Poverty," *The Journal of Genetic Psychology,* 128 (1978), 3-6.

63. Richards, Hilda, "The Role of the Nurse in the Therapy of the Lower Socioeconomic Psychiatric Client," *Perspectives in Psychiatric Care,* 5, no. 2 (1967), 82-91.

64. Scheff, Thomas, ed., *Mental Illness and Social Process.* New York: Harper & Row, Publishers, Inc., 1967.

65. Serrano, Alberto, and Guadalupe Gibson, "Mental Health Services to the Mexican-American Community in San Antonio, Texas," *American Journal of Public Health,* 63, no. 12 (1973), 1057.

66. Sills, Grayce, "Social Systems and Mental Health Services," in Elaine Goldman, ed. *Community Mental Health Nursing,* p. 205. New York: Appleton-Century-Crofts, 1972.

67. "Social Factors in Mental Disorders in Texas," *Social Problems,* 4 (1957), 322.

68. Spector, Rachel, "Health and Illness among Ethnic People of Color," *Nurse Educator,* 2, no. 3 (1977), 10-13.

69. Spratlen, Lois, "Introducing Ethnic-Cultural Factors in Nursing: Some Mental Health Implications," *Journal of Nursing Education,* 15, no. 2 (1976), 23-29.

70. Sullivan, Harry Stack, *The Interpersonal Theory of Psychiatry,* pp. 32-33. New York: W. W. Norton & Co., Inc., 1953.

71. Thomas, Alexander, and Samuel Sillen, *Racism and Psychiatry.* New York: Brunner/Mazel, Inc., 1972.

72. Thuy, Vuong, *Getting to Know the Vietnamese and Their Culture.* New York: Frederick Ungar Publishing Co., Inc., 1976.

73. Torrey, E. F., "The Irrelevancy of Traditional Mental Health Services for Urban Mexican-Americans." Paper presented at the American Orthopsychiatry Association, San Francisco, March 1970.

74. Trotter, Robert II, and Juan Antonio Chavira, *The Gift of Healing,* p. 3. Edinburgh, Texas: Pan American University, 1975.

75. Van den Berghe, Pierre, *Intergroup Relations: Sociological Perspectives.* New York: Basic Books, Inc., 1972.

76. Weaver, Jerry, *National Health Policies and the Underserved: Ethnic Minorities, Women, and the Elderly.* St. Louis: The C. V. Mosby Company, 1976.

77. Wechsler, Henry, Leonard Solomon, and Bernard Kramer, *Social Psychology and Mental Health.* New York: Holt, Rinehart and Winston, 1970.

78. White, Ernestine, "Giving Health Care to Minority Patients," *Nursing Clinics of North America,* 12, no. 1 (1977), 27-40.

79. Yamamato, J. J., C. Quinton, and N. Pally, "Cultural Problems in Psychiatric Therapy," in C. A. Hernandez, M. J. Haug, and N. N. Wagner, eds. *Chicanos: Social and Psychological Perspectives,* 2nd ed., pp. 217-22. St. Louis: The C. V. Mosby Company, 1976.

10

The Family as a Client

Study of this chapter will assist you to:

1. Define a family, both in an objective and subjective sense, and describe commonly occurring family constellations.

2. Describe Family Systems Theory and the characteristics of a family system.

3. Assess family characteristics, functions, patterns, strengths, and weaknesses.

4. Formulate nursing diagnoses based on assessment of the family.

5. Determine goals of treatment with the family.

6. Implement nursing intervention measures pertinent to nursing diagnoses and goals and the family's needs.

7. Increase the effectiveness of your interactions with families.

8. Evaluate the contribution of your care to family mental health.

This chapter contributed by Joyce Brockhaus, R.N., Ph.D. and Gail Stringer, R.N., M.S.N. Portions of this chapter also contributed by Ruth Murray, R.N., M.S.N.

Throughout generations and in all cultures, the family has been the primary agent for human development. The family is the universal institution for childrearing and for the transfer of cultural and social norms and values. All of us are products of our family, the time we live in, and our community. Sense of self, awareness of reality, and methods by which we have or have not become self-actualized and fulfilled are traceable to our earliest years. Personal methods of coping with stresses, openness to others, and capacity to adapt to change are conditioned within the family unit (59). What we bring from our family of origin is taken with us as we form new family units and is in turn passed on to our offspring, who will carry the learnings with them into the next generation.

Developmental tasks that the family is expected to perform in all cultures and that directly or indirectly contribute to emotional health of the person are to (1, 12, 26, 79):

1. Provide for physical safety and economic needs of its members and obtain enough goods, services, and resources to survive.

2. Help members to develop emotionally and intellectually as well as to develop a personal and family identity.

3. Provide social togetherness simultaneously with division of labor or patterning of sexual roles.

4. Reproduce and socialize the child(ren), inculcating values and appropriate behavior, providing adult role models, and fostering motivation, morale, and a positive self-concept and self-esteem in the child(ren).

5. Help the members cope with the demands of and become integrated into society and the organizations in which they must function.

6. Utilize social organizations for special needs.

7. Create satisfaction and a mentally healthy environment for the family's well-being.

8. Maintain order, authority, and decision making, with an acknowledged head of the family representing society to family members and the family unit to society.

9. Release family members into the larger society — school, church, organizations, work, politics.

10. Develop a philosophical, moral, or spiritual framework in keeping with cultural values and personal needs.

THE NURSE'S ROLE WITH THE FAMILY

For the past three decades there has been an ever-increasing shift in health focus and practice away from treating the individual in isolation to treating the person within the family context: thus the family becomes the client. Contact with families is not a new phenomenon within nursing. Nurses have always been involved to some extent with family members. Often the contact occurs with families that are experiencing change, crisis, or difficult situations. At other times the family has been experiencing an ongoing or long-term dysfunction.

This chapter acknowledges the family's importance in terms of the client's health and well-being and focuses on the counseling role of the nurse. Other chapters include the nurse's supportive roles as he/she works with the family in a program of care and teaching.

As in other psychiatric treatment modalities, therapeutic interventions with families rely on the use of yourself as your own best tool. Thus, you will need to maintain your emotional and physical health, openness, and empathy. To work effectively with families, you must also equip yourself with a theoretical frame of reference for the assessment and care of family systems. The extent to which you offer therapeutic aid to a family or refer the family to appropriate resources is dependent on the extent to which you have established a knowledge base and developed your clinical skills.

Do not underestimate your abilities. Many of the skills needed to do mental health work with families are not foreign to you as a nurse. For example, communication skills have already been acquired. You are a skilled observer, and much of family phenomena is observable and describable. Voice inflections, postural presentation, and double or assumed messages are readily seen and heard when you become sensitive to them (5).

Also do not underestimate your own influence and impact on families. Society and families cast the nurse in various roles, such as mother surrogate, teacher, counselor, technician, or manager. The nurse is expected to improve family dysfunction. Families expect advocacy on their behalf within the health care system, as well as preventive, supportive, and therapeutic intervention. In many situations the nurse is the only professional contact the family has with whom they feel comfortable in discussing problems.

The focus of this chapter is not to teach you how to become a family therapist. Rather, the focus is on providing you with a knowledge base to understand and assess family characteristics, functions, strengths, and weaknesses—in order to make your interactions with families effective.

DEFINITIONS OF FAMILY

In building upon your understanding and ability to assess and assist families, you need some idea as to your personal definition of a family. What is your idea of a family? Do you believe that only those who are blood-related belong to a family? Is a family composed only of parents and children? Do you believe that all families are loving, nurturing, and communicative?

The *family is defined as two or more persons who reside together, who share economic resources, who are "related by birth, marriage, or adoption, and who have commitments to each other over time* (45). The authors define *family* as *a grouping of interdependent persons who are bonded together by some form or order into a recognizable unit.*

No one definition of the word *family* fits all families. Acknowledge what you believe a family to be. However, do not thrust your beliefs on the families you encounter; objectively focus on *their* family constellations, values, beliefs, and customs and assess *their* closeness, communication, authority, problem-solving skills, and autonomy.

Although families differ in terms of composition of members, some commonly occurring family constellations have been identified. The *nuclear family* is two-generational, time-limited, and usually designates a married couple and their children by birth or adoption who cooperatively interact for the purpose of attaining common goals (50). The *nuclear dyad* consists of a husband and wife living together who are either childless or whose children are not living at home. The *extended family* encom-

passes the nuclear family plus other relatives, whether by birth, adoption, or marriage. The **alternative family** *may consist of adults of a single generation or a combination of adults and children who choose to live together without social sanction of marriage.* The alternative family could be a communal arrangement or composed of roommates who are homosexual or heterosexual. The **single parent** **family** *consists of one adult who, due to death, divorce, separation, or abandonment, is alone with children.* This could also be a single adult who has adopted a child. The **reconstituted or blended** **family** *occurs by remarriage of one or both spouses to create a situation where parents, step-parents, children, and stepchildren live together.*

SYSTEMS CONCEPT OF FAMILIES

Family Systems Theory

The family can be conceptualized as a behavioral system with unique properties. A close interrelationship exists between the psychosocial functioning of the family as a group and the emotional adaptation of its individual members. The link between disorders of family living and disorders of family members can best be understood in the context of Systems Theory. Systems Theory, as it relates to the family unit, will better help you assess and intervene with the family. Refer to Chapter 2 for further information on Systems Theory, and see other references at the end of this chapter.

Systems Theory is an orientation that recognizes people by defining who they are within the context of their relationships with family, friends, and the society in which they live. Third Force theorists teach us that thoughts, emotions, and actions take their meanings not only from the intention of the person to whom they belong but also from the meaning that is given to them by people and institutions. This broad view creates a unique outlook on mental illness and its treatment. Thus the person who is labeled as mentally or emotionally ill is not considered totally responsible for a problem or for trying to solve it. The source of the problem lies not only within the person but also within the interface between the individual and the social environment. The feelings of distress are experienced by all who live together. Therefore, the approach to a solution includes not only treating the individual identified as emotionally disturbed but also treating other people who share in the problem.

Because the family is the social unit that is most closely experienced as a part of a person's identity, and because the family tends to have the most influence on behavior, any assessment of problems and their treatment should include the family, if at all possible. For example, a child experiencing behavioral problems in school, such as hurting other children or being disruptive in the classroom, may actually be reacting to marital conflicts between his/her parents. Thus helping the parents to more effectively cope with their conflicts may clear up the child's problem in school.

Just as the child is viewed in the context of the family, rather than being treated as a product in isolation, the family itself is viewed in the context of the environment in which it is functioning. The family interacts with other systems, such as the school, church, work world, and community agencies; and these other systems have an impact on the family's daily life. This approach to emotional disturbance not only provides more reliable information about the source of the disturbance but also offers the full resources of the individual, family, and other institutions in attacking the problem.

A *family system is defined as a grouping of interdependent persons who are bonded together by some form or order into a recognizable unit.* The family system may itself be a *subsystem, a unit of a larger system.* The family system may also have subsystems within it and may be related to a number of other systems. For example, a nuclear family is a subsystem of an extended family and also a subsystem of a community. The subsystems of the nuclear family are the individual members. Each of these subsystems exchanges matter or material goods, psychic energy, and information back and forth between social institutions or systems; and this provides the opportunity for change to occur both inside and outside the subsystem and system.

Characteristics of a Family System

Interdependent Units

The basic interdependent units of a family system are the individual members. Change by or within one person, which is an inevitable part of life, affects the entire family. For example, if one family member becomes physically or emotionally ill, the entire family will be changed in some way. Change in family membership as a result of a birth, divorce, death, hospitalization, leaving home for college, or marriage will result in a degree of disequilibrium within the system. Since all changes bring about disruption and disequilibrium in the system, the dynamic characteristics of the system must be utilized to permit the family system to return to equilibrium, as matter, energy, and information are exchanged (48, 69).

Environment

The family system has an environment. *Internal environment refers to the social and physical world within the family boundaries,* the quality of which is reflected by factors such as: (a) the marital relationship, (b) location of power, (c) closeness of members, (d) communication patterns, (e) problem-solving abilities, (f) free expression of feelings, (g) ability to deal with loss, (h) family values, and (i) degree of intimacy and autonomy of members. The *external environment refers to the social and physical world outside of the family unit,* such as church, neighbors, extended family, school, friends, work, health care system, political systems, and recreation (48, 69).

Boundary

The *boundary is an imaginary line or area of demarcation that keeps the family system separate from its external environment.* Energy, in the form of information, material goods, and feeling states, is exchanged between family members and the external environment. The *openness* or *closedness* of the specific family system is determined by the nature of the boundary and the degree of information/energy the family allows to cross its boundaries from other systems. Each member or grouping, within the family, is also open to various degrees of influence from other members of the family. The

information entering the family system provides it with data about the environment and about its own functioning in the environment. The family can accept or reject the incoming information. If energy/information is accepted, it can be utilized to formulate and respond to environmental conditions, to restore energy, and to repair breakdowns or disequilibrium in the family that occurred as a result of illness, stress, or crisis situations. Energy/information entering the family system can also be stored to prevent it from becoming depleted of resources. This reserved energy will be readily available to the system when it is needed (48, 69).

The amount of energy/information that enters and leaves a system must be balanced within certain limits in order to maintain a steady state of functioning (homeostasis) or proper adaptation of the system. A system can become dysfunctional by being either too open or too closed. If a family were totally open, it would probably lose its identity as a system separate from other systems to which family members belong. The family members could suffer from alienation, rootlessness, and a lack of belonging. At the other extreme, where the boundaries are rigid and closed, family members become enmeshed, fixed, and unable to move out, grow, or change.

Communication

Communication is the verbal and nonverbal interaction between family members that is required in order to send and receive information and energy. A number of factors contribute to a family's pattern of communication: (a) the extent to which the family encourages a clear exchange of words, (b) how much each member takes responsibility for expressing individual feelings, thoughts, and actions in a constructive way, and (c) the pattern of members acknowledging each other's verbal and nonverbal messages, talking spontaneously, and allowing family members to speak for themselves. Family members are bonded together by the form of communication that flows between them.

Roles

Roles are the patterns of wants, goals, beliefs, feelings, attitudes, and actions by which family members place expectations on themselves and others. Roles are assigned and acquired; they specify what individuals must do, and they promote family functioning (67). Each family member has a part to play. Roles are often dependent on cultural or social-class norms. Roles are dynamic and should change and adapt as growth and development, crisis, or health needs dictate.

By recognizing the role(s) that a person is playing, you can gain increased understanding of what is occurring between the members of a family system. No role is carried out in isolation. Roles are reciprocal; for each role there is a complementary role. For example, to fulfill the role of mother there must be someone willing to accept the role of child. If both persons were relating as mothers, tension and confusion would result. There are specific behaviors for each person in the reciprocal arrangement; each knows how to behave and what behaviors to expect from another. The family's (i.e., the system's) equilibrium or balance depends on how well roles reciprocate each other (67).

Role-taking is influenced by various factors. Some roles are influenced by characteristics or attributes of individual family members. Temperament, height, weight, gender, birth order, age, and health status are some of the attributes that affect role. For example, a female can fill any of the following roles: sister, daughter, wife, mother, or girlfriend. Other roles are factors of performance. Roles such as breadwinner, homemaker, cook, handyman, or gardener are dependent on the person's ability to perform certain tasks. Emotional roles such as leader, nurturer, scapegoat, caretaker, jester, arbitrator, or martyr are adopted at certain times as a means of adjusting to the demands of family life, an extended family crisis such as congenital and long-term illnesses, or long-term family conflict (53). Although the function of emotional roles is to reduce conflict between members and temporarily promote adaptation, consistent use may impair adaptation. For example, one member, often the oldest child, may assume the role of family caretaker, supporting other members and arbitrating disputes. As this member is an achiever who succeeds in most endeavors, he/she also represents the family's self-worth, which is expressed in the attitude, "We can't be doing too bad; look what we were able to produce." The family supporter appears strong and capable and has the unrealistic feeling, "I can't fail; I can't be weak." This person is functioning under pressure to be perfect but may have feelings of self-doubt and fear.

Family Organization

Family organization requires structuring of functions and goals. Families are not static but dynamic, endlessly adaptable, and continually evolving, both in structure and function. The function of any family is somewhat dependent on the individual needs and wants of its members. A family is a place where needs get met, and if they are not, pain is felt and confusion exists. American society directs its families to be self-perpetuating and to be the primary system for the transfer of social values and norms.

The two primary goals of the family are: (1) encouragement and nurturance of each individual's personality, and (2) production of autonomous, healthy children (48). Marital partners are expected to be supportive and protective of each other and to have a sense of meaning and emotional closeness within their relationship so that the goal of personality development can be accomplished. The hurts and conflicts that people acquire early in life are brought with them into marriage and into the new family. The resulting perceptions, patterns of behavior, and limitations may be accepted as characteristics of the person or may be corrected in the sense that past traumas and hurts are constructively resolved. The quest to fulfill one's potential is encouraged in families when parents are able to continue their personality development. However, in families that do not have supportive relationships, the limitations become disabilities, and realization of the first goal (encouragement and nurturance of each individual) is not attainable. The second goal, production of autonomous, healthy children, involves encouraging and allowing each child to develop and experience his/her individuality and eventually leave the family in order to love another. The family encourages the children toward separateness, individuality, and autonomy by enabling the child to have his/her own ideas, feelings, and life direction, to sense both similarities and differences from others, and to be able to initiate activities (48).

Patterns of relationships within the family determine the degree to which the family will accomplish the two primary goals or tasks. Some families fail in accomplishing these goals. Psychiatric disturbances, incomplete maturation of children, and ultimately, disintegration of the family system result. Utilization of adaptive mechanisms, on the other hand, will permit the family to maintain an internal equilibrium so that it can fulfill its goals and deal with stress and crisis. Adaptive mechanisms are dependent on: (a) communication skills within the family, (b) individual contributions of members to family welfare, (c) amount of care, respect and love within the family, (d) the kinds of stresses encountered, (e) the family's response patterns to stressors in the internal and external environment, and (f) the kinds of opportunities and support or resources available to the family (1).

Four Levels of Functioning

Family organization and levels of functioning are conceptualized in Fig. 10-1. Four levels of functioning are identified in increasingly abstract levels: (I) family functions and activities, (II) intrafamilial interactions, (III) interpersonal relationships, and (IV) the family system (71).

Level I deals with the daily affairs and functions, the tangible, pragmatic activities that are either observable or fairly easily identified and that family members are comfortable in discussing. Four categories of family functioning are in Level I:

1. Activities of daily living. The provision of physical safety and economic resources, and the ability of family members to obtain goods and services, such as food, clothing, shelter, and assistance for health and nonhealth crises, to ensure the physical survival of its members.
2. Ability of the family to help each other develop emotionally and intellectually and to attain a personal as well as a family identity.
3. Reproduction, socialization, and release of

children, which is closely aligned with transmission of cultural and subcultural roles and values.
4. Integration between the family, its culture, and society, and the ability to utilize external environmental resources for support and feedback.

Areas of functioning and how the family has managed to meet, over a period of time, the functions identified in Level I, are part of family process. The levels of functioning become increasingly abstract and are often less readily identified or discussed by family members. However, the importance of these levels cannot be underestimated.

Level II deals with communication or interactions among family members: what is said, how it is said, patterns of communication that have evolved over time, quality of communication skills, and how information is communicated among its members and to persons outside the family.

Level III moves from interactions into relationships that are occurring within the family constellation. Dimensions of closeness and power and the amount of empathy, support, and commitment existing between family members are important. How the family functions in decision making and problem solving is included.

Level IV addresses the concepts of family system and how the family functions as a system. This is the most abstract area of family functioning and encompasses the concepts of wholeness, openness/closedness, homeostasis, and rules (71).

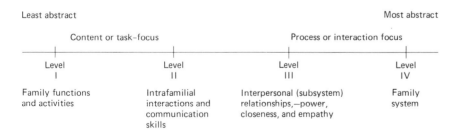

FIGURE 10-1   Conceptual scheme of family organization and functional levels of analysis. [Data from R. Schneider (71).]

Diagrams of Family Relationships

The concepts of Family Systems Theory can be compared with the functioning of a mobile (69). Each part of the mobile, like each family member, is separate and yet in connection with the other. Change or movement in one part will result in change and movement in all other parts. The internal environment of the mobile is determined by how the parts are spaced and related to each other. There are unlimited variations in terms of the number, shape, and weight of the parts. Several levels can be added to create and add dimension, and various groupings or subsystems can be arranged. The key, however, is in how each part relates to the other—in the placement, closeness, and distribution of weight. Each part has its role and must interact in a certain way to maintain equilibrium of the mobile. There are also boundaries in terms of how free each part can be in its movement and still allow for balance of the whole. Furthermore, the most perfectly designed mobile is unable to function without influence from the external environment. Movement of air is essential. It is then a matter of how much air movement: Too much air movement (too open) would create chaos; whereas inability to respond to air movement (too closed) would result in static appearance. In either case, the beauty of the mobile would be lost. Movement and balance are the goals in creating a mobile for purpose of decoration, sound, or reflection of light. Utilization of a mobile to describe basic aspects of a family system is helpful in working with families, especially to communicate the significance of the interrelationships between members and how these dynamics are important to understand if change is to occur.

In Figure 10-2, each object of the mobile is an individual family member with specific attributes and relationships with other members. A change or movement in one member of the family system will result in change and movement in all the other members. The entire system is affected, and adaptation is required to return the system to equilibrium.

In Figure 10-3, subsystems within the family can be identified: marital, sibling, parent-child, mother-daughter, and father-son. Other subsystems could include relatives of each spouse. Energy or information is exchanged within and between the internal or external environments. The boundaries can be imagined as encompassing the family structure. The structure or organization of the system can be seen by moving the physical arrangement of the individuals in relation to one another.

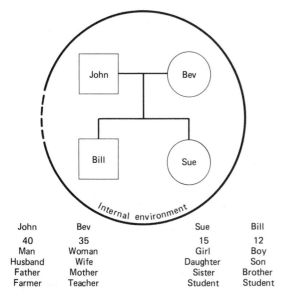

John	Bev		Sue	Bill
40	35		15	12
Man	Woman		Girl	Boy
Husband	Wife		Daughter	Son
Father	Mother		Sister	Brother
Farmer	Teacher		Student	Student

FIGURE 10-2   Units and attributes of the nuclear family.

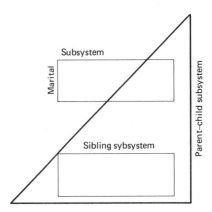

FIGURE 10-3   Subsystems of the family. Note: Other subsystems, such as grandparent-parent, grandparent–grandchild, or aunt-mother, may exist in the extended family. The family system may consist only of siblings, of homosexuals, or of a communal group of friends, all with subsystems within the total group.

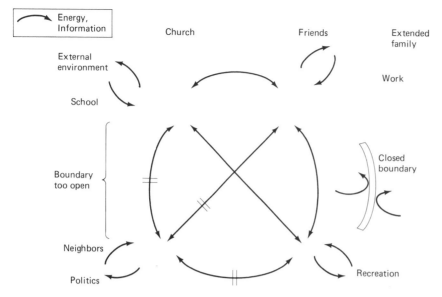

FIGURE 10-4 Interaction of family system with other systems.

Figure 10-4 shows systems outside of the family with which the family system interacts. Family boundaries may be too open or too closed, which would affect the flow of energy or information, as shown in the diagram. The quality of communication between individual members, for example, stressful or supportive, can be shown on the communication lines connecting individuals in the family.

The Family Systems Theory has been presented in this chapter as the primary theoretical model for understanding families. Other theoretical views of family therapy include structural family therapy (6, 55), communication therapy (36, 81), and psychodynamic family therapy (19, 47). Various authors give information on family dynamics that is useful in understanding behavior in a family. The treatment approach that will be most effective with a family is primarily a function of the particular family and your theoretical orientation. Typically, you will utilize techniques of various models as they seem appropriate to the specific situation. Most important, however, is that you blend the philosophies, techniques, and styles from a variety of theorists into an approach that is comfortable and genuine for you.

FAMILY ASSESSMENT

A great deal of variance exists in terms of how much and in what way information is gathered and assessment is done by professionals who work with families. The extent and manner of your assessment will depend on the development of your skills, the extent to which you are working with families, and the needs of your particular work setting.

Some who work with families choose to deal only with the present problem of the observable current behavior and communication patterns. The assumption is that history repeats itself, and disruptive family patterns will surface repeatedly. In this case, little or no background information is obtained, and the focus is primarily on what is *now* happening within the family unit.

Alternative assessment methods are based on gathering information about the family's internal environment, the family's genogram or history, and the family's relationship to its external environment. These three areas will be explored and guidelines for assessment formats are suggested.

Regardless of the theory base that you use, assessment involves collection of the following specific information about the family:

1. Relationships that individual members of the family have with one another.
2. Relationships that the family has with the environment.
3. Sources of support in the family's environment.
4. Strengths and limitations of the family system.

This information is then utilized in developing client-care goals, a plan of care, and appropriate interventions.

From a humanistic framework, you will use the family's perspective and perceptions in your assessment rather than assigning behaviors or labels to the family members. You will not necessarily see all of the behaviors in any one family in the following definitions of family types. The family may also describe some particular feelings or behavior that is not included in any of the four types. Realize, too, that although you or any health professional may assess Type C as dominated or conflictual or Type D as chaotic, the family members may not perceive their unit or their behavior in that way. Let the family first describe and label, and with that information you can then move to the professional language and categories that you must use as you work with other professionals. But always keep the family's perceptions in mind, especially as you intervene in the ways described later in this chapter.

Assessing the Internal Environment of the Family: Four Types of Families

The family's internal environment is described in terms of competency levels in accomplishing the two major goals of the family: (1) encouragement and nurturance of each member's personality, and (2) production of autonomous, healthy children.

The following dimensions can be used to assess the quality of the family's internal environment and thus the family's degree of competence: (a) the parental marriage, (b) power, (c) closeness, (d) communication, (e) problem solving, (f) feelings, (g) dealing with loss/change, (h) family values, and (i) intimacy and autonomy. Families can be grouped into four major types based on the information obtained in these nine areas (48).

Type A

Type A family pattern shows a relationship between the marital dyad that is close, personal, and warm. The spouses feel self-esteem and express love and admiration for one another; they experience intimacy with respect for each other. Listening to one another is an important and enjoyable component of their communication system. Personal thoughts and feelings are shared. There are no secrets. Difficulties in the relationship are discussed openly, then negotiated and resolved either by compromise or through acceptance of the differences that exist between them. They discuss mutual and individual goals. Their individual goals complement one another; they share interests and activities. Both spouses spontaneously answer questions about themselves and their marriage, conveying respect and love for self and each other, and both view the sexual relationship as satisfactory.

The couple's relationship with their parents is spontaneous, enjoyable, and free from major conflicts. Mutual friends enhance their relationship, and their children are enjoyed and unite the couple. The leadership is shared between parents, changing with the nature of the interaction.

As with any family, the quality of the marital relationship determines the emotional atmosphere and competency of the family as a system. In the Type A family pattern, there is a strong sense of closeness with distinct boundaries among the family members. The power structure or pecking order in the family is easy to determine. There is a strong parental coalition. The family is efficient in negotiation and problem solving. The expression of individual thoughts and feelings is clear. The members regularly are able to voice responsibility for individual actions. There is little evidence of invasions; members do not speak for one another or make mind-reading statements. The members are usually open and receptive to the statements and direct expression of feelings of other family members. The family's interaction is usually warm, affectionate, humorous, and optimistic. There is little unresolved conflict. There is sensitivity to and understanding of each other's feelings within this family. This family is fun to belong to.

However, no family is perfect, and neither is this family. The family members will experience arguments, tears, disagreements, frustration, stress, and crisis. But the interaction pattern is such that the love for one another enables them to work things through at the time of the situation and to feel loved and stronger as a result.

Type B

Type B family patterns shows a marital relationship that is polite but without an intense warmth or affection expressed between spouses. There is a lack of strong feelings of intimacy, but the partners love and care about each other. There is some evidence of conflict between spouses, although family functioning is not impaired. Listening is perceived to be important in the communication pattern between the spouses. Most personal thoughts and feelings are shared; the spouses have difficulty talking about negative feelings or difficulties but make an effort to do so. Both spouses talk about some mutual and complementary goals and share a moderate amount of interests and activities. The sexual relationship is satisfactory for one member of the couple but not necessarily for the other. Both can enjoy intercourse at times, but sexual satisfaction is variable. There is occasional fighting and arguing, but resolution is achieved with some discussion and negotiation. Both feel arguing lets off steam and leads to making up. There is an absence of self-depreciation; questions about themselves and their marriage are answered positively but with reservation. They are confident in most situations.

Their relationship with their parents is usually pleasant, but specific problems are present. Mutual friends usually enhance their relationship, and children are enjoyed most of the time. There is a tendency toward dominance and submission, but most of the interaction is through respectful negotiation. Although there is an empathic responsiveness to one another, obvious conflicts and resistance are also present. The major problems in this family tend to center around developmental stages and tasks. Crisis may immobilize the family, but it has the ability to adapt to change, enjoy the present, and plan for the future.

Type C

Type C family pattern shows two subtypes of family patterns: dominated and conflicted. The *dominated family pattern exists when the parental relationship is clearly one of dominance and submission.* The dominant parent exerts control and

authority over the other spouse and children. The submissive spouse may form coalitions with the children, parents, or someone outside the family in order to gain a sense of intimacy that is definitely lacking in the couple's relationship. The *conflicted family pattern exists when both spouses desire to exert control and authority: neither person is willing to accept a submissive role.* Tension, manipulation, and sarcasm are common in this pattern.

The relationship between the marital dyad in the Type C family pattern (both dominated and conflicted patterns) is impersonal. The spouses express disfavor, mixed feelings, or uncertainty about one another. They may also express dislike, hate, or fear. They are isolated and alienated from each other. Talking occurs, but neither listens well to the other. Personal thoughts and feelings are rarely expressed because of the fear of consequences and feelings of increased vulnerability to attack. Expression of feelings often leads to arguments and fights, which are frequent but only occasionally resolved. Both partners feel that fighting and arguments are harmful to the relationship. The couple does not talk about mutual or individual goals that complement each other. They spend a minimal amount of time sharing common interests; however, they do participate in activities together even though this may be stressful. A sexual relationship exists that is usually free from specific sexual problems, but both partners feel it is not close or happy in feeling tone. They do not discuss their sexual relationship with one another, and both wish the partner would pay more attention to this component of their relationship. Both spouses are ambiguous about liking self, each other, and the marriage. There is a moderate lack of self-confidence in themselves and their marriage. There are more negative than positive opinions expressed. One member is typically more negative than the other about self and the marriage.

One set of parents, either his or hers, usually interferes and produces conflict or avoidance. Some friends produce conflict, as do the children. Overinvolvement of one spouse with the children is common; there is a weak parental coalition. Isolation and distancing behaviors are evident with family members. Members sometimes voice responsibility for individual actions, but tactics also include blaming others or speaking in the third person or plural. Although some feelings are expressed, there is masking or obvious restriction in the expression of most feelings. Interactions between members are overtly hostile. There is definite conflict in the family with moderate impairment of family functioning. The family is unable to support and promote development of its members and often appears defensive, fearful, and unable to change.

The family needs much assistance before members are able to acknowledge problems realistically. Yet this family may stay together because there is some caring about each other and because unconscious as well as tangible needs are being met, even in an atmosphere of submission or argument. The members are likely to rally to each other's aid at least temporarily when a severe situation is encountered.

Type D

Type D family pattern shows a relationship between the marital dyad that lacks any sense of intimacy and is chaotic. A strong pattern of disruption, upheaval, alienation, and isolation exists between spouses. Both partners state that listening is not important. Listening is an effort; they only pretend to listen. They do not share personal thoughts or talk about feelings or their relationship. They talk about no mutual or individual goals that complement each other. They do not share interests or activities, *or* they interact as one unit in a symbiotic manner in which no individuation is permitted. Physical fights, screaming, throwing things, holding grudges, refusal to talk, and walking out are typical in the chaotic family. The members of this dyad do not like themselves as individuals or as a couple. The relationship is marked by self-depreciation and complete lack of self-confidence as a couple. The individuals are ineffectual in marriage, in relations with others, and in everyday activities. Sexual intercourse is negligible. Signs of specific sexual incompatibility, such as frigidity, vaginismus, and deviations, are common.

The couple's parents interfere, and both partners attempt to avoid them. They are not close to either set of parents. Conflicts about friends are common. The children are perceived to be burdens. Arguments about the children lead to increased distance between the couple.

The family is basically leaderless. No one has enough power to structure the interaction; parent-child coalitions frequently occur. Amorphous, vague, and indistinct boundaries exist among members. The family is extremely inefficient in negotiation and problem solving; seldom does anyone clearly or directly disclose feelings and thoughts. Members rarely voice responsibility for individual actions. There are many attempts of members to speak for one another. Members are unreceptive to statements of other family members. The feeling tone of this family's interaction is cynical, hopeless, and pessimistic. They live from day to day without any orientation to the future. The family may be barely able to meet needs for security and physical survival. There are difficulties in securing adequate wages or housing, in budgeting money, or in maintaining adequate nutrition, clothing, and other basic needs. There is severe conflict in the family with severe impairment of the family's functioning.

You may wonder why these people continue to live together. Sometimes they don't. Sometimes they seek help and improve their happiness a little. Often they do not seek help but continue to live together out of habit, or they are fearful of change and unconscious needs are being met. The individual may feel too helpless to leave or has no resources (financial or people) to assist in establishing a new life style. Also if the family of origin lived this way, members may assume that this is what family life is supposed to be like. Sometimes members stay together out of a sense of obligation, although there is no real affection or happiness. Some individuals will claim they remain because he/she knows that the family members will at least try to give assistance when essential, and there is no guarantee that outsiders will.

Refer to Table 10-1 for a more comprehensive comparison of the various family patterns. Be aware when you assess the family for the behaviors described in Table 10-1 that the larger or more extended the family, the more complex and interdependent is the behavior—and your assessment.

Questions Specific to Assessing the Internal Environment of the Family

The questions in Table 10-2 can be asked to elicit information from the family in the specific areas described: parental marriage, power, closeness, communication, problem solving, feelings, dealing with loss and change, family values, intimacy and autonomy. We are *not* suggesting that you ask all of these questions, nor that you ask them in the

TABLE 10-1. Types of Family Based on Competence Levels
and Quality of Family Interactions

TYPE A

Outcome

Optimal development in each member.
Production of autonomous children.

I. *Parental Marriage*

Spouses are good friends; personalities not fused.
Individual characteristics, interests, and activities encouraged.
Differences valued; resentment and competition are absent.
Feelings freely expressed; high level of empathy.
Conflicts/problems dealt with effectively.
Tension from unresolved problems short-lived.
Sexual relations satisfying.
No powerful triangles or alliances outside parental marriage.

II. *Power*

Shared by parents; easy leadership style; not authoritarian.
Clear differentiation between roles of parents and children.

III. *Closeness/Boundaries*

High levels of individuality and closeness.

IV. *Communication*

Clear; members listen to each other.
Individual responsibility for own thoughts and feelings.
Differences respected and viewed as normal.
Individual thoughts, feelings, opinions, and suggestions are encouraged and respected.
Warmth, humor, and concern for others.
No blaming or scapegoating.

V. *Problem Solving*

Identification of problem.
Consensus; compromise; negotiation.
Alternatives and solutions by family unit.

VI. *Feelings*

Expression of *all* feelings encouraged.
Empathic response by members to each other's expression of feelings.
Nonjudgmental attitude; warmth, humor, and concern.

VII. *Dealing with Loss/Change*

Members express openly feelings of sadness and loss.
Flexibility of system allows for coping with loss and change.

VIII. *Family Values*

People are mostly good; to err is human.
Human behavior is complex and needs to be examined and reexamined periodically.
Change is normal and healthy.
Well-established personal philosophy and standards of right and wrong.

IX. *Intimacy and autonomy*

Intimacy and autonomy are possible and are encouraged.

TABLE 10-1. Continued

TYPE B

Outcome

Some growth in parents.
Pain in parental relationship due to failure to achieve intimate level of communication.
Production of autonomous children.

I. *Parental Marriage*

Emotional needs of neither spouse fully met.
Unhappiness, disappointment; dissatisfaction; anger; sadness are felt at times.
Typically depressed and demanding wife; detached isolated husband.
Both blame each other for distressed relationship.
Both fucus on meeting needs of children.
Problems of relationship typically assigned to wife; she may become the "patient."
Wife starved for affection, not sexual relations.
Sexual relations are somewhat mechanical.
Coalitions (△) may develop.

II. *Power*

One-parent dominance.

III. *Closeness/Boundaries*

High level of individuality and separateness without accompanying levels of closeness.

IV. *Communication*

Like Type A family; all members communicate thoughts and ideas clearly.
Individual responsibility for own thoughts and feelings.

V. *Problem Solving*

Like Type A family; dominant parent more apt to be problem solver.
Less negotiation than with Type A family.

VI. *Feelings*

Less open expression of feelings; feelings masked to prevent parental conflict.
Less spontaneous expression; sense of inhibition.
Occasional expression of empathy.

VII. *Dealing with Loss/Change*

Family copes effectively with loss and change.

VIII. *Family Values*

Values similar to Type A family but not as integrated into system.

IX. *Intimacy and Autonomy*

Environment not as conducive to development of intimacy.

TYPE C

Outcome

A. *Dominated family pattern:* Disturbance in development of members and production of autonomous children.

B. *Conflicted family pattern:* Same as in dominated family pattern.

TABLE 10-1. Continued

TYPE C

I. *Parental Marriage*

  A. *Dominance-submission pattern*

    Powerful control and authority by one parent in marital dyad.

    Submissive parent permits pattern to develop and continue.

    Coalitions (△) between submissive parent and others.

  B. *Conflicted family pattern*

    Each parent struggles openly to control the other.

    Neither parent accepts submissive role.

    Constant warfare, struggle, and competition.

    Relationship based on conflict.

II. *Power*

  A. *Dominance-submission pattern*

    One parent is dominant; power extended in all areas.

    Rigid rules prevail.

  B. *Conflicted family pattern*

    Parents unable to share power.

    No stable set of rules about power, authority, and responsibility.

III. *Closeness/Boundaries*

  A. *Dominance-submission pattern*

    Focus of all relationships becomes power rather than closeness.

    Disclosure and closeness are too risky.

  B. *Conflicted family pattern*

    Closeness is too risky—provides ammunition for spouse to use in an attack.

    Coalitions (△) are common.

IV. *Communication*

  A. *Dominance-submission pattern*

    Influenced by dominant parent.

    Avoidance of responsibility for thoughts, feelings, actions.

    Blaming; scapegoating.

    Protect self from dominant spouse/parent.

    Lack of spontaneity.

    Insensitivity to others' needs.

  B. *Conflicted family pattern*

    Power is most important; confict is normal.

    Cautiousness, distance, and blaming are typical.

    Avoidance of responsibility for thoughts, feelings, actions.

    All members listen and acknowledge what others say; this provides more ammunition for attacks.

V. *Problem Solving*

  A. *Dominance-submission pattern*

    Little negotiation, consensus, or compromise.

    Dominant parent is authoritarian decision maker.

TABLE 10-1. Continued

TYPE C

B. *Conflicted family pattern*
Marked by disagreements, lack of negotiation.
Attack-counterattack pattern between parents.

VI. *Feelings*

A. *Dominance-submission pattern*
Disapproval of expressions of anger, hurt, sadness.
Constant undercurrent of resentment of dominant parent—not expressed openly.
Feelings of affection, joy, and happiness are stifled.

B. *Conflicted family pattern*
Free expression of angry feelings.
Expressions of affection, sadness, and tenderness are masked to decrease one's
    vulnerability.

VII. *Dealing with Loss/Change*

A. *Dominance-submission pattern*
Inflexibility and rigidness of system make dealing with loss and change difficult.

B. *Conflicted family pattern*
High levels of anger reduce ability to deal with loss and change.

VIII. *Family Values*

A. *Dominance-submission pattern*
Authoritarian style; expression of feelings is dangerous.
Dominant parent makes and enforces rules; rules are not to be broken.
Mistakes are not tolerated.

B. *Conflicted family pattern*
Intense competition.
Anything is justified to achieve victory.

IX. *Intimacy and Autonomy*

A. *Dominance-submission pattern*
Environment not conducive to development of intimacy or autonomy.

B. *Conflicted family pattern*
Same as dominance-submission pattern.

TYPE D

Outcome
Failure of development in members.
Failure of the production of autonomous children.

I. *Parental Marriage*
Disorganization in all areas; severely distressed marital patterns.
Fused marriage or complete sense of togetherness between spouses.
Burned-out marriage with long-standing emotional divorce.

TABLE 10-1. Continued

TYPE D

Immature parents; unable to assume adult roles.

Child abuse and neglect.

Coalitions (△) common.

II. *Power*

Chaos, distortion and confusion of roles in family.

Insufficient power within family to provide structure and organization.

Emotionally ill child may have more influence than either parent.

Children may take over tasks and roles of nonfunctioning parents.

III. *Closeness/Boundaries*

Family clings together like a glob of protoplasm.

IV. *Communication*

Flow of ideas, thoughts, feelings, and meanings of such are obscure and difficult to follow.

Inability to hear others.

V. *Problem Solving*

Problems are disregarded as if not to exist.

VI. *Feelings*

Feelings expressed indirectly through despair, hopelessness, or cyncism.

Feelings of failure; depression; feelings often denied.

VII. *Dealing with Loss/Change*

Losses are often completely denied.

Insecurity of family prevents change.

Change, even maturational change, is difficult to cope with.

Defensiveness and distortion used to keep others from getting near enough to cause change.

Adolescent treated as if preschooler; family not capable of providing emotional support necessary to deal with change and loss.

VIII. *Family Values*

Individuals are expected to remain enmeshed in family system indefinitely.

Individuality, autonomy, and change are not valued.

Distrust of outsiders.

IX. *Intimacy and Autonomy*

Intimacy should not be confused with enmeshment of family members with each other.

Autonomy not possible.

Hostile and resistant to offers of help.

Unable to use community resources and services; alienation from the community.

TABLE 10-2. Questions to Assess Internal Environment of Family

PARENTAL MARRIAGE

1. How did you meet your present husband/wife?
2. Do you like each other? How close do you feel to each other?
3. How long did you date before you began to discuss marriage?
4. What qualities about this person made you want to marry him/her?
5. What qualities about this person make you want to stay married?
6. How has marriage changed you? What is the best thing you've gotten out of marriage? Worst thing?
7. What do you especially like about your husband/wife? Not like?
8. What would you like to change about your husband/wife? How have you tried? Did it work?
9. Have you been married before?
   (If indicated: I'm wondering about how it was with your other marriage. Could you tell me about your previous marriage(s)? Dates? Children? When and why did this marriage end? What did you learn from this experience?)
10. What do you and your spouse agree/disagree about?
11. When do you and your spouse spend time together? Doing what?
12. Would you prefer to spend more time, less time, or about the same amount of time together? More time alone? What would you do?
13. How do you and your husband/wife negotiate?
14. In your relationship, do you listen to what your spouse wishes to talk about? Is talking an important part of your relationship? Do you find yourself listening easily to what the other person is saying, or is it an effort? Do you sometimes only pretend to listen?
15. Are there some things about yourself that you would not want to tell your spouse or anyone else?
16. Do you talk about feelings, even if they are negative feelings? Can you talk about your personal relationship if there are difficulties?
17. What would make you consider divorcing your husband/wife?
18. How might your spouse make your marriage better/worse? What is your fear? Fantasy?
19. What problems do you have handling money?
20. What kinds of things do you like to do? Not like to do?
21. How would you describe your current relationship with your parents (over the past month)? Are you close? Do you avoid them? Is the relationship spontaneous? Do they interfere? Is your relationship enjoyable?
22. Do members of your extended family live nearby?
23. People talk about the feeling of closeness with words, such as warmth or coldness, personal or impersonal, caring or uncaring, affection, or other terms. How much and what type of closeness do you experience?
24. Hugging, kissing, sexual intercourse, and other displays of physical affection are an important part of all couples' relationships. Over the past month, how satisfactory has your sexual relationship been?
25. Could your partner pay more attention to you? Do you discuss your sexual pref-

TABLE 10-2. Continued

PARENTAL MARRIAGE

ference? Is the frequency of intercourse satisfactory? Are there specific problems? Frigidity? Impotence?

POWER

1. Who is the boss? Does everyone always agree with the boss?
2. Do any family members avoid making decisions?
3. What happens to the maverick in the family?
4. What is expected of each member of the family by him/herself and by others?
5. How satisifed are members with the arrangement?
6. Can you tell me the roles of different family members? For example: Who is the boss in the family? Who is the peacemaker? What roles and jobs do you and others perform in your family?
7. Is the behavior of family members consistent with their roles?
8. Do all family members agree on the roles assigned to them? Tell me about any disagreements.

CLOSENESS

1. Who are the members of your family? List from oldest to youngest.
2. Do your family members share common goals?
3. Does your family work together cooperatively, or does each person go his/her own way?
4. What do your family members enjoy doing together?
5. How are they related to one another? (blood ties or friendship)
6. How often do they see one another?
7. What are the dependency-independency patterns in your family system? Who is dependent or independent of whom? (e.g., financial/emotional)
8. What is your family's pattern of separateness or togetherness? Are you close or distant?
9. Do difficulties bring the family together or push it apart?
10. What are the boundaries of experience in your family? For example, do you travel a lot? How often has your family moved? How often do you touch one another?

COMMUNICATION

1. Is the communication system open?
2. Are all family members included in the communication system?
3. Do family members understand through communication what other family members are thinking, feeling, and doing?

TABLE 10-2. Continued

COMMUNICATION

4. What are the communication patterns in your family? Who talks to whom about what? How frequently? What types of feedback occur?
5. What topics are not openly discussed? What topics are most difficult?
6. What problems are discussed most in your family?
7. Do your family members seem to be able to decipher one another's hidden messages?
8. What are the patterns of nonverbal behavior that occur in your family?
9. Does double-binding communication occur in which you get opposite messages about what you are, can do, or are not to do?
10. Does your family focus on you when there is conflict or tension going on?

PROBLEM SOLVING

1. How do family members express their differences of opinion?
2. If I had seen the last disagreement, what would it have looked like? How do you usually stop? How would it have sounded?
3. Everyone who lives together has disagreements. What precipitates disagreements?
4. What kind of discipline is used with the children in your home?
5. How does your family system handle conflicts or crisis?
6. Are there ever times when the members of your family seem to work against one another? Tell me about them.
7. How does the family go about solving problems? Is it an individual or group process? Who are the decision makers? Do you consider the problem solving process to be effective? If so, why? If not, why?
8. Do you discuss the differences in your personal relationship? Do you compromise? Negotiate? Fight verbally or physically? Do you refuse to discuss differences? Avoid differences?

FEELINGS

1. What kinds of feelings are pleasurable for you? How does this come about? Examples.
2. What kinds of feelings are uncomfortable for you? How does this come about? Examples.
3. How do family members show affection toward each other?
4. What happens when someone does not agree with the boss of the family?
5. What kinds of things do you laugh about?
6. How does your spouse deal with upsetting situations? Can you give me an example?

DEALING WITH LOSS/CHANGE

1. Have you ever lost someone close to you? Tell me about the experience.

TABLE 10-2. Continued

DEALING WITH LOSS/CHANGE

---

2. What have been the major crises or changes in your life? How did you react to them?

3. How open is your family to new ideas and people?

4. How does your family react to illness or the threat of illness of a family member?

5. What changes have there been in your family within the past five years?

6. How does your family cope with crises? Changes? Moves? Deaths?

7. Who does your household jobs when you cannot do them?

8. How does your family function when one family member is out of the home—i.e., who fills in when someone is in the hospital, on a trip, etc.?

9. How have your roles changed since you have been married? In your family of origin? With close friends? As a community member?

FAMILY VALUES

---

1. What goals and accomplishments would you expect your child to achieve? What would happen if he/she was unable to achieve these goals or your expectations?

2. What gratifications or rewards do you seek from parenthood?

3. What things could you absolutely not tolerate in a child?

4. How do you reward yourself?

5. What have been the biggest events in your life?

6. What do you like about each person in your home? What don't you like?

7. Does your family think you act your age and behave as a male or female should? If not, what do they say?

8. Are there family goals that all the members of your family pursue—e.g., a college education for all members?

9. What is the role of religion in your family?

10. What strengths do you see in yourself? Your family?

11. Tell me about your family's central concern or theme, e.g., success.

12. How compatible are members of your family in terms of shared beliefs (religious, political, etc.); mutual goals (children, house, etc.); shared interests (friends, reading, etc.); and shared activities (sports, church, etc.)?

INTIMACY AND AUTONOMY

---

1. Do your family members support each other in individual goals?

2. How do your family members show affection to persons outside of the family?

3. Do you think things are done to you? Do you feel you have control over your life, or that others control you and your life?

4. How are you affected by what others say about you? Feel about you? Do to you?

5. What are some of the risks you have taken in life?

TABLE 10-2.   Continued

INTIMACY AND AUTONOMY

6. How do you spend your money? Earn it? Save it?
7. What kinds of things have you seen as a challenge in your life?
8. Are you allowed to pursue individual goals even though they might not be in agreement with family goals? Tell me about it.
9. Who do you go to for help with decisions?
10. Who do you cry with?
11. Who do you turn to when you are afraid?
12. Who do you spend time with? Who do you have fun with?
13. What is your opinion of yourself? How confident do you feel about yourself?
14. How would you describe the current relationships between the parents and children in your family?
15. How would you describe your current relationships with friends?

format presented. The questions are simply presented as a guide to assist you in developing your own style of interviewing and talking with families. If the family is extended or nontraditional, the questions will have to be modified in accordance with the situation.

Assessing the Family in Time

We have looked at the family as it is immersed in its present internal environment and as it interacts with the various members in the present life space. However, the family not only exists in space, it has also developed through time. Thus the family history will help you to understand the current life of the individual and the family since the main source of each person's identity is formed in the saga of his/her family.

The starting point of this approach is an assumption that all people are deeply immersed in their family of origin and past history. Family history affects peoples' perception of who they are, how they think and communicate, and how they see themselves and others. It influences what they choose to do and be, whom they choose to be with and to love and marry, and how they choose to structure their new family.

The Genogram

A genogram is a useful way of gathering and organizing a family history or of obtaining information about an extended or reconstituted family. (See Figure 10-6.) A *genogram is a family tree or a map of three or more generations of a family that records genealogical relationships, major family events, occupations, losses, family migrations and dispersals, identifications and role assignments, and information about alignments and communication patterns* (14, 19, 32). The skeleton of the genogram tends to follow the conventions of genetic and genealogical charts. The following symbols are used in a genogram.

Male   Female   Unknown sex

The triangle is used when a person says, "I think there were seven children in my grandfather's family, but I have no idea whether they were males or females." Or "My mother lost a full-term child five years before I was born, but I don't know what sex it was."

A marital pair is indicated by

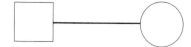

and it is useful to add the marriage date

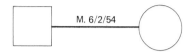

Offspring are shown in Figure 10-5.

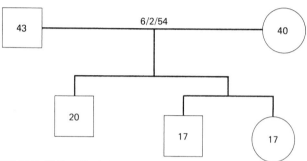

FIGURE 10-5   Marital pair and offspring.

The offspring are generally lined up according to age, starting with the oldest on the left. The above family has an older son followed by a set of twins.

A divorce is generally portrayed by a dotted line, and again it is useful to include dates.

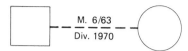

A family member no longer living is generally shown by the symbol,

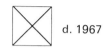

Thus a complex, but not untypical, reconstituted family may be drawn as shown in Figure 10-6. It is useful to draw a dotted line around the family members who compose the household. Incidentally, such a family chart enables the nurse to quickly grasp "who's who" in complicated reconstituted families.

With these basic building blocks expanded horizontally to depict the contemporary generation of siblings and cousins and vertically to chart the generations through time, it is possible to chart any family, given sufficient paper, patience, and information. As you chart the relationship structure of the family, it is also important to fill this out with the rich and varied data that portray the saga of the particular family.

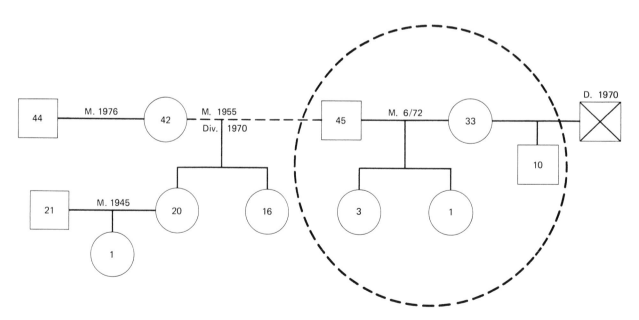

FIGURE 10-6.   Genogram of a reconstituted family.

The genogram is helpful in the following ways:

1. Given names, both first and middle, will identify family members, and will indicate naming patterns and surface identification.
2. Dates of birth and death will identify when members joined the family, and will indicate longevity and family losses.
3. Birth dates will also indicate the ages of family members when important historical and cultural events occurred, and will identify each individual's place in the family.
4. Place of birth and current place of residence will show movement of the family through space. Such information charts the family's patterns of dispersal and the major immigrations, and brings attention to periods of loss, change, or upheaval. This information may also indicate that generations of a family have stayed within a fairly small geographical radius. Picturing the family's movement through space may communicate a good deal about the family boundaries and norms concerning mobility. Is this a family that "holds on" or "lets go"? Locating family members in space begins to tap the extent to which the family continues to be intimately connected with extended family members. Is the extended family available and interested?
5. Occupations of family members will tell about interests and talents, successes and failures, and the varied socioeconomic levels that are found in most families. Occupational patterns may also point to intrafamily identifications, and often will portray family life prescriptions and expectations.
6. Facts about family members' health and causes of death will provide an overall family health history and also may say a good deal about the way a family views health, illness, and handicaps.

The most important and valuable thing about constructing the genogram is that it is an orderly way of obtaining a family history and organizing that history so that you and the family can look at it together. Drawing the genogram makes sure that the right questions are asked and that primary family patterns, myths, losses, illnesses and other important issues are discussed. This approach provides a nurse and family a visual basis for identifica- of problems, alternatives, and possible solutions.

The list of questions in Table 10-3 can help to assess family history and add data to the genogram. You probably will not ask all of these questions, but any of them are pertinent. Listen to the family members as they talk to you and among themselves, for they are likely to answer some of these questions without your asking.

TABLE 10-3.   Questions to Assess Family History

FAMILY OF ORIGIN AND YOUNG YEARS

1. When you think of your mother, what three words come to mind?
2. When you think of your father, what three words come to mind?
3. Are you more like your mother or father? In what ways?
4. What did your parents do? (occupation)
5. How would you describe the family you grew up with? (parents, brothers, sisters, and others) Ages? Your position in the family?
6. Who are you closest to in your family of origin?
7. What three words best describe your parents' marriage?
8. What was the best thing for you about being: oldest, middle, only, youngest? Worst thing?
9. What did you learn about marriage from your parents? Do you still believe it?
10. In what religion were you raised? How do your feelings about religion affect your life now?
11. How did your mother and father let you know you did something right? Wrong?

TABLE 10-3. Continued

FAMILY OF ORIGIN AND YOUNG YEARS

12. What decisions have you made about their discipline approach?
13. How do you get along with the people in your family of origin now? With the people of your husband's/wife's family?
14. What good experiences did you have in school? With friends?
15. What bad experiences did you have in school? With your friends?
16. What was dating like for you?
17. How old were you when you left home? Where did you go? Your family's reaction?
18. Has your family of origin had any history of certain illnesses? Hospitalizations?
19. Have you had any major problems to work out in the past? How did you work those out?

PRESENT FAMILY

1. Who are the persons in your home? What is their age, sex, physical description? Describe their personalities, interests, characteristics.
2. What images or perceptions do you have of various family members?
3. Are the images of your family members and yourself similar?
4. What are the occupations of various family members?
5. What pets are in the family?
6. Has your family by marriage had a history of certain illnesses?
7. Does your family perceive itself as healthy or sick?
8. How are your physical needs met within your family? Explain.
9. Is this your first illness? If not, list past illnesses and hospitalizations.
10. What do you think your family members are communicating about your illness?
11. Are you the only family member who is ill at the present time?
12. How long have you had the present symptom(s) before seeking help?
13. Have you received family counseling or psychological therapy? What was the nature of the problem? How was this resolved?
14. What is ___ reaction to your decision to ___?
15. How have things changed in the family since ___ was born?
16. How might the ___ be good for ___? Bad for this person?
17. What does ___ need from you? What problems do you share?
18. Who in the family helps with ___'s care?
19. How can I be helpful to you as a family?
20. Is ___ acting as you thought he/she would?
21. How does ___ get along with father, mother, siblings, teacher, friends?
22. How does ___ manage his/her activities of daily living?
23. Tell me about ___'s childhood illnesses. (hospitalizations, operations, clinic appointments, etc.)

TABLE 10-3.   Continued

PERCEPTIONS OF SELF

1. What three words best describe you physically?
2. What three words best describe your personality?
3. What do you like about yourself? What do you want to change?
4. Who did/do you get along with easily? Not easily? Why?
5. How can you love somebody and not necessarily like what they do?
6. When do you feel like a good person? Husband/wife? Father/mother? Son/daughter? When do you feel bad?
7. What makes you feel like you are having a good day? A bad day?
8. When you feel bad, how do you help yourself feel better?
9. Have you had any disease/disability?
10. How do you feel family members view you?
11. Are you a high-energy person?
12. How do you organize your time? With whom do you spend time?
13. How do you think you have been managing?
14. What problems have you been having? What problems do you anticipate?

Assessment of the Family's External Environment

Ecology is the study of the sensitive balance that exists between living things and their environment and the ways in which this balance can be enhanced and maintained. An ecological perspective recognizes that all living things are dependent on their environment and on each other for support. Changes in one element of the environment cannot be made without disruption of the overall environmental balance.

The ecological model for family assessment focuses on the relationships between the family and the environment. No family is an island. Consider what a family needs from the environment to survive, grow, develop, and enhance the quality of life. Look at sources of support in a family's environment, the relationships the family has with the environment, and the relationships individual members of the family have with one another and with units in the environment.

The EcoMap

The *EcoMap, an interviewing and assessment tool that captures and organizes the complex ecological system that includes the family and the total environment and the transactional relationships between that family and the environment,* is one method of assessing the family ecology (7, 31). An EcoMap may be done using a structured map similar to Figure 10-7. This diagram is called a *map* because the key units of a family environment and the relationships or paths between the family and environmental units can be identified. You will note some similarities between the environmental components of the family in Figure 10-5 and the systems with which a family interacts, as shown in Figure 10-4. The map (Figure 10-7) illustrates how family needs and resources, both tangible and intangible, interact in the environment. These needs are not the same for all people; a need for one person is not a need for another.

It is important to know not only a family's needs and the resources available to meet these needs, but also the existing social and cultural values that influence how needs are defined and how they will be met. Values also influence the kinds of resources available to meet needs.

The EcoMap can be utilized in the following way. Within the large rectangle in the middle of

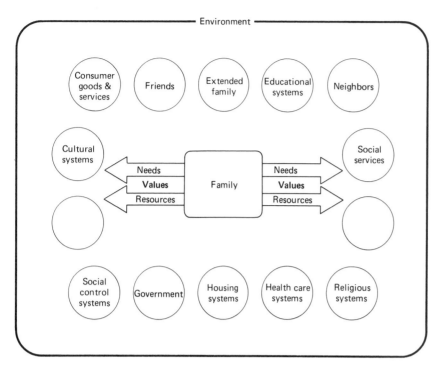

FIGURE 10-7   An ecological map (EcoMap).

the EcoMap, chart the members of the household. The symbols are the same as those used in the genogram. A married couple with two children living at home are portrayed as follows

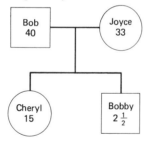

It is often useful to add their names and ages.

A single parent, divorced, mother of one son, and living with her parents would be pictured as follows:

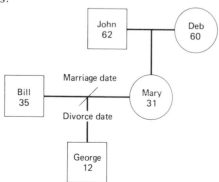

If the disruption of the marriage was the result of the death of the husband, it would be indicated by:

The mapping of more complex family systems has been demonstrated in the previous discussion of genograms.

Having pictured the household within the large rectangle in the middle of the EcoMap, the next step is to begin to draw in the connections between the family and the different parts of the ecological environment. Some of the common systems in the lives of most families have been labeled in Figure 10-7. Other circles have been left undesignated so that the map is sufficiently flexible to be individualized for different families.

Connections between the family and the various systems are indicated by drawing lines between the family and those systems. The nature of the connection may be expressed by the type of line drawn. A solid or thick line indicates an important or strong connection. A broken line indicates a tenuous connection. A hatched line shows a stressful or conflicted relationship. The direction of the flow of resources, energy, information or interests can be shown by drawing arrows along the connecting lines.

The use of these various kinds of lines to describe relationships is an efficient form of shorthand when you use the EcoMap procedure as an analytic tool without the family's direct participation. When using the map as an interviewing tool, however, it may be more helpful to ask family members to describe the nature of the connection and then qualify that connection by writing a descriptive word or two along the connecting line.

Some of the connections may be drawn to the family or household as a whole when such lines are intended to portray the total group's relationship with some system in the environment. Other connections may be drawn between a particular individual and an outside system when that person is the only one involved, or when different family members are involved with an outside system in different ways. This differentiation enables the map to contrast the way various family members are connected with the world.

It is easy to learn to do the EcoMap, and it is important to become comfortable with it before using it with clients. A simple way to learn is to do your own EcoMap. You may also practice with a friend or two. Pertinent questions for completing an EcoMap include those listed in Table 10-4.

After completion of reading this section on assessment of the family, you may wish to formulate your own assessment tool for the family unit, using the guidelines presented previously.

TABLE 10-4.   Questions to Assess the Family's External Environment

1. What do you like best about your house and your neighbors? Like least?

2. Is there anything that you would like to change? Can change?

3. What magazines come into your home?

4. Do you rely on anyone outside of the home for advice/solace? Who is it? Tell me about him/her.

5. What community resources are available to you for spiritual, recreational, educational, and medical needs? Do you avail yourself of these services?

6. Where do family members go for help when they feel ill? How did the family decide to go there? How does the family get there? What has been each member's experiences in getting health care when he/she needed it?

FORMULATING A NURSING DIAGNOSIS

The nursing diagnosis(es) is your descriptive statement(s) of the family as a living unit. What are the patterns within the family—its strengths, weaknesses, deficits? What are the behaviors that support your statement? What restricts and promotes growth and what could be done to alter, modify, or enhance the process that is occurring? The information you have gathered may seem voluminous and overwhelming because some data interrelate and some problems overlap. Your ability to identify dysfunctional patterns in any family unit is dependent on the quality of the data that have been collected, your understanding and application of related theory, and the amount of expertise you possess. Whenever possible, establish the nursing diagnosis from the viewpoint of the family, although you will use professional terms in developing your care plan.

In a general hospital setting, where you are including the family unit as part of your care of the client, your nursing diagnosis may be general, or family issues may be included in the client's nursing diagnosis. For example, you may state a nursing diagnosis as follows:

1. Anxiety in client related to lack of family contact.

2. Family's denial of client's disease and of need for special diet and hygiene measures is related to lack of understanding on the part of the family.

Examples of a nursing diagnosis may be derived from some of the material presented earlier in the chapter. Using Family Systems Theory, you may state your nursing diagnosis(es) in the following ways:

1. *Family system insufficiently open to internal (or external) environment* related to *inability of members to express feelings* (or *impaired ability to interact with neighbors*).
2. *Impaired communication processes in family system* related to *power struggles.*
3. *Family goals and functions unmet* related to *disorganized life-style patterns of members.*
4. *Dysfunctional family system* related to *limited communication between family members, including extended family.*

Using Fig. 10-1, you may state your *nursing diagnosis(es)* as follows:

1. *Impairment in fulfilling family functions and activities* related to *inadequate material resources.*
2. *Impaired intrafamily interactions and lack of communication* related to *abusive behavior between spouses.*
3. *Disruptive family interpersonal relationships* related to *power conflicts and lack of closeness.*

Using knowledge about the four types of family patterns, you may state your *nursing diagnosis(es)* as follows:

1. *Conflicted family pattern* related to *power struggles between spouses.*
2. *Impaired family relationship* related to *domination by —— in family interaction.*
3. *Alienation between family members* related to *chaotic interactional patterns and lack of leadership.*
4. *Dysfunctional family interactions* related to *parental struggles for dominance.*

Using a genogram or EcoMap, you may state your *nursing diagnosis(es)* as follows:

1. *Altered family relationships* related to *mourning of death of parent (or divorce, remarriage, or coalitions between stepchildren against wife's children, or death of another family member).*
2. *Unachieved family goals* related to *inability of family to utilize environmental resources.*

You will think of other ways to formulate nursing diagnosis(es) so that the statements are meaningful to you and to other nurses.

FORMULATION OF CLIENT-CARE GOALS AND PLAN OF CARE

The primary *goal* in working with families is to use yourself and your assessment in a way that allows the family to: (1) bring issues into the open, (2) gain a new awareness, (3) learn new ways to facilitate balance in the family system, and (4) fulfill family functions in a more healthful way. Having diagnosed a dysfunctional pattern(s) within a family system, your specific goal(s) in conjunction with the family is to determine what changes can be effected to create a more constructive pattern(s).

Short-term client-care goals could be stated as follows:

1. The family system will convey support to the ill member through daily visits and empathic conversation.
2. Family members will be able to describe special dietary needs and other self-care measures essential to client recovery.
3. Family member (specific person) will demonstrate correct techniques for rehabilitative care of client.
4. Family members will admit each person's contribution to disruptive communication and life-style patterns.
5. Family members will formulate a contract for 20 minutes of conversation each day where feelings can be expressed honestly and without argument (or fear, blame, scapegoating, derision, etc.).
6. Husband and wife will discuss dominance/submission patterns and ways to share in decision making.

7. The family system will utilize community agency (name specific one) as a support while adjusting to changes produced by ——.

Long-term client-care goals are appropriate if you will be working with a family over a period of time. Such goals could include the following:

1. The family system will accurately identify key issues that contribute to hostile communication and withdrawal of members from participation in family life.
2. Family members will practice daily (for an increasing amount of time) communication methods that promote cohesion.
3. Parents will discuss and adhere consistently to effective disciplinary measures of child(ren).

4. The nuclear family will reestablish harmonious relationships with the extended family.
5. The spouse will be less authoritarian in interactions with the partner and child(ren).
6. The husband/wife will contribute toward completion of daily activities related to homemaking, instead of using illness to escape these family functions.
7. The husband will avoid seductive behavior toward his daughter and relate affectionately toward his wife.

You will write goals specific to the family systems with which you are working. Perhaps the above examples will stimulate your thinking.

NURSING INTERVENTION

Principles for Humanistic Care

As in other treatment modalities, self-awareness is essential. Effective family intervention is dependent on your ability to attain and maintain an awareness of your definition of family, your values, and your own life style, and to then examine and accept the differences between yourself and the families you encounter. Differences could be in terms of values, cultural backgrounds, beliefs, living or communication patterns, or sexual practices. Be cognizant also of your personal goals in working with families.

Recognize that your presence with members of a family, or within a family unit, is in itself an intervention. You become a physical part of the system, and change occurs within the system because you are active within the process. You are a participant observer in the family system. Your role is one of being empathetic, nonjudgmental, and supportive while assisting the family to make adjustments related to having an ill member or to make necessary changes in the behavior of the entire unit. Feedback to the family members regarding their activities is essential.

Look at the family's behavior and goals for change from their perspective. Seemingly simple matters may arise that can become major issues between family members and potentially between yourself and the family unless you remain objec-

tive. Mealtime issues, for example, could relate to the number and time of meals per day, the type of meals, and who should be present at meals. Sexual practices raise several issues: attitudes about frequency and time of day/month for intercourse, preferences in techniques, and forms and frequency of expressions of love and intimacy. Any area of concern or life-style practice is influenced by individual preference, culture, and the historical time in which the person lives. Without the ability to ignore your beliefs, you could find yourself taking sides and identifying yourself with one family member at the expense of another. Or the family might try to institute your value or norm in an effort to please you without any sense of appropriateness or improvement in overall family function. You must remain perceptive of your beliefs about being a family member, separate from the family with whom you are working, in order to avoid: (1) imposing your own values, (2) satisfying your own needs at the expense of the family's needs, (3) siding with family members, (4) playing judge, or (5) making a hurried assessment and inappropriate intervention.

Personal Goals and Competencies in Intervention

In order to use the humanistic approach and interact therapeutically with families, you must first set some goals for yourself. Personal goals useful in working with families would include to:

1. Increase your understanding of yourself and your family of origin.
2. Clarify your nursing role to yourself and to others.
3. Increase your ability to be empathic, patient, consistent, and able to set limits.
4. Understand Systems Theory as it relates to the family.
5. Gain increasing depth and breadth in clinical skills, both technological and interpersonal.
6. Increase your ability to utilize other team members in your own growth and as referral resources.
7. Become knowledgeable about community resources for families.
8. Obtain supervision for your family interventions.

In working with families, questions will arise about how much support or intervention is needed? You may ask: Am I capable of intervening with this family? Should I make a referral to another resource?

In your encounters with and assessments of families, there will be times when you decide not to intervene and to leave the family to its own resources. Or you may suggest a referral to another coworker or to a community resource. There will be times, however, when you do choose to intervene, and then you must determine which interventions would be therapeutic and which would not be appropriate. Whenever you work with a family unit, it will be helpful to have another professional with whom you can confer for validation and supervision.

Two assessment aids can assist you in determining whether and how much you will intervene. First, decide which type of family you are encountering. (See family types.) Type A families are equipped to deal with difficulties, change, or crisis with minimal disequilibrium. Supports and coping strategies are well-established, and little intervention is needed. You also may encounter Type B families who are generally functioning in an adaptive way. However, because they are encountering temporary disequilibrium related to a threatening experience such as birth, death, or health crisis, they may require external support and resources in addition to the resources they have already established. Your intervention will help this type of family recover equilibrium. Type C and D families have more extensive and chronic dysfunction and will be unable to cope with change or crisis or to seek or accept support from outside resources. These families require the worker to possess considerable skill and expertise in nursing intervention.

Second, use the conceptual scheme of family organization and function shown in Figure 10-1, which aids in: (1) organizing your observation, thoughts, and data concerning the family's functioning, (2) determining the complexity of the issues the family wants to address, (3) determining your ability to meet these needs, and (4) focusing your interventions. The levels from I to IV (see Figure 10-1) indicate a progression from less abstract issues to more abstract, complex, and illusive issues. When you begin to work with families, focus your interventions first on those issues identified in Level I. If goals for change are not met, then it is time to evaluate the need to address issues on another level. Issues identified in levels II, III, or IV require a greater knowledge of family dynamics, additional theoretical frameworks, and more clinical expertise and supervision than were needed in Level I (71).

Also refer to Chapter 12 for discussion about working with the family who has a member who is acutely or chronically ill or is experiencing role impairment.

Intervention Measures

Certain measures will help you to meet the client-care goals previously stated. These measures include the following:

1. *Develop a therapeutic relationship.* Establish rapport and trust between yourself and the family through use of therapeutic communication previously described. Use the family's language, but be a model for clear, effective communication. Remember the trust, influence, and impact that you, in your role of nurse, have on the family unit. Be empathic, supportive, and impartial as you give feedback to the family. Thus you will enable the family members to identify and modify patterns that cause dysfunction and discomfort.
2. *Identify issues with the family.* Subjective

issues are what the family members perceive as problem areas. Objective issues are what you see as limits or problems. Each family member should list or identify what he/she sees as a problem and what needs to be changed. Refrain from challenging or questioning the accuracy of anyone's values or statements of problem areas. Do not side with any one particular member. Encourage family members to also explore those areas that you see as dysfunctional.

3. *Encourage and assist members in their communication skills,* to listen to each other, to talk kindly, and to clarify their own perceptions and each other's feelings, thoughts, and behaviors. You gently confront and are a mirror for the family members so that they can gain increased understanding of themselves as a unit. As they learn to talk honestly to each other, members will have less need to deny the pain they feel or deny hurtful behaviors practiced in family living.

4. *Establish a teaching plan for the family unit if it is appropriate,* either for the client as a member of the family or for the family as a whole. Help each one find appropriate resources in his/her external environment as well as to identify his/her own strengths for managing a situation. Encourage the family to find ways to adapt the life style or home situation to better manage an illness or crisis.

5. *Determine willingness of family members to participate in counseling and change.* Keep in mind that families, according to Systems Theory, strive to maintain their balance and are frightened and ambivalent about negotiating and enacting change. Having each member participate in defining the problem and in making the decision for change will enable family members to feel more in control of what is occurring and more willing to participate. Even so, some members may continue to be resistant to change during counseling or may choose not to participate at all. It is essential for you to remain objective, re-

assuring, and supportive. Considerable theoretical knowledge, communication skill, and supervised practice are necessary before you will be able to work with deep, long-term, or complex problems; resistant behavior; power struggles; or coalitions.

6. *Negotiate a contract as to the goals for treatment.* (See Chapter 4 for guidelines for contracting.) Goals must be formulated with the family and in terms that the members understand and can achieve. Identify with the family one or two goals that are crucial to work toward, in order to begin to achieve some happiness and smoother function. Later, other goals may be added to the list. It is better to set small achievable goals that the family perceives as worthwhile than to inhibit family change through an extensive list of statements about what it will eventually do or which are unrealistic. Although a family frequently expresses goals in terms of changes it would like to see in a particular family member, remember that the behavior of any one family member is a symptom of a problem in the family system in the interface of the individual with the other family members.

7. *Negotiate a contract about specific behavioral changes that can be accomplished* and that will encourage family members to interact or behave in ways that break dysfunctional patterns or rigid structures. Assist members to disagree constructively and to contract with one another for change. Help the family to anticipate problem areas, work through alternatives, and explore consequences of the alternatives.

8. *Be patient.* Do not expect great change. The family may change its behavior, but only to the point that is comfortable and tolerable to all. Regression to previous patterns will occur. Your consistent kindness and encouragement may be the main factors in the family coping with stressors or crises, adjusting daily routines to the needs of an ill member, or staying with therapy and trying to modify behavior.

EVALUATION

You will be able to evaluate the accuracy of your assessment and nursing diagnosis, as well as the effective use of nursing measures, as you attend to the family's behavior over a period of time. Listen for changes in the conversation. You may also notice changes in previously troublesome behavior, fewer arguments, more agreements, more smiles, and fewer frowns. You can validate your observations with the family members, reinforcing their own development as you evaluate.

There may be times that you will not work with a family long enough to be able to determine the extent of your helpfulness. In this case, perhaps you can query a colleague or contact the referral agency to determine if your initial intervention laid the groundwork for another professional's therapy. Do not underestimate the importance of your initial contacts in helping a family to later resolve its difficulties.

There may be times when you can get no feedback, or the feedback you do get may indicate that the family did not accept your referral and did not follow your suggestions. Do not become discouraged by what may seem like a failure. Promoting effective growth in one individual is quite a nursing challenge and responsibility, and this challenge and responsibility are multiplied when you work with the additional persons that make up a family unit. You may need more experience or knowledge before you can be effective in working with everyone you try to help—often for reasons unknown or out of your control. However, you can learn from the experience and try again, knowing that the chances are great that you will be perceived as helpful and that the feelings of satisfaction are worth your efforts.

REFERENCES

1. Ackerman, Nathan, *The Psychodynamics of Family Life.* New York: Basic Books, Inc., 1958.

2. ____, "A Dynamic Frame for the Clinical Approach to Family Conflict," in *Exploring the Base for Family Therapy,* eds. N. Ackerman, F. Beatman, and S. Sherman. New York: Jewish Family Services, 1961.

3. ____, *Treating the Troubled Family.* New York: Basic Books, Inc., 1966.

4. Altneave, C., "Social Networks as the Unit of Attention," in *Family Therapy,* ed. P. Guerin. New York: Gardner Press, Inc., 1976.

5. Anderson, D. B., "Nursing Therapy with Families," *Perspectives in Psychiatric Care,* 7 (1969), 2-27.

6. Aponte, Harry, "Underorganization in the Poor Family," in *Family Therapy,* ed. P. Guerin. New York: Gardner Press, Inc., 1976.

7. Averswald, E., "Families, Change, and the Ecological Perspective," in *The Book of Family Therapy,* ed. A. Ferber. Boston: Houghton Mifflin Company, 1973.

8. Barnhill, L., "Dimensions of Healthy Family Interaction." Ph.D. dissertation. Southern Illinois University, Carbondale, Ill. 1975.

9. ____, "Healthy Family Systems," *Family Coordinator,* 28 (1979), 94-100.

10. Bertalanffy, L., "General System Theory and Psychiatry," in *American Handbook of Psychiatry,* vol. III, ed. S. Arieti. New York: Basic Books, Inc., 1966.

11. Black, Sister Kathleen, "Teaching Family Process and Intervention," *Nursing Outlook,* 18, no. 6 (1970), 54-58.

12. Bossard, James, and Eleanor Boll, *The Sociology of Child Development,* 4th ed. New York: Harper & Row, Publishers, Inc., 1966.

13. Boszormenyi, I., and J. Franco, eds., *Intensive Family Therapy.* New York: Harper & Row, Publishers, Inc., 1965.

14. Bowen, M., "The Family as the Unit of Study and Treatment," *American Journal of Orthopsychiatry,* 31 (1961), 40-60.

15. ____, "Family Psychotherapy with Schizophrenia in the Hospital and in Private Practice," in *Intensive Family Therapy,* eds. I. Boszormenyi-Nagy, and J. Framo, pp. 213-44. Harper & Row, Publishers, Inc., 1965.

16. ____, "The Use of Family Theory in Clinical Practice," in *Changing Families: A Family Therapy Reader,* ed. J. Haley, pp. 159-92. New York: Grune & Stratton, Inc., 1971.

17. ____, "Toward the Differentiation of a Self in One's Family of Origin," in *Georgetown Family Symposia: A Collection of Selected Papers, I.,* eds. F. Andres and J. Lorio. Washington, D.C.: Georgetown University Medical Center, 1974.

18. ____, "Theory in the Practice of Psychotherapy," in *Family Therapy: Theory and Practice,* ed. P. Guerin, pp. 42-90. New York: Gardner Press, Inc., 1976.

19. ____, "Principles and Techniques of Multiple Family Therapy," in *Family Therapy: Theory and Practice,* ed. P. Guerin, pp. 388-404. New York: Gardner Press, Inc., 1976.

20. ____, *Family Therapy in Clinical Practice*. New York: Jason Aronson, Inc., 1978.

21. Bradt, J., and C. Moynihan, *Systems Theory, Selected Papers: Theory, Technique, Research*. Washington, D.C.: Groome Child Center, 1971.

22. Bulbulyan, A. A., "The Psychiatric Nurse as Family Therapist," *Perspectives in Psychiatric Care*, 7, no. 2 (1969), 58–68.

23. Bundler, Richard, John Grender, and Virginia Satir, *Changing with Families*. Palo Alto, Calif.: Science and Behavior Books, Inc., 1976.

24. Clement, J., "Family Therapy: The Transferability of Theory to Practice," *Journal of Psychiatric Nursing and Mental Health Services*, 15, no. 8 (1977), 33–37, 42–43.

25. Curtis, W. R., "Community Human Service Networks: New Roles for Mental Health Workers," *Psychiatric Annals*, 3 (1973), 23–42.

26. Duvall, Evelyn, *Family Development*, 4th ed. Philadelphia: J. B. Lippincott Company, 1971.

27. Egan, C., and M. Cowan, *People in Systems*. Monterey, Calif.: Brooks/Cole Publishing Company, 1979.

28. Eichel, E., "Assessment with a Family Focus," *Journal of Psychiatric Nursing and Mental Health Services*, 16 (1978), 11–14.

29. Foley, V., *An Introduction to Family Therapy*. New York: Grune & Stratton, Inc., 1974.

30. Garrish, M., "The Family Therapist Is a Nurse," *American Journal of Nursing*, 68 (1968), 320–23.

31. Germain, C., "An Ecological Perspective in Casework Practice," *Social Casework*, 54, no. 6 (1973), 323–30.

32. Guerin, P. J., and P. Pendergast, "Evaluation of Family Systems and the Genogram," in *Family Therapy*, ed. P. J. Guerin. New York: Gardner Press, Inc., 1976.

33. Haley, J., *Strategies of Psychotherapy*. New York: Grune & Stratton, Inc., 1963.

34. ____, *Changing Families*. New York: Grune & Stratton, Inc., 1971.

35. ____, *Uncommon Therapy: The Psychiatric Techniques of Milton H. Erickson, M.D.* New York: W. W. Norton & Co., Inc., 1973.

36. ____, *Problem-Solving Therapy*. San Francisco: Jossey Bass, Inc., Publishers, 1976.

37. Haley, J., and Lynn Hoffman, *Techniques of Family Therapy*. New York: Basic Books, Inc., 1967.

38. Hall, Joanne, and Barbara Weaver, *Nursing of Families in Crisis*. Philadelphia: J. B. Lippincott Company, 1974.

39. Haller, L. L., "Family Systems Theory in Psychiatric Intervention," *American Journal of Nursing*, 74 (1974), 462–63.

40. Henrion, R. P., "Family Nurse Therapist: A Model of Communication," *Journal of Psychiatric Nursing and Mental Health Services*, 12, no. 6 (1974), 10–13.

41. Hill, Martha, "When the Patient Is the Family," *American Journal of Nursing*, 81, no. 3 (1981), 536–38.

42. Jackson, D. D., "The Study of the Family," *Family Process*, 4 (1965), 1–20.

43. ____, "The Question of Family Homeostasis," in *Communication, Family, and Marriage*, ed. D. Jackson, Palo Alto, Calif.: Science and Behavior Books, Inc., 1968.

44. Kleigman, J., "Enmeshment and Fusion," *Family Process*, 15 (1976), 321–23.

45. Kleiman, Carol, "When a Family Is Not a Family to Us." Paper presented at Adoption Builds Families Conference, St. Louis, Mo., May 1980.

46. Koehne-Kaplan, Nancy, "The Use of Self as a Family Therapist," *Perspectives in Psychiatric Care*, 14, no. 1 (1976), 29–33.

47. Kramer, Charles, *Becoming a Family Therapist*. New York: Human Sciences Press, 1980.

48. Lewis, Jerry, *How's Your Family?* New York: Brunner/Mazel, Inc., 1979.

49. Lidz, T., *The Family and Human Adaptation*. New York: International Universities Press, 1963.

50. Longo, Dianne, and Reg Williams, *Clinical Practice in Psychosocial Nursing: Assessment and Intervention*. New York: Appleton-Century-Crofts, 1978.

51. Martin, B., "Family Interaction Associated with Child Disturbance: Assessment and Modification," *Psychotherapy*, 4 (1967), 30–36.

52. Mereness, D., "Family Therapy: An Evolving Role for the Psychiatric Nurse," *Perspectives in Psychiatric Care*, 8 (1968), 256–59.

53. Messer, Alfred, *The Individual in His Family*. Springfield, Ill.: Charles C Thomas, Publisher, 1970.

54. Minuchin, S., "Conflict-Resolution Family Therapy," *Psychiatry*, 28 (1965), 278–386.

55. ____, *Families and Family Therapy*. Cambridge, Mass.: Harvard University Press, 1974.

56. Minuchin, S. et al., *Families of the Slums: An Exploration of Their Structure and Treatment*. New York: Basic Books, Inc., 1967.

57. Minuchin, S., B. Rosman, and L. Baker, *Psychosomatic Families: Anorexia Nervosa in Context*. Cambridge, Mass.: Harvard University Press, 1978.

58. Monea, H. P., "A Family in Trouble," *Perspectives in Psychiatric Care*, 8 (1968), 256–59.

59. Morgan, S. A., and M. J. Macey, "Three Assessment

Tools for Family Therapy," *Journal of Psychiatric Nursing and Mental Health Services,* 16 (1978), 39–42.

60. Murray, Ruth, and Judith Zentner, *Nursing Concepts for Health Promotion,* 2nd ed. Englewood Cliffs, N.J.: Prentice-Hall, Inc., 1979.

61. Napier, A. Y., and C. A. Whitaker, "Problems of the Beginning Family Therapist," *Seminars in Psychiatry,* vol. 5 (1973).

62. ——, *The Family Crucible.* New York: Harper & Row, Publishers, Inc., 1978.

63. Nelson, Elof, *Prime Time.* Owatonna, Minn.: Journal Chronicle Company, 1972.

64. Rappaport, A. F., "Conjugal Relationship Enhancement Program," in *Treating Relationships,* ed. D. H. L. Olson. Lake Mills, Iowa: Graphic Publishers, 1976.

65. Rice, D. G., W. F. Fly, and J. G. Kepecs, "Therapist Experience and Style as Factors in CoTherapy," *Family Process,* 11 (1972), 1–12.

66. Rice, D. G., A. S. Gurman, and A. M. Rozin, "Therapist Sex, Style, and Theoretical Orientation," *Journal of Nervous and Mental Diseases,* 159 (1974), 413–21.

67. Robischon, Paulette, and Diane Scott, "Role Theory and Its Application in Family Nursing," *Nursing Outlook,* 17, no. 7 (1969), 52–57.

68. Satir, Virginia, *Conjoint Family Therapy.* Palo Alto, Calif.: Science and Behavior Books, Inc., 1967.

69. ——, *Peoplemaking.* Palo Alto, Calif.: Science and Behavior Books, Inc., 1972.

70. Satir, Virginia, J. Stachowiak, and H. A. Taschman, *Helping Families to Change.* New York: Jason Aronson, Inc., 1975.

71. Schneider, Robert, "Conceptual Scheme of Family Or-ganization and Function." Paper presented at St. Louis University Medical Center Conference, St. Louis, Mo., June 1980.

72. Sedgewick, Rae, "The Family as a System: A Network of Relationships," *Journal of Psychiatric Nursing and Mental Health Services,* 12, no. 2 (1974), 17–20.

73. ——, *Family Mental Health: Theory and Practice.* St. Louis: The C. V. Mosby Company, 1981.

74. Shapiro, R., "Some Implications of Training Psychiatric Nurses in Family Therapy," *Journal of Marriage and Family Counseling,* 1 (1975), 323–30.

75. Sharp, L., and J. E. Lantz, "Relabeling in Conjoint Family Therapy," *Journal of Psychiatric Nursing and Mental Health Services,* 14, no. 7 (1976), 23–28.

76. Skinner, S. W., *Family Therapy: The Treatment of Natural Systems.* London: Routledge & Kegan Paul Ltd., 1976.

77. Smoyak, Shirley, ed., *The Psychiatric Nurse as a Family Therapist.* New York: John Wiley & Sons, Inc., 1975.

78. Speck, R. V., "Family Therapy in the Home," *Journal of Marriage and Family Living,* 26 (1964), 72–76.

79. Torman, M., *Family Constellations.* New York: Springer Publishing Co., Inc., 1972.

80. Waldrond-Skinner, S. W., *Family Therapy: The Treatment of Natural Systems.* London: Routledge & Kegan Paul Ltd., 1976.

81. Watzlawick, Paul, *Language of Change.* New York: Basic Books, Inc., 1978.

82. Watzlawick, P., J. H. Weakland, and R. Fisch, *Change: Principles of Problem Formation and Problem Resolution.* New York: W. W. Norton & Co., Inc., 1974.

11

The Group as Client: Group Dynamics and Caring Processes

Study of this chapter will assist you to:

1. Discuss the historical development of group work and the implications for present-day group work with psychiatric patients.

2. Define *group* and differentiate between primary and secondary groups.

3. Discuss purposes and benefits of group work for clients in any health care setting and with any kind of illness.

4. Analyze the group as a system.

5. Explore behavioral characteristics and forces that contribute to group process.

6. List phases of group development, and describe characteristic behaviors of group members and the leader's responsibilities in each phase.

7. Describe effective behaviors of the group leader, including during each phase.

8. List and define the members' task and maintenance functions that characterize group process, and the roles of recorder and observer.

9. Compare and contrast effective versus obstructive individual behavior of group members.

10. Contrast the purposes and formats of various types of groups that can be used with clients.

11. Initiate and maintain a group experience for selected clients, utilizing knowledge from this chapter and the guidance of a skilled supervisor.

12. Evaluate your leadership style and ability to fulfill responsibilities in each phase.

13. Work with the recorder, observer, and group members to analyze effectiveness of members in the group process.

14. Evaluate benefits of the group experience for the clients.

This chapter contributed by M. Marilyn Huelskoetter, R.N., M.S.N.
Portions of this chapter contributed by Ruth Murray, R.N., M.S.N.

OVERVIEW AND DEFINITIONS

Since the beginning of man, groups have been in existence. Early in time, primitive groups were used to promote safety and to protect and maintain life. As time progressed, groups became more organized and social and were used for control, companionship, progress, and accomplishment. Now we live in what some people call the Age of the Group. With advanced knowledge and technological skills, we have become less personalized and less intimate. This industrialized, urbanized age has brought us to new experiences and pleasures but also to a greater vulnerability to loneliness. There are fewer extended family ties and fewer long-standing community groups. Many people seek a sense of belonging, security, and contact in group experiences, experiences that can furnish opportunities for personal fulfillment and growth. The group has become an accepted and commonplace environment for experience.

This chapter will help you understand general group development and process; it will introduce you to the group experience and encourage you to adapt this knowledge to group work with your clients in a variety of settings.

What is a Group?

E. Durkheim described the *group* as *a collective representation with an identity of its own* (43). G. C. Homans defines the *group* as *a limited number of persons who communicate with one another often, over a period of time, and face-to-face rather than secondhand through each other* (43). R. Anderson and I. Carter define *group* as *a system, a constellation or cluster of individuals, which is a whole entity in itself separate from its environment, and fulfills the criteria of a system* (1). The group also includes patterns of associations and activity in which most people engage daily.

Groups are either primary or secondary, depending on the importance of the group to the person. A *primary group* is like a family; it has considerable influence upon the person, especially upon affective functions. In the *secondary group, people react to each other as role occupants or in a formalized manner.* As the group becomes more goal-specific, more narrow in its range of influence, and more formalized, the closer it is to being a secondary group and becoming like an organization (1).

Groups are narcissistic or generative; they provide for self-gratification of one or more of their members, or they facilitate a commitment to group goals. Narcissistic groups are rigidly structured; no provision is made for internal and external adjust-ments in order to protect against threat or the passage of time. A generative group is engaged in mutually constructive interchange with its environment (1).

BENEFITS OF GROUP EXPERIENCE

The group experience can be used in primary prevention to prevent illness and to promote health, as well as to provide avenues for involvement, discussion, sharing feelings, and working through problems of living. Group interactions broaden the perceptions of self, life situations, other people, and potential solutions to problems because of multiple sources of feedback. Such groups might be found in day-care centers, community centers, girl scout groups, schools, and churches—any place where a group of people can meet and talk face-to-face over a period of time. As a nurse, you will be working with groups of functioning, healthy, adjusted people as well as with groups of emotionally ill clients. Some groups may be composed of professional team members and other health care personnel; other groups may include the family as well as the patient. These groups may be formal or informal, ranging from a structured team conference, a weekly support group, a daily meeting with a client's family, or an on-the-spot discussion with a group of clients concerning the day's activity.

Groups may provide for intensive experiences, such as the encounter, sensitivity training, sensory awareness, team building, or Gestalt groups. These groups are for people who are functioning normally, but they want to improve their capacity for living with their own set of relationships. In such groups the leader acts as a facilitator to establish a safe climate, and he/she helps people become more open to and expressive of inner feelings, more spontaneous in their reactions, more flexible, and more genuine in their interpersonal relationships. As a result of these characteristics, the participants may also be more vulnerable to the hurts of others (76, 77). Self-help groups emphasize the power of organized people to work out their own destinies and include groups for battered women, ostomy clubs, groups for terminally ill people, Synanon, Parents-without-Partners, and community-organization and welfare-rights groups concerned primarily with failures of environmental and social systems (1).

The group experience is also useful in secondary and tertiary prevention. The emotionally ill person with whom you will be working is especially in need of group experiences. The pain involved in any mental illness is often accentuated by experiences of rejection, loneliness, and detachment from others. Therefore a group experience for these clients can provide more involvement with others and can give the advantages of social contact, as well as providing a treatment tool for healing and growth. Intensive group therapy for the emotionally ill person often involves meeting for an hour weekly over a period of time, or intensive week, month, or weekend experiences may also be used. In such groups the leader functions as therapist (78).

Many writers have reported effective group work among emotionally ill. Research has been done with groups, and successful results have been documented. A. Silver noted improvement in morale, cleanliness, and general behavior after group work with 17 psychotic elderly patients (89). M. Linden worked over a two-year period with 51 institutionalized women and found old values regained importance, hunger for social relationship returned, regression was halted, and an urge to contribute to group cohesion emerged (52). A. Goldfarb and H. Turner treated 150 elderly residents in a nursing home; 49 percent improved with an average of 8.5 sessions (36). Nurses, including I. Burnside (16, 19), M. Loomis (55), G. Marram (58), J. Werner (101), and F. Terrazas (108), have also reported the effectiveness of group work. However, there are still many unanswered questions concerning the effectiveness of group work for health care clients, and more research is needed (55).

Psychiatric nurses have been involved in group work for a long time. They have synthesized Psychoanalytic, Interpersonal, Communication, Group Dynamics, Gestalt, and Behavior Modification Frameworks into an eclectic orientation and a broad base. First, study the theorists and group approaches summarized in Table 11-1. Study also research and other literature on group process. Try out a variety of approaches until you are familiar with the concepts and styles. Talk to other group workers. Then build a flexible framework that will work for you (58), utilizing a Humanistic Framework with other theoretical frameworks.

TABLE 11-1.   Summary of Major Group Methods and the Founders.

DATE	FOUNDER	GROUP METHOD	DESCRIPTION
1912	Joseph Moreno	Psychodrama	A type of therapy whereby the person expresses feelings by acting out various roles on a stage. The audience becomes a participant vicariously and is asked to make comments and interpretations to the individuals acting the roles.
1920	Trigant Burrow, S. H. Foulkes	Group Psycho-analysis	A type of group approach that applies the understanding and theories of individual psychoanalysis to a group. The concepts of transference and resolution of resistances are emphasized.
1935	C. Diederich	Alcoholics Anonymous	A type of inspirational group whereby alcoholics are directed, cared for, and admonished by leaders and by group members who themselves are former alcoholics. With twelve steps toward abstinence, dependence on God and fellow man, and support by the group, the individual struggling with alcoholic addiction is treated.
1937	Abraham Low	Recovery, Inc.	A type of directive and inspirational group composed of former hospitalized psychiatric patients. The groups are led by the members with the guidance of the book by Abraham Low, *Mental Health Through Will-Training*, 20th ed. (West Hanover, Mass.: Christopher Publishers, 1976).
1930–1940	Leon Festinger, Kurt Lewin, R. White	Group Dynamics Theory	A type of group approach that uses an understanding of group interaction, Group Dynamics Theory, based on the systematic and scientific study of groups. Group cohesiveness or closeness, expression of feelings, and interaction are emphasized.
1940	Maxwell Jones	Therapeutic community	A type of group approach that considers individual needs in relation to the group needs and uses the health-promoting environment as an agent for treatment. The concept of Milieu Therapy, a surrounding environment conducive to

TABLE 11-1. Continued

DATE	FOUNDER	GROUP METHOD	DESCRIPTION
			emotional growth and healing of the patient, includes the total hospital environment, physical milieu, emotional atmosphere, ward policies, staff members, patients, and their participation. This approach initiates and encourages unit government by patients, open-door policies, and mutual responsibilities.
1950	Martin Buber	Existential groups	A type of group approach based on existentialism, the philosophy that man's being is contained only in community and relationships. Lonely, alienated, isolated people meet together to seek meaning in life, gain spontaneity, and share self with others. Group members and therapists participate mutually.
1950	W. R. Bion	Tavistock Conference	A holistic approach to group therapy first developed during World War II at Tavistock Clinic in England. Focus is on the group's common problem or tension. The group is a system; thus the therapist attempts to seek out similar kinds of problems within the members of the group. Examples of a common theme operating within the group might be doubt, trust, rejection, fear, loss, hopelessness, or dependency.
1960	Nathan Ackerman, Theodore Lidz, Carl Whitaker, Donald Jackson	Family dynamics	The study of the family as a group was the basis for developing the "double bind" theory relating to the families of schizophrenics. The family dynamics approach, study of communication and functioning of members within a family system, has evolved from this research.
1960		T-Group movement	An intense method begun in the 1940s that gained emphasis later as a training method to help mental health workers become more sensitive, knowledgeable, and capable as group leaders and therapists. Encounter, Sensitivity, T.A., and other groups were developed as a means for socially overcoming distance and alienation between people.
1960	Eric Berne	Transactional Analysis (T.A.)	A type of group approach that utilizes psychoanalytic theory and focuses on

TABLE 11-1.   Continued

DATE	FOUNDER	GROUP METHOD	DESCRIPTION
			symbolic reenactment of the past in present relationships. Members' participation is analyzed according to adult, child, and parent roles, since members symbolically reenact former problems by relating to others in the role of parent or child. The group leader helps the person understand the nature of the interaction and to alter behavior by choosing the adult role.
1960	Lawrence Tirnauer	Encounter group	A type of group approach that is theme-centered, intense in emotion, short-lived, and focuses on group process rather than technique. The workshops vary from a weekend marathon to two-hour sessions and were developed especially to promote personal growth of people in the helping professions.
1960	Carl Rogers	Basic encounter	A type of sensitivity training group that emphasizes the nondirective, empathic approach to establishing a congruent relationship so that the client may express feelings in an open, permissive atmosphere. The individual within the group is the focus rather than the group as a phenomenon.
1960	Fritz Perls	Gestalt	Group method begun in the late 1940s–1950s, but more prominent in the 1960s. Focuses on the individual within the group. The technique of having a person "on the hot seat" is used to concentrate on a person's problems and on ways to make changes in his/her life. Role-playing, personal experimentation, and exploration of individual feelings, fantasies, and dreams are used in the group.

HISTORICAL PERSPECTIVE

The study of group function has long been of interest to many philosophers, scientists, sociologists, psychologists, and educators; but it has achieved particular prominence in the twentieth century, possibly related to breakdown of primary group relationships. Group work began in 1905 as Joseph Pratt, a physician, gathered together a group of tubercular patients in order to teach them self-care and at the same time elevate their morale and mood. Since that time, various group techniques, leaders, and purposes of group work have evolved. Table 11-1 summarizes some of these leaders and their methods.

Group work is now diverse in leadership, purpose, and approach. For example, a physician or a housewife might be found leading similar types of groups. Goals or objectives of individual groups are equally diverse. Objectives might include personality reconstruction, promotion of insight, remotivation, problem solving, reality orientation, emotional support, or education. Objectives depend on the skills and interests of the leader or therapist and on the needs of the group members (58).

Although individual group leaders use a variety of methods, approaches, and philosophies, these groups can be currently divided into three major categories (92):

1. *Evocative*—to encourage spontaneous expression of feelings in an atmosphere of acceptance and understanding.
2. *Directive*—to indoctrinate or give advice, with emphasis on proper attitudes and conduct, using an authoritarian approach.
3. *Didactic*—to educate through a class or seminar.

THE GROUP AS A SYSTEM

A group, like a family, is dependent on particular persons and is affected by changes in members more so than other systems. Formation and disintegration of a group are more likely to occur during an observer's or member's lifetime than are the formation and disintegration of other systems.

Steady State in the Group

Groups, like organisms, are characterized by a *steady state, a sense of balance or equilibrium that is maintained even as the group changes.* Groups form, grow, and reach a state of maturity. The group begins with a set of elements—individuals with unique personalities, needs, ideas, potentials, and limits. In the course of development, a pattern of behavior and a set of norms, beliefs, and values evolve. Parts become differentiated; each member assumes special functions (1).

As a group reaches maturity, it becomes increasingly complex, differentiated, interdependent, and integrated. The group has a subculture and identity of its own; the commonly experienced meanings, definitions, norms, and behavior all make up the subculture of the group (1).

The group can evolve toward one of two steady states—either instrumental or expressive. The *instrumental group has clear, time-related, specific objectives, and seeks specific results; the organization is vertical in relationships.* In the *expressive group,* objectives or goals are diffuse and unspecific, and the organization is horizontal in relationships, *resulting in harmonious sentiments.* Other terms for such states could be *adaptive* versus *integrative.* The instrumental group shows optimal adaptation to the outer situation at the cost of internal integration; the expressive group demonstrates optimal internal integration at the cost of adaptation to the outer situation. However, these polarities are not mutually exclusive. The instrumental or adaptive group must consider relationships at least minimally in order to accomplish tasks. The expressive or integrative group is unlikely to remain together without some task, however minimal—for example, choosing meeting dates and places (1, 65).

Two components of a group's steady state are consensus and goal attainment. *Consensus refers to the agreement about goals, norms, roles, and other aspects of the group.* Cohesiveness results when such agreements foster mutual satisfaction of group members' important needs, mutual responsibility of each toward the other, and sharing of a common fate. Each person is under obligation to cooperate with the other, so that another's needs become as important as one's personal needs. Such a group bond occurs on one of three levels: (1) as a conscious purpose, such as with sociability or friendship, (2) as an assumed objective, such as seeking achievement, status, or ego expansion, or (3) as an unconscious purpose, including sanctioned release of aggression, escape from reality, and sublimation of erotic impulses. Having a goal or purpose that is mutually defined and valued also promotes the steady state of the group. Group members must distinguish between affective and goal-seeking behavior, must divide activity between the two aspects, and will receive separate rewards for each (1).

Behavioral Aspects of the Group

Steady state requires that all group behavior must have some bearing on securing and expending energy externally. Problem-solving and decision-making activity and the production of some service will help to keep a group adaptive (1).

Socialization or integration furnishes energy to the group and reduces the likelihood of conflict. Socialization into the group is based on some match between the person's needs and the group's offerings. Groups are often used by the person to gain security or acceptance, to make friends, and to learn about other people's life styles; or to prepare for entrance into other groups, an occupation, or different life style (1). Socialization may occur in one of the following processes:

Compliance—the person conforms without believing or accepting the group's view.

Internalization—the person adopts the group's view because it agrees with his own or solves a problem for him.

Identification—the person adopts the group's view through internalizing and making it part of himself.

The adaptation of the person and the integrative behavior of the system must be mutual, or socialization will fail.

The group achieves an identity by setting a standard or norm and then shaping its members' behavior through approval and reinforcement or by threat of ridicule, disapproval, exclusion, or punishment. For example, traditionally, Robert's Rules have been used in formal meetings to control when and how members speak.

Conflict and social control occur in any group. An important part of social control in groups is management of conflict. Conflict, the response when there is an emotional gap between what people need and want and the support and warmth that is available, is inherent in group experience. For a group to form, members must be free to change to some degree. Further, the group as a whole may accept and reward some members more fully than others, which is a form of central control over members. For the member to give up old behavior and learn new behavior may be a source of conflict until

the member is reassured about the value and effectiveness of the new behavior (1).

Communication is essential to maintain a system. Although any group activity could be a form of communication, actually communication is the exchange of messages or energy to accomplish adaptation, integration, social control, or goal attainment for the system. Frequently, the use of effective communication in the group helps members to improve their communication skills and to transfer them to other systems (1).

Structural Aspects of the Group

Boundaries, autonomy, role differentiation, and hierarchy are characteristics of the group as a system. The boundaries of the group are determined by the group members and refer to the interaction among members and with the external environment. Groups have more or less autonomy from their environment, so that the degree of support and control given the group will vary depending on the agency, the leader, and the external environment (1).

As the group evolves, roles are developed among its members to promote adaptation, integration, and task and maintenance functions. The member filling a role is evaluated by other group members, both as a person and as a role, and in the evaluation will be placed above or below other group members in influence. In secondary groups, members tend to respond primarily to the role of the other; whereas in primary groups, the person is considered more important than the role he/she plays. When such rankings of each other as persons and roles reach a consensus among group members, the group is described as *stratified* (1, 65).

Some roles are standard within most groups and persist regardless of who occupies them, such as: (1) scapegoat, the receiver of group hostility, (2) clown, the giver or butt of humor, (3) peacemaker, the reducer of conflict, and (4) idol, the moral or social standard bearer. The clown role serves an important expressive function; the peacemaker serves an important integrative or social function (43).

The evolutionary process of a group as a system can be described in the following steps (1):

1. The group adapts to its environment; in response to adaptive behavior, members develop activities, sentiments, and interactions.

2. The group develops activities, sentiments, and interaction beyond necessary adaptations through goal-directed behavior.
3. As the group system elaborates, the group develops bonds, cohesiveness, norms, statuses, and roles.

4. In feedback fashion, adaptation is affected by the environment and by the direction of development of group members as a whole.
5. The group as a whole in turn modifies the functioning of its members. Members' behavior and sentiments become more alike.

PRINCIPLES RELATED TO GROUP PROCESS

Behavior Has Meaning

Everything that goes on in a group has some meaning. All activity of each member has significance — everything that is said, all of the movements made, and all of the verbal and nonverbal communication. It is impossible to attend to all of this behavior; however, it is just as problematic to attend only to the obvious. You need to recognize, as much as possible, the full dimension of what is happening within the group and to focus on the pattern of behavior that is appropriate at the time to the understanding and development of the person and the group.

Behavior Occurs on Different Levels

Behavior within the group takes place on two levels simultaneously — the cognitive and the affective. *Cognitive behavior refers to the intellectual understanding involved with the content of the task, conscious discussion of facts, information given for completion of designated goals or tasks, discussion of factual issues and topics about the members or others, and attention to procedural questions* (7). For example: How shall the group get started? What is the agenda for group sessions? What are the general rules for operation?

Affective behavior refers to the group morale and participation, influence of emotions upon members, nonverbal interaction within the group, interpersonal atmosphere and relationships, influence of members upon each other, styles and struggles of leadership, and degree of conflict, competition, and cooperation (7). A pertinent question to ask is, What is happening within the group? Group members seldom notice or recognize the affective level of group functioning, yet the affective level of the group frequently makes or breaks a group's effectiveness.

The cognitive level of functioning is relatively easy to recognize, but sensitivity and awareness are needed to observe affective behavior. Ask yourself the following questions to analyze affective behavior:

1. What is my general impression of the group?
2. What is the feeling generated within the group?
3. What feelings am I aware of within myself and the group generally: interest, boredom, anger, hopelessness, sadness, suspicion, guilt, loneliness, happiness, hope, distrust, disgust, or caution?
4. What are the clues that give me this impression? Am I aware of voice tone, facial expressions, body posture, gestures, and other nonverbal expressions?
5. What expressions of anxiety are present in myself and others? You must also be able to pick up indications of anxiety within the individual as difficult topics and experiences are dealt with, as well as anxiety within the group. Look for symptoms of anxiety when:
   a. The person manifests or complains of physical symptoms described in Chapter 12.
   b. The person frequently leaves the group, shifts in his/her chair, paces in the room, or demonstrates a variety of motor behaviors.
   c. The person appears inattentive, repeatedly asks for clarifications or restatements, is unable to follow directions, does not respond to another person's statements, seems unable to remember major points, or is ambivalent about planning.
   d. The person expresses irritability, mood changes, impatience, and impaired relationship with family, friends, or the group.

Being aware of feelings and manifestations of anxiety within yourself can be indication of the general anxiety level of the group.

The Existence of Dynamic Forces

Certain dynamic forces—intrapersonal, interpersonal, and environmental—operate within the group to facilitate communication, collaboration, understanding, commitment. These forces constitute group process. Ask yourself what is happening during the meeting. Try to envision the forces that bring about change.

Intrapsychic forces refer to energy that originates within the person—thoughts, feelings, ideas, fears, defensive maneuvers—as a result of the group's interaction. These forces will affect the person's behavior and development within the group, and therefore indirectly or directly will affect the entire group.

Interpersonal forces refer to energy and movement among the persons involved in the group as they move toward or away from each other, as they seek, avoid, support, or ignore each other. All members and the total group function will be affected by the interpersonal dyads or triads that develop, by the irritability or concern that members feel for each other, and by the willingness to listen, share, and compromise with one another.

Environmental forces refer to the external events or stimuli that reach and affect the person. Such stimuli could include a member's worries about his/her family or job; noise in a surrounding area; room temperature or decor; appearance, behavior, or smell of another group member; number of group members; or home or weather conditions. External events may seem minor, yet they can profoundly affect the person and the group process.

Principles of Group Dynamics

General principles of group dynamics that are important for you to know before you work with your own group include the following (98):

1. Attitudes of the person have anchorage in a group. It may be easier to change a person's attitudes by changing the group climate than by attempting to directly change the person.
2. Groups demand a certain degree of conformity from members. The closer and more cohesive the group, the more power it has over members' behavior.
3. Decisions made by a group obtain greater commitment from members than decisions arbitrarily imposed from outside the group.

4. Groups that are highly cohesive can overcome greater difficulties and frustrations in pursuit of group goals than can less cohesive groups.
5. Group cohesiveness is related to the degree to which members feel the group is meeting their needs.
6. People tend to be more effective learners when they are acting as group members than if they are acting as individuals in an audience situation.
7. Amount and nature of verbal interaction among members are a function of group factors. For example, in cohesive groups, views, opinions, and behaviors that are quite deviant from the consensus of the group are likely to be ignored, rejected, or punished.
8. Cooperation and communication are increased in groups where goals are mutually defined, accepted, and understood by the members.
9. Group climate or style of group life has an important impact on the personalities of members. The behavior of members may differ greatly from one group climate to another. The person who is hostile, aggressive, or disruptive in one group situation may behave very differently in another situation where the group climate is different.

Other principles related to using group process to change group behavior are:

1. Those who are to be changed and those who are attempting to influence change must have a strong sense of belonging to the same group —if the group is to be an effective medium for behavioral change.
2. The more relevant a person's attitudes, values, or behavior are to the purpose of the group, the more influence the group will exert on him/her in order to bring about change.
3. The greater the group member's prestige in the eyes of the other members, the greater the influence he/she can exert on the group.
4. Efforts to change a person's behavior so as to deviate from group norms will encounter strong resistance from the person.

All of these principles seem deceptively simple and self-evident, yet they are frequently violated, in attempts to achieve behavior change (23).

STAGES OF GROUP DEVELOPMENT

Every group, like the persons who make up the group, is unique and develops an individual style and identity. Research with therapy groups and observational studies of sensitivity groups indicate that the group has a broad pattern of development, divided into the following states of group movement:

Phase I — Formation of the Group

When several people initially come together with varied experiences and backgrounds, with or without previous contact, they usually come wanting to hide their real selves from others — in order to protect themselves. Each person within the group is unique and brings to the group everything he/she is, has been, and hopes to be. Each person has unique patterns of behavior; different emotional and intellectual needs; and individual defenses, feelings, expectations, and goals — yet all have more or less similar reasons for being in the group. Most group members are fearful of disclosure and are only willing to risk getting to know and be known after periods of testing. However, from the beginning, members will make decisions concerning group involvement based on the desire to be included (1).

At this point the group is an aggregation or a collection of individuals where members are independent and self-centered, with little affection and no real commitment for one another. Every member responds in his/her own way to the group experience but often feels isolated or lonely. The group, in varying times and ways, will be perceived as threatening to most individuals within the group; these individuals will then respond with a usual pattern to stress, such as aggression, withdrawal, competition, or vacillation (1).

Carl Rogers describes five steps or patterns that make up the first major phase (78):

1. *Milling around* — Initially there is a period of frustration; confusion; awkward silence; polite, superficial, or irrelevant conversation; self-preoccupation; intellectualization; and lack of continuity. The person may search for status or power, resist authority, or pair off or "gang up" with another.
2. *Resistance to personal expression or exploration* — Some people reveal rather personal atti-

tudes initially, which causes great ambivalence in the other members. Then gradually, although with fear and ambivalence, everyone will begin to reveal something about his/her private self.
3. *Description of past feelings* — Expression of feelings begins to assume a large proportion of the discussion.
4. *Expression of negative feelings* — Anger directed toward the group leader or group members is usually the first significant expression of feelings. Deeply positive feelings are more difficult and dangerous to express. The member may feel no one is interested in his/her problem at this early stage.
5. *Expression and exploration of personally meaningful material* — At this point, a member begins to reveal aspects of self in a significant way, a painful process that is directed inward to the self. The entire group may not always be receptive to the member's sharing of deep feelings.

During Phase I, members discuss structure of the group, what "freedom" means within the group, and how others interpret what the leader says. Each person struggles for security, as well as to maintain a personal identity, to regain equilibrium, and to adapt to the new situation. Later members gradually share their life experiences and permit others to enter their own personal territory. Conscious or unconscious agreement among members that each person has a unique place and that feelings, thoughts, and opinions are to be tolerated is essential in order to begin open discussion and move toward a group identity and a subculture (1).

Phase II — Change within the Group

In Phase II, the emphasis shifts from personal needs, goals, and desires to more collective identity with an expanded sense of self. The mood of the individual member changes. The members engage in more genuine, meaningful, open communication. Each one attempts to find a place within the group, and tries to evaluate the power he/she has, as well as the expectations of the group. The members gradually become more patient, respectful, cooperative, supportive, and oriented to planning. Members may seek or offer assistance. The leader must be supportive of the affective state and cognitive shift (1).

Every member begins to deal with the trust of self and others. Most people want to trust freely but are blocked by fears of rejection, betrayal, and exposure. These fears may have been generated by past experience and hurt with significant others, which has caused a lack of self-esteem and of self-trust. Trust might be defined as *risk*. Every member, as he/she is able to step out and risk self with the other members, begins to develop a feeling of trust and confidence. If this develops, the members move toward a deeper sense of safety and security. The more a member can trust, the more extensive will be the experience, and the more responsive he/she will be to himself and others.

As members begin to share important and private feelings and ideas about themselves, a change occurs within the group:

1. Members experience feelings of intimacy and closeness.
2. Members show the real self; this results in further expressions of feelings, both positive and negative. Each begins to perceive others as they really are.
3. Members show more empathy and concern for each other and are more confrontive as well as supportive.
4. Members feel more at ease with one another, and as a result the group will experience changes, new insights, new understandings, and a growing, healing process.
5. Members begin to learn and share more and to become more productive.

Into Phase II would fit five steps described by Rogers (78):

1. *Expression of immediate interpersonal feelings in the group*—The person states a feeling response positively or negatively to the speaker.
2. *Development of healing capacity in the group*—The person spontaneously shows a capacity for being helpful and therapeutic to others in emotional pain.
3. *Self-acceptance and the beginning of change*—The person shows more insight into self and own behavior and discusses goals for behavioral change.

4. *Cracking of facade*—Each person gently or savagely demands that all the others be the real self, drop the facade, and be more open and spontaneous. Defenses are torn down by the members working with each other.
5. *Individual receives feedback*—Each person expresses honest reactions about behavior.

Now the group members are socialized into the group; they accept and have internalized norms of caring and expression of feelings. They have sorted out the roles of facilitator (not always the group leader), conciliator, and others. The members begin to heal each other as they show caring for each other; members who do not show caring and patience are constrained by other members. Intimacy and cohesiveness are achieved as thoughts, feelings, and behavior are expressed; outsiders will be emotionally and physically rejected by the group. During this phase the group moves toward a goal if a goal has been established (1).

Phase III—Crisis within the Group

Phase III may occur at any time in the life of the group, or it may not occur at all. Because of the nature of the group process, the group may now regress back to an earlier stage, resolve the issue, or manage the issue somehow so it can proceed. Intense encounters of this phase are described by Rogers (65, 78):

1. *Confrontation*—Members express deep negative feelings very honestly, forcefully, and spontaneously as feedback to each other. Both the member speaking and the one being spoken to will need support from the group members and leader. Because of the directness, other group members may feel as rejected or anxious as the member who was spoken to.
2. *Helping relationship outside the group*—Members seek out each other between group sessions to show support, understanding, and caring, or to share experience. Such relationships also need to be shared within the group or the purpose of the group is no longer functional.
3. *Basic encounter*—Members change in interaction. This is one of the most central, intense, emotionally charged, and behavior-changing steps of group experience. Although negative

feelings were previously expressed to each other in an honest way, the relationship has grown and is now characterized by deep acceptance and warmth. Mutual exchanges of deep, positive, and caring feelings cause group members to feel acceptance from others and thus of themselves.

4. *Expression of positive feelings and closeness continues.*

5. *Behavior changes in the group*—Members change behaviorally because of the group process. The voice tone becomes less harsh and stronger in quality. The person acts with less facade and with more feeling. Members show considerable thoughtfulness to each other. This is the stage of affection among group members. However, if such positive outcomes do not occur, conflict in the group may cause disintegration or termination, since confrontation with caring is a basic function of the group. If positive caring attitudes are not present in the group, the group may use one of the following methods to resolve the ensuing negative feelings and conflict:

   a. *Elimination*—Members force the opposing person to withdraw from the group.

   b. *Subjugation or domination*—Members who are influential force others to accept their viewpoints.

   c. *Compromise*—Members who have formed factions give up something to safeguard the common interest of the group.

   d. *Alliance formation*—Members unite to form a partnership or speak for each other against another member.

e. *Integration*—Members of the group arrive at a solution that is satisfying to each member and more productive and creative than any single member's suggestion of solution. This is the height of group experience.

In this phase, conflict may be reduced by concentration on a supraordinate problem such as an external threat to the group. When the group achieves integration, both the components (individual members) and the system (the entire group) have their needs satisfied and goals met.

Phase IV — Termination of the Group

If there is no preceding Phase III of crisis, the group may proceed directly to the Termination Phase.

Separation of a group must be planned and prepared for in advance. If the group experience has been meaningful, there will usually be feelings of separation anxiety, loss, rejection, and abandonment. These feelings must be dealt with in the same manner as any other crisis or difficulties were dealt with. Through individual expression and mutual sharing, the resolution can promote personality growth and a strengthening of the person's ability to deal with stress and life itself, even while this experience comes to a close (1).

The group experience is difficult to describe; so much of it is in the realm of feelings. Only a positive group experience can help the person know the warm, safe emotional climate that encourages a deep sharing, a broader scope of thinking, and attitudinal changes.

GROUP GOALS AND FUNCTIONS

Group Goals

All groups are trying to reach at least one *goal, a target, aim, or long-range task that gives direction.* The group attempts to develop a product or an idea, or facilitates achievement of personal development. The major goal may be as simple as companionship or as specific as planning a party.

The focus of the group you work with depends on your objectives and encompasses the ability and

interest of each member to the extent possible. Frequently, the leader considers his/her goals so important that they tend to overwhelm the members' goals. The goals for the group should be: (1) known to the group, (2) attainable by the group, (3) rational, and (4) directed toward change. Additionally, the group might set up *secondary goals, short-term objectives that must be reached in order to accomplish the overall task.* For example, a specific goal for a group of hospitalized patients might be to prepare for an openhouse on the psychiatric unit. Secondary goals would include: (1) setting up a time schedule, (2) planning an outline, and (3) preparing pictures. An effective group has a clear understanding of its purposes and goals and is flexible in selecting its procedures as it works toward its goals (54).

One specific type of group, a therapy group, includes individuals who are having difficulty in coping with emotional stress and who have chosen to participate in a group situation led by a mental health expert to receive treatment. A therapy group is relatively unstructured; thus specific goals are different for each member and are difficult to set. However, in this instance, the primary objective of the group might be personal development and growth. The secondary goals may be unknown or may evolve as the group relationship develops and as members feel more secure (2).

As the group changes, the goals will change from unrealistic, absolutistic goals to more rational, attainable, growth-producing goals. The group may become a launching pad to assist the members to develop new ways of solving problems, not only within the group but also outside in other areas of living.

Group Functions

Careful analysis of any group will show *task functions, behaviors directed toward selecting and achieving the specific and primary goals of the group,* and *maintenance functions, activities that assist and support the welfare, morale, harmony, and relationship of the group* (54, 65). Task functions, which get a job done, include the behaviors shown in Table 11-2. Maintenance functions, which increase feelings of security, include the behaviors shown in Table 11-3.

Qualities That Enhance Group Functioning

Group development, maintenance, and goal achievement are enhanced by the following qualities: (1) constructive openness, (2) accepting atmosphere, (3) relatedness, and (4) responsibility.

Constructive openness refers to being open, to being able to disclose, share, facilitate, allow freedom, or expose oneself. Rarely when two or more

TABLE 11-2.   Task Functions of a Group

1. Initiating activity: The person suggests new ideas, solutions, or ways of handling a problem or organizing the group.
2. Seeking information: The person asks for clarification, information, or facts pertinent to the discussion.
3. Seeking opinion: The person asks for an expression of feelings, values or ideas.
4. Giving information: The person offers generalizations, facts, beliefs, or statements of personal experience in order to push what he/she thinks should become the group's view.
5. Giving opinion: The person states an opinion or belief about a suggestion or piece of information, based on personal values rather than facts.
6. Clarifying or elaborating: The person gives examples or develops meanings to help the group envision how a proposed solution might work.
7. Coordinating: The person shows relationships among various ideas or suggestions, pulling together new ideas or various activities.
8. Summarizing: The person restates suggestions, ideas, or proposed solutions after the group has discussed them.
9. Testing: The person examines the practicality of ideas, makes application of suggested solutions to real situations, and pre-evaluates.

TABLE 11-3.   Maintenance Functions of a Group

1. Encouraging: The person is warm, friendly, responsive to others, praises others and their ideas, agrees with or accepts another's ideas and statements, and pushes for group solidarity.
2. Expressing group feelings: The person summarizes the group feeling and reactions.
3. Harmonizing: The person mediates differences between other members or relieves tension and conflict through use of humor or pleasantries.
4. Compromising: The person yields, admits error, or moves from his/her original position in order to work out a conflict.
5. Gatekeeping: The person makes it possible for another member to contribute to the group by calling on him/her or by suggesting a time limit for talking to another. Thus communication channels are kept open.
6. Setting standards: The person states standards for the group to use in choosing a task, procedure, or solution. He/she reminds the group to avoid decisions that conflict with group standards.

people talk do they interact in such a manner that we could even use the term *open*. Most of us withhold our feelings, thoughts, and information about ourselves. If the person can be open and self-disclosing, he/she gains a new freedom to be his/her real self—to drop the facade—and to feel the pleasure of his/her own personality. Others respond to the openness as the person shares something about the self. Relationships begin and grow.

Openness involves risk taking. The degree of risk depends on a variety of factors. One factor might include the nature and intensity of the disclosed material. If the disclosure is of a highly personal nature, emotionally charged, and previously undisclosed, the risk is obviously greater than for a lesser issue. A second factor is whether the listener will receive the disclosure as the person intends. The risk is diminished if the discloser is certain that the receiver shares similar concerns and is sensitive to his/her needs. A third factor would be whether the receiver will react as the person intends. Too little self-disclosure results in limited opportunity for growth; however, self-disclosure that is too intense, too much, too fast, or too early can also have negative results. If the person is unable to discriminate when he/she or the relationship is ready for self-disclosure, his/her group position is jeopardized. Many times, group members who reveal material before they are emotionally ready will drop out of the group.

The risk of being rejected, exposed, or hurt is minimized by two qualities—an accepting environment and the degree of relatedness or involvement. The fear of being open is often great because of past experiences, patterns, and insecurities; thus the person may be unwilling to take a chance even though the desire to share is present. Time and patience are important. The group must wait until the member can share without coercion and without undue pressure. Rapid self-disclosure does not necessarily mean progress or growth; often too early self-disclosure achieves nothing except bruised feelings (104).

Accepting atmosphere relates to a climate that is psychologically safe for the group members. The leader sets the tone by conveying in every way possible that there is respect for each person as a unique human being and that all the members of the group are separate, special, and valued. The dignity of the person is respected. Even if all of the person's behavior is not acceptable, he/she is accepted. In turn, the person responds to such an environment, and potential for growth is seen in the person's attitude and capacity to change in response to the group.

Relatedness is defined as the emotional, perceptual, and cognitive capacity of a person to become involved with another (84). Relatedness refers to the realm of feelings and is more than the spoken word. Expression of feelings encourages the development of closeness and cohesiveness—a bond—within the group. Certainly relatedness or involvement is important for maintenance functioning.

Responsibility relates to the sense of obligation and dependability of members within the group and of the group as a whole entity. As the group becomes more open and involved, there must be a reciprocal honesty, reliability, accountability, and confidentiality between each participant. If there is to be continued growth and a sense of trust, the group must be trustworthy. The leader or other members should intervene so that no member is manipulated, probed, or denigrated by another.

CHARACTERISTICS OF AN EFFECTIVE GROUP

When is an assemblage of people a real group? When do these persons join together and work toward achieving the goals they have set up? A group exists when it:

1. Knows why it exists.
2. Has created an atmosphere in which its work can be done.
3. Has developed guidelines for making decisions.
4. Has established conditions under which each member can make a unique contribution.
5. Has achieved communication among its members.
6. Has developed a process whereby members give and receive help.
7. Has helped members to cope with conflict.
8. Can diagnose its processes and can improve its functioning through its members.

As a group progresses and grows together, achieving its major goals, it becomes increasingly effective. Effective groups have responsible, facilitating leaders as well as committed, working group members.

Emotionally Responsive and Facilitating Leader

The leader is the key to a successful group. The leader may set a democratic, autocratic, or laissez-faire climate. R. White and R. Lippett investigated the effects of these three styles on group performance and found that the democratic style resulted in increased friendliness and more group-mindedness, motivation, and originality (103). Certainly different leaders will promote different climates. Therefore, be aware of the type of leadership you create and be sensitive enough to observe the results of your methods. The leader is not a passive member but a role model for the members.

If the group has co-leaders, it is essential that their styles are not so different as to create conflict within the group. Smooth working relationships between co-leaders can provide a model for the group on how to relate and solve problems together. The combined personality strengths of co-leaders can strengthen the group.

Leadership may be either task (instrumental, adaptive) or social-emotional (expressive, integrative) in style. However, regardless of style, several rules must be followed by the leader. The leader will need to (1, 65):

1. Maintain the leadership role.
2. Live up to group norms; the higher the conformity, the higher the rank as a member.
3. Avoid giving orders that cannot or will not be obeyed, in order to avoid losing face.
4. Use established channels in giving directions.
5. Listen attentively to each member and the group as a whole.
6. Demonstrate self-knowledge as a model for the group and to avoid causing conflict in the group.

The form of leadership will determine the type of communication within the group. All communications may originate with a leader who is abrupt and forceful. Or communication between the leader and members can be slow, relaxed, and dispersed, so that leadership is decentralized. Energy changes between the leader and group members will determine which form of leadership is functional to the group system (1).

No leader is perfect. However, certain qualities contribute to group comfort. The first quality is security, since the more security you have within you (as leader), the more secure the group members will be with you. A sense of security also helps members to accept human nature and their own deficiencies if they see you are comfortable with your own limitations. Group members will certainly be able to recognize your strengths and your weaknesses. They will also be aware of the qualities you have as a person, what you say and what you don't say, and who you are. The more of life you have encountered and dealt with successfully, the more you will help the group members mature. What you are outside of the group influences what you bring to the group, and what you learn within the group will influence your behavior outside the group. You may not change life itself or the struggles and pain associated with it, but you can become more successful in coping and in living life more fully, and in turn, become more helpful to group members.

Another important quality of a leader is acceptance, warmth, and concern for others. This is hard to describe; there is no blueprint because much of this quality lies in the realm of feelings. If you have experienced talking to an accepting, empathetic person or had an empathetic group experience, you will understand the emotional impact. Perhaps the most important knowledge the person gains from experiencing empathy and acceptance is the conviction that he/she is important, unique, and worthwhile. This quality of acceptance will help carry a group through periods of frustration, hostility, and confrontation in the beginning and early-middle phases. Expression of negative feelings is neither encouraged nor discouraged; an open, accepting leader will enable the members to express any feelings they are experiencing, encouraging them to deal with the feelings honestly, and then to profit from the experience.

An equally important characteristic of a leader is listening with a "third ear," or for the unspoken word. A sensitive person listens with all senses and tunes into the feelings of others. To be sensitive means to be acutely aware of any and all of the messages sent by another in a variety of ways, to assess these messages, and to be able to find meaning in them. Practice using your total self to be sensitive to what the members and the group are saying.

In addition to a sense of security, acceptance and empathy, and sensitivity, you must have a capacity to love, laugh, and cry; spontaneity, yet restraint; compassion, yet objectivity; capacity to be assertive, yet to listen; perceptive of reality, yet creative and open to change.

Objectives and Responsibilities of the Leader

It is not enough to speak of the characteristics of a group leader. The leader is not only responsive but is also responsible. When you begin a group of any kind, you are accountable from the beginning and up to and through the last day and termination. Not only do you have the responsibility to share with the group what you are personally, but you have the responsibility to fulfill certain objectives to the best of your ability.

Advance Planning

As a leader, you are responsible for careful planning before the group begins. The following questions should be asked prior to making decisions about the group:

1. What type of group do I want—one that focuses on activity, support, insight, discussion, or reality orientation?

2. How does my agency regard group therapy? Will the group have agency support?

3. What are my strengths and weaknesses? Am I prepared to do group work? How can I learn more about leading groups?

4. Do I need a co-therapist? What are the advantages—validation or support from another person or another role model for the group?

5. Would I benefit from a supervisor or counselor who could help me validate group processes, rethink my leadership style, and help me become more effective in the group experience?

6. How will I choose group members? Should the group be homogenous, with all members having a similar problem? Should the group be heterogeneous, with a variety of problems presented? Can I handle the heterogeneous group, which is more lifelike? Is the group experience best for the client? Some people are not likely to function well in a group situation: for example, the manic-depressive patient who is very elated, the person with severe organic brain damage, the person who is

severely hearing impaired, or the person who has a lifetime pattern of being totally alone and depressed.

7. What are the members' needs? Will I have the time and opportunity to interview each one before the first meeting?

Orientation

The leader should orient the group members to the general purpose and plan of the group sessions and to the expectations of the members before the first meeting. Although this information must be repeated at the first session, the members should have some understanding prior to the meeting as to why they were chosen; they have the right to make the final decision about attending. The first session will also be less disorganized if members have received information previously about the group.

Physical Arrangements

The leader is responsible for physical and structural arrangements. Sessions may be held daily, or once, twice, or three times weekly. Starting time, duration of session, and place should be consistent. Whether the sessions are open or closed often depends on the format of the group and on the kind of clients and type of agency. In an *open format, new members are continually added and other members leave.* In a **closed format**, *the membership remains the same for the duration of the group.* Visitors to the group sessions are usually discouraged, so members should not bring their family or friends. The size of the group ideally should be between eight and twelve people so that all have an opportunity to interact. During the meetings, the seating arrangement should allow all members to see each other face to face; a circular arrangement is usually best. Mechanical equipment, such as movie or slide projector or tape recorders, is used for certain types of groups. Equipment should be obtained in advance and be in proper working order.

Appointment of Recorder and Observer

The leader decides whether or not to have a group recorder and observer. The *recorder takes notes of the session's proceedings; the observer does not participate but analyzes the group process with the leader.* These two service team members can validate with you as the leader about group process and thus enable the group to function more productively. Need for a recorder and observer will depend on the size, type, and goals of the group and on the leader's expertise.

Implementation

After the above considerations, you can begin your plan for group work. Be as prepared as possible, but once you begin, the best way to become skillful is to plunge ahead. Trust the group process and trust yourself. You are human and will make mistakes, but that very factor will draw you closer to your group.

During the formation of establishment phase of the group, you are responsible to (69, 107, 108):

1. Help the group get acquainted by defining the problem or reason for meeting.
2. Establish a group contract. It is up to you whether or not to have a contract, that is, an agreement between you and the members. The contract can be general or specific, depending on how it is established. Irving Yalom suggests that the leader contracts with the members concerning regular attendance, promptness, and completion of group experience. Confidentiality should be clearly understood. Open discussion of the contract and of all the feelings concerning any aspect of it is essential.
3. Help the group establish ground rules about appropriate behavior.
4. Invite trust gently, allowing distance when necessary.
5. Help members discuss feelings and thoughts about their expectations, misconceptions, or group experiences generally.
6. Redirect questions so that they are answered by members.
7. Help all members participate, calling on them if necessary.
8. Keep members' attention on goals, evaluating the group process as you go along.
9. Clarify issues as they arise.
10. Assist the recorder and observer in their roles, and clarify their roles to the group.

During the change or working phase, you are responsible to (58, 69, 107):

1. Call on the group to clarify, analyze, and summarize problems.
2. Permit verbal rebellion or expression of negative feelings. Ventilation and catharsis are useful. Through expressing feelings, the group member gains comfort, insights, and tools for relieving pent-up feelings of anxiety, guilt, and anger. Through this release and the sharing of feelings, thoughts, fantasies, and experiences, group members become better acquainted with one another. They learn to care about each other because of the mutually shared feelings and experiences.
3. Provide for security of the members and safety of property.
4. Clarify feelings, encouraging all members to state their feelings.
5. Help the group to move toward goals.
6. Encourage involvement, cooperative activity, and mutual support. As the group works and grows together, cohesiveness—a sense of belonging and togetherness—develops. The members get to know one another; this broadens into loyalty and closeness. The members begin to value one another and are then willing to work together more closely toward group goals. Cohesiveness creates a curative quality, relieving the feelings of isolation and loneliness. Once cohesive feelings have been firmly established, identification with the group begins. Members begin to share their feelings and learn from one another. Cohesiveness seems to be a significant factor in successful group outcome.
7. Observe for forces that block change or growth within the members. Obstructive manuevers include using silence, yawning repeatedly, moving around, assuming the therapist role, talking about the environment, overreacting to others' statements, acting out, monopolizing, being absent or late repeatedly, or making tangential associations.

Intervention to Avoid Blocking

Other forces that block change are individual role behaviors, resistance, transference, and counter-transference. Table 11-4 summarizes types of individual role behaviors, dynamics, and leader intervention. *Resistance can be defined as any psychological maneuver on the part of a group member to resist self-awareness, personal growth, change, or relationship with the group and other group members.* Feelings of apathy, hostility, or fear may be the cause of resistance. Defense mechanisms such as denial, projection, or isolation may be used. Resistance may result in a person breaking away from the group or destroying its progress. D. Benton describes the detrimental results when staff members are resistive in group therapy, especially when resistance is shown through absence or overt efforts to meet personal needs (6). The dynamics of resistance in group members are very similar to the dynamics encountered in the nurse-client relationship discussed in Chapter 6.

Transference refers to unconscious attachments directed to the leader or group members whereby feelings, attitudes, and experiences will be expressed that are appropriate to parental or other authority figures from the past. These feelings can be used to better understand the individual and his/her relationships and patterns of living. Transference behavior may be seen as over-acceptance, hostility, aggression, or distortion of others' statements. The transference phenomenon is used most frequently in insight therapy, but knowledge of it can be used superficially as a tool for understanding the emotional life of group members. Dynamics of transference behavior will be similar to what was discussed in Chapter 6.

Countertransference relates to the leader's unconscious or conscious emotional reaction to the individual group members. The leader may respond to certain members as he/she did previously to other people outside the group. These feelings may be positive or negative, and they may interfere with group change and growth. You will need to identify these feelings, especially the negative ones, such as boredom, fear, anxiety, apathy, or hostility toward the group or individual members. Counter-transference may be demonstrated by authoritarianism, overpermissiveness, overprotectiveness, or power struggling. These questions are appropriate to ask yourself:

1. What am I doing to cause these emotions?
2. Do any of the group members remind me of anyone I know or have known?

3. What do I feel about the individual group members?

4. What can I do about these feelings?

Dynamics of countertransference will be similar to those described under the nurse-client relationship in Chapter 6.

TABLE 11-4.   Summary of Dynamics of Individual Role Behavior and Leader Intervention.

INDIVIDUAL ROLE	THE "WHY" OF BEHAVIOR	INTERVENTION BY LEADER
Aggressor Attacks, disapproves, and expresses anger verbally; takes credit for other's ideas; shows envy.	Gaining distance from others. Ventilation of anxiety. Attacking own projections. Rejects others before being rejected by others.	Do not engage in verbal combat. Promote sense of security. Support other group members. Try to understand theme that has set off behavior and explore reasons for it. Reinforce for less aggressive behavior.
Blocker Resistant and stubborn. Blocks without reason; goes off on tangent. Argues; rejects others' ideas.	Passive expression of hostility. Fear of proceeding. Immobilized by anxiety. Attention-seeking.	Interpret hostility if appropriate. Support and clarify feelings to promote understanding. Give attention to positive behavior. Involve individual in process so he/she can receive reward for appropriate behavior.
Help-Seeker Tries to get sympathetic response by maneuvering others with statements of self-depreciation, insecurity, and confusion.	Example of emotional needs. Behavior is meaningful. Avoidance of problem.	Provide empathy and security. Acknowledge feelings. Promote group support. Clarify problem.
Playboy Lack of involvement in the group. Cynicism, clowning, flirting, mimicking, and joking around.	Sexual insecurity. Feelings of isolation. Insecurity with self; lack of knowledge and skill in carrying out identity.	Support. Evaluate own feelings. Remain matter-of-fact. Empathize. Help person to clarify self-identity and work through how to use positive aspects of personality in various situations.
Self-Confessor Expresses personal points of view, feelings, or themes irrelevant to group.	Unable to become involved with others. Lack of self-awareness. Seeking attention.	Reintegrate into group. Avoid promoting guilt. Clarify for yourself and others. Help group members work through resentment to person. Give attention to more appropriate behavior.

TABLE 11-4.   Continued

INDIVIDUAL ROLE	THE "WHY" OF BEHAVIOR	INTERVENTION BY LEADER
Dominator		
Asserts authority or superiority by monopolizing or manipulating members through flattery, interruptions, or giving directions.	Need to control. Feelings of inferiority. Seeking involvement by inappropriate behavior. Manipulation of others.	Encourage expression of fears. Enhance security. Involve individual in being helpful. Encourage group to be receptive. Clarify why person needs to manipulate. Assist group in coping with person. Reinforce individual for less dominating, listening, helpful behavior.
Special interest-pleader		
Introduces or supports suggestions related to personal concerns and philosophy.	Preoccupied with own conflicts. Avoidance of other problems. Demand for sympathy. Need to control ("do things my way").	Align group to assist in understanding person's conflicts. Focus on real issues. Give instructive attention and provide nurturance. Help person compromise, cooperate, and relinquish control.
Competitor		
Competes with others to produce best idea, be the best one, or gain leader's favors.	Personal insecurity. Because of fear, person cannot be cooperative.	Promote security. Explain how to be a cooperative member and to become involved.
Blackmailer		
Intimidates others into going along with personal schemes; threatens confidential content will be discussed outside group or that members will suffer harm.	Fearful. Inability to handle aggression. Desire for pseudocloseness.	Clarify fear in supportive way. Support individual to prevent his/her becoming increasingly fearful. Help with constructive use of aggressive energy. Provide real intimacy over time through group experiences.

Termination and Evaluation

During termination, you are responsible to:

1. Prepare the group for the time of termination and separation.
2. Help the group review, summarize, and evaluate the group existence.
3. Help the group separate physically and let go emotionally from each other.

Termination of the group occurs either when members have obtained optimal results from the therapy or when special circumstances occur with the leader, client, or agency. Termination should be talked about prior to the date set. Further treatment groups can be discussed with the members as well. Common reactions of the group member include:

1. Pride in accomplishment of behavioral change and increased self-worth.

2. Doubts about one's ability to carry on without the group.
3. Hostility toward the leader, demonstrated by open anger or through increased dependency. The whole group may be hostile, or the members may plan a ceremony similar to a graduation in order to formally mourn the felt loss and to separate.

As the leader, you also may find termination difficult. You may doubt the ability of the group members to get along and thus foster overdependency or feelings of rejection. Ideally, you should recognize the accomplishments of the group, help members to recognize their growth, and realize that optimal function of members was the original goal of the group. Hostility is likely to be felt by members (as well as by the leader) if the group must terminate for some reason beyond its control, or before the members feel they have resolved the problems of the group or of the individual members.

As the leader, you are responsible for evaluating yourself throughout the duration of the group. The checklist in Table 11-5 can be used. You will probably never be able to answer yes to every question on this list, but if your answers progress from "sometimes" to "often" to "usually," you will experience rewards from observing growth in group members and in realizing your own increasing effectiveness as a group leader. Working with a supervisor also helps to evaluate yourself, using the above questions. Clarifying with the group recorder and observer can further help you to evaluate your skill.

TABLE 11-5.   Self-Evaluation Form for Group Leader

1. Am I successful in reducing the member's anxiety about participating in this group?
   a. Do I encourage a warm-up period, with members becoming acquainted with me before the meeting begins?
   b. Do I relate with warmth, supportiveness, and nonthreatening humor?
   c. Do I arrange for a comfortable meeting environment?
   d. Do I have a matter-of-fact, businesslike approach if the group has many suspicious or unfriendly members?
2. Do I reward participation and promote progress toward group goals by verbal conditioning, smiling, or nodding my head?
3. Have I conveyed to the members during the orientation phase that participation is a group norm? Or do I talk too much and for too long?
4. Do I encourage all members to participate by doing the following:
   a. Accept contributions and work them into the group discussion so that the statement has meaning to the group?
   b. Make reluctant members feel their ideas are wanted and needed?
   c. Prevent talkative members from monopolizing or dominating without conveying rejection of them?
   d. Keep discussion and activity moving forward?
   e. Accept feelings and attitudes of all members as valid points for consideration?
   f. Protect persons whom other group members attack verbally?
   g. Accept conflict or disagreement as therapeutic if it is expressed reasonably and appropriately?
5. Can I keep quiet during pauses, so that group members realize their responsibility toward the group discussion?
6. Do I hear ideas and feelings expressed by members and restate them accurately in a more concise, clear form, thus conveying acceptance, attention, respect, and understanding—without necessarily indicating agreement?
7. Am I sensitive to nonverbal communication from group members? Am I empathic to sadness, apathy, hostility, or intense concentration?

TABLE 11-5. Continued

8. Do I ask questions that stimulate problem solving by clarifying situations, inquiring about feelings, raising alternative choices, and remaining nonthreatening?

9. Did I learn enough about each member before the group started? Do I keep sufficient contact with members between group sessions in order to promote a sense of trust and group cohesiveness and to be able to ask pertinent questions about a member's behavior?

10. Do I summarize periodically to move the discussion forward, to indicate progress, to restate the problem in a new light, or to point up differences that exist in the group?

11. Do I receive genuine feedback verbally, or do members tell me what they think I want to hear?

12. Do I keep the group interested by asking questions that are difficult enough, encouraging tasks that are neither too easy nor too hard, using a variety of techniques and formats for meetings, and promoting a sense of momentum by encouraging members to perform tasks or solve problems rather than personally doing all the work?

13. Do I use every possible opportunity to give the group real power to make choices? Do I consider that patient groups tend to be more conservative than staff in decisions and can usually be trusted about matters related to them?

14. Do I turn responsibility over to the group as soon as possible and take back from them as needed?

15. Am I relating to group deviants (or those with different opinions) wisely, conveying respect, providing for their emotional safety, and preventing scapegoating by members? When scapegoating appears, am I comfortable enough to look for and deal with members' feelings of worthlessness, fear of weakness, and fear of similarity to the deviant?

16. Am I contributing to group cohesiveness by encouraging members to make choices, agree on goals and norms and the means to achieve them, talk out and resolve differences, and review and alter goals as necessary so that the group remains therapeutic?

17. What is my leadership style?

18. Am I developing and rewarding qualities of leadership among the members? Do I support members who have the ability to draw out others? Do I encourage members to direct statements and questions to each other, not only to me? Am I quiet whenever possible?

19. Is the group moving toward its goals and am I facilitating progress by helping the group remain aware of its goals and the gains the members are making?

20. Am I flexible enough to revise goals as members progress or as circumstances change?

Role of the Recorder

The role of the recorder is to make notes on the ideas of the group. This will provide data for a content summary as well as help members to be more involved without the distraction of taking their own notes. The general theme of the discussion, quotes, specific content, sources, and summaries may be included. This information may be reported to the group from time to time as needed. A summary may be given at the end of each group session, or it can be typed and distributed at a later date. This information can also be used to clarify misconceptions or to give evaluations as needed. This information should be properly identified with the leader's name, group title, topic, date, number of group session, and recorder's name.

Role of the Observer

The role of the observer is to act as evaluator of the group process. This person should observe the manner in which the group works. Usually he/she does not participate in the general discussion but tries to be sensitive and empathic to the feelings without losing objectivity. The observer evaluates the group atmosphere, participation of members, effectiveness of leadership, group cohesiveness and productivity, and general flow of forces operating from moment to moment. The observer must also evaluate the nature and progression of the discussion. The observer should be aware of the group goals and should analyze how successful the group is in maintaining direction toward such goals, as well as describe achievement of these goals. The observer may use various tools, such as a graph, checklist, or sociogram, to assist in demonstrating dynamics to the group. Figure 11-1 is an example of a report form that may be used.

Leader's name: Observer's name: Group:

Date: Number of sessions:

Group size: Meeting time:

Physical facilities:

Group atmosphere: (mark on a scale of 1 to 5, with 1 being the highest score)

    Accepting   1   2   3   4   5   Rejecting   1   2   3   4   5

    Cohesive   1   2   3   4   5   Individualistic   1   2   3   4   5

Group stage of development:

Group goals:

    Movement in the direction of goals:

    Clarity of goals:

    Commitment to goals:

    Content toward goal achievement:

Leadership style: (check one)

    Democratic: Autocratic   Laissez-faire:

Leader effectiveness: (mark on a scale of 1 to 5)

    Participation   1   2   3   4   5   Resistance   1   2   3   4   5

Communication pattern:

Observer response:

FIGURE 11-1   Report of group process.

Committed, Working Group Members

Group members, as well as the leader and service members, have a responsibility to the group. All group members must assume responsibility for the way a group functions. The members' activities and behaviors contribute to group maintenance, move the group to its goals, and help the member achieve personal goals, *or* they block the group's performance.

Individual goals of a member may serve only

that member's self-interest, often at the expense of the group's productivity. Behavior that is irrelevant or destructive to group function includes a group member's lack of self-esteem, negative self-concept, inability to communicate appropriately with others, faulty interpersonal relationships, or anxiety related to the group situation. Table 11-4 summarized more specific dynamics behind individual role behavior and appropriate leader intervention.

The group member should prepare carefully before the meeting so that he/she can think through a problem, come to a conclusion, and then speak ideas clearly and concisely. Individual contributions may include expressing attitudes, facts, feelings, illustrations, examples, viewpoints, and questions. Each member should ask for clarification if statements are not clear; then he/she can summarize after a period of discussion, or ask the leader or another group member to summarize as necessary. The member should speak when he/she has something to say but listen attentively when others are contributing.

Observation of the group process and maintenance of an accepting climate are also the responsibility of group members. Each member should keep in touch with self and the group, contribute, prepare, observe, suggest, and support the total functioning of the group.

Figure 11-2 is a form that may help the group member to periodically analyze his/her behavior as a group member.

Evaluation of myself before group:

Evaluation of where I would like to go:
   Long-range goal:
      What can I do to achieve this goal?

Evaluation of group goals:

My participation in the group:
(Rate each of the behaviors listed on the following scale)
   1. Always
   2. Usually
   3. Often
   4. Sometimes
   5. Never

Behaviors:

	1	2	3	4	5
1. Make clear open statements.					
2. Paraphrase others' comments.					
3. Direct my comments to group members.					
4. Encourage others to participate.					
5. Listen attentively to other members.					
6. Share openly my feelings with the group.					
7. Give feedback.					
8. Help summarize.					
9. Work toward productivity.					
10. Check out perceptions.					
11. Support others in group.					
12. Stay actively involved.					

FIGURE 11-2   Group member self-evaluation form.

TYPES OF GROUPS

Whether you are knowledgeable in group process and accustomed to group work, or whether you are reading about group function for the first time, you should approach the task of group work as a new experience. Certainly all of your past knowledge is important, and it strengthens and deepens your ability to build a group. However, any group you work with, in any setting, is unique. Each group is a different experience in spite of similarities, because the group responds out of its own inner resources and experiences and has its own objectives.

The following pages discuss a variety of groups that you could initiate and maintain with emotionally ill clients in a variety of settings.

Reality Orientation Group

The purpose of reality orientation is to maintain reality contact and to reverse or halt the confusion, disorientation, social withdrawal, and apathy characteristic of residents in institutions (40). Reality orientation should be not only a technique to prevent confusion or disorientation but also a philosophy—a way of thinking about care of the patient. As a philosophy, reality orientation helps the staff recognize that regressive phenomena do not occur automatically in mental illness or old age and that expecting regression and treating the person as an infant will only reinforce such behavior.

Reality orientation has three components that

can be used simultaneously: (1) a 24-hour daily routine, (2) supplementary classroom experience, and (3) attitude therapy (40).

Twenty-four-hour reality orientation involves using every staff-patient contact to help the person know who and where he/she is, the time of day, the day of year, and the people who are present. Basic, current, and personal information is presented repeatedly to the person. Clocks with large numbers are in plain view. Calendars with big print are displayed and are checked off. Each person wears a readable name tag. Large lettering on doors and color codes on floors, walls, and doors help the person find his/her room and other areas on the ward. Any realistic response is reinforced with a smile, praise, or supportive statements. Staff members state what they are doing in all activities with the person. Repetition of information and reinforcing are essential. A sense of constancy and familiarity is maintained in order to help the person cope with daily living and unusual stressors (31, 40).

Supplementary classroom reality orientation is a simple form of small group work for severely confused and disoriented persons. A group of four to six residents meets daily for 30 minutes with a staff member who is familiar with each individual's total nursing care plan and needs. The immediate goal is to teach the group basic person-time-place information and to establish group participation in a structured setting. The classroom setting provides for personal attention in a firm, supportive environment. Classroom reality orientation for six weeks has been reported effective in reversing signs of memory loss, confusion, and disorientation for patients over 80 years of age (40).

Attitude therapy is basic to all reality orientation. A consistent attitude and approach maintained by all staff members when they care for the person or lead the group are essential to convey to the resident what is expected. One or a combination of the following five attitudes is prescribed as part of the treatment: active friendliness, passive friendliness, matter-of-fact, kind firmness, and no demand (40).

Reality orientation has been proven effective. After one year of treatment, hospitalized patients have achieved markedly improved behavior by showing more self-pride, greater socialization, improved manners, more interest in radio or television, and more concern with general appearance. Several studies have shown that 76 percent of regressed patients have improved (31, 40).

Reality orientation programs are useful in that some residents improve considerably in behavior, and all can be maintained at the functioning level that was observed on their admission to the institution. Thus regression typical of institutionalization can be prevented.

One reality orientation program with women in a state hospital helped the patients to again respond to their names. They also increased conversational and socialization skills, called other residents and attendants by name, followed directions, and increased accuracy of time orientation (40).

Reality orientation programs show that the elderly are capable of more physical and mental activity than commonly believed. A relationship certainly exists between expectancies and behavioral change. The attention given to residents through this kind of program reinforces appropriate behavior as well as the desire to be appropriate (40).

Staff involved in reality orientation programs usually consider themselves, and are considered, to be a special group, which increases their morale and thus improves their performance with and care for the residents (64).

The first reality orientation program was proposed and implemented by the Veterans Administration Hospital in Tuscaloosa, Alabama. Further information and training material may be obtained from the hospital.

Sample session

As each patient enters the day room, the nurse shakes his/her hand and greets the patient by name. "Good morning Mary" and "Hello Ann." Each person is given a large, easily seen name tag, which is pinned in a prominent place. Orientation to the room and one another is done with clearly stated words and adequate time. The pace is slow; eye contact for even a moment is considered important. Simple-level discussion about each person is done to clarify identity. Orientation to time, day, and place is done creatively, using visual materials such as newspapers, clocks, and calendars. The meeting time is kept short and without pressure. Comments can be made about weather, current events, and special days in order to orient the person to reality. Staff leading the group and group membership must be consistent to promote reality. Sessions last 20 to 30 minutes and should be continued on a regular basis as long as necessary.

Remotivation Group

Remotivation is a simple form of group work that

can be used in a community home, hospital, or senior day-care center. It is often used in combination with reality orientation groups. The goal of this therapy is to prevent disengagement, increase interest in reality, and stimulate thinking as the person focuses on simple objective aspects of everyday life. Institutionalized patients of any age may suffer the effects of emotional, social, and sensory deprivation, or withdrawal, depression, loneliness, alienation, confusion, disorientation, or disturbed thinking resulting from the loss of familiar faces and the new setting.

Remotivation sessions involve five specific steps (61):

1. *Creating a climate of acceptance.* About 5 minutes are spent greeting each person by name, expressing pleasure at his/her presence, and making encouraging remarks.

2. *Creating a bridge to the world.* About 15 minutes are spent talking about a topic of general interest that was chosen by the group at the previous session. Each person is encouraged to respond.

3. *Sharing the world we live in.* About 15 minutes are spent in further developing the topic just discussed. Visual aids are used in this step.

4. *Appreciating the work of the world.* About 15 minutes are used to discuss jobs that relate to the topic, how a commodity is produced, and the types of related jobs done in the past.

5. *Creating a climate of appreciation.* About 5 to 10 minutes are spent expressing pleasure in the person's attendance and contribution. Plans are made for the next meeting, which provides continuity and something to look forward to.

The group is usually limited to twelve sessions, one hour per session, with as many as fifteen people in a group. The leader can be a nursing attendant or lay person, although a professional nurse leader can add to the depth of the group. Nurses working with patients have reported change in life satisfaction after a series of remotivation groups. Remotivation kits may be obtained from the American Psychiatric Association in Washington, D.C.

Sample session

Refreshments of punch and cake are served in the Day Room as twelve to fourteen patients wander into the room. Each is greeted in a different way. Some are escorted and served a drink; others are greeted and encouraged to get whatever they would like. This beginning sets a *climate of acceptance.* People sit in a semicircle. The leader stands in the center and conducts the group in an organized classroom style. A simple topic is chosen and presented to the group. Today the topic is to be "green leaves." (The topic could be structured around an animal, nature study, poem, game, or any topic of interest that promotes reality.) The leader mentions the topic and that this subject was chosen by the group at the last meeting. Simple concrete statements are made, such as: "Leaves cover a tree," "Leaves are green," or "There are veins in leaves." Baskets of leaves are passed, and the patients smell, feel, and look. The leader stands in a circle talking to the group as well as speaking to individuals, thus trying to create a *bridge to the world.* Several patients tell about trees they like *(sharing the world we live in).* Questions are directed to the group to encourage continuation of the discussion. For example: "Trees grow fruit," or "Some people sit under trees." One person discusses a tree he knew when "he was a kid." Patients are encouraged to talk about past experiences to appreciate the *work of the world.* The leader comments about the responsiveness of each person. Patients begin to talk more as the session progresses. At the end of 45 minutes, the leader closes with summarizing remarks. Good-byes are said, and each name is stated. The leader expresses appreciation for their coming. Members are reminded of the next session. Thus a *climate of appreciation* is created as the session ends.

Activity Group

The goal of the activity group is to set up the structure and provide the direction of task accomplishment (82). The leader of this group, through support and encouragement, helps people cope with stress through an activity. Reality awareness, physical ability or dexterity, and learning abilities are enhanced (64).

The activity should also enable the people to experience accomplishment, sensory and cognitive stimulation, and encounters with others. The needs, characteristics, and interests of the clients, instead of those of the therapist, must be considered in planning the group. How often have you seen the activity director engrossed in making a doll or having a party while members of the group seem bored or uncomfortable? It is helpful for the leader to have a consistent group so that relationships can be developed. The leader can then plan activities based on knowledge of the group. The activity groups might be involved in such tasks as having a party, modeling with clay, doing exercises, or sketching a large picture together.

Activity groups can be useful with regressed, withdrawn, and immobilized clients when tasks are planned to meet specific needs. However, not all patients need an activity group. For example, activity groups are very popular in institutions for long-term or chronic illness, but the emphasis is often only on the physical task. Here every group has to be doing something, even if it is only physical exercises. Every group has to be a happy, cheery one. Apparently staff members may be more comfortable with activity rather than with feelings, *doing* rather than *being,* treating the superficial rather than the more honest deeper thoughts and encounters. Unfortunately, such staff members may not realize the feelings of pain, resentment, and frustration that can underlie the happy facade. In such a group, the patients learn not to talk about feelings. Possibly the leader is not able to tolerate the pain, loneliness, and suffering. The clients' feelings may come out in physical complaints, hopelessness, or further withdrawal. Thus activity groups should be planned to meet emotional and social as well as physical needs.

Sample session

The leader greets six chronically ill schizophrenic patients as they enter the Activity Room. The group has been meeting for 24 sessions, so several patients speak to or nod to one another. After a period of greeting and social talk to adjust to one another and the new setting, the activity begins. The leader has prepared a sheet of paper and several colored crayons for each person on a large table. The leader asks each member to draw a picture about anything he/she wishes. Several begin to work; others need encouragement. Some pictures are colorful; others somber. One patient draws straight lines carefully and with reluctance. Each patient is encouraged to talk about his/her picture, telling what and who it represents. One large sheet is laid on another table and patients are told they can draw a picture on a group mural if they wish. Several patients look at the sheet without touching it. One draws a small picture in the corner. Another feels secure enough about his identity so that he draws a small face. Time is called. Refreshments are served while members haltingly discuss their pictures. One member is mute and eats the candy vigorously. Others are able to talk about their feelings. Little is said as the clients leave, except for the leader who praises each for coming and gives encouragement for them to return.

Reminiscing Group

The goal of the reminiscing group is to allow members an opportunity to share their thoughts and feelings about their past life. Members are usually elderly, but some could also be younger and facing death through terminal illness. R. Butler spoke of the life review as a common process in the elderly, especially as death becomes more imminent. As this process occurs, the past is considered and dealt with in preparation for death (21). The reminiscing process is natural, universal, and adaptive.

A reminiscing group is useful to the aged because members share experiences and participate with one another, gain a new perception of self and others, and review historical and significant events of their time (30).

Reminiscing groups may be long-term or short-term, formal or informal, structured or spontaneous. A democratic climate is essential. The leader might plan a topic for the session, such as travel, foods, animals, or historical eras. Pictures, records, music, or various objects could be used to stimulate discussion. Or members could spontaneously discuss whatever topic is of interest. As the group grows in trust, conversation moves from the superficial to more intimate and emotionally loaded levels.

For example, one 89-year-old man in a reminiscing group told the author, who was the group leader, about five short events; each event related to rejection by or loss of a loved one. As he reminisced, he became increasingly tearful. The leader responded by asking if he was concerned about what would happen to his relationship within the group. The discussion that followed centered on trusting the leader and the group.

If you truly accept the elderly or terminally ill, you will acknowledge and be interested in his/her past life. Most of what this person is lies in the past and present, for not a great deal of future remains. Encouraging this person to talk about the past promotes better acceptance of self and the current situation. The sense of self-worth increases as the leader acknowledges the person's past experience and wisdom.

Sample session

The leader begins the group by asking, "What comes

to your mind for discussion today?" The members are accustomed to the broad opening and are comfortable with the leader and with each other.

One petite lady with beribboned, silver-gray hair begins by telling the group she saw a robin that morning. This is a fairly neutral topic. An Italian man replies, "That means spring is on the way." This leads into a discussion of previous springs. Jerry, a spry Irishman, laughs and replies, "It was the spring of 1892 when I was working through New England selling violins. I was a pusher of instruments, just like Music Man." As he tells the group about his lucrative position, the other members laugh, and he joins in. He obviously enjoys telling the story.

Feelings of joy, pleasure, humor, and sadness are evident in the group. The group sits quietly, and the leader asks if anyone could say what he/she is feeling. Mary answers, "It was good to hear, but the sadness is that it's gone." Jerry states, "Yes, but there is each day to be lived." After a few more minutes of discussion, the group ends the session with coffee or tea and cookies. With the sharing of events and memories, a closeness prevails (64).

The sharing of memories is adaptive and promotes a bonding with others. It reaffirms individual identity, position, and personal worth, and in turn reduces loneliness and isolation.

Support Group

The primary goals of the support group are to present information about normal changes in life and crises of living and, through informal group contact, to bring about individual growth and the ability to cope with these changes. A pilot Geriatric Arthritis Program was set up at the University of Michigan Hospital. Four support groups were formed; themes like depression, social isolation, and sensory losses were discussed repeatedly. Brainstorming covered such topics as memory, vision, hearing, interpersonal relationships, health management, housing and relocation, dying and death, and how to anticipate or cope with various situations. Role-playing, group techniques, and group exercises were used to encourage expression, experience, and problem solving.

Increasingly health care agencies are sponsoring groups for people with emotional illness, heart disease, strokes, cancer, diabetes, ostomies, cystic fibrosis, or other illnesses in order to allow the identified patients and their families to meet regularly, as long as needed, to talk through their feel-

ings, concerns, and problems of adjustment, and to give support to each other. Some agencies sponsor groups for widows or widowers. Often a psychiatric nurse is the leader of a group. Support groups can be maintained for clients during hospitalization, predischarge, and after discharge.

Sample session

A group of people of varying ages arrives at the center, and each one finds a comfortable chair in the circle in the group room. The atmosphere seems subdued and quiet. Talking is minimal. Some members appear physically ill; others do not. Several appear to be adolescents; others are young adults; and four or five are middle-aged. The leader asks the members, "What do you want to talk about today?" Several members begin talking at once; all are alert and interested. This is the tenth session of a group of people suffering varying stages of advanced cancer. The group is in the working stage of development and trust, and relationships are well established. Sharing physical complaints and experiences are common. Several persons have more immediate needs, and time is given to their crises and difficulties: "I really had a difficult week." "They couldn't get in with their needles." "My body feels like it is heavy and bloated." More feelings are expressed: "I'm scared." "I get so down; feel like I'm going into Hell." Other members are quick to support one another and to offer words of concern and help. The group moves from expression about physical complaints to emotional levels of belonging, guidance, support, nurturing, caring, and love. Some members hug and cry. The expression of feelings is open and demonstrative. Topics of life, death, loss, rejection, and family problems are discussed. The feeling of depression and heaviness lifts; the closeness is uplifting. The time to close comes too soon, and members comment, "Life is hard but when there is togetherness, it can be so much better." "I feel so much more relaxed—like living again." The group breaks for the evening, but the members are very much together in spirit and support, which will help sustain them for the coming week.

A major benefit of a support group is to help members realize the universality of their problems. Most older or ill people feel that no one has the same difficulties as they experience. When they hear that others share in the same dilemma, it can be a "discovery of not being alone." Also, as the topic is discussed and solutions to the problem are given, some people might be able to find answers to their own problem.

Loss is a universal theme. A group of elderly patients led by this author for one and one-half years discussed the theme of loss repeatedly. At one session there were two empty chairs: one member had died and one had been discharged since the last meeting. No one would sit in the two chairs formerly occupied by the two lost members. The other members immediately spoke of the two missing persons. As the group discussed the two men, the experiences associated with them, and the jokes told by them, the group members appeared more and more depressed. Apparently they were allowing themselves to experience the feelings they had previously tried to deny. One man stated, "Well, it's like when you are in the Army. Your buddy goes to the front line and never comes back. You learn never to have a buddy again." In essence, he was saying it hurts to lose a friend. Rather than be hurt again, he wanted to protect himself and not become involved again. However, after much discussion, the members agreed it was unwise to withdraw. As one 80-year-old man said somberly, "Without others, you are very lonely." Another gave the group hope when he said, "As one door closes, others will open up."

Closely related to loss is the subject of death. This subject frequently comes up in group sessions. One of the author's groups began with twelve patients. Over the course of two years, six patients died. Every group member was aware of the decreasing size of the group, but several times members voted not to allow new members to join. One patient said to the leader, "One day you'll be the only one left." This statement indicated that he thought death was only for the elderly. Death is the end, a wrap-up of what life has meant, a closure, and a judgment. One patient, almost 95-years old, stated, "Death is like summing up a column of numbers and coming up with a total." Contrary to the attitude of younger people, older people realize that their chances are few to redo life or to give life new meaning. One patient said, "To give my life meaning, I need something to do, someone to love, something to look forward to." From this statement we can understand the sense of hopelessness and worthlessness that many elderly people are likely to experience.

Group Process Group

The major goal of the group process group is one of personal growth and team building. The group

promotes resolution of motives and conflicts, and this brings about personality change (5, 44). The members come together with personal motives, a desire to develop, disclose, and be more open. At the same time, there is a holding back and a fear that the disclosure will be foolish. The restrictive solution is to withdraw, keep quiet, or pull back. The enabling solution is to risk involvement although there is fear that it will not be safe emotionally (5). This describes the forward and backward process that occurs in any successful group. This kind of group discusses the motives and fears and becomes aware of the conflict situations.

The approach of J. M. French (32) and D. Whitaker and M. Lieberman (102) discusses the fear responses of group members to conflict situations. See also Banet (5) and Rosenbaum and Snolowsky (82). This focal conflict can be a here-and-now behavior stemming from past conflicts developed early in life.

The facilitator may ask the members to describe their wishes. These wishes may include to be happier, to be closer to others, to be approved of, or to be loved. Members also talk about fears, such as fear of holding back, being rejected or laughed at, feeling stupid, losing control, or making others angry (5). Such wishes and motives can evoke feelings of fear; but arriving at solutions and sharing feelings or becoming involved will decrease the fearful feelings and can help the person mature.

Sample session

John, the leader begins the eighth session of the group by asking the members to discuss their thoughts and feelings. Mary responds by telling John she is beginning to care for him but has been reluctant to say this. As John asks her to tell more about her feelings, she begins to blame herself, "I feel so dumb. It's so easy to be angry, to tell you what I don't like, but these new feelings are beginning to come out." (Expressions of feelings of warmth and love usually come later in the development of a group and may be more frightening than negative expressions.) John asks about Mary's fears; he asks her to describe her feelings and how she pictured what would happen if she told him. Other members relate their experiences with the same feelings. Most members become involved in the discussion and are able to share feelings. The feelings generated by an enabling solution and discussed because of Mary's willingness to risk bring a sense of closeness and security within the group and increased self-esteem for individual members.

Growth Group

The goal of the growth group is to increase the personal growth of the members, depending on personal needs and level of experience. The focus is on developing a person's potential and increasing his/her personal sensitivity and ability to problem solve. Growth groups may be comprised of new mothers, pastors, teachers, clients with psychiatric or other diseases, or nursing or medical students. A variety of roles, professions, and common bonds can enable a group of people to join together for a group experience to promote self-acceptance, self-awareness, and increased self-esteem. The common bond enables the group to have similar stressors or issues to discuss. D. Walton found a significant positive change in personal growth of college students who participated in fourteen one-hour growth group sessions (99).

M. Coleman and P. Glofka studied senior nursing students in their psychiatric experience and found positive growth with increased self-esteem (25). Similar results have been found by others (28, 29).

The leader encourages the members to discuss stressful situations and feelings about their own experiences as well as give to and receive support from others. At times, intervention is based on the human relations approach and emphasizes conscious phenomena and emotional expression.

Psychotherapy Group

The goal of the psychotherapy group is to heal the troubled mind or to achieve major personality change with treatment in a group setting. This may mean that classical or modified analytic methods are used by the therapist. The treatment is not carried out by the group interaction but by the relating of life, historical development, resolution of transference phenomena, neutralization of resistance, interpretation of dreams, and resolution of intrapsychic conflicts. Regression and dependency are allowed, and symbolic reactions are analyzed to

be understood. Ventilation of feelings without gaining deeper understanding is discouraged (82).

Sample session

A group of six persons has come together for a group session that meets three times a week. The leader asks who would like to start today. The group session begins with the members giving an account of disagreeable situations or symptoms they have been suffering. The primary goal at this point is relief and greater comfort. Each member tells his/her difficulty. For example: "I get poor grades." "My daughter is leaving home and I can't handle it." "I fight with my husband all the time." "I don't have any problems, but my head aches." John seems to have more insight as he states, "My problem is my relationship with my parents; I have some real conflicts." He does not know precipitating reasons for the conflicts, but as he looks for answers, he discovers some. The group is relatively at ease; so one by one, they discuss in more detail their life situations. Finally John says, "You guys said what you had to say real well. I've had symptoms too, including ulcers and high blood pressure. I went to school and didn't finish. Went into the Army and became disinterested. I've been bouncing around the last three years—even got married to a pretty fine girl, but that didn't solve my problems. There were bouts of drink, travel, highs, and lows. Now I'm low and I thought maybe you guys could help. I feel like I've had too much mother." A general voicing of resentment toward mothers follows, which is interrupted when the leader says, "Well, we need to close for the day. We didn't get around to everyone having a chance to talk. We have to continue to work next session."

Thus the leader acknowledges through a summary of the session that the group participation was meaningful and that the group would continue. Therapy is a learning process. The first step toward insight has been taken. Insight is the perception of relationships—the affective and intellectual understanding of behavior, which may follow an interpretation by a therapist, or at least the person looking into him/herself. The leader shares insights with group members when he/she feels the member can assimilate the interpretation. Insight and interpretation follow clarification and support.

REFERENCES

1. Anderson, Ralph, and Irl Carter, *Human Behavior in the Social Environment.* Chicago: Aldine Publishing Co., 1974.

2. Arnhart, Emelia A., "Establishing Group Work in a Psychiatric Unit of a General Hospital," *Journal of Psychiatric Nursing and Mental Health Services,* 13, no. 1 (1975), 5–9.

3. Bains, J., "Effects of Reality Orientation Classroom

on Memory Loss, Confusion, and Disorientation in Geriatric Patients," *The Gerontologist,* 14 (1974), 138–42.

4. Balgopal, P., "Variations in Sensitivity Training Groups," *Perspectives in Psychiatric Care,* 11, no. 2 (1973), 80–86.

5. Banet, Anthony C., "Wishes and Fears," in Ed Jones, John Pfeiffer, and J. William Pfeiffer, eds., *The 1975 Annual Handbook for Group Facilitators,* pp. 118–19. La Jolla, Calif.: University Associates, Inc., 1975.

6. Benton, Denise, "The Significance of the Absent Member in Milieu Therapy," *Perspectives in Psychiatric Care,* 18, no. 1 (1980), 21–25.

7. Blocher, Donald, *Developmental Counseling.* New York: The Ronald Press Company, 1966.

8. Bormann, Ernest, *Discussion and Group Methods: Theory and Practice.* New York: Harper & Row, Publishers, Inc., 1969.

9. Boucher, Michael, "Personal Space and Chronicity in the Mental Hospital," *Perspectives in Psychiatric Care,* 11, no. 5 (1971), 206–10.

10. Boylin, William, S. Gordon, and M. Nehrke, "Reminiscing and Ego Integrity in Institutionalized Elderly Males," *Gerontologist,* 16, no. 2 (1976), 118–24.

11. Bradford L., and Dorothy Mial, "When Is a Group?" *Educational Leadership,* 21 (1963), 147–51.

12. Brown, Frances, "Therapeutic Group Discussions," *American Journal of Nursing,* 58, no. 6 (1958), 836–39.

13. Browne, Louise, and Jennie Ritter, "Reality Therapy for the Geriatric Psychiatric Patient," *Perspectives in Psychiatric Care,* 10, no. 3 (1972), 135–39.

14. Burgess, Ann, and Aaron Lazare, "Nursing Management of Feelings, Thoughts and Behavior," *Journal of Psychiatric Nursing and Mental Health Services,* 10, no. 6 (1972), 7–11.

15. Burnside, Irene M., "The Patient I Didn't Want," *American Journal of Nursing,* 68, no. 8 (1968), 1666–69.

16. ——, "Group Work among the Aged," *Nursing Outlook,* 17, no. 6 (1969), 68–71.

17. ——, "Group Work with Aged," *Gerontologist,* 10 (1970), 241–46.

18. ——, *Psychosocial Nursing Care of the Aged.* New York: McGraw-Hill Book Company, 1973.

19. ——, "Overview of Group Work with the Aged," *Journal of Gerontological Nursing,* 2, no. 6 (1976), 14–17.

20. ——, *Nursing and the Aged.* New York: McGraw-Hill Book Company, 1976.

21. Butler, Robert, "Intensive Psychotherapy for the Hospitalized Aged," *Geriatrics,* 15 (1960), 644–53.

22. ——, "The Life Review: An Interpretation of Reminiscence in the Aged," *Psychiatry,* 26, no. 1 (1963), 65–76.

23. Cartwright, D., "Achieving Change in People: Some Applications of Group Dynamics Theory," *Human Relations,* 3 (1951), 381–92.

24. Citrin, Richard, and David Dixon, "Reality Orientation—A Milieu Therapy Used in an Institution for the Aged," *The Gerontologist,* 17, no. 1 (1977), 39–43.

25. Coleman, Margaret, and Peter Glofka, "Effect of Group Therapy on Self-Concept of Senior Nursing Students," *Nursing Research,* 18, no. 3 (1969), 274–75.

26. Culbert, S. A., "The Interpersonal Process of Self-Disclosure: It Takes Two to See One," *Explorations in Applied Behavioral Science.* New York: Renaissance Editors, 1967.

27. Durkin, Helen, *The Group in Depth.* New York: International Universities Press, 1964.

28. Dye, Celeste F., "Self-Concept, Anxiety, and Group Participation: As Affected by Human Relations Training," *Nursing Research,* 23, no. 4 (1974), 301–6.

29. Dyer, E. et al., "What Are the Relationships of Quality Patient Care to Nurses' Performance, Biographical and Personality Variables," *Psychological Reports,* 36, no. 1 (1975), 255–66.

30. Ebersole, P., "From Despair to Integrity through Reminiscing with the Aged," in *A.N.A. Clinical Sessions.* New York: Appleton-Century-Crofts, 1975.

31. Folsom, J., "Reality Orientation for the Elderly Mental Patient," *Geriatric Psychiatry* (Spring 1968), pp. 291–307.

32. French, J. M., *The Integration of Behavior,* vols. 1 and 2. Chicago: University of Chicago Press, 1952 and 1954.

33. Giambra, Leonard, "Daydreaming about the Past: The Time Setting of Spontaneous Thought Intrusions," *The Gerontologist,* 17, no. 1 (1977), 35–38.

34. Giffin, Kim, "Adulthood and Old Age," *The Gerontologist,* 9, no. 4 (1969), 286–92.

35. Goldberg, Carl, *Encounter: Group Sensitivity Training Experience.* New York: Science House, Inc., 1970.

36. Goldfarb, A., and H. Turner, "Psychotherapy of Aged Persons—Utilization and Effectiveness of Brief Therapy," *American Journal of Psychiatry,* 109 (1953), 916–21.

37. Guinan, James, and Melvin Faulds, "Marathon Group:

Facilitator of Personal Growth?" *Journal of Counseling Psychology,* 17 (1970), 145–49.

38. Hallowitz, E. et al., "Small-Group Process in Teaching Human Sexuality," *Health Social Work,* 3, no. 11 (1978), 131–51.

39. Harris, C., "The Florida State Hospital Patient Behavior Rating Sheet," in J. Cane and R. Hawkins, eds., *Behavior Assessment: New Directions in Clinical Psychology.* New York: Brunner & Mazel, Inc., 1976.

40. Harris, Clarke, and Peter Ivory, "An Outcome Evaluation of Reality Orientation Therapy with Geriatric Patients in a State Mental Hospital," *The Gerontologist,* 16, no. 6 (1976), 469–503.

41. Harris, Gloria, ed., *The Group Treatment of Human Problems.* New York: Grune & Stratton, Inc., 1977.

42. Hinckley, Robert, and Lydia Hermann, *Group Treatment in Psychotherapy.* Minneapolis: University of Minnesota Press, 1951.

43. Homans, George C., *The Human Group.* New York: Harcourt Brace Jovanovich, Inc., 1950.

44. Jones, John, and J. William Pfeiffer, *The 1975 Annual Handbook for Group Facilitators.* La Jolla, Calif.: University Associates, Inc., 1975.

45. Kalkman, Marion, and Anne Davis, *New Dimensions in Mental Health Psychiatric Nursing.* New York: McGraw-Hill Book Company, 1974.

46. Kastenbaum, Robert, *New Thoughts on Old Age.* New York: Springer Publishing Co., Inc., 1964.

47. Kellerman, Henry, *Group Psychotherapy and Personality Intersecting Structures.* New York: Grune & Stratton, Inc., 1979.

48. Lazarus, Lawrence W., "A Program for the Elderly at a Private Psychiatric Hospital," *The Gerontologist,* 16, no. 2 (1976), 125–31.

49. Lewin, Kurt, "Frontiers in Group Dynamics: Concept, Method and Reality in Social Science; Social Equilibria and Social Change," *Human Relations,* 1 (1947), 5–42.

50. Lewis, C. N., "Reminiscing and Self-Concept in Old Age," *Journal of Gerontology,* 26 (1971), 240–43.

51. Lieberman, M., and J. Falk, "The Remembered Past as a Source of Data for Research on the Life Cycle," *Human Development,* 14 (1971), 132–41.

52. Linden, M., "Group Psychotherapy with Institutionalized Senile Women," *International Journal of Group Psychotherapy,* 3 (1953), 150–70.

53. ——, "Transference in Gerontologic Group Psychotherapy," *International Journal of Group Psychotherapy,* 5 (1955), 61–79.

54. Lippitt, Gordon, and Edith Seashore, *The Leader and Group Effectiveness.* New York: Association Press, 1962.

55. Loomis, Maxine E., *Group Process for Nurses.* St. Louis: The C. V. Mosby Company, 1973.

56. Luft, Joseph, *Group Process: An Introduction to Group Dynamics.* Palo Alto, Calif.: National Press Books, 1970.

57. Manaster, Al, "Therapy with the 'Senile' Geriatric Patient," *The International Journal of Group Psychotherapy,* 22 (April 1972), 250–57.

58. Marram, Gwen, *The Group Approach in Nursing Practice.* St. Louis: The C. V. Mosby Company, 1973.

59. Masnik, R. W., et al., "Coffee Groups; A Nine-Year Follow-up Study," *American Journal of Psychiatry,* 137, no. 1 (1980), 91–93.

60. Matheson, Wayne E., "Which Patient for Which Therapeutic Group," *Journal of Psychiatric Nursing and Mental Health Services,* 12, no. 3 (1974), 10–13.

61. McClelland, Lucille, *Textbook for Psychiatric Technicians.* St. Louis: The C. V. Mosby Company, 1971.

62. McCordie, Wm., and Sharon Blom, "Life Review Therapy: Psychotherapy for the Elderly," *Perspectives in Psychiatric Care,* 17, no. 4 (1979), 162–66.

63. McMahon, A., and P. Rhudick, *Psychodynamic Studies on Aging: Creativity, Reminiscing, and Dying.* New York: International Universities Press, 1967.

64. Meerloo, J., "Modes of Psychotherapy in the Aged," *Journal of the American Geriatrics Society,* 9 (1961), 225–34.

65. Mills, Theodore, *The Sociology of Small Groups.* Englewood Cliffs, N.J.: Prentice-Hall, Inc., 1967.

66. Moody, Linda, Virginia Baron, and Grace Monk, "Moving the Past into the Present," *American Journal of Nursing,* 70, no. 11 (1970), 2353–56.

67. Morrison, Malcolm, "A Human Relations Approach to Problem Solving," *The Gerontologist,* 16, no. 2 (1976), 185–86.

68. Murray, Hazel R., "Group Work with Aged Blind Japanese in the Nursing Home and in the Community," *The New Outlook for the Blind,* 69, no. 4 (1975), 160–64.

69. Murray, Ruth, M. Marilyn Huelskoetter, and Dorothy O'Driscoll, *The Nursing Process in Later Maturity.* Englewood Cliffs, N.J.: Prentice-Hall, Inc., 1980.

70. Nordmark, Madelyn, and Anne Rohweder, *Scientific Foundations of Nursing,* 2nd ed. Philadelphia: J. B. Lippincott Company, 1967.

71. O'Dell, Stan, and Gary Seilir, "The Effects of Short-Term Personal Growth Groups on Anxiety and Self-

Perception," *Small Group Behavior,* 6, no. 3 (1975) 251-69.

72. Ofske, Richard J., *Interpersonal Behavior in Small Groups.* Englewood Cliffs, N.J.: Prentice-Hall, Inc., 1973.

73. Ohlsen, Merle, *Group Counseling.* New York: Holt, Rinehart and Winston, 1970.

74. Petty, Beryl, T. Moeller, and R. Campbell, "Support Groups for Elderly Persons in the Community," *The Gerontologist,* 15, no. 6 (1976), 522-28.

75. Powdermaker, Florence, and Jerome Frank, *Group Psychotherapy, Studies in Methodology of Research and Therapy.* Cambridge, Mass.: Harvard University Press, 1953.

76. Rogers, Carl, *On Becoming a Person.* Boston: Houghton Mifflin Company, 1961.

77. ____, "The Process of the Basic Encounter Group," in *Challenge of Humanistic Psychology,* ed. J. F. T. Bugenthal, pp. 260-76. New York: McGraw-Hill Book Company, 1967.

78. ____, *Carl Rogers on Encounter Groups.* New York: Harper & Row, Publishers, Inc., 1970.

79. ____, "Carl Rogers Describes His Way of Facilitating Encounter Groups," *American Journal of Nursing,* 71, no. 2 (1971), 215-19.

80. Robin, Herbert, and Max Rosenbaum, *How to Begin a Psychotherapy Group: Six Approaches.* New York: Gordon & Breach, Science Publishers, Inc. 1976.

81. Rohrbaugh, Michael, and Bryon Bartels, "Participants' Perceptions of 'Curative Factors' in Therapy and Growth Groups," *Small Group Behavior,* 6, no. 4 (1975).

82. Rosenbaum, Max, and Alvin Snolowsky, *The Intensive Group Experience.* New York: The Free Press, 1976.

83. Rounsaville, B., et al., "The Natural History of a Psychotherapy Group for Battered Women," *Psychiatry,* 42, no. 2 (1979), 73-78.

84. Rouslin, Sheila, "Relatedness in Group Psychotherapy," *Perspectives in Psychiatric Care,* 11, no. 4 (1973), 165-71.

85. Sanderson, Marilynn, and Judith Blackley, "Problems Displayed in Vivi—A Particular Advantage of Group Therapy," *Perspectives in Psychiatric Care,* 17, no. 4 (1979), 176-86.

86. Scott, M. Louise, "To Learn to Work with the Elderly," *The American Journal of Nursing,* 73, no. 4 (1973), 662-64.

87. Shepherd, Clovis, *Small Groups.* San Francisco: Chandler Publishing Co., 1964.

88. Shere, E., "Group Therapy with the Very Old," in R. Kastenbaum, ed., *New Thoughts on Old Age.* New York: Springer Publishing Co., Inc., 1964.

89. Silver, A., "Group Psychotherapy with Senile Psychotic Patients," *Geriatrics,* 5 (1950), 147-50.

90. Smith, E. Frances, "Teaching Group Therapy in an Undergraduate Curriculum," *Perspectives in Psychiatric Care,* 11, no. 2 (1973), 70-74.

91. Smith, Loretta, "Finding Your Leadership Style in Groups," *American Journal of Nursing,* 80, no. 7 (1980), 1301-3.

92. Solomon, Philip, and Vernon Patch, *Handbook of Psychiatry.* Los Altos, Calif.: Lange Medical Publications, 1971.

93. Spotnitz, Hyman, *The Couch and the Aide.* New York: Alfred A. Knopf, Inc. 1961.

94. Stevens, Leonard, "Nurse-Patient Discussion Groups," *American Journal of Nursing,* 63, no. 12 (1963), 67-69.

95. Swanson, Mary, "A Check List for Group Leaders," *Perspectives in Psychiatric Care,* 7, no. 3 (1969), 120-26.

96. Thralon, Joan, and Charles Watson, "Remotivation for Geriatric Patients Using Elementary School Students," *Nursing Digest,* 5, no. 4 (1975), 48-49.

97. Toffler, Alvin, *Future Shock.* New York: Bantam Books, Inc., 1970.

98. Trow, W. et al. "Psychology of Group Behavior: The Class as a Group," *Journal of Educational Psychology,* 41 (1950), 322-88.

99. Walton, Dan, "Effects of Personal Growth Groups on Self-Actualization and Creative Personality," *Journal of College Student Personnel,* 20, no. 6 (1973), 490-94.

100. Water, Jane, *Group Guidance, Principles and Practices.* New York: McGraw-Hill Book Company, 1960.

101. Werner, Jean, "Relating Group Theory to Nursing Practice," *Perspectives in Psychiatric Care,* 5, no. 6 (1970), 248-61.

102. Whitaker, Dorothy, and Morton Lieberman, *Psychotherapy through the Group Process.* New York: Atherton Press, 1964.

103. White, R., and R. Lippett, "Leader Behavior and Member Reaction in Three Social Climates," in D. Cartwright and A. Zander, eds., *Group Dynamics,* Chapter 40. Evanston, Ill.: Row Peterson, 1953.

104. Wicks, Robert J., *Counseling Strategies and Intervention Techniques for the Human Services.* Philadelphia: J. B. Lippincott Company, 1977.

105. Wolff, K., "Treatment of the Geriatric Patient in a Mental Hospital," *Journal of the American Geriatrics Society,* 4 (1956), 472–76.

106. ____, "Group Psychotherapy with Geriatric Patients in a Mental Hospital," *Journal of the American Geriatrics Society*, 5 (1957) 13–19.

107. Yalom, Irvin D., *The Theory and Practice of Group Psychotherapy.* New York: Basic Books, Inc., 1970.

108. Yalom, Irvin, and Florence Terrazas, "Group Therapy for Psychotic Elderly Patients," *American Journal of Nursing,* 68, no. 8 (1968), 1690–98.

IV

Nursing Diagnoses and the Nursing Process

12

The Person on the Health-Illness Continuum: Promoting Adaptation to the Stress Response

Study of this chapter will assist you to:

1. Define emotional health and illness as they relate to the health-illness continuum.

2. Discuss factors that influence definitions of health and illness.

3. Compare and contrast factors that contribute to health or illness.

4. Differentiate between *stress, stressor,* and *distress* and relate the concept of stress to health and illness.

5. Contrast physiological, cognitive, and emotional manifestations of the Alarm, Resistance, and Exhaustion Stages of the General Adaptation Syndrome that may occur in self or client.

6. Describe anxiety and relate the concept of anxiety to the concept of stress.

7. Identify manifestations of each level of anxiety that may occur in self or client and relate levels of anxiety to the health-illness continuum.

8. Determine factors that contribute to anxiety and a distressed emotional status.

9. Describe the psychosomatic concept and the effects of the emotional status on physiological status and disease processes.

10. Contrast somatopsychic and psychosomatic concepts.

11. Explain the concept of sick role and common feelings and behaviors in response to physical illness and treatment in the health care system.

12. Examine the potential meaning of physical versus psychiatric illness to the client and differences in individual and family reactions to each type of illness.

This chapter contributed by Ruth Murray, R.N., M.S.N.

13. Discuss the concept of impaired role and the effects of disability or chronic illness on the emotional status of the client and family.

14. Utilize concepts of stress and anxiety to assess your response to physiological, mental, emotional, and social stressors.

15. Assess physiological, mental, emotional, and social manifestations of the stress response and anxiety in the client.

16. Formulate nursing diagnosis(es) and goals of care specific to the unique reactions and needs of your clients.

17. Practice various coping strategies and relaxa-tion techniques in order to more effectively teach them to clients.

18. Intervene with clients to promote coping with and adaptation to stressors as well as relaxation in the presence of the stress response.

19. Intervene to assist the client through the sick role and convalescence.

20. Intervene with the disabled or chronically ill client and family to promote adaptation to the impaired role.

21. Evaluate effectiveness of your emotional care, using criteria based on established goals.

In psychiatric/mental health nursing, you care for people who are physically as well as emotionally ill. The stress response and illness in one sphere affect the health status of all components of the person. This chapter discusses effects of the interplay between mind and body, with application to the nursing process.

THE CONCEPTS OF HEALTH AND ILLNESS

Definitions of the Health-Illness Continuum

In the same way as the literature speaks of the health-illness continuum, definitions of health range on a continuum from the absence of symptoms, to optimal functioning, to a utopian ideal of complete physical, mental, emotional, spiritual, and social well-being (39).

R. Dubois views health as adaptation, a function of adjustment. He believes a utopian state of health can never be reached because the person will never be so perfectly adapted to the environment that life will not involve struggle, failure, and suffering. Humans can adapt to environmental conditions or change the environment, but each new adaptation produces new problems that demand new solutions (37).

H. S. Hayman defines health as a state of feeling sound in body, mind, and spirit, with a sense of reserve power. This perception of health is based on normal functioning of the body's physiological processes, understanding of the principles of healthful living, and an attitude that regards health not as an end of survival and self-fulfillment in itself but as a means to a creative social adjustment and a richer, fuller life as measured in constructive service to mankind (74).

H. Blum defines health as the person's capacity to function in a way to maximize potential; to maintain a balance appropriate to age and social needs; to be reasonably free of gross dissatisfaction, discomfort, disease, or disability; and to behave in ways that promote survival as well as self-fulfillment or enjoyment (14).

F. and E. Rathbone formulate health as a wholeness of function, movement toward self-actualization, relating effective, creative use of potential, realistic interpretation of experiences, and coordination of attitudinal, physiological, and behavioral adaptations. This definition is directly pertinent to psychiatric/mental health nursing (151).

Although health can be viewed as a medical model (freedom from symptoms), a utopian ideal, or a cultural norm, in psychiatric/mental health nursing, health can be viewed as a *process. Health in the affective domain means that the feelings, emotions, interests, motivations, attitudes, and values of the person continue to mature and change over a lifetime, as the person engages in transactions with other people and the broader environment, manifests both flexibility and stability in adaptive abilities, accomplishes the developmental tasks appropriate to the life era and age, and fulfills social roles with a maximum of effectiveness and happiness* (1). Health is a multidimensional process and includes physical, intellectual, developmental, emotional, spiritual, and sociocultural components.

Illness is more than signs and symptoms. It is a process and an experience. *Illness is failure of the person's adaptive powers to maintain physical and emotional balance and to utilize the usual health-promoting resources in the face of internal or external stressors. It is an experience that exists when there is disturbance or failure in the bio-psychosocial development or adaptation of the person, with observable or felt changes, discomforts, or impaired ability to carry out minimal physical, psychological, or social behavioral expectations appropriate to customary roles and status* (211).

H. S. Sullivan defines **mental or emotional illness** *as inappropriate interpersonal behavior or behavior that is inadequate for the social context.* Sullivan believes that each person has some small degree of illness—physical or emotional—even when he/she feels and looks well. The illness may be minor aches, temper flares, inappropriate forgetfulness, or overuse of certain defense mechanisms such as rationalization or forgetfulness. Similarly, the emotionally ill person manifests some degree of health—some appropriate thinking and behavior (194). See the health-illness continuum depicted by Figure 12-1.

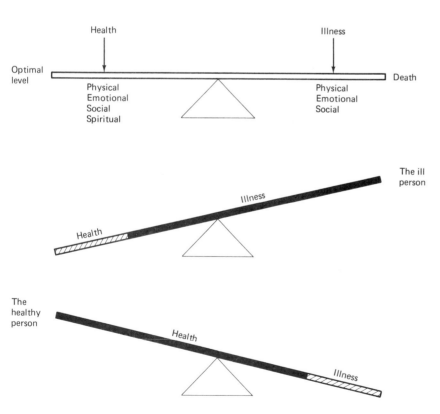

FIGURE 12-1   The health-illness continuum.

Factors That Influence the Definitions of Health and Illness

Culture and historical era (as shown in Table 2-1, Chapter 2) define health and illness. Thus there are many definitions of health and illness since each family interprets the culture to the child. The definitions of physical and emotional illness are learned in the family.

Health is perceived uniquely by the person and may vary from day to day and even within a day. According to Third Force theorists, described in Chapter 2, health and illness are defined differently by each person, although the definitions are generally in line with cultural definitions. Health in all its components is dynamic in that it includes the degree of fitness and adaptation that varies from one time period to another. There is a continual interaction between the physical, mental, spiritual, and social components (74).

Men and women may define health and illness differently. Women in the United States report more illnesses and disabilities, visit the physician more, and are hospitalized more often, including for emotional illnesses, although there is no great difference between men and women in the incidence of psychosis. Women also have longer life expectancies than men (135). The illnesses and disabilities reported by women often do not seem to be major ailments. Perhaps the seeking of health care reflects: (1) a different perception of what men and women consider illness or disability, (2) different cultural norms about health care behavior of men and women, (3) different responses to sex-role conflicts (described in Chapter 23), or (4) differences in diagnostic and treatment services for men and women. All these factors may be operating. The longer life expectancy of women may be the result of early diagnosis and treatment, of inherent sex-linked resistance to disease, or of different exposure to noxious physical and social stressors (18, 84).

Married and unmarried persons differ in their health status according to W. Gore (61, 62, 63), I. Hauenstein et al. (73), M. Ibrahim (84), and A. Nathanson (135). Married men and women have lower morbidity rates for physical illness, use health services less frequently, and live longer than unmarried people. Although married women have higher incidence of emotional illness than married men, single women have less incidence of emotional illness than single men. Married, employed women exhibit fewer psychiatric symptoms (even less hypertension) than married, nonemployed women. Single men are at greater risk for both physical and emotional illness. Sex role expectations and life style, as well as resultant affective states, may be factors behind these statistics.

A person's age influences the definition of health. J. Natapoff found that children do not define health in the same way as adults do (134). Children define health positively—as feeling good and being able to participate in desired activities. Children's ideas about health progress from a specific, concrete concern for health practices to future-oriented interests in optimal development and societal problems. Six-year-olds view health as completely different from illness and as a series of specific health practices, such as eating nutritional foods, getting exercise, and keeping clean. Nine-year-olds are less concerned with specific health practices and are more concerned with total body states, such as feeling good or being "in shape." To them, health means being physically fit to do the activities of daily living; it is impossible to be partly healthy and partly unhealthy. Twelve-year-olds, who Piaget theorizes are in the Formal Operations Stage of cognitive development, view health as long-term feeling good, not being sick, participating in desired activities, and including mental as well as physical components. Some children include a fit environment as part of health (58).

In contrast, adults typically define health as a state enabling them to perform at least minimal daily activities and including physical, mental, spiritual, and social components (134). The adult's perception as well as life situation will influence the definition of health. B. Bauman (8) and L. Pratt (147) found that the poor person defines health as being able to do necessary daily activities. Yet many adults define themselves as ill when minor symptoms are experienced, even though those symptoms do not interfere with work or interpersonal relations.

Factors That Contribute to Health and Illness

Many forces and variables contribute to health and illness, including environmental circumstances, genetic endowment, constitutional predisposition, personal experiences, general health and behavioral habits, life style, personality status, presence of interpersonal harmony or conflict, or presence of internal pathology.

To remain emotionally healthy, the person must be with people who are healthy and in a group climate that contributes to developing one's optimal potential. Emotional health implies the capacity to love, learn, live fully, and share with others in the adventure of life. The emotionally ill person comes from an environment where there is excessive tension, a barrier to emotional communication, an isolation between people, and where emotional and social needs are not met. The emotional illness of one person in the family/group spills over so that all members are to some degree unhealthy. Any change in one member's attitudes and behavior alters the reciprocal behavior of all other members, and in turn the initial family/group member is affected (1).

Perception and evaluation of the environment can be crucial since there is usually a relationship between the frequency of a person's illness episodes and the perception of life situations. Those who perceive their life experiences as excessively challenging or demanding and conflict-laden suffer more disturbances of bodily processes, mood, thought, and behavior than those who do not. Risk of emotional as well as physical illness can be predicted from the amount and meaning of change to the person and his/her response to change (see Chapter 8). Susceptibility to illness may also be influenced by age since adaptive defenses are not as well developed in the very young and are less effective in the very old. Developmental level also influences perception and response to environmental demands (8, 79, 140, 147). Social roles are significant to health since they place various demands on the person and call for shifts and flexibility in attitude and behavior. At times the kind and nature of roles in which the person is involved are demanding or stressful to the point of contributing to physical and emotional illness. The occupational role is important. Whether the person is a farmer, nurse, psychiatrist, coal miner, executive, or an office clerk predisposes the person to different kinds of stressors and illness.

The family contributes not only to genetic predisposition but also to the actual etiology of specific diseases through the transmission of social values, the socialization process of the child, and the family pattern of daily living and behavior.

Many of the variables that affect the developing person's health and illness were referred to in Chapter 3, and theories about emotional health and illness, as well as causative factors, were described in Chapter 2. Causative or contributing factors related to each nursing diagnosis are discussed in this Part on the use of the nursing process with the person who is emotionally ill. Primary prevention, related to the health end of the continuum, and secondary and tertiary prevention, related to the illness end of the continuum, will be discussed in Chapter 25.

Because a major factor in health and illness is response to stress and the anxiety it engenders, this chapter will include the concepts of stress and anxiety, their manifestations, and the nursing process pertinent to their management.

STRESS: RELATIONSHIP TO HEALTH, ADAPTATION, AND ILLNESS

Basic Concepts

Stress is a physical and emotional state always present in the person as a result of living; it is intensified in a nonspecific response to an internal or external environmental change or threat. Stress reactions are purposeful and initially protective; the manifestations are physiological and psychological, structural and functional, overt and covert (24, 174, 175). On the positive side, stress helps to maintain equilibrium as well as to increase motivation, learning, creativity, development, productivity, and satisfaction. Complete freedom from stress is death or a nonexistent state. In contrast, *distress is negative, noxious, unpleasant, or damaging stress.* Distress occurs when needs cannot be met or when well-being and integrity are threatened. Each period of distress leaves psychological and emotional wear and tear, which is sometimes irreversible (176). The terms *stress* and *distress* are often used interchangeably, although all stress is not negative.

The person's survival and health status depends on the intensity, duration, and location of the stress and on the adaptive capacity of the person. Various emotional and physical adaptive mechanisms are in constant operation, adjusting the body to a changing number and nature of **stressors**, *tension-producing internal or external stimuli, agents, or factors causing intensification of the stress state and disequilibrium.* Table 12-1 lists stressors (stress agents) that may have emotional consequences.

TABLE 12-1. Stimuli That Are Stressors

1. *Physical*: excessive or intense cold or heat, sound, light, motion, gravity, or electrical current.
2. *Chemical*: alkalies, acids, drugs, toxic substances, hormones, gases, or food and water pollutants.
3. *Microbiological*: viruses, bacteria, molds, parasites, or other infectious organisms.
4. *Physiological*: disease processes, surgery, immobilization, mechanical trauma, fever, organ hypo- or hyperfunction, or pain.
5. *Psychological*: anticipated marriage or death, imagined events, intense emotional involvement, anxiety or other unpleasant feelings, distortions of body image, threats to self-concept, others' expectations of behavior, rejection by or separation from loved ones, role changes, memory of negative past experiences, actual or perceived failures.
6. *Developmental*: genetic endowment, prematurity, immaturity, maturational impairment, or the aging process.
7. *Sociocultural*: sociocultural background and pressures, unharmonious interpersonal relationships, demands of our technological society, social mobility, changing social mores, job pressures, economic worries, child-rearing practices, redefinition of sex roles, or minority status.
8. *Environmental*: unemployment, air and water pollution, overcrowding, disasters, war, or crime.

Stressors can have a constructive effect as long as regulatory mechanisms are able to function and few symptoms result. The exaggerated stress state occurs when stressors are excessive or intense, limits of adaptation are exceeded, and the person cannot cope with the stressor's demands.

What is considered a stressor by one person may be considered pleasurable by another. The amount of stress in the immediate environment cannot be determined by examining only the stressor or source of stress. However, there are certain principles that apply to most people (56, 176, 177, 179):

1. Most stressors in the environment occur at levels below that which would cause immediate physical or emotional damage. The impact is cumulative.
2. Circumstances alter the impact or harm done by a stressor. The social and emotional context of an event and the attitude and previous experiences of the person are as important as physical properties of the stimuli.
3. People are remarkably adaptable. Each person has evolved a normal range of response or a unique pattern of defense. What may at first be considered uncomfortable or intolerable may eventually be perceived as normal routine. The immediate impact of a stressor is apparently different from long-term or indirect consequences, which are more difficult to detect.
4. Various psychological or social factors can ease or exaggerate the effects of a stressor. If a stressor is predictable, it will not be as harmful as an unpredictable one. If the person feels in control of the situation or can relate positively or directly to the stressor, the effects are less negative. For example, the person in a noisy environment suffers less startle reaction

if sudden noises come regularly and are anticipated. Those who work in a noisy environment without the ability to control the noise show low frustration tolerance, uncooperative behavior, and more errors on reading and arithmetic problems. Studies also show less stress response when people feel and actually have control over a stressful environment.

5. There are definite low points when stressors are poorly tolerated. Time of day affects stress response. For example, in most people, hydrocortisone secretion normally peaks in the early morning and decreases through the day, until it is almost undetectable at night. Although diurnal rhythms vary from person to person, stressors may be better tolerated early in the day.

6. Conditioning is an important protection. The person whose heart, lungs, and skeletal muscles are conditioned by exercise can withstand cardiovascular and respiratory effects of the Alarm Stage (see below) better than someone who leads a sedentary life.

7. Responses to stress throughout life are both local and general. The Local Adaptation Syndrome, typified by the inflammatory response, is the method used to wall off and locally control the effects of physical stressors. When the stressor cannot be handled locally, the whole body responds to protect itself and ensure survival in the best way possible through the General Adaptation Syndrome.

The General Adaptation Syndrome is characterized by the Alarm and Resistance stages and when body resistance is not maintained, by the end stage, Exhaustion (174, 175, 176, 177, 178, 179).

The General Adaptation Syndrome

The *Alarm Stage is an instantaneous, short-term, life-preserving, and total sympathetic nervous system response that occurs when the person consciously or unconsciously perceives a stressor and feels helpless, insecure, or biologically uncomfortable. This stage is typified by a "fight-or-flight" reaction* (174). Perception of the stressor—the alarm reaction—stimulates the hypothalamus, which in turn stimulates the anterior pituitary to increase production of adrenocorticotropic hor-

mone (ACTH). The adrenal cortex is stimulated by ACTH to increase production of glucocorticoids, primarily hydrocortisone, or cortisol, and mineralo-corticoids, primarily aldosterone. Catecholamine release triggers increased sympathetic nervous system activity, which stimulates production of epinephrine and nonrepinephrine by the adrenal medulla and release at the adrenergic nerve endings. The alarm reaction also stimulates the posterior pituitary to release increased Anti-Diuretic Hormone. Because of these changes, the person is generally physiologically prepared to act, to be more mentally alert, and to adapt. Emotionally, the person feels mild to moderate anxiety, and certain defense mechanisms will be unconsciously used. The physiological responses that occur when the sympathetic nervous system is stimulated are shown in Figure 12-2.

To complicate assessment, there are times when parts of the parasympathetic division of the autonomic nervous system are inadvertently stimulated during a stressful state because of the proximity of sympathetic and parasympathetic nerve fibers. Also, because of the influence of the cerebral cortex, memory of past experiences, present perceptions or special training override the normal effects of the sympathetic nervous system. Figure 12-3 shows parasympathetic nervous system responses that may occur during the General Adaptation Syndrome.

R. Lazarus identified three psychological stages that occur during the Alarm Stage: (1) threat, (2) warning, and (3) impact (102). The psychological processes that occur when the stress state is intensified begin with appraisal of the *threat* or potential degree of harm (*warning*). This process is cognitive and affective and involves perception, memory, thought, and a feeling response to the *meaning of the impact* of the threat, such as anxiety, fear, anger, guilt, or shame.

The *Stage of Resistance is the body's way of adapting through an adrenocortical response to the disequilibrium caused by the stressors of life* (174). Because of the adrenocortical response, many changes occur to sustain the body's fight for preservation, including: increased use of body resources, endurance, and strength; tissue anabolism; antibody production; hormonal secretion; changes in blood sugar levels and blood volume, including hemodilution; and hyperchloremia (81, 174, 175, 178). Moderate anxiety is felt; habitual ego defenses are unconsciously used. Responses eventually return

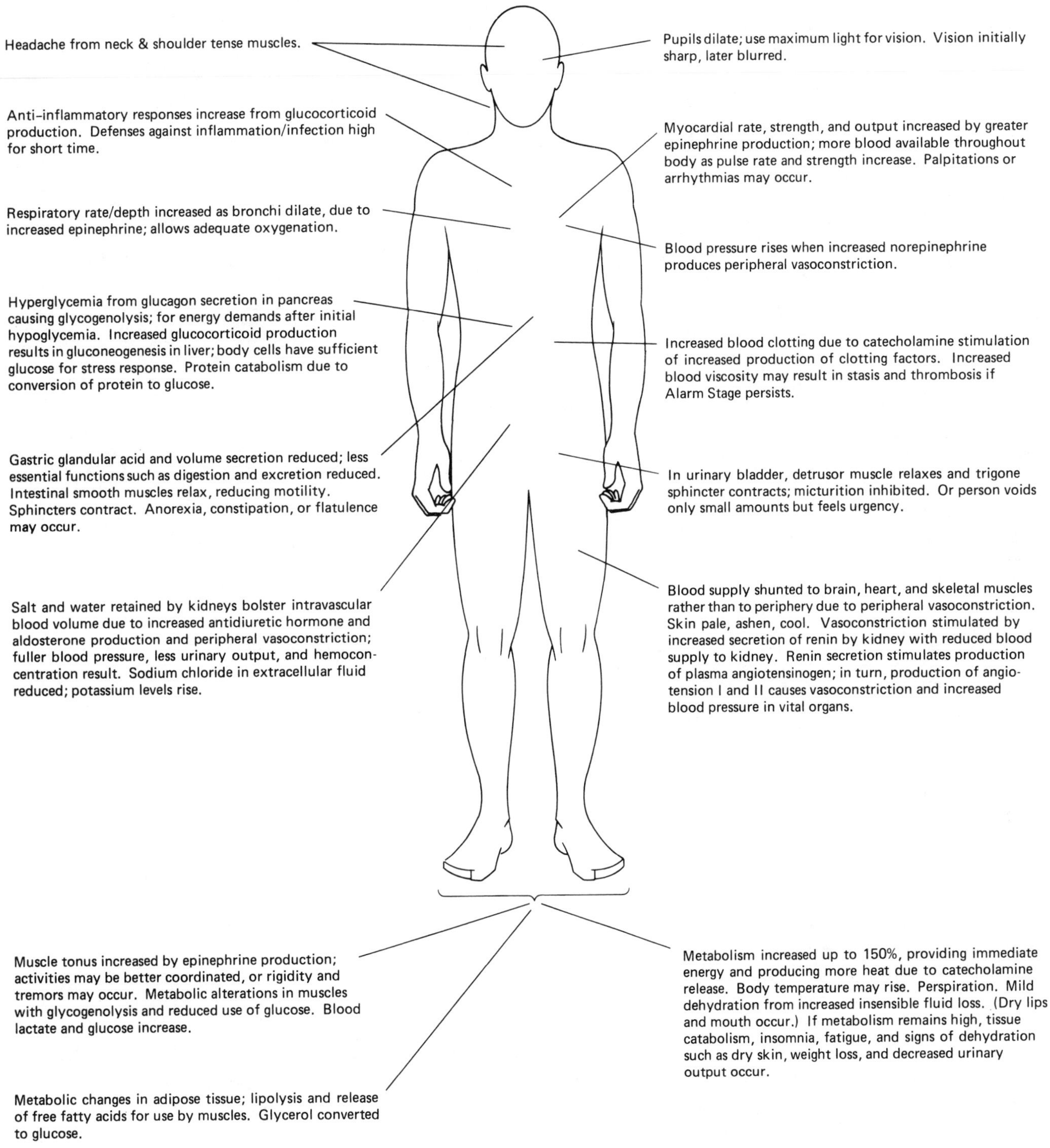

Headache from neck & shoulder tense muscles.

Anti-inflammatory responses increase from glucocorticoid production. Defenses against inflammation/infection high for short time.

Respiratory rate/depth increased as bronchi dilate, due to increased epinephrine; allows adequate oxygenation.

Hyperglycemia from glucagon secretion in pancreas causing glycogenolysis; for energy demands after initial hypoglycemia. Increased glucocorticoid production results in gluconeogenesis in liver; body cells have sufficient glucose for stress response. Protein catabolism due to conversion of protein to glucose.

Gastric glandular acid and volume secretion reduced; less essential functions such as digestion and excretion reduced. Intestinal smooth muscles relax, reducing motility. Sphincters contract. Anorexia, constipation, or flatulence may occur.

Salt and water retained by kidneys bolster intravascular blood volume due to increased antidiuretic hormone and aldosterone production and peripheral vasoconstriction; fuller blood pressure, less urinary output, and hemoconcentration result. Sodium chloride in extracellular fluid reduced; potassium levels rise.

Muscle tonus increased by epinephrine production; activities may be better coordinated, or rigidity and tremors may occur. Metabolic alterations in muscles with glycogenolysis and reduced use of glucose. Blood lactate and glucose increase.

Metabolic changes in adipose tissue; lipolysis and release of free fatty acids for use by muscles. Glycerol converted to glucose.

Pupils dilate; use maximum light for vision. Vision initially sharp, later blurred.

Myocardial rate, strength, and output increased by greater epinephrine production; more blood available throughout body as pulse rate and strength increase. Palpitations or arrhythmias may occur.

Blood pressure rises when increased norepinephrine produces peripheral vasoconstriction.

Increased blood clotting due to catecholamine stimulation of increased production of clotting factors. Increased blood viscosity may result in stasis and thrombosis if Alarm Stage persists.

In urinary bladder, detrusor muscle relaxes and trigone sphincter contracts; micturition inhibited. Or person voids only small amounts but feels urgency.

Blood supply shunted to brain, heart, and skeletal muscles rather than to periphery due to peripheral vasoconstriction. Skin pale, ashen, cool. Vasoconstriction stimulated by increased secretion of renin by kidney with reduced blood supply to kidney. Renin secretion stimulates production of plasma angiotensinogen; in turn, production of angiotension I and II causes vasoconstriction and increased blood pressure in vital organs.

Metabolism increased up to 150%, providing immediate energy and producing more heat due to catecholamine release. Body temperature may rise. Perspiration. Mild dehydration from increased insensible fluid loss. (Dry lips and mouth occur.) If metabolism remains high, tissue catabolism, insomnia, fatigue, and signs of dehydration such as dry skin, weight loss, and decreased urinary output occur.

FIGURE 12-2 The alarm stage of the General Adaptation Syndrome showing physiological responses to sympathetic nervous system stimulation. [Data from A. Chut (28), A. Guyton (68), M. Horowitz (81), M. Marcinek (114), H. Selye (174, 175, 178, 180), and C. Stephenson (190).]

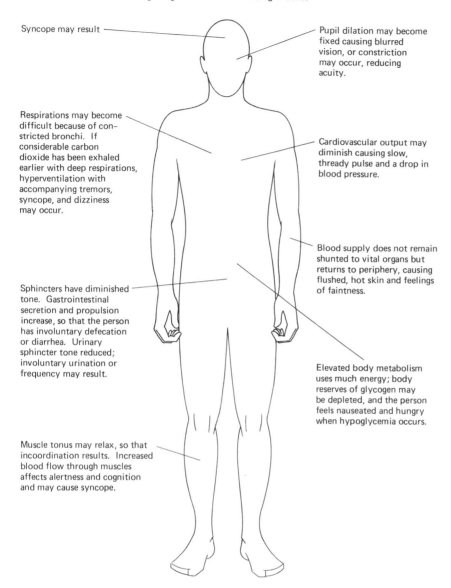

Syncope may result

Pupil dilation may become fixed causing blurred vision, or constriction may occur, reducing acuity.

Respirations may become difficult because of constricted bronchi. If considerable carbon dioxide has been exhaled earlier with deep respirations, hyperventilation with accompanying tremors, syncope, and dizziness may occur.

Cardiovascular output may diminish causing slow, thready pulse and a drop in blood pressure.

Blood supply does not remain shunted to vital organs but returns to periphery, causing flushed, hot skin and feelings of faintness.

Sphincters have diminished tone. Gastrointestinal secretion and propulsion increase, so that the person has involuntary defecation or diarrhea. Urinary sphincter tone reduced; involuntary urination or frequency may result.

Elevated body metabolism uses much energy; body reserves of glycogen may be depleted, and the person feels nauseated and hungry when hypoglycemia occurs.

Muscle tonus may relax, so that incoordination results. Increased blood flow through muscles affects alertness and cognition and may cause syncope.

FIGURE 12-3 The alarm stage of the General Adaptation Syndrome showing physiological responses to parasympathetic nervous system stimulation. [Data from A. Guyton (68), M. Horowitz (81), H. Selye (174, 175, 178, 180), and C. Stephenson (190).]

to normal when stressors diminish or when the person has found adaptive mechanisms that meet emotional needs and physical demands.

Stressors that are sudden in onset cause Alarm Stage physiological reactions, along with feelings of anxiety, but when the perception of stress is reduced, the person returns to parasympathetic nervous system functioning (Stage of Resistance). The adaptive response may be temporarily weakened but soon recovers unless the stress is of intense magnitude (178). (See Figure 12-4.) The person

may use a variety of ego adaptive mechanisms in response to sudden or short-term stressors.

If biological, psychological, or social stressors,

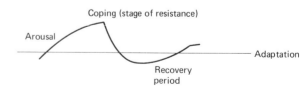

FIGURE 12-4 Reaction pattern in acute stress.

single or in combination, occur over a long period without adequate relief, the Stage of Resistance is maintained. With continued stressors, the person becomes distressed and manifests objective and subjective emotional, intellectual, and physiological responses, as shown in Figures 12-5 and 12-6. Finally, physical and emotional adaptive limits are reached. Resources become depleted. Use of ego defense mechanisms is excessive and rigid. The person cannot cope with even the slightest additional stress (Stage of Exhaustion). The longer the stressors are present, the more severe the effects. Long-lasting or irreversible damage may occur, although each body part and each person suffers to a unique and different degree.

The *Stage of Exhaustion occurs when the person is unable to continue to adapt to internal and external environmental demands or when adaptive mechanisms are inadequate* (174). Physical or emotional disease, or death, results because the body can no longer compensate for or correct homeostatic imbalances. Manifestations of this stage are similar to those of the Alarm Stage except that all reactions first intensify and then diminish in response and show no ability to return to an effective level of function. Frequent or prolonged General Adaptation Syndrome response triggers disease, which in turn predisposes the person to further emotional response. The Stage of Exhaustion is also related to the person's low points of the biorhythm cycle (81, 174, 175, 178). Emotionally, the moderate anxiety seen in the Stage of Resistance becomes severe, sometimes to the point of panic, neurosis, or psychosis.

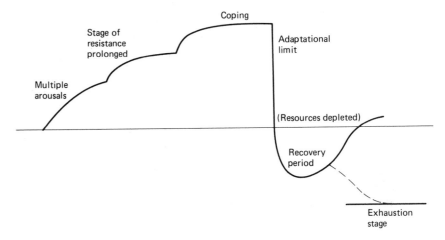

FIGURE 12-5   Reaction pattern in chronic stress. [Data obtained from M. Horowitz (81), D. Munz (130), S. Roberts (158), and H. Selye (175, 178).]

Factors that Influence the Stress Response*

Some experience with stressors may help the organism cope with stress and be protective against stress-induced disease. Animal studies indicate that ACTH somehow enhances effects of fear as a motivator for behavior during stressful periods, so that avoidance of stressors results. Development of an endocrine system that effectively deals with avoidance of stressors depends on critical environmental events in early life. In animal studies, young rats that were handled and exposed to low levels of

*Throughout the chapter, the asterisk refers to sections that may be optional reading for the student in psychiatric/mental health nursing.

stress developed faster than the controls and were better able to handle a stressor when mature. In these animals, hormone secretion response was more efficient and returned to normal more quickly when danger was past (108).

Research with people shows that early experiences with stress and the social environment seem to affect susceptibility to disease. The intensity of stress appears less important than the way it is handled. Certain coping methods, feeling in command of the situation, and strong family and social ties can help a person to suffer less deleterious effects of stress. Breaking ties by separating from the group or a loved one, divorce, mobility, or death, and the resultant sense of loss, rejection,

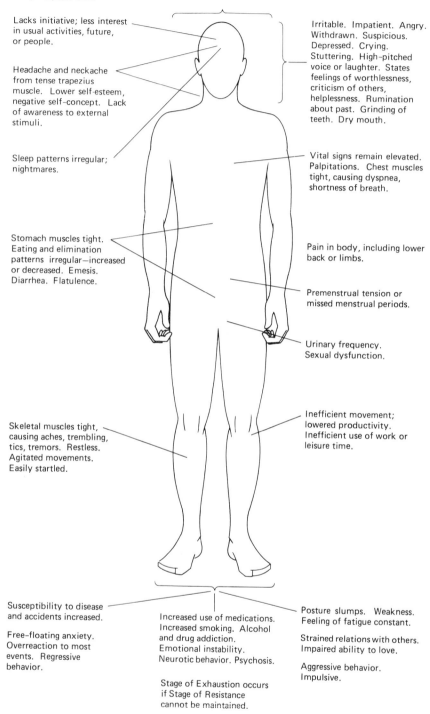

Preoccupied. Forgetful. Disoriented. Confused. Low tolerance for ambiguity. Errors in judgment in relation to work, distance, grammar, or mathematics. Misidentification of people. Inability to concentrate, to solve problems, or to plan. Inattention to detail or instructions. Reduced fantasy, creativity, and perceptual field.

Lacks initiative; less interest in usual activities, future, or people.

Headache and neckache from tense trapezius muscle. Lower self-esteem, negative self-concept. Lack of awareness to external stimuli.

Sleep patterns irregular; nightmares.

Irritable. Impatient. Angry. Withdrawn. Suspicious. Depressed. Crying. Stuttering. High-pitched voice or laughter. States feelings of worthlessness, criticism of others, helplessness. Rumination about past. Grinding of teeth. Dry mouth.

Vital signs remain elevated. Palpitations. Chest muscles tight, causing dyspnea, shortness of breath.

Stomach muscles tight. Eating and elimination patterns irregular—increased or decreased. Emesis. Diarrhea. Flatulence.

Pain in body, including lower back or limbs.

Premenstrual tension or missed menstrual periods.

Urinary frequency. Sexual dysfunction.

Skeletal muscles tight, causing aches, trembling, tics, tremors. Restless. Agitated movements. Easily startled.

Inefficient movement; lowered productivity. Inefficient use of work or leisure time.

Susceptibility to disease and accidents increased.

Free-floating anxiety. Overreaction to most events. Regressive behavior.

Increased use of medications. Increased smoking. Alcohol and drug addiction. Emotional instability. Neurotic behavior. Psychosis.

Stage of Exhaustion occurs if Stage of Resistance cannot be maintained.

Posture slumps. Weakness. Feeling of fatigue constant.

Strained relations with others. Impaired ability to love.

Aggressive behavior. Impulsive.

FIGURE 12-6 The stage of resistance in the General Adaptation Syndrome showing signs of emotional, intellectual, and physiological distress.

and loneliness predispose a person to disease and death (2).

All behavior is an attempt at adaptation to meet basic needs. *Adaptation is the physiological, psychological, or sociological responses or changes in or by a person to limit the site of, lessen the impact of, or neutralize the effects of stress.* Adaptation involves the ability to change self or the environment or to compromise when necessary, in response to internal or external stimuli, in order to meet basic needs. Adaptations are innate or acquired and may be involuntary (unconscious) or conscious (deliberate). Automatic or habitual behavior is never fully adequate. Adaptation may be efficient or inefficient, slow or rapid, and may result in temporary or permanent change, or create new stresses to which further responses are necessary. Adaptations are either directly or indirectly related to the stressor, and are either primary (an initial result of stressors), or secondary (a response to earlier inefficient stress reaction) (169). Adaptation involves increasing autonomy of the organism, whereby with self-determination external influences are resisted and the forces of the physical and social environment are subordinated to a personal sphere of influence.

During *critical periods, when accelerated physical growth and personality development are occurring and the capacity to adapt to stressors is underdeveloped,* the normal growth processes are already placing tremendous demands on the organism. Thus the person is more vulnerable to stressors. Critical periods exist throughout the life span. Adaptive processes are taxed and may not be sufficient for health or survival.

RELATIONSHIP OF ANXIETY TO THE STRESS RESPONSE

The Concept of Anxiety

During the Alarm, Resistance, and Exhaustion Stages of the General Adaptation Syndrome, anxiety may be felt in various degrees and be manifested in a variety of ways. Everyone feels anxiety in response to stressors at some time in life.

Anxiety is an ubiquitous emotional state that is experienced when the self-identity or essential values are threatened but which has no specific object. The feeling state is characterized by a subjective sense of dread, apprehension, threat, failure, helplessness, or impending disaster; by a sense of losing control, becoming disoriented, or committing a destructive act; or by a fear of sudden death. In contrast, *fear is a feeling of apprehension or disaster in response to a specific object* (66). Well and ill people experience both feelings.

Normal anxiety is the degree of arousal appropriate to a situation, as validated by others familiar with the situation. Whenever the person is placed in a new situation or one demanding more than the usual performance, mild or moderate anxiety is experienced, with increased alertness, muscular tension, elevated vital signs, perspiration, and internal trembling. Often performance is improved with mild or even moderate anxiety (66). In the face of acute stressors, the person may temporarily experience severe anxiety or panic, and this is considered normal if the feeling is appropriate and temporary.

Anxiety can be categorized in other ways since the person's experience differs to some extent with each anxiety state. *State anxiety refers to the temporary state the person is in when the anxiety episode occurs and sympathetic arousal results. Trait anxiety refers to habitual or chronic anxiety or arousal;* the person with habitual (trait) anxiety is also prone to attacks of acute, severe anxiety. Chapter 13 discusses further the ineffective behavior that results from excessive, habitual (trait) anxiety. *Psychic anxiety refers to an emotional state and includes muscular tension and worry. Somatic anxiety refers to use of somatic (physical) complaints to discharge feelings and mental distress. Morbid anxiety is severe anxiety or panic that is incapacitating, causing the person to be unable to function effectively.* Inability to cope is based in part on misperception of the situation (66, 72, 167, 214). Chapter 13 explores morbid anxiety in relation to the various nursing diagnoses.

Anxiety and fear are different. Anxiety is experienced by the child before language is acquired and, therefore, is experienced as a vague, global, often unnamed feeling. Later the person experiences anxiety as a strong sense of impending doom without a specific cause; thus direct action is difficult to take, and helpless, isolated, and insecure feelings result. Fear occurs developmentally later than anxiety, when the young child encounters specific situations or objects that cause harm; therefore the experience can be named and managed. The subjective feeling is that life or limb is threatened by an external danger; direct action to escape, to remove the danger, or to relieve the pain and discomfort are seen as solutions. Fear and anxiety often occur together and may potentiate each other (66).

Anxiety is a word that has many meanings (214):

1. *Affect*—vague, uncomfortable feeling.
2. *Etiology*—cause of behavior: for example, overeating or withdrawal.
3. *Motivator*—drive or reason for behavior: for example, anxious (or eager) to participate in an activity.
4. *Personality state or response*—specific response to specific situational stimuli: for example, a job or school.
5. *Personality trait*—inherent and habitual mode of responding.
6. *Emotional disorder*—free floating, nonsituational, generalized, and nonspecific distress, diagnosed as anxiety disorders, anxiety neurosis, or anxiety reaction. (See Chapter 13 for discussion of anxiety as an emotional disorder.)

Etiologic Theories

Refer to Chapter 2 for a discussion about theories of anxiety, as proposed by Freud (48), Sullivan (194), Rank, Horney, and May (72, 167). Hildegarde Peplau shared Sullivan's view that anxiety is aroused in the interpersonal situation when interactions with people are unpleasant and there is an absence of tenderness (144).

Anxiety is a natural compensatory or adaptive feeling state that involves every aspect of the person. Anxiety arises from the following developmental threats: (1) separation from or loss of significant others, including mother in infancy, (2) physical injury when mastery of environment and self-assertive powers are valued, or (3) loss of self-esteem or of social approval because of restrictions against egoistic strivings or related to superego formation (115). The child may react with anxiety to illness, sudden deprivations, birth of a sibling, tension in the home or school, or sudden environmental changes.

Other sources of anxiety include feelings of helplessness or dependency in relation to another, anticipated disapproval, an evaluation of not measuring up to personal ideals or the ideals or performance of another, a perceived lack of warmth or tenderness from others, or apprehension about expressing feelings such as anger to another. A sense of helplessness and anxiety may be triggered by the enforced immobility of illness, injury, or surgery, or the intrusive procedures associated with diagnosis and treatment, which may arouse feelings of being attacked since self-esteem and feelings of worth may depend on being active, independent, or engaged in work (43). Anxiety is the basis for caution; for comparison of goals with capabilities; for regulation of drive; and for motivation, aspiration, and protection of the self (ego) (121). Anxiety promotes emotional development but may also cause dysfunctional behavior. Anxiety is associated with all of the nursing diagnoses that are discussed in this unit.

Some research studies claim a biological basis for onset of anxiety. First Force theorists claim that anxiety is an innate and biological response to stimuli that threaten survival. The biochemical and neural chain of events that causes anxiety feelings or the effects of anxiety continues to be studied, but these studies are not conclusive in all subjects (108, 120, 145, 153). Some studies of families with anxious patients infer a genetic predisposition to anxiety (30). Other studies support an intrafamily resemblance in anxiety behavior (20, 31, 185). Studies of monozygotic and dizygotic twins provide support for a genetic predisposition to anxiety as well as other mental diseases (212). However, the constitutional predisposition toward anxiety is only one component of personality; the expression of anxiety also depends on complex interactions with other people and with the environment (42, 72, 167). Biological studies on anxiety do not control for the variables of past experience, parental care measures, or learned ways of coping with stress.

Levels and Manifestations of Anxiety

The levels of anxiety tend to be progressive or sequential in their development; often you observe increases ranging from mild to moderate, severe, or panicked. However, the characteristics of each level may overlap, and the person may reach a state of panic without ever having exhibited some of the manifestations of previous levels. In some cases, anxiety may not progress past the moderate stage.

The levels of anxiety and their manifestations that you may encounter in a variety of clients are described in Table 12-2.

Expressions of anxiety may differ according to age or developmental level, sex, or cultural background. Expressions of anxiety in the child depend on developmental age as well as the situation. The infant, aged 7 to 9 months, the toddler of 18 and 24 months, and the three-year-old all experience separation or *stranger anxiety, acute anxiety when separated from the mother or approached by a stranger.* Crying, clinging to the parent, apathy, irritability, withdrawal, regression to earlier behavior, nightmares, and depression are not uncommon manifestations of anxiety in the young child. The child who is hospitalized or separated for some time from the mother will display anxiety associated with the *grief process: initially the child will protest, then despair, and finally will exhibit apathy and disinterest in the mother.*

Older children may present signs of restlessness, agitation, fearfulness, and physical complaints.

Behavioral regression, such as enuresis; school phobia, or hysteria, may occur (76).

Older persons may manifest anxiety in ways different from young adults. Instead of stating feelings, the older person may report more fatigue, various somatic symptoms, or increased muscular tension; be overly demanding or compliant; show agitated or avoidance activity; withhold verbal responses; or be unable to make decisions. The older person may be less likely to recognize, admit, or report anxiety.

Men are different from women in some measures of anxiety: for example, free fatty acids in the bloodstream are higher in anxious older men than in women. The overt behavior of men may also differ. In Western cultures, men are more likely to channel anxiety into aggressive behavior: women are more likely to channel anxiety into depressive behavior (41).

The life style of the person, his/her experience with multiple losses or crises, his/her coping or adaptive mechanisms, and polydrug use also may alter response to anxiety and should be assessed before diagnosis and treatment (41).

TABLE 12-2.   Levels of Anxiety and Their Manifestations

Mild	Physiological —	Tension of needs motivates behavior.
		Adaptive to variety of internal and external stimuli.
	Cognitive —	Attentive, alert, perceptive to variety of stimuli; effective problem solving.
	Emotional —	No intense feelings; self-concept not threatened.
		Use of ego adaptive mechanisms minimal, flexible.
		Behavior appropriate to situation.
Moderate	Physiological —	Some symptoms may be present.
	Cognitive —	Perceptual field narrows; responds to directions.
		Tangible problems solved fairly effectively, at least with direction and support.
		Selective inattention — focus is on stimuli that do not add to anxiety.
	Emotional —	Impatient, irritable, forgetful, demanding, crying, angry.
		Uses any adaptive mechanism described in Table 2-3 to protect from feelings and meaning of behavior.
	(Physiological, cognitive, and emotional changes of Alarm and Resistance States. (See Figures 12-2 and 12-6.) Individual functions in normal pattern, but may not feel as healthy physically or emotionally as usual. Illness may result if feeling persists.)	
Severe	Physiological —	Alarm Stage changes intensify, and Stage of Resistance may progress to Stage of Exhaustion. (See Figure 12-2.)

TABLE 12-2.   Continued

	Cognitive—	Perceptual field narrows; stimuli distorted; focus is on scattered details.
		Selective inattention prevails.
		Learning and problem solving ineffective.
		Clarification or restatement needed repeatedly.
		Misinterprets statements.
		Unable to follow directions or remember main points.
		Unable to plan or make decisions; needs assistance with details.
		Consciousness and lucidity reduced.
	Emotional—	Self-concept threatened; sense of helplessness; mood changes.
		Behavior erratic or inappropriate; may be aware of inappropriate behavior but unable to improve.
		Many ego defense mechanisms used; dissociation and amnesia may be used.
		Disorientation, confusion, hallucinations, and delusions may be present.
		(Psychoses or physical illness or injury may result.)
Panic	Physiological—	Severe symptoms of Exhaustion Stage may be ignored.
	Cognitive—	Sensory ability and attention reduced so that only object of anxiety noticed.
		May fail to notice specific object of concern or disastrous event but will be preoccupied with trivial detail.
	Emotional—	Self-concept overwhelmed.
		Ego defense mechanisms ineffective; behavior often inappropriate and uncontrollable.
		Behavior focused on finding relief; may scream, cry, pray, thrash limbs, run, hit others, hurt self.
		Often easily distracted; cannot attend or concentrate.
		No learning, problem solving, decision making, or realistic judgments.
		May become immobilized, assume fetal position, or become mute, or be unresponsive to directions. Needs protection.
		(Psychoses may occur.)

PSYCHOPHYSIOLOGICAL RESPONSE TO STRESS AND ANXIETY

The Concept of Mind-Body Relationship

The relationship between the mind (soul) and body and its effect on health have been explained in various ways for thousands of years. The earliest Greeks possessed no fully developed concept of the body as a whole entity or of the soul as a separate entity. Rather, they believed that individual will, responsibility, and personal decisions did not belong to the person but to the gods, and that people should listen to and obey the gods if they wished to be alive and healthy (182).

Hippocrates was the first to espouse the idea

that disease results from more than spiritual causes and that mental life results from brain function rather than from the heart. The Romans then carried on the beliefs begun by the Greeks (182).

The cultural forces of the Middle Ages and the conflicts between Christian theology and science set the stage for developing modern ideas about the human. Knowledge about the body was reserved for scientific scrutiny; the nonmaterial soul belonged to the church. Pasteur's germ theory and Pinel's work to extend the concept of disease to behavioral disturbances influenced others to focus more on the body as a machine and on disease rather than on the person (182). Adolph Meyer in the late 1800s again emphasized the idea that the person is a unit and not a mind-body dualism (182). He recognized not only physical aspects of disorders but also psychological, socioeconomic, and environmental factors. Subsequent development of Western religious and philosophical systems caused the discovery that the person can be aware of self as an individual and is responsible for using the mind (182).

In the twentieth century, we have again recognized that all parts of the human system are coordinated, that mental and physical phenomena are interrelated, and that illness is more than being attacked by external destructive agents. Mind and body function as one; what happens in one part affects the whole. Illness, therefore, affects the whole person.

The Psychogenic Theory of Disease

The Psychogenic Theory of disease is based on Freud's postulate that emotional conditions render people susceptible to illness. If emotional conflicts are present or if emotional outlets are blocked, the subsequent internalization of feelings may result in physiological dysfunction.

Disease initiated by the psychogenic process is real; it does not exist purely in the mind. It is as real as any other disease and can be just as dangerous. Psychogenic disorders are sometimes misunderstood because the term is derived from *psyche, meaning mind,* and *gene, meaning beginning or originating in the mind.* It is possibly better to use the word *psychosomatic* or *psychophysiological, which literally means that both the mind and body are involved (psyche—mind; soma—physiological or body).* The *psychosomatic disorders are those in which psychic elements are significant for initiating chemical, physiological, or structural alterations, which in turn create the symptoms responsible for the person's complaints.* Psychosomatic medicine regards the body, mind, and sociocultural influences as closely related. Emotional stress, frequently resulting from anxiety, fear, worry, or overt or repressed anger, cause a number of physical illnesses. *Somatization refers to using physiological processes to express emotions that are blocked from expression in more direct ways* (112, 182).

Pathophysiology of psychosomatic disorders*

The pathophysiology of psychosomatic disorders is related in part to the fact that emotional stress finds expression in the vascular structures during and after the period of distress (in both the Alarm and Resistance Stages). Vasospasms and vasoconstriction cause ischemic effects on the arterial wall and result in local edema and atrophy, possible vascular thrombosis, degeneration of tissues, necrosis, hemorrhage, aneurysm formation, and rupture. (The vasodilation that follows relief from stress response predisposes to aneurysm formation and potential rupture of the vessel.) Capillary changes include increased permeability and the passage of proteins and finally, of red blood cells. In the brain, necrosis is followed by cyst formation and gliosis. In the stomach, where hydrochloric acid secretion increases, other mucouslike structures, ulceration, and scarring follow as a result of this process (16, 115). Vasospasm, with or without thrombosis, is an important factor in brain disease and migraine headache, and may be important in a number of neurological disorders, including epilepsy, and even some of the schizophrenia-like illnesses. Repeated ischemic cell damage from vasospasm is also a possible factor initiating autoimmune disease and cancer (16) and in noise-induced hearing loss (85). Intermittent hypomagnesemia may occur in persons under stress since free fatty-acid levels in the plasma are increased by stress, which in turn causes deficiency of magnesium in the blood. Extracellular magnesium also decreases, causing blood vessels to increase tone and constriction. The resultant vasospasm contributes to ischemia and tissue necrosis, especially in the heart. Coronary vasculature is especially sensitive to magnesium deficiency.

Organic changes

Organic changes and various diseases with psychogenic factors include: peptic ulcers, ulcerative colitis, hypertension, cardiovascular disease, migraine headache, diabetes, asthma and other allergic conditions, eczema and other skin rashes, arthritis, muscle and joint conditions, insomnia, premenstrual tension, and menstrual disorders. Some of these diseases can predispose to more serious conditions; for example, hypertension can predispose to heart failure, cerebral vascular accident, or renal damage. It is also possible that most illnesses, including cancer, infections, the common cold, gingivitis, and dental caries, have their basis in psychological factors. Various references at the end of the chapter describe these psychophysiological illnesses and their effects in adults. Children as well as adults may suffer psychosomatic illnesses (76).

Sites and symptoms

The site and types of symptoms do not necessarily remain the same in the person over time (198). A symptom may have different effects for the same person at different times in life and in different family, group, or cultural circumstances. The Theory of Somatic Weakness explains why emotional stress affects each person differently, or some not at all. Genetic inheritance, previous illness in a body organ, prior strain of a body system, and learned behavior responses all influence which organ/body system will be vulnerable to symptoms or disease when the person experiences distress. A person is more likely to develop a psychosomatic disorder if there is a previous family history of such a disorder. Or a person may develop a psychosomatic disorder by observing and learning a pattern from another family member with the same disorder (110).

The main issue is not the form of symptom but the way in which the person's integrative capacity deals with the emotional conflict, as well as the effect of family and social relationships on the person. The final health outcome depends on the person's resources for handling the conflict and symptoms, the integrative potential of the personality, and the psychological character of the family/group. The adaptive relationships that exist between the person's emotional status and the family, group, or environmental situation influence precipitation and the course of illness, recovery, and possible relapse (1).

Correlation between Emotional Status or Personality Type and Physical Status or Disease

Early research on psychosomatic processes and empirical data have linked certain personality types or attributes to specific diseases (e.g., repressed anger to arthritis) (89, 122, 123, 124). Type A personality or behavior pattern has been linked to atherosclerosis and coronary heart disease in many past studies (6, 89, 161). The Type A personality is described as dominant, aggressive, extrovertive, competitive, ambitious, fast-paced, abrupt in gesture and speech, unable to relax, impatient, time-conscious, prone to do more than one activity at a time (50, 161), and more successful in career than social relations (199). Contrary to this finding, other research, using more refined statistical methods and diverse subjects such as students, various ethnic groups, persons who are depressed, and people who had experienced myocardial infarction or moderate or severe exertional angina, has indicated that no such direct correlation exists between specific physical disease and personality type, not even for the Type A personality and coronary disease.

For further information, refer to A. Antonovsky (5), J. Dimsdale et al. (35), E. Goldberg et al. (59), R. Keith et al. (94), H. Klein and O. Parsons (95), R. Koenig et al. (98), R. Marinelli and A. Dell Orto (115), R. Moos and G. Solomon (123, 124), A. Mordkoff and R. Golas (125), A. Mordkoff and O. Parsons (126), E. Rim and M. Bonami (157), F. Shontz (182), K. Smyth et al. (187), I. Waldron et al. (200), and L. Warren and D. Weiss (202).

However, research does show that emotions, affective states, and covert or repressed traits (157) can cause organic changes that disturb the body's adaptive functions, and in turn predispose to disease (9, 40, 182, 205).

Temperament

Temperament, rather than separate personality characteristics, appears to be a variable that is predictive of individual stamina and vulnerability to premature disease and death. Persons characterized by an uneven, moody, tense temperament and irregular living patterns showed, in a 30-year study, lower stamina and greater incidence of premature disease and death than persons characterized by a stable, calm temperament and either a regularly slow- or rapid-moving behavior pattern. Thus, youthful reactions to stress are linked with future health or disease (11, 195).

Environment*

Interplay between certain personality attributes and the environmental and cultural milieu result in Type A behavior; it is apparently not an innate temperament type (32, 161, 200, 201). Fifty percent of urban samples are classified as Type A personality; fifty percent are classified as other personality types (32). For example, the Type A personality may become more susceptible to coronary atherosclerosis, hypertension, and coronary disease if the person continues to live, work, or study in an adverse or stressful environmental climate (32, 67, 161, 200, 201). Various factors contributing to development of the Type A personality are as follows:

1. Parental and child-rearing behaviors involving severe and frequent physical punishment, which contribute to anger and aggression in the child.
2. Emphasis in the urban, middle-class American home on the cultural values of mastery and controlling challenges.
3. Academic pressures on students—non-Type A students are converted to Type A at the end of a scholastically stressful semester.
4. Professional and managerial occupational levels, especially when the person has had comparatively little education for the position and has worked very hard to succeed.
5. Emphasis on work rather than on home and family to meet emotional needs.
6. Middle age, when home and job demands and responsibilities are heavy.
7. Daily stress of employment for both sexes.

For further reading on the subject, see M. Chesney and R. Rosenman (27), M. Davidson and C. Cooper (32), S. Haynes and M. Feinleib (75), J. House (82), J. Howard, D. Cunningham, and P. Rechnitzer (83), S. Kobasa (96), K. Matthews and F. Soal (116), P. Townsend (197), I. Waldron (199), and I. Waldron et al. (200, 201).

Employment*

Employment and the work environment contribute heavily toward manifestation of Type A behavior, especially for working women who experience more job mobility, daily stress, and marital dissatisfaction than working men (27, 75, 199, 200). Most working women with children also bear major responsibility for child care. Thus women are not only exposed to the same physical and emotional hazards of the work environment as men, but in addition, they are also exposed to the stressors created by multiple roles and conflicting expectations of self, family, and others. The health consequences of these dramatic and rapid changes are complex and not yet well known (84). Although hypertension is less prevalent in married, employed women who are happy in their multiple roles, when the woman is excessively committed to the work role, and thus has greater conflict related to the roles associated with home, wife, and parent, hypertension incidence increases (73). Overall, working women do not have significantly higher incidence of coronary heart disease than housewives. But women working in clerical occupations, married, and raising three or more children are at increased risk of coronary heart disease; and clerical women workers married to blue-collar workers are at highest risk (75). Thus the complexity of psychological and social factors are evidenced by an eight-year study by S. Haynes and M. Feinleib (75).

The following job stressors can make a relaxed Type B into a Type A, or a lower scoring Type A into a more exaggerated Type A personality, and may contribute to coronary heart or other diseases:

1. Chronic and unpredictable stress.
2. Intense job involvement; expected high levels of conscientiousness.
3. Time and speed pressures; work overload.
4. Perceived lack of control over the situation; lack of participation in decision making.
5. Responsibility for people and things.
6. Role ambiguity or role conflict.

7. Overpromotion and feared inability to perform.
8. Poor interpersonal relationships.
9. Working alone or without a support system.
10. Feeling dissatisfied with subordinates or being misunderstood by superiors.
11. General job dissatisfaction.

Occupational stressors can increase catecholamine levels and can cause other physiological effects in Type B persons to the same extent as in Type A persons. But Type A persons tend to initially suppress fatigue, hostility, and other bodily symptoms, including those of early coronary disease, so that preventive measures may be ignored. People who do not become ill in the presence of occupational stresses have an attitude of vigor toward the environment, a stronger commitment to self than the job, and an internal locus of control (25, 27, 32, 57, 83, 116, 200).

Crisis and Change

Correlations between environmental changes and illness were noted in the early 1900s by Adolf Meyer (111), and more recently have been made explicit in the Social Readjustment Rating Scale (also known as the Life change Unit Scale) developed by T. H. Holmes and R. H. Rahe (79). (See Table 8-1 in Chapter 8.) If the stressors are very intense for a short time or are milder but overly prolonged, the usual emotional coping mechanisms and parasympathetic nervous system responses may prove inadequate, and increased primitive regulatory behaviors of each organ system are utilized. Organic changes and disease may result. (Refer to Figures 12-4, 12-5, and 12-6 earlier in this chapter.) Seventy percent of people experiencing severe crisis become ill, whereas only 37 percent of people experiencing moderate or mild crisis become ill. The rate of change, rather than the specific type of change, is especially significant (78, 110).

L. Hinkle found that illness occurs when people perceive their lives as being overdemanding, unsatisfying, and full of change and conflict and when they feel unable to adapt to life situations. According to Hinkle, illness patterns are established early and are often maintained throughout life. He pointed out that not all persons exposed to microorganisms or noxious substances become ill; 30 percent of the population have 70 percent

of the illness. Often an individual has multiple body systems involved in symptoms or illnesses. Even minor health problems, such as cuts, bruises, colds, headaches, and backaches, are more likely to occur on days that have greater than average stressors or life changes. Depressed people experience nearly three times as many life changes than the general population (77, 78).

Persons who are at high-level emotional health tend to remain physically well, even in an environment that is unfavorable to health or is rapidly changing (36). In a study of two groups of executives who were exposed to comparably high degrees of stress over a three-year period, the executives who demonstrated less illness were those who perceived themselves to be in control, who felt committed to their positions, and who perceived stress and change as a challenge (96, 97). Another study showed little illness manifestation in a population that had low stress and was generally well-adjusted (12).

Emotional Status

Emotional status or feeling states have been linked to organic changes that may result in disease. For example, suppression of hostility is a coping mechanism whereby negative feelings are not expressed when the person is in conflict with another person who is considered powerful or in authority, such as a parent, boss, landlord, or policeman. If hostility is shown to the attacker, guilt feelings can result. Chronic suppression of hostility has also been related to hypertension in both white and black people. But Negroes who had the blackest skin and who also live in high-stress urban areas—areas that are characterized by low socioeconomic status and high crime, high population density, high residential mobility, and high marital dissolution—had the highest average blood pressure when compared to blacks living in low-stress areas or Caucasians living in high- or low-stress areas. Although more studies are needed to determine the physiological relationship between dark skin and blood pressure, there is little current evidence to support the above proposition. However, from a sociopsychological view, the darker the skin, the more likely the person is to have less education, lower occupational status, and lower income, all of which are stressors contributing to organic changes (71). Thus high unmet need for power is related to chronic sympathetic nervous system overactivity, which in turn has an immunosuppressive effect, making the person more susceptible to frequent and severe illness, as shown in a study of college males (118).

Subjective Perceptions

Mental perceptions, feelings, social or environmental conditions, and physical health are closely interrelated, as demonstrated in one prospective study of an entire community. The following variables were related to a ten-year incidence of cancer and internal diseases (67):

Blocked expression of feelings and needs.

Psychosocial stress in the form of either lasting depression and hopelessness or lasting anger and irritation.

Idealization, with negation of self or low self-worth.

Explosive behavior or hyperactivity.

Exposure to adverse environmental conditions.

Ignoring signs of illness.

Correlation between Emotional Status and Death Incidence

Studies on psychosomatic disease indicate that stressful relationships may speed up death, whereas healthy relationships slow the terminal process. For example, voodoo or spontaneous deaths are well documented as occurring when the person either wills to die because he/she has broken one of the cultural taboos or is the victim of a hex or of an enemy pointing a bone. Only the medicine man coming at the right time can save the person. The medicine man organizes and directs the community's attitude toward the ill person. His ultimate diagnosis and attitude are important. If he feels the patient can be cured, he mobilizes the community's attitude in a positive and supportive way. In a short time, the individual usually improves and is accepted by the community as a vital member. However, if the ill person broke taboos or if the medicine man considers the person incurable, negative attitudes are directed to him/her. Support is withdrawn from the person, even by the family. Social relationships collapse, and the person is left alone to die. The person feels death is deserved, and dies (15, 23, 37, 70, 100, 127).

Other animal and human studies have shown that fears about life, belief that death will occur at a certain time, the loss of hope or of the will to live, or the loss of the desire to fight stressors—all may contribute to sudden death. Refer to Y. Binik et al. (13), J. Langone (100), O. Mowrer and R. Vick (129), C. Richter (155), M. Seligman (173), A. Weisman (203), and S. Wolf (207). For example, rats have died a parasympathetic death (cardiac arrest) when they suffered restraint and could not fight against aversive stimuli. M. Seligman's experiments with dogs showed that they would become inert in the face of aversive stimuli if they sensed no way to escape (173). Other studies show the relationship between a sense of helplessness, loss of internal control, depression, and death (40, 70, 107, 115). Persons who are highly anxious, agitated, or depressed prior to radical surgery are less likely to survive than those who have a favorable outlook (23, 45, 190), whereas persons with internal locus of control are less likely to exhibit anxiety or depression in response to stressors and therefore can better cope with disease and various treatment measures (108).

Perhaps our elderly and ill persons sometimes die because they sense that medical and nursing personnel have withdrawn support. M. Dubree and R. Vogelpohl describe a person who lost hope and as a result was resigned to death, isolated himself from the staff, and turned anger inward into a profound depression. The turning point was the loss of a significant relationship (37). Research has shown that dying persons often sense that their illnesses and deaths are somehow their own faults, which may contribute to their deaths (23, 43, 70).

A number of biographies also tell of how people choose a target date or specific time as the goal for the life span. For example, Mark Twain died on his target date, April 21, 1910. Just as some people die when they have a will to, others survive when medical science predicts death because the determination to live is so strong that it overrides the physical condition. Others live until shortly after a very important event, such as a birth, anniversary, wedding, holiday, or return of a loved one.

The importance of warm, supportive relationships in sustaining health has been demonstrated by the Hutterites in Canada and the western United States. When a member of the group begins to act bizarre—mentally ill—it is a signal to the community to intensify the warm supportive relationships within the whole community. As supportive relationships are maintained, the opposite of voodoo death occurs; the person continues to be a functioning, working individual and often makes remarkable improvement. If the sick behavior has stabilized, the person works toward his capacity and is accepted as an integral part of the community. Attitudes of support apparently help to maintain health, as shown by the low incidence of intense emotional illnesses among the Hutterites (127).

Social science studies suggest that even though hospitals are necessary for medical and therapeutic efficiency, the patient may do worse in these strange settings when he/she is cut off from loved ones than he/she would do at home. Being hospi-talized or removed from the community may hasten death (a fact that American Indians, Orientals, Chicanos, and the elderly have "known" for some time) because of impersonal treatment, dehumaniz-ing care, and overly scientific attitudes of the medical personnel (127).

If human relations and interactions can slow the death process, then a return to home care must be considered whenever possible. If home care is not possible, efforts must be made to create an authentic community in the institutional setting (127). Significant human relationships must be sustained from birth to death because they appear vital for social, emotional, and physical well-being (127).

SOMATOPSYCHIC RESPONSE: EMOTIONAL REACTIONS TO THE STRESS OF ILLNESS

Just as emotional status causes certain physiological and organic responses, defined as the psychophysiological or psychosomatic process, so does the opposite occur. The *somatopsychic process refers to the emotional responses that occur as a result of physical illness or disability.* In this section, some of the reactions to illness and treatment by the health care system are described. In psychiatric/mental health nursing, you may care for people who are suffering from the emotional consequences of acute or chronic physical illness.

People in American society perceive illness as an obstacle to goal achievement, a personal crisis, a frustration of normal life patterns and enjoyments, a disruption in social relations, or a punishment for misdeeds (211). Thus illness is considered a deviant role because the culture enforces an unusually high level of activity, independence, and responsibility on the person. Illness is perceived as related to childhood dependency. Moreover, resorting too frequently to illness as an escape poses a threat to the stability of social systems. Thus, the institutionalized role of illness involves important mechanisms of social control. During illness, certain behaviors are expected of the sick person and of the caretakers (60, 139, 140, 211).

The Sick Role

Illness forces the person to assume an unaccustomed social posture, called the *sick role* by T. Parsons (139, 140) and H. Lederer (104). In the sick role, the patient comes into contact with the caretakers— doctors, nurses, or other health workers—whose jobs are defined by society. In addition, society defines who is sick and who is well.

In the sick role, the person has declared him/ herself to be incompetent to some degree and in a position in which he/she must be taken care of; this is reinforced by society and the health care system. The sick role frees the person from responsibility for the illness and his/her behavior. For example, even if the person has committed murder, if the presence of psychiatric illness at the time of the crime can be proven the person is not held legally or morally responsible but is given treatment. But the sick role also carries the obligation to cooperate with caretakers. The person is freed from ordinary duties, obligations, and responsibilities while working to return to an independent, healthy status. Thus the sick person's two rights are: (1) exemption from usual responsibilities, and (2) absolution of blame for illness and behavior. His/her three obligations are to: (1) view illness as undesirable, (2) want to get well, and (3) seek competent help from and cooperate with caretakers (104, 139, 140).

Certain behaviors normally unacceptable to society are common during physical or emotional illness and are considered helpful in promoting rest and recovery. By accepting illness, the structure of the person's world becomes simpler and more constricted. Initially the person becomes somewhat dependent and regressed: (1) because of unpleasant sensations of physical illness or the physical weakness and helplessness caused by somatic manifestations of the emotional illness; (2) because of Western society's expectations that certain emotions or behaviors must be expressed before the person can get well; or (3) because of egocentricity or the inability to maintain more mature adaptive and coping patterns. Typical feelings and behaviors of the sick person include:

Withdrawal into self rather than interest in others.
Negative self-concept and low feelings of self-esteem.
Mild depression, anger, frustration, fear, and anxiety.
Reduced ability to concentrate and think abstractly.
Avoidance of normal routines.

The ill person is simultaneously in a position of great power and of extreme weakness. This combination of domination and dependence provides a difficult inner conflict, a certain ambivalence similar to what young children feel at times. The person may come to love the authority figure (the nurse or doctor) for taking care of him/her, and simultaneously feel angry toward the health care worker for being powerful while he/she is essentially helpless and dependent (121, 211).

Deviant Behaviors

Certain deviant or maladaptive behaviors in the sick role may occur and be so labeled by the medical team since the behaviors do not assist the person in getting physically, emotionally, or socially well or in regaining independence. When the person uses illness for secondary gain, attention, escape from responsibility, control, or manipulation of others in the environment, he/she does not move through the sick role to return to health at the expected pace or in the expected way (211). For example, this person may hinder progress by becoming apathetic about recovery. Overly compliant, submissive, docile behavior should not be mistaken for cooperation with the treatment plan. The person's feelings of powerlessness and hopelessness, inability to accept the situation or

the feelings involved, lack of initiative and enthusiasm, signs of physical and emotional depression, and inability to reestablish family and social ties — all interfere with working through the emotional or physical illness. Other defenses, such as counterphobic behaviors that include verbal denial of the illness, independent or aggressive acts, or continuing to be on the job contrary to treatment regimen, will interfere with recovery and are considered maladaptive. The compulsive patient may also show maladaptive behavior since he/she is likely to keep especially busy and maintain control with demands or efforts to keep organized and orderly (33, 42).

In the past, sick role behaviors, including dependency, were promoted by health care workers. The patient was expected to do as he was told, even if counsel was inappropriate to the situation. However, in recent years, a more sophisticated public and enlightened health care workers have questioned the negative aspects of the sick role. Now the emphasis is on the client helping to make decisions about the health care treatment, about counseling, and about discharge plans. The client is not only a passive recipient of care but an active participant in his/her own behalf, which may reduce some of the somatopsychic responses to illness. However, it is important to remember that most people need help and are dependent at some point in their illness. Overemphasis on client self-care may indicate that the health care worker cannot tolerate or is fearful of the patient's dependency.

Reactions to Psychiatric Illness and Treatment

The feelings in the previous section may be aroused by entering the health care system for psychiatric treatment. The person *feels* especially vulnerable if he/she is a child or adolescent, is aged, is from a minority culture, or has been mistreated or abused.

Because of society's low tolerance for behavior that falls outside so-called normal limits, families tend to place a disturbed member into an institution as quickly as possible.

The emotionally ill person may feel and be perceived by health care workers, consciously or unconsciously, as a lower form of human, a nonperson, bad or inferior. The ill person may feel, or may be perceived to be, incompetent and unable to take charge of personal affairs, even when he/

she has not been declared legally incompetent by the courts. Even if this person is in contact with reality and has only minor symptoms or few behavioral changes, the label "patient" may signify to others that the person is out of control, unreliable, or in need of improvement. Such responses from caretakers and the climate of the treatment setting are demoralizing for both the person and the family.

Fortunately psychiatric care has improved in the past several decades. There is no longer any excuse for labeling and derision of the emotionally ill person. Our understanding of behavior is adequate so that no person should be perceived in the negative way just described. The therapeutic milieu described in Chapter 4 and other chapters does indeed exist. Yet, in a therapeutic setting and with nurturing caretakers, some clients will feel accepted and respected, but others will feel insecure, inferior, and castigated because of their own previously held stereotypes about emotional illness or their unique personality and psychopathology.

Reactions to Physical Illness or Disease Processes

Understanding the whole person is important in understanding reactions to physical illness. This includes understanding the psychological and social aspects of illness, which requires knowledge about many things: the disease condition; the physical, emotional, and social effects of the condition; the influence of these effects on perception, learning, coping, body image, and self-esteem; and the interaction of these physical and psychological factors with animate and inanimate objects, organizations, and institutions (115).

Effect of Previous Experience and Prior Personality

The individual's personality prior to development of the disturbed structural and physiological functioning will affect response to the illness. Previous experiences that influence how he/she is affected by the changes include (115):

Physical and psychological developmental experiences.
Family, social, and cultural influences.
Special symbolic meaning of the experiences.

Motivation, level of aspiration, and tolerance for frustration developed as a result of past experience.

The prior personality may determine the special meaning of a somatic disturbance; an example is the different types of reactions to a dermatological lesion, such as sebaceous adenoma. The obsessive-compulsive person might interpret it as a beginning cancer; the person with repressed sexual masturbatory tendencies might finger it as if it were a phallus; and the person with a need to prove strength, perfection, and effectiveness might completely ignore its existence as if it were not present (115).

Effect of Defenses

Various defenses may be used simultaneously. For example, denial is a significant defensive mechanism in somatic illness or disability. Regression and yielding to the defect or developing an overcompensated, consciously contrived, preferred behavior may also constitute attempts to manage the anxiety produced by the somatic changes. The degree to which any particular defense is unconsciously utilized helps determine the nature of the psychological reaction (115).

Symbolic Meaning of Injury

The symbolic meaning of the disturbance has far-reaching implications for behavior. In general, the greater the tissue injury, disfigurement, and loss of effective function, the more likely it is that somatopsychic influences will be felt. The loss of a toe, for instance, may have special symbolic significance that may lead to disability disproportionate to the functional loss. Body image concepts are intimately tied to the symbolic significance of any change in body structure and to the mind-body relationship. Whenever the body image is disturbed by disease, amputation, or disfigurement, the person may need special recognition, or he/she may deny loss of parts that are invested with considerable emotional feeling. If the person values beauty and physical wholeness, he/she will feel rejected and unloved. When a limb is amputated, the "phantom limb" may occur; i.e., the person has the illusion that the extremity is present. Neurologically, the phantom represents the organized impression of the person's image of the body before the loss of the limb, and this should disappear when the stimuli that produced the organized sensory impressions of the limb in the parieto-temporal center of the brain are no longer present. The phantom feeling normally shrinks with time. A wish-fulfilling perception, however, may retain the limb indefinitely and illustrates how one type of somatic disturbance can alter mental functioning. The painful phantom, through intractable pain, may serve a need to expiate feelings of guilt. The person may also feel that the organ that offended was the organ punished, according to the talion principle of an eye for an eye and a tooth for a tooth, so that loss of a body part is punishment for past misdeeds (115).

The experience of any physical loss goes beyond the painful distortion of the body image, beyond image of self as a physical being. It involves the image of self as a social being whose family, social relationships, occupation, and hobbies may become altered from a cherished ideal. Independence, self-sufficiency, and autonomy may have to be surrendered (115).

Effect of Timing and Special Circumstances

The time, circumstances, extent, type, and speed of onset of the immediate somatic disturbance are also important. For example, a soldier with an injury may show continuous improvement in physical well-being as he moves further from the battlefield but have an exacerbation of symptoms if confronted with the need to return to the battlefield. In contrast, a civilian with a similar injury may show progressive disability as he/she moves from home to the physician's office and then to the hospital. Also children with chronic illnesses that do not seriously impede locomotion may have a psychic conflict between the desire to be active and the wish to be passive in order to satisfy an overprotective mother, especially where such overprotection has been excessively determined by the mother's guilt (115).

Effect of Alteration in Brain Structure or Chemistry *

Brain changes, whether from fever, alcoholism, drugs, toxins, cardiovascular accident, arteriosclerosis, injury, or infection, can cause psychological disturbances in perception and sensory function, learning and concept formation, orientation, memory, judgment, mood, and behavior. Slowing of speech and decreased motor function often accompany these changes. Psychological reactions to brain injury are dependent on the nature, extent, and location of the lesion and when, during life, the lesion occurs. The type of pathology, whether tumor, trauma, infection, metabolic disorder, toxic agent, thermal, electrical, vascular, or degenerative, may not be as significant with regard to specific effects as the speed with which the etiologic agent affects the nervous system. For instance, fast-growing tumors in a certain location may create disturbances that are quite different from slow-growing tumors in the same area. And infections may superimpose symptoms that result from the invasion by a unique organism and the specific brain response to that particular organism, for example, cell body degeneration in poliomyelitis or perivascular infiltration with syphilis (115).

Direct sequelae of damage to a specific region of the brain include signs and symptoms of headache; dizziness; convulsions; peripheral sensory defects; weakness; paralysis or disorganization of motor control (tremors, tics, choreiform or dystonic movements, clonus, nystagmus); speech, language, and sense organ defects; and a tendency of perseveration and repetition.

Bilateral frontal lobe pathology, when extensive, is associated with impaired attention, distractability, poor retention and learning, poor emotional restraint, euphoria, boasting, impaired abstraction and judgment, slowness, stereotypy, and impulsiveness. Temporal lobe pathology, especially when associated with a discharging type of lesion, may create clinical pictures confused at times with schizophrenic reactions. Attacks may begin with chewing, smacking of lips, or tasting movements, and progress to motor activity performed automatically; aggressive reactions; hallucinations and distortions in perceiving the size and distance of objects and body parts; *déjà-vu* phenomena; fear; and depression. Parietal lobe lesions affect positional and tactile discriminations and cause difficulty in speech reception, dyslexia, dysphasia, and sensory and visual inattention. Corpus callosum tumors commonly cause apathy, drowsiness, depression, and memory defect (115).

Somatopsychic Influences on the Aging Person

Somatopsychic influences on the aging include awareness of loss of prestige, lovability, and sexual potency, and fear of rejection, as well as attempts to deny the aging process, disease, or loss of integrity of body and mind. The need to develop defenses such as regression, dependency, depressive behavior, and demanding, irritable aggressivity is an attempt to restore a sense of mastery and self-worth. Further complications are brought about by the disturbances in memory, recall, retention, and a more profound breakdown in the integrative functioning of the brain (115).

Positive Effect of Somatic Influences on the Mentally Ill

Somatic influences on mental illness may be dramatic. It is not at all uncommon to see a severely psychotic patient suddenly manifest complete remission from overt psychotic manifestations when some acute illness, surgical intervention, or severe trauma intrudes on the patient's disordered psyche. A threat to vital life processes can mobilize latent constructive forces to deal with the new problem because the conflict that maintained the psychotic state is no longer the major problem. The particular symbolic meaning to the patient of illnesses, structural alterations, and physical treatment may also be a factor for improvement from mental dysfunction. Any process affecting the psyche so as to create a new state of balance or necessitating reactivation of psychic functioning on a more mature level may be followed by improvement in the mental state (115).

Reactions to Hospitalization and Treatment

Treatment for physical or emotional illness cannot always be accomplished in an outpatient setting. Hospitalization may be required.

In the best of settings, the person is overwhelmed with many strange, foreboding, conflicting, or frightening feelings. In spite of the many people around, he/she may feel isolated and lonely. In fact, lack of privacy, with the intrusion of the many health care workers into his/her room, often unannounced, is a frequent complaint. Compartmentalization of care and constraints of bureaucracy combine to strip the identified patient of a sense of individuality, identity, decision making, self-responsibility, and significant communication. An

often rigid schedule, ritualistic routines, and staff who appear to hurry or who leave questions unanswered, talk too fast, or use words that are not understood—all contribute to a sense of isolation (211).

The hospital usually means separation from family and other valued persons, objects, and activities. It may be perceived as a place that inflicts undesirable controls and forced conformity, or as a place of punishment for inappropriate behavior. There is endless waiting, and the patient is overwhelmed with feelings of boredom, aimlessness, and sameness every day, even with the planned therapies or activities such as physical, occupational, or group therapy. To others, the hospital may be perceived as a source of relief. It may seem a secure place, with its emergency equipment and trained concerned personnel, where basic needs can be met without effort of self. For still others, the hospital is a place to die (211).

Other possible undesirable effects of hospitalization on the individual include (211):

Enforced dependency on strange authority figures.

Dramatic changes in the physical environment.

Disruption of daily routines, preferences, and at times, biological rhythm.

Different behavioral expectations imposed by the sick role.

Forced adjustment to an interaction with a variety of strangers at a highly vulnerable time.

Depersonalization, loss of privacy and freedom, and fostered regression.

Increased anxiety from all of these effects, which may cause further physical and mental changes and further impede progression toward wellness.

The family also initially feels inadequate to offset or protect its member from these undesirable effects. The family finds itself dependent on the whims of strange authority figures, and it undergoes changes in daily routine as the ill person's responsibilities are absorbed by the members and visits to the sick person are fit into a schedule. The family may be less functional with the sick person out of the home, missing either authoritative or dependent behavior or missing his/her normally healthy disposition or the role of scapegoat for family difficulties. The family may feel threatened by assessment, resenting intrusion into private matters, or fearing that family secrets will be divulged.

Thus illness, especially if it necessitates hospitalization, is a crisis for the person and family (see also Chapter 8). The person is moving from familiar into strange territory, and the usual patterns of behavior are not adequate to cope in the strange situation. The crisis is greater when as a result of illness, the person and family suffer financial strain or value, goal, role, job, or social changes; or when the person and family must adjust to life with a chronic debilitating or disabling condition or an altered body structure or function.

IMPAIRED ROLE BEHAVIOR RELATED TO ILLNESS

The Concept of Impaired Role

Following illness or surgery, the person may not regain complete health or may remain chronically ill. The person reaches a state, *the impaired role, where there is no improvement, but the person is no longer viewed by self or society as being ill in the usual sense of the word. Yet the condition may impose restrictions on activity and life style* and may provoke social prejudice and stigma. Or the person may have an acquired or congenital disability or be socially ineffective because of chronic emotional illness (210).

Often the terms *disability* and *handicap* are used interchangeably, but they are not the same. **Disability** *describes some medically diagnosable condition, either physical or emotional.* **Handicap** *implies a disadvantage in obtaining some desired life goal.* Not all disabilities are handicapping, nor are individuals who may be disadvantaged in achieving some life goal necessarily disabled. Whether the disability becomes a handicap or not is partly related to how a person perceives self and how society responds. It is more accurate to say "a person with a disability" than "a disabled person (40, 210)." **Chronic illness** *is a long-term illness that begins when the acute stage of disease is over and may be characterized by remissions and exacerbations.*

Examples of conditions resulting in some degree of impaired role include blindness, deafness, paralysis, and cases in which some body part or function is congenitally or surgically absent or malfunctioning. *The disability may or may not be obvious, and the person considers him/herself well most of the time. The crisis that surrounded the disability has been resolved, but the ability to carry on usual roles and responsibilities remains limited to some degree.* For the disabled person who is not experiencing illness, social pressures serve to aid in maintaining normal behavior within the limits of potential. This situation is called *impaired role behavior* (60).

The behavior of the person depends on self-perception of the disability as well as on the perceptions of others. Some persons who are chronically ill or congenitally or surgically disabled will remain in the sick role indefinitely. Such persons have not resolved the crisis; the person with impaired role behavior has (60). (See Chapter 8.)

The primary reason for discussing impaired role behavior is that with increased use of technology, medical advances, and heroic measures, the person may have survived a serious or life-threatening illness but then must still adjust to the challenges imposed by continuing to live with the sequelae or an irreversible process. The person is considered neither ill—and therefore governed by sick-role norms—nor healthy in the usual sense. The disabled or chronically ill person who is well-adjusted views him/herself as physically or psychosocially restricted rather than ill (40, 210). The person who is not well-adjusted to role impairment will be in need of emotional care.

Characteristics of Impaired Role Behavior

E. Thomas suggests that *impaired role behavior is an extension of the sick role. The disabled or chronically ill person, however, is not considered by society to be exempt from normal behavior or responsibilities within the limits of the condition. He/she is expected, as far as possible, to improve or modify the life situation in light of the condition, to make the most of remaining capabilities to overcome it, and to accept realistic limits* (196).

The person is then considered to be rehabilitated or under medical control and no longer in the sick role.

The behavioral responses of the disabled chronically ill person also depend on feelings of being accepted or rejected. The disabled or chronically ill person desires and needs to have some close relationships with well persons and needs to be accepted by others for what he/she is, in spite of the condition (171).

Disability often forces the person to modify self-concept and self-image. New and different body sensations, changed appearance or body functions, and changed or reduced abilities challenge the person's self-confidence. Feelings of shame, worthlessness, and inferiority result, often to a degree not justified by the condition. Negative responses from others intensify low self-esteem, and a negative self-image results (40, 210).

The disabled/chronically ill person often gets a mixed message. He/she is expected to be rehabilitated and independent; and yet at times he/she is also expected to be dependent on others—in spite of the American cultural emphasis on self-reliance and independence. The person is expected to share in the management of the medical condition and to be involved in decisions regarding treatment and care. He/she will be asked to explain the condition to others, often revealing considerable personal information and accepting self as an object of curiosity, medically and socially. Yet these explanations can help to reduce social stigma, pity, and prejudice, and will eventually provide opportunities to realize the person's full potentialities (40, 210).

Disability or chronic illness affects all spheres of the person and all aspects of family life. Attempts to remaster the environment and establish a comfortable life style may take considerable time and effort. The house plans or furnishings may have to be changed or rearranged. Living habits, including sleep patterns, may be disrupted. Savings are spent. Vacation plans are cancelled. Future education and job opportunities may be altered (55, 80, 188, 192). The degree of incapacity and related losses, the stage of emotional maturity and developmental level of the person, the nature of previous skills of occupation and their value, and the kinds of resources—including family—available to the person are all important variables in determining capacity to deal with the problem. Persons with mild conditions may have a more difficult time adjusting because they are almost normal. They may try to hide or deny the deficit because it is marginal (115, 168).

Reactions of the Family

After the initial diagnosis of disability or physical or emotional chronic illness in the adult or child, the family may rally to the crisis. However, some families may never completely accept the diagnosis and implications of the condition. Some individuals and families are more successful at learning to cope than others. For these others, the limitations imposed by the health problem are not incorporated into the life style, and the treatment or care plan is not followed.

Threat to Self-Esteem and Family Stability

The self-esteem of members and the sense of family stability may be threatened by the illness of one family member. Roles change. Divorce is more likely, as are problems with the children. Other members of the family may become ill, develop learning or work problems, or forego achievement of their own developmental tasks as they assume others' roles and responsibilities. Family members and the in-laws often blame each other for the conditions, for neglect that may have predisposed to it, or for delay in treatment. When members blame each other, they do not use each other as support. A chronically ill child can become a wedge between the spouses and between parents and other children. One parent may spend most of the time with the ill child; the other may take over responsibilities of job, home, and the other children. One spouse may spend so much time in care of the other spouse that relationships with friends, neighbors, or relatives suffer. Other relatives of the extended family—grandparents, aunts, uncles and cousins—as well as friends, can be a help or a hindrance. Reactions will vary in intensity and kind. Relatives may deny, demand reassurance, and question adequacy of care, rather than give emotional support or assistance with care or finances. To grandparents, a deformed or ill child may represent another loss at a time when many other losses are occurring and cannot be handled (55, 64, 107, 168, 210).

Chronic Sorrow

Chronic illness or disability means chronic

sorrow. At various times the family may feel grief similar to that felt at the onset of the health problem. There is a mourning period for a child who is not born normal, or grief for the present illness or disability and eventual loss of a member, as well as sadness over the loss of hopes, expectations, and dreams for the person. Such grief will be rekindled at the time when the person should be accomplishing some developmental task, such as walking, school entry, graduation, marriage, or childbearing. Sadness and depression occur when expectations cannot be reached. Family members frequently may have to modify hopes, ideals, expectations, and dreams. Grief involves an intermingling of anger, sadness, and despair. Suicidal thoughts may occur. The world looks gray, uninteresting, disorganized. The grieving family member has difficulty making decisions and feels irritable and fatigued, as if he/she is coming apart at the seams, and at a distance from others (64, 109, 168). Refer to Chapter 8 for additional discussion on the grief–mourning process.

Fear and Apprehension

Fear, apprehension, and worry are common. Parents have fears about the consequences of their child not being normal, and they may have concerns about transmitting a genetic disorder to future children. The grieving family members may fear they are going crazy when they are unable to think and make decisions. They, as well as the ill person, fear loss of control and incompetence. Healthy members worry about becoming ill and being unable to care for the ill person, even though they may resent the caretaking. Family members may feel inadequate, fear making mistakes or using poor judgment, and fear financial crises and job loss. Also, if well children are overprotected, their own fears about becoming ill may heighten (146, 168).

Denial

Family defenses will influence whether the disability or chronic illness is viewed realistically and how well members cope with associated stresses. Denial is a common response. The family may disguise facts, hear the words of explanation but not understand or recall, refuse to ask for additional explanation or to admit the forgetting, or

go to another health worker for help. Denial may be seen when the parent, especially the father, shirks responsibility. The members need to go at their own pace to come to grips with the situation.

Anger

Anger is a common response to chronic illness. It is difficult to fight a disease or diagnosis; thus health workers may become the target. Anger may also be displaced as complaints about or bitterness toward God, the church, or other family members. Parents may direct anger at the healthy children or resent the healthy children having fun while another child is ill, and thus set unreasonable limits. The angry family member may internalize his/her feelings, become stoic, be accused of being noncaring by other family members or health workers, and become alienated and isolated at a time when support from others is most needed. Angry or stoic members are as concerned as anyone about their loved ones, but they are reacting differently from others. In turn, the ill person may react to the family's anger and anxiety and become demanding and irritable. However, anger can also be sublimated positively. Families can direct their fighting for the person by becoming involved in the treatment, mastering techniques with fastidiousness, planning for the person's future needs, and joining with other people to promote education, research, or fund raising.

Guilt

Guilt occurs in parents who expect to keep the child safe but, in the face of disability or chronic illness, cannot do so. Thus, they blame themselves. Parents may feel they should be ill instead of the child. Family members may feel guilt and responsibility if previously they felt anger or resentment at the ill person; or the parents may feel guilty if they did not want the child; or a person may feel guilty if he/she has been unfaithful to his/her spouse. The ill person may also feel guilt because of the extra responsibilities, expenses, or constraints placed on the family because of the chronic illness. Fantasies, both in the well and ill, about how different the situation could be, are not uncommon and may cause guilt. Or the ill person may feel that the condition is deserved because of past behavior.

Reaction of Siblings

Siblings of the disabled/ill child are likely to become more withdrawn, irritable, inhibited, and immature. They mourn the loss of an idealized perfect baby and fantasize that they may have caused the defect. They may be angry and resentful about the attention given to the ill child. They note the change in family routines, that fun-filled activities are seldom pursued, and that desired or needed articles cannot be purchased because of medical expenses. Friends may be lost, or never acquired, because of the situation. The children may become so resentful, jealous, or angry at the ill sibling that they declare the child is not a sibling, refuse to be seen with the ill child, or state that they wish the child would die. Guilt or psychosomatic illness may follow. School phobia or poor school performance may also result (168).

Hope

Hope arises anew as the family receives help from professionals, expands knowledge, and expresses feelings. Hope is demonstrated as the family becomes more energetic, starts to make plans, describes a sense of direction, seeks more facts, reaches out to others, and expresses feelings of competence, control, and mastery of the difficulty. Hope is when the impossible seems possible. Hope is not a drifting or comfortable setting; rather it is like steering a ship in a gale. Hope can be fostered if the family unit (including the client) can perceive itself as steering the ship rather than being at the mercy of the winds of the impaired role.

Reactions of the Individual

The person can never be defined by his/her illness. Within a diagnostic category, a wide range of variables will converge to contribute to unique reactions in each person. There is also no simple or direct link between physical disease and psychological behavior (136). Radical changes in body structure may have little or no effect on personality; personality disturbance is more likely to occur when disability is mild or marginal. Personality disorganization is usually transient, if it occurs at all (115).

The psychological impact is determined by the person's stage of development, the degree and visibility of the condition, the meaning and experience of the impaired role, the pain and restrictions, the frequency and duration of hospitalization, the amount of remission, and the person's relationships with family and peers.

The chronically ill person or disabled person is vulnerable to the following types of psychological stress, all of which have their roots in early childhood: (1) threat to self-esteem, (2) fear of strangers, (3) separation anxiety, (4) fear of loss of love, (5) fear of loss of control of developmentally achieved functions, (6) fear of loss of, or injury to, body parts, (7) guilt and fear of retaliation, and (8) fear of pain, which cuts across all of the other stresses. Other psychological reactions to chronic illness include regression, conflict, and inevitable distortions in object relationships (136, 192).

The Infant

The infant needs consistent gratification, appropriate environmental stimulation; and opportunities for play and body exploration; these needs may be interfered with by a defect or serious illness. The infant is totally unequipped to deal with noxious or painful stimuli emanating either from outside the body, in the form of treatment procedures, or from distress within the body, for example, hunger or respiratory illness. Separation from the mother may interfere with attachment formation and object relationships. Thus illness and hospitalization in infancy can have a serious impact on the development of a child's sense of confidence and trust in self and environment (136).

The Toddler

The toddler seeks increasing autonomy and opportunities for exploration and mastery of environment. A continual close, positive relationship with the mother builds upon the developmental foundations provided earlier. Separation anxiety, which peaks at two years of age, is the central emotion for toddlers experiencing illness and hospitalization. In addition, conditions of the neuromuscular system will significantly alter opportunities for developing autonomy in terms of mobility and mastery of the body. Sensory impairments will hinder cognitive and speech development (136).

The Preschooler

The preschooler is developing a sense of initiative. The world is fascinating; parents are seen as omnipotent; thinking is egocentric and fantasy-filled. The fantasy of the child's feelings are frightening because of inability to understand the difference between feeling and action. The experience of illness and hospitalization is filled with fantasy and causes fears of multilation and body damage. The experience may be perceived as punishment for bad thoughts and deeds, and the child may become fixed with guilt, fear, and hostility. These feelings will become part of his/her character unless there is an opportunity to work them through in play, talking, and art (136). The effect of disability or chronic illness may influence the self-concept and gender role identity well into adulthood.

The School-Age Child

The school years are a time for consolidating earlier development. The child normally has effective motor control, sufficient ego structure for the use of defense mechanisms, and skills for reality testing. Energy is normally available for relatively conflict-free activities of learning, exploring and developing deeper relationships with peers and adults. The disabled or chronically ill school-age child is particularly vulnerable to developing a sense of inferiority. Loss of time from school impedes learning, interferes with a sense of achievement, and alters peer relationships. Physical discomfort, growth retardation, and anxiety about health can reduce the child's energy, which is essential to mastering important tasks of this period. The child's growing realization of the chronicity of the condition is balanced by increasing cognitive understanding, capacity to use language, and ability to cope with the reality of the situation. The child needs to learn how to cope with peer reactions, to develop industrious study habits, to compensate for inability to compete physically in adolescence and adulthood, and to develop a hobby or skill at which he/she can excel and gain a sense of achievement and self-worth (53, 136).

The Adolescent

Adolescence is often characterized as a period of fluctuations between extreme opposites. The importance of physique, the marked increase in the intensity of the sexual drive, a new capacity for abstract thinking, and the changing relationships with peers and family all contribute to making adolescence the proving ground of earlier development. A sense of identity is established in the process of finding acceptance by peers, making a career choice, consolidating sexual identity, and forming a system of values. Chronic illness may alter physical growth and bodily appearance and can interfere with a sense of femininity, masculinity, or attractiveness. Potential for finding a partner may be seriously affected, and career choices may be limited. At a time when the person needs to establish increasing independence from parents, progressive conditions such as muscular dystrophy will force increased dependence as the disability progresses. Both the disability/illness and treatment regimens restrict freedom. Conflicts with parents may be acted out in risk-taking or failure to comply with treatment regimens. The female who has been taking medications must deal with the potential danger of their effects on a fetus, should she choose to become pregnant. The possibility of death may be present in conditions such as cystic fibrosis and muscular dystrophy at a time when the person needs to feel some sense of omnipotence and hope for the future (40, 53, 136, 213).

The child and adolescent tend to develop the same attitudes toward disability and chronicity that parents, other adults, and peers demonstrate. The importance of others' acceptance thus becomes clear. Acceptance connotes not only acceptance of the disease, however. The child must ultimately achieve a mature self-concept and realize potential for being an adult, and therefore he/she must be allowed opportunities for growth-stimulating experiences. Age-appropriate challenge and stress are essential to growth. Negative experiences in the general community, where acceptance is less readily available, can be especially threatening and may serve to increase parental overprotectiveness (53).

The Adult

The adult is influenced by the American values of youth, vitality, beauty, physical intactness, and strength. Further, people who value physical stature and motor activity often express their emotional conflicts and insecurities through physical activity; the disabled or chronically ill person may not be able to demonstrate these values. The disabled adult has to continue reworking body image and self-concept as he/she sees reflections of him/herself in the mirror, tries to master skills expected of adults, copes with the changing physical condition, makes or relinquishes various social or occupational contacts, and gains or loses support systems. Self-esteem may decrease because expectations of self or others can no longer be met and because of poor physical condition and function. If the person does not measure up to expectations, he/she is stigmatized, and sense of social worth decreases. The more visible the disability or effect of chronic illness, the greater the stigma faced. If the person had denied the disability all along, he/she will probably continue to disown the body part or wait for a miracle cure. Then no effective rehabilitation can occur (17, 40, 210).

Adult paraplegics, after hospital discharge, usually show a marked reduction in: (a) number of social contacts with others in the community, (b) frequency in entering community settings, and (c) number of roles that they play. However, most paraplegics eventually show some increase in these three activities. All paraplegics face problems that evolve from the *stigma of disability.* In the hospital,

medical personnel try to help paraplegics develop a self-image of independence and personal worth. However, it is easier to establish and maintain this self-image in the sheltered social environment of the hospital than in the world outside (29). As adult paraplegics resume social relationships in the community, they choose individuals who support their independence and social worth. These relationships are sequentially timed. First, paraplegics phase out and seldom resume relationships with pretrauma friends; pretrauma friends see the paraplegic as he/she once was, so that the paraplegic frequently has difficulty establishing a new identity with people who are unable to relate to a disabled person. Second, paraplegics may begin to associate with individuals of lower social status. By choosing friends of lower status, paraplegics are able to balance the negative definitions of disability against some negative characteristic of the other person. If, in these relationships, paraplegics become successful in projecting themselves as persons of worth and become skilled in eliciting this definition from others, they will proceed to more advanced relationships. Finally, they begin to associate with individuals of equal status who may not be disabled (29).

THE NURSING PROCESS WITH A CLIENT WHO IS EXPERIENCING STRESS

Self-Assessment

Throughout the book we shall be emphasizing self-assessment as the first step in giving emotional care. When caring for clients who are in emotional pain, your self-assessment should precede client assessment.

Just as patients and families experience various emotional reactions, the stress of being a health care provider can also provoke anxiety. You may identify with the client because of age, sex, disease type, or professional or cultural background. Perhaps you are in a health care field as a counterphobic reaction, as a way to deal with your fears and anxieties related to illness. You may also become very attached to the client and feel a sense of loss upon discharge or death. Concerns about failure in doing the job correctly, causing damage to the client and receiving criticism from colleagues, are

common sources of anxiety (33). Chapters 1 and 24 describe more fully feelings, concerns, and stressors that you may encounter as student or professional nurse. Anticipating stressors and their effects, and realizing that you are not the only nurse who feels anxious, is an important step in your stress management and in coping with your anxiety and other unpleasant emotions. If you can identify in yourself the effects of stress—physiological, emotional, and intellectual—depicted in Figures 12-2, 12-3, and 12-6, you will be able to more readily assess these stress responses in others. If you are aware of your level of anxiety and its manifestations, you will more readily understand your client who is describing anxiety and related feelings and behavior.

You are a model of health to your clients. If you cannot cope effectively with stressors, you will not be effective in teaching stress management techniques to others. If you have learned some ways of coping with stressors and anxiety, you can share these with your clients.

Be aware of excessive stressors and related stress response and anxiety in your personal and professional life that may contribute to another's feeling of anxiety, or to your own unhappy or destructive life style, disease, and eventually premature death. If you have a chronic stress response, you may become increasingly ineffective in your performance at school, work, and home. You may feel a low morale and self-confidence, and the physical concomitants to emotional stress may result in tardiness or absenteeism as well as higher health care costs. Further, if your client sees you engaged in a self-destructive life style, you will not be perceived as a model for health. Instead, the client will pick up your feelings of distress.

You can use Table 12-3 to score your vulnerability or response to stress.

TABLE 12-3.   Self-Assessment: What Do You Know About Stress?

This is a four-part test. The first three parts are designed to measure your vulnerability to certain types of stress and to increase your awareness of stress and how it affects you. The fourth part will give you some idea of how well you cope with stressful situations.

Stress Test — Part One

Read and circle the most appropriate answer (a, b, c, or d) for each of the ten questions as they actually pertain to you.

	ALMOST ALWAYS TRUE	USUALLY TRUE	USUALLY FALSE	ALMOST ALWAYS FALSE
1. When I can't do something "my way," I simply adjust to do it the easiest way.	a	b	c	d
2. I get "upset" when someone in front of me drives slowly.	a	b	c	d
3. It bothers me when my plans are dependent on others.	a	b	c	d
4. Whenever possible, I tend to avoid large crowds.	a	b	c	d
5. I am uncomfortable having to stand in long lines.	a	b	c	d
6. Arguments upset me.	a	b	c	d
7. When my plans don't "flow smoothly," I become anxious.	a	b	c	d
8. I require a lot of room (space) to live and work in.	a	b	c	d
9. When I am busy at some task, I hate to be disturbed.	a	b	c	d
10. I believe that "all good things are worth waiting for."	a	b	c	d

TABLE 12-3.   Continued

Stress Test—Part Two

Circle the letter of the response option that best answers the following ten questions. How often do you . . .

	ALMOST ALWAYS	VERY OFTEN	SELDOM	NEVER
1. Find yourself with insufficient time to complete your work?	a	b	c	d
2. Find yourself becoming confused and unable to think clearly because too many things are happening at once?	a	b	c	d
3. Wish you had help to get everything done?	a	b	c	d
4. Feel your boss simply expects too much from you?	a	b	c	d
5. Feel your family/friends expect too much from you?	a	b	c	d
6. Find your work infringing upon your leisure hours?	a	b	c	d
7. Find yourself doing extra work to set an example to those around you?	a	b	c	d
8. Find yourself doing extra work to impress your superiors?	a	b	c	d
9. Have to skip a meal so that you can get work completed?	a	b	c	d
10. Feel that you have too much responsibility?	a	b	c	d

Stress Test—Part Three

Circle the response option that is generally true for you.

	ALMOST ALWAYS TRUE	USUALLY TRUE	SELDOM TRUE	NEVER TRUE
1. I hate to wait in lines.	a	b	c	d
2. I often find myself "racing" against the clock to save time.	a	b	c	d
3. I become upset if I think something is taking too long.	a	b	c	d

TABLE 12-3. Continued

	ALMOST ALWAYS TRUE	USUALLY TRUE	USUALLY FALSE	ALMOST ALWAYS FALSE
4. When under pressure I tend to lose my temper.	a	b	c	d
5. My friends tell me that I tend to get irritated easily.	a	b	c	d
6. I seldom like to do anything unless I can make it competitive.	a	b	c	d
7. When something needs to be done, I'm the first to begin, even though the details may still need to be worked out.	a	b	c	d
8. When I make a mistake, it is usually because I've rushed into something without giving it enough thought and planning.	a	b	c	d
9. Whenever possible I will try to do two things at once, like eating while working or planning while driving or bathing.	a	b	c	d
10. When I go on a vacation, I usually take some work along just in case I get a chance.	a	b	c	d

Scoring—Parts One, Two, and Three

Part One: Questions 1 and 10   a = 1 pt.; b = 2 pts.; c = 3 pts.; d = 4 pts.
            Questions 2 through 9 a = 4 pts.; b = 3 pts.; c = 2 pts.; d = 1 pt.
            This test measures your vulnerability to stress from being "frustrated," i.e., inhibited. Scores in excess of 25 seem to suggest some vulnerability to this source of stress.

Part Two: a = 4 pts.; b = 3 pts.; c = 2 pts.; d = 1 pt.
            This test measures your vulnerability to "overload," i.e., having too much to do. Scores in excess of 25 seem to indicate vulnerability to this source of stress.

Part Three: a = 4 pts.; b = 3 pts.; c = 2 pts.; d = 1 pt.
            This test measures the presence of compulsive, time-urgent, and excessively aggressive behavioral traits. Scores in excess of 25 suggest the presence of one or more of these traits.

Stress Test—Part Four

Some coping strategies may actually be as harmful as the stress they are used to alleviate. This scale informs you of ways in which you can effectively and healthfully cope with the stress in your life, while at the same time, through a point system, give you some indication of the relative desirability of the coping strategies you are currently using.

Simply follow the instructions given for each of the 14 items listed on following page. When you have completed all of the items, total your points and place that score in the box provided.

TABLE 12-3.   Continued

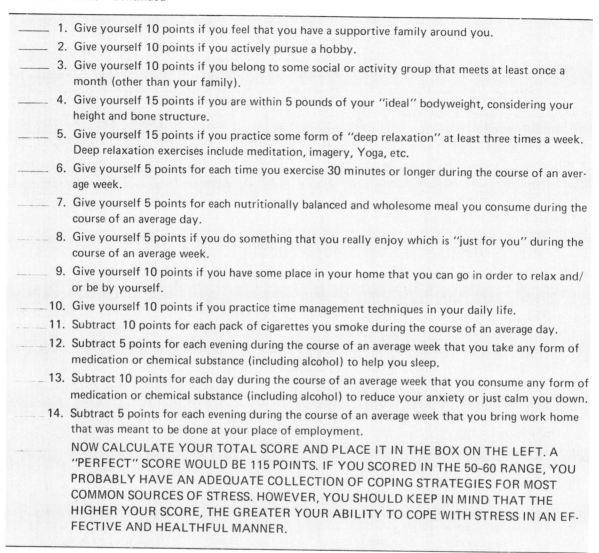

_____ 1. Give yourself 10 points if you feel that you have a supportive family around you.

_____ 2. Give yourself 10 points if you actively pursue a hobby.

_____ 3. Give yourself 10 points if you belong to some social or activity group that meets at least once a month (other than your family).

_____ 4. Give yourself 15 points if you are within 5 pounds of your "ideal" bodyweight, considering your height and bone structure.

_____ 5. Give yourself 15 points if you practice some form of "deep relaxation" at least three times a week. Deep relaxation exercises include meditation, imagery, Yoga, etc.

_____ 6. Give yourself 5 points for each time you exercise 30 minutes or longer during the course of an average week.

_____ 7. Give yourself 5 points for each nutritionally balanced and wholesome meal you consume during the course of an average day.

_____ 8. Give yourself 5 points if you do something that you really enjoy which is "just for you" during the course of an average week.

_____ 9. Give yourself 10 points if you have some place in your home that you can go in order to relax and/or be by yourself.

_____ 10. Give yourself 10 points if you practice time management techniques in your daily life.

_____ 11. Subtract 10 points for each pack of cigarettes you smoke during the course of an average day.

_____ 12. Subtract 5 points for each evening during the course of an average week that you take any form of medication or chemical substance (including alcohol) to help you sleep.

_____ 13. Subtract 10 points for each day during the course of an average week that you consume any form of medication or chemical substance (including alcohol) to reduce your anxiety or just calm you down.

_____ 14. Subtract 5 points for each evening during the course of an average week that you bring work home that was meant to be done at your place of employment.

_____   NOW CALCULATE YOUR TOTAL SCORE AND PLACE IT IN THE BOX ON THE LEFT. A "PERFECT" SCORE WOULD BE 115 POINTS. IF YOU SCORED IN THE 50–60 RANGE, YOU PROBABLY HAVE AN ADEQUATE COLLECTION OF COPING STRATEGIES FOR MOST COMMON SOURCES OF STRESS. HOWEVER, YOU SHOULD KEEP IN MIND THAT THE HIGHER YOUR SCORE, THE GREATER YOUR ABILITY TO COPE WITH STRESS IN AN EFFECTIVE AND HEALTHFUL MANNER.

Source: Table based on data from Daniel Girdano and George Everly, *Controlling Stress and Tension: A Holistic Approach* (Englewood Cliffs, N.J., 1979), pp. 62, 67–68, 72–73. Used with permission of Prentice-Hall, Inc. (54).

Assessment of the Client

Be aware of the health-illness continuum, individual definitions of health and illness, and the many factors that contribute to health and illness as you begin your assessment. Be able to identify stressors and sources of anxiety as your client gives a health history. Assess all components of the person—physiological, emotional, intellectual, developmental, spiritual, and sociocultural—since any or all of these spheres can manifest the stress response and signs of anxiety. Do not overlook the physiological symptoms of the General Adaptation Syndrome in the psychiatric client, or the signs of anxiety in a medical-surgical client. However, the human cannot be easily compartmentalized. Physical lesions and disease affect psychological adjustment, and, in turn, physical abilities are affected by emotional and perceptual states. Moreover, physical illness may be misdiagnosed as psychiatric, and vice versa. Any disease causes some of the same emotional effects as any other disease. Psychological conflicts may facilitate the development of body disorders in people who are physically vulnerable, have low resistance, or are constitutionally predisposed to illness in certain body systems. Multiple causation is a major factor in the development of any physical or emotional illness and must be considered in assessment (115, 182).

When predicting or analyzing stress and anxiety responses in the client, his/her perception or interpretation of the stressful event, as well as the manner in which the individual interacts with the environment, is of primary consideration, rather than just the magnitude of the stressor. Other factors, such as the presence of infectious organisms, poor nutrition, physical overexertion, or temperature extremes all contribute toward depletion of adaptive resources and toward the breakdown and/or disease of organs or tissues. However, the meaning of the stressors, the person's feelings about self, and his/her distorted cognition may be the major contributors to exaggerated behavior patterns for physical or emotional illness.

Figures 12-2, 12-3, and 12-6 have depicted current knowledge about effects of stress and anxiety, and the text has described current knowledge of psychological and somatopsychic processes. In addition, there are many journals that give specific information about the psychological influences of the effects of illness and disability. These periodicals include: *American Journal of Psychiatry, Archives of Physical Medicine and Rehabilitation, Chemical Psychology, Journal of Abnormal Psychology, Journal of Chronic Disease, Journal of Nervous and Mental Disease, Journal of Personality, Journal of Psychosomatic Research, Psychosomatic Medicine,* and *Psychosomatics.*

Certainly knowledge of the content in this chapter is important for accurate assessment. Equally essential is your own ability to empathize—to pick up the meaning of what the person is saying—and to detect nonverbal manifestations of stress and anxiety as well as to hear the client's verbal descriptions.

Various scales and techniques exist to assess stress and anxiety. You may use the scales in Table 12-1 for client assessment as well as for self-assessment. You may also utilize Table 8-1 in Chapter 8 for your client assessment. Besides observation and use of an unstructured or structured interview to learn of the client's self-report of stress symptoms and anxious feelings, you may use other tools for subjective assessment. These tools include: (1) projective tests, such as the Rorschach Test, (2) self-rating tools, such as the Self-Rating Anxiety Scale or Multiple Affect Adjective Check List, (3) tools that quantitatively rate signs and symp-

toms, and (4) laboratory instruments to objectively measure somatic reactivity associated with anxiety.

Physiological Assessment*

Physiological measurements of various organ systems that can indicate anxiety (and the devices for measuring) include the following (44, 214):

Central nervous system—electroencephalogram.

Cardiovascular system—electrocardiogram and blood pressure readings.

Respiratory system—respiratory rate and depth.

Gastrointestinal system—stomach mobility and pH.

Genitourinary system—penile circumference in males and vaginal blood volume in females.

Musculoskeletal system—electromyogram.

Skin—palmar sweat response and galvanic skin response.

Numerous variables affect physiological measurements, such as intellect, emotional set, motivation and cooperation, introspection or self-awareness, and arousal or attention level. These variables are in turn influenced by age, drug effects, illness state, environmental conditions, premorbid personality, cultural background, social relations, and overall physical condition or presence of specific diseases. These variables influence the results and cannot be controlled. Other variables also affect the person's response to physiological measurements and can influence the results; these include the learning that comes from repeated testing, the kind of test construction, and the list of target signs and symptoms used to select on a rating scale. Finally, there are those unique aspects of the person and his/her preceptual state that are like a residue that cannot be measured or explained but which will influence behavior.

Data from various affective-subjective, motor-behavioral, and physiological measures do not correlate well with each other; they may be interrelated but not in a linear fashion. The lack of high correlation reflects the uniqueness of individual differences in response patterns and the multidimensional aspect of anxiety. W. Zung describes validity and reliability of several tests for anxiety (214).

In summary, your ability to accurately empathize, observe, and listen remains the consistently most important way to gain pertinent assessment data from your client. Avoid labeling behavior, especially as either maladaptive or sick. Rather, look at behavior from the client's viewpoint. Place yourself in the role of the client or family member, or try to see the situation as if you were a member of the cultural group that is represented.

Formulation of Nursing Diagnosis and Client-Care Goals

After assessment of the client, using information about the General Adaption Syndrome, levels of anxiety, psychophysiological and somatopsychic processes, sick role, convalescence, impaired role, and chronic illness/disability, your *nursing diagnosis* could be any of the following:

1. *Acute response to stress, Alarm State*, related to _____.
   (stressor)
2. *Acute response to stress, Resistance Stage, with adaptation being maintained.*
3. *Chronic response to stress, diminishing Resistance Stage*, related to _____.
   (stressor)
4. *Anxiety, severe level*, related to _____ (interpersonal or _____ environmental situation).

After each of the above items, specific etiologic stressors and specific signs/symptoms should be stated. Other diagnoses are:

5. _____ related (organic change or problem, physical disease) to (or increased by) _____.
   (emotional status)
6. _____ related to presence of _____ (emotional reaction)   (physio-
   _____.
   logical change, acute or chronic disease, disability)

Specific information should be used for each nursing diagnosis: for example, numbers 5 and 6 above could read:

5. *Somatization of anger, expressed in immobility of arthritis*, related to *feelings in the employment situation.*
6. *Self-imposed social isolation* related to presence of *muscular dystrophy.*

Although you can do little, as a nurse, about the medical diagnosis of arthritis or muscular dystrophy, you can help a client to manage the effects of such illnesses. That is the focus of your nursing diagnoses.

General and long-term goals arrived at mutually with the client may be as follows:

1. Identify stressful aspects of the life style to reduce frequency of the stress response or to avoid stressors when possible.
2. Determine ways to enjoy selected stressors as a challenge by learning more about self or the mechanisms involved in the stress situation, and by adjusting personal philosophy or behavioral patterns accordingly.
3. Manage the stress response by practicing one (or more) relaxation techniques when manifestations of stress or anxiety are anticipated, experienced, or identified.
4. Maintain life style and emotional as well as physical health practices that will aid in disease prevention.
5. Admit the presence of emotional or physical illness; accept assistance, care, and treatment appropriate to the sick role; and carry out measures to return to health.
6. Admit presence of the impaired role and mobilize and expand healthy characteristics that exist, avoiding use of disability or chronic illness as a refuge.
7. Communicate and resolve feelings and thoughts related to the stress response, anxiety state, sick role, impaired role, and the dependency-independency conflicts that are pertinent to the psychophysiological or somatopsychic processes.
8. Demonstrate behavior that is increasingly integrated, socially acceptable, and reflective of a positive self-concept.

Each of these goals is very broad. Therefore, when using the Humanistic Framework, work with the client as a unique person in determining his/her personal needs and goals from the clients's perspective. Some of these goals will incorporate the ideas in the eight goals that are listed above. You will also need to formulate some short-term goals that will assist in meeting these broad, long-term goals.

Nursing Interventions for Eight Client-Centered Care Goals

Strategies for adaptation to stressors and anxiety include biological mechanisms, psychological adaptive or defense mechanisms, coping behaviors, and mastery of skills. There are intrapsychic, interpersonal, and system or institutionalized ways of coping with stressors. You will assist clients to develop and use these strategies through (1) direct care, (2) exploration with the client, (3) teaching or counseling of the client, or (4) creating changes in the person, family, group, health care agency, or the client's environment. Approach intervention from a *holistic* philosophy; mind, body, and culture are a fully unified system, and a variety of approaches can be used to prevent or treat illness.

Biological coping mechanisms and responses of the endocrine, neurological, cellular, and biochemical regulatory systems occur in the Alarm Stage and help the person to maintain the Resistance Stage, recover from disease, and have the energy level necessary to maintain other adaptive strategies. These responses were shown in Figures 12-2, 12-3, and 12-6, and have been described briefly in this chapter. More information can be gained from any physiological textbook.

Psychological adaptive/defense mechanisms, shown in Chapter 2, Table 2-3, are unconsciously but commonly used in response to stress to block the resultant anxiety from awareness and to maintain self-integrity. All of these mechanisms, which can be inferred from observing behavior, help us adapt and are at times necessary. However, they become defensive if any one or all are used repetitively or excessively, if the same mechanism is used in many different kinds of situations, if the duration of use of these mechanisms causes an inflexible personality structure, or if the person is unable to become aware of or admit the use of these mechanisms, even with the help of counseling.

Coping strategies refer to any conscious, observable response or method for handling external life strains, changes, threats, or stressors—in order to prevent, avoid, or control anxiety and emotional distress and to master a task through active problem solving (131, 132, 142). The repertoire of coping behaviors becomes a part of the person's pattern of functioning.

Adaptional strategies depend on securing adequate information about the environment, maintaining autonomy or freedom of movement, having time for development (204), and utilizing social and psychological resources (142).

Resources refer to what is available to the person in developing coping repertoires. Cultural resources are the learned values, customs, and norms of behavior prescribed for survival of the group and well-being of the individual in the group. Social resources are interpersonal networks, such as family, friends, neighbors, work colleagues, the church, and various community groups, associations, or organizations. *Psychological resources are internal personality characteristics, independent of social roles, that help the person withstand threats imposed by events and objects in environment.* These include a sense of self-esteem, mastery abilities, and use of various defense mechanisms, tendencies to escapism, or movement to or away from people (142). *Spiritual resources refer to belief in a Supreme Being, a sense of faith that a deity (God, Jesus Christ, Allah, or others) is guiding you and your life, a practice of prayer, a pattern of practices or rituals associated with your religious beliefs, or membership in an organized religious group.*

People tend to develop modal styles of dealing with life strains that transcend role or situational boundaries. However, inner personality resources as well as available external supportive resources will be needed for coping with certain stressors. No single response or resource is effective against all types of stress situations. Coping depends not only on what but how much the person does. Using only a few responses and possessing few resources will increase the probability that role strains will result in emotional stress (142).

The developmental level of the person is a factor in the ability to cope. All people encounter some problems as they go through the developmental life span of infancy to old age. The difference between those who are healthy (normal) and those who are seriously disturbed is in the way in which problems have been handled, rather than in the presence or absence of problems. Detailed explanations of coping strategies in children, along with critical adaptational periods and the contribution of the mother, are described by L. Murphy (131). Early adolescence, during the junior high-school years, is also a period of great stress, and the young adolescent is vulnerable to stress because of a lack of well-developed coping skills. Hormonal, cognitive, and cultural factors influence the developing self-image and coping skills, and the differential impacts of maturational rate and sex add to the stress (69).

Social roles in adulthood can create certain life strains that are experienced by many people; the coping mechanisms shown by people who are in the same social roles are often similar (142).

The following measures discussed under each goal are useful in coping with stressors, the stress response, and anxiety and other feelings engendered by stressors. These measures are effective for you to use personally as well as to explore with and teach to clients. Only a limited number of measures are described, but others exist. You should explore the many periodicals and books that can be found in professional and public libraries that cover the topic of stress management.

Goal 1: Identify stressful aspects of the life style to reduce frequency of the stress response or to avoid stressors when possible.

Intervention

Teach the client self-assessment. The way you take the client's psychosocial history can help the client determine stressful aspects of his/her life style. Use of the self-assessment scales in Table 12-3 can stimulate thinking about stressors as well as stress response. Anticipating the stressful situation will allow time to prepare for the stressor. When stressors are identified, explore with the client those that can be decreased through direct action and those that can be avoided.

Facilitate the client's *use of an action plan on the identified stressor or problem in order to lessen or remove it.* Any of the following actions could be explored with the client: drop an activity, change jobs, or make a geographic move in order to leave behind that which is stressful and cannot be changed in spite of deliberate efforts. Confront the alcoholic spouse about his/her behavior. Set limits on the children's behavior. Look for resources to allow leaving an abusive spouse. Be assertive with a family member or supervisor. Become involved with a consumer advocacy group or an organization that is working on a special problem. Negotiate with others to find ways to lessen identified stressors at home, school, job, or in the community group. Change the methods you use to get a job done.

Temporary avoidance of identified stressors can be useful at times for regaining strength, energy, and ideas on how to cope. Help the client retreat in a constructive way. Find a place of temporary quiet and isolation. Have a special retreat area, whether it is a room, a special chair, a garden area, or a chapel for prayer, reflection, and thinking calm and beautiful thoughts. Take time to watch the birds, a sunrise, sunset, moonrise, a starry sky, or to look at and smell the flowers. See a television show or movie, drive on a scenic route or take a vacation trip, even for a weekend. Spend an evening with light reading, rather than reading what is necessary for education or a job. Enjoy a window-shopping tour or a shopping spree that can be afforded. Spend an evening a week with the spouse, children, or other loved ones, ignoring all distractions. Encourage the person to choose an activity that is enjoyable—a quiet place, a sport, a game, a good book. The choice should be geared to what works for the particular person.

Goal 2: Determine ways to enjoy selected stressors as a challenge by learning more about self or the mechanisms involved in the stress situation, and by adjusting personal philosophy or behavioral patterns accordingly.

Intervention

Perhaps the most basic rule for coping with stress is to *accept that we live, and will continue to live, in a stressful environment*—although the stressors may change from time to time. If it is possible to enjoy some stressors, life will be less troublesome.

Perception, cognition, stressors, and behavior, and their interrelationships, can be explored with the client. Apparently people experience stressors and cope with stress in a way characteristic of their own cognitive style. The person's perception of the stressor, problem-solving and decision-making ability, ideas and beliefs—all alter the way in which stressors are experienced and coped with. Work with the client to change perceptually the meaning of an experience in order to neutralize its problematic character, so that a situation can be seen as routine, positive, useful, necessary, or challenging rather than threatening. Examples include: (1) comparing self positively to another or judging the personal situation equal to, or better than another's; (2) seeing the present situation as better than the past; (3) ignoring the negative and focusing on positive aspects of the situation; and (4) reordering life priorities (184).

I. Janis found that people who engage in the work of worry or give considerable thought to possible negative experiences they might suffer are less apt to exhibit inappropriate extremes of distress subsequent to a stressful event than are people who either ignore potential stressors/crises or are overly vigilant or excessively worried about life events. Mental role-playing of potential happenings can reduce anxiety and distress and can increase coping ability (87). Richard Lazarus found that the autonomic responses to stress could be reduced through problem solving, intellectualization, or maintaining a detached perspective through which the stressful event could be interpreted (103).

Help the client understand that aversive events are experienced in accord with the perceived degree of control over those events. Apparently the knowledge that one can cognitively structure or exert control over an event increases self-confidence and alters the impact of an aversive event (57, 107). Try to regularize the environment. The same stressors are less harmful if they occur predictably, or if the schedule can be arranged to fit in the stressful events. Determine the client's sense of internal locus of control. *Locus of control refers to ways in which causation of experience is attributed. Internal locus of control refers to a belief that outcomes of interactions between persons and events that befall them are determined, at least in part, by self-action; this belief involves a sense of autonomy or self-controls. External locus of control refers to the belief that events occur for reasons irrelevant to personal action, such as luck, fate, other people, the gods, or nature, and are beyond attempts at controlling them* (163). Persons with internal locus are attentive to information about a situation and maintain an active stance toward stress and crises in both daily actions and dreams. They assimilate information more rapidly about changing events in the environment, maintain a greater degree of vitality, remain alert to the possible roles and behavior to meet demands of the stress or crisis, and do not deliberate as long with difficult choices. Such a person is perceived by others as demon-

strating courage, hope, or self-reliance (105, 106, 162, 163, 164). Persons with internal locus are also more likely to rely on humor to soften abrasive events, and they engage in achievement-oriented daydreams, which in turn contribute to a positive perception of the stressor and promote successful coping (107).

Orient the client to correlations between life changes (as stressors) and illness, so that decisions can be made to either purposefully initiate, structure, direct, or avoid threatening changes. Explore the meaning of change and the feelings that are experienced. Examine ways to adjust to change and anticipated life events. Timing of change decisions should be considered. The accomplishment of a task should be viewed positively as a part of daily living and not as a time for letdown (205).

Holding self responsible for accidents, illness, crisis, or distressing events is an adaptive mechanism that allows the client to perceive the stressor as a challenge and him/herself as in charge of the event. Feeling responsible for recovery and coping will help the person seek assistance and cooperate with necessary procedures. Holding self responsible, along with an unwillingness to become despondent and apathetic despite misfortune, can be observed in persons with internal locus, whereas a tendency to blame others and less adaptive behavior are associated with external locus (23).

Assertiveness as part of a behavioral pattern can be used by the client to reduce effects of stress. *Assertiveness means to take responsibility for defining and meeting personal needs and rights and for communicating with others in an honest, clear, open manner, without becoming angry or aggressive, or without using displacement or projection.* The assertive person listens carefully and respectfully to what others say and speaks in such a way that others will want to listen. Respect of self and personal rights and responsibilities, as well as of the other person and his/her rights and responsibilities, fosters a sense for when to say yes, no or engage in compromise. Sometimes being assertive means to decide *not* to exercise control over stressors, or not to assume responsibility for an event or its consequences. Respect for the feelings of others helps to avoid aggressive behavior that uses any means to gain the end result, achieved at the expense of or control over others, and which may entail verbal or physical abuse.

Encourage the client to validate opinions with friends and professional colleagues, to seek their viewpoints and constructive criticism, to share personal concerns and feelings, and to ask for and accept help when necessary. Getting outside of the self is often useful for looking at stressors from another perspective. Discuss and role-play an anger or anxiety-provoking work situation with a client, taking the role of the person who is creating stress. The client who receives help can in turn extend support or a helping hand to others who experience stress or need help on a specific task, which reaffirms his/her strengths, abilities, and maturity. Stressors loom less large when there is contact between people and when the life philosophy includes sharing with and doing for other people.

Fulfillment of emotional need is essential for coping with stress. Through contact with others, the person can assure that his/her needs for positive attention, recognition, and appreciation are being met on a consistent basis. This is essential to maintain a positive perspective toward life and stressors. People can give themselves positive feedback by acknowledging their own uniqueness, talents, and worth as persons who are good and do good things. Positive comments should also be given to others whenever occasion permits. Encourage the client to feel free to reject negative comments from another and to accept affirmations and compliments from others. A sense of humor and the perspective that goes with it are also great reducers of stress and foster a positive personal outlook. Another resource for need fulfillment is to start or maintain a hobby, devoting enough hours to it weekly so that it remains interesting and satisfies creative needs. Hobbies can be sedentary or active. They may be done alone, such as needlework, leatherwork, cooking, painting, gardening, or photography. Or they can involve a group, such as classes working with clay or ceramics, singing in a choir, doing volunteer work at a local hospital or institution, or joining a garden club.

Achieving attitudinal and behavioral changes that involve a positive set of attitudes toward self, others, and situations, which in turn brings about desired or required results, is the consequence of trying some of the previous suggestions for handling stressors. Creating new personal and professional goals can assist in examining what is really important. Acceptance of the truth, even when it includes behaviors, thoughts, and feelings that could be viewed with alarm, is easier to live with than uncertainty or falsehoods. Part of the truth is awareness of personal strengths, limits, adaptive mechanisms, coping strategies, and resources for assistance. The ability to forgive, to totally cancel whatever blocks one from holding self and others as anything less than totally worthy human beings, is a reformation of attitude that can release stress. Closely related to this is developing the ability to understand the needs and circumstances of others as they see them.

Goal 3: Manage the stress response by practicing one (or more) relaxation techniques when manifestations of stress or anxiety are anticipated, experienced, or identified.

Intervention

Relaxation techniques include cognitive, physical, and emotional responses.

Conscious Cognitive Coping Responses for Relaxation. Deliberately thinking in a certain way is one way to handle stressful situations effectively. Some people develop one or more *thought strategies* as a pattern so that the cognitive process and attitude of relaxation are part of the personality. These mental coping responses are summarized in Table 12-4.

TABLE 12-4.   Various Thought Strategies to Handle Stress and Their Rationale

MENTAL RESPONSE	*DEFINITION AND RATIONALE*
1. Use of knowledge	Learn causes of stress and ways to prevent/manage situation.
2. Objectivity (reality orientation)	Sort out, compare, and validate events, ideas, and emotions to get a total perspective and better understanding on basis of facts, not just feelings; maintain realistic perception.

TABLE 12-4.   Continued

MENTAL RESPONSE	DEFINITION AND RATIONALE
3. Analysis	Study logically and systematically the component parts of a situation to arrive at realistic explanations and answers; manage part if not all of situation.
4. Concentration (mental self-control)	Set aside deliberately thoughts and feelings unrelated to the situation to master tension, save energy, find answers, and necessary decisions for the task at hand.
5. Planning	Think through situation prior to action to release tension, promote problem solving, and avoid unnecessary use of energy, error, and consequent frustration.
6. Fantasize (daydream)	Visualize release of tension and successful achievement rather than dwelling on fear of failure, in order to plan strategy, ensure goal-directed action, cope with stressors, and relieve tension.
7. Rehearsal	Fantasize or anticipate event or another's response prior to stressful event in order to practice coping mentally or behaviorally and to gain confidence in ability to manage.
8. Substitution of thoughts and emotions	State ideas and feelings that are different than real ones in order to avoid adding to stressful situation or to meet demands of the situation.
9. Suppression	Hold thoughts and emotions in abeyance or momentarily forget, in order to wait until it is more timely to change behavior, attack a problem, or implement a solution.
10. Valuing	Establish or reaffirm religious or sociocultural values to foster sense of balance and relaxation in face of stressors.
11. Empathy	Imagine how others in the situation are feeling so that behavior can take these feelings into account.
12. Humor	Point out inconsistencies in situation, laugh at self, and use past feelings, ideas, and behavior in order to be playful, keep objective distance from a problem, reduce anxiety, maintain self-identity, enrich solution, and add enjoyment to life.
13. Tolerance of ambiguity	Function in a way that lays the basis for eventual effective solutions when the situation is so complex that it cannot be fully understood or clear choices cannot be made now.

Research is beginning to show what the ancients know—that *fantasy, visualization, or imagery* can be used with clients to help them overcome disease as well as other stressors. For example, cancer patients who imagine their cancer cells as weak and confused, attacked by medications, and overcome by chemotherapy tend to have fewer symptoms and less pain than people who have ominous visions of cancer, who tend to regress and die sooner than expected (93, 108, 165, 166).

The following exercise uses visualization to enhance healing. Help the client develop a relaxed state of mind and follow these steps. (1) Imagine all of the disease symptoms becoming bubbles. (2) Then imagine all of these bubbles being blown from the body and mind until they are no longer seen.

(3) Then imagine being in a favorite place—the beach, desert, flower garden, church—with a heightened feeling of being alive, comfortable, and healthy, surrounded by clear, bright light. Allow the light to flow into the body, bringing brightness, energy, and health. Relax and enjoy this feeling. (4) Return to normal consciousness with good feelings about self and others (46, 165, 166). This process can also be used to overcome anger or ill feelings to others.

Concentration exercises, both active and receptive, are described by M. Samuels and N. Samuels (166). These exercises can help direct attention at will, overcome distractions, and master a relationship with an object, person, or event. The focused mind has great power. Self-hypnosis and other altered states of consciousness that promote relaxation are described by E. Rosenfeld (160) and other authors.

The following *verbal techniques* are linked to cognitive abilities that release tension and promote relaxation (22):

1. *Talking* about the stressful situation and personal feelings, which enables the person to call for help, do problem solving, consider alternate actions, work through related feelings, and release tension.
2. *Laughing and joking* in order to reduce tension.
3. *Crying,* which elicits support and assistance from others and releases tension.
4. *Praying and spiritual worship.*

Cognitive reprogramming involves using techniques to look at life from a different vantage point of reality and some of the "positive thinking" described by Norman Vincent Peale (141). *Semantic reprogramming* is one form of cognitive reprogramming. Assumptions and belief systems are analyzed because they influence actions. Objective data, including stressors, are made to fit into the belief system. There is a difference in feeling about any situation that is perceived and described as:

"I must do ___."
"I need to do ___."
"I want to do ___."

When the person *wants* to do something, life becomes a challenge or enjoyable, instead of a burden (130).

Use of alibis and rationalizations should be discouraged. Alibis and excuses keep us from seeing reality. An excuse for not managing better can always be found. Analyze the concept of "enough." Realize that there may never be enough money, time, energy, or knowledge for living happily or for avoiding stressors, unless the person adopts a positive attitude of:

I have enough—
or more than enough—money, time, energy, knowledge—
or much more than enough of the necessary resources—
in order to direct or adjust to the situation, to live happily (130).

Internal dialogue, or *talking to the self,* is done many times throughout the day. Often negative ideas, self-doubts, and nagging from the past continue to run through the mind. The person can be taught to: (1) be aware of such ruminations, (2) identify the energy consumed by and the stressful effects of unhappy thoughts, as well as the energizing, freeing effects of positive thoughts, (3) reorient self to thinking pleasurable, self-fulfilling, purposeful thoughts rather than petty, argumentative, conflictual, doubtful thoughts, and (4) keep thoughts focused on the present rather than on past admonitions from others, misgivings, hurts, or problems (130).

A realistic time perspective is also helpful. Focus on the present, rather than expending energy over past situations or future worries.

Physical Methods for Coping with Stress: Relaxation Techniques. Progressive relaxation techniques were first taught by Dr. Edmund Jacobsen in the early 1920s (86). Since then, use of relaxation measures has become increasingly popular.

Dr. Herbert Bensen says that everyone has *a natural and innate protective mechanism against the stress response* called a **relaxation response.** The relaxation response allows us to turn off harmful bodily effects caused by stress: by achieving a decrease in metabolism, pulse, and respiration rates, thus bringing the body into a healthier balance. A number of techniques, as described below, can be used to foster the relaxation response (10).

Change of pace or scenery can bring about immediate stress relief. Taking a brief walk outside; looking at the sky, flowers, or birds; carefully washing hands and face; massaging the face and forearms briefly; listening to music for a few minutes; looking out a window at a tree or clouds in the sky—all are examples of brief moments of interruption that can help reduce stress temporarily, if they are done with intent and attention.

Postural release of tension is the most basic movement of the body and helps the body to regain natural movement patterns and balance and to integrate all body parts. At the beginning of any movement or act, pull the head upward and away from the body, and let the whole body lengthen by following that upward direction (130).

Deep abdominal breathing is done by standing in a comfortable position, head up and level, neck relaxed, arms and shoulders relaxed, knee joints straight but not locked, and feet a little more than shoulder width apart. Close the eyes and practice slow, deep, abdominal breathing for ten cycles. The chest should be relaxed and ribs allowed to move naturally. As the diaphragm moves downward on inhalation, the abdomen will move outward. Conscious control of breathing patterns

helps to maintain a calm, but alert, mental state and control over body movement (46, 191).

Tense and relax muscles systematically while sitting in a comfortable position. Contrast the sensation of tension with that of letting go. Eventually learn to tense and release body muscles from head to toe. Practice this technique to feel the rippling effect (191).

A modification of the above exercise is the following method. Sit in a comfortable chair, feet uncrossed on the floor, hands lying relaxed in your lap. Or lie on your back on a flat, comfortable, but firm surface. Close your eyes. Take a deep breath. Hold your breath for a moment, then exhale slowly. Do this three times or more. Allow your body to become more and more fully relaxed. Now breathe normally. Breathe in a comfortable, relaxed rhythm. For best results, put the instructions shown in Table 12-5 on tape. As each part of the body is named, inhale. Then on exhalation, imagine the breath being sent to whatever part of the body is tense.

TABLE 12-5. A Total Body Relaxation Technique

Inhale. Send breath down to your toes and relax them. Send breath to the soles of your feet and ankles, and relax them. Exhale. Your feet are now fully relaxed.

Inhale. Send breath to your muscles of the lower legs from the ankles to the knees and relax them. First the left leg; then the right leg. Exhale. Feel the relaxation from your toes to the tops of your legs.

Inhale. Send breath to your buttocks and groin and relax them. Exhale.

Inhale. Send breath to your stomach and lower back muscles. Relax them. Exhale.

Inhale. Send breath to your chest and upper back muscles. Relax them. Exhale.

Inhale. Send breath to your shoulders to the tips of your fingers. Relax them. Exhale.

Inhale. Send breath to your forehead, cheeks, eyelids, and jaw muscles. Let jaw drop. Feel a comfortable letting go as these muscles are relaxed. Let this feeling of deep relaxation spread to your neck, throat, and tongue muscles. Exhale.

Breathe very slowly and easily throughout this exercise, allowing breathing to match rhythms of the relaxed body.

Exercise can be used to relax the neck and back muscles and the lumbar spine. See Table 12-6. The exercise is done in three parts.

Exercise or massage of a specific body area can also promote relaxation. *Rotation of the head in a circular motion* while maintaining relaxed shoulders with arms hanging at the side may allow relaxation of the neck muscles and can relieve a

headache. You can also rotate the shoulders backward in a circular, shrugging motion. This will stretch the muscles of the chest that tend to shorten and cause round shoulders. Back, shoulder, neck, and foot massage promote relaxed muscles and a calm mind.

Additionally, the use of *touch* can be perceived as supportive, calming, and strengthening. Holistic

TABLE 12-6.   Exercise Routine for Relaxation of Neck and Back Muscles

Part One:

First, lie on your back on the floor. Lift your knees so your feet are flat on the floor. Arms lie comfortably a little less than 90° from the sides of your body. Cross your right leg over your left leg at the knee. Take in a deep abdominal breath; on exhalation, the legs are allowed to drop by gravity to the right. Relax for a moment. With the next inhalation, bring your legs up to a crossed knee position. Repeat five or ten times. Switch leg positions and repeat to the other side. Slowly extend your legs to lie flat on the floor. Notice that the lumbar region of your back is now touching the floor, or is not as arched as before the exercise.

Part Two:

Next, lie flat and lift both arms above your chest and clasp your fingers together. A triangle is formed by your arms at each side with your shoulders and chest as the base. Maintain this triangle as the exercise in Part One is repeated. Your shoulders will be gently pulled off the floor during the exercise. Notice more of a stretch from shoulder to hip this time. Repeat five to ten times with crossed knees and legs falling first to the right, then to the left.

Part Three:

Finally, bring your arms back to a central position above your body, unfold your hands, and allow your elbows and forearms to slowly touch the floor. Allow both knees to fall to the side and extend legs slowly to the floor. Move to a side-lying position and then push to a sitting position. (Do not sit erect by pulling the torso vertically after this or any exercise that is done while lying on the floor.)

---

health workers emphasize the importance of touch, massage, and anywhere from four to twenty hugs daily for mental and physical health (46, 165).

Some relaxation methods can be done simultaneously with other tasks or while at work. For example: while sitting, raise your legs until they are parallel with the floor. Then alternate bringing your feet back toward the upper torso and then pointing them straight out while curling your toes. When talking on the phone or reading, elevate your feet. This will aid circulation by redistributing the blood that tends to pool in the legs and feet after prolonged sitting. Stand up and stretch two or three times a day, perhaps when breaking for coffee and lunch. Find ways to increase physical activity while going to and from work. Park the car or get off the bus a few blocks from your destination and walk the rest of the way. Avoid the elevator or escalator in going up and down two or three flights of stairs. Or get off the elevator two or three floors below the destination and use the stairs. Try taking steps two at a time.

Autogenic training was first developed by a European doctor, Johannes Schulz, about 1910. Autohypnotic suggestion, visualization, breathing, concentration on physical feelings, touch, and stroking a body area are used to become aware of body parts and to induce certain physical changes that normally occur when we are quiet. These responses include a heavy feeling, generalized warmth, regular pulse and respirations, warmth in the diaphragm, and coolness in the forehead. With practice, relaxed breathing and resultant relaxed musculature become a part of daily life. The person is then able to stop response to tension (46, 165). More information is available in the reference by B. Geba (52).

Transcendental meditation, from which other meditation methods derive, combines physical and cognitive methods and involves self-mastery of mental functioning. Meditation is practiced 15 to 20 minutes twice daily, preferably in the early morning and in the evening before meals. The technique can be practiced by anyone from any culture, religion, or belief (46). Meditation causes decreased oxygen consumption and increased skin resistance and alpha brain waves, indicating a state of deep relaxation and rest, different from sleep in that the person remains aware of surroundings. When the body is at optimum rest, the muscles are relaxed and the mind becomes more clear, alert, creative, stable, and less tense and depressed. Decreased anxiety, greater resistance to stress and pain, increased inner control, better job performance and interpersonal relationships, and a sense of joy about life can re-

sult. Physical health improves. Psychophysiological illnesses, such as peptic ulcer or hypertension, are reduced. The resulting relaxation may help the person gradually decrease his/her need for alcohol, drugs, and cigarettes. Research studies indicate a faster reaction time, more energy, and higher scores on self-actualization in persons who meditate (46, 54, 181). The method described in Table 12-7 is only one of several effective techniques of medication.

TABLE 12-7.   A Meditation Technique

1. Find a quiet place. Avoid interruptions.
2. Sit in a comfortable position in a chair or on the floor. Maintain good posture with your back straight.
3. Select a sound or word to use as a mental device (*mantra*) (God, One, Allah, Buddha).
4. Gently close your eyes and notice how extraneous thoughts leave the mind. Passively disregard distracting thoughts in favor of the mantra. Continue to disregard any distracting thoughts; now is not the time to deal with them.
5. After about 15 or 20 minutes have passed, allow the mantra to fade away. As the mind increases its activity and thoughts come freely, sit quietly for a few minutes before slowly opening your eyes.
6. Remain seated and observe the changes that have taken place, including the following:
   a. Changes in breath rate or heart rate.
   b. Shift in the quality of mental functioning, perhaps more perceptive and relaxed.
   c. Loss of sense of time.
   d. Release of physical tensions.
   e. Shift in sense of body boundaries.

Biofeedback training is a process that helps the person to learn about causes and consequences, and to control stressors and acquire skills in coping with stress via biofeedback autogenic training and progressive relaxation techniques. With this technique, the individual can learn to regulate some aspects of normally involuntary physiological activity. A health and social history are taken to determine various factors that may contribute to the presenting problem. Baseline physiological measurements are taken. The person is first taught to relax through deep breathing and other techniques, and then to use sophisticated measuring devices to further relax in response to visual or auditory cues. The goal is to listen to the body. For example, a sensitive electrode is placed on the

forehead to relay the changing tension of the forehead muscles, which is heard as a series of clicks. With practice, control over the muscle tension is gained. Control of body temperature through biofeedback can also be used to increase blood vessel relaxation, to change blood flow, to quiet the autonomic nervous system, and to reduce headache and other pain (46).

Biofeedback therapy may be useful for persons who suffer the stress response through various psychophysiological disorders, including muscle contraction (tension) headaches, migraine (vascular) headaches, essential hypertension, certain circulatory disorders (such as Raynaud's phenomenon), some gastrointestinal disorders, some disorders related to stroke or spinal-cord injury, certain types of low-back or other chronic pain, bruxism (teeth-grinding), temperomandibular joint pain, and certain anxiety states. As a result of the improved capacity to relax, reliance on medication is often decreased. Several authors give additional information about this therapy; see J. Basmajian et al. (7), D. Girdano and G. Everly (54), A. Putt (148), and M. Samuels and H. Beurett (165).

Emotional Methods for Relaxation. Some of the methods already discussed involve emotional commitment and promote emotional changes that facilitate relaxation. It is useful to keep emotional consequences of problems within manageable bounds through certain accommodations. Examples include living the proverbial clichés, such as: "Try not to worry; time solves problems"; "Accept hardship because it is meant to be"; "Avoid confrontation"; Take the good with the bad"; "The good person will be rewarded in time"; "Everything works out for the best"; and "The endurance of unavoidable hardships represents moral virtues." Denial, passive acceptance, withdrawal, magical thinking, hopefulness bordering on blind faith, religious faith, and believing that avoidance of worry and tension is the same as problem solving are all life orientations that help reduce emotional consequences of stressors for some people (103, 142, 158).

> *Goal 4: Maintain life style and emotional as well as physical health practices that will aid in disease prevention.*

Intervention

Healthful habits can be taught to the client to promote resistance against the organic effects of stress and to provide energy for using various coping strategies. Adequate nutrition—avoiding caffeine and excessive sugar, fat, and overall food intake, and ingesting adequate vitamins, minerals, fluids, fiber, and nutrients are essential (46, 165). Avoid unnecessary chemical additives to food. Adequate sleep is essential for tissue healing and cell multiplication as well as for an alert mind and positive feelings. The amount of sleep time needed varies with the individual but should be of sufficient duration to allow for dreaming, which is one

way of releasing stress. Take time for special skin care and grooming. Exercise that is vigorous and engaged in regularly, at least three times a week, such as jogging, swimming, tennis, racquetball, dancing, or fast-paced walking, to the point of tolerance and double the resting heart rate, promotes all body functions and relieves tension. Physical activity, such as washing the car, mowing the yard, gardening, washing windows, painting walls, swimming, walking, jogging, a game of tennis or golf, helps to relieve feelings of stress if the activity is done with attention and purpose; pleasure is gained from the results, and the labor itself does not add to or cause frustration.

A *hobby or avocation* that allows for creativity and fun is another stress-reduction outlet. No matter what the activity, it must be given full attention and must provide enjoyment while doing it, even if it is only for a few minutes a day. Having time and a safe place in which to physically and creatively express feelings that would otherwise go unexpressed is also important.

Behavior modification, based on Skinner's operant conditioning theory (see Chapter 2), can be used in teaching clients to stop unhealthful practices such as excessive smoking, or to overcome phobias or inappropriate behavior. In a behavior modification program, the inappropriate behavior is identified, the appropriate or desirable behavior is determined, and a learning program to accomplish the replacement is devised. Considerable emphasis is placed on external environmental events that can be used to alter behavior. Circumstances that frequently occurred before, with, or after the client's specific undesirable behavior are avoided, since these situations help to maintain the client's deviant behavior. You can work with the client to increase his/her antecedent, concurrent, or consequent behaviors; to clarify reasons why he/she wishes to stop the deviant behavior; and to establish goals that will maintain motivation to continue the program. The client should play a major role in determining the direction of the behavioral change, and you can assist in formulating a plan. You are a resource person or facilitator. The client acts as his/her own change agent. The client is encouraged to take one day at a time with the new regimen, to set specific short-term goals, and to identify ways to make it difficult to carry out the undesired behavior. Self-reinforcement and self-punishment techniques are used to help the client administer consequences to the self contingent upon behavior rather than receiving consequences from an external agent. The behavior must conform to the person's specific needs and be simple enough so that achievement is possible (45).

Goal 5: Admit the presence of emotional or physical illness; accept assistance, care, and treatment appropriate to the sick role; and carry out measures to return to health.

Intervention

You will be concerned with *promoting the Resistance Stage and preventing or reversing the Exhaustion Stage,* whether through drugs, bed rest, medical treatments, crisis intervention, psychotherapy, or social action. Ideally, you should identify potential stressors that the person might encounter and determine how to alter the stressors or best support the person's adaptive mechanisms and physical, emotional, and social resources, since the person will respond as a whole entity to the stressor. The relationship of stress to life crises or changes is discussed in Chapter 8 and must be considered whenever you are doing health promotion measures as well as when you intervene with the ill person.

The importance of giving care that is accurate and comprehensive is emphasized by an anonymous author—a former patient. The article describes numerous omissions and commissions by nurses, physicians, and aides that made two weeks of hospital care depersonalized, inhumane, and even dangerous. Although the situation described is that of a surgical patient, many of the potential errors described could as easily be observed in a psychiatric or other setting (4).

Studies show that the most important factor for client and family cooperation with the treatment plan is the *relationship with a caring person (107).* Often the nurse is the one person who has the most consistent contact and relationship with a client, especially in the urban, technologically oriented hospital.

Acceptance of illness occurs when the person feels the reality and impact of the illness, acknowledges the illness, seeks validation from significant others, seeks help from a caretaker, and enters into the sick role. During illness, a mourning process for loss of body function or structure may occur, even if such loss is temporary. During this time the person has many worries—job, finances, ability of the family to manage without him/her, fidelity of the spouse, child care, and loss of status. The client may become aggressive or haughty, displacing anger on others, even though he/she feels weak or inadequate. Or the person may be passive in order to hide fear and anger. The stigma, embarrassment, or shame, along with emasculating or defeminizing effects felt as part of the illness, are gradually worked through. Feelings of rejection, of being abandoned, and self-pity diminish.

Different body parts and certain body functions may have great significance to the client. If these have been altered by illness or the treatment plan, the distortion in body image that occurs must be resolved before the patient can enter the last stage of illness, convalescence. Gradually the coping mechanisms are reorganized, and perception becomes more realistic.

The way you talk with and care for the person contributes to his/her ability to accept the sick role and then move toward health.

Establishing a frame of reference is helpful in preparing the client for diagnostic, treatment, or care measures, which are often perceived as threatening, intrusive, or mutilating. If he/she can compare a familiar event or sensation to the event about to be experienced, the event will seem less strange. The person will feel less threatened and more in control of the situation, and the illness can be better tolerated and perceived more realistically. Of course, the frame of reference must have meaning for the patient. For example, a breast biopsy could be compared to the removal of a mole. If the procedure is going to hurt, the sensation should be described to the patient—like the feeling of pain from a burn from a hot stove, a needle prick, a toothache, or abdominal pressure from having overeaten. Group therapy sessions could be compared to serious "rap sessions" with significant people. Electroconvulsive therapy could be compared to going to sleep and then awakening with a feeling as if the sleep position had been uncomfortable, in that there will probably be some grogginess and muscle soreness. A client usually will not engage in a comparison of the sensation or experience of illness without prompting; his/her main concern is to get relief from it. However, if the person is curious, mental anticipation can lessen anxiety.

If the person has been *prepared intellectually* to expect certain consequences, such as the possible outcome of a diagnostic procedure or the complexity of a tentative treatment plan, the emotional reaction will be less disorganized when he/she learns that the possibilities have become reality. If the possibilities of what might happen can be anticipated, behavioral mechanisms can be used to help cope with potential or actual danger. The client's behavior will become more cooperative with the health care team, whereas when the person's perception of the diagnostic or treatment plan is anxiety-laden and negative, behavior is more likely to be negative and uncooperative (87, 88). You will be the health team member best qualified to do this preparation.

Help the client adjust to the sick role by: (1) explaining generally what is expected of the person and family during hospitalization, (2) giving individualized care, (3) preparing the individual and family for various procedures; (4) coordinating all aspects of care to avoid error, fragmentation, and depersonalization, (5) listening to and observing for the person's unique responses, and (6) engaging in person-centered rather than superficial social conversation (90).

Giving clients information that describes what they will see, hear, taste, smell, and experience during health care events, such as electroconvulsive therapy, cast removal, endoscopy examination, or gall bladder removal, reduces stress level more than the traditionally prescribed procedural information that tells what is going to be done, which often heightens the stress (88). Experiments with adults and children have demonstrated that information that helps the client's expectations to mesh more closely with the real experience is effective in lowering stress levels during potentially anxiety-producing situations. Nursing interventions based on Jean Johnson's research have not only reduced stress but also the hospital stay by about one day (88). The results support the cost effectiveness of nursing care.

Consider the less obvious but equally important needs of clients, such as esthetic needs. Eliminate or at least control unpleasant sights, sounds, and odors whenever possible. Consider the likes and dislikes of client and family; let them make

decisions about "the little things that count"— as long as these decisions do not interfere with the treatment plan. Help the person maintain identity by addressing him/her by proper title and name. Encourage bringing some personal possessions from home, and instruct the patient and family about hospital routines and policies in order to reduce feelings of strangeness, isolation, and powerlessness. Flexible visiting hours can reduce loneliness and anxiety related to separation from loved ones.

Convalescence is analogous to the adaptation or resolution phase of crisis. Now the person returns to health. Or, in the case where there is permanent disability and no further physical improvement is possible, convalescence marks a gradual increase in satisfying experiences. The new sense of worth and reduced anxiety enable the client to utilize abilities typical of physical and emotional health. This period is like moving from adolescence to adulthood. The person is reassessing the meaning of life and is becoming increasingly independent, stable, outward-looking, and involved in decision making (137).

There are many variations in convalescence. Convalescence from physical disease frequently occurs before emotional convalescence or resolution of the crisis. The client's level of maturity, the kind of crisis intervention given, the environment in which the person must function, and whether or not the person has a family to return to combine to determine progress. If others encourage constructive activity instead of passive, less adaptive behavior, the person can more easily resolve feelings about having been ill.

In some cases, health may represent more of a threat than illness because of the pressures of life. If illness justifies irresponsible behavior, provides an escape from obligations, or satisfies emotional or financial needs, then the person may actively (although perhaps unconsciously) resist convalescence.

Tasks of convalescence must be accomplished in addition to solving the practical problems of returning home from the hospital. The minor adaptations to the physical environment of the home and daily routine can usually be easily made. But once home, the family and friends expect the newly discharged client to be grateful for recovery and for what they have done for him/her, to be cheerful about rejoining loved ones, and to be eager to return to the usual way of life. However, they may soon find the person is unable to live up to these expectations. Before the client can resume usual activities and make the transition back to health, he/she must first accomplish the three tasks of convalescence described by C. Norris and presented in Table 12-8 (137).

TABLE 12-8. Tasks of Convalescence

I. Reassessment of life's meaning	Goals, purposes, and meaning of life and death are reexamined.
II. Reintegration of body image	Changes in appearance, structure, or function; removal of valued organs; or admission to psychiatric unit must be dealt with and be integrated into the self-concept. Feelings of being dependent, dirty, repulsive, unattractive, unacceptable must be overcome.
III. Resolution of role changes or reversals	Adaptation must be made to changed body, relationships, or roles. Client moves from dependency and self-interest to independency and self-assertion. Returns gradually to normal pattern of living and reassumes roles to extent possible. Behavior increasingly predictable with family and others. Patient returns to optimal level of health as possible.

The *tasks of convalescence* can best be accomplished when client, family, and nurse collaborate, with the client doing most of the work. Promote realistic adaptation by exploring with client and family the meaning of the crisis of illness and the tasks of convalescence. With shorter hospitalization the rule today, some resolution of feelings traditionally accomplished in the hospital must now be done at home. Be supportive and accepting; help the client and family prepare for the tasks of convalescence to be managed at home after discharge. Ask about the client's situation so that realistic planning can be done. This preparation is as important as the discharge planning that helps the client make necessary physical adaptations or learn self-care (133).

Therapeutic communication is essential in helping the person resolve convalescence (see Chapter 5). Foster communication between the client and family members about changes in daily routine, priorities, goals, life-style patterns, and perceptions about self and each other. Help the client and family utilize other resources and explain the benefits of community services, for example, the benefits of a stroke, ostomy, or mental health club. Pick up the subtle meaning of verbal cues. Reflect pertinent statements. Do not feel you must give answers. Encourage exploration of thoughts and feelings so that the person will arrive at his/her own answers.

The person who has a fatal illness will not truly convalesce, yet he/she may enjoy periods of essentially good physical health. His/her reaction must be understood in terms of numerous and sometimes conflicting factors, taking into account previous relationships and previous experiences with crisis, particularly illness and loss. There must be an understanding of the significance of family, social group, occupation, and religion, as well as of the other sources of love, comfort, and support. The person's self-concept and body image, ability to recognize and cope with reality, and responses to dependency, pain, and uncertainty will influence the overall reaction. Other crucial factors are the nature of the specific illness; the organ or body system affected, along with its symbolic as well as real significance to the person; the type of treatment required; and the degree of functional loss and disfigurement.

Final discharge planning and preparing for *termination* of the nurse-client relationship should be started long before the day of discharge. Work though feelings about termination with the client.

(Refer to Chapter 6.) Explore ways to increase the client's sense of interdependence with others and a sense of belonging to the community. Convalescence and the crisis of illness have frequently been resolved when the person can talk about the illness, hospitalization, or surgery with equanimity and acceptance and again feel concern for others. However, convalescence is not resolved when the person needs to talk continuously about the illness experience or states that he/she "never did get over it." You can help to prevent or minimize such responses.

Goal 6: Admit the presence of the impaired role and mobilize and expand healthy characteristics that exist, avoiding use of disability or chronic illness as a refuge.

Intervention

The most striking feature of disability or chronic illness is that it is unrelenting, adding enormous complexity and psychosocial stress to the life of the affected child or adult and the family. As a nurse, you see only the "tip of the iceberg" in relation to their experiences. The disabled or chronically ill, except for those with very severe conditions, will spend most of their lives in the general office, hospital, or clinic. When the client comes in for a checkup, you should discuss his/her status not only with the client but also with each family member individually in order to grasp the total effect of the person's chronic physical or emotional disease on the family. Each family places a different value on physical ability, appearance, and cognitive and emotional functioning. For some families or individuals, impairment of physical ability is devastating. Others can adjust to physical disability as long as cognitive and emotional functioning remain intact (136). Chronic emotional illness often causes the family to give up and to break ties with the client. Thus you and other health workers may become "the family" for the chronic psychiatric client.

Recognize the dynamic nature of development and family life; periodically reassess each family's knowledge, current difficulties, and coping. Each stage of development has its own risks, problems, and responses that affect the quality of life. For example, parents who are aware that their chronically ill or mentally retarded toddler will always be moderately dependent on them will experience this knowledge in a new and profound way ten or fifteen years later. Although the diagnosis does not change, the meaning and effect of the illness will vary as parents and child mature (136).

Family members, particularly early in the illness, may have difficulty in coping with and learning to maximize the help available in the health care setting. You can intervene early by making people aware of their right to comprehensive, optimal care. Specific help, for example, in identifying questions they should be asking and in encouraging them to ask or write questions, can ease anxiety and can facilitate a beginning and continuing sense of competence (136). Families should also know which health team member is the main coordinator of care and who assures that all areas of care are being provided. Problems are also minimized when follow-up home visits are made, with the nurse and other health professionals assisting in a sustained, caring, creative, client-centered way (168).

The greater the responsibility the ill member and his/her family can take, the greater the sense of mastery and autonomy. Responsibility for care should be assumed at the most basic level possible. It is important to recognize that disabled and chronically ill children and adults and their families are often able to teach professionals how to be more helpful to them and to other families with similar problems (136).

Family members of the ill person may become so disease-oriented or so focused on the disability that it may be difficult for them to recognize and appreciate the strengths and abilities of the patient. The person's changing developmental needs also may be overlooked. For example, it is very painful for parents to have their child struggle to achieve what siblings or peers have done with ease. Parents need help in understanding and anticipating the developmental needs of their growing child, so that they can learn to set age-appropriate expectations and limits and appreciate the constructive value of stress in promoting growth and mastery. Also in the case of a disabled adult, others often cannot watch while the person struggles with a task; the *urge to do for* the disabled, *rather than at the person's request*, is great indeed.

Recognize that acceptance will come slowly and will be intermixed with rejection at various times and in various situations. Sharing this understanding with the family and ill person can help to reduce the pain of these periods. Disabled persons should be assisted to learn the skills necessary to reduce stigma from others, to enter a new world resulting from the disability, to reestablish an identity, to establish social relationships, and to overcome loneliness and isolation.

You can work to limit effects of the *spread phenomenon,* the belief that if one function is impaired the person *is unable to perform any functions.* When in the presence of a person with a physical disability or chronic emotional illness, make conscious efforts not to generalize or make assumptions about abilities. Remind yourself to address the person directly rather than through another person. Finally, teach the individual with the disability about the spread process so that it does not come as a surprise and so that plans can be developed for handling such situations (26).

Several guidelines to the development of healthy attitudes toward the impaired role can be stated as follows:

1. *Enlarge the scope of values. Extend horizons beyond the condition and self. There are values besides physique or high intelligence that are sufficiently attractive.* There are a variety of interests and vocations to pursue. Where one path is closed because of a disability, other paths adapted to the needs and abilities of the person can be found. Other values can assume greater potency in the person's life, such as doing what one can, or being understanding and helpful to others.

2. *Contain disability effects, preventing spread of limitations of a disability into nondisability-connected areas.* This is particularly important in the case of a visible disability, but it is also important that the emotionally healthy areas of the personality remain intact.

3. *Uphold asset evaluation. Emphasize what the person can do.* The evaluation takes place in terms of the requirements of the situation rather than in terms of an inappropriate "normal" standard. Attention to what the person cannot do may be appropriate to situational requirements, but the limitations do not thereby come to represent the essence of the person.

Help the person in the impaired role get back into the family system, and help the family secure emotional, social, spiritual, and financial support from other systems in the community as needed.

Help the family members find self-forgiveness by working through feelings of blame and talking about events they think brought on the chronic illness or disability. Encourage catharsis and talking through self-reproach. Give information about etiology, when known. Review all positive aspects in relationships of family members, and show how the positive outweighs the negative. Explain that no human relationship is free of negative feelings. If guilt is especially intense, the feeling may be related to something in the past. Refer family members for professional counseling when needed.

If parents of a disabled or chronically ill child can talk about their feelings, the marriage can be stronger. Otherwise, separation and divorce may occur. Parents have difficulty with and need help in how to tell their other children about the sick child and how to convey that the other children will be safe and not also become ill. Questions about the death of the child should be anticipated and answered honestly; for example, "I can't give an exact answer," or "Bobby is very sick but is getting treatment and is as comfortable as possible."

Help families determine how to utilize grandparents or other relatives, if possible. Relatives can help with transportation, can provide relief at home with daily chores, can supply special activities for the ill member or healthy children, or can help with baby-sitting so that parents can get away at times. Help parents gain ideas on how to prevent a show of favoritism to a well or ill child and how to handle the situation when others talk about the ill person as if he/she is not present.

What happens to the family if and when the chronically ill member dies will depend on family dynamics while the person was alive. If the family accepted the condition and its consequences, they will be prepared to cope with the grief and mourning. If they denied the consequences, the family will need much initial assistance and support and later counseling.

Work with the family and ill member as a unit on ways to buffer the person in the impaired role from the external environment when necessary. Clients may profit from an understanding of the reactions and behavioral patterns of other people that will be encountered in social situations and why they tend to occur. Anticipation of unpleasant events may increase anxiety, but anticipation also allows time to prepare for these events. Practice in handling situations is useful for the person who is in the impaired role emotionally or physically. Practice may include mental rehearsal, watching others (modeling), role-playing, discussing alternatives, or going into the community to encounter and practice handling the situations that arise (26).

Although initial response to treatment or rehabilitation programs may be slow, the disabled person may later become involved in social activities and in an occupation and be a fully contributing citizen. B. Cogswell found that maintaining encouragement and contact with paraplegic clients and families for several years was important (29). Paraplegics were at first unwilling to resume full-time work, but repeated opportunity for job training or placement helped them move into the community and employment. Therefore, do not despair if initial rehabilitation efforts do not result in action or if the client tests your patience.

Goal 7: Communicate and resolve feelings and thoughts related to the stress response, anxiety state, sick role, impaired role, and the dependency-independency conflicts that are pertinent to the psychophysiological or somatopsychic processes.

Intervention

The principles of therapeutic communication and the helping relationship discussed in Chapters 5 and 6 are pertinent to intervention for this goal. Through use of these principles, you can help the client talk about feelings related to stress and illness, relate the emotional distress to physical symptoms/disease, develop a realistic optimism, gain awareness of his/her strengths, recognize positive alternatives and try those that are feasible, and set short- and long-term goals (38).

Intervention with anxiety depends on the level and situation. The anxious person can first talk about actions, then thoughts, and finally feelings. Behavior or concrete events are more easily discussed than ideas or abstractions because cognitive and perceptual tasks are more demanding in energy and concentration. This direction also

parallels the child's development of speech, and under stress we tend to fall back on earlier patterns of behavior. Thus communication and relationship with an anxious person are facilitated if you focus first on a description of client behaviors, then on related thoughts, and then on feelings. Concrete, direct questions elicit more information and help the person gain a sense of self-control. For example, the following questions can be asked: Who are you? Where were you? What happened? When did it happen? What did you do? Who was there? What did he/she say? What did you reply? Avoid questions that ask for description of opinions, feelings, or reasons, such as "Why did you do that?" Observe the person as he/she talks; nonverbal cues reflecting anxiety, fear, hope, and other feelings will be seen (66).

The following guidelines are useful for the severely anxious client (66):

1. *Provide means for expenditure of physical energy.* In conjunction with an interview, you may walk or jog around the grounds or around a gymnasium or pound a punching bag with the client. The client may also yell, scream, or sing as a way to release tension (warn others about what's happening).

2. *Keep communication simple and direct.* Speak in short sentences; avoid detailed explanations. Complex, analytic, cognitive function is impossible at this time.

3. *Decrease situational stimuli.* Take the person to a quiet, calm environment and away from groups of people.

4. *Allow ample personal space* for the person. There is a direct correlation between the amount of personal space needed and the level of anxiety. This is usually not a time for closeness and touching. However, occasionally a highly panicky person may be helped to control extreme restlessness by being held gently but firmly by a nurse quietly expressing reassurance.

5. *Create diversion* if necessary. If asking the client to focus on behavior increases anxiety, offer an alternate focus of awareness until the anxiety decreases to moderate anxiety, when he/she can focus on your statements and on self.

6. *Medication may be required* in some situations where anxiety mounts so rapidly and circum-

stances are so unfavorable that use of the interpersonal relationship is not sufficient alone. This can help reduce the anxiety to a level at which the person can deal with it and its concomitant manifestations.

7. *When the client is under control, work with him/her* to describe the situation—what happened and when, who was there, what was said, and the client's behavior and feelings.

Anxiety states may be treated by various means. For more detail on the use of short-term psychotherapy and behavioral therapy, see references at the end of this chapter. Refer to J. de la Torre (34), F. Frankel (47), and J. Wolpe (209), as well as other authors.

Goal 8: Demonstrate behavior that is increasingly integrated, socially acceptable, and reflective of a positive self-concept.

Intervention

Help the client realize that he/she has adapted to stressful events in the past and can accomplish similar goals in the present or future, which increases his/her self-esteem and self-confidence. In turn, the person becomes motivated by internal goals, desires, values, and ideas, and he/she develops new potential.

When the client is able to internalize the guidelines and measures that have been described above and that are pertinent to him/her, then a positive self-concept and changed attitude and behavioral pattern will be seen. The person will have moved to a higher level of maturity because of your intervention. And in the process of intervening, you also will have become more mature.

Evaluation

The information about evaluation presented in Chapter 4 is applicable in determining your effectiveness in promoting stress reduction.

Part of evaluation of care involves evaluating your own ability to cope with stressors as you care for clients. Share your feelings and talk about your coping skills. You will need someone who values you as a person, not just as a worker—someone who sees you as more than nurse, job, position, or nurturer, and who can help you put stressful work situations into perspective. Strive to develop a sense of autonomy in your own life and circumstances, a feeling that you can exert some direction over what happens to you by the way you view yourself and adjust your own behavior. When you can cope with your own work-related and other stressors, then you can help patients and their families to be adaptive. Refer to Chapters 1 and 24 for more information pertinent to self-evaluation as a student and nurse.

Also evaluate where the client is on the health-illness continuum, but realize that factors within the client or his/her situation may prevent restoration to or maintenance of an improved health status. Any of the criteria given in Table 12-9 could assist with evaluation of the effectiveness of your assessment, teaching, counseling, and goal setting, and other nursing interventions. You may think of other criteria.

You will evaluate care in a variety of settings: while the client is in the hospital or extended care facility; during follow-up home visits; during return visits to the clinic or doctor's office or through telephone contacts or survey questionnaires. You should always determine who is the coordinator of care and whether the care appears comprehensive or fragmented in order to avoid inadequate care for future clients (168).

TABLE 12-9.   Criteria for Evaluation of Intervention Related to Stress Management

1. Client can identify stressors, stressful relationships, and life style that interfered with personal functioning and interpersonal relationships.
2. Client can identify physical (psychosomatic) manifestations of stress that warrants self or other intervention.
3. Client can describe feelings related to anxiety state and can accept assistance in coping with anxiety as necessary.

TABLE 12-9. Continued

4. Client can describe and use at least one strategy to reduce frequency of stress response.

5. Client can describe and demonstrate at least one strategy to avoid a stressor.

6. Client can describe at least one situation whereby he/she has changed perspective about life and stressful situations, so that a situation is perceived as challenging or positive rather than distressful.

7. Client practices at least one of each of the following: (a) conscious mental coping mechanism, (b) verbal response to release tension, (c) physical relaxation method, and (d) emotional method of relaxation.

8. Client describes and practices one positive health habit and one other method to prevent disease and promote health.

9. Client demonstrates behaviors that reflect tasks of convalescence: (a) reassessment of life's meaning, (b) reintegration of body image, (c) role resolution.

10. Client demonstrates _____taught in preparation for discharge.
    (specific tasks)

11. Client functions in impaired role, using maximum potential as indicated by demonstration of strategies to cope with disability/chronic disease.

12. Client's behavior changes from panic or severe anxiety to behavior typical of moderate or mild anxiety.

13. Client describes positive characteristics about self and life style.

14. Client demonstrates improved interpersonal relationships; changed behavior is validated by significant others.

15. Client sets priorities and goals appropriate to developmental stage and life situation and that do not predispose to excessive stress.

REFERENCES

1. Ackerman, Nathan, *Psychodynamics of Family Life.* New York: Basic Books, Inc., 1958.

2. Adler, Jerry, and Mariana Gosnell, "Stress: How It Can Hurt," *Newsweek*, April 21, 1980, pp. 106–8.

3. Altura, B., "Type A Behavior and Coronary Vasospasm: A Possible Role of Hypomagnesemia," *Medical Hypotheses*, 6, no. 7 (1980), 753–57.

4. Anonymous, "A Consumer Speaks Out about Hospital Care," *American Journal of Nursing*, 76, no. 9 (1976), 1443–44.

5. Antonovsky, A., "Social Class and the Major Cardiovascular Diseases," *Journal of Chronic Diseases*, 21 (1968), 65–106.

6. Bartner, R., and R. Rosenman, "The Measurement of Pattern A Behavior," *Journal of Chronic Diseases*, 20 (1967), 525–33.

7. Basmajian, J. V. et al., "Rehabilitating Stroke Patients with Biofeedback," *Geriatrics*, 32, July 1977, pp. 85–88.

8. Bauman, B., "Diversities in Conceptions of Health and Physical Fitness," *Journal of Health and Human Behavior*, 2, no. 1 (1961), 39–46.

9. Bellak, Leopold, *Psychology of Physical Illness.* New York: Grune & Stratton, Inc., 1951.

10. Benson, H. et al., *The Relaxation Response.* New York: William Morrow & Co., Inc., 1975.

11. Betz, B., and C. Thomas, "Individual Temperament as a Predictor of Health or Premature Disease," *Johns Hopkins Medical Journal*, 144, no. 3 (1979), 81–89.

12. Bieliauskas, L., "Life Events, 17-OHCS Measures and Psychological Defensiveness in Relation to Aid Seeking," *Journal of Human Stress*, 6, no. 1 (1980), 28–36.

13. Binik, Y., G. Theriault, and B. Shustack, "Sudden Death in the Laboratory Rat: Cardiac Function, Sen-

sory and Experiential Factors in Swimming Deaths," *Psychosomatic Medicine*, 28 (1970), 576–85.

14. Blum, Henrik, *Planning for Health.* New York: Human Sciences Press, 1974.

15. Bowers, Margaretta et al., *Counseling the Dying.* New York: Jason Aronson, Inc., 1975.

16. Boyd, G., "Stress and Disease: The Missing Link. A Vasospastic Theory: Part III. Stress, Vasospasm, and General Disease," *Medical Hypotheses,* 4, no. 5 (1978), 432–44.

17. Brinkman, J. R., and T. Hoskins, "Physical Conditioning and Altered Self-concept in Rehabilitated Hemiplegic Patients," *Physical Therapy,* 59, no. 7 (1979), 859–65.

18. Briscoe, M. E., "Sex Differences in Perception of Illness and Expressed Life Satisfaction," *Psychological Medicine,* 8, no. 2 (1978), 339–45.

19. Brody, J. V. et al., "Avoidance Behavior and the Development of Gastro-duodenal Ulcers," *Journal of Experimental Analysis of Behavior,* 1 (1958), 69–72.

20. Brown, F. W., "Heredity in the Psychoneurosis," *Proceedings of Royal Society of Medicine,* 35 (1942), 785–90.

21. Bulman, R., and C. Wortman, "Attributes of Blame and Coping in the Real World," *Journal of Personality and Social Psychology,* 35 (1977), 351–63.

22. Burgess, Ann, and Aaron Lazare, *Psychiatric Nursing in the Hospital and the Community.* Englewood Cliffs, N.J.: Prentice-Hall, Inc., 1981.

23. Burgess, Karen, "The Influence of Will on Life and Death," *Nursing Forum,* 15, no. 3 (1976), 238–58.

24. Byrne, M., and L. Thompson, *Key Concepts for the Study and Practice of Nursing.* St. Louis: The C. V. Mosby Company, 1972.

25. Caplan, R., and K. Jones, "Effects of Workload, Role Ambiguity, and Type A Personality on Anxiety, Depression, and Heart Rate," *Journal of Applied Psychology,* 60 (1975), 713–19.

26. Carlson, Carolyn, "Psychosocial Aspects of Neurologic Disability," *Nursing Clinics of North America,* 15, no. 2 (1980), 309–20.

27. Chesney, M. A., and R. H. Rosenman, "Type A Behavior in the Work Setting," in *Current Concerns in Occupational Stress,* eds., C. Cooper and T. Payne, pp. 187–212. New York: John Wiley & Sons, Inc., 1980.

28. Chut, A. et al., "Reduction of Plasma Triglyceride Concentration by Acute Stress in Man," *Metabolism,* 28, no. 5 (1979), 553–61.

29. Cogswell, Betty, "Self-Socialization: Readjustment of Paraplegics in the Community," in *The Psychological and Social Impact of Physical Disability,* eds. Robert Marinelli and Arthur Dell Orto, pp. 151–59. New York: Springer Publishing Co., Inc., 1977.

30. Cohn, Lucille, "Coping with Anxiety: A Step-by-Step Guide," *Nursing '79,* 9, no. 12 (1979), 34–37.

31. Cooper, A. J., V. Cowie, and E. Slater, "Familial Aspects of Neuroticism and Extraversion," *British Journal of Psychiatry,* III (1975), 70–83.

32. Davidson, M. J., and C. L. Cooper, "Type A Coronary-Prone Behavior in the Work Environment," *Journal of Occupational Medicine,* 22, no. 6 (1980), 375–83.

33. Decker, Norman, "Anxiety in the General Hospital," in *Phenomenology and Treatment of Anxiety,* eds. W. Fann, et al., pp. 287–98. New York: Spectrum Publications, Inc., 1979.

34. de la Torre, Jorge, "Anxiety States and Short-Term Psychotherapy," in *Phenomenology and Treatment of Anxiety,* eds. W. Fann, et al., pp. 377–88. New York: Spectrum Publications, Inc., 1979.

35. Dimsdale, J. et al., "The Risk of Type A Mediated Coronary Artery Disease in Different Populations," *Psychosomatic Medicine,* 42, no. 1 (1980), 55–62.

36. Dorfman, W., "Psychosomatic Medicine: Some Past and Current Concepts," *Psychotherapy and Psychosomatics,* 31, no. 1–4 (1979), 33–37.

37. Dubois, R., *Man Adapting.* New Haven, Conn.: Yale University Press, 1965.

38. Dubree, Marilyn, and Ruth Vogelpohl, "When Hope Dies—So Might the Patient," *American Journal of Nursing,* 80, no. 11 (1980), 2046–49.

39. Dunn, H. L., *High Level Wellness.* Washington, D.C.: Mount Vernon Publishing Company, 1961.

40. Eisenberg, M. G., *Psychological Aspects of Physical Disability.* New York: National League for Nursing, 1977.

41. Eisendorfer, Carl, "Anxiety in the Aged," in *Phenomenology and Treatment of Anxiety,* eds. W. Fann, et al., pp. 43–49. New York: Spectrum Publications, Inc., 1979.

42. Enelow, Allen, and Scott Swisher, *Interviewing and Patient Care,* 2nd ed. New York: Oxford University Press, 1979.

43. Feifel, Herman, ed., *The Meaning of Death.* New York: McGraw-Hill Book Company, 1959.

44. Fink, Max, "Anxiety, Anxiolytics, and the Human EEG," in *Phenomenology and Treatment of Anxiety,* eds. W. Fann, et al., pp. 237–50. New York: Spectrum Publications, Inc., 1979.

45. Fisher, Mary Lou, "Helping Acutely Ill Patients Put Out the Fire," *American Journal of Nursing,* 79, no. 6 (1979), 1104–5.

46. Flynn, Patricia, *Holistic Health: The Art and Science of Care.* Bowie, Md.: Robert J. Brady Co., 1980.

47. Frankel, Fred, "Hypnotic Procedures in Treatment of Anxiety," in *Phenomenology and Treatment of Anxiety,* eds. W. Fann, et al., pp. 389–97. New York: Spectrum Publications, Inc., 1979.

48. Freud, Sigmund, *The Problem of Anxiety.* New York: W. W. Norton & Co., Inc., 1936.

49. Friedman, B., and B. Knight, "Running for Life, Health, and Pleasure," *American Journal of Nursing,* 78, no. 4 (1978), 602–7.

50. Friedman, M., and R. H. Rosenman, *Type A Behavior and Your Heart.* London: Wildwood House, 1974.

51. Garrett, James, and Edna Levine, *Psychological Practices with the Physically Disabled.* New York: Columbia University Press, 1962.

52. Geba, Bruno, *Breathe Your Tensions Away.* New York: Random House, Inc., 1974.

53. Geist, R. A., "Onset of Chronic Illness in Children and Adolescents: Psychotherapeutic and Consultative Intervention," *American Journal of Orthopsychiatry,* 49, no. 1 (1979), 4–23.

54. Girdano, Daniel, and George Everly, *Controlling Stress and Tension: A Holistic Approach.* Englewood Cliffs, N.J.: Prentice-Hall, Inc., 1979.

55. Glaser, Anselm, *Chronic Illness and the Quality of Life.* St. Louis: The C. V. Mosby Company, 1975.

56. Glass, D. C., and J. E. Singer, *Urban Stress: Experimentation Noise and Social Stressors.* New York: Academic Press, Inc., 1972.

57. Glass, I., "Pattern A Behavior and Uncontrollable Stress," in *Coronary Prone Behavior,* eds., T. Dembroski et al. New York: Springer-Verlag, Inc., 1978.

58. Gochman, D., "Some Correlates of Children's Health Beliefs and Potential Health Behavior," *Journal of Health and Social Behavior,* 12, no. 3 (1971), 148–54.

59. Goldberg, E., G. Comstock, and R. Hornstra, "Depressed Mood and Subsequent Physical Illness," *American Journal of Psychiatry,* 136, no. 4B (1979), 530–34.

60. Gordon, Gerald, *Role Theory and Illness.* New Haven, Conn.: College and University Press, 1966.

61. Gore, W., "The Relationship between Sex Roles, Marital Status, and Mental Illness," *Social Forces,* 51 (1972), 34–44.

62. ——, "Adult Sex Roles and Mental Illness," *American Journal of Sociology,* 78, no. 4 (1973), 812–35.

63. ——, "The Effect of Children and Employment on the Mental Health of Married Men and Women," *Social Forces,* 56, no. 1 (1977), 67–76.

64. Grace, Helen, "Symposium on Crisis Intervention," *Nursing Clinics of North America,* 9, no. 1 (1974), 1–9.

65. Grasha, Anthony, *Practical Applications of Psychology.* Cambridge, Mass.: Winthrop Publishers, Inc., 1978.

66. Graves, Helen, and Elaine Thompson, "Anxiety: A Mental Health Vital Sign," in *Clinical Practice in Psychosocial Nursing: Assessment and Intervention,* Dianne Longo and Reg Arthur Williams, eds., pp. 87–104. New York: Appleton-Century-Crofts, 1978.

67. Grosserth-Maticek, P., "Psychosocial Predictors of Cancer and Internal Disease: An Overview," *Psychotherapy and Psychosomatics,* 33, no. 3 (1980), 122–28.

68. Guyton, A. C., *Basic Human Physiology: Normal Function and Mechanisms of Defense,* 2nd ed. Philadelphia: W. B. Saunders Company, 1977.

69. Hamburg, Beatrix, "Early Adolescence: A Specific and Stressful Stage of the Life Cycle," in *Coping and Adaptation,* eds. George Coelho, David Hamburg, and John Adams, pp. 101–24. New York: Basic Books, Inc., 1974.

70. Hand, Wayland, eds., *American Folk Medicine: A Symposium.* Los Angeles, Calif.: University of California Press, 1976.

71. Harburg, Ernest et al., "Socio-Ecological Stress, Suppressed Hostility, Skin Color, and Black-White Male Blood Pressure: Detroit," *Psychosomatic Medicine,* 35, no. 4 (1973), 275–96.

72. Harmatz, Morton, *Abnormal Psychology.* Englewood Cliffs, N.J.: Prentice-Hall, Inc., 1978.

73. Hauenstein, E. et al., "Work Status, Work Satisfaction, and Blood Pressure among Married Black and White Women," *Psychology of Women Quarterly,* 1, no. 4 (1977), 334–39.

74. Hayman, H. S., "An Ecologic View of Health and Health Education," *Journal of School Health,* 35 (1965), 3.

75. Haynes, Suzanne, and Manning Feinleib, "Women, Work, and Coronary Heart Disease: Prospective

Findings from the Framingham Heart Study," *American Journal of Public Health,* 70, no. 2 (1980), 133–41.

76. Heagarty, Margaret et al., *Child Health: Basics for Primary Care.* New York: Appleton-Century-Crofts, 1980.

77. Hinkle, Lawrence et al., "An Investigation of the Relation between Life Experience, Personality Characteristics, and General Susceptibility to Illness," *Psychosomatic Medicine,* 20, no. 4 (1958), 278–95.

78. ——, "Ecological Observations of the Relation of Physical Illness, Mental Illness, and the Social Environment," *Psychosomatic Medicine,* 23, no. 4 (1961), 289–97.

79. Holmes, T. H., and R. H. Rahe, "The Social Readjustment Rating Scale," *Journal of Psychosomatic Medicine,* 11, no. 8 (1967), 213–18.

80. Holroyd, J., and D. Guthrie, "Stress in Families of Children with Neuromuscular Disease," *Journal of Clinical Psychology,* 35, no. 4 (1979), 734–39.

81. Horowitz, Mardi, *Stress Response Syndromes.* New York: Jason Aronson, Inc., 1976.

82. House, J., "Occupational Stress and Coronary Heart Disease: A Review and Theoretical Integration," *Journal of Health and Social Behavior,* 15 (1974), 12–27.

83. Howard, J. H., D. A. Cunningham, and P. A. Rechnitzer, "Work Patterns Associated with Type A Behavior: A Managerial Population," *Human Relations,* 30 (1977), 825–36.

84. Ibrahim, Michel, "The Changing Health State of Women," *American Journal of Public Health,* 70, no. 2 (1980), 120–21.

85. Iches, W., and J. Espili, "Pattern A Personality and Noise-Induced Vasoconstriction," *Journal of Speech and Hearing Research,* 22, no. 2 (1979), 334–42.

86. Jacobson, Edmund, *Anxiety and Tension Control.* Philadelphia: J. B. Lippincott Company, 1964.

87. Janis, I., *Psychological Stress.* New York: John Wiley & Sons, Inc., 1958.

88. "Jean Johnson Researches Stress Reduction," *American Journal of Nursing,* 78, no. 1 (1978), 128–29.

89. Jenkins, C., R. Rosenman, and M. Friedman, "Development of an Objective Psychological Test for the Determination of the Coronary-Prone Behavior Pattern in Employed Men," *Journal of Chronic Diseases,* 20 (1967), 371–79.

90. Johnson, Dorothy, "Cardiovascular Care in the First Person," in *ANA Clinical Sessions,* pp. 127–34. New York: Appleton-Century-Crofts, 1972.

91. Johnson, Jean, "Effects of Restructuring Patients' Expectations of Their Reactions to Threatening Events," *Nursing Research,* 21, no. 6 (1972), 499–504.

92. Karp, S., and H. Pardes, "Psychological Differentiation (Field Dependence) in Obese Women," *Psychosomatic Medicine,* 27 (1965), 238–44.

93. Kaufman, Art, "Can Imagination Conquer Cancer?" *St. Louis Globe Democrat,* October 30, 1978, Sec. 13A, p. 1.

94. Keith, R., B. Lown, and F. Stare, "Coronary Heart Disease and Behavior Patterns," *Psychosomatic Medicine,* 27 (1965), 424–34.

95. Klein, H., and O. Parsons," Self-Descriptions of Patients with Coronary Disease," *Perceptual and Motor Skills,* 26 (1968), 1099.

96. Kobasa, S., "Stressful Life Events, Personality and Health: An Inquiry into Hardiness," *Journal of Personal and Social Psychology,* 37 (1979), 1–11.

97. ——, "Personality and Resistance to Illness," *American Journal of Community Psychology,* 7, no. 4 (1979), 413–23.

98. Koenig, R., S. Levin, and M. Brennan, "The Emotional Status of Cancer Patients as Measured by a Psychological Test," *Journal of Chronic Diseases,* 20 (1967), 923–30.

99. Kutash, Irvin, Louis Schlesinger, and Associates, *Handbook on Stress and Anxiety.* San Francisco: Josey-Bass, Inc., Publishers, 1980.

100. Langone, John, "When Hopelessness Kills," *Discover,* October 1980, p. 116.

101. Lavigne, J., and M. Ryan, "Psychologic Adjustment of Siblings of Children with Chronic Illness," *Pediatrics,* 63, no. 4 (1979), 616–27.

102. Lazarus, Richard, *Psychological Stress and the Coping Process.* New York: McGraw-Hill Book Company, 1966.

103. ——, "Positive Denial: The Case for Not Facing Reality," *Psychology Today,* 12, no. 6 (1979), 44–60.

104. Lederer, Henry, "How the Sick View Their World," *Journal of Social Issues,* 8 (1952), 4–15.

105. Lefcourt, Herbert, "Locus of Control and Coping with Life Events," in *Personality: Basic Aspects and Current Research,* ed. Ervin Staub. Englewood Cliffs, N.J.: Prentice-Hall, Inc., 1980.

106. Lefcourt, H., L. Lewis, and I. Silverman, "Internal Versus External Control of Reinforcement and Attention in Decision-Making Tasks," *Journal of Personality,* 36 (1968), 663–82.

107. Levinstein, S., "The Psychological Management of the Patient with Chronic Illness and His Family," *South African Medical Journal,* 57, no. 10 (1980), 361-62.

108. Levinthal, Charles, *The Physiological Approach in Psychology,* pp. 84-111. Englewood Cliffs, N.J.: Prentice-Hall, Inc., 1979.

109. Levy, N., "The Chronically Ill Patient," *Psychiatric Quarterly,* 51, no. 3 (1979), 189-97.

110. Lewis, Howard, and Martha Lewis, *Psychosomatics: How Your Emotions Can Damage Your Health.* New York: The Viking Press, 1972.

111. Lief, Harold, "Anxiety, Sexual Dysfunction, and Therapy," in *Phenomenology and Treatment of Anxiety,* eds. W. Fann, et al., pp. 311-24. New York: Spectrum Publications, Inc., 1979.

112. Longo, Dianne, "Communications and Human Behavior," in *Clinical Practice in Psychosocial Nursing: Assessment and Intervention,* eds. Dianne Longo and Reg Williams, pp. 1-21. New York: Appleton-Century-Crofts, 1978.

113. Mailick, M., "The Impact of Severe Illness on the Individual and Family: An Overview," *Social Work and Health Care,* 5, no. 2 (1979), 117-28.

114. Marcinek, Margaret, "Stress in the Surgical Patient," *American Journal of Nursing,* 77, no. 11 (1977), 1809-11.

115. Marinelli, Robert, and Arthur Dell Orto, eds., *The Psychological and Social Impact of Physical Disability.* New York: Springer Publishing Co., Inc., 1977.

116. Matthews, K., and F. Soal, "Relationship of the Type A Coronary-Prone Behavior Pattern to Achievement, Power, and Affiliation Motives," *Psychosomatic Medicine,* 40 (1978), 631-37.

117. May, Rollo, *Existential Psychology.* New York: Random House, Inc., 1960.

118. McClelland, D. et al., "Stressed Power Motivation, Sympathetic Activation, Immune Function, and Illness, *Journal of Human Stress,* 6, no. 2 (1980), 11-19.

119. Mechanic, D., "The Concept of Illness Behavior," *Journal of Chronic Diseases,* 15 (1962), 184-94.

120. Mefferd, Roy, "The Developing Biological Concept of Anxiety," in *Phenomenology and Treatment of Anxiety,* eds. W. Fann, et al., pp. 111-24. New York: Spectrum Publications, Inc., 1979.

121. ——, "How Much Anxiety Is Normal?" in *Phenomenology and Treatment of Anxiety,* eds. W. Fann, et al., pp. 59-77. New York: Spectrum Publications, Inc., 1979.

122. Moos, R., and G. Solomon, "MMPI Response Patterns in Patients with Rheumatoid Arthritis, *Journal of Psychosomatic Research,* 8 (1964), 17-28.

123. ——, "Psychologic Comparisons between Women with Rheumatoid Arthritis and Their Nonarthritic Sisters: I. Personality Tests and Interview Rating Data," *Psychosomatic Medicine,* 27 (1965), 135-49.

124. ——, "Psychologic Comparisons between Women with Rheumatoid Arthritis and Their Nonarthritic Sisters: II. Content Analysis of Interviews," *Psychosomatic Medicine,* 27 (1965), 150-64.

125. Mordkoff, A., and R. Golas, "Coronary Artery Disease and Responses to the Rosenzweig Picture-Frustration Study," *Journal of Abnormal Psychology,* 73 (1968), 381-86.

126. Mordkoff, A., and O. Parsons, "The Coronary Personality: A Critique," *Psychosomatic Medicine,* 29 (1967), 1-14.

127. Morgenson, Donald, "Death and Interpersonal Failure," *Canada's Mental Health,* 21, no. 3-4 (1973), 10-12.

128. Morris, Carolyn, "Stress: Relaxation Therapy in a Clinic," *American Journal of Nursing,* 79, no. 11 (1979), 1958-59.

129. Mowrer, O. H., and P. Vick, "An Experimental Analogue of Fear from a Sense of Helplessness," *Journal of Abnormal and Social Psychology,* 43 (1948), 193-200.

130. Munz, David, "Stress Management Technique." Paper presented at Conference on Managing Stress, St. Louis University, February 16, 1980.

131. Murphy, Lois, "Coping, Vulnerability, and Resilience in Childhood," in *Coping and Adaptation,* eds. George Coelhi, David Hamburg, and John Adams, pp. 69-100. New York: Basic Books, Inc., 1974.

132. Murphy, Lois Barclay, and Alice Morearty, *Vulnerability, Coping, and Growth.* New Haven, Conn.: Yale University Press, 1976.

133. Murray, Ruth, and Judith Zentner, *Nursing Concepts for Health Promotion,* 2nd ed. Englewood Cliffs, N.J.: Prentice-Hall, Inc., 1979.

134. Natapoff, Janet, "Children's View of Health: A Developmental Study," *American Journal of Public Health,* 68, no. 10 (1978), 995-1000.

135. Nathanson, A., "Sex, Illness, and Medical Care: A Review of Data, Theory, and Method," *Social Science and Medicine,* 11 (1977), 13-25.

136. Neill, Kathleen, "Behavior in Chronic Physical Disease," *Nursing Clinics of North America,* 14, no. 3 (1979), 443-56.

137. Norris, Catherine, "The Work of Getting Well," *American Journal of Nursing,* 69, no. 10 (1969), 2118-21.

138. O'Flynn-Comiskey, Alice, "Stress—The Type A Individual," *American Journal of Nursing,* 79, no. 11 (1979), 1956-58.

139. Parsons, Talcott, *The Social System.* New York: The Free Press, 1951.

140. ——, "Definitions of Health and Illness in Light of American Values and Social Structure," in *Patients, Physicians, and Illness,* ed. E. Jaco. New York: The Free Press, 1972.

141. Peale, Norman Vincent, *The Power of Positive Thinking.* Norwalk, Conn.: Gibson Publishers, 1970.

142. Pearlin, Leonard, and Carmi Schooler, "The Structure of Coping," *Journal of Health and Social Behavior,* 19, no. 3 (1978), 2-21.

143. Pelletier, Kenneth, *Mind as Healer, Mind as Slayer.* New York: Dell Publishing Co., Inc., 1979.

144. Peplau, Hildegarde, *Interpersonal Relations in Nursing.* New York: G. P. Putnam's Sons, 1952.

145. Pitts, Ferris, and Robert Allen, "Biochemical Induction of Anxiety," in *Phenomenology and Treatment of Anxiety,* eds. W. Fann, et al., pp. 125-40. New York: Spectrum Publications, Inc., 1979.

146. Pond, H., "Parental Attitudes toward Children with a Chronic Medical Disorder: Special Reference to Diabetes Mellitus," *Diabetes Care,* 2, no. 5 (1979), 425-31.

147. Pratt, L., "The Relationship of Socioeconomic Status to Health," *American Journal of Public Health,* 61, no. 3 (1971), 281-91.

148. Putt, Arlene, "A Biofeedback Service by Nurses," *American Journal of Nursing,* 79, no. 1 (1979), 88-89.

149. Rahe, Richard, "Life Change Events and Mental Illness: An Overview," *Journal of Human Stress,* 5, no. 9 (1979), 2-10.

150. Rahe, Richard, and R. J. Arthur, "Life Change Patterns Surrounding Illness Experience," *Journal of Psychosomatic Research,* 11 (1968), 341-45.

151. Rathbone, F., and E. Rathbone, *Health and the Nature of Man.* New York: McGraw-Hill Book Company, 1971.

152. Ray, J., and R. Bozek, "Dissecting the A-B Personality Type," *British Journal of Medical Psychology,* 53, no. 2 (1980), 181-86.

153. Redmond, O. E., "New and Old Evidence for the Involvement of a Brain Norepinephrine System in Anxiety," in *Phenomenology and Treatment of Anxiety,* eds. W. Fann, et al., pp. 153-203. New York: Spectrum Publications, Inc., 1979.

154. "Relationship of Psychosocial Factors to Coronary Heart Disease in the Framingham Study. I. Methods and Risk Factors," *American Journal of Epidemiology,* 107, no. 5 (1978), 367-83.

155. Richter, Curt, "The Phenomenon of Unexplained Sudden Death in Animals and Man," in *The Meaning of Death,* ed. H. Feifel. New York: McGraw-Hill Book Company, 1959.

156. Richter, Judith, and Rebecca Sloan, "Stress: A Relaxation Technique," *American Journal of Nursing,* 79, no. 11 (1979), 1960-64.

157. Rim, E., and M. Bonami, "Overt and Covert Personality Traits Associated with Coronary Heart Disease," *British Journal of Medical Psychology,* 52, no. 1 (1979), 77-84.

158. Roberts, Sharon, *Behavioral Concepts and Nursing throughout the Life Span.* Englewood Cliffs, N.J.: Prentice-Hall, Inc., 1978.

159. Roessler, Robert, and Jerry Lester, "Vocal Patterns in Anxiety," in *Phenomenology and Treatment of Anxiety,* eds. W. Fann, et al., pp. 225-35. New York: Spectrum Publications, Inc., 1979.

160. Rosenfeld, Edward, *The Book of Highs.* New York: Quadrangle/The New York Times Book Co., Inc., 1973.

161. Rosenman, R., and M. Chesney, "The Relationship of Type A Behavior Pattern to Coronary Heart Disease," *Acta Nerv Super,* 22, no. 1 (1980), 1-45.

162. Rotter, J. B., *Social Learning and Clinical Psychology.* Englewood Cliffs, N.J.: Prentice-Hall, Inc., 1954.

163. ——, "Generalized Expectancies for Internal Versus External Control of Reinforcements," *Psychological Monographs,* vol. 80 (1966).

164. Rotter, J. B., J. E. Chance, and E. J. Phares, *Applications of a Social Learning Theory of Personality.* New York: Holt, Rinehart and Winston, 1972.

165. Samuels, Mike, and Hal Bennett, *The Well Body Book.* New York: Random House, Inc., 1973.

166. Samuels, Mike, and Nancy Samuels, *Seeing with the Mind's Eye.* New York: Random House, Inc., 1975.

167. Saranson, Irvin, and Barbara Saranson, *Abnormal Psychology: The Problem of Adaptive Behavior,* 3rd ed. Englewood Cliffs, N.J.: Prentice-Hall, Inc., 1980.

168. Satterwhite, B., "Impact of Chronic Illness on Child and Family: An Overview Based on Five Surveys with Implications for Management," *Interpersonal Journal of Rehabilitation Research,* 1, no. 1 (1978), 7-17.

169. Saxton, Dolores, and Patricia Hyland, *Planning and Implementing Nursing Intervention.* St. Louis: The C. V. Mosby Company, 1975.

170. Schultz, Terri, "What Science Is Discovering about the Potential Benefits of Meditation," *Today's Health,* 50, no. 4 (1972), 44.

171. Schutz, William, *FIRO: A Three-Dimensional Theory of Interpersonal Behavior.* New York: Holt, Rinehart and Winston, 1960.

172. Schweizer, Laurence, and George Adams, "The Diagnosis and Management of Anxiety for Primary Care Physicians," in *Phenomenology and Treatment of Anxiety,* eds. W. Fann, et al., pp. 19–42. New York: Spectrum Publications, Inc., 1979.

173. Seligman, M., *Helplessness.* San Francisco: W. H. Freeman Publishers, 1975.

174. Seyle, Hans, *The Stress of Life.* New York: McGraw-Hill Book Company, 1956.

175. ——, "Stress Syndrome," *American Journal of Nursing,* 65, no. 3 (1965), 97–99.

176. ——, *Stress without Distress.* Philadelphia: J. B. Lippincott Company, 1974.

177. ——, "Implications of Stress Concept," *New York State Journal of Medicine,* October 1975, pp. 2139–45.

178. ——, *The Stress of Life,* rev. ed. New York: McGraw-Hill Book Company, 1976.

179. ——, "Forty Years of Stress Research: Principal Remaining Problems and Misconceptions," *Canadian Medical Association Journal,* 115 (July 3, 1976), 53–56.

180. ——, "Stress and the Reduction of Distress," *Primary Cardiology,* 5, no. 8 (1979), 22–30.

181. Shapiro, Deane, *Meditation: A Scientific/Personal Exploration.* New York: Behavioral Science Book Service, 1980.

182. Shontz, Franklin, *The Psychological Aspects of Physical Illness and Disability.* New York: MacMillan Publishing Co., Inc., 1975.

183. Silbrenner, Joanne, "Experimental Evidence: Stress Has a Role in Atherosclerosis," *Medical News,* June 7, 1980, 7.

184. Singer, Jerome, and David Glass, "Making Your World More Livable," in *Stress, A Blue Cross Report,* pp. 59–65. Chicago: Blue Cross Association, 1974.

185. Slater, E., and J. Shields, "Genetical Aspects of Anxiety," *British Journal of Psychiatry,* Special Publication No. 3 (1967), pp. 62–71.

186. Smith, M., and Hans Selye, "Stress: Reducing the Negative Effects of Stress," *American Journal of Nursing,* 79, no. 11 (1979), 1953–55.

187. Smyth, Kathleen et al., "Type A Behavior Pattern and Hypertension among Inner-City Black Women," *Nursing Research,* 27, no. 1 (1978), 30–35.

188. Sparacino, J., S. Hansell, and K. Smyth, "Type A (Coronary-Prone) Behavior and Transient Blood Pressure Change," *Nursing Research,* 28, no. 4 (1979), 198–204.

189. Stein, R., and C. Riessman, "The Development of an Impact-on-Family Scale: Preliminary Findings," *Medical Care,* 18, no. 4 (1980), 465–72.

190. Stephenson, Carol, "Stress in Critically Ill Patients," *American Journal of Nursing,* 77, no. 11 (1977), 1806–9.

191. Stewart, E., "To Lessen Pain: Relaxation and Rhythmic Breathing," *American Journal of Nursing,* 76, no. 6 (1976), 958–59.

192. Strain, J., "Psychological Reactions to Chronic Medical Illness," *Psychiatric Quarterly,* 51, no. 3 (1979), 173–83.

193. "Stress and Illness," *Journal of American Medical Association,* 242, no. 5 (August 3, 1979), 417–18.

194. Sullivan, Harry S., *Conceptions of Modern Psychiatry.* New York: W. W. Norton & Co., Inc., 1953.

195. Thomas, C., and D. McCabe, "Precursors of Premature Disease and Death: Habits of Nervous Tension," *Johns Hopkins Medical Journal,* 147, no. 4 (1980), 137–45.

196. Thomas, Edwin, "Problems of Disability from the Perspective of Role Theory," *Journal of Health and Human Behavior,* 7, no. 1 (1966), 2–14.

197. Townsend, P., "Inequality at the Work Place: How White Collar Always Wins," *New Society,* 50 (1979), 120–23.

198. Vaillant, G., "Natural History of Male Psychological Health: IV. What Kinds of Men Do Not Get Psychosomatic Illness," *Psychosomatic Medicine,* 40, no. 5 (1978), 420–31.

199. Waldron, I., "Type A Behavior Pattern and Coronary Heart Disease in Men and Women," *Social Science and Medicine,* 128 (1978), 167–70.

200. Waldron I. et al., "The Coronary-Prone Behavior Pattern in Employed Men and Women," *Journal of Human Stress,* 3 (1977), 2–18.

201. ——, "Type A Behavior Pattern: Relationship to Variation in Blood Pressure, Parental Characteristics, and Academic and Social Activities of Students," *Journal of Human Stress,* 6, no. 1 (1980), 16–27.

202. Warren, L., and D. Weiss, "Relationship between Disability Type and Measured Personality Characteristics," *Proceedings, 77th Annual Convention, American Psychological Association,* (Washington, D.C. 1969). Pp. 773–74.

203. Weisman, A. D., "Predilection to Death: Death and Dying as a Psychiatric Problem," *Psychosomatic Medicine,* 23 (1961), 232–56.

204. White, Robert, "Strategies of Adaptation: An Attempt at Systematic Description," in *Coping and Adaptation,* eds. G. Coelho, D. Hamburg, and J. Adams, pp. 47–68. New York: Basic Books, Inc., 1974.

205. Williams, Cindy, and Thomas Holmes, "Life Change, Human Adaptation, and Onset of Illness," in *Clinical Practice in Psychosocial Nursing: Assessment and Intervention,* eds. Dianne Longo and Reg Williams, pp. 69–85. New York: Appleton-Century-Crofts, 1978.

206. Williams, R. et al., "Disturbed Sleep and Anxiety," in *Phenomenology and Treatment of Anxiety,* eds. W. Fann, et al., pp. 211–23. New York: Spectrum Publications, Inc., 1979.

207. Wolf, S., "The End of the Rope: The Role of the Brain in Cardiac Death," *Journal of Canadian Medical Association,* 97 (1976), 1022–25.

208. Wolf, S., and J. Ducette, "International Performance and Incidental Learning as a Function of Personality and Task Directions," *Journal of Personality and Social Psychology,* 29 (1974), 90–101.

209. Wolpe, Joseph, "Behavior Analysis and the Elimination of Anxiety Response Habits," in *Phenomenology and Treatment of Anxiety,* eds. W. Fann, et al., pp. 369–87. New York: Spectrum Publications, Inc., 1979.

210. Wright, Beatrice, *Physical Disability: A Psychological Approach.* New York: Harper & Row, Publishers, Inc., 1960.

211. Wu, Ruth, *Behavior and Illness.* Englewood Cliffs, N.J.: Prentice-Hall, Inc., 1973.

212. Young, J. P. R., G. W. Fenton, and M. H. Lader, "The Inheritance of Neurotic Traits: A Twin Study of the Middlesex Hospital Questionnaire," *British Journal of Psychiatry,* 119 (1971), 393–408.

213. Zeltzer, L. et al., "Psychologic Effects of Illness in Adolescence. II. Impact of Illness in Adolescents—Crucial Issues and Coping Styles," *Journal of Pediatrics,* 97, no. 1 (1980), 132–38.

214. Zung, William, "Assessment of Anxiety Disorder: Qualitative and Quantitative Approaches," in *Phenomenology and Treatment of Anxiety,* eds. W. Fann et al., pp. 1-17. New York: Spectrum Publications, Inc., 1979.

13

The Person Who Uses Dysfunctional Coping Patterns

Study of this chapter will assist you to:

1. Relate stress and anxiety to dysfunctional, maladaptive, or neurotic behavior.

2. Compare and contrast psychoneurosis and psychosis.

3. Relate nursing diagnosis to psychoneurosis.

4. Assess signs and symptoms that express chronic anxiety, including the obsessive-compulsive behavior patterns, phobic symptoms, somatization through conversion or hypochondriasis, and dissociation.

5. Examine the importance of the nurse-client relationship in intervention with the chronically anxious person.

6. Describe other interventions useful in reducing expressions of chronic anxiety.

This chapter contributed by M. Marilyn Huelskoetter, R.N., M.S.N.

DYSFUNCTIONAL BEHAVIOR AND EMOTIONAL ILLNESS—RESPONSE TO STRESS AND ANXIETY

Anxiety as a signal of psychological function is the counterpart to pain as a signal of physiological function. At least a minimal level of anxiety exists in everyone most of the time: arousal is appropriate to the situation and can be validated by others familiar with the situation. Even moderate anxiety may be present and can be tolerated for a relatively short period of time. Anxiety is usually seen as part of a pattern of emotions; it rarely exists alone. Various behavioral responses, including motor activity, unconscious adaptive mechanisms, and purposeful coping strategies, are used to disguise or ward off anxiety and other feelings. See Figure 13-1 and refer to Chapter 2, Table 2-3, and Chapter 12.

Severe anxiety can be tolerated physically and behaviorally for only a short interval. If severe anxiety persists, the person cannot cope with or defend against the intense feelings, and ineffective or dysfunctional behavior results. The person's behavior may be ineffective in one or two areas of life, such as in family relations or job performance, or many aspects of life may be affected. If family, work, and social relations are sufficiently disrupted,

or if the person's intense feeling state and behavior persist and are perceived by self or others as being a nuisance, unusual, deviant, or dysfunctional—*abnormal* as defined by the culture and social group—then the person is diagnosed as being emotionally (mentally) ill.

There are many medical labels or diagnoses of emotional or psychiatric illness: see Appendix I of this text, taken from the *Diagnostic and Statistical Manual,* 3rd ed. (*DSM-III*) (5).

In this Part we discuss behavioral patterns that are nursing diagnoses related to emotional illness as well as the various psychiatric diagnostic labels. One set of dysfunctional behaviors is generally grouped under the label *neurosis,* a term you have probably heard. You may have used it to describe the age we live in or the behavior of a friend. You may even have wondered at times if you were neurotic as you experienced the stress, anxiety, and frustration of life. Neurosis is a commonly used concept and has held an important place in the history of psychiatry over the years.

Although "neurosis" is not listed in the third

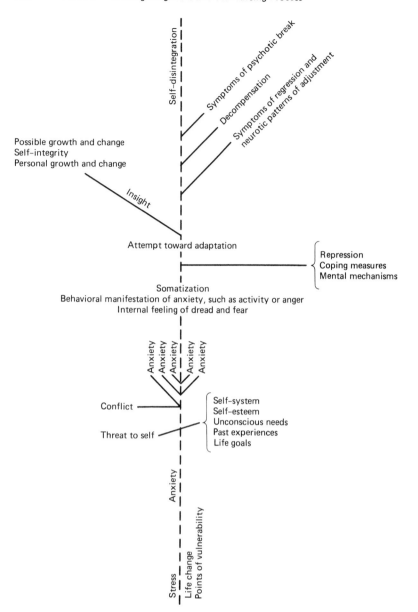

FIGURE 13-1   Dynamic model of anxiety and progression to illness.

edition of the *Diagnostic and Statistical Manual* (in contrast to earlier editions), behavior that is non-psychotic but dysfunctional, maladaptive, or neuro-tic still exists. Thus, neurosis is discussed in this text because you will be caring for these people in nonpsychiatric as well as psychiatric settings.

HISTORICAL PERSPECTIVE OF THE CONCEPT OF NEUROSIS

The term *neurosis* was first used in 1769 by William Cullen (1710–1790). Cullen, founder of a medical school in Edinburgh, Scotland, developed a classification of mental illness according to balance principles, divided into genera and species. He postulated that the brain was the animal life organ producing a fluid supplying the nerves and body with available energy. Depending on this fluid, there would be an increase or decrease in the tonus of the nervous system, resulting in health or illness. He used *neurosis* as synonymous with *nervous system disease* (34).

The German psychiatrist Emil Kraepelin (1856–1926) was one of the first to systematize mental illness. He developed a series of classifications based on descriptive outcomes of mental illness. This was an important step in psychiatry, for this brought the study of mental disease closer to medicine. He presented such thorough and defined descriptions of mental illness that some are still in use today. The less severe types of disorders were not mentioned, but he set the stage for further progress.

A German physician, Adolf Meyer (1866–1950) developed a less static nomenclature than Kraepelin and said that behavior was a force acting upon the individual. He emphasized the more dynamic approach and stressed the movement of forces impinging on the person. Meyer included in his nomenclature a separate description of neurosis, psychoses, affective states, organic brain disease, and subnormality.

The Austrian physician and neurologist, Sigmund Freud (1856–1939), studied hysteria, a form of neurosis, and with the assistance of a colleague, Joseph Bleuler (1841–1925), wrote *Studies on Hysteria*, giving a description, cause, and treatment of neurosis (29). Freud developed a classification of neurosis, and his concepts about neurosis have formed the foundation of psychoanalytic thought.

He saw neurosis arising out of three basic problem areas: (1) traumatic experiences in childhood; (2) transfer of id drives to later developmental stages; and (3) weakened ego unable to keep id material repressed and thus creating conflict (23). Refer to Chapter 2, pp. 40, for further discussion of Freud's concept of neurosis.

Jonathan Cohen, an American psychiatrist, currently hypothesizes that our defenses work to keep out of awareness the instinctual wishes that were originally, or are potentially, sources of pleasure (19). Other theorists propose other views about neurosis and their concepts can be found in Chapter 2: Rank, pp. 51–52, Bandura, p. 55, Maslow, p. 68, Rogers, p. 69, and May, p. 70.

Through the years, various classifications of neuroses have been formulated along both descriptive and dynamic lines. In 1952, *DSM-I, Diagnostic Criteria Classification* appeared, representing an important step in the organization of psychiatric thinking (3). The neurotic disorders listed therein each bore the accompanying term *reaction*, a Meyerian concept. *DSM-II* in 1968 dropped the term *reaction* and utilized a somewhat more detailed listing of types of neurosis (4). *DSM-III* in 1980 (see Appendix I of this text) has officially dropped the term *neurosis* but continues to allow its parenthetical use (5). The rationale behind this change is that the term *neurosis* implies the theoretical direction of dynamic psychiatry, a meaning that is widely held in both America and abroad. However, some theorists have objected to this emphasis, hence the change in *DSM-III*.

THE CONCEPT OF NEUROSIS

Prevalence of Neurosis

There are an immense number of people suffering from disorders relating to stress and anxiety disorders, although the exact figures are unknown. In addition to clients who have officially been diagnosed as suffering from anxiety and dissociative disorders, there are many others with physical complaints who seek psychiatric care. Thirty to 50 percent of the persons admitted to a general hospital are considered to have neurotic illnesses (41). There is also no way to estimate the anxiety and stress disorders of persons suffering from alcohol and

drug problems. Furthermore, many people never seek assistance for their symptoms; they may be ashamed or feel that their symptoms are too minor to seek treatment. Much will depend on the social, economic, and cultural characteristics of the person. Usually those who seek treatment for emotional illnesses are in the middle or upper social classes, whereas those who seek treatment of emotional problems manifested in physical symptoms are in the lower middle or lower stratum of economic society. Some writers even state that the symptoms a person experiences are culturally and economically determined (41).

The Meaning of Neurosis

Neurosis is commonly thought of as less severe than other emotional disorders; however, the anxiety and other disturbing feelings and behaviors can be incapacitating. Since everyone at times experiences and suffers from painful emotions, such as anxiety, fear, guilt, shame, depression, hopelessness, helplessness, anger, and panic, it is difficult to differentiate between adjusted adaptive states and nonadjusted behavior or maladaptive states. A person able to adjust will experience disturbing feelings but will be able to handle related stress, express feelings, cope with the situation, and return to a more comfortable equilibrium and adjustment. A person may be said to be *neurotic when he/she is unable to adjust to the feelings that are experienced or to cope with the situations causing the feelings.* The feelings states are quantitatively more severe or the accompanying behavior is qualitatively more aberrant for the neurotic as compared to the nonneurotic person.

Many believe anxiety is the major symptom in any neurotic illness. Anxiety may be manifested directly in an anxiety attack or panic, or indirectly in psychomotor or autonomic nervous system manifestations or in a covert, compromised set of defenses (see Chapter 12 and Table 2-3).

When is anxiety a symptom of health and when is it a symptom of illness? To differentiate, consider the appropriateness of the anxiety. Is the person's reaction appropriate to the stress or threat? How is the degree or level of anxiety experienced and evidenced? How does the person respond? Is there disorganization in any area? What effect does anxiety have on the person holistically (46)? For example, if the person experiences a panic level of anxiety in response to the opening of school, with severe disorganization of thinking, you would assume that the response of the individual is not normal anxiety but a pathological state.

Stress Can Precipitate Neurotic Impairment

As described in Chapters 8 and 12, stress frequently precedes both psychological and physical illness. Suicide attempts (54), schizophrenia (12), and depressive onsets (54), as well as neurotic illness, have been shown to have been preceded by increased stress. C. Tennant and G. Andrews, in a study on life event stress in neurotic impairment, reported

that the distressing quality of the event rather than the cumulative life change scale is significant to the pathogenic onset of neurosis (65). Third force theorists have also suggested that what makes life changes distressing to one person and not to another is related to individual perception (Chapter 2). In summary, it appears that the significance of the stress event depends on a variety of factors: the stress event, the importance of the stressor, the number or accumulation of events, and the type and amount of change. The reaction of the individual to the stress event is also important. Some people are more vulnerable to certain events than others, depending on "vulnerability points" in their organ systems, background, life stage, biorhythms, and self-esteem.

Stress produces varying levels of anxiety. (see Chapter 12, Table 12-2). Figure 13-1 on p. 436 showed the dynamic formulation of anxiety and the behavioral consequences open to the person. Psychoanalytic theorists believe this process is an unconscious rather than a problem-solving exploration; i.e., the person does not always select the direction for his/her life. Instead, the person makes a psychological adjustment to a position that will work best at the time. To deal with the precipitating stress (conflict), the individual must develop a variety of coping measures or defense mechanisms in order to feel more comfortable and make an adjustment. If the person is able to develop insight about behavior, there is possibility for deeper maturity and higher levels of integration. However, more research is needed in this area (18). If the person is unable to handle the impact of the stress or/and all of its related feelings, he/she will adjust at a lower level of integration. This lack of adjustment may bring a decompensation of personality, with a lower degree of personality functioning, a psychotic break, or a pattern of functioning with neurotic impairment or withdrawal. The functioning of the personality is complex and dynamic. It cannot be compartmentalized and simplified—except for efforts at understanding and description. You must be aware of the uniqueness of each person and the complexity of the mind and emotions.

Anxiety frequently arises out of conflict. Conflicts can arise from opposing forces in any level of the need hierarchy or from opposing goals and can be conscious, unconscious, or partly unconscious (see Chapter 3). Conflicts, as described by analytical theorists, arise from the instinctual (id) desires and the conscience (superego) standards, and are involved in the psychogenic problem of neurosis. Repression occurs in an attempt to resolve the conflict. Thus the anxiety may be totally or partially submerged. Then, whenever the conflict seeks release, the person experiences anxiety. The repressed conflict or anxiety, unless resolved or dealt with, will lead ultimately to symptom formation.

All anxiety, however, is not born out of conflict. Everyone feels anxiety at some time in life. Kirkegarde wrote about existential anxiety that arises from some of the human qualities that most people are afraid to admit in themselves and from the frightening aspects of life that we can only partially understand (40). As we face death, illness, pain, vulnerability, and our inability to wrestle with and solve the realistic problems of life and nature, we deal with anxiety as a human experience (see Third Force Theory in Chapter 2).

Types of Neurotic Disorders

The Diagnostic Criteria from *DSM-III* (see Appendix I of this text) provide three major categories for the neurotic disorders: Anxiety Disorders, Somatoform Disorders, and Dissociative Disorders (5). The seven major symptoms (dysfunctional behavior patterns) found in these disorders will be defined and related to assessment, nursing diagnosis, goal setting, intervention, and evaluation. These seven, described as nursing diagnoses, are:

> Anxiety
> Obsession
> Compulsion
> Phobia

Somatization through conversion symptoms
Somatization through hypochrondiasis
Dissociation

Depression could be included here but will be discussed in Chapter 15 instead.

General Symptoms and Signs of Neurosis

The neurotic person you will be working with will describe symptoms of emotional pain, intruding thoughts, fears, and other complaints. You may notice behavioral signs of panic, nervousness, restlessness, or evidence of lack of self-confidence. Many times the symptoms will be the same as if there were a physical illness or deficit. Therefore an organic illness must first be ruled out by physical examination, tests, and clinical judgment. With evidence of an emotional basis and lack of an organic basis, the underlying conflict or struggle must be dealt with. This is not an easy task. Both the symptoms and their reasons are elusive and are not easily understood. The client may even resist help. He/she usually wants to feel better but may not want to change well-established living patterns, based on conscious needs. The person will probably not understand the reasons for the illness and not understand how improvement can occur. Consciously he/she wants to be healthy. Unconsciously the illness serves a purpose. Therefore a major goal in the treatment of these illnesses is to assist the person in conflict resolution, which can relieve symptoms.

CONTRAST OF PSYCHONEUROSIS WITH PSYCHOSIS

Some say mental health and illness symptoms can be envisioned on a continuum, with neurosis identified as a less severe illness in the middle area of the continuum, and psychosis as a more severe illness found at the far end. Others say there is no evidence to support the distinction between neurosis and psychosis and that these groupings are vague and unscientific. Yet others feel that the terms are irrelevant and instead seek concrete lists of behaviors to diagnose. Psychiatry should be seen as similar to, yet different from other specialties of medicine.

In physical medicine, concrete, overt, observable symptoms are necessary to make a diagnosis of heart disease and diabetes, whereas in psychiatry, observations can also be made with important conclusions drawn, but the data are not always black and white. Actually, the diagnosis of heart disease or diabetes may also be enhanced by attention to covert factors and subtle signs.

Psychosis and psychoneurosis can be differentiated into two major groups, but the symptoms found in the two groups will not be mutually exclusive (see Table 13-1). The major distinction that can be made between neurosis and psychosis is determined by the extent to which the illness impinges on the total personality. The personality of the neurotic person is organized, intact, and usually suffers from constriction and rigidity rather than disorganization. The psychotic has a personality that tends to disorganize easily. When the psychotic person is threatened or experiences anxiety, the self falls apart or loosens. The "glue" (identity, values, attitudes, beliefs) holding the person together appears to dissolve and disorganize. The client may say, "I am going apart," "I don't feel together." In contrast, when the neurotic person is threatened or experiences high anxiety, he/she

merely builds additional walls; defenses get tighter, and patterns of defensive behavior found successful in the past are used. Most neurotic persons use a variety of defenses or show mixed features, but they will rely largely on one major defense to control anxiety. Therefore, one predominant symptom is usually seen. The clients you will work with may have a variety of symptoms but will express more difficulty with one particular symptom, such as phobia, obsession, or compulsion. Generally, the person with greater diversity of available defenses, as well as greater flexibility in their use, is more successfully adaptive. Similarly the person who utilizes what are developmentally more mature defenses is better equipped to deal with life (41).

TABLE 13-1.   Comparison between Psychosis and Neurosis

NEUROSIS	*PSYCHOSIS*
Personality organization intact.	Personality organization less formed.
Restricted thinking.	Dereistic thinking.
Associations clear.	Associations loosened.
Interest in world retained.	Interest in world frequently lost.
Some insight into illness.	Little insight.
Object relations maintained.	Object relations impaired.
Reality testing sound.	Reality testing impaired.
Defenses substitutive.	Defenses extreme or ineffectively used.
Regression less frequent.	Regression more severe.
Repression maintained.	Projection of wishes and fears in forms of delusions and hallucinations.
Social functioning organized.	Social functioning disorganized.
Affect unchanged (except depression).	Affect inappropriate, lability increased.
Frequently secondary gains from illness.	Seldom secondary gains from illness.
Sexual relations constricted.	Sexual relations confused.
	More evidence of biochemical factors.

DYSFUNCTIONAL OR CHRONIC (NEUROTIC) ANXIETY STATE

Assessment and Nursing Diagnosis

Assessment parameters for the *nursing diagnosis, dysfunctional chronic anxiety state* related to *non-*

specific stress response and ineffective coping with conflict focus on anxiety and its manifestations. The anxiety may be felt directly, without defense or maneuvers to capture, control, or convert it.

The direct, uncontrolled feeling of anxiety becomes the outstanding feature of the person's illness. The ego has attempted unsuccessfully to repress the surging feeling, so that the individual overtly looks, acts, and feels anxious. As the level of anxiety increases, so does the intensity of the experience and the effect on the person. Moderate to severe anxiety is predominant in this state, although moderate to severe anxiety may also be experienced in hyperthroidism, drug withdrawal or intoxication, hypoglycemia, pheochromocytoma, other physical illnesses, and severe psychotic illness such as schizophrenia (5). The levels of anxiety may vary with the person, situation, and duration of precipitating events. The anxiety may come in waves, or it may be *free floating anxiety, a vague fearful experience without an observable object or cause,* as Freud called it (29). People will experience and describe anxiety differently. Many authors create outlines of anxiety symptoms and these are helpful. (See Chapter 12 for a description of levels of anxiety.) Remember the symptoms are numerous and varied and are sometimes difficult to pinpoint in the person. Talk to people you are working with about their anxiety experience. One patient described it as follows:

> I had never experienced a feeling like this before. It was more pronounced when I was quiet, sitting, or trying to sleep. It hurt, was unsettling, and frightening. I was cold, my heart beat fast, and my stomach fluttered. I tried to think of something pleasant so the feeling would go away. It hovered over my body and soul like a shroud. I felt heavy, unsure, afraid of something happening but knew of nothing. I felt afraid.

A generalized long-lasting or chronic state of anxiety occurs when a person lives continuously with a pervading feeling of anxiety. This person may experience occasional panic states or intense attacks lasting from a few minutes to several hours, but usually he/she complains of a variety of persisting symptoms: trembling, fearfulness, apprehension, feeling of a viselike band around the head or throat, and other physical discomforts. The person is worrisome and self-absorbed, overreacts to situations, and may develop psychosomatic illness (41). Frequently the anxious person hyperventilates, which is a common physiological expression of the acute anxiety state. The person begins to breath rapidly, at first ever so slightly in degree, depth, and rhythm. The rapid breathing becomes deeper, and the carbon dioxide content of arterial blood, along with blood bicarbonate, is reduced. When the carbon dioxide level is inadequate to trigger respirations, lightheadedness, incoordination, palpitations, and sensations of air hunger, pain, and pressure occur. Accompanying perspiration, fear, tremors, and paresthesia occur. Unless the condition is terminated by breathing carbon dioxide (for example, by breathing into and out of a paper bag), the person may faint. If the condition progresses, severe convulsions, and in time, death could occur (41).

Assess signs and symptoms of the anxiety syndrome. Look for obvious physical symptoms. Feel the client's pulse. Note perspiration and respiration. Shake his/her hand or touch the skin. Look for pupil dilation. Listen to objective complaints. He/she may complain of heart symptoms or diarrhea but will not necessarily suffer heart disease or an intestinal virus. Listen to subjective complaints, fears, dreams, and worries. Frequently the person will express significantly meaningful information with descriptions of how awful he/she feels; the emotionally laden words that describe fears, dreams, and worries can tell a great deal. Usually the person only knows about the symptoms—not what is happening, nor the reasons for the feelings.

Look for nonverbal clues concerning feelings as the person describes the event and what he/she was experiencing and thinking before the anxiety increased. Get as much information as you can. Who was present? What was the situation like? Has the person been in a situation like that before? The words are important, but also note how the words are stated. Listen for reflections in voice, pitch, tone, urgency, hesitations.

Assess your own feelings of anxiety as you observe the client. Since anxiety is catching, you will probably sense your client's anxiety. At times people cover up anxiety with a facade or smile. Your only clue to your client's anxiety may be your own feelings. Listen to the clue or hunch within yourself; try to validate your hunch. Do not confront the person with an interpretation. Rather ask another question. For example, "This may not seem important, but have you ever had the same thoughts before? Did you feel anxious then?" As the person talks, conscious and unconscious data will be given. The feelings conveyed and the words used will confirm the nursing diagnosis.

Client-Care Goals and Related Nursing Interventions

Goal: Describe relief from distress of chronic state.

Intervention

As with any person in pain, methods should be attempted to relieve the emotional pain of anxiety. *Immediate emotional support* and the presence of another person can be comforting. Speak in a calm voice in short understandable sentences. Make supportive statements, such as, "You have people here to help," "You are trying hard," "There is no reason for you not to improve." State words of support and hope with kindness, warmth, and honesty. Provide firmness if the person is having trouble with decisions. Touch may be reassuring. Communicate care and concern nonverbally with an attitude of positive assurance. Control the manifestations of your own anxiety or cope with your feelings, for an anxious nurse can increase the fear and anxiety of a client.

Verbal communication is an effective means of alleviating distress and anxiety. If the person can "say the words," using clarifying, descriptive statements, with an accompanying release of feelings, there can be increased comfort. Allow the client to lead, but ask related questions. Slow the conversation if the client is having difficulty thinking or stating feelings. Reflect feeling in your face to encourage his/her involvement as well as to let the person know you are listening. For other principles of communication with the anxious client, see Chapter 5.

Recognize the source of the anxiety and deal with the conflict if the person is able to discuss the problem and is in a less severe state. Associate present feelings with past feelings (23). A face-to-face discussion of conscious reality may be helpful. The client with severe conflicts needs counseling that takes into consideration the meaning of symptoms, recurring stress and vulnerability, past experiences, feelings, and attitudes (41). Nurses with psychiatric experience and formal education are prepared to do insight therapy with an anxious patient.

Cognitive methods of relieving anxiety, using a problem-solving approach to uncover realistic fears, personal concerns, and anxieties, can be helpful (see Chapter 12). A person with chronic anxiety may experience a panic state with any added tension and pressure. This client may feel better when given a clear, honest statement of fact about the situation than if given a tranquilizer. A client may feel relieved when told, "You are having an anxiety attack. Your heart is not damaged; it was beating faster because of stress." Or a person experiencing hyperventilation may be very relieved to hear the symptoms are reversible.

Other measures to relieve dysfunctional anxiety may be helpful. For example, an activity may provide a temporary release, and the activity time can be used to develop a relationship and talk. Dancing, jogging, walking, hammering, playing an active game, or cleaning may be used. Sometimes medication may be necessary to give relief and to assist the person to relax enough to talk (see Table 13-2). Many hospitalized patients receive negative feedback and contempt for stating fears and feelings and may be hesitant to talk. Reduce demands on the person. Try to meet and anticipate other needs. Teaching relaxation techniques can give the person a tool to use during future stressful periods and to promote self-direction and self-control. Refer to the goals and interventions described in Chapter 12. Many of these are applicable to the person with chronic anxiety.

EXPRESSION OF ANXIETY THROUGH PERSISTENT, INEFFECTIVE THOUGHTS AND ACTIONS (OBSESSIVE AND COMPULSIVE BEHAVIOR PATTERNS)

An *obsession is a recurring thought, image, idea, or impulse that returns to conscious thinking without the person's ability to ignore or suppress it.* The obsession is *a magical thought, symbolic in that it is a substitute for an even more alarming thought that is being repressed.* Obsessions may be distressing or unwanted, such as thoughts about being dirty, unclean, or repugnant. The obsessions may urge the person to act in a certain way, such as to attack, fight, or even kill, and these thoughts are fearful. The obsessive person may seem delusional but knows the thoughts are senseless and without foundation and is unable to control them.

A *compulsion is the need to act in a repetitive*

TABLE 13-2. Summary of Minor Tranquilizers

GENERIC NAME	TRADE NAME	AVERAGE DAILY DOSE	SIDE EFFECTS/ TOXIC EFFECTS	NURSING IMPLICATIONS
Propanediol group Meprobamate Synthetic drug. Acts as a muscle relaxant and anticonvulsant.	Miltown, Equanil	200–1200 mg. Large dose may produce state like barbiturate intoxication.	Skin rash, itching, hives. Drowsiness. Tolerance and dependence on drug not unusual. Withdrawal should be gradual.	Notify physician of side effects; drug may be discontinued and/or antihistamines given. Teach patients that alcohol potentiates drug. If prolonged use with abrupt cessation, look for withdrawal symptoms, including convulsions.
Benzodiazepine Group Most widely used drugs. Infrequently causes central nervous system depression. Have disinhibiting effect; may release hostilities and anger.				
Diazepam	Valium	4–10 mg. Metabolized slowly—as long as 50 hours with some people. Concentrations and increased cumulative effect occur after 5–10 days.	Weakness. Ataxia. Drowsiness. Fatigue. At times can cause nightmares and sleep disturbances. If given IM or IV, injection may cause local pain and irritation and phlebitis.	Caution persons to be careful working with machinery, equipment, or driving automobile. Be aware of sleep habits and any changes in patterns of behavior. Question any complaints of skin, muscle, or local pain.
Oxazepam	Serax	30–200 mg. Particularly valuable to the elderly. Metabolized more rapidly than Diazepam.	Possible agranulocytosis and jaundice. Severe withdrawal symptoms may occur.	Be aware of and teach client need to take drug for cumulative build-up.
Cloraxepate dipotassium	Tranxene	7.5–60 mg.	Occasionally blurred vision, constipation, singultus, confusion, depression, euphoria.	Use safety precautions. Observe mood; adapt approach. Long-term therapy may result in psychic and

TABLE 13-2. Continued

GENERIC NAME	TRADE NAME	AVERAGE DAILY DOSE	SIDE EFFECTS/ TOXIC EFFECTS	NURSING IMPLICATIONS
				physical dependence. Observe length of time drug is given.
Chlordiazepoxide hydrochloride	Librium, Libritabs	15–300 mg. Frequently used in non-psychiatric settings, particularly for psychosomatic conditions. Complaints of decreased libido not uncommon.	Occasionally blurred vision, constipation, singultus, confusion, depression. Hypotension and syncope have occurred with large doses. Regular doses have been noted to exacerbate ventilatory failure due to chronic bronchitis.	Long-term therapy with larger doses may result in psychic and physical dependence. Observe blood pressure. Use safety precautions, including for postural hypotension. Use with caution for patient with chronic pulmonary disease. Do not discontinue abruptly. Withdrawal symptoms may develop slowly upon cessation; convulsions may occur.
Diphenylmethane Group				
Hydroxyzine hydrochloride	Atarax	50–400 mg.	Side effects low. Drowsiness tends to be transient without major difficulty. Potentiates opiates and barbiturates. Some may complain of dry mouth. Ataxia. Bradycardia. Increased gastric motility and diarrhea. Antiemetic reaction with increased appetite may produce weight gain.	May be helpful in producing sleep if used with barbiturates. Dose should be noted and reactions observed. Use safety measures. Ice chips or mints help dry mouth. Observe elimination patterns and weight. Devise dietary plan to promote normal pattern if necessary.
Hydroxyzine pamoate	Vistaril	50–400 mg.	Side effects low. Drowsiness transient.	Withdrawal reactions not observed.
Benactyzine hydrochloride	Suavitil	3–10 mg. Should not be given to patients receiving E.S.T. or suffering from glaucoma or prostatic hypertrophy.	No apparent sedative or hypnotic action. Some people experience difficulty in concentration, strange sense of unreality, or open hostility.	Be observant of patient.

and seemingly purposeful way; the act is carried out to relieve tension and helplessness and to prevent loss of control or exposure. Failure to carry out the act increases anxiety and tension. The behavior may be repeated and elaborated into a ritual or ceremony. The act may seem simple; yet when carried out in a certain order and in a formalized manner, it carries considerable significance. Common compulsions are handwashing, touching, bathing, or checking equipment, doors, and appliances. Compulsions may be as complex and ritualized as that of an eleven-year-old boy described by Freud. Before bedtime the child told his mother details of the day, cleaned the floor, pushed the bed against the wall, kicked his legs, and then turned on his side (28).

All people use obsessions and compulsions at times in order to cope with anxiety. Transient obsessions and compulsions are common among children, especially during the school years. If the obsessions are severe, or if they remain over time and interfere with the child's social life and normal functioning, the child should be referred for evaluation and treatment. But it is important not to alarm the parents, creating even more anxiety in the child. If obsessions and compulsions begin in adolescence or early adulthood, the prognosis is more questionable. There may be a period in early schizophrenia predominated by obsessions and compulsions (see Chapter 16).

Dynamics

The obsessive-compulsive person learns in childhood that it is imperative to control self and feelings. Usually power struggles with parents have occurred over a variety of emotionally laden issues. The young child needs to gain a sense of autonomy and exert self, and in this process, parental love may be lost and rejection occur. The parents of these clients usually have had difficulties and conflicts with control, and they have encouraged the child to inhibit feelings through overt control measures, denial, concealment, intellectualization, rationalization, conscious suppression, unconscious repression, diversion, and displacement (46).

As the child grows, a realistic appraisal of self does not develop, so that the person reaches adulthood with a low level of self-esteem. Low self-value brings about self-doubt and self-criticism and consequent defensive operations to maintain and build up self.

Strategies to build a low self-esteem include comparing and rating self with others, striving for positions of respect or prestige, competing to win or be better than others, and striving for approval. Other defenses such as reaction formation, denial, regression, projection, and isolation are commonly used to maintain equilibrium. Undoing, symbolization, substitution, and displacement are employed in the service of compulsive acts. A strong sense of right and wrong, strict rules and principles, and a strong sense of responsibility all add to the standards that push toward comformity and being critical, which is part of the obsessive thinking pattern.

Assessment and Nursing Diagnosis

Assessment parameters for the *nursing diagnosis, persistent ineffective thought patterns* (obsessions) *and actions* (compulsions) related to *multiple conflicts, chronic anxiety, and dysfunctional coping* focus on the content of thinking and persistence of behavior. David Miller distinguished obsessive-compulsive patients from other neurotic persons by their negative, isolated view of self (51). The person suffering from obsessive-compulsive symptoms also experiences anxiety. Most of the anxiety is bound up or captured by the defenses in an attempt to neutralize the conflict; however, anxiety is still present and increases with stress. It is as if a cap covered over the turmoil of feelings and anxieties, converting the feelings into thoughts (obsessions) and actions (compulsions).

Signs and symptoms of obsessions and compulsions are easy to recognize, but the individual personality conflicts and problems that the person must deal with are far more complex and difficult to understand. When you meet this person for the interview you will usually be presented with a meticulously well-groomed person—unless he/she is regressed. All of the pleasantries of a casual conversation will be present. You may wonder if the individual has any difficulties at all. However, the difficulties will shortly appear. Three of the major problem areas will be: (1) lack of emotional contact, (2) need for control, and (3) struggle with a variety of conflicts.

Avoidance of emotional contact is present when you feel disinterest or boredom as you talk to the client; he/she is usually working hard to maintain distance and emotional and social isolation (11). Looking away, bringing up details, keeping notes, and a variety of other measures are the client's way of unconsciously putting emotional space between him/herself and you. The closeness of involvement is frightening to this person, and further contact might disclose his/her needs for love and attention, as well as his/her fears and a sense of vulnerability that the person is trying to conceal. A vicious circle might be noted: the person's increasing need for people also increases the sense of vulnerability, which may lead to a withdrawal from and a greater distance from people, which in turn increases need for interaction without satisfaction (46).

You can observe in the client a desire for control of self, you, and the environment. The more the risk involved, the more the need to control. Watch for body rigidity, a tense set of the jaw, a closed body position, a deliberate use of words, and statements of command. You might notice the person overcontrolling feelings, such as holding back anger, expressing a false politeness, or showing a lack of spontaneity and warmth. You may also feel you are pushed and directed and that decisions are being made for you, with the client leading the way by asking questions or directing the interview. This individual thinks in terms of "I should," "I must," and "I will," and in so doing there is a control, a limiting, and a suppression of others. You may feel very frustrated or angry as the feeling of being controlled takes over; remember these are symptoms of an inhibited person with low self-esteem and much doubt. This is not a person with aggressive, grandiose feelings.

Struggle with conflicts gives rise to anxiety. This person has a multitude of conflicts; you will note the ambivalence, tension, and struggle within the person. Conflicts are manifested by the following behaviors: (1) polite behavior mixed with evidence of anger and rage, (2) a sense of superiority and competitiveness and interspersed with self-doubt and criticism, (3) a desire for cleanliness and order, yet a spotty but unmistakable sloppiness, (4) manifestations of independence, but evidence of dependency desires, (5) defiance, yet submissiveness. Such ambivalence leads to confusion and uncertainty, which is usually dealt with in the obsessive style of sureness, control, and attention to detail.

This person lives hampered by anxiety, recurring thoughts, rituals, and loss of spontaneity and pleasure, although he/she usually does not manifest acute episodes. The person remains in a life style that is bounded by restricted emotions,

perfectionism, indecisiveness, and rigidity, but his/her emotional status does not progress to full-blown emotional illness or neurosis. However, if the external demands and internal stresses become greater than the individual's adaptive capability, he/she may move from the obsessive-compulsive personality style to a neurotic disorder. The person may then seek help from a physician, usually for a secondary problem or symptom. For example, he/she may complain of psychosomatic problems, such as colitis, ulcers, asthma, tachycardia, hypertension, phobias, and sometimes depression. Addictive problems with drugs, food, gambling, or alcohol may also center around an obsessive-compulsive disorder.

Occasionally you may contact a patient suffering from a full-blown obsessive-compulsive disorder in the hospital. The client may be hampered by compulsiveness, by spending the entire day checking, cleaning, touching, gesturing, washing, or showering. He/she often has ruminating, obsessive thoughts to the point of being miserable. Many times the client may have waited, suffering for months before seeking help. The skin may be abraised from rubbing and bathing. This person may have lost his/her job because of the use of certain rituals. When the family insists that he/she be hospitalized, *other related nursing diagnoses* are evidenced, such as, *impaired nutrition, impaired skin integrity, fatigue,* and *dehydration,* as exemplified by the following cases:

> John was admitted to the hospital with anxiety, fears, and compulsiveness. He spent twelve hours a day shoveling one pile of dirt back and forth. He seldom socialized with others because he was embarrassed and secretive about his activity. He did not take time for sufficient ingestion of food and fluids.

> Mary's skin was bleeding and cracked. She had been showering for several hours at a time, three times a day, for over a year. As she prepared to shower, she touched all the knobs in the room two times. Her movements were slow and methodical; her expression was bland and concentrating.

Many researchers have attempted to assess the major complaints of the person who is obsessive-compulsive. R. Hodgson and S. Rochman have devised a scale for assessment, and they established two major complaints (checking and washing) and two minor complaints (slowness and doubting). The majority of the people had more than one complaint: 76 percent of those who did checking complained of doubting, 58 percent of slowness, and 55 percent complained of washing. Of the people who complained of slowness, 65 percent also complained of doubting, 60 percent complained of checking, and 50 percent complained of cleaning problems (36).

Client-Care Goals and Related Nursing Interventions

Many of the characteristics and qualities of the obsessive personality are valued in our culture. Preciseness, sense of responsibility, emotional control, orderliness, and detailed thinking can be useful traits in most occupations, but when these become excessive in quality or persistence, they become a liability. Because of the success of many obsessive-compulsive people, it is sometimes difficult for the person to want to change. For a successful treatment program the individual must be willing to try to be involved in the treatment process and must want to modify behavior. Many times the client will want to feel better but does not want to behave differently.

Self-awareness is crucial to approaching this client. The obsessive-compulsive person will stimulate your conflicts; it is easy to "act out" in response. All of us demonstrate resistance to being controlled. We resent being pushed around, bossed, and maneuvered. When your client tries to direct the interview, it is difficult not to respond with anger. A natural response might be to lash out and express your feelings, as an expression of your own needs. This is not helpful to the person. Never get involved in a power struggle or quarrel. H. S. Sullivan warned against the power struggle since the therapy time becomes converted into a near nothing (64). Do not judge the person by his/her ruminating thoughts or sticky behavior. Look to the person's potentials and strengths to help neutralize your anger. Many times these clients are ridiculed in the hospital. Consider the pain of such persons. Their inappropriate patterns and thoughts are as repugnant to them as they are to you and others. Another reaction might be for you to want to quickly break the ritualistic patterns. This is a pertinent goal but should come from the quieting of inner problems rather than as a response to your direction. Avoid countercontrol of this person; he/she already has a problem with control.

Goal: Demonstrate some increase in warmth and spontaneity through a developing relationship that allows relinquishing controlling and ritualistic behavior.

Intervention

Be available to this person, carefully *creating an atmosphere* where the client can be secure enough to make some emotional contact. He/she may move a step forward and touch, and then move backward. However, contact is rewarding to this emotionally deprived person, so he/she will reach out again. Frequently the person initially talks without feeling or ruminates around the issue without any sense of involvement. Nurture any flicker of feeling you observe; realize how frightening warmth and emotionality are to this person. How carefully you maintain distance should be guided by his/her fearfulness. Be sensitive to it. The obsessive person lives through an experience in his/her mind, in logical thinking (intellectualization) rather than being emotionally involved in the event or even life itself. Encourage spontaneity through your own behavior. Foster trust and safety by approaching the person with an attitude of openness and a desire to understand. Look beyond the symptoms to who the person is, not what he/she is doing.

Determine the symbolization behind the symptoms and vary your approach accordingly. Symptoms of washing, checking, slowness, doubting, and others create pain. *Limits may be set,* such as encouraging a washing for only a set period of time. *An activity schedule may be made,* and usually the person is comfortable with it if it is not strictly imposed. However, the main focus is to look beyond the symptoms to the puzzle the symptoms are representing. The client is dominated by the symbols represented by symptoms, but he/she does not understand what they mean. Clients frequently say, "I don't know why I am doing this." Try to unravel the meaning by listening to the words used and watching the nonverbal expressions of feeling. Observe how the client lives and how he/she relates to you. What the person is in real life will give you clues to the conflicts and problems, although the client is a master at closeting self and covering his/her feelings and problems. The behavioral facade of pleasantries and activities needs to be noted, but respond to the unique individual underneath. This takes an informed sense of compassion.

Guidelines for communicating with the obsessive-compulsive person include the following:

1. *Speak in a gentle voice,* presenting a calm, accepting atmosphere to decrease anxiety.

2. *Listen carefully and with patience.* Words, details, and endless irrelevant information are used to *not* communicate and to maintain distance. Try to hear the feelings within the flood of words, and speak to the feelings as the significant information.

3. *Be a genuine person* to the client. Tell the client you want to understand but cannot when he/she whispers, mumbles, lectures, screams, or avoids eye contact in an attempt to avoid you. An unexpected caring remark from you may break the maneuvering, controlling defenses. Spontaneity on your part may promote a feeling of connection.

4. *Avoid argument or angry discussion.* If the client is provoking you, comment on the feelings and change the subject to one pertinent to the client. Your anger will only cause the client to feel attacked and to further withdraw.

5. *Silence should be studied and not maintained* for a long period. Silence can be used by some clients for thinking, concentrating on an experience, or sorting out a problem. In this case, however, silence is used by the person to control or as a distancing manuever. Silence is not difficult for this client. Ask what he/she is thinking about. The person may reply, "Nothing," and you may need to gently confront. But if the person responds with feeling, focus on the feelings conveyed to try to reduce emotional distance.

The persistent thoughts and ritualistic behavior will gradually decrease as the client gains increased self-confidence, security, and self-esteem. He/she will become more at ease with people as conflicts are resolved. With an inner sense of control, the person does not have to rely on overt behaviors to control self or others. I. Bennun assisted clients with obsessive slowness and slow rituals by setting up a list of action in three phases, with each phase having a target completion date. The self-pacing allowed a feeling of self-control and task completion (11).

EXPRESSION OF ANXIETY THROUGH EXCESSIVE FEAR (PHOBIC BEHAVIOR PATTERNS)

Phobia is an irrational, abnormal fear of an object or situation that is out of proportion to the circumstances involved. Many objects or situations may be feared, including snakes, insects, cancer, heights, closed spaces, dogs, water, elevators, and even school. Phobic objects are often culturally determined and come and go in fads. The objects are frequently such an integral part of the person's life that avoidance may be difficult, although if the individual fears tornadoes, there may not be much activity restriction, i.e., to avoid storms, except in rare instances. But usually the feared object is close and difficult to avoid. For example, a person living in an apartment may fear elevators, dogs, heights, and closed places. This person will spend much time each day avoiding these objects, which takes considerable energy. The fears may change as the external focus of the difficulty shifts. A person fearful of one object may begin to fear a greater number of objects. For example, a person afraid of elevators later may become afraid of getting close to all buildings with elevators. Intellectually the phobic person knows that the object is not a real source of danger, but emotionally and experientially he/she continues to feel fear.

Many people experience phobias. It is not an unusual occurrence for normal preschool and early school-age children to have some fears (36). Some adults without any pronounced emotional difficulties also complain of mild phobias. The phobia may be short-termed or an integral part of the person's related illness, such as a fear associated with psychotic or neurotic illness (49). Phobic neurosis occurs when fear and maneuvers to avoid the fear are the primary symptoms or when the phobia becomes the primary means of handling anxiety. The duration of the time the fear is present and the severity of the symptom will indicate the extent of the difficulty.

The diagnostic criteria from *DSM-III* (see

Appendix I of this text) list phobias as an anxiety disorder (5). The most common one listed is *agoraphobia, fear of being alone or in public places without escape.* Other types include agoraphobia with and without panic attacks, social phobia, and simple phobia. The Greeks wrote of a variety of phobias (58). Freud often wrote of phobias, declaring a definite relationship to both obsessive thinking and hysteria. In writing the case of the famous child phobic, Freud saw phobia as belonging to the anxiety neurosis (29).

Dynamics

The phobia is a defensive maneuver used by the person to externalize anxiety from within to a source outside of self. Displacement is used to detach the anxiety to a specific object, idea, or situation in daily life (41). Symbolization is used as the person treats the object as if it were the threat. Intensity of the fear or feeling associated with the phobia is usually of the same intensity associated with the internal conflict. A client with intense fears is usually equally troubled with unresolved internal conflicts. Common conflicts center around sexual and dependency problems, although it is difficult to categorize because each phobia is so individualized. The primary objective or gain is the transfer of anxiety related to a threatening conflict into fear of a certain object. This transfer handles most of the anxiety and enables the person to function without becoming incapacitated. A second gain from the symptom is receiving attention, special support, or treatment. S. Arieti saw these secondary gains as very difficult to give up (8).

Assessment and Nursing Diagnosis

Assessment parameters for the *nursing diagnosis excessive fears (phobic behavior patterns)* related to *chronic anxiety and conflicts* focus on the actions of the person. A phobic symptom is easy to recognize: the individual is extremely afraid of a certain object or situation. The person readily tells you what the problem is. Usually the person responds quickly, makes contact with you, and wants assistance (48). The person will be cooperative and pleasant, but superficial, during the initial interview. Let the phobic person talk. Explore fears and worries. Get a picture of the life the person leads. Get some perspective on the extent of the difficulty. Try

to determine reasons for the type of phobia and the situations that precipitate the attack. The phobia may be such that the person will not be hampered. However, the phobia may be such that the person is unable to enjoy life or is even completely incapacitated.

After getting a general picture, fill in the details. Ask about the first time the difficulty occurred. Try to move away from the primary topic. Ask "what if" questions, such as, "What would you have done if you were alone in the room?" or "What do you do when you encounter the _____ situation?" Ask related questions. Explore related feelings. Ask about the people associated with the problem situation or about other significant people in the person's life. Assess the person's family adjustment as well as his/her personal adjustments in relation to each of the phobias. W. Arrindel demonstrated that all phobias were related to emotional and social adjustment, but especially so for agoraphobia (9).

As you begin to explore further and deeper, this person will probably maneuver to avoid further discussion of conflicted areas. Avoidance is usually a lifetime pattern to handle anxiety and life difficulties.

Client-Care Goals and Related Nursing Interventions

> *Goal: Become desensitized to the phobic object or situation.*

Intervention

Focus on the person, since emphasis has been on the fears and symptoms. While you unravel the reasons for the phobias, be empathetic and concerned with the person's feelings. Some authors found the most critical intervention for reducing phobias was the *nurse-client relationship.* Work with the client to establish rapport and trust. As you reach out and as the client and you begin to know each other better, there will be a firmer foundation for continued maturing. Asking questions is assessment but also a means to resolution. You will want to explore the person's feelings, not only about him/herself but also about his/her personal relationships, important people, life situations, and events. The client may never have thought much about feelings or any exploration about life and how stressors and life situations are avoided. At first the client will try to avoid this discussion, but through continued intervention, you can nurture a straightforward approach to facing conflicts and life itself. The client must understand the symbolic significance of the recent events in his/her life and must try to alter the family environment and routines so that fear need not be transferred (8).

As anxiety lessens, the person will be ready to face more easily the phobic situation by *desensitization, an experience of gradual exposure, relearning, and retraining, whereby the person places self near or in the feared situation by small steps and degrees until the fear is overcome.* At first, the client's anxiety may increase even to the point of panic. Your own anxiety may also increase. You may start by presenting pictures or sounds related to the feared object or situation to the client. As the person becomes more comfortable with the idea of the phobic object, prepare the person to encounter it. Accompany the client at first when he/she is in proximity to the feared object or event. Support the person. Involve the family in supporting and accompanying the person. Gradually anxiety will lessen to the point that the client can encounter the phobic object or event alone, without intense fear and symptoms (8). You may collaborate with a psychiatrist, psychologist, or a treatment program in a behavioristic desensitization approach.

SOMATIZATION THROUGH CONVERSION SYMPTOMS RELATED TO CHRONIC ANXIETY AND CONFLICT

Somatization is the expression of an emotional turmoil or conflict through a physical symptom with a loss or alteration of physical functioning which is *not under voluntary control and is not otherwise explained by a known physical disorder* (5). *Somatization* refers to the *persisting abnormal autonomic discharge caused by anxiety which is experienced as a physical symptom. Conversion is defined as the unconscious process through which anxiety is converted or transmuted into a physical, physiologic, or psychologic symptom* (46). The psychiatric nomenclature for somatization includes "conversion," "psychogenic pain," "hypochondriasis," "chronic physical symptoms," and "atypical symptoms (5)."

Dynamics

The use of the body for expression of conflict is a kind of body language that is not intended to convey any specific word meaning but frequently manifests a definite symbolic meaning. In any physiologic symptom of psychophysiologic illness, such as colitis, asthma, ulcer, or migraine headache, there is nonverbal communication and primitive expressions of need (46). These illnesses might be thought of as being on one end of a continuum, and nonfunctional illnesses without organic cause, such as conversion symptoms, are on the other end of the continuum.

Conversion symptoms are expressed through motor and sensory symptoms and relate to increased stress, repressed or disowned ideas and feelings, and maladaptive coping methods. For example, a client hospitalized for depression who needs monetary assistance from his parents but has a conflict about asking for help loses the use of his arm before he can write to them asking for help.

The conversion disorders are symptoms without an organic cause and tend to be related to the hysterical personality. In contrast, psychophysiological disorders involve organic changes, although they are also an expression of anxiety. In conversion, the person invests a large amount of energy and interest in the illness so that the illness is the main preoccupation. The person becomes the illness.

Assessment and Nursing Diagnosis

Assessment parameters for the *nursing diagnosis, somatization through conversive symptoms* related to *chronic anxiety and unresolved conflicts* focus on personality factors as well as on physical symptoms, the precipitating stress prior to symptom onset, and the emotional needs met by the symptoms.

The client will complain to you bitterly about the symptoms, which may resemble a specific physical illness, such as multiple sclerosis or epilepsy, or there may be isolated symptoms. The range is limitless. Commonly encountered manifestations are dyskinesias, ataxia, contractures, paralysis, blindness, deafness, numbness, tingling, itching, and vomiting. A physical examination, health history, and diagnostic studies should be done to make sure the illness has no physiological basis (45). Many clients have been said to have conversion and were later found to be suffering from cancer or an equally serious illness.

The client will be invested in or preoccupied with the symptom, spending time and effort to describe, complain, and go over in detail every change in symptoms. Yet the significance that the illness plays in the person's life is of no great concern. Pierre Janet first called this *la belle indifference*; the significance, implication, or incapacity of the symptom is not given the importance it would be ordinarily. For example, the blind person is not concerned about blindness when he/she is describing the loss of sight (46).

Look for the histrionic personality, the immature, shallow person who is prone to have conversion symptoms. Many clinicians feel the personality basis is important in diagnosis since certain hysterical behaviors are used extensively to solve problems in living (37). P. Chaloff and H. Lyons established seven criteria for recognizing hysteria based upon observable behavior (17). These criteria include the following characteristics:

Vain and egocentric
Labile and excitable
Shallow affect
Dramatic attention-seeking
Conscious of sex, sexually provocative, yet with sexual problems
Demanding
Dishonest

The diagnosis is more apt to be appropriate when you note four or five of these behavioral traits.

Frequently the person seems very warm at the first meeting, is demonstrative, uses dramatic gestures and words, and is emotional. You like this person and feel some contact. His/her personal appearance is usually pleasing and attractive. However, the emotional response is frequently defensive; the client keeps the interaction on a distorted, superficial level, away from feelings of loneliness, depression, and anxiety (70). The person may flatter you and beguile you into talking about yourself, or

joke about irrelevant topics rather than talk about him/herself. He/she is frequently manipulative, using other people to meet personal needs; and controlling, or dominating, trying to have power over you. He/she is suggestible. For example, if you ask about a physical symptom, such as a rash or itching, the person may begin to itch and scratch.

You may feel you want to take care of the person as he/she talks to you. Dependency traits are a major characteristic. The client often communicates to others in a variety of ways that he/she cannot help the self (37). Projection, blaming others, repression, denial, and not accepting responsibility are commonly used mechanisms. The person says through behavior, "I am not a responsible person," or "I cannot take care of myself (35). Many times the conversion symptom itself will demand that society or family take care of the person. ("I cannot walk; you must care for me.") Regression is a large part of the symptom formation, requiring the person to be helpless and dependent. The histrionic person may decompensate under stress and appear extremely ill, even psychotic, and then recovers in a short time (70).

Other traits include the following (46):

Egocentricity
Lack of inhibitions
Acting out impulsive behavior with little regard for consequences
Limited drive toward intellectuality
Personality compartmentalization
Potential for dissociation

Understand the cultural background of the client. There is a varying incidence of conversion in different cultural groups, and physical expression of conflict and stress may be acceptable as a cultural pattern in some groups (45) (for example, some American Indians or black Americans). Hysteria is also common in lower economic groups of people. Briquet found in his ten-year study of 430 cases that people who had been habitually maltreated or parented harshly and in fear had a higher incidence of conversion hysteria (49). Incidence of hysteria is also related to area. In a recent study in Japan, hysteria was higher in the suburbs and lower in the inner city and country, possibly because of the loss of sociocultural ties for those moving from the city or country to the suburbs (45).

Client-Care Goal and Related Nursing Interventions

Goal: Expresses anxiety and conflicts verbally rather than physically.

Intervention

The person with conversion segments self: he/she becomes the symptom. Do not relate just to the symptom and further disjoint the person. The problem symptom takes on the intensity of the need and urgency of the conflict, as if the person is fighting for survival. Accept the need for the symptom; do not strip the person of his/her defense by confrontation. The person is fighting to maintain integrity and identity and needs the defensive symptom to retain a feeling of wholeness. Relate to the person's uniqueness and sense of identity and integrity. Call the person by name. Talk about life experiences.

Help the person see the significance and connection between needs and conflicts and the symptom in terms of his/her life. Help the client use words rather than symbols to explore feelings, such as loneliness and isolation. Many times the person will discuss intimate topics without outward expression of feeling. You might comment on this. What the person says is not so important as what is omitted (40). Listen between the lines and respond with realistic feedback to the feelings and the meaning of symptoms.

Show understanding and patience. Do not be punitive or condemn. Have a sense of your own anger. It is difficult to work with a person who has symptoms of illness without an organic basis, but he/she feels pain. Also be aware of the contempt that many health care workers have for this client. Serve as a client advocate with other staff members. The person is not consciously trying to be sick or to get out of work. He/she is not lying or planning consciously to avoid responsibility.

Minimize the sick role. Do not reinforce the illness by giving a great deal of attention to the physical complaints. For example, a client came to the clinic weekly, always fainting at the emergency room door. After a period of assessment, the team collaborated on an approach in which no attention would be given to the person after fainting. This was difficult for the staff, but consistency was essential.

Sometimes staff will respond with anger to the client. A danger in the care of this person is the stress on the staff. If the staff is unable to understand the client's needs and responds with anger, he/she feels more threatened and alone. In this case, as in past stress situations, the client will fall back on the symptom and will cement the relationship with the symptom.

Encourage the client to make decisions and to be responsible and capable when possible. Reduce demands made on the client when anxiety is too great. When he/she becomes anxious with responsibility, give support and assist with decision making. Encourage the family to be involved. Explore with the client helpful community resources.

SOMATIZATION THROUGH HYPOCHONDRIASIS RELATED TO CHRONIC ANXIETY

Dynamics

Hypochondriasis is the expression of excessive anxiety about physical concerns and fears of deteriorating health. As feelings of isolation, loneliness, and lack of gratification with other people increase, the hypochondriacal person begins to turn all his/her energy inward. The person regresses to an earlier narcissistic level of development. As inner preoccupations become greater and energy investment in external factors lessens, fears increase about illness, change in organs, and death. Usually the person spends all his/her time concentrating on concerns,

indicating a lack of worth or self-esteem and further contributing to rejection by others.

Assessment and Nursing Diagnosis

Assessment parameters for the *nursing diagnosis, somatization through hypochondriasis* related to *chronic anxiety* focus on emotional status rather than on physical symptoms.

Freud named character traits of the hypochondriacal person: orderliness, stinginess, and obstinacy (29). Meister observed that this person is egocentric, miserly, very reliable, conscientious in performing petty duties, irascible, and distrustful (52). These characteristics are similar to those of the obsessive-compulsive personality with one major difference: the hypochondriac has an unusual concern about body image and size. Body image is important to the hypochondriac since he/she is overly concerned with the physical self and maintains continual self-observation.

Some see this condition placed on a continuum, as follows (50):

Stage 1. Mild—Excessive or fanatical preoccupation with and care of the body without presence of physical symptoms, such as jogging or use of health foods to the extreme.

Stage 2. Moderately severe—Excessive preoccupation with the physical condition and a firm belief that one or more illnesses are present.

Stage 3. Most severe—Considerable time is spent thinking and talking repeatedly about illness. Some people seek medical help; others do not.

In a study of 300 hypochondriacs and through validation with other health professionals, Meister found another kind of hypochondriac—the client who seeks medical help by contacting one physician after another. Meister also discovered the "closet" hypochondriac who is almost never seen by physicians or by other health care workers. This person treats self because he/she lacks confidence or trust in others (50). P. Fyrer and co-workers stated in their research that this person focuses on an increased awareness of body functions and conditions, not just on the body functions and conditions themselves (31). Meister cited a hypochondriac who checked her body out for 30 minutes, three times a day, at exact hours. She examined her entire body surface by palpation and observation. Twice daily she gave herself a gynecological examination. She was certainly aware of or in touch with her body, but what a high price to pay in terms of time, effort, relationships, and life style (50).

Client-Care Goal and Nursing Interventions

Goal: Demonstrate less concern with body function and symptoms and direct attention to other people and events.

Intervention

First, *listen thoroughly to the person's symptoms.* It does not take long to learn what he/she is complaining about; for if you give the client an opportunity, he/she will repetitiously describe the symptoms. Question: "What is this person saying with his/her symptoms? Why these somatic fears?" The client usually appears more ill than he/she really is because of the fear and concern expressed in his/her description. Listen in a neutral manner to the person's ruminating conversation. It is usually difficult to encourage discussion on any topic other than the symptoms. Do not minimize the symptoms, but do not focus excessively on them either. If this is the first medical contact, some diagnostic studies may be necessary, depending on the symptoms described. However, repeated diagnostic workups should be avoided.

Listen to the life story, the person's history. Frequently fear is responsible for the symptoms that are expressed. For example, a client whose mother died of cancer of the breast was afraid that her nipples were rotting and that her breasts were turning hard. She would cry and ask for reassurances that she was all right. By far the majority of the fears are based on experiences with parents or the environment. Give related information when appropriate about why such fears are unfounded.

Try to develop a relationship. Reward and give special attention when the person talks about something other than symptoms. There is a tremendous need for attention and love. The repetitious complaints and emotional pulling from you make the relationship a difficult one. Try to see through the behavior to the real person and relate to, reinforce, and support healthy behaviors. Through your relationship, help the person become interested or invest first in you, and then in others. Explore ways to make friends since this person has few. Work with the family who also find it difficult to relate to the client. By your example, let the person know what he/she is missing in relationships with other people. Very gradually this client can be helped to develop interest in other activities and people beside him/herself.

PERSONALITY CHANGE THROUGH DISSOCIATIVE SYMPTOMS RELATED TO SEVERE ANXIETY

Dynamics

Dissociation is a symptom whereby anxiety is dealt with by a splitting off of one portion of the personality and a breaking up of the whole sense of self. Association means to join or connect. In contrast, *dissociation means to separate, split off, break apart, or disjoin.* In dissociation, there is an unconscious separation of an idea, wish, function, segment of attention, behavior, or sense of awareness from the main stream of consciousness (46). Dissociation includes an alteration of consciousness and a change in level of reality, awareness of self, surroundings, or body parts when the anxiety in-

creases to an unbearable level or when the person cannot tolerate what is happening.

Refer to Table 13-3 for descriptions of the various types of dissociative reactions. These various reactions seem interesting and bizarre. Each state is in some sense different from each of the other states. However, all of these behaviors represent an escape, a running away from anxiety, stress, and crisis. At times the running is physical, and the person may suddenly find him/herself in a bus station, police station, or distant geographic area, running away psychologically from a conflict or stress.

TABLE 13-3.   Types of Dissociative Reactions

SYMPTOM	DESCRIPTION	DISSOCIATIVE RESPONSE
Amnesia	Inability to remember; complete forgetting of a period of time. Cause is both organic (alcoholism, neuronal deterioration, trauma, brain lesions) and psychological difficulties.	Dissociation of information or an experience that becomes inaccessible to the recollection of the person. Can be sudden and massive in that a large portion of life and behavior cannot be recalled because of repression. Evidenced by statements and behavior of the person. Person may act surprised to find self in current situation with no recall of events leading up to the situation.
Depersonalization	Experience of unrealness; feelings of separation, isolation, unreality; loss of feeling and personal identity.	Dissociation of parts of self that become strange or unreal. Mild to severe symptoms and usually transient. Evidenced by the report of the person. May state that limb feels like concrete or is not attached to body. May report numbness or paresthesia.
Fainting	Sudden complete, involuntary, temporary loss of consciousness.	Dissociation of the person from reality. Nonpsychotic break, a primitive defense seen less frequently today; symptoms used more when culturally acceptable. Evidenced by report of family, friends, or associates.

TABLE 13-3. Continued

SYMPTOM	DESCRIPTION	DISSOCIATIVE RESPONSE
Fugue states	Major change in personality with confusion, loss of personality organization, and flight to another geographic area.	Massive dissociation of personality, causing amnesia and physical running away. Hallucinations and depression decrease with amnesia. Feels like in another world. May last days to months. May be found by police.
Somnambulism	Walking while asleep. Usually associated with dreaming where the person becomes physically active, acting out sleep fantasy or conflict.	Dissociation during sleep. Indicative of pathological conflict in adult years. Common in children. Observed by other persons. May or may not be remembered by the person.
Multiple Personality	Living two or more lives independently without awareness of the other(s). A self-hypnosis wish-fulfillment for alter ego or another self-identity.	Major complete dissociative process whereby personality or identity separates, with some symbolic significance. More advanced dissociative state. Rare. Sometimes difficult to identify unless person is closely observed over time.

Assessment and Nursing Diagnosis

Assessment parameters for the *nursing diagnosis, personality change through dissociative symptoms,* related to *severe anxiety,* focus on personality type and change in behavior.

Since the histrionic personality previously mentioned carries the highest vulnerability for both conversion and dissociative symptoms, first study the personality of the client. Do you note characteristics and behaviors common to the hysterical person? Second, assess the symptoms that followed the crisis or stress situation. Has the client told you of symptoms reflecting "breaking off behavior," such as sleepwalking, trance states, and forgetting? Do you notice changes in level of consciousness, awareness states, eye expression, or facial appearance? Sometime you may have a feeling that the person is no longer with you in thought or feeling. The client may describe feelings of unreality, estrangement, detachment, of being outside the body looking in on his/her own life. The person may be unable to remember an event, or just fall asleep at a highly anxious time. Behaviors include dreams, fainting, hypnotic trances, fugue states, amnesia, multiple personalities, and sleep reactions.

The following patient history is an example of the dissociative symptom:

Mary Edwards came to the mental health clinic seeking help. She stated she was fearful of hurting her nine-month old baby. Several times she twisted his arm and bounced him on the bed until he cried. Mary was short, heavy set, and pleasant in appearance. She was dramatic in her speech, friendly, made contact easily, yet lacked depth in affect. She was assigned a nurse specialist and soon was seeing the nurse regularly. On the eighth visit she was discussing her relationship with her father, and her eyes became trancelike. She did not respond to the nurse's touch, yet she continued talking. The nurse called her name and she did not answer. After 2 to 3 minutes, she regained conscious awareness, having no memory of the earlier discussion.

The nursing diagnosis of dissociative symptoms may be difficult until you have had experience. Validate with a supervisor. Assessment of behaviors described in Table 13-3 will be pertinent to your diagnosis.

Client-Care Goal and Related Nursing Interventions

Goal: Help client experience and describe decrease in anxiety with increased awareness of self and life.

Intervention

Review the nursing care of the client with somatization through conversion symptoms; the approach is similar since the basic personality type is similar (see pp. 454–456). *Relate to the person as a whole. Encourage staff consistency in approach and limit setting.* Do what is necessary to *relieve anxiety* and *meet dependency needs,* including to provide a *safe, protected environment.* Try not to be manipulated into doing what the client can do for him/herself.

The major focus of communication should be aimed at uncovering the affect and reality of conflicted areas. Explore the dynamics of the problem.

Learn the life story, the defense mechanisms used, and the stressful event that precipitated the symptom. Uncovering the basic problem areas will be important but difficult. Expect the client to test you.

A relationship of trust and security comes slowly but eventually will allow the client greater comfort in release of true feelings. The relationship allows for teaching and support as the client struggles toward greater maturity and stability. Support his/her self-esteem.

Explore with the client how to relate to others. Encourage greater autonomy through controlling impulses, thinking before acting, and developing greater skills in solving problems. Encourage new interests and development of long-term goals and strategies for living with anxiety and stress. Goals and guidelines for intervention discussed in Chapters 8 and 12 can be useful for the long-term therapy needed by this client.

Medications can be a helpful method to relieve anxiety or to induce relaxation. The anti-anxiety agents are frequently referred to as "minor tranquilizers." Meprobate was the first to be used in the early 1960s but has lost popularity because of the addictive quality and decreasing tolerance. The most commonly used drugs today are Librium and Valium (10). Barbiturates and antihistamines are sometimes used. Refer to Table 13-2 for further information.

EVALUATION

Indices of how client is progressing can be based on the number, intensity, and extent of observed behavioral manifestations of anxiety. The person may share with you in the relationship how he/she is feeling and doing. If the person does not have the insight to describe feelings, validate your observations with other health team members. As the person recovers, he/she will demonstrate fewer dysfunctional behaviors, will have the ability to handle more stress without defensive behavior, will make more statements of self-confidence and autonomous development, and will enjoy more the everyday experiences of life.

REFERENCES

1. Akhtar, S., "Obsessional Neurosis, Marriage, Sex and Fertility: Some Transcultural Comparisons," *International Journal of Social Psychiatry,* 241, no. 3 (1978), 164–66.

2. Akhtar, S. et al., "Socio-Cultural and Clinical Determinants of Symptomatology in Obsessional Neurosis," *International Journal of Social Psychiatry,* 24, no. 3 (1978), 157–62.

3. American Psychiatric Association, Committee on Nomenclative and Statistics, *Diagnostic and Statistical*

Manual of Mental Disorders-I. Washington, D.C.: American Psychiatric Association, 1952.

4. ___, *Diagnostic and Statistical Manual of Mental Disorders-II.* Washington, D.C.: American Psychiatric Association, 1968.

5. ___, *Diagnostic and Statistical Manual of Mental Disorders-III.* Washington, D.C.: American Psychiatric Association, 1980.

6. Anderson, Robert, *Stress Power.* New York: Human Sciences Press, 1978.

7. Arieti, Silvenia, "Man's Spirituality and Potential for Creativity as Revealed in Mental Illness," *Comprehensive Psychiatry,* 21, no. 6 (1980), 436–43.

8. ___, "New Views on the Psychodynamics of Phobias," *American Journal of Psychotherapy,* 33, no. 1 (1979), 82–95.

9. Arrindel, Willem, "Dimensional Structure and Psychopathology Correlates of the Fear Survey Schedule in a Phobic Population: A Factorial Definition of Agoraphobia," *Behavior Research and Therapy,* 18, no. 4 (1980), 229–42.

10. Baldessarini, Rose, *Chemotherapy in Psychiatry.* Cambridge, Mass.: Harvard University Press, 1977.

11. Bennun, I., "Obsessional Slowness: A Replication and Extension," *Behavior Research and Therapy,* 18 (1980), 595–98.

12. Birley, J. L. T., and G. W. Brown, "Crises and Life Changes Preceding the Onset or Relapse of Acute Schizophrenia: Clinical Aspects," *British Journal of Psychiatry,* 116 (1970), 327–33.

13. Bliss, Eugene, "Multiple Personalities," *Archives of General Psychiatry,* 37 (1980), 1388–97.

14. Brooker, C., "Nursing Care Study: The Behavioural Management of a Complex Case," *Nursing Times,* 76, no. 9 (February 28, 1980), 267–69.

15. Buber, M., *I and Thou.* Edinburgh: Clark Publishing, 1953.

16. Cameron, Norman, *The Psychology of Behavioral Disorders.* Boston: Houghton Mifflin Company, 1947.

17. Chaloff, P., and H. Lyons, "Hysteria, the Hysterical Personality and Hysterical Conversion," *American Journal of Psychiatry,* 114 (1958), 734–40.

18. Chiriboga, David, and Hannah Dean, "Dimensions of Stress: Perspectives from a Longitudinal Study," *Journal of Psychosomatic Research,* 22 (1978), 47–55.

19. Cohen, Jonathon, "Structural Consequences of Psychic Trauma: A New Look at Beyond the Pleasure Principle," *International Journal of Psychoanalysis,* 61, no. 3 (1980), 421–32.

20. Connelley, J., "Obsessions—The Psychiatric Nurse as Therapist," *Nursing Mirror,* 142, no. 3 (March 16, 1973), pp. 25–26.

21. Cooper, W., "Don't Write Us Off as Neurotics," *Nursing Mirror,* 147, no. 24 (December 19, 1978), 21–22.

22. Deakin, H. G., "Phobias," *Nursing,* 10, no. 11 (1980), 815–18.

23. Dean, P. R., "The Neurotic Process: An Overview and Its Application to Nursing," *Journal of Psychiatric Nursing,* 17, no. 12 (1979), 35–37.

24. Emmelkamp, Paul, "Agoraphobics, Interpersonal Problems. Their Role in the Effects of Exposure in Vivo Therapy," *Archives of General Psychiatry,* 37, no. 11 (1980), 1303–6.

25. Fenichel, Otto, *The Psychoanalytical Theory of Neurosis.* New York: W. W. Norton & Co., Inc., 1945.

26. Freeman, D. F., and T. P. Cornwall, "Hyperactivity and Neurosis," *American Journal of Orthopsychiatry,* 50, no. 4 (1980), 704–11.

27. Freud, Anna, "Fears, Anxieties, and Phobic Phenomena," *Psychoanalytic Study of the Child,* 32 (1977), 85–90.

28. Freud, Sigmund, "Analysis of Phobia in a Five-Year-Old Boy, 1909," in *Collected Papers, vol. III,* pp. 149–289. New York: Basic Books, Inc., 1959.

29. ___, *Collected Papers, Volume II.* London: Hogarth Press Ltd., 1950.

30. Fukuda, K. et al., "Hysteria and Urbanization Letter," *British Journal of Psychiatry,* 137, no. 9 (1980), 300–301.

31. Fyrer, Peter, Ian Lee, and John Alexander, "Awareness of Cardiac Function in Anxious, Phobic and Hypochondriacal Patients," *Psychosomatic Medicine,* 10, no. 1 (1980), 171–74.

32. Garrison M., "A New Look at Little Hans," *Psychoanalytic Review,* 65, no. 1 (1978), 523–32.

33. Gorman, J., "Dissociation and Play Therapy: A Case Study," *Journal of Psychiatric Nursing and Mental Health Services,* 10, no. 2 (1972), 23–25.

34. Groy, Melvin, *Neurosis: A Comprehensive and Critical View.* New York: Van Nostrand Reinhold Company, 1978.

35. Heagarty, M. et al., *Child Health: Basics for Primary Care.* New York: Appleton-Century-Crofts, 1980.

36. Hodgson, R., and S. Rachman, "Obsessional-Compulsive Complaints," *Behavior Research and Therapy,* 15 (1977), 389–95.

37. Holleck, Seymour, "Hysterical Personality Traits," *Archives of General Psychiatry,* 16, no. 6 (1967), 750–57.

38. Holmes, T., and R. Rahe, "The Social Readjustment Rating Scale," *Journal Psychosomatic Research,* 11 (1967), 213-18.

39. Horton, P., and D. Miller, "The Etiology of Multiple Personality," *Comprehensive Psychiatry,* 13, no. 3 (1972), 151-59.

40. Kalkman, Marion, *Psychiatric Nursing,* 3rd ed. New York: McGraw-Hill Book Company, 1967.

41. Kolb, Lawrence, *Modern Clinical Psychiatry.* Philadelphia: W. B. Saunders Company, 1977.

42. Koles, Anthony et al., "Somnambulism," *Archives of General Psychiatry,* 37, no. 21 (1980), 1406-7.

43. Krohn A., "Hysteria: The Elusive Neurosis," *Psychological Issues,* 12, Nos. 1-2 (1978), 7.

44. Jamieson, B., "Agree to Live Dangerously," *Nursing,* 10, no. 11 (1980), pp. 819-21.

45. Jones, Molly, "Conversion Reaction: Anachronism or Evolutionary Form, A Review of the Neurologic, Behavioral, and Psychoanalytic Literature," *Psychological Bulletin,* 87, no. 3 (1980), 427-41.

46. Laughlin, Henry, *The Neuroses.* London: Butterworth and Co., 1967.

47. Liebowitz, M. R., and D. F. Klein, "Case 1. Assessment and Treatment of Phobic Anxiety," *Journal of Clinical Psychiatry,* 40, no. 11 (1979), 486-92.

48. MacKinnon, Roger, and Robert Michels, *The Psychiatric Interview.* Philadelphia: W. B. Saunders Company, 1971.

49. Mai, F. M., and H. Merskey, "Briquets Treatise on Hysteria, A Synopsis and Commentary," *Archives of General Psychiatry,* 37, no. 12 (1980), 1401-5.

50. Meister, Robert, "Closet Hypochondriacs," *Psychology Today,* 14, no. 8 (1980), 29-37.

51. Miller, D. G., "A Repertory Grid Study of Obsessionality: Distinctive Cognitive Structure or Distinctive Cognitive Content," *British Journal of Medical Psychology,* 53, no. 1 (1980), 59-66.

52. Nichols, Barbara, "Dealing with Conflict," *Journal of Continuing Education in Nursing,* 10, no. 6 (1979), 24-27.

53. Pasquali, E. et al., *Mental Health Nursing: A Bio-Psycho-Cultural Approach.* St. Louis: The C. V. Mosby Company, 1981.

54. Paykel, E. S. et al., "Life Events and Depression," *Archives of General Psychiatry,* 21 (1969), 753-60.

55. Rendon, M., "Discussion of Horney's Theory of Neurosis: A Developmental-Structuralist Interpretation," *American Journal of Psychoanalysis,* 39, no. 1 (1979), 37-39.

56. Roy, A., "Hysteria: A Case Note Study," *Canadian Journal of Psychiatry,* 24, no. 2 (1979), 157-60.

57. ———, "Hysteria," *Journal of Psychosomatic Research,* 24, no. 2 (1980), 53-56.

58. Salzman, Leo, *The Obsessive Personality.* New York: Science House, 1968.

59. Seif, M. N., and A. L. Atkins, "Some Defensive and Cognitive Aspects of Phobias," *Journal of Abnormal Psychology,* 88, no. 1 (1979), 42-51.

60. Shapiro, David, "Obsessive-Compulsive Style," in *Stress and Coping: An Anthology,* eds. Alan Monat and Richard Lazarus. New York: Columbia University Press, 1977.

61. Skevington, Suzanne M., "Stress and Anxiety Neurosis: A Study of Recovery," *Journal of Psychiatric Research,* 14 (1977), pp. 439-49.

62. Stegman, R. L., and W. T. McReynolds, "Learned Helplessness, Learned Hopefulness, and Learned Obsessiveness: Effects of Varying Contingencies on Escape Responding," Part I, *Psychological Reports,* 43, no. 3 (1978), 795-801.

63. Stephenson, Carol, "Stress in Critically Ill Patients," *American Journal of Nursing,* 77, no. 11 (1977), 1806-9.

64. Sullivan, Harry Stack, *The Interpersonal Theory of Psychiatry.* New York: W. W. Norton & Co., Inc., 1953.

65. Tennant, Christopher, and Gavin Andrews, "The Pathogenic Quality of Life Event Stress in Neurotic Impairment," *Archives of General Psychiatry,* 35, no. 7 (1978), 859-63.

66. Von Rad, M. et al., "Alexithymia: Anxiety and Hostility in Psychosomatic and Psychoneurotic Patients," *Psychotherapy and Psychosomatics,* 31, nos. 1-4 (1979), 223-24.

67. Wallace, C., "Nursing the Hysterical Patient," *Nursing Mirror,* 42, April 27, 1973, pp. 40-41.

68. Watson, J., "Phobic Disorders—Management," *Nursing Mirror,* 141, March 10, 1972, pp. 32-33.

69. Weinberg, S. Kirson, *The Sociology of Mental Disorders.* Chicago: Aldine Publishing Co., 1967.

70. Weiss, J. R., and J. M. Rhoads, "Brief Reactive Psychosis: A Psychodynamic Interpretation," *Journal of Clinical Psychiatry,* 40, no. 10 (1979), 440-43.

14

The Person
Who
Abuses Substances

Study of this chapter will assist you to:

1. Increase empathy for the person who abuses substances, describing him/her as a unique individual of worth who has a chronic disease.

2. Define terms pertinent to alcoholism and other drug abuse and obesity.

3. Describe the incidence and scope of substance abuse as a health problem.

4. Relate the psychological, physiological, and sociological factors that contribute to the origin and maintenance of substance abuse.

5. Compare and contrast progressive physical, psychological, and sociocultural effects of alcohol and other drugs.

6. Assess the person who suffers from alcoholism, other drug abuse, polydrug abuse, or obesity.

7. Assess the impact of substance abuse on the family and how it affects their needs and problems.

8. Formulate nursing diagnoses, based on assessment of the substance abuser.

9. Determine mutually the care goals with the client and his/her family.

10. Implement nursing intervention measures pertinent to nursing diagnoses and goals and the client's phases of recovery.

11. Intervene as indicated with the client's family.

12. Become a support system for the client and family and facilitate the development and use of other support systems.

13. Evaluate the contribution of your care to the maintenance of the wholeness, dignity, and health of the client and family.

This chapter contributed by Phyllis Jacobs, R.N., M.S.N. and Gail Stringer, R.N., M.S.N.

Who is the substance abuser? The substance abuser *does* include the skid row alcoholic whose permanent residence may be several blocks within a major metropolitan area. The substance abuser *does* include the heroin addict whose entire life centers around procuring enough money for the next fix. The substance abuser also *does* include the person who may be 150 pounds overweight and eats mountains of food that would make most other people sick. But these are only a small minority of the people who abuse substances. At some point in time, you, I, our families, and those we work with may become substance abusers. In other words, the majority of people who abuse substances are functional within society and are not only those few who are drastically different from you or me. Of the 12 million alcoholics in our country, only 3 to 5 percent are found on skid row; the other 95 to 97 percent are persons who are employed or are employable (46).

SUBSTANCE ABUSE: HISTORICAL AND CURRENT PROBLEM

Ours is a drug-oriented society, but this is not a new phenomenon. Drugs have been around since the Stone Age when fermented drinks were made from plant saps and wild fruits. As early as 8000 B.C., wine was a popular drink. In Egypt, in 3000 B.C., specialized classes of artesans developed brewing techniques. Distilled liquors date back to the twelfth century and beer to the fifteenth century (66). The famous artists of the Renaissance depicted that overweight women were certainly considered desirable. Smoking and drinking have been accepted activities for centuries. However, just because alcohol, drugs, smoking, and excessive food intake have been part of society for so long does not diminish the intensity of the present problem. But substance abuse is being discussed more openly now than twenty years ago, and perhaps there is more concern over the short- and long-term effects on life. Today's emphasis on preventative, holistic health care may help focus on the relationship between substance abuse and health problems.

Apparently the use of drugs, including alcohol, began as part of a tribal ritual. Then, as people became aware of the tension-reducing and relaxing properties of these substances, their use for this purpose became increasingly individualized. Today, people use drugs to overcome their feelings of anxiety or frustrations, to cope with tensions, or just because it makes them feel happy and free from pain and trouble. As a result of the continued use of these substances, some people become ill (29).

Alcohol is the number one drug problem in the world today, although this does not lessen the magnitude of the other drugs that are abused. Society has always had a direct influence on the magnitude of alcohol and drug abuse. For example, alcohol ingestion has long been associated with masculinity. The stimulant drugs came into use in the 1940s when truck drivers, students, and others were looking for something to help them stay awake for long periods of time. Today the abuse of stimulants, especially among teen-agers, remains widespread. Also, for some years now, barbiturates and other sedatives and tranquilizers have been readily prescribed by the medical profession to alleviate complaints of anxiety, stress, or sleeplessness. Causative factors for these complaints have seldom been explored. The extremely widespread prescription of minor tranquilizers and barbiturates is such that middle-class society considers this normal behavior and does not seem aware of their habit-forming properties, withdrawal symptoms, and lethal potential when combined with alcohol. Sniffing of solvents and use of alcohol are increasingly common among preadolescents as well as among adolescents. This group is particularly vulnerable to group pressure and is less aware than older people of the long-term ramifications of this behavior. Marijuana and psychedelic drug abusers are commonly found among young adults of middle-class background with some college experience. The motivation seems to come from a variety of sources; including peer pressure, a feeling that they are not vulnerable to addiction, and a desire for fun or for quick and easy personal psychologic insight, expanded consciousness, or a peak experience (8).

Nicotine is an addicting drug. Today about 120 countries are growing tobacco, and cigarette sales are rapidly increasing in developing countries (15). Cigarettes are readily available, and peer pressure to begin smoking exists among school-age children despite the many educational campaigns against smoking.

Although not as lethal as some of the other substances abused, food may be the substance most abused. Obesity is seen in all age groups, from the young child to the elderly, and at all levels of society. Approximately 30 million Americans are overweight!

For some people, turning to an external substance to solve a problem has been a learned behavior ever since they were toddlers, for example, being given candy to quiet crying after a fall, or receiving a reward of dessert for eating all of the meal. America is a problem-solving society in that we feel the need to *do* something in response to events. There *must* be something that can be done, and we readily turn to something that is accessible, immediate, and painless. For example, it is easier to take a diet pill in order to do something about a weight problem than it is to realize that two pieces of dessert always follow being upset with one's husband. Or how much easier to have a couple of cocktails before lunch to prepare for a difficult afternoon business meeting than to work through anxiety about the possible confrontation and attempt to find a solution other than drinking. Changing reactions to stressors is often painful, and it is not unusual for a person, when trying to stop dependence on one substance, to move to dependence on other substances or activities such as drugs, food, nicotine, or even sex, gambling, and work. For many, there is a need to be dependent on something external. Without treatment, these persons will continue replacing one substance with another.

It is very difficult to look at your own behavior and see dependence on an external substance, although we may readily criticize such behavior in others. We may think of the drug abuser as the high-school dropout who lives on the fringes of society and exists from one "fix" to the next. And although we may deplore this behavior, this life style may have certain appeal for some people. For example, the outsider looking at the drug culture may feel an attraction to a group that seems to be responsible to no one and doing whatever it wishes. However, neither the suburban housewife, nor the occasional drug abuser understands the compulsion and one-track dimension in the life of the addict.

In this chapter, the abuse of alcohol, narcotics, sedatives, barbiturates, minor tranquilizers, stimulants, hallucinogens, marijauna, hashish, inhalants, nicotine, caffeine, and food will be discussed. The scope of substance abuse, etiologic theories of dependence on substances, and physical and emotional effects of abuse of particular substances will be explored. Major emphasis will be on factors you need to assess in order to provide comprehensive care of the client. Since assessment of the client is only the beginning step, probable nursing diagnoses and some short-term and long-term nursing care goals will be suggested in terms of the client's psychological, sociocultural, and spiritual well-being.

Because the substance abuser has a chronic illness with a high recidivism rate, you will often have continued contact with the client over a long period of time. And even when the client has withdrawn from his/her dependence on a substance, it is not necessarily the end of treatment. He/she will have to continually work to maintain an awareness of thoughts, feelings, and actions to avoid resuming substance abuse again. And your attitude needs to remain caring throughout the entire recovery process.

Alcoholism will be the main focus in this chapter since it is the greatest drug problem in the United States. However, much of the information on alcoholism also applies to abuse of other substances (drugs, food) in terms of etiology and psychodynamics. Methods of interacting with all clients who abuse substances are also very similar. Therefore information on specific drugs and on excessive eating will be discussed only in those areas where the effects of their overuse differs from the effects of alcoholism. How the dynamics of overuse of drugs and food differ from the dynamics of alcoholism will be emphasized.

DEFINITIONS OF TERMS

Terms related to the abuse of substances are often used very loosely and interchangeably, which leads to misunderstanding and confusion. You need to know the meaning of the following terms when caring for a substance abuser (10, 23):

Substance: Refers to alcohol, drugs, and food that are ingested for reasons unrelated to health.

Substance Abuse: Excessive or unhealthy use of harmful substances, such as alcohol, tobacco, or drugs, or use of products, such as food, that becomes unhealthy when excessive amounts are ingested.

Drug Use: Ingesting in any manner a chemical substance that has an effect on the body. This definition applies to all drugs taken legally and illegally, both for medical and nonmedical usage.

Drug Abuse: Persistent or sporadic excessive drug use inconsistent with or unrelated to acceptable medical practice. This definition includes *all* drug intake that is not prescribed for medical use or is not within the generally accepted context of taking nonprescription medications for a specific health problem, such as a headache or gastrointestinal upset.

Tolerance: The declining effect of the same drug dose when it is taken repeatedly over time. There is evidence that tolerance is an adaptive mechanism of the brain to repeated doses of a drug. This leads to taking greater amounts of the substance to obtain the same effect.

Habituation: A psychological dependence on the use of a drug. Since the drug gives relief from tension and emotional discomfort, it is repeatedly used despite the detrimental effects, such as loss of job or family problems.

Addiction: Physical dependence on a substance, causing an altered physiological state because of repeated use of a substance. The drug must be continued to avoid physical symptoms of withdrawal, which vary from moderate, such as muscular pain or increased perspiration, to life-threatening, such as convulsions. The brain cells have become adapted to functioning with the substance and for a period of time cannot function properly without it.

Chemical Dependence: A state of psychic and/or physical dependence on a substance following its administration on a periodic or continuing basis. This definition combines habituation and addiction. Over the years these two terms have often been used interchangeably and inappropriately.

Even though terms related to drug use are used very loosely, it is important that you understand the proper meaning of the terms and *use* the proper meaning in talking with both clients and colleagues.

CARE OF THE PERSON WHOSE USE OF ALCOHOL IS OUT OF CONTROL

Scope of the Problem

You will be caring for alcoholic clients in a wide variety of settings and must be aware of the possibility of alcoholism when caring for anyone. It has been estimated that one-third of the patients in most general hospitals have a drinking problem (70), although the patient is seldom admitted with the diagnosis of alcoholism. The diagnosis may be peptic ulcer or cardiac disease. Also alcoholism as a family problem may be a factor when a child is admitted because of having been abused. Or alcoholism may be a complicating factor when a patient is hospitalized for elective surgery. Therefore always be alert for withdrawal symptoms related to alcohol or other drug abuse. Always ask about alcohol consumption.

You may be surprised to learn that alcoholism is the fourth largest public health problem following cardiovascular disease, cancer, and mental illness. One adult in ten in the United States is a problem drinker or an alcoholic, and this person's drinking affects the lives of at least four other people. In addition to adult drinkers, there are an estimated 3.3 million problem drinkers among the 14- to 17-year age range (69). Insurance statistics show that there is a 10- to 12-year decrease in life expectancy among alcoholics. Nearly one-third of all cases handled in child guidance clinics show that one or both parents are alcoholic. One-fourth of all suicides are alcohol-related. Approximately two-thirds of all homicides are alcohol-related. And 50 percent of auto accidents that are fatal to the driver are also alcohol-related (46). Current media reports indicate that alcoholism and related problems are particularly widespread among minorities, poor men under 25 years of age, city residents, persons who have moved from rural areas or small towns to large cities, and those with childhood disruptions such as broken homes or alcoholic parents.

The rate of alcoholism is increasing! From these statistics you can readily see the magnitude of alcoholism as a social problem without even considering the anguish alcoholism causes in individual lives and among families. It is a major health problem not only in the United States but also worldwide, especially in developing countries. Money in these countries that is spent on alcohol often means a lack of money for food, shelter, and other basic life necessities. Some feel that there is a universal lack of effort to combat alcoholism (15). As a nurse using the Humanistic Framework, you will attempt to reduce the problem through teaching, political action, and your personal modeling behavior.

Properties of Alcohol

Ethyl alcohol is a clear, colorless liquid with a strong, burning taste. It does not have to be digested but exerts its action directly on the body in its original state. The rate of absorption of alcohol into the bloodstream is more rapid than its elimination; thus, if a person is drinking rapidly, a high concentration of alcohol may exist in the bloodstream.

The rate of absorption is dependent on the concentration of alcohol in the beverage. Beer usually is about 4 percent alcohol; wines usually range from 12 to 16 percent, and distilled beverages are usually about 50 percent alcohol. Figure 14-1 shows alcoholic equivalency in beverages:

4 oz of wine, 12% alcohol   12 oz of beer, 4% alcohol   1 oz of distilled beverage, 48% alcohol

FIGURE 14-1   Alcoholic equivalency in selected beverages.

Absorption of alcohol into the bloodstream is slower if there is food in the stomach to delay the contents emptying into the small intestine. Proteins and fats in the stomach are more effective in slowing down emptying of the stomach than carbohydrates. Once alcohol has passed into the duodenum, rapid absorption into the bloodstream occurs. A small amount is excreted in the urine, and a small amount is exhaled; but the majority is oxidized in the body by the liver. The main steps of this oxidation process are:

Breakdown of alcohol $\longrightarrow$ acetaldehyde $\longrightarrow$ $\longrightarrow$ acetic acid $\longrightarrow$ carbon dioxide and water

Energy in the form of heat is given off during this oxidation process at a rate of 7.1 calories per gram.

As alcohol travels throughout the body, it exerts a toxic effect on the organs, especially on the brain and central nervous system. In sufficient dosage, alcohol has a depressant effect. The apparent stimulating effect of alcohol is caused by the loss of inhibition and control as it depresses the central nervous system. A concentration of 100–150 mg of alcohol/100 ml of blood results from about four drinks in a three-hour period; this should be considered intoxication. Legal intoxication is usually defined as 80 or 100 mg of alcohol/100 ml of blood. The person with 200–250 mg of alcohol/100 ml blood may be ataxic, go to sleep, or have confused thought processes, fine muscle incoordination, and disturbed speech and vision. At 300 mg/100 ml of blood, the person may lose consciousness, and a concentration of 500 mg/100 ml of blood can be fatal. There is some individual variance of symptoms according to increased tolerance.

Definition of Alcoholism

There are many definitions of alcoholism. Some emphasize a particular symptom of alcoholism, such as loss of control. Others emphasize the physiologic aspects or the withdrawal symptoms that occur when someone abruptly decreases or discontinues use of alcohol. According to the American Medical Association, *alcoholism is an illness characterized by significant impairment that is directly associated with persistent and excessive use of alcohol.* Impairment may involve physiological, psychological, or social dysfunction (46). A simpler, general definition of alcoholism is *the use of alcoholic beverages to the point of causing damage to the individual, society, or both.* The definition can be summed up as WART: With Alcohol-Repeated Trouble. Thus alcoholism should not be defined by the amount of consumption or by the frequency of consumption. Such methods would exclude many alcoholics and would include many people who are not alcoholics. The manner in which a client drinks, such as drinking alone or morning drinking, is significant in assessing the client; but this does not define alcoholism.

Theories of Etiology

What brings the alcoholic to the point of being unable to control drinking? How does this person differ from the one who drinks socially?

Theories of causation are generally divided among three basic areas: psychological, physiological, and sociocultural. Actually, the cause of alcoholism appears to be a *combination* of psychological, physiological, and sociocultural factors. However, each factor does not have the same influence in each person's life.

When caring for an alcoholic client, be open to a variety of causative factors, although knowing the causation is not necessary for treatment, and much time can be wasted on theorizing what led a particular person to alcoholism. If you are aware of the effect environment can have, such as the drinking patterns in the early home environment, you can ascertain this information in the nursing assessment. The *how* of the person's drinking (the development and progression) will be a factor to consider in planning treatment with the client, even though the *why* is not known.

Psychological Theories of Causation

There are several psychological theories of causation. Many theorists feel that the alcoholic drinks because of problems with psychological development, which result in a need for an external crutch. In this case, alcohol is the crutch that is used to substitute for healthy coping skills that were never developed.

Several researchers have studied the family background of alcoholic patients; H. J. Clinebell's study is representative (12). He interviewed 76 alcoholic patients regarding their home lives as children and found that 57 percent came from homes that could be regarded as severely inadequate. The four major parental characteristics in these homes were authoritarianism, success-worship, moralism, and overt rejection. Because the home environment obstructed the development of healthy coping skills, alcohol became an alternative for coping.

Psychoanalytic theorists hypothesize that the alcoholic has been fixated at the oral level of psychosexual development. The person is seeking a union with a fantasized all-caring mother figure and symbolically achieves it via the bottle. Often the family histories of alcoholic persons demonstrate a variety of pathological relationships. One in particular is an overindulgent mother who encourages infantile oral demands, and when these demands become excessive to her, she meets them inconsistently. The child, bewildered by this inconsistency, becomes a passive-dependent person with needs that cannot be expressed. There are feelings of anger, betrayal, and a wish to destroy the parents, combined with the simultaneous fear of losing them, which causes the person to keep the rage inside. As an adult, the unacceptable dependency feelings cause other feelings of frustration, guilt, and resentment. Because the ego function has not developed sufficiently to allow for appropriate expression of feelings, the aggression may be expressed outwardly, or it may be vented inwardly. Drinking is then used to cover the guilt felt over anger expressed toward others and to compensate for the decreased feelings of self-worth from the anger being turned inward (36).

Need for self-punishment and feelings of worthlessness are accepted over the years, but getting drunk helps the person to temporarily forget such feelings. Later in life, other factors, situations, or people substitute for the role that the parents once filled. The perception of being rejected, neglected, or unloved will be part of most of these relationships. Alcohol continues to be the crutch that is used in order to meet needs when other relationships fail to do so or to alleviate feelings of guilt and anger.

Learning theorists suggest that drinking alcohol is a reflex response to some stimulus and a way of reducing inner drives such as anxiety (72). For many people, alcohol relieves the anxiety, guilt, and fear they feel. The reward is the reduction of the stressful feelings. Alcohol becomes a conditioned response to stressors, and the response is strengthened each time by the decrease in anxiety through the loss of inhibitions that occur when drinking. An example would be the man who is to make a formal presentation in his job. His superiors will be there, evaluating him, and he wants to get ahead in the company. He is apprehensive about making a poor presentation. Therefore he has a stiff drink at lunch to prepare for the afternoon meeting and then makes a successful presentation. Thus he feels the use of alcohol has worked, and he begins to use it more often to prepare for stressful events. The alcohol has become the conditioned response to stress, and it is the learned behavior he uses in a majority of situations.

The alcoholic personality has been studied extensively. Since the clients studied are already alcoholic, it has not been determined whether the person had these personality characteristics before becoming an alcoholic, or if these characteristics developed as a result of the illness. No specific personality type associated with alcoholism has been found. However, certain characteristics *are* quite common among alcoholics, although these characteristics are not exclusively found in alcoholics. The alcoholic typically portrays the following characteristics (10):

Angry overdependency: Is painfully aware of an excessive need for attention, affection, and praise; feels chronic anger that these excessive needs are not met to the extent desired.

Inability to express emotions adequately: Has difficulty talking about feelings; either holds them inside or explosively lets them out. Alcohol intake may begin as an aid in releasing these feelings.

High anxiety in interpersonal relationships: Uses alcohol to calm anxiety at social gatherings, and to relax and have fun, especially early in the disease.

Emotional immaturity: Is often self-centered, moody; must have needs met promptly.

Ambivalence toward authority: Struggles between being dependent and being dominant.

Low frustration tolerance: Has limited ability to withstand frustration.

Grandiosity: Demonstrates attitude of superiority, which serves as a defense against the guilt that is felt.

Low self-esteem: Feels he/she has never really been loved and is not worth loving.

Feelings of isolation: Has problems getting along with others. As drinking increases, social isolation increases.

Perfectionism and compulsiveness: Needs to see self as better than others because of low self-esteem.

Sex role confusion: Questions manliness or womanliness. Alcohol increases sexual feelings and so tends to dissipate the questioning of one's sexual identity. However, alcohol does not increase potency or performance.

Physiological or Biological Theories of Causation

Physiological or biological theories of causation are numerous, and some have gained prominence at different periods. Certain theories have survived for years, but none have received widespread acceptance. However, there does seem to be agreement that physiological factors do contribute to the origin of alcoholism, although no specific factors have been identified to date (46). Physiological theories claim that the alcoholic has some metabolic abnormality, such as an endocrine imbalance, that predisposes the person to becoming an alcoholic. Some theorists believe there is an abnormal metabolism of sugar. Others suggest that the alcoholic has a nutritional deficiency of certain substances, such as vitamins, zinc, and magnesium. Additional causes may be an undetermined sensitivity to a basic foodstuff, the symptoms of which are relieved by alcohol, or an acquired allergy to alcohol itself.

Presently, a major area of study of biologic origin is whether alcohol addiction has a hereditary component. There is a high correlation between family history of alcoholism and the incidence of alcoholism in offspring. E. M. Jellinek's study found an overall average of 52 percent of alcoholics had at least one alcoholic parent (29). When at least one parent is an alcoholic, the expectancy rate of alcoholism in the children is 20 to 30 percent, whereas the expectancy rate in the general population is only 2 to 3 percent (29). D. Goodwin studied subjects, who had been adopted at birth and raised by nonalcoholic parents, but who had a biologic parent who was an alcoholic. He found that the chances of adopted offspring having serious drinking problems are four times greater when one of the biologic parents was alcoholic, in contrast to adopted children with nonalcoholic biologic parents. He also found that sons of alcoholics were no more likely to become alcoholics if reared by the biologic parent than if separated at birth and reared elsewhere. Goodwin concluded that the more severe types of alcoholism seem to be influenced by heredity (21).

The fact that alcoholism tends to run in families may indicate biological, psychological, and sociological causes. Genes are transmitted via families and predispose the person to developing alcoholism if the family's values and habits promote drinking alcoholic beverages. In turn, the family environment and interaction patterns may influence the development of alcoholism as a way to cope with stressors.

Sociocultural Theories of Causation

Sociocultural theories of causation acknowledge that the incidence of alcoholism varies among groups and from society to society. Patterns of drinking and attitudes about drinking have been found to differ widely among different cultures, partly because alcohol tends to serve different functions among various subcultures or ethnic and religious groups. High rates of alcoholism are reported among the northern French, Americans, Swedes, Poles, and northern Russians. Cultural groups that show a low incidence of alcoholism are the Italians, some Chinese groups, Orthodox Jews, and the southern French (72). Interestingly enough, it is not that these cultures do not use alcohol, but rather that its use is confined to meals and/or religious rituals, and excessive drinking is condemned. The population tends to conform its behavior to the accepted attitudes, although this does not exclude a variance of drinking patterns within a particular society.

Attitudes about the use of alcohol can be divided into four broad categories (46):

1. *Total abstinence:* Little distinction is made between the social drinker and the chronic alcoholic. Here alcoholism is rarely seen.
2. *Ambivalence:* There is a high degree of variability and inconsistency of feelings regarding the use of alcohol. This is true of much of the United States. Alcoholism is usually a common problem where there is such a variation of attitudes.
3. *Permissiveness:* Frequently the child is introduced to alcohol very early, but the drinking occurs only within the family setting. Often there is much custom and tradition surrounding alcohol intake. Thus permissiveness may be allowed only within a specific framework of drinking patterns. The incidence of alcoholism is usually lower where there are more controls.
4. *Total permissiveness:* Any type of drinking is tolerated, and the behavior that results from it would also be tolerated. For example, in the United States, there are certain occasions or specific settings where society would accept drinking, such as at a bachelor party. In a totally permissive society, alcoholism is prevalent.

In the United States, attitudes toward drinking differ according to age. In most states, an adolescent can legally begin to drink between ages 18 and 21. It is assumed that on the day adolescents become "of age" they will be ready to assume the responsibilities that go with drinking. It is further assumed that they will not drink until they become that age, which is usually *not* the case. Increased drinking is seen today among teen-agers, especially among girls (46). Alcohol seems to be the drug of choice among teen-agers, although many who drink also use other drugs, which must be considered when assessing a teen-age client. Teen-agers may drink because drinking is symbolic of adulthood. They may feel that they are already an adult but are not accorded what they consider the "privileges" of adulthood. Drinking in adolescence may be a way of getting back at authority by shunning its laws. The fact that drinking of alcoholic beverages is illegal for teen-agers may increase its attractiveness. Drinking is also very often condoned by parents. Although some parents may admonish the teen-ager or preadolescent not to drink, the parents often use alcohol themselves—as an apparent solution to many problems.

Sex is another factor that influences our attitudes. Our society seems much less tolerant of an intoxicated female than a male, which might explain the secrecy surrounding the female alcoholic. The current ratio is 1:1 for women and men treated for alcoholism in private hospitals and private office practices (23). However, alcoholism among women is rapidly increasing, with the highest incidence of heavy drinking among women being in the 30- to 50-year age group; among men, the highest incidence of heavy drinking is in the twenties (46). Women tend to drink more at home. They usually begin heavy drinking later than men, but the stages of alcoholism development are often telescoped in women, so that women become alcoholics after fewer years of heavy drinking. Alcoholism in women is also frequently associated with depression (23).

Social position affects reaction of others to the person who drinks. For example, the person in a high social position who is arrested for being intoxicated may receive preferential treatment from the courts as compared to the disheveled skid row alcoholic. More people in urban areas tend to drink than those who live in rural areas. Alcoholism is also more prevalent among the higher socioeconomic groups who are better educated and hold better jobs than it is among the lesser privileged. The alcoholic is often a college graduate who functions in the business world. Alcoholism also tends to be higher among divorced and unmarried persons than among married couples (19).

The media play a role in that the person who is shown drinking in television, magazine, and newspaper advertising is depicted as a sophisticated, beautiful young person who is surrounded by friends. The implied message is that if you drink, you will surely be like that person.

As with the other two major etiologic theories (psychological and physiological), sociological factors cannot be considered *the* causative agent, but these factors are certainly influential in the development of alcoholism. Actually all three major areas must be considered in determining what has influenced the client to become an alcoholic.

Physical Effects of Alcohol

The physical effects and medical problems associated with alcohol use, abuse, and addiction are extensive. Alcohol is a central nervous system depressant, an irritant, and an inflammatory agent, so that some diseases are caused directly by the toxic effects on various organs and tissues. For example, these effects can damage the nervous system and compromise brain function. Cardiac disease, muscle impairment, alcoholic hepatitis, and cirrhosis may also result. Large doses of alcohol also depress the respiratory system, which in turn may lead to pneumonia or other respiratory infections (34, 65).

Alcohol contributes to nutritional deficiency when it is substituted for adequate food intake because alcohol metabolizes 7.1 calories per ml of alcohol. Peripheral neuropathy results from thiamine deficiency, and hematological abnormalities are attributed to either dietary deficiency or the direct toxic action of alcohol in blood cell formation sites. Alcoholic hepatitis and cirrhosis are also related to nutritional deficiency (34, 65). Sometimes the combined effects of toxicity, malnutrition, and metabolic defects are thought to result in tissue damage, including cardiomyopathy.

The irritant effects of alcohol on the stomach, along with the increased production of hydrochloric acid from alcohol intake, contribute to acute esophagitis, gastritis, inflammation, or peptic and duodenal ulcer. Alcohol intake also changes pancreatic secretions, causing acute and chronic recurring pancreatitis (34, 65).

Because the effects of alcohol on the physical status of the body are so extensive, only those illnesses that are frequently associated with alcoholism will be discussed here. For an extensive review of physical illnesses related to alcoholism, consult a medical nursing text. Figure 14-2 depicts the major organ and tissue damage and the resulting symptoms. Abstinence and improved diet can overcome some chronic effects of alcoholism and can reverse myopathy, gastrointestinal symptoms, liver damage and the resulting symptoms, and reproductive, respiratory, and hematologic effects (34, 65).

Since the effects of alcohol on the central nervous system and brain are extensive and are directly related to psychiatric/mental health nursing, we will present a detailed description here of the following: alcoholic intoxication, alcohol withdrawal syndrome, and Wernicke/Korsakoff Syndrome.

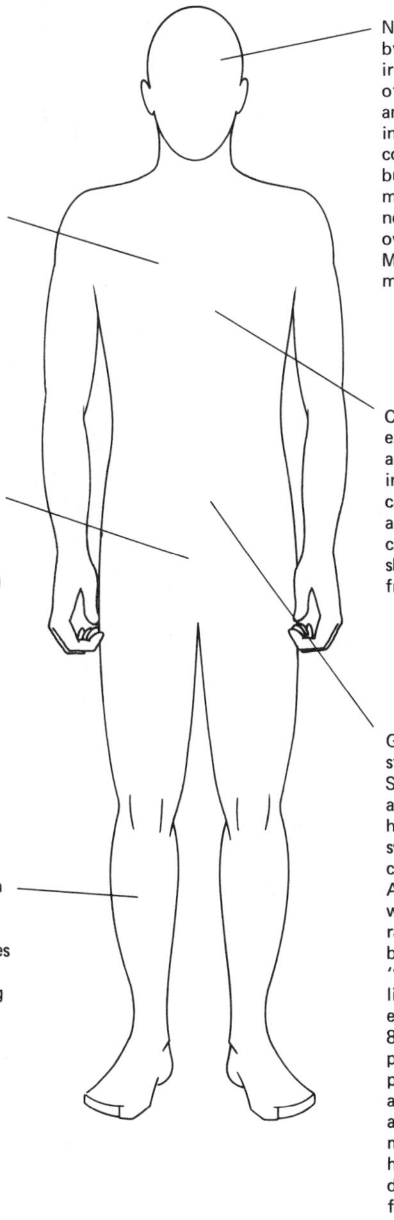

NERVOUS SYSTEM AND BRAIN function compromised by alcohol intake. Alcohol is a sedative, depressant, irritant, and inflammatory agent. See text for discussion of alcohol intoxication, alcohol withdrawal syndrome, and Wernicke's/Korsakoff's Syndrome. Excessive alcohol intake causes peripheral neuropathy, defects in nerve conduction, with tingling, numbness, prickly sensations, burning, itching, weakness, paralysis, or gastrocnemius muscle and foot pains. Changes in gait due to peripheral nerve damage. Nerve palsies due to prolonged pressure over the nerve sites, perhaps while in alcoholic stupor. Myopathy, with severe pain and tenderness of skeletal musculature and edema in the lower extremities.

RESPIRATORY SYSTEM depression due to large doses of alcohol, causing decreased respiratory rate and cough reflex, pooling of secretions, and increased susceptibility to infection and trauma. Ascites from liver damage reduces vital capacity, as do injuries to rib cage from falls or fights. Incidence of tuberculosis is higher in alcoholic population.

CARDIAC tissue damage due to effects of alcohol on excitability and contractility of heart muscle. Intoxicating amounts of alcohol affect cardiac rate and output and increase both systolic and pulse pressures. Toxicity a causative factor in hypertension. Alcohol contributes to a weakened heart muscle and heart failure. Alcoholic cardiomyopathy, a severe condition with heart failure, shortness of breath, and enlargement of the heart, frequently seen in long-term chronic alcoholics.

REPRODUCTIVE SYSTEM affected. In males, alcohol can cause swelling of prostate gland, leading to prostatitis and interference with voiding or sexual functioning. Complaints of impotence not uncommon. In females, counseling concerning intake of alcoholic beverages during pregnancy especially important. Intake of more than 2 oz of absolute alcohol per day involves risk. Fetal Alcohol Syndrome is the third leading cause of mental retardation. Newborn also characterized by facial malformation, cardiac problems, hyperactivity, growth deficiency, microencephaly, joint abnormalities, and fine motor dysfunction.

GASTROINTESTINAL complications common; the stomach, pancreas, and liver are affected. Acute gastritis. Symptoms of morning nausea and vomiting common, along with abdominal distention, pain, belching, and hematemesis. If esophagus is irritated, pain occurs on swallowing. Also mid-chest or epigastric pain. Alcohol contributes to or aggravates stomach or duodenal ulcers. Acute pancreatitis and chronic reoccurring pancreatitis, with nausea, vomiting, and severe upper abdominal pain radiating to back. Liver structure and function changed by excessive alcohol intake, causing swollen, enlarged, "fatty" liver. Alcoholic hepatitis—inflammation of liver, with fever, jaundice, abdominal swelling, and foot edema. Alcoholic hepatitis is a precurser of cirrhosis; 8% of alcoholics develop irreversible cirrhosis with progression from mild liver damage to liver failure. With progressive liver damage, there is protein, carbohydrate, and vitamin metabolism defects, bleeding tendencies, and severe jaundice. Dilation of veins, secondary to malfunctioning liver, leads to esophageal varices, hemorrhoids, and ascites. Secondary sex characteristics develop in the male when liver unable to destroy the female hormones he produces.

HEMATOLOGICAL abnormalities numerous. Production of red and white blood cells affected, leading to anemia and increased risk of infections. Platelets destroyed; lack of vitamin K production because of gastrointestinal changes causes bleeding tendencies. Alteration in bone marrow function leads to increased bruising and decreased clotting time.

FIGURE 14-2 The effect of alcohol on major tissues and body organs.

Alcoholic Intoxication

Alcoholic intoxication is exhibited by varying degrees of exhilaration, excitement, loss of self-control, behavior changes, speech pattern changes, lack of coordination, irritability, drowsiness, and in advanced cases, stupor and coma. Coma due to alcoholic intoxication is a medical emergency because of the danger of respiratory suppression. Symptoms include subnormal body temperature, decreased respiratory rate, stertorous breathing, weakened pulse, contraction or dilation of pupils, decreased or absent reflexes, pale or cyanotic skin, and possible incontinence or retention of urine (65).

Alcohol Withdrawal Syndrome

Although alcohol is a depressant, its rebound or aftereffects are that of an irritant and can result in Alcohol Withdrawal Syndrome. If you have ever had a hangover, you may recall how jumpy, irritable, and edgy you felt. The irritation effect outlasts the sedative effect of alcohol. Chronic alcohol use can lead to physical dependence and addiction, which is marked by the development of tolerance and withdrawal symptoms (34, 65). A person with a physical addiction who has had a sustained period of chronic intoxication will have withdrawal symptoms whenever the intake of alcohol is abruptly stopped or sharply reduced. This can include the binge drinker as well as the daily drinker. Some withdrawal symptoms are direct effects of depriving the dependent nervous system of alcohol; others are indirect effects of the nutritional disturbances that affect the brain.

The withdrawal syndrome is comprised of four major manifestations: (1) tremulousness, (2) hallucinosis, (3) convulsive seizures, and (4) delirium tremens. Each of these manifestations may occur separately from the others or in various combinations, but for the sake of clarity, they will be discussed individually below.

Tremulousness

Tremulousness is the most common manifestation of alcohol withdrawal. Tremors, also known as "the shakes" or "the jitters," occur within the first 24 to 48 hours and can range from mild to severe. The client may complain of feeling shaky inside, or visible tremors may be so severe that speaking is difficult or the person must have assis-

tance to hold a glass of water. The person may be easily startled, irritable, and unpleasant. Often there is a fast pulse, sweating, dilated pupils, and a flushed face. Complaints of nausea and vomiting or of disturbed sleep or insomnia are also common. Memory for recent events may be poor, but there is no serious confusion. The client is aware of his/her surroundings and the nature of the illness (65).

If withdrawal symptoms do not progress further, the tremors will subside in two or three days; peak intensity is 24 to 36 hours after drinking stops. However, discomfort, irritability, and sleep difficulties can persist for two or three weeks or longer (34).

Hallucinosis

Hallucinosis refers to symptoms of disordered perception and hallucinations that occur in about one-fourth of those suffering withdrawal from alcohol. In disordered perception, sounds and shadows may be misinterpreted, or familiar objects may be distorted and assume unreal forms. Bad dreams or nightmares are common and are associated with disturbed sleep patterns. Hallucinations are auditory, visual, or tactile, and may occur separately or in combination with each other. Auditory hallucinations are often sounds such as buzzing, ringing, or clicking; they may be in the form of voices, which may be pleasant or threatening and disturbing. Visual hallucinations are often of people, animals, or insects, and can be very hideous and frightening. Tactile hallucinations are frequently of insects, especially spiders crawling on the body. The hallucinations occur even in persons who are lucid, oriented, and have an intact memory. The sounds, voices, visions, or tactile sensations are real and vivid. The person cannot separate the illusion from reality. For example, the police may be called to provide protection from "intruders" who are threatening harm. Suicide may be attempted to avoid what the voices threaten. Only when improvement in condition occurs is the person able to begin to doubt the hallucinations. He/she usually remembers the experience clearly but may be reluctant to talk about it since it seems so unusual.

Convulsive seizures

Convulsive seizures, also known as "rum fits," may occur within 7 to 48 hours or longer after alcohol intake is markedly lowered or discontinued;

they can occur up to one week after the last drink. The seizures are grand mal in type, involving major generalized convulsions with loss of consciousness. Usually only one or two seizures occur, although there may be more. Occasionally the person develops status epilepticus, a severe and continuous type of convulsion with many potential complications. One-third of the clients with seizures develop delirium tremens.

Delirium tremens

Delirium tremens (DTs) are characterized by profound confusion, delusions, vivid hallucinations, tremor, agitation, sleeplessness, dilated pupils, fever, tachycardia, and profuse perspiration. Someone who develops the DTs will also have had all the symptoms described for tremulousness. Instead of clearing by the second or third day, the symptoms continue and get worse. The hallucinations and delusions are usually terrifying. The episode generally ends after several days of wakefulness and relentless activity, when the client falls into a deep sleep. On awakening, the client is lucid and there is rarely any memory of the events of the delirious period. The period lasts for up to 72 hours for 80 percent of those who experience it in a single episode. For others, relapses can occur. Delirium tremens are a medical emergency; even with treatment there is a 20 percent fatality rate (65).

Wernicke/Korsakoff Syndrome

Wernicke/Korsakoff Syndrome is a nutritional disease of the nervous system found in alcoholics, caused primarily by the deficiency of thiamine and niacin as a result of alcohol intake. The Syndrome is characterized by significant cerebral deterioration and actual brain cell death with chronic, permanent impairment. Korsakoff's Syndrome is characterized by progressive memory loss, disorientation, confabulation, and an outward appearance of cheerfulness. With Wernicke's Syndrome, the person is emotionally labile, moody, apathetic, weak, and easily fatigued (29, 65).

Progression of Alcoholism

Jellinek assigns a definite pattern to the appearance and progression of the symptoms of alcoholism in terms of increasing dysfunction as a person moves through the stages of psychologic dependence and physical addiction. The four phases are the prealcoholic, prodromal, crucial, and chronic (35). Although there are signposts that mark the progression of the illness, great variance occurs from person to person. For example, the amount of time required can vary dramatically; what may be a process of years for one person may take only months for another. Also sometimes it is difficult to determine where one phase ends and another begins and some symptoms may occur in a random order.

A case-study description of progression of the alcoholic during each phase and a description of what is occurring to those persons who are closely associated with the alcoholic is presented. This case study has also been used to clarify the progression of the illness as the person, called "Jennie" remembers it occurring in her life (73).

Prealcoholic Phase

In the prealcoholic phase, the person's drinking occurs in social situations. With the discovery that alcohol provides psychological relief and a pleasant, often euphoric feeling, more such experiences are sought out, and the choice of friends and activities becomes dominated by whether or not alcohol will be involved. There is discomfort if alcohol is not available. More and more, alcohol is used for relief and becomes a primary means of coping with stress and insecurity. An *increase in tolerance* to alcohol begins to develop. Often a person drinks rapidly to hasten the euphoric feelings or swallows a few drinks prior to an activity to "loosen up" (34).

Those closely associated with the alcoholic are beginning to feel that the emphasis on, frequency, and amount of drinking are extreme but decline to say so, or they rationalize and find excuses for the drinking. Later this may give way to nagging and making attempts to manage or control the person's drinking (55).

Prealcoholic Phase.   Aside from being given sips from my parents' drinks and sneaking into our parent's supply with my friends for a few gulps and a few grins, my memories of drinking pretty much begin when I was in high school. My mother made an effort to teach me about alcohol. We would sit and have one or two beers; she believed it was important for me to experience the effects of alcohol and to learn my limits. I continued with my "alcohol education" at high-school parties. I found that when I drank, I'd get high but would be the one who could drive others home — I could hold it pretty well! I liked the way it changed me. Usually I was real quiet, but when I drank, I wasn't quiet anymore. That was when I first started to like it. My friends would say, "Oh, man, you're not usually like this!" They really enjoyed me and I felt really well liked. I was known as a person who enjoyed a party, who knew where to get the alcohol and who could hold it. The guy I dated drank and when we went out on the weekend, there would always be alcohol; we just never considered doing anything that didn't involve alcohol. All my friends drank; if you didn't drink you were weird. Sometimes I would sneak a quick gulp at home from my parent's supply so I could loosen up before a party.

I only remember being drunk once. One night my boyfriend and I were driving around and there was some beer; I just kept drinking one right after the other and didn't feel how drunk I was getting. I kept drinking until I passed out. The next thing I knew, I was sitting in the shower. Boy, was I embarrassed. My parents laughed when I got home. It was a big joke at the time. [73]

Prodromal Phase

Movement into the prodromal phase is often marked by the occurrence of blackouts. Blackouts are often confused or used synonymously with passing out. A *blackout*, however, *is an episode where a person has continued to engage in or function in conversations or activities but is unable to remember the occurrence,* or perhaps remembers only bits and pieces. The information is usually never available to the person, although on occasion memory has returned during a subsequent drunken episode. In this phase, alcohol goes from being just a beverage to becoming a need in the person's life; drinking becomes serious business. Sneaking extra drinks is common, as is bolstering oneself with a few drinks before entering a social drinking situation. The person is beginning to experience some guilt and uneasiness, which leads to a loss of self-esteem. Promises to alter behavior are made, and lies are told to oneself and others about the drinking. Drinking is not seen as being responsible for the decreasing discomfort. Denial increases, and detailed explanations are given for drinking (34).

Those closely associated with the alcoholic begin to feel embarrassed or humiliated by the person's behavior and are confused about what is happening. They question if they are to blame for the difficulties and the drinking. More efforts are made to pressure the person to drink less; denial is used to hide the problem (55).

Prodromal Phase. I was accepted into college following my junior year at high school. My goal was to be a dentist, so I knew I had to make good grades, but other than that, there were no controls. My parents were in another state.

I continued to drink to get a buzz on and to feel different. I didn't really like myself too much; I didn't like the way I was when I wasn't drinking. I was also drinking once in awhile during the week but I had to be careful so it didn't affect my grades. By this time, I had graduated from beer to hard stuff — cherry vodka! I was gradually drinking more and kept a bottle in my room. Taking a belt or two before a party was routine, as I was getting drunk without realizing I was getting drunk.

By the beginning of the second semester, I was becoming more self-conscious of my drinking. I would get drunk and really down and out. I started drinking alone on the weekend if I wasn't going out and also during the week if I didn't have any difficult class the next day. Drinking by myself was kind of strange and would really get me down at times. I didn't feel adequate in many ways, even though I did make good grades. There was a point I really got down. I was very drunk and made a stupid attempt at slitting my wrists with a dull steak knife. It wasn't at all effective and I think I was trying to get attention. I didn't know what I wanted to do. Somebody, help me please. I was embarrassed about this later. Two of my friends noticed my wrists and asked what had happened. I told them the truth and I remember them looking at me kind of puzzled and asking why I would do such a thing.

My drinking to drunkenness has gotten progressively more frequent. I had my first blackout and it scared the shit out of me. I was talking long distance to my boyfriend one night and woke up six hours later sitting on the floor in the hallway of the dorm holding the phone. I could remember the conversation to a point but then nothing. Had I passed out? I made a telephone call to my boyfriend and found out that we'd had a long conversation which I couldn't remember and which had ended because he couldn't make any sense out of what I was saying. I was angry with my roommate for leaving me in the hall all night, and I was afraid of what I might have said on the phone. It was scary. I thought, "Maybe something is wrong with me."

A month later, I bought some books on alcoholism, mostly, I think, because I was curious, but I was also remembering a comment my mother had jokingly made to me when I'd left for school. She'd said, "You'd better keep an eye on your drinking; you may become an alcoholic." The books scared me because they talked about some of the things that I was experiencing. But, I told myself that someone my age (eighteen) could never be an alcoholic because it took fifteen or twenty years of drinking. So even though the description fit, this couldn't really be what was happening to me. I hid those books in a trunk in my closet never to be read again (73).

Crucial Phase

In the crucial phase, the person feels increasingly self-conscious, guilty, confused, and angry; self-esteem is very low. Denial is used to fend off much of the discomfort and to keep a lid on the awareness that is ever-threatening within. Rationalizations, alibis, and isolation are also used. Reality is increasingly distorted. Often employment, marital, or geographical changes are made in an effort to bring life back into order. Personality changes are increasing. Irritability, resentfulness, aggressiveness, irresponsibility, nervousness, and depression are some of the more common changes. Other people are seen as avoiding, blaming, and being unfair. Morning drinking or having an "eye-opener" is often necessary to relieve the unpleasantness of a hangover and to "begin the day." *Loss of control,* which is a cardinal symptom of alcoholism, begins to occur. Loss of control means that the person loses the ability to predict how much alcohol will be consumed. The person can control taking the first drink, but once the drink is taken, he/she is no longer in control. Often the person changes the pattern of drinking or goes "on the wagon" (abstains) to prove that alcoholism is not the problem, but after the first drink, the bottle regains control. Previous levels of drinking will be reestablished either the day drinking was resumed or within a short period of time (34).

Those close to the alcoholic also increasingly distort reality through denial, rationalization, and minimization. Covering-up continues by attempting to correct the damage, overprotecting, or assuming responsibility for the alcoholic's inappropriate behavior. Extreme measures are taken as a means to pressure the person to drink less. Often the actions extend from one end of the continuum to the other. One night might be spent dumping all the alcohol in the house down the drain and then the next night purchasing and consuming alcohol until drunkenness occurs in an effort to show the alcoholic how obnoxious the behavior becomes. The family still feels that perhaps they themselves are to blame for driving the other person to drink; often their own self-worth and sanity are questioned. Living becomes increasingly centered around the alcoholic person and drinking. Feelings of insecurity, fear, and anxiety increase and often lead to headaches, ulcers, nervousness, apathy, withdrawal, overinvolvement in outside activities, or possibly an attempt to obtain a divorce or get professional help (55).

Crucial Phase

I was starting to become more self-conscious of how much I was drinking. I could see that my drinking wasn't like others. I was getting a reputation for being someone who liked to party and I was known as the person who would always go for a drink or two. It wasn't the same as in high school. The "Yeh, she kinda likes the booze" comments weren't positive and complimentary anymore. Others were seeing me as different and that didn't make me feel good. Still, no one said I had a drinking problem.

My blackouts were becoming more frequent. I kept a log and often would find things written there that I didn't remember writing. This became less upsetting to me as I got used to it. I would try filling in the gaps by asking others, "How did I get home? What happened last night?" Sometimes I found out that I had fallen down a flight of stairs, and occasionally someone would offer me some advice to cut down.

I began looking for reasons to excuse my drinking, such as my unhappiness at school and my confusion about what I wanted to do with my life. I also tried to cut down on what I was drinking so I wouldn't be so embarrassed. I would resolve not to drink so much or not to get drunk, but I would. I couldn't control not getting drunk.

I began staying in on Saturday nights and drinking by myself. My drinking through the week was also increasing. I would tell myself that I could study better if I were more relaxed or that with a few drinks I could increase my creativity and write better. I was drinking about three fifths of vodka a week; cherry vodka had long ago been abandoned for the regular stuff. One of my roommates told me that I was drinking to much, but I didn't agree nor did I respect her opinion.

During my sophomore year at college, I pulled away from others more and more. Covering up from my roommates meant hiding all the empty bottles and watching for the trash man. When we'd go out, I'd have a strong one before going; but, usually, I didn't join in on outings. I didn't want anyone to know how much I was drinking. I kept feeling worse about myself. I still didn't admit it was my drinking; it was because as an all-around person I just didn't feel I was worth much. Even drinking I felt inadequate. Alcohol wasn't taking this feeling away; it was no longer giving me the euphoria it used to. I would drink to hit that high but would overshoot it into drunkenness or passing out.

The summer following my sophomore year I enrolled in summer school to take chemistry. When I didn't pull my usual A on the first test, I got fed up and dropped the course. I began to feel that I was going to school to satisfy my father rather than myself. So, instead of resuming my goal to be a dentist, I enrolled at a college at home with physical education as my major. My parents became aware that I had been partying more than they had thought, but I had maintained my grades. And I was so young; my mom thought I was going through a phase and didn't know what I wanted to do; that became my identified problem.

My grades began to drop. I told myself it was because I really didn't care for what I was doing. I began drinking before class or would skip morning class and then go to afternoon classes with a soda laced with vodka. I remember thinking this was a riot. I had two incompletes that semester.

I decided to quit school and got a job as a waitress. Even though I wasn't of age, I had a free supply available to me from the restaurant's bar. Initially, I was fairly responsible, but after I learned the ins and outs, I loosened up and took advantage of the situation. The turnover of managers was so great that by the time one would begin to realize that too much alcohol was missing, he would leave and a new one would start.

By summer, I wasn't remembering driving home most nights. Frequently I wouldn't even make it to my room and my parents would find me sprawled somewhere in the house. There were times when I had even been incontinent during the night. My parents were getting worried and would threaten to admit me for psychiatric treatment if I did it one more time. Of course, I did it several more times and they threatened several more times, but I was never admitted.

Other than work, I was almost always by myself now. I slept until it was time to go to work and would drink a double shot while driving there to get rid of my blah feeling and to get me ready for work. I was feeling worse and worse about me; in the back of my mind I knew I had a problem but denied it vehemently and angrily to my parents. I still tried to tell myself that I was too young to be an alcoholic and

that when I decided what I wanted to do with my life, I wouldn't need alcohol anymore.

By August of that year, my parents had contacted an alcohol treatment center and had made arrangements for admission. My mother had taken a course on alcoholism and now knew more about the problem. I was beginning to admit there was a problem; things weren't getting any better and I was causing a lot of problems. I also wanted them off my back; maybe the "pros" would say my problem wasn't alcohol anyway. Maybe it was as my parents had said; it was just a phase I was going through until I knew what I wanted to do.

On the day I was to go to the hospital, I was frightened and angry. I didn't know what to expect and didn't really believe I belonged there. I surely didn't want to be an alcoholic. I arrived at the treatment center drunk (73).

Chronic Phase

In the chronic phase, the alcoholic is drinking earlier in the day to relieve the withdrawal discomfort that is being experienced after a night's sleep. The person awakens "shaky." The first drink must be obtained with no delay; the bottle is kept by the bedside. The person is existing in an intoxicated state all day long, every day as long as money can be obtained to buy a bottle. Prolonged binges or weekend bouts are most frequent. Extreme fears and hallucinations may be experienced. The primary motivation is to keep the supply of alcohol coming. The alcoholic avoids contact with others, isolates self, or chooses to associate with those who are in a similar condition. Functioning is on the fringes of society. Deterioration has occurred in all areas: physical, spiritual, emotional, and social. Eventually the person's tolerance for alcohol drops and a few drinks will bring on a stuporous state. The final outcome, if the person continues to deteriorate, is brain damage, alcoholic psychosis, or death (34).

For those closely associated with the alcoholic person, the feelings of insecurity, fear, and anxiety have led them to take extreme measures, some of the more common actions are to: (1) leave the alcoholic and avoid any further contact, (2) develop a life style that is very demanding and rigid and allows them to function in the same setting but with extreme isolation from the alcoholic, (3) retaliate by having affairs or neglecting the family, or (4) develop severe physical or psychological problems themselves (55).

ASSESSMENT FOR ALCOHOLISM

You will encounter the alcoholic person in a variety of settings. Assessing for alcoholism is not an easy task. The nursing assessment must include physical status, emotional status, and the socioeconomic circumstances the client is presently living in or will be returning to upon discharge.

Barriers to effective assessment are found within our own belief and value system. Alcoholism is not a disease that anyone wants to be diagnosed with or that you want to diagnose in someone else; it continues to be viewed by many as a sinful condition or as a sign of being weak-willed. To be an alcoholic is to be stigmatized. Diagnoses of gastritis, hepatitis, or peripheral neuropathy are preferable. Depression or marital, financial, legal, or employment difficulties are also preferable to being an alcoholic. Such attitudes contribute to clients being diagnosed with problems that are actually secondary to alcoholism, with the alcoholism not being diagnosed or treated at all. Another barrier is a commonly held value that a person's drinking habits are his own business. If you believe this, then inquiring into someone's drinking habits seems to be prying and intrusive, and you opt not to obtain this information. Further, use of alcohol is accepted, socially and legally, in our society. You may value this drug as an appropriate way to relax, celebrate, socialize, or pass the time; overindulgence once in awhile is considered all right. Finally, if you do suspect an alcohol problem in a client, you may feel you will be ineffective and that nothing can be done anyway. You may feel that this older person can be helped only if he/she wants to be, so why bother if help has not been asked for? If you wish to be effective in assisting the alcoholic client, you must be aware of your personal values that may interfere with the client's care.

Increase your effectiveness in assessment of alcoholism by keeping your definition of alcoholism loose and by building a good knowledge base of the disease, the phases of its progression, and the faces it presents. The person who is admitted to the agency with an illness closely associated with alcohol, such as peptic ulcer, hepatitis, pancreatitis, cardiomyopathy, or neuropathy, may not exhibit symptoms of alcohol addiction but may still be an alcoholic. Alcohol intake is life-threatening to this person; yet he/she continues to drink. Use of alcohol by a person to cope with life's stresses to the point of atrophy or nondevelopment of other coping techniques means the person is psychologically dependent on alcohol and is an alcoholic. In addition to psychological dependence, a person may also exhibit physical dependence or addiction to alcohol. Remember, when alcohol is absent, the withdrawal syndrome previously described is experienced. Assessment should include a history of drinking patterns, other drug usage, family history, legal or employment problems, sobriety patterns, mental status, and prior treatment, both psychiatric and medical.

Obtaining an accurate history of drinking patterns is a routine part of assessment. Remember that your values, attitudes, and comfort level influence the person's feelings and have a bearing on interview reliability. Being nonjudgmental and objective are essential. If the client perceives that you are uncomfortable in asking questions about drinking, the answers may be contrived to please you. Or if the client perceives that you assume alcoholism is a problem his/her answers may be tailored to prove that alcoholism does not exist. The goal is to get a clear picture of alcohol usage and to ascertain whether or not it is a problem. Questions concerning alcohol usage asked along with questions related to general physical or mental health and past medical history will usually be accepted by the client as standard procedure. The person's status at the time of the interview influence how extensive a drinking history can be obtained. His/her responses will also determine how much exploration is necessary. If alcohol use is denied and you perceive no suggestion of inaccuracy, your assessment is finished.

What? How much? and When? are essential questions but answers may be difficult to get. If alcohol usage is present, identify type of alcohol and how much of each kind is consumed on any one occasion. In problem drinkers or alcoholics, a pattern of drinking is evident in terms of daily, weekend, or binge drinking; therefore, how often and in what way alcohol is used are important factors. Ascertain length of the drinking pattern to determine possible dependence and tolerance. Recent changes in alcohol use may also give additional information regarding life crises and adjustment problems.

Onset of problem drinking gives information about several aspects of alcoholism. Does the client perceive his/her drinking as being different from that of others or as causing any problems? If so, in what way and for how long? These questions give some indication of the client's awareness of the problem and willingness to seek help.

If the client or family member indicates that there may be some problem with alcohol, or if you perceive a problem based on interview information or from observing the client, proceed with obtaining more information, as noted below.

Ask about withdrawal symptoms. Ascertain what reactions the person has experienced in the past while drinking or when alcohol intake has been decreased or stopped. This information is significant for determining the stage of illness, the absence or presence of addiction, and the probability of the client experiencing withdrawal problems during the current treatment period. Define your terms and pose questions clearly. The following list of questions could serve as an example.

1. Has there been an experience of *tremors*—being jittery or having the shakes?

2. Have there been *blackouts*—times when it has been impossible to remember getting home, where one had been, or what the conversation had been? Has there been the experience of finding out about a conversation or argument that was not remembered?

3. Have there ever been *seizures* (convulsions/fits)? The client should describe this, as seizures are often confused with the shakes or with passing out.

4. Has there been an experience when sounds or voices were heard that did not make sense or when there was no one or nothing there that could have made the sound or produced the voice (*auditory hallucination*)?

5. Was there an experience when something or someone was seen that others could not see or that later was proven not to have been there (*visual hallucination*)?

6. Has there ever been a time when it felt like there was something crawling on the skin, such as spiders or spider webs that could not be removed (*tactile hallucination*)?

7. Was there ever an experience when you firmly believed something to be fact when others did not, and then found out they were right (*delusion*)?

If the client's responses are positive to *auditory, visual,* or *tactile hallucinations,* or *delusion,* obtain

a description of the experience: What was it like? How did the person feel? How often has this occurred? Did it occur during intoxication or while sober?

Recent drinking history is also important to obtain. When was the client's last drink and what has been the daily intake of alcohol for the past five days? Has there been a recent reduction in the amount of alcohol used?

Other drug usage is pertinent information that is often overlooked. Is the client using other drugs or has there been a history of other drug usage? Of special interest is use of other mood-altering drugs such as marijuana, or addictive substances such as minor tranquilizers or opiates. Poly-drug abuse is a growing problem in our society, and use of other drugs can influence the treatment regime as well as retard recovery.

Family history will help you determine present support systems and who is significant to the client. What is the client's marital status and for how long? Are there children in the family? How many? Age? Has there been separation or divorce in the past? Is there currently disruption in the family? Is there an interest in family involvement in treatment? Who does the client consider to be helpful or supportive?

Legal problems associated with drinking should be explored. Often the nurse is hesitant to explore this area because of the double stigma—alcoholism and arrest. Driving while intoxicated or charges of drunk and disorderly conduct or assault can substantiate the identification of a drinking problem.

Employment problems such as frequent job changes or lack of employment may indicate an alcohol problem. If the client is employed, are there any problems at work? Have there been frequent absences? The job situation is often the last area to be affected by alcoholism, so steady employment for a number of years is not unusual with the alcoholic client.

Periods of sobriety should be determined. Has the client ever had a period of **sobriety**—*abstinence from alcohol for a period of time?* When? For how long?

Prior treatment for alcoholism should be determined. Has the client ever been treated for an alcohol problem before? Attended Alcoholics Anonymous? If so, when, and what was the experience like?

Asking about *past medical and psychiatric*

treatment may be a way to lead to questions about coexistent psychiatric disorders and current mental status. Depression and suicidal rates are often associated with alcoholism. Questions starting with past history and working up to the present physical and mental status are often less threatening. In this way you are more likely to gain accurate information.

Emergency assessment is done if the client's status is such that an extensive interview is prohibited. Ascertain how much alcohol has been drunk, for how long, when the last drink was taken, any physical problems present, and what reactions have occurred when drinking was stopped in the past. Also, determine if any other drugs are being taken. Make sure the assessment is completed when the client's status permits.

Table 14-1 is a suggested assessment form to be used as part of an emergency room or admission assessment. The most essential questions are indicated.

TABLE 14-1. Summary of Assessment of the Alcoholic

1. Do you drink alcoholic beverages?
2. How often do you drink?
3. What kind of alcohol do you drink?
4. How much of each kind do you drink?
5. How long have you been drinking this amount this often?
6. How is your drinking different from what it used to be?
7. Has drinking been causing you problems? What kind?
8. Have you ever experienced blackouts? For how long? How often?
*9. Have you ever had tremors? When and for how long?
*10. Have you ever had seizures? Describe.
*11. Have you ever had hallucinations (auditory, visual, tactile)? What was the experience like? How often has this occurred? Were you drinking or had you stopped or cut down?
*12. Have you ever had DTs? Describe.
*13. When was your last drink? Amount?
*14. What has been your daily intake of alcohol for the past five years?
*15. Has there been any recent change in your drinking habits in terms of frequency or amount?
*16. Are you currently taking any prescribed or unprescribed drugs? Amount? Frequency?
17. Do you have a history of past drug usage? Describe.
18. What is your marital status and for how long? Who do you live with? Do you have children? Has anyone close to you felt you had a problem with alcohol? Explain.
19. Have you ever had a DWI (driving while intoxicated)? How many? When? Have you had any other arrests? When and for what?
20. Are you employed? (If unemployed, for how long?) Have you been having any problems at work?
21. Have you ever had a period of sobriety? When and for how long?
22. Have you had previous treatment for drinking?
23. Have you ever attended Alcoholics Anonymous?
24. Have you had past medical or psychiatric help? Describe.
25. Do you currently have any medical or emotional problems? (Assess current mental status including suicidal potential.)

*Emergency assessment.

FORMULATION OF NURSING DIAGNOSES

The nursing diagnosis of *alcohol usage out of control* is made when the person manifests the physical effects of excessive alcohol intake; signs of alcohol intoxication; the alcohol withdrawal syndrome with tremulousness, hallucinosis, convulsive seizures, and delirium tremens; or Wernicke/Korsakoff Syndrome. The duration of excessive alcohol usage will be demonstrated by signs and symptoms and by a history of the prealcoholic, prodromal, crucial, or chronic phases.

Nursing diagnoses for the inebriated alcoholic in an emergency room or for the client in a detoxification center in acute alcohol withdrawal includes physiological disorders or physical disease. There may be evidence of physical injury, such as broken bones, bruises, or head trauma. The possibility of seizures must always be considered. Dehydration, overhydration, or poor nutritional status may be a problem. Vital signs may be dangerously elevated.

Nursing diagnoses may include altered emotional status; fear and agitation may be present. A nursing diagnosis of "cognitive disturbance" is made if the client is disoriented, delusioned, or hallucinating and having nightmares that cannot be separated from reality. Other nursing diagnoses may relate to the family. If the children or spouse accompany the alcoholic, there may be signs that they have been beaten and are fearful, ashamed, confused, and in need of counseling on how to either live with or leave the alcoholic person.

Your nursing diagnoses must reflect the physical, emotional, cognitive, and social needs of the client and family, but priority diagnoses must first be made based on the client's and family's most immediate problems.

NURSING INTERVENTIONS RELATED TO CLIENT-CARE GOALS DURING THE ACUTE PHASE

Principles of care during alcohol withdrawal include early detection of alcohol addiction, establishing the probability of withdrawal symptoms, and initiating treatment before the client is in a state of impending delirium tremens (DTs). The episode can be prevented even though the client previously has had a history of seizures, hallucinations, and DTs. Physical and psychological support during alcohol withdrawal are necessary so that the client returns to a stable health state.

The alcohol in the system is replaced with a drug. Librium is often used with vitamins (especially thiamine), so that the nervous system does not react with a rebound effect as alcohol content is reduced. Then the withdrawal of the drug from the system is monitored in the transition from physical dependence on a drug to becoming drug-free. Various dosages are used, but whatever level is begun with is slowly reduced. Any abrupt stoppage of the drug can initiate with withdrawal syndrome since drug omission represents an insult to a nervous system that is drug-dependent.

Detoxification is usually conducted in an inpatient setting, although it may also be done safely on an outpatient basis if the client is experiencing only mild-to-moderate withdrawal symptoms. The nonhospitalized client must be supervised daily. The client and family must be given specific instructions regarding what medication to take and the need for abstinence from alcohol. Usually detoxification can be accomplished in seven days. You are then dealing with a person who may have sleeping and eating difficulties and irritability. Alcohol interferes with REM (rapid eye movement) sleep, and reduced REM sleep results in impaired concentration, anxiety fatigue, irritability, and nightmares (67). During detoxification, no drugs containing alcohol should be prescribed or administered, including elixers, cough syrups, and mouth wash. Hair tonic also needs to be considered. The alcohol content of some hair tonics is high enough that the person may drink it instead of putting it on the hair, as the craving for alcohol during this time is often very strong.

Nursing care goals during alcohol withdrawal are as follows:

1. Promote adequate food intake to restore nutritional balance.

2. Promote and maintain adequate fluid and electrolyte balance.

3. Promote safety and protection of the client who is disoriented and impulsive.

4. Decrease anxiety and promote comfort, relaxation, and orientation to reality.

5. Promote restful sleep.

6. Prevent seizures and decrease agitation.

7. Stabilize vital signs and overall physical condition. (Fluctuating vital signs can indicate increased agitation or complications.)

Nursing interventions related to each of the above goals are listed in Table 14-2.

TABLE 14-2.   Care Plan for the Alcoholic Client

NURSING GOALS	CLIENT-CARE GOALS	NURSING INTERVENTIONS
Goal 1: Promote adequate food intake to restore nutritional balance.	Demonstrates increased appetite and food intake, weight gain, and coordination. Craving for alcohol reduced.	1. Provide high-protein, high-vitamin diet. 2. Promote pleasant mealtime environment. 3. Assist tremulous client with eating. 4. Provide frequent small feedings that are attractive, on time, and compatible with client's preferences. 5. Encourage mouth care, other hygienic care, and grooming as aids to increase appetite and food intake. 6. Provide alternative beverages and snacks to substitute for need for drinking. 7. Provide sweet, fast-energy foods to help decrease physical craving for alcohol. 8. Observe client for effects of and caution against high caffeine intake (no coffee, tea, cola, or chocolate drinks). 9. Provide nutritional counseling to client and family if needed.
Goal 2: Promote and maintain adequate fluid and electrolyte balance.	Demonstrates increasingly taut skin turgor, normal urine pH, and nearer normal blood electrolyte values.	1. Determine level of hydration from skin condition and urine pH and quantity. 2. Determine reason for abnormal hydration status: a. Overhydration from consuming large amounts of liquor and/or the effect of alcohol on anti-diuretic hormone (ADH). b. Dehydration from vomiting and diarrhea. 3. Record intake and output and weight for several days. 4. Offer fluids frequently. 5. If forcing fluids, have variety of flavored fluids available. 6. Administer medications for vomiting and diarrhea, if present.
Goal 3: Promote safety	Is oriented for person, place,	1. Observe for symptoms of injury sustained prior to admission such as from falls, fights,

TABLE 14-2. Continued

NURSING GOALS	CLIENT-CARE GOALS	NURSING INTERVENTIONS
and protection of the client who is disoriented and impulsive.	time. Shows no evidence of injury or elopement.	or self-injury, and give treatment as indicated.
		2. Encourage expression of feelings; give information as indicated.
		3. Provide close observation or constant supervision if necessary to prevent self-injury or client attempting to leave unit.
		4. Provide orientation to surroundings in quiet, caring manner; do not whisper to avoid misinterpretation.
		5. Provide safety measures, such as padded side rails, if needed.
		6. Remove hazardous articles. (A high correlation between alcohol and suicide exists.)
		7. Assist with ambulation; remove hazardous or excessive furnishings.
		8. Avoid use of physical restraints if possible.
		9. If client is being withdrawn from alcohol as an out-patient, prepare client and family for withdrawal symptoms that may occur and instruct them to go to nearest emergency room at any sign of unusual reaction or complication.
Goal 4: Decrease anxiety and promote comfort, relaxation, and orientation to reality.	Demonstrates increasing physical relaxation and decreasing anxiety level.	1. Be present with the client as behavior indicates; be calm, empathic, and pleasant.
		2. Encourage expression of feelings verbally and through appropriate activity.
		3. Keep light on in client's room; shadows and reflections may distort perceptions and increase fears.
		4. Reorient client to surroundings as needed.
		5. Provide quiet environment. Decrease environmental stimuli such as television, radio, and stereo.
		6. Do not support hallucinations or illusions by asking a lot of questions about them.
Goal 5: Promote restful sleep.	Sleeps without disturbance during the night. States feels rested.	1. Provide for periods of uninterrupted sleep; reduce extraneous noises and adjust room temperature.
		2. Give back rub or utilize physical and emotional techniques described in Chapter 12.
		3. A warm, nonalcoholic, noncaffeine drink before sleep may promote relaxation.
		4. Use a hypnotic only as a last resort.

TABLE 14-2.   Continued

NURSING GOALS	CLIENT-CARE GOALS	NURSING INTERVENTIONS
Goal 6: Prevent seizures and decrease agitation.	Demonstrates no seizures or agitated behavior.	1. Provide calm, supportive, quiet environment. 2. Provide adequate sedation without over-medication. 3. Have padded tongue blade taped to head of bed and others easily accessible on unit if client has history of seizures or is very tremulous. (Padded tongue blade should be used only when it can be easily inserted, so that there is no damage to teeth, mouth tissue, or to the jaw.)
Goal 7: Stabilize vital and overall physical condition.	Manifests increasingly normal vital signs and other signs of improved health status.	1. Take and record blood pressure, temperature, pulse, and respirations as indicated. 2. Conduct neurological checks upon admission and as indicated. 3. Provide measures to normalize vital signs (i.e., fluids for increased temperature and quiet environment for elevated pulse and blood pressure). 4. Check for signs of injury. 5. Prevent stasis of secretions by having client turn, cough, breathe deeply, and sit up; have client ambulate when possible. 6. Monitor bowel and bladder function.

NURSING INTERVENTIONS RELATED TO CLIENT-CARE GOALS DURING THE RECOVERY PHASE

Detoxification from alcohol is only the beginning of treatment, not the end. When the client has been restored to a stable physiological state, learning must occur in terms of life management without drinking. This is a major long-term and lifelong goal. Helping the person learn to live without alcohol is not something done one time. Sobriety is maintained on a day-to-day basis and is dependent on the client's ability to recognize and change those living patterns that trigger drinking behavior.

The overall, long-term goal is to help the person live a full life and be a fully functioning member of society without the use of alcohol. Specific goals include the following:

1. Client identifies the drinking problem.

2. Client identifies changes in living patterns that are necessary.

3. Client explores the alternatives to drinking.

4. Client makes efforts at change, using support of nurses and other personnel.

5. Client assumes responsibility for self and develops interdependence with others.

6. Client states increased feelings of self-worth.

7. Client develops or redevelops a support system of family, employer, and nonalcoholic friends.

You will be actively involved in carrying out these goals throughout the phases of recovery. Nursing and medical interventions are designed to introduce the client to a sober, drug-free existence. The philosophical goal of most treatment facilities, including Alcoholics Anonymous, is total abstinence. There is no universal mode of treatment for the alcoholic: individual, group, education, and family therapies, assertiveness training, relaxation techniques, stress management, and meditation are some of the more common methods. Recovery is a process that can be broken into phases, although it is often difficult to know where one phase ends and another begins.

Phase I: Preliminary or Introductory Phase of Recovery

Goal 1: Identifies the drinking problem.

Intervention

Assessment of the physical, emotional, and social status of the client, together with information obtained from the drinking history, should provide you with the pieces necessary to determine whether or not alcohol is a problem in the client's life. If your nursing diagnosis is that alcohol is a problem, your goals are to: (1) share with the client your impression of the problem, presenting in an accurate, nonjudgmental manner the factual data that you have used in making your diagnosis, (2) identify the drinking problem, and (3) explore the alternatives. Often the client has never put the problems together in an organized way and viewed them as emanating from one source — alcohol. Because of the client's distortion of reality and denial system, the problems have been used as excuses to drink rather than seen as symptoms of a disease.

Denial and dependence are two treatment issues that occur throughout the entire recovery process. Denial of alcoholism and of the problems related to it is one of the most difficult defenses to deal with. Operating on an unconscious level, the defense mechanism of denial saves the client from the painful acknowledgment that he/she is sick, has feelings of inadequacy and low self-esteem, and is dependent on a drug. An elaborate system of rationalizations, falsifications, and alibis has developed. Because the alcoholic has become so adept at making excuses and alibis and manipulating others, the label of "con-artist" or the diagnosis of "character disorder" may be applied. Although there may be an underlying psychiatric illness that coexists with the drinking problem, it is also important to realize that you may be dealing with behaviors that have been well developed and are adaptive in the alcoholic's attempt to avoid or deny reality. Denial and its associated behaviors need to be dealt with objectively. Present your assessment with supporting evidence to the client. Avoid engaging in an argument; the alcoholic is extremely skilled at manipulation and debate. Your goal is to present the alcoholic with the facts as you see them. Your confrontation does not mean attack; it just means putting information together to assist a person in identifying a problem. This may be all you can do. It is the client's choice and responsibility to determine how much, if any, of the information will be used and when. Breaking through the denial system requires your openness, honesty, patience, and hope. Required also is the realization that denial is useful in preventing the person from being overwhelmed with anxiety. The nurse needs to assess what should be confronted and when. The client cannot face all the facts at one time. The client's skills for dealing with anxiety in other ways than by drinking need to be developed. In addition to assessing the client's readiness to accept those things that have been so strongly denied for such a long time, you must also assess when there is too much resistance and avoid any confrontations that only stiffen the denial.

Dependence is a frequently identified issue with the alcoholic person. Assess how much dependence is therapeutic and realize that the degree of dependence decreases as recovery is accomplished. The *long-term goal* is for the client to assume responsibility for self and to develop healthy interdependence with others, but this goal is accomplished through a series of *short-term goals* that slowly place responsibility for choices and behavior on the person. Initially, you may need to allow the client to be very dependent; you act as a guide and may need to give much assistance and support to the client. As the client progresses and has gained more awareness, effective adaptive behaviors, and problem-solving skills, your role becomes one of a resource person. To keep the relationship therapeutic requires constant assessment as to what responsibilities the client is able to assume. Too much independence and too much responsibility too fast can be overwhelming and herald relapse; too little can foster dependence and retard the client's growth.

Plant the seed of reality. You may feel that

the person will quit drinking when ready and not before. You are right in that the alcoholic must see the drinking as a problem and choose sobriety. Your goal is to place responsibility on the person for making an informed choice. You provide an opportunity for the alcoholic to look at the reality of the situation; you take the first step in breaking through the denial system of the alcoholic. Perhaps this is as far as the client will progress; there may be no readiness to take any additional steps. The response you get may be insulting and hostile. The progress you *have* made, however, is to plant the seed. Perhaps this is all you can do at this time. Many alcoholics come into treatment after having heard often from other health professionals that the presenting problems or symptoms were due to alcohol. The alcoholic starts to think that maybe there is something to what others are saying. That "maybe" is a big breakthrough; the seed is growing!

Timing is of great importance in confronting the alcoholic with the reality of the situation. The nurse in any setting has many valuable, well-timed opportunities to plant the seed or to nurture one that has been planted in the past. Often you have access to the sober alcoholic who is suffering physical or emotional pain, a pain that is directly related to drinking. In this case, the respectivity of the alcoholic is high. A solution to the pain is wanted. It is not important that the client admit to being an alcoholic nor that you put that label on the person. What is important at this point is that the physical or emotional pain is seen as being associated with drinking.

Referral is being introduced at this point of recovery because for many nurses there is little opportunity to go beyond the referral of the client to the other steps that are involved in treatment and recovery. Perhaps others before you have utilized opportunities to plant a seed, and your client expresses a desire to further explore the problem of alcoholism. Nurses in any areas need to be aware of the available resources in the community for the alcoholic. Where are public and private treatment programs located? What is the telephone number for Alcoholics Anonymous? Is there a branch of the National Council of Alcoholism in your area? If possible, find the client a resource who can be used to further explore the problem. You may even make the first telephone call. The client at this phase of recovery requires a great deal of guidance and direction. Provide an initial plan for the client to follow. This gives the person an option, and with a plan in hand, the responsibility to follow through. Although you may not be able to follow through with all the interventions for the alcoholic, through referral you can realize your goal of assisting the client to develop a support system.

Nurture the seed of reality. The recovery process starts when the client expresses a desire for help. Your goals for helping the client assume self-responsibility and increase self-esteem are pertinent here. The client has made the connection that alcohol is a problem. Often this connection is shaky and needs to be reinforced—through your encouragement, support, belief that change is possible, and restatement of reality in terms of how alcohol is at the core of the client's difficulties. Borrowing these supports from the nurse enables the person to believe and hope that recovery is possible, that the pain of being an alcoholic can stop.

The client does not need to be happy about choosing sobriety; in fact, the thought is usually quite depressing because it is an agreement to lose something that is very significant. Often the client's goal at this point is not sobriety but how to learn to drink socially again—how to regain control over alcohol.

The person entering treatment feels defensive, frightened, lost, guilty, alone, vulnerable, and very ambivalent. How can it be possible for this person to discontinue and walk away from the strongest attachment that he/she has ever made? Is it possible to leave such an influential friend, one that has had more importance than deteriorating health, family, employment, and financial difficulties? Alcohol has become for many the focus of existence. You might as well be asking for the client to agree to the amputation of both arms. For the alcoholic, life without alcohol is life without defenses, without being able to cope, without an escape from unendurable pain. Therefore, until the client's commitment to recovery strengthens, the client will be ambivalent; he/she will approach and avoid, will often reject help, and will possibly return to drinking.

For recovery to progress, it is essential that the connection between the client's problems and alcohol be strengthened from *within* the alcoholic. The "maybe there is a problem" becomes an acknowledgment in the client's heart that the problem is alcohol. This has been described as acceptance and as surrender; that is, the alcoholic admits defeat to alcohol. At this point the label of "alcoholic" is self-applied. Once the client has acknowledged being an alcoholic, the next phase of recovery begins.

The *nurse's role in the preliminary phase of recovery is one of being open, honest, patient, and nonjudgmental.* Provide reality when you see that the alcoholic's thinking in terms of alcohol is distorted. Provide hope that things can change. Provide the guidelines for change. Help the alcoholic to feel self-worth and dignity. Keep in mind that recovery takes time. Your patience, tolerance, understanding, and direction are essential for the client's recovery.

Phase II: Active Treatment Phase

Goal 2: Identifies necessary changes in living patterns.

Intervention

A *honeymoon period* often occurs with initial sobriety. The person at first believes that with cessation of drinking there will be no more problems. All the implications that alcoholism has on life are denied. Depending on how far the illness had progressed, alcohol has had a dramatic effect on the client's life style, personality, social life (family, friends), employment, and financial and physical status. Realistically, many alcoholics might be seen as Rip Van Winkles in that during their years of alcoholism their world has changed; those they love have changed; their own bodies have changed; aging has occurred. Many activities of daily living feel new or strange. The concept of time is being experienced anew, and there seems to be either too much of it or too little. The now sober mind is reawakening its ability to think and plan. Things sound, look, and taste different. There are choices to be made in terms of living through each day, choices that have not been made for a long time. Partial or total life reorientation and reconstruction are required. To many alcoholics, everything is beautiful; getting sober is seen as an end rather than as the beginning it really is (34).

Dry drunk is a phenomenon similar to the honeymoon period. The person has gotten sober, but the necessity for any further changes has been denied. The person "bites the bullet," so to speak, and attempts to exist with little means for adapting to life's pains and frustrations. The low self-esteem, irritability, isolation, and other emotional charac-

teristics of the active alcoholic remain. Those associated with this person frequently feel that drinking might as well have continued since the behaviors are still impossible and unpleasant to deal with.

Until acknowledgment (surrender, acceptance) is made by the alcoholic that further work is necessary, *the recovery cannot progress.* A return to drinking is often seen at this point of recovery. In the recovery process, it helps to know that resumption of drinking (relapses, slips) does not mean failure either for the client or for the nurse. These relapses only indicate that treatment has been insufficient and that more learning is needed.

The role of the nurse remains consistent. Although your goal at this point of recovery is to help the client to identify and acknowledge those other life changes that are necessary, you continue to provide support, encouragement, and hope. You continue to provide the reality of the situation in an open, honest, patient, and nonjudgmental manner. You assist in the identification of problems, the setting of priorities, the exploration of alternatives, and the making of plans. You are a guide who, because you are aware of the terrain, can provide directions as to how to proceed.

The *life changes* that are necessary *vary from client to client.* Recovery can be sought at any point during the progression of the illness. Not only do you need to assess the problems, but priorities must be set. In the beginning of recovery the alcoholic is without many healthy adaptive behaviors; alcohol has replaced these over the years. Stress management has been achieved through the use of alcohol. Self-confidence is low. It is essential that initially you assist the alcoholic with simplifying life and breaking it into manageable pieces. Much direction needs to be given. Each day of sobriety brings increased confidence and self-esteem as well as the development of unused or new adaptive behaviors for the client to rely on.

Education about the disease helps the alcoholic discover that many of the embarrassing, bizarre, and shameful behaviors that were experienced while drinking were actually symptoms of alcoholism. This is a relief; suddenly things make sense. All the crazy behavior is actually normal for a drinking alcoholic. This relevation does much to alleviate the tremendous guilt the alcoholic experiences, and self-esteem increases.

The recovering alcoholic is thirsty for knowledge and needs to be given the facts about alcohol, alcoholism, and the implications of being an alcoholic. Through education, new attitudes are instilled that help the client in the management of alcoholism.

> *Goal 3: Client explores the alternatives to drinking.*

> *Goal 4: Client makes efforts at change, using support of nurses and other personnel.*

Intervention

Finding alternatives to drinking behavior occurs by reaching back into the past and dusting off skills that have atrophied because of excessive reliance on drinking. New adaptive behaviors are learned through exploration and trial and error. Often new behaviors are blocked because what is being sensed, thought, felt, wanted, or done is not being reevaluated in terms of the present situation and goals.

Emotions in the past have usually been dealt with by repression or through acting out. The alcoholic needs to learn how to recognize emotions and how to deal appropriately with them. The client's belief that alcohol is needed to anticipate or get through anything stressful should be challenged, evaluated, and eventually replaced. Wants and desires must be analyzed, goals set, reality of goals determined, and goal achievement planned. Old habits or automatic reactions are still used. For example, going to a favorite liquor store to purchase some batteries needs to be evaluated in terms of what this action means. The alcoholic person needs assistance in recognizing and anticipating situations that will be stressful, and he/she needs help in planning alternative behaviors.

By increasing the client's awareness of what goes into the decisions that are made, you assist in the movement away from the repetition of old behaviors that lead to drinking, and move toward alternatives for living without drinking. The more alternatives of action the alcoholic is aware of, the greater the probability of making decisions that aid in the recovery process.

With each day of sobriety, the alcoholic has been gaining skills and confidence. There is now the ability to identify problems, explore alternatives, and identify possible outcomes of each alternative. The basic tools for living sober have been acquired. A shift occurs in the therapeutic relationship; you become a resource person rather than a guide.

Phase III: Continuing Treatment Phase

> *Goals 5: Client assumes responsibility for self and and develops interdependence with others.*

> *Goal 6: Client states increased feelings of self-worth.*

> *Goal 7: Client develops or redevelops a support system of family, employer, and nonalcoholic friends.*

Intervention

The final phase of recovery requires that the client maintain a *continuing* awareness, understanding, and monitoring of self. Those persons who are most successful in recovery accept the fact that alcoholism is a chronic illness and remain active in individual or group therapy with an alcoholic treatment facility or remain involved with Alcoholics Anonymous (AA). The maintenance phase of the nurse-client relationship described in Chapter 6 would be applicable to this client. With ongoing therapy, the client first develops interdependence with the therapist, then other staff members, and finally with family, work colleagues, and friends. The interdependence involves being helpful to others, such as being a buddy in AA, and being able to ask for and accept help from those interested in his/her recovery. As the period of sobriety lengthens, relations with others improve, and the person remains employed, sociable, and able to meet the hierarchy of needs. He/she increasingly feels self-respect, self-worth, and self-confidence.

The Recovery of Jennie. In my treatment and recovery process the first big milestone was acceptance. You *feel* a change in yourself and start acting different. My attitude changed; I wasn't negative anymore. It's not just getting off alcohol. That does make you feel better. It's also being able to say to yourself, "Hey, maybe I'll get better—there's a way out!" For me this elation lasted until my expectations that things were going to be different clashed with the fact that things weren't different. I just wasn't drinking. It kind of smacks you in the face.

Things were still really tense with my parents. I had a lot of resentments. I resented for a long time the fact that they had shoved me into treatment. I was grateful, but I was angry too. At home I could also sense their dilemma. They weren't sure how hard to push me in terms of getting a job or of starting to function normally again. How much pressure could they put on me? I left treatment with the intention of getting a job, but I didn't really want to. The thought of going back to school for three to four years wasn't too appealing either. Long-term things seemed to turn me off. As long as I thought in terms of years, I couldn't mobilize myself; it was just too much. My parents saw me as irresponsible and lazy.

It was the New Year's Eve explosion that somehow broke up the log jam, so to speak. My parents and I had this big fight, and I understood their position quite clearly. They were not going to watch me just sit around anymore. It was either get with it or get out. I got with it and followed through on something I'd been tossing around in my head, even in my waitress days. I applied to nursing school. I was accepted and that was another milestone for me. I started flowing again, I had a plan, I was starting to head somewhere, but, one day at a time.

To fill in my time before the semester started, I started doing volunteer work at the treatment center. That really helped; my friends were there and at AA. Since I surrounded myself with nondrinking people, I got a lot of experiences with having fun without alcohol.

I did contact one old friend and I was kind of worried how she would react to what I was doing and where I had been. I wasn't sure how to tell someone who knew me before that I was an alcoholic. What would the reaction be? She accepted it okay. That was neat! Sometimes I choose to tell people I'm on a diet, but I now know that friends don't really care what you're drinking.

It's been three years now since I was in treatment. I have reached many of my goals—becoming a nurse being one of them. There were many things that I had to really work on to change—like my relationship with my parents. I am still attending weekly AA meetings and that support really helps. When you start feeling sorry for yourself and old ways of thinking start creeping back, people are there to point that out to you and tell you to cut it out. Without that it would be hard to do on your own (73).

Family treatment is as essential as individual treatment. Alcoholism has been called the "family disease." Those close to the alcoholic are also in need of help for themselves, for *their* problems. Often they will be the first ones asking for assistance while the alcoholic continues to drink. The presenting problems are not only those that were discussed during the progression of the illness. The cessation of drinking also creates disequilibrium in those who are closely associated with the alcoholic. For example, the drinking member may have long ago abandoned responsibility in terms of the management of the home; now with sobriety the client is expecting to step in and become a fully participating member again. This often is met with resentment and resistance from those who had assumed the duties and who may not want to share or relinquish any of the responsibilities or power. The family needs assistance and support in working through this and other problems.

In many ways the recovery of those associated with the alcoholic parallels the recovery of the alcoholic. There needs to be acceptance that alcoholism is a disease and that no matter how much you love an alcoholic, you have *no* control over the drinking or the resumption of drinking. There needs to be education about alcohol, alcoholism, and the implications of being an alcoholic and of being close to one. There needs to be identification, evaluation, and change of behaviors that: (1) fit into or perpetuate the alcoholic's drinking, and (2) prevent family members from living their own lives to the fullest potential possible despite the alcoholic.

Al-Anon and Alateen are successful self-help groups for family members and siblings or friends of alcoholics and serve as good referral resources for the nurse.

Disulferam (Antabuse) administration may provide a deterrent to drinking. The drug is inert in the body until alcohol is introduced and then it interferes with the metabolism of alcohol. Acetaldehyde builds up in the body, resulting in a severely uncomfortable reaction. The alcoholic needs to be told that the reaction includes an intense, throbbing headache, severe flushing, extreme nausea, vomiting, palpitations, falling blood pressure, labored breathing, and blurred vision. Antabuse treatment should be initiated when there is no alcohol in the client's system. The antabuse is effective for several days after it is taken; therefore, the client cannot suddenly stop taking it and immediately start drinking. The use of Antabuse is most effective in the management of a client who returns to drinking impulsively or who has had a history of spree or binge drinking (65).

EVALUATION

Since recovery from alcoholism is a long process, it is imperative that you continually evaluate the progress made. If evaluation of progress toward the goals is not done frequently, valuable time could be lost in working on something that is actually at a stalemate. Ask the following questions:

Did the client move toward the goal, and in what way? If not, why didn't the client move toward the goal?

If progress has been made, is it continuing? For example, is the client able to interact rationally with his wife most of the time when discussing problems? Or did that just occur soon after discharge, with the client now reverting back to old behaviors?

What other approaches could have been used or may now need to be used? Perhaps an intervention needs to be modified, or it may need to be discarded and a new approach used. Maybe the living arrangements the client has set up are not working out and moving may be the only answer.

Did the client deviate from the determined plan? Perhaps the living arrangements are not working out because the client refuses to participate in cooking and cleaning as was originally planned.

Are there new problem areas that require intervention? If the client is attempting to develop new nonalcoholic relationships, there may be unanticipated problems. Mutually agreed-upon priorities may need revision as changes in the client's life style occur. Even though you may have worked with the client for a period of years, potential new problems must be assessed to prevent resumption of drinking.

CARE OF THE PERSON WHOSE USE OF OTHER DRUGS IS OUT OF CONTROL

Scope of the Problem

Substance abuse is often equated with illicit drug usage. Therefore over-the-counter drugs and medically prescribed drugs that are abused are often overlooked. Alcohol, the drug that is most widely used and causes most of the medical problems, has already been discussed.

Theories of Etiology

The theories of causation of drug abuse closely parallel those of alcoholism. Therefore, only those aspects in the development of drug abuse that seem to differ from the development of alcoholism will be discussed here. Drug abuse, like alcoholism, develops from a complex interaction of sociological and psychological factors and drug characteristics and is stimulated by the easy availability of drugs.

Sociological Factors in Causation

Sociological factors vary with the type of drug abused. For example, the majority of heroin addicts in the United States involve groups dwelling in the central city section of metropolitan areas. Here wages are often the lowest, housing the poorest, and rates of delinquency the highest (26). On college campuses, young people are prone to abusing marijuana, hallucinogens, and amphetamines. These students are in the process of becoming adults, which involves the unlearning of some behaviors that were appropriate in childhood and the learning of new behaviors aligned with how society defines an adult (56). This definition of adulthood, along with learning what behavior is appropriate, can be very difficult for youth today. Therefore, the use of hallucinogenic drugs may have appeal to these young people, offering a solace in this sometimes frustrating process.

The whole socializing process of adolescence seems to contribute to drug abuse. Peers and their values are particularly strong influences. As the drug user comes in contact with other people in the drug world, there are often strong pressures to experiment with various drugs. Drug availability is also conducive to experimentation. Curiosity, rebellion against parents or against other authorities, imitation, peer pressure, boredom, the wish to escape from some distress, or the expectation of ultimate pleasure all motivate the individual to try a drug (36). Once the drug has been introduced, the environmental situation tends to sustain its use. The individual may be addicted to the drug, but he/she is also addicted to the process of addiction and the life style it involves. Life centers around the taking of drugs, and for many dependent on drugs, this style seems to offer a much more predictable way of life than the uncertainties of the real world (53).

What is even more alarming, we find heroin, marijuana, cocaine, and other addictive drugs increasingly dispensed at adult social gatherings of affluent and professional people. The number of well-educated and medical persons who engage in such drug use indicates clearly how societal attitudes have changed in the last decade.

Psychological Factors in Causation

Whether a person initiates drug use and possibly becomes socialized into the drug life style depends on individual personality characteristics. As is true with the alcoholic, a particular personality type associated with drug dependence has not been found, although many theorists consider drug abusers to be fixated at an oral or infantile level of development. However, there are certain personality characteristics that are often seen in people dependent on drugs. These include: low frustration tolerance, antisocial tendencies and feelings of inferiority associated with overt behaviors of superiority, fearfulness, and dependency (72). Again, studies do not clarify whether the addiction fostered the development of these characteristics or whether these characteristics fostered the addiction; the person being studied is already addicted.

L. Kolb feels that the majority of narcotic addicts are antisocial personalities who are emotionally immature, hostile, and aggressive persons and take drugs to get relief from tension. Other narcotic addicts, he feels, are neurotic people with anxiety and obsessive-compulsive or psychophysiological symptoms that are relieved by drugs (36).

Easy Availability of Drugs

Obviously, the easy availability of drugs stimulates the development of drug dependence. Hypno-tics, sedatives, and stimulants are available in large part because of their widespread use in medical practice. Thus some people may become addicted when narcotics or other medications are prescribed for pain during an illness or after surgery. Psychologic dependence can develop in a few days. Other drugs under strict legal controls, such as cocaine and herion, may be attractive because their procurement symbolizes rebellion. Furthermore, the abuse of one drug frequently leads to the abuse of another. Thus drug-dependent people may abuse several drugs simultaneously, and they switch from one drug to another, depending on availability (26).

Because of the high cost of drugs, drug abuse and addiction is not limited to the inner-city poor. It is also a disease of the affluent and educated. Further, drug abuse frequently creates economic hardship, which in turn fosters a life of crime, whether white-collar crime in business or prostitution are used as the means to maintain the habit.

Interplay of Causative Factors

Once the addiction has developed, various physiological, psychological, and sociological factors tend to support and perpetuate it. These are the addictive properties of the drugs used, the desire to avoid withdrawal symptoms, attraction to the comfort of the addiction in terms of feeling one's needs are met, the pull of the ritual of addiction, social support by the drug-using community, fear of survival in the straight world, and the lack of preparation for leading a "straight" life. However, there are also certain factors that motivate the person to seek help. These include: encounters with the law or fear of it, deteriorating physical health or fear of it, disgust or disenchantment with the addiction, pressure from family or friends, and the desire to cut back the habit for financial reasons (47). The factors that support addiction as well as those that bring the client in for help must be assessed to help determine how involved the client is in the addiction and how motivated he/she is to change.

Detoxification is the easiest part of the client's rehabilitation. The more difficult part is helping the person develop a life style in which there is no need to depend on drugs. For some drug abusers, this may mean finding new friends, a totally different place to live, and some means to fill the time that was formerly centered around drugs. For example, the heroin addict may have existed in a sub-culture of drug addiction, isolated and alienated from general society. It is fairly easy to stop taking drugs when hospitalized for drug withdrawal, but much more difficult to remain off drugs when the person returns to that same subculture where the pressure to resume taking drugs is extreme and the nondrug abuser is often considered abnormal (42).

Nursing Assessment of the Drug-Dependent Person

Ask the client for specific information about drug use in *all* cases of suspected substance abuse. Ascertain the following:

1. What drug is being used.
2. Time, kind, and amount of last use and if this is typical of client's current usage pattern.
3. Length of current abuse cycle.
4. What combination of drugs is being used.
5. How long client has been without proper nutrition or general physical care, if condition warrants the question.
6. Previous seizure history.

A thorough physical, psychological, and social assessment should be done (see Chapter 4) to determine the client's present health state and signs of drug abuse. Assess not only the problems; also determine strengths of the drug abuser/addict. All the areas that must be assessed in the alcoholic client apply when assessing the drug abuser.

Formulation of Nursing Diagnosis

The nursing diagnosis of *drug usage out of control* must include the kind of drug(s) the client is dependent on, the severity of dependence, and the factors motivating the client to continue or discontinue the abuse of drugs. For example, the client is motivated to continue drug abuse when he/she: (1) shares a room with others who are drug-dependent; (2) has never held a job for more than a few weeks at a time and has little legitimate means of support, (3) began taking excessive amounts of drugs by doctor's prescription after elective surgery or during an especially stressful period on the job. One positive factor that may motivate the client to stop using drugs is when the client is sent to a treatment center instead of jail. Attempting to avoid jail can be a strong motivator. Or perhaps the client's husband is very supportive in helping his wife discontinue daily amphetamines.

The three major areas that must be considered in the nursing diagnosis include: (1) physical problems resulting from drug dependence, (2) psychological problems that support drug dependence, and (3) sociological factors.

Client-Care Goals

Recovery from drug dependence closely parallels recovery from alcohol addiction. It is usually a long process with many relapses. Be prepared to deal with the client over a fairly long time and do not give up if the client temporarily returns to drugs or becomes dependent on a different drug. Goals must be realistic in terms of what the client is capable of at this point in time.

Immediate client-care goals include to assist the client to:

Withdraw from the drug without complications.

Return to a stable state of health.

Learn proper health habits.

Seek further specialized treatment.

Depending on the drug and the client's physical and psychological condition, withdrawal may be done on either an inpatient or an outpatient basis. After the client has been detoxified, treatment is often discontinued if the client feels able to stay drug-free without support. However, this can be very difficult because of the pressures encountered when the client returns to the pretreatment environment where drugs are prevalent. The client is usually rapidly back on drugs. You will need to be creative in and committed to achieving the goal of further treatment for the client.

Longer-term client-care goals include assisting the client to:

Restructure patterns of living so that life is no longer centered around drugs.

Develop a stable life situation with employment and a stable support system with family or others.

Maintain abstinence from addictive drugs after the treatment program has ended.

Nursing Interventions Related to Acute Effects of Drug Abuse

Table 14-3 summarizes information pertinent to assessment and nursing diagnosis and related to key nursing interventions for commonly abused legal and illegal drugs. In addition to identifying these drugs by drug type and street name, the table also summarizes: (1) the drug's action, (2) duration of action, (3) effect sought by the user, (4) method of administration, (5) physical and emotional effects of the drug, (6) potential for tolerance, physical dependence, and psychological dependence, (7) characteristics of withdrawal/detoxification, if applicable, and (8) recommended nursing care.

TABLE 14-3. Summary of Legal and Illegal Drugs Related To Nursing Assessment and Intervention

DRUG TYPE/NAME	STREET NAMES	ACTION & DURATION OF ACTION	ADMINISTRATION	EFFECT SOUGHT BY USER	PHYSICAL & EMOTIONAL EFFECTS/COMPLICATIONS
Narcotics Opiates opium, morphine, heroin, codeine Synthetic nonopiates Methadone, Demerol	Snow, stuff, H, junk, smack, scag, dreamer.	Central nervous system depressant: 3–24 hours.	Oral; smoked; sniffed; injected under skin (skin popping); intramuscular (IM); intravenous (IV).	Euphoria. Prevention of withdrawal discomfort.	Drowsiness, sedation (nodding), stupor. Euphoria. Relief of pain. Impaired intellectual functioning and coordination. Constricted pupils that do not respond to light. Excessive itching. Constipation. Loss of sexual desire, temporary impotence or sterility. Slow pulse and respiration(s); death from overdosage caused by respiratory and cardiovascular depression and collapse. Severe infection at injection sites (needle marks and tracks).
Barbiturates Nembutal, Seconal, Amytal	Sleepers, downers, goofballs, redbirds, yellow jackets, heavens, red devils, barbs.	Central nervous system depressant: 1–16 hours.	Oral, or injected IM or IV.	Relaxation and euphoria	Relief of anxiety and muscular tension, relaxation, sleep. Euphoria. Impaired emotional control, judgment, and coordination. Irritability. Weight loss. Death from overdose. Psychosis, possible convulsions or death, from abrupt withdrawal of barbiturates.
Sedatives Doriden, Chloral hydrate, Miltown, Equanil, Quaalude *Minor Tranquilizers* Valium, Librium					
Inhalants (Glue sniffing, aero-		Central nervous system depres-	Inhaled.	Intoxication, relaxation,	Excess nasal secretion. Watering of eyes. Poor muscular con-

Evaluation

Since recovery from drug addiction and dependence is a long process, you must continually be alert to the same questions that were asked under the section on evaluation of the person who is an alcoholic. Determine your own feelings and values as you work with the client. Try to determine the affects of significant others and the general environment upon the client's rehabilitation progress. Do not become discouraged if progress is slow and if relapses occur. A sustained relationship between you and the client may be one of the important factors in eventual rehabilitation of the client.

TOLERANCE POTENTIAL	PHYSICAL DEPENDENCE	PSYCHOLOGICAL DEPENDENCE	WITHDRAWAL CHARACTERISTICS	NURSING CARE
Yes	Yes	Yes	Abdominal pain. Muscle cramps. tremors, spasms. Nausea, vomiting, diarrhea. Lacrimaition, watery eyes. Goose bumps, sweating, chills. Hypertension, tachycardia, increased respirations. Anxiety, irritability, depression. Craving for drugs.	(1) Observe for symptoms of withdrawal and report to physician. (2) Give medications prescribed to suppress withdrawal symptoms. (3) Monitor for vital signs at least q.i.d. for first 72 hours following admission. (4) Carry out nursing measures to promote safety, general health, and sense of security.
Yes	Yes	Yes	Nausea, vomiting, diarrhea. Bleeding, Tremors. Diaphoresis. Hypertension or hypotension. Temperature above 99.6 F. Irritability, hostility, restlessness, agitation. Sleep disturbance. Impaired cognitive function. Acute brain syndrome. Seizures.	(1) Observe for withdrawal symptoms and report to physician. (2) Give prescribed medication to suppress symptoms. (3) Provide calm, quiet, safe environment, as free of external stimuli as possible, for acute/severe withdrawal symptoms. (4) Observe for insomnia and nightmares and provide nursing measures to promote sleep. (5) Observe and take precaution for seizure activity. (6) Promote general health and sense of security.
Yes	No	Yes	Withdrawal symptoms have not been recorded.	(1) Emergency care for respiratory damage or neurological

TABLE 14-3. Continued

DRUG TYPE/NAME	STREET NAMES	ACTION & DURATION OF ACTION	ADMINISTRATION	EFFECT SOUGHT BY USER	PHYSICAL & EMOTIONAL EFFECTS/COMPLICATIONS
sols, airplane glue, amyl nitrate, nitrous oxide.)		sant: 1–3 hours.		euphoria.	trol, lack of coordination. Appears dreamy or blank. Impaired perception and judgment. Possibility of violent behavior. Damage to lungs, nervous system, brain, liver. Death through suffocation, choking, or overdose.
Stimulants					
Amphetamines	Pep pills, uppers, speed, crystal, dexies.	Central nervous system stimulant. Varies in duration of action.	Oral; or injected under skin or IV; cocaine also sniffed.	Alertness, feelings of activity and increased initiative. Excitation.	Giggling, silliness. Rapid speech. Dilated pupils. Hypertension, tachycardia. Loss of appetite, loss of weight. Extreme fatigue. Dry mouth, bad breath. Chills, sweating, increased muscle tension; shakiness, tremors, restlessness. Irritability. Confused thinking. Mood swings. Aggressive behavior. Feelings of persecution. Delusions. Hallucinations. Toxic psychosis. Possible seizures. Tachycardia may cause heart damage or heart attack. Death from cardiac damage, hypertensive crisis, or overdose.
Cocaine	Leaf, snow, speedballs.	2–4 hours.			
Caffeine (Found in tea, coffee, cocoa, cola and tablet form, including many over-the-counter drugs.)		Central nervous system stimulant. Cardiac stimulant. 2–4 hours.	Oral	A "pick-up"; to increase alertness and decrease fatigue. More rapid, clearer flow of thoughts.	Restlessness. Disturbed sleep or insomnia. Nausea, abdominal distention. Myocardial stimulation, palpitation, and tachycardia. Large amounts have led to irrational or hysterical behavior.
Hallucinogens					
Synthetic D-lysergic acid (LSD) 4-methyl-2 (STP, DOM)	Acid, Bid D, sugar, trips, cubes., Serenity, tranquility, peace.	Hallucinogenic varies: LSD 10–12 hours; STP 6–8 hours.	Primarily oral; some some are inhaled or injected.	Insight. Distortion of senses. Exhilaration. Increased energy.	Severe hallucinations, feelings of persecution and detachment. Incoherent speech. Laughing, crying. Exhilaration, depression, or panic. Suicidal or homicidal tendencies. Cold, sweaty hands and feet; shivering, chills. Vomiting. Irregular breathing. Exhaustion. Brain damage from chronic use. Accidental death. Flashbacks. May intensify existing psychosis; long-lasting mental illness has resulted. Symptoms may
Dimethyltryptamine (DMT)	Businessman's special.				
Natural Cactus (mescaline) Mushroom (psilocybin)		Mescaline 12–24 hours.			

TOLERANCE POTENTIAL	PHYSICAL DEPENDENCE	PSYCHOLOGICAL DEPENDENCE	WITHDRAWAL CHARACTERISTICS	NURSING CARE
				complication. (2) Provide for safety. (3) Implement other nursing measures related to presenting symptoms, especially if this drug has been used in combination with others.
Yes	No	Yes	Tremors. Neurological hyperactivity. Paranoia. Assaultive behavior. Depression. Possible suicidal behavior. Tachycardia, hypertension. Oversensitivity to stimuli. Insomnia.	(1) Observe for symptoms of withdrawal and report to physician. (2) Give medication as prescribed to suppress agitated state and prevent exhaustion. (3) Take precautions for staff and client safety according to client's paranoia and depression. (4) Monitor vital signs at least q.i.d. for first 72 hours following admissions. (5) Provide calm, unthreatening, quiet environment and sense of security. (6) Provide for sleep and nutrition.
Yes	Strongly possible	Yes	In moderately heavy users, there may be headache, irritability, nervousness.	(1) Introduce substitute decaffeinated beverage. (2) Provide for general health needs and teaching.
Yes	No	Possible	Severe apprehension, fear, or panic. Perceptual distortions and hallucinations. Hyperactivity. Diaphoresis. Tachycardia.	(1) Have someone who is close to client stay with client at all times to provide support and comfort. (2) Provide nonthreatening environment with subdued, pleasant stimuli. (3) Provide orientation and diversion to pleasant experiences. (4) Avoid use of sedative/ tranquilizers, if possible. (5) Monitor vital signs. (6) Provide for general health needs.

TABLE 14-3.   Continued

DRUG TYPE/NAME	STREET NAMES	ACTION & DURATION OF ACTION	ADMINISTRATION	EFFECT SOUGHT BY USER	PHYSICAL & EMOTIONAL EFFECTS/COMPLICATIONS
					persist for an indefinite period after discontinuation of drug.
Marijuana

Hashish | Joints, reefers, pot, grass.

Hash. | Mixed: central nervous system depressant and stimulant. Great variance in duration: 2–12 hours. | Smoked or swallowed. | Euphoria. Relaxation. Increased perception. Escape. | Relaxation or euphoria. Pupils dilation, conjunctivitis. Incoordination of walk. Increased appetite and craving for sweets. Mood swings from joy to extreme anxiety or depression; erratic behavior. Withdrawn. Impaired memory, judgment, or problem solving. Distortions of time and space. Possible cause for bronchitis. Acute panic or hallucinations are symptoms of overdose. |
| Nicotine (Found in cigarettes, cigars, pipe and chewing tobacco, and snuff.) | | Variable action. Central nervous system toxin. Can act as stimulant or depressant: 15 minutes–2 hours. | Smoked, sniffed, chewed. | Calmness, sociability. | Can have stimulating and/or calming effect. Factor in lung cancer. coronary artery disease, circulatory impairment, peptic ulcer, and emphysema. |

CARE OF THE PERSON WHOSE USE OF FOOD IS OUT OF CONTROL

Scope of the Problem

It is generally accepted that obesity is the most important nutrition problem in the United States today: 15 million Americans are overweight to the point that it shortens their life; and more than one-third of middle-aged Americans are at least 20 percent overweight (25). In spite of these epidemic proportions, little has been done to determine the risk involved in being overweight.

Food is one of the major aspects of our lives. We spend at least an hour a day eating, and for many of us it is more than that. The person in a family who prepares meals three times a day spends many hours a week planning meals, purchasing food, preparing meals, and, of course, cleaning up after meals. Furthermore, much of the entertainment we participate in centers around a meal. Particularly for women, a lot of time is often spent talking about food and also how to lose the excess pounds after you have eaten the food.

Food should not be considered only for its biologic aspects, that is, the consumption of calories to provide energy. All societies endow food with certain values, and since much of life is centered around food, eating habits and food traditions have become a large part of our culture and we pass these along from generation to generation. Some people eat to live; others live to eat. Food may symbolize love, reward, protection, or a defense from others.

Anorexia nervosa is an abuse of food wherein the client does not eat because of the fears of gaining weight. Another manifestation of the disease is

TOLERANCE POTENTIAL	PHYSICAL DEPENDENCE	PSYCHOLOGICAL DEPENDENCE	WITHDRAWAL CHARACTERISTICS	NURSING CARE
No	No	Probable	Withdrawal symptoms have not been recorded.	Not usually admitted to acute care settings unless this drug has been used in combination with others, so that a mixed effect occurs. Implement nursing measures listed above under Hallucinogens. Likely to see increasing numbers of children and adolescents with physical effects from chronic use or injuries from accidents; appropriate medical and surgical nursing care should be given.
Yes	Possible to yes	Yes	Headache. Anorexia, irritability, nervousness. Decreased ability to concentrate. Craving for cigarette. Energy loss. Fatigue. Dizziness. Sweating. Tremor and palpitations.	(1) Provide support. (2) Explore behavioral changes necessary to quit smoking as well as provide information as to available self-help groups. (3) Provide for general health needs.

binge eating and then forcing oneself to vomit. Anorexia nervosa is a disease that primarily affects girls following puberty. See Chapter 21 for a discussion of this abuse of food.

Those who regularly ingest an excess of food usually are obese. Obesity is caused by energy intake that is greater than energy expenditure, resulting in the storage of excess energy in the form of fat. *Obesity can be defined as excessive adipose tissue that results in a person being at least 10 percent in excess of normal or desirable weight. Excessive obesity is when the person is 20 percent in excess of the desirable weight. Morbid obesity is present when the person is 30 percent over desirable weight* (13).

Theories of Etiology

What causes some people to eat excess calories? If there is an increased drive to eat, is this drive caused from physiological factors, psychological aspects, or our sociocultural heritage? As with other substance abuse, the most probable cause is a complex interrelationship of all of these factors.

Physiological Factors

Physiological factors are responsible for only a small percentage of obesity cases. In these cases, obesity is caused by endocrine abnormalities, hypothyroidism, hypothalamic injury, or genetic disorders (25). Other physiological cause theories have been postulated, and research is yielding much new information about the endocrine and biochemical role in obesity.

For example, a wide variety of physiological circumstances may exert a carbohydrate saving action so that the obese person converts large amounts of carbohydrates into fat and stores it. Obesity may be either a causal factor or a result of these physiological changes. Changes in the neuro-regulatory mechanisms of the brain also seem to affect eating. Animal studies show that damage to the hypothalamus can create an increased appetite (13). Research is only beginning to show the very complex interactions of the neuroregulatory mechanism of the brain.

There is a high familial incidence of obesity. Studies have found that if neither parent is obese, 7 percent of the offspring will be obese. If one parent is obese, 40 percent of offspring will be obese. If both parents are obese, 80 percent of offspring will be obese (25). This may support a genetic theory, although obesity is also complicated by environmental factors such as family eating habits. However, studies of identical twins raised apart were shown to be closer in weight than dizygotic twins reared together. Also weights of adopted children showed no correlation with those of their adopting parents (13).

Recent studies indicate that juvenile-onset obesity results from an elevated number of fat cells. Early infancy seems to be one of the periods when excessive caloric intake leads to an increase in cell division and in total fat cell numbers. Four-fifths of fat babies become fat adults, and 50 percent of excessively obese adults (250 pounds and over) were obese infants (24). Dieting decreases the size of fat cells but does not decrease the number of fat cells. It may be that these people have a higher baseline of body fat. Being overweight is the condition of equilibrium their bodies attempt to return to. The hypothalamus attempts to maintain this set point (5). Early-onset obesity has been found to be much more difficult to treat than adult-onset obesity, perhaps because the body continually attempts to return to its "normal" weight for that individual.

Sociological Factors

Sociological factors must also be considered as contributory, and are interwoven with biological and psychological causes. Obesity is not evenly distributed throughout our culture. The living conditions of various sections of the culture and the differing priorities of certain socioeconomic groups may support the development of obesity. A study of obesity in the City of New York showed that 5 percent of upper-class women were obese as compared with 30 percent of lower-class women. It follows that obesity is less likely to be found in families who are upwardly mobile in socioeconomic status (32). Wealthier families can afford the more expensive foods necessary for dieting; whereas "fattening" food such as starches and sweets are more readily available to people in lower socioeconomic settings, and they are cheaper than meats, fresh fruits, and vegetables. Also the slim appearance of the woman may be considered important for the husband's success in business in the higher social classes. The pursuit of exercise and athletics, which takes time and money, is also more readily available in the upper social classes.

Recent immigrants to the United States have a higher incidence of obesity, perhaps because of lower initial socioeconomic status and memories of recent hunger in their countries of origin (13). The longer the person has been in the United States, the lower is the incidence of obesity. The country of origin may also be a factor in obesity. The incidence of obesity increases as one moves eastward across Europe, starting with Great Britain.

Our way of living may contribute to obesity. Television and spectator sports have made Americans more sedentary. Labor-saving devices at home and at work decrease exercise. Even food preparation requires less energy expenditure.

Another factor is that many children have been brought up according to the adage of "clean your plate." It doesn't make any difference if the person is already satiated or does not like the food to be consumed. For some, refusing a second helping or refusing dessert may imply bad manners. Eating may also be a way of filling unplanned leisure time.

Women diet more often than men, perhaps because the self-concept of women is more closely tied to physical desirability. The physical appearance of men is important, but the male's financial status, educational achievement, and occupation receive more emphasis. Less emphasis is placed on these characteristics in a female. Another cultural influence is the shape of women's clothing, which is designed to reveal body configuration, whereas men's clothing is more concealing. Peer pressures may also be a contributory factor. Adolescents diet more than adults because physical appearance is of great importance during the adolescent years and they do not want to deviate from their peers (33).

Psychological Factors

Psychological factors are of major importance

in obesity. Patterns of eating develop in early infancy. Some theorists suggest that awareness of hunger and satiation are related to the relationship with the mothering person and how the infant's demands are met instead of being related to an internal process (7). Obesity tends to develop in children whose parents compensate for their own frustration and disappointment through their attachment to the child. The mother has very high expectations for the child, and as the aims of the parent predominate, the child cannot develop independence and self-esteem. On the surface the child may seem submissive. But the child's demands in the family are met with food instead of love (36). As the child grows, frustration is handled by eating. Food symbolizes love. People who are obese are not necessarily more anxious or depressed than nonobese people, but eating does tend to relieve feelings of anxiety or depression (13). Food represents such feelings as pleasure, security, and affection. Dieting denies the client the pleasure that eating represents, and feelings of anxiety, irritability, and depression may result. During these periods it is very easy for the person to discontinue dieting.

As with the other addictions, no particular personality type has been found. Psychological problems may be the result of obesity rather than the cause. Our society stresses thinness and the obese are discriminated against; this factor alone may account for psychological problems.

The Stigma of Being Obese

Many obese people are treated with hostility and negative feelings. They are judged on the basis of the obesity and not on their personality or ability. For example, obese applicants to college were found to be less likely to be accepted than the nonobese, even though there was no measurable difference in academic achievement, social class, and motivation (33) Also physicians have been found to have negative attitudes toward the obese. One study found that physicians often considered the obese incurable or only slightly amenable toward help. This expectation of failure by physicians may account in part for the low success rate when treating the obese.

Justification given for these negative attitudes includes the following two arguments: (1) that success depends on physical attractiveness, and (2) that excess weight is detrimental to health, which

is a measure of status and security. The Protestant ethic has also emphasized the need to control impulses; the obese person is viewed as not having control over his/her impulses. Thus the individual is held responsible for being overweight—even though the real cause may be beyond his/her control!

The negative attitudes of others may come to be accepted as fact by the obese because the intimidating social environment helps distort the obese person's self-concept. Feelings of self-worth decrease because of the prejudice to which the person is subjected (45). The body image may be distorted. Some obese persons are overwhelmingly preoccupied with the image of their body. They often look at themselves as being grotesque and loathesome and feel that others look at them with the same feelings. A. Stunkard and M. Mendelson feel this disturbed body image in the obese occurs when the person: (1) became obese in childhood, (2) has some additional emotional disturbance, and (3) experiences a detrimental parental evaluation of the obesity as a child (63). This finding underscores the importance of prevention of obesity during childhood.

Loss of weight can improve body image, but it can also result in some perceptual distortions during the weight loss period. For example, if being a large person has come to represent strength and power to the person, or a protection from the hostile world, weight loss may symbolize loss of these defenses. Or if eating substitutes for a feeling of being loved, eating less may make one feel unloved. Thus the weight may soon be regained to decrease feelings of vulnerability. Also the reactions of others to the person's weight loss may be such that a disturbance occurs in the relationship. New patterns of relating to others may have to be developed in response to the changed appearance (58). Or in order to reestablish balance, the person may feel he/she has to regain the weight.

Eating Characteristics of the Obese

Obese individuals tend to respond to food differently than normal weight individuals. S. Schachter's studies of eating behavior found that overweight people were more affected than nonobese people by external cues such as the sight of food, its availability, and the apparent passage of time; whereas normal weight individuals were motivated to eat by physiological cues such as hunger feelings. Overweight people ate more rapidly and ate more at a given sitting. Obese people were found to be more highly taste-responsive; they ate very large quantities of good-tasting food. Obese people also never seemed to reach a point of satiety; they could always eat more when another food was presented, even though they had just had a lot to eat (60).

Schachter described the Night Eating Syndrome, a cycle that occurs frequently in obese people (60). The person overeats at the evening meal, and may gorge until bedtime, even getting up during the night to eat. Consequently the person is anorexic in the morning and skips breakfast, may have a small lunch, and again is ravenously hungry by evening when exercise after meals is decreased.

Another type is the Binge Eater. This behavior is a sudden, uncontrolled ingestion of very large amounts of food in a very short time, followed by self-condemnation. The binge represents a reaction to stress or occurs in response to a slight insult or disappointment (7).

The extreme form of binge eating results in reactive obesity, which develops in response to an emotional trauma, such as the death of a loved one or when fear of death or injury is aroused. Overeating and obesity may serve the function of warding off depression, as the situations reacted to are those in which others might react with despair. It is useful to note that the suicide rate in obese persons is low unless the person is pushed excessively to diet. Some people become depressed and suicidal when they lose considerable weight. Overeating would certainly be a less destructive reaction (7).

Nursing Assessment of the Obese Client

Many obese people have tried all kinds of diets on their own, only to readily return to their previous weight after they stopped dieting. Many people see their physicians for a diet or anorexic drugs. Types of drugs that have been given for weight loss include gonadotropic hormones, amphetamines, thyroxine, diuretics, and laxatives. There are still no good long-range studies showing the value of these drugs for aiding and then maintaining weight reduction. Weight that is lost with medication always seems to be regained when the medication is discontinued (25). This may teach the client that weight loss can only be accomplished with medication. Realistically the problem involves readjustment in the entire

eating pattern as well as working through related emotional and social factors. This readjustment begins with the client's exploration of eating patterns and the meaning and effect of the obesity.

Areas to assess include the following:

1. *Client's current height and weight, compared with normal values.*
2. *Birth weight and rate of weight gain during early childhood,* if known.
3. *Eating patterns and food intake during early childhood and currently.* Attempt to ascertain when obesity began to develop.
4. *Weight during adolescence and client's remembrance of feelings if overweight during this time.*
5. *Family history.* Height and weight of parents and siblings, compared with normal weights. There is a high correlation between overweight parents and overweight children.
6. *Social and cultural history, including employment history, leisure activities, exercise, and cultural patterns.* Determine if the person has had difficulty obtaining or maintaining employment because of weight. Does weight affect the client's ability to function on the job, such as getting into small spaces or operating certain machinery? Does the area of employment have an effect on the client's weight, such as having to take customers to lunch or dinner frequently?

   Explore use of leisure time. Is going out avoided because of physical appearance? Are occasions avoided where food will be served? Is the evening spent with television and snacks? What is the use of alcoholic beverages?

   The amount and frequency of exercise must be assessed. Does weight interfere with physical exercise or the tasks of daily living, such as meal preparation or driving a car?
7. *Past medical history,* particularly illnesses related to obesity.
8. *Previous weight fluctuations and attempts to lose weight.* How has the client's weight fluctuated? What was occurring in his/her life, such as stressful events, during periods of weight gain? Are these stressful events occurring at present? Times of crisis are not the time to consider weight reduction. What experience has the client had with dieting, weight loss

medications, or participation in group weight-loss programs? Why does the client feel these attempts were or were not successful?

9. *Emotional feelings and motivation.* Does the client eat when anxious? Have previous attempts to lose weight led to feelings of anxiety or depression? The client's motivation is very important. Weight loss must be highly desired to be successful. Parents may be motivated to have an obese child lose weight, but if the child shows little interest, weight reduction will be difficult.

10. *Nutritional history and eating patterns.* What are specific food habits of the person's culture? Does the client adhere to these? What is the meaning of food? Are there special foods for certain occasions or stresses? What is the most common way of preparing food: frying, broiling, baking, boiling? When and where does eating take place? How much time is spent eating? What is being done while eating? Who does the person eat with? What are feelings before eating? What quantities are eaten? How does the person feel after eating? Determine exactly what foods are eaten. The client can be asked to list all that has been eaten during the previous three-day period to get more specific information about quantity of food and eating patterns. Ascertain the client's nutritional knowledge.

11. *Physical appearance.* Distribution of weight should be assessed. The obese person may wear ill-fitting clothes because of the expense of larger-sized clothes. Perhaps no attention is paid to how clothes fit since weight has been gained. Body odor may also be a problem for the obese person.

Formulation of Nursing Diagnosis

The nursing diagnosis, *obesity or food consumption out of control*, indicates the need for significant weight loss, which usually takes quite a long time. Permanent weight loss cannot be expected without examining the factors in the client's life situation that may have contributed to the weight gain. The client may eat frequently throughout the day, carrying food along with him/her. Perhaps huge amounts are eaten during the evening hours after a stressful day at work. Or you may learn that the client cooks excessive amounts for meals, although there are only two people to cook for, and therefore leftovers are eaten by the client the next day. It is important that these factors be dealt with at the same time a weight-control regime is started. Plan for the client to have contact with you over a long period. Priorities must be established regarding those areas that present the greatest problems for the patient.

Examples of *nursing diagnoses* related to the nursing diagnosis of obesity (food consumption out of control) are:

1. Client avoids social contact because of embarrassment and disgust about obesity and physical appearance.
2. Client describes distortion of body image related to weight gain and loss.

Client-Care Goals

Goals for an obese client are long-term since weight reduction takes place over a long period of time. Goals must be addressed toward the weight loss and the changes in life style that need to be initiated. Reinforcement as weight loss occurs is also necessary to keep the client motivated to continue the program. The following are examples of goals for this client:

1. Readjusts food and drink consumption habits to promote realistic weight loss.
2. Presents an attitude of achieving success in weight loss.
3. Describes a positive self-image.
4. Demonstrates self-sufficiency in changing eating habits so that weight loss can be maintained without continued reliance on the nurse.
5. Increases level of activity.
6. Increases social interactions and comfort level during social interactions.

Nursing Interventions Related to Client-Care Goals

Intervention related to each of the above six goals will be discussed below.

Goal 1: Readjusts food and drink consumption habits to promote realistic weight loss.

Intervention

1. Have client record eating habits for at least a week including when, what, and where food is eaten, what is done while eating, and feelings before and after eating.
2. Instruct client to eat meals slowly so that they last at least 20 minutes; chew each mouthful of food ten times, and place the utensils on the plate between mouthfuls.
3. Instruct client to decrease the size of food portions and to serve the meals restaurant-style.
4. Instruct client to leave small portions of food on the plate at each meal and to discard left-over food immediately after meal is completed.
5. Encourage client to avoid keeping prepared snack food in the house.
6. Explore ways to alter the composition of foods to be lower in caloric content. For example, over a period of days, decrease the amount of bread used to make a sandwich.
7. Encourage use of low-calorie substitutes for meals and low-calorie sodas.
8. Encourage client to shop for groceries after eating a full meal and to shop from a prepared grocery list.
9. Instruct client to turn off the light bulb in the refrigerator so that food cannot be seen so easily.
10. Instruct client to keep all foods in covered containers so that they are less enticing.
11. Encourage client to eat only in one room and in one chair.
12. Encourage client to avoid carrying out house-hold and personal activities, such as telephone calls or letter writing, in the kitchen.
13. Encourage client and family to establish nonfood reward for appropriate dietary behavior (32).
14. Encourage family members and friends to provide positive reinforcement in addition to your reinforcement to give client a feeling of accomplishment, even for a small weight loss.
15. Encourage verbalization of feelings of frustra-

tion and/or depression. Depression commonly occurs during the first twelve months of weight reduction (35).
16. Teach client to utilize an effective reducing diet that includes the following characteristics:
    a. Satisfies all nutrient needs except energy or calories (26).
    b. Is adapted as closely as possible to the client's tastes and habits.
    c. Protects the client from between-meal hunger and leaves client with a sense of well-being and a minimum of fatigue.
    d. Is easy for client to obtain at home or away from home without feeling different.
    e. Readjusts eating habits, which may be followed over time so that with suitable caloric additions can become a pattern for lifetime eating (2).
17. Encourage group interaction if it seems war-ranted for particular client in readjusting eating habits. Examples of organized groups are Weight Watchers, TOPS (Take Off Pounds Sensibly), and Overeaters Anonymous. These organizations can provide sound educational information about weight control and group support and reinforcement.
18. Educate mothers about the vulnerable periods of weight gain (infancy and adolescence). A fat baby is not necessarily synonymous with a healthy baby or later with a healthy adult. Proper diet, planned exercise, and recreational programs should be emphasized with children of all ages, including adolescents.

Goal 2: Presents an attitude of achieving success in weight loss.

Intervention

1. Encourage client to "see self" achieving suc-cessful results in weight loss and to establish a mental set of being successful.
2. Emphasize small changes in behavior and give positive reinforcement for these.
3. Avoid authoritarian instructions.
4. Emphasize the positive aspects of changed appearance and how much better client will feel when weight is lost.

*Goal 3: Describes a positive
self-image.*

Intervention

1. Encourage verbalization about feelings related to changing self-image and how changed self relates to image of "fat" self.
2. Help client be assertive in maintaining dietary goals if others try to undermine efforts through their remarks or statements.
3. Support client so that he/she is able to accept and receive positive feedback for any accomplishment in weight reduction.
4. Explore with client how to wear clothes that do not accentuate body size.
5. Explore ways to maintain good personal hygiene.

*Goal 4: Demonstrates
self-sufficiency in changing
eating habits so that weight
loss can be maintained without
continued reliance on the
nurse.*

Intervention

1. Have client keep an accurate record of what is eaten to develop self-awareness of eating patterns.
2. Be accepting of the client; authoritarian behavior will develop controls from an external source instead of internal controls on eating patterns, which are necessary for maintaining weight loss.
3. Encourage client to become aware of what cues lead to overeating, such as opening the refrigerator and seeing small amounts of food.

*Goal 5: Increases level
of activity.*

Intervention

1. Review daily routine to find areas where activity can be increased, such as climbing the stairs instead of riding the elevator.
2. Explore with client recreational activities that are accessible, fun, and provide exercise.

3. Instruct about the value of exercise in weight loss.

*Goal 6: Increases social
interactions and comfort level
during social interactions.*

Intervention

1. Encourage participation in social functions; loneliness may contribute to eating.
2. Help client develop strategies for eating behavior when attending social functions, such as not standing near the buffet table, leaving small amounts of food on the plate, and planning beforehand what will be eaten at the social function (43).
3. Encourage client to maintain an attractive appearance and invest in new outfit a size smaller as an incentive to reduce eating.

Evaluation

Evaluation of nursing intervention cannot be made solely on the client's weight loss. The degree of weight loss varies widely. Many clients will have quite a rapid loss initially and then taper off as the body seems to become more efficient in energy usage. Determine if there is a change in the client's eating habits. The client's appearance should provide clues to the client's self-image. The person may need additional instruction about personal hygiene or some direction in how to alter clothes while weight loss occurs. The client may not want to purchase new clothes before the weight reduction goal is attained, but self-image may suffer if clothes are ill-fitting during this time. Review the daily routine to determine increase in activity. Observe for increased attendance at social functions and comfort at these. Listen for increased verbalization of pride in appearance and increased self-worth. Determine also how the family is working with the client in the therapy regime.

Weight reduction is often a very slow process. The client may become discouraged and give up on the program. You must give a lot of positive reinforcement to the client's accomplishment. You can also support the family in their efforts to assist the client in following a treatment plan and maintaining weight control. If the family purchases and cooks what the client should not eat, or conveys verbally or nonverbally that they do not value the client's efforts toward weight loss, the client will be sabotaged and may lose motivation to continue self-care measures.

You must be very aware of personal attitudes toward obesity. Be sure that you do not become discouraged and give up on the client. Your attitudes may be what deters the client from continued efforts at weight reduction.

REFERENCES

1. Adams-Woodward, Carolyn, "Wernicke-Korsakoff Syndrome: A Case Approach," *Journal of Psychiatric Nursing and Mental Health Services,* 16, no. 4 (1978), 38–41.

2. Asher, Wilmer Lee, ed., *Treating the Obese.* New York: Medcom Press, 1974.

3. Bakdash, Diane, "Essentials the Nurse Should Know about Chemical Dependency," *Journal of Psychiatric Nursing and Mental Health Services,* 16, no. 10 (1978), 33–37.

4. Berg, Nancy, Sue Williams, and Barbara Sutherland, "Behavior Modification in a Weight Control Program," *Family and Community Health,* 1, no. 2 (1979), 41–51.

5. Bray, George, and John Bethune, eds., *Treatment and Management of Obesity.* New York: Harper & Row, Publishers, Inc., 1974.

6. Brecher, Edward, and the editors of Consumer Reports, *Licit and Illicit Drugs.* Boston: Little, Brown & Company, 1972.

7. Bruch, Hilde, *Eating Disorders: Obesity, Anorexia Nervosa and the Person Within.* New York: Basic Books, Inc., 1973.

8. Burgess, Ann, and Aaron Lazare, *Psychiatric Nursing in the Hospital and the Community.* Englewood Cliffs, N.J.: Prentice-Hall, Inc., 1976.

9. Burkhalter, Pamela, *Nursing Care of the Alcoholic and Drug Abuser.* New York: McGraw-Hill Book Company, 1975.

10. Catanzarro, Ronald, ed., *Alcoholism, The Total Treatment Approach.* Springfield, Ill.: Charles C Thomas, Publisher, 1968.

11. Clement, Jeanne, and Carol Notaro, "Nursing Intervention in the Alcohol Detoxification Process," *Alcohol Health and Research World,* 1, no. 2 (1975), 27–29.

12. Clinebell, H. J., Jr., *Understanding and Counseling the Alcoholic.* Nashville, Tenn.: Abingdon Press, 1956.

13. Craddock, Denis, *Obesity and Its Management.* Edinburgh: E. & S. Livingston Ltd., 1969.

14. Criteria Committee, National Council on Alcoholism, "Criteria for the Diagnosis of Alcoholism," *American Journal of Psychiatry,* 129, no. 2 (1972), 12–20.

15. Edwards, Griffith, "Alcohol: No Excuse for Inaction," *World Health,* 6, no. 6 (1979), 14–17.

16. Estes, Nada, Kathleen Smith-DiJulio, and M. Edith Heineman, *Nursing Diagnosis of the Alcoholic Person.* St. Louis: The C. V. Mosby Company, 1980.

17. Ferneau, Ernest, Jr., and Elvera Morton, "Nursing Personnel and Alcoholism," *Nursing Research,* 17, no. 2 (1968), 174–77.

18. Fitch, Kenneth, H. Chandler Elliott, and Perry Johnson, *Life Science and Man: A Biological Approach to Health.* New York: Holt, Rinehart and Winston, 1973.

19. Francis, Gloria, and Barbara Munjas, *Manual of Social-Psychologic Assessment.* New York: Appleton-Century-Crofts, 1976.

20. Fultz, J. et al., "When a Narcotic Addict is Hospitalized," *American Journal of Nursing,* 80, no. 3 (1980), 478–81.

21. Goodwin, Donald, *Is Alcoholism Hereditary?* London: Oxford University Press, 1976.

22. Grace, Helen, Janice Layton, and Dorothy Camilleri, *Mental Health Nursing: A Socio-Psychological Approach.* Dubuque, Iowa: William C. Brown Company, Publishers, 1977.

23. Greenblatt, Milton, and Marc Schuckit, eds., *Alcoholism Problems in Women and Children.* New York: Grune & Stratton, Inc., 1976.

24. Heinemann, Edith, and Nada Estes, "Assessing Alcoholic Patients," *American Journal of Nursing,* 76, no. 5 (1976), 785–89.

25. Howard, Lyn, "Obesity: A Feasible Approach to a Formidable Problem," *Nursing Digest,* 4, no. 4 (1976), 86–90.

26. Isbell, Harris, "Characteristics of the Different Types of Drug Dependence: Pharmacologic and Physiologic Considerations," *Southern Medical Bulletin,* 55, no. 6 (1967), 9–20.

27. Jacob, Moire S., and M. Edward Sellers, "Emergency

Management of Alcohol Withdrawal," *Drug Therapy,* no. 4 (1977), pp. 28–34.

28. Janowsky, D. S. et al., "Interpersonal Effects of Marijuana," *Archives of General Psychiatry,* 36, no. 7 (1979), 781–851.

29. Jellinek, E. M., *The Disease Concept of Alcoholism.* New Haven, Conn.: College and University Press, 1960.

30. Jessor, R., J. Chase, and J. Donovan, "Psychosocial Correlates of Marijuana Use and Problem Drinking in a National Sample of Adolescents," *American Journal of Public Health,* 70, no. 6 (1980), 604–13.

31. Johnson, Vernon E., *I'll Quit Tomorrow.* New York: Harper & Row, Publishers, Inc., 1973.

32. Jordon, H., L. Levitz, and G. Kimbrall, "Managing Obesity—Why Diet Is Not Enough," *Postgraduate Medicine,* 49, no. 4 (1976), 183–86.

33. Kalisch, Beatrice, "The Stigma of Obesity," *American Journal of Nursing,* 72, no. 6 (1972), 1124–27.

34. Kinney, Jean, and Gwen Leaton, *Loosening the Grip.* St. Louis: The C. V. Mosby Company, 1978.

35. Knauert, Arthur, "The Treatment of Alcoholism in a Community Setting," *Family and Community Health,* 2, no. 2 (1979), 91–102.

36. Kolb, Lawrence, *Modern Clinical Psychiatry.* Philadelphia: W. B. Saunders Company, 1977.

37. Kornguth, Mary, "When Your Client Has a Weight Problem: Nursing Management," *American Journal of Nursing,* 81, no. 3 (1981), 553–54.

38. Lambert, Vickie, and Clinton Lambert, *The Impact of Physical Illness and Related Mental Health Concepts.* Englewood Cliffs, N.J.: Prentice-Hall, Inc., 1979.

39. Langford, Rae, "Teenagers and Obesity," *American Journal of Nursing,* 81, no. 3 (1981), 556–59.

40. Lee, K. et al., "Alcohol-Induced Brain Damage and Liver Damage in Young Males," *Lancet,* October 13, 1979, pp. 759–61.

41. Leon, L., "Personality and Morbid Obesity: Implications for Dietary Management through Behavior Modification," *Surgical Clinics of North America,* 59, no. 6 (1979), 1007–15.

42. Lewin, David, "Care of the Drug-Dependent Patient," *Nursing Times,* 74, no. 4 (1978), 621–24.

43. Lewis, Carol, "Body Image and Obesity," *Journal of Psychiatric Nursing and Mental Health Services,* 16, no. 1 (1978), 22–24.

44. Little, Ruth, F. Schultz, and W. Mandell, "Drinking during Pregnancy," *Journal of Studies on Alcohol,* 37 (1976), 375–79.

45. Longo, Dianne, and Reg Arthur Williams, *Clinical Practice in Psychosocial Nursing: Assessment and Intervention.* New York: Appleton-Century-Crofts, 1978.

46. *Manual on Alcoholism.* Chicago: American Medical Association, 1977.

47. "Marijuana Use Believed Spreading among Subteeners," *Medical News Report,* January 7, 1980, p. 21.

48. Marks, Vida, "Health Teaching for Recovering Alcoholic Patients," *American Journal of Nursing,* 80, no. 11 (1980), 2058–61.

49. McElmeel, Evy, and Pamela DiDente, "Alcohol Withdrawal," *The Nurse Practitioner,* 5, no. 1 (1980), 18–26.

50. Miller, Barbara, "Jejuno-Ileal Bypass: A Drastic Weight Control Measure," *American Journal of Nursing,* 81, no. 3 (1981), 564–58.

51. "Mind over Platter," *Imprint,* 26, no. 2 (1979), 46–47.

52. Mojzisik, Cathy, and Edward Martin, "Gastric Partitioning: The Latest Surgical Means to Control Morbid Obesity," *American Journal of Nursing,* 81, no. 3 (1981), 569–72.

53. Morgan, Arthur, and Judith Moreno, *The Practice of Mental Health Nursing: A Community Approach.* Philadelphia: J. B. Lippincott Company, 1973.

54. Morton, Paula, "Assessment and Management of the Self-Destructive Concept of Alcoholism," *Journal of Psychiatric Nursing and Mental Health Services,* 17, no. 11 (1979), 8–13.

55. National Council on Alcoholism, "The Progression of Alcoholism within The Family." St. Louis, Mo., 1975.

56. Nowles, Helen, "Why Students Use Drugs," *American Journal of Nursing,* 68, no. 8 (1968), 1680–85.

57. "Overeaters Anonymous," *American Journal of Nursing,* 81, no. 3 (1981), 560–63.

58. Pescatore, Edward, "Personal Reaction to Weight Loss," *American Journal of Nursing,* 74, no. 12 (1974), 2227–28.

59. Pittman, David J., ed., *Alcoholism.* New York: Harper & Row, Publishers, Inc., 1967.

60. Schachter, Stanley, "Eat, Eat," *Psychology Today,* 5, no. 4 (1971), 45–81.

61. Silverstone, Trevor, ed., *Obesity: Its Pathogenesis and Management.* Littleton, Mass.: Publishing Sciences Group, Inc., 1975.

62. Streissguth, Ann, "Maternal Alcoholism and the Outcome of Pregnancy: A Review of the Fetal Alcohol Syndrome," in M. Greenblatt and M. Schuckit, eds.,

Alcoholism Problems in Women and Children. New York: Grune & Stratton, Inc., 1976.

63. Stunkard, Albert, and Myer Mendelson, "Disturbances in Body Image of Some Obese Persons," *Journal of the American Dietetic Association,* 38, no. 4 (1961), 328–31.

64. Thompson, W. Leigh, "Management of Alcohol Withdrawal Syndrome," *Archives of Internal Medicine,* 138, no. 2 (1978), 278–83.

65. Thorn, George W. et al., eds., *Harrison's Principles of Internal Medicine,* 8th ed. New York: McGraw-Hill Book Company, 1977.

66. Trémoliéres, J., section ed., *International Encyclopedia of Pharmacology and Therapeutics, Section 20. Volume I, Alcohol and Derivates.* Elmsford, N.Y.: Pergamon Press, Inc., 1970.

67. U.S. Department of Health, Education and Welfare, *The First Special Report on Alcohol and Health from the Secretary of N.E.W.,* rev. ed. Washington, D.C.: U.S. Govt. Printing Office, 1972.

68. ____, *The Third Special Report to the U.S. Congress on Alcohol and Health from the Secretary of H.E.W.* Washington, D.C.: U.S. Govt. Printing Office, June 1978.

69. White, Jane, and Mary Ann Schroeder, "When Your Client Has a Weight Problem: Nursing Assessment," *American Journal of Nursing,* 81, no. 3 (1981), 550–53.

70. Williams, Ann, "The Student and the Alcoholic Patient," *Nursing Outlook,* 27, no. 7 (1979), 470–72.

71. Woodell, Jeff, "The Alcohol Withdrawal Syndrome," *Family and Community Health,* 2, no. 8 (1979), 23–30.

72. Worick, Wayne, and Warren Schaller, *Alcohol, Tobacco, and Drugs, Their Use and Abuse.* Englewood Cliffs, N.J.: Prentice-Hall, Inc., 1977.

INTERVIEWS

73. Jennie, recovering alcoholic, January 1980.

15

The Depressed Person

Study of this chapter will assist you to:

1. Define and classify various types of depression.

2. Explore the meaning and feelings of depression for the person.

3. Discuss the psychodynamics of depression.

4. Assess a depressed person, using the parameters discussed in this chapter.

5. Differentiate behaviors of cognitively impaired and depressed persons.

6. Formulate client-care goals related to assessment and nursing diagnosis.

7. Care for the depressed person using guidelines for intervention described in this chapter.

8. Work with suicidal client, using an understanding of the dynamics and appropriate care measures.

9. Work with the family and health team members as a part of client care.

10. Evaluate effectiveness of your care.

11. Promote community resources and programs to assist the person in coping with loss and depression.

This chapter contributed by M. Marilyn Huelskoetter, R.N., M.S.N.

SCOPE OF THE PROBLEM

Depression is a common problem. *Depression can be defined as an emotional reaction, altered mood state, and physical symptom complex accompanied by negative self-concept and lowered self-esteem and associated with regressive and self-punitive wishes* (6). Hippocrates first described depression and called it *melancholy* (51, 83).

A longitudinal study by M. M. Weissman and J. K. Myers reviewed 1095 subjects; 18 percent of the subjects were moderately depressed (106). Rates of the depression were highest in women less than 35 years of age; lowest rates were in men less than 35 years. Depression also increased among those with disadvantaged life situation—poor, uneducated, and unemployed persons (106). J. Mendels found 5 percent of adults significantly depressed at some time in their lives (67). Thirty-eight percent of an elderly population admitted to the hospital for the first time had a depressive disorder (18). Depression is also a problem in adolescence and childhood, although it may be masked. It is a major health problem because of the numbers affected, the reduced productivity, the intense experience of psychic pain, and human suffering endured by the person (95). You can often see the pain if you look for it.

The many faces of depression speak through drawn, taut expressions, stiff smiles, hopeless and helpless looks, angry frowns, and sorrowful weeping. Many other signs and symptoms also have depression as the underlying factor, as shown by the following case:

> Mrs. B. was a woman in her late forties. Her face was somber and sad. Her forehead was pinched and tight. Her eyes were downcast; her mouth was taut. She spoke of negative topics and seldom laughed. She stated she felt heavy, as if she were carrying a weight. She felt useless, alone, and without hope. This feeling was most severe in the morning but improved during the day. She complained of sleeplessness, increasingly poor appetite, and a clutching, viselike pain in her chest. She saw her family doctor frequently for such symptoms as headaches, leg cramps, back pain, and fatigue.

This chapter will help you to differentiate

between normal grief work and different types of pathological depression, to recognize the many overt and masked symptoms, and to intervene appropriately.

ETIOLOGY OF DEPRESSION

Freud, in *Mourning and Melancholia,* described the cause of depression as a turning inward of angry, ambivalent feelings that are directed toward a lost love object (38).

K. Abraham described manic-depressive illness as he compared normal grief with depression. He built upon Freud's psychosexual stages of development, stating that adult depression was a reenactment of the strivings of the infantile loss during the oral phase (1). R. Spitz wrote about anaclitic depression of the infant who failed to thrive, which manifested itself in protest, despair, and detachment (96). M. Klein spoke of depression as a position of development the child must resolve. She described this as a normal depressive position of sadness, fear, and guilt when the child becomes angry, hating the good mother. With this anger there is a fear of destroying the mother, who is also loved. Guilt and loss of self-esteem result (53). Edward Behring saw the loss of self-esteem as the vital element in depression, and Therese Benedik described the depressive constellation as a state of emotional relationship between mother and child (67).

S. Arieti and J. R. Bemporad posed three basic underlying patterns initiated early in life that later in adult life created a vulnerability to depression (4). These are:

1. *Dominant other*—The person relies on others to give meaning and esteem to self and life. Characteristic behavior includes being manipulative, clinging, passive, and fearful of anger.
2. *Dominant goal type*—The person relies on achievement of high goals. This person has always been pressed by the parents and has difficulty with self-imposed objectives. Characteristic behavior includes overachieving and feeling that the reaching of goals will satisfy fantasies of importance. The person manifests seclusive, arrogant, and obsessive behavior.
3. *Chronic depressive feelings*—The person is unable to develop deep relationships, has few gratifications, and constantly feels hopeless and empty. Characteristic behavior includes

periods of depression and feeling that life is meaningless.

Researchers have also noted a significant family tendency in depression, particularly the bipolar illnesses, such as manic-depressive psychosis (32, 49).

Many writers, however, continue to believe depression stems from environmental and childhood experiences (30, 76). The well-known writings of M. A. Cohen et al. documenting the life histories of twelve manic-depressive patients in middle-class American families revealed a strong sense of duty, punishment through shaming, and emphasis on conformity and achievement as influential in the illness (22).

The studies of Arieti and Bemporad found that characteristically the family of the depressed person had one dominant parent, with the rest of the family in a submissive role with little tolerance for differences from an expected norm. In all cases, the depressed clients had experienced a nurturance during childhood that changed into a conditional love being given for good behavior. Parents were characteristically critical and moralistic toward the child (4).

Several studies have found that parental loss before seventeen years of age increases the development of neurotic depression (15, 88). Alec Roy studied 102 depressed patients: 39 had parental loss before seventeen years of age (27 losses were by separation and 12 by death). Nondepressed psychiatric patients were used as controls. The study found that parental loss creates a vulnerability point specific to depression (88).

Other studies have researched social factors in depression. Studies by T. Harris showed that level of intimacy, employment, number of children at home, and early loss of mother were significant in development of depression (45).

Dr. Aaron Beck of the Depression Research Unit at Philadelphia General Hospital emphasized that all people have a certain pattern or framework of thinking (6). His clinical observations reveal that depressed people have abnormal thinking patterns. He analyzed their primary thinking patterns and characterized them as having: low self-regard; ideas of deprivation, self-criticism, and self-blame; exaggerated ideas of duty and responsibility; frequent self-command and injunctions; and escapist and suicidal wishes. From his theories and other behavioristic theories, certain cognitive and behavior therapies were developed for the treatment of depression. These therapies are directive, structured, goal-directed, and time-limited. They encourage the client in active collaboration and behavioristic techniques combined with homework skill assignments (55).

Currently the majority of publications on depression emphasize the biological approach. Numerous studies have shown a biological cause of depression, with a number of biological changes occurring in the metabolism related to the adrenocortical hormone, electrolytes, calcium, and biogenic amines. Temperature and other changes also occur (57, 67, 69).

The successful use of drug therapy gives some credit to the theory that some depression is caused by some kind of biochemical changes. Certain drugs contribute to feelings of depression. Reserpine, used for high blood pressure in the 1950s, frequently caused depressive symptoms. In contrast, Iproniazid given to tuberculous patients caused euphoria. Research concluded these drugs affected the neurotransmitters in the brain, the chemicals that carry impulses from cell to cell. Iproniazid increased the neurotransmitters; reserpine depleted them. Some antidepressants used today block the action of the enzyme monoamine oxidase that breaks down norepinephrine. Tricyclic antidepressants prevent breakdown of serotonin, another neurotransmitter (25). Further research is needed to differentiate whether chronic stress experiences cause changes in the cortisol and norepinephrine metabolism.

The classification and terms used in depression can be confusing. Table 15-1 summarizes the descriptive terms used by various authors.

TABLE 15-1.   Classification of Depressive States

CLASSIFICATION BY	TYPES OF DEPRESSION	
Etiology	*Exogenous* Symptoms from reaction to loss; cause outside of person. Reaction to loss excessive in duration and degree because of meaning of loss.	*Endogenous* Symptoms without overt precipitating cause. Due to multiple factors, including long-time faulty life patterns, hormonal, nutritional, chemical imbalance, other disease status.
Symptom	*Reactive* Symptoms a reaction to bereavement. Person more responsive to psychotherapy.	*Endogenous* Symptoms autonomous, without obvious cause. Research concerning biochemical disturbance being done. More evidence of family history. Person more responsive to somatic treatment (electroshock and drug therapy).
Activity	*Retarded* Reduced motor or cognitive function.	*Agitated* Psychomotor restlessness.
Mood Change	*Unipolar* One extreme only of mood, usually depression.	*Bipolar* Circular mood swings of elation (mania) alternating with depression.

TABLE 15-1.   Continued

CLASSIFICATION BY	TYPES OF DEPRESSION	
Reality testing	*Neurotic* Aware of reality. Inappropriate response in relation to feelings about self. No secondary symptoms.	*Psychotic* Inappropriate or faulty aware-ness of reality in relation to self, others, and the environ-ment. Secondary symptoms of delusions and hallucinations.
History	*Primary* First episode; no known psychi-atric history of depression. De-pression major problem.	*Secondary* Previous episodes of psychiatric depression. Depression re-sponse to another illness.
Disease entity according to *DSM-III*	Major affective disorders..	Manic episode. Major depressive episode.
	Bipolar disorder. Major depression. Other affective disorders.	Cyclothymic depressive neurosis.

Source: Murray, et al. *Nursing Process in Later Maturity* (Prentice-Hall; © 1980), Table 21.1. Used with permis-sion, Prentice-Hall, Inc., Englewood Cliffs, N.J.

THE MEANING OF DEPRESSION

Loss, separation from a loved object, a person, thing, status, or place to which the person is at-tached, is the most common precipitant of depres-sion. The loss may be real, such as loss of health, spouse, or job through retirement. The loss may be fantasized; e.g., the person may imagine that he/she is less attractive to others as aging occurs. The loss may also be symbolic; e.g., the person may feel less feminine after a hysterectomy or less masculine after a prostatectomy.

Differentiation between Grief and Depression

Grief and depression have been experienced by everyone to some degree. An acute depressive reac-tion occurs whenever there is crisis or loss, as discussed in Chapter 8. *Grief is the feeling of sad-ness related to an objective loss or separation; it occurs in predictable phases, varies in degree, and is self-limited.* The physical symptoms that accom-pany grief are not so intense or long in duration as the symptoms of depression. In grief the person

suffers less from a distorted self-concept or damaged self-esteem than in depression. The person's mood may shift from sadness to a more normal state when others show interest or new stimuli confront him/her. The person may be able to smile or laugh a little, respond briefly to something genuinely funny, and respond to reassurance and warmth. Friends and relatives usually feel interest in and empathy for the grieving person, but they may feel irritation with the depressed person because of the lack of response to them and the lack of an appar-ent reason for his/her depressed behavior. Depres-sion may be unrelated to a specific loss or to an objective situation. If the client does not receive help, a long-term perceived defect in self, with accompanying low feelings and related symptoms, is intensified as the person ages, and the depression becomes fixed. Refer to Chapter 8 for further dis-cussion of the grief-mourning process.

Dynamics of Depression

In depression, the person reacts to perceived loss

with intense feelings of decreased self-confidence, loss of self-esteem, and negative self-concept. The person feels damaged, diminished, worthless, and ashamed, and blames self for the loss or for what was not achieved, apparently because of long-established high ideals and expectations of self. An important part of the self is gone; a feeling of emptiness occurs. The person experiences feelings of rejection, abandonment, and loneliness related not only to this loss but also to past losses, past failures, or past experiences with important people. Further, anger at the lost object for deserting him/her is intense, although the anger is repressed because of guilt feelings. Perception of self becomes increasingly distorted; finally relationships with others and the ability to function in daily living become ineffective (7).

An example of this cycle was seen in the man who became severely depressed after the death of his wife. He frequently commented, "She left me; she left me." His tone of voice and enunciation conveyed anger. Yet, he felt very guilty and ashamed because his anger was unacceptable to him. The resulting ambivalent, guilty, and angry feelings were turned inward into self-accusation and depression.

When the person perceives self as failing, when he/she thinks less of self and is angry, the adaptive abilities are diminished, and the person resorts to more primitive mechanisms to try to restore a sense of security and adjustment. He/she may withdraw from others; or deny depressive feelings or that anything has changed; or project anger onto others so that he/she conveys that others are angry with him/her. Or the person develops physical symptoms (somatization). The person may also respond with global anxiety, expressing it openly and to anyone, much as a young child does. Sarcasm, blaming, or criticism may be directed at another, especially when that other considers crying or other obvious expressions of sadness and anger as inappropriate (18).

ASSESSMENT OF THE DEPRESSED PERSON

When you first meet the person, he/she may not appear depressed and may even wear a smile. However, he/she does not usually look happy (50). Observe carefully the nonverbal behavior; listen to the manner of speech as well as to what is said; be aware of your own reaction. Continue your assessment over time so that you will be accurate.

As you interview, you may begin to feel depressed yourself; Depressive feelings can be sensed as easily as anxiety. Or you may feel apathetic or hopeless. Be alert to your feelings. Sometimes the client will deny feelings of depression, but your ability to sense your own feelings as well as the client's feelings may help you determine the nursing diagnosis.

Appearance

Notice the person's general appearance. Often the person's clothing and hair appear disheveled, as if they have received little attention. Clothing may be ill-fitting or somber in color. Facial makeup, if worn, is often not apparent or is sloppily applied. Shoes may be scuffed or inappropriate for the other clothing. Posture is stooped; movement is usually heavy and slow. Facial appearance is sad: dull expression, furrowed brow, worried frown, turned-down corners of the mouth, reddened eyes from crying. Weight loss, poor muscle tone, dry skin, weakness, and general malaise may be apparent. He/she may look ten years older than the chronological age. The person may have tears in his/her eyes as if ready to cry, or he/she may have frequent crying spells (39).

If the person is agitated, you will see rapid, restless, jerking movements and walk. He/she may wring his/her hands, cry without shedding tears, or laugh inappropriately. The skin may be scratched or bruised from picking at it. He/she may pull at his/her hair or clothes and may be unable to sit still while talking with you.

Nonverbal behaviors were found to be indicative of level of depression in a recent study. The most consistent behaviors that were noted as different from normal were duration and consistency of mouth smile, of body contact and body-focused movements, and of looking behaviors, with increased eye contact (50).

Verbal Response

Open the conversation with a broad statement; note how the person responds. Be conscious of the topics initiated. The client may ask, "What is the world coming to?'' or "Life isn't what it used to be, is it?''

The pace of conversation will be slow and halting, with long pauses between phrases or sentences. Do not hurry the client if responses include silence or agitation. There may be disinterest in you or in the interview. The person frequently loses the trend of the conversation or looks preoccupied, confused, or angry. He/she may lack the energy or motivation to talk or to recall events. Ask direct, simple questions, such as, ''Where do you live?'' or ''Where are you now?'' to determine his/her ability to answer. The client may give you a one-syllable answer very softly, or may look at you and shrug his/her shoulders. Yet, the person is capable of answering if given time; the depressive person thinks very slowly.

In acute reaction to loss, less emotional upset and less verbal retardation are seen (59).

Physical Symptoms

During the interview the client may have many physical complaints. Some of these symptoms may be related to the person's depression since depression is a systemic disease. As emotional processes slow down, so do autonomic, neuromuscular, chemical, metabolic, and circulatory processes. Thus, constipation and anorexia may be a problem. The depressed person may occasionally overeat; the elderly depressed person is less likely to overeat than is the young one. The depressed person may have dry mouth, headache, hypotension, weight loss, sleep disturbances, fatigue, and lowered libido. Vague aches and pains may rotate from one body site to another. The person may either have difficulty going to sleep or may awaken about 3:00 A.M. or 4:00 A.M.; therefore, he/she does not get the required amount of sleep. In psychotic depression, the person feels worse in the morning, with symptoms improving during the day. In neurotic depression, the person may feel better in the morning than later in the day. Or the pattern may be reversed; the person may be most depressed in the evening. Note the depressed insomniac's response to hypnotics, which is not the same as in other clients who suffer from sleep disturbances. Also barbiturates do not help the depressed person to sleep; rather, they may increase the depth of depression and even release feelings of suicide and

aggression against self (78). The person is normally depressed physically and emotionally by barbiturates; therefore, respiratory depression and confusion may be severe.

Since the slowing process is related to all body processes, the immune body system is also affected. The person is more susceptible to illness, including: colds, pneumonia, ulcers, urinary tract infections, viral infections, boils, decubiti, and other infectious illnesses. Thus, frequent infections may be another clue to a depressive state.

Since anxiety is many times a precursor of depression, the person may describe symptoms related to anxiety, such as muscular weakness, vague aches, tightness in the chest, stomach cramps, shaking, dizziness, palpitations, lump in the throat, sweating, and diarrhea. Anxiety tends to increase as the illness progresses and is the underlying force of agitation.

The depressed person may have hypochondriacal complaints that have no organic basis but mimic a specific illness. Since he/she is more prone to physical illness, complaints should be carefully evaluated. Differential diagnosis is important, but often in the depressed client the more you explore the symptoms, the less differentiated the illness appears to be (18).

The person may deny depressed feelings and may attribute his/her mood to the symptoms that he/she is experiencing. The client may say, "Nurse, this pain is sure getting me down." He/she cannot perceive that the depression is causing the physical symptoms. The client believes that the hopeless feelings are related to the lack of symptom improvement (18).

The person may have a *hypochondriacal preoccupation, a strong, intense, almost morbid preoccupation with health.* He/she frequently seems to be concerned with the gastrointestinal tract and cardiovascular system (17). The complaints may have a bizarre quality; the client may say that his/her organs are not working right, the brain is all upset, or pain is stirring up the bowels. Many times these complaints are the beginning of *nibilistic or somatic delusions, false ideas concerning bodily function or annihilation of self or organs.* The person may state, "My stomach is turned to stone," or "My heart is eaten away." A common statement today is, "Cancer is eating up my entire body."

In acute reaction to loss, physical symptoms and physical retardation will be less severe (59).

Masked Symptoms

Masked or *covert symptoms* are symptoms experienced by the client that appear to be something other than depression. Many people are likely to deny any symptom of depression as unacceptable. They feel that to have an emotional problem is weak or ungodly. However, physical symptoms may be acceptable to the client, family, and community. How do you feel about the person who complains of headache and stomach cramps? About the one you hear complaining of "feeling no good," who is crying and condemning self? A subtle rejection is frequently noted among professionals concerning psychological symptoms, and this attitude may be found even more so among the older generation of friends and family of the client. It is no wonder that at a time in life when it is normal and acceptable to have physical problems, the older client tends to express depression with physical complaints. These vegetative signs of depression, including anorexia, weight loss, constipation, amenorrhea, and insomnia, may be indicative of severe depression (47).

Behavior

The person's verbal response indicates the level of alertness, interest, and distorted thinking. The depressed person has little interest in the surroundings and neglects usual interests and responsibilities. The poverty of ideas is shown by limited conversational response. He/she has difficulty with concentration and is preoccupied with self and feelings. At times he/she may become mildly aggressive or agitated, but probably will not do anything impulsive unless it is a self-destructive act. In recent studies, depression was found to lower scores on the Wechsler Memory Scale, impair performance on psychological tests, and reduce short-term memory. Thus the depressed person may be misdiagnosed as cognitively impaired since persons with irreversible organic brain disease and depression have similar verbal response patterns and overt behaviors. In comparison to the depressed client, the person with cognitive impairment suffers greater confusion, becomes lost in words, and is unable to respond appropriately even when given time. Memory for remote or recent events is not intact. In the cognitively impaired person, you will observe emotional lability instead of the consistently dejected mood. Physical complaints are also less prominent. Further, the person is not so self-accusatory and suicidal as the depressed person (77).

Agitated behavior is very common with the severely depressed client. The person may pace, wring hands, pick at himself or herself, beg for support or reassurance, and appear totally miserable. It is not uncommon as you try to assess or understand the symptoms that the agitated client answers by begging you to help him/her to feel better. A basic problem is that in the attempt to gain relief from pain, the attention-seeking behavior of the client pushes away the people most needed.

Other symptoms, not easily recognized but having their source in the core problem of depression, relate to daily living. The person might be drawn away from religious beliefs, complain of an uninteresting job, break up relationships that have been meaningful, begin compulsive drinking or gambling, or get in frequent fights with friends and family members. The person may be uninterested in grooming and habits of body care that gave him/her a great deal of pleasure in the past. Some changes may be caused by the inability to concentrate or to make a decision. Sense of responsibility is usually reduced and energy level is low. Disinterest in self relates to negative self-concept and angry feelings toward the self.

Feelings

Note the person's affect. The depressed person's mood is very sad and dejected, as evidenced by appearance and behavior: irritability; lack of humor; apathy; exhaustion; disappointment in self; sense of shame; lack of self-confidence and self-respect; statements about being worthless, empty, and a burden to everyone; and blaming self for anything that goes wrong. He/she expresses ambivalence, pessimism, and hopelessness in most situations. Depression may be expressed in the following ways:

"I feel sad." (direct report)
"I feel heavy." (descriptive report)
"I feel stripped of pleasure." (action—depression report)
"I feel like a dragging chain." (metaphor—descriptive report)

The depressed person may know intellectually that he/she loves the family, but he/she cannot feel love for or attachment to them. He/she loses caring behaviors for the spouse, relatives, friends, pets, and home. The person may say, "I don't care about anything anymore," and feels no joy as he/she thinks of previous pleasures. The person has many fears, especially of being alone. These behaviors over a period of time tend to isolate him/her from others.

The depressed person expresses in every way loss of self-esteem and negative self-concept. The person may state that he/she is empty or vacant, in reference to *sense* of self. He/she looks at self in the mirror with disgust, criticizes or condemns self for insignificant behavior, and may say, "I feel so guilty," even when he/she has done no great misdeeds. The person may have made many important contributions but *feels* useless. Ask the person to tell you about recent events; he/she will select the saddest news to report. "Nothing is any good anymore. There's nothing left in life for me." He/she feels there is no future for self and that the world has no future either. The severely depressed patient may move beyond the negative self-feeling to self-destructive behavior.

In acute reaction to loss, the intensity of hopelessness, regression, self-criticism, self-depreciation, and suicidal motivation are less severe (59).

Other Symptoms

In a major depression, the symptoms just described may be manifested intensely and for a longer duration. A nursing history may reveal a labile personality characterized by depressive episodes. Other symptoms may also be present, including delusions, hallucinations, severe slowing (retardation) of emotional and physical processes, severe agitation, and intense, unrealistic, and morbid feelings of guilt and remorse (59). The person may say, "I have committed every sin in the world."

Table 15-2 summarizes symptoms of depression.

Symptoms of Depression with Suicide Ideation

Suicidal thinking can occur in a variety of life situations and mental illnesses. It is more prevalent in more severe forms of depression.

TABLE 15-2.   Summary of Symptoms of Depression

SOMATIC SYMPTOMS	WORK AND OTHER INTERESTS
Anorexia	Apathy about work
Fatigue	and learning
Muscle aches	Decreased work capa-
Lower libido	city
Insomnia	Social disinterest
Weight loss	Underestimates com-
Early morning awakening	petence
Diarrhea or constipation	
Vague pains	
Hallucinations	

MOTOR SYMPTOMS	MOOD
Agitation or retardation	Irritability
Seeks physical contact,	Seeks approval
proximity, or touch	Apathy
	Cries easily
	Feels sad
	Feels empty

IDEAS	FEELINGS
Cognitive processes	Anxiety
slowed	Guilt
Memory loss	Pessimistic
Self-preoccupation	Hopelessness
Focus on negative	Helplessness
aspects of life	Loneliness
Loss of insight	Fear
	Depersonalization
	Anger

Suicide is a direct purposeful action taken by a person to end his own life. Suicide is a significant health problem; it ranks second to accidents as the leading cause for loss of life in Americans under 24 years of age (100). Nine young people in 100,000 take their own life. Other statistics include (63, 81, 100):

1. Women attempt suicide two to three times more than men.
2. Men kill themselves more than women.
3. Minorities have a higher suicide rate than Caucasians.
4. Elderly persons are more likely to kill themselves than any other age group.
5. People experience significantly more stress in the months preceding suicide.

Depression is present in 80 percent of suicidal attempts in persons over 60 years, and 12 percent of the attempters will try suicide again within 2 years, usually in an identical setting (41).

Many factors contribute to suicide in the elderly: physical illness, perceived mental decline, intense loneliness, hopelessness, a deprived living situation and economic insecurity, and severe guilt reactions following loss of a loved one. Suicide may be seen as a way to rejoin deceased loved ones. The anniversary date of an important loss is frequently a time for a suicide attempt. In paranoid states the suicide may be an attempt to escape tormenting delusions. The person may attempt suicide as a way of controlling or beating death; suicide does not necessarily mean death to the person. Or the elderly person may try suicide in order to die while he/she is still physically and mentally able to be in charge of self, especially if there is a debilitating, terminal illness and the person is alone. Even if early moral and religious training taught the person that suicide is wrong, the belief that he/she has a right to choose when and how to die may overcome guilt feelings. The person may also attempt suicide to gain attention from loved ones who have abandoned him/her.

The most common internal conflicts in a suicidal person are those associated with murderous impulses toward a loved person arising out of actual or imagined rejection or abandonment (98). The person who has attempted suicide before, is alcoholic, or psychotic, has had recent surgery, has a depression that is lifting, is hypochondriacal, or is having sleep problems is likely to attempt suicide (40, 41). The more hopeless the person feels in any situation, the more likely he/she is to try suicide (7). The older white male is especially at risk because he reacts adversely to many situations that accompany aging (8).

Karl Menninger's theory of suicidal behavior is that people have a wish for revenge, a wish to kill; a wish to be killed, with feelings of hopelessness; and fantasies of death and reunion with a wish to die (68). A study based on this theory reported that the first two wishes decrease with age, but the third wish increases (33).

Rarely is suicide a gesture in the elderly person, who is more likely to succeed in suicide, especially if plans include a violent method and a note is left. He/she is more likely to use a truly dangerous method, such as taking coma-producing drugs, using cutting or piercing instruments, inhaling gas, jumping from heights, or attempting drowning (7, 41). However, less severe attempts also occur, including subtle methods of self-destruction, such as self-neglect, refusal to eat, and withdrawal, in which the person resigns self, stoically and undramatically, to die (98, 99). Other indirect self-destructive behaviors might include high-risk sports, destructive eating habits, gambling, smoking, drug use, and excessive drinking and eating (33).

Every person has at some time thought about suicide. Some have openly stated this wish. The depressed person who states the wish to die is certainly at high risk. Statements such as, "I am tired of living; I find no joy in going on; I want to die," or "I am no good; I am worthless; I want to kill myself," should be taken seriously. A death wish may also be stated in a more subtle form, such as, "You shouldn't bother about me; I'm a burden to everyone." Or, "Don't do anything special, nurse; it's over anyway." Encourage the person to talk. After listening to cues, and when he/she seems less anxious, gently ask, "Have you ever thought of taking your life?" If the answer is yes, ask if he/she is thinking of suicide now. You will not put suicidal ideas into the person's head by stating the word *death* or encouraging the person to describe feelings and plans. Learn of others who care for the person. Your invitation to share enhances your assessment and may reduce the chance of a suicide attempt. Respond with an empathic statement so that the client can see you as a helping person.

Depressed clients are usually ambivalent about the desire to die in spite of their overt attempts. In a research study investigating communication with family members of 134 elderly persons who had succeeded in taking their own lives, 60 percent of the elderly group had talked about committing suicide, but 25 percent of the listeners felt the communication was not serious (85).

If the person has a sense of ego integrity, life is worth defending against physical, social, and economic threats. But a lack of ego-integrity combined with a negative self-concept cause a sense of despair, hopelessness, and depression. Suicide may then seem to be the only answer.

A recent study in a small rural community with eight suicides found all of the people to be socially isolated, with negative self-esteem, a tendency to internalize feelings, and overly dependent on family (104).

Table 15-3 compares facts and myths about suicide (94).

TABLE 15-3.   Facts and Myths About Suicide

Myth:	People who talk about suicide don't commit suicide.
Fact:	Of any ten people who kill themselves, eight have given definite warnings of their suicidal intentions.
Myth:	Suicide happens without warning.
Fact:	Studies reveal that the suicidal person gives many clues and warnings regarding suicidal intentions.
Myth:	Suicidal people are fully intent on dying.
Fact:	Most suicidal people are undecided about living and dying, and they "gamble with death," leaving it to others to save them. Almost no one commits suicide without letting others know how he/she is feeling.
Myth:	Once a person is suicidal, he/she is suicidal forever.
Fact:	Individuals who wish to kill themselves are suicidal only for a limited period of time.
Myth:	Improvement following a suicidal crisis means that the suicidal risk is over.
Fact:	Most suicides occur within about three months after the beginning of "improvement," when the individual has the energy to put morbid thoughts and feelings into effect.
Myth:	Suicide strikes much more often among the rich—or, conversely, it occurs most exclusively among the poor.
Fact:	Suicide is neither the rich man's disease nor the poor man's curse. Suicide is very "democratic" and is represented proportionately among all levels of society.
Myth:	Suicide is inherited or "runs in the family."
Fact:	Suicide does not run in families. It is an individual pattern.
Myth:	All suicidal individuals are mentally ill, and suicide always is the act of a psychotic person.
Fact:	Studies of hundreds of genuine suicide notes indicate that although the suicidal person is extremely unhappy, he/she is not necessarily mentally ill.

NURSING DIAGNOSIS AND FORMULATION OF CLIENT-CARE GOALS

Nursing Diagnosis

Your *nursing diagnosis of depression with or without suicidal ideation* may include a childhood history of loss, disturbed family relationships, and a history of characteristic thought, personality, and behavior patterns that increase vulnerability to depression. Or there may currently be a crisis or loss to which the client is responding with an acute depression.

Other assessments that may contribute to the nursing diagnosis include:

1. Verbal responses indicating low self-esteem,

negative self-concept, guilt feelings, and self-accusation.

2. Varying degrees of altered mood state; feelings of dejection, hopelessness, helplessness, emptiness, and anger.

3. Changes in physical appearance and general health status in a negative direction.

4. Verbal responses and behavior indicating slowing of cognitive processes and inability to produce ideas.

5. Complaints of various physical symptoms and manifestation of physical signs that accompany depression, such as fatigue and low energy level in a variety of situations.

6. Decreased interest in personal, social, interpersonal, spiritual, financial, and occupational activities.

7. Statements of self-destructive wishes or plans.

Thus your nursing diagnosis relates to the quality, meaning, and degree of depression, which are expressed by a wide variety of signs and symptoms that are not always easily assessed (26).

Client-Care Goals

Long-term goals for the client could include the following:

1. Statements and behavior demonstrate acceptance of self and a positive self-concept.

2. Behavior with others shows appropriate interdependence.

3. Statements and behavior express hope and a desire to live.

Short-term goals could include:

1. Personal hygiene is managed without assistance.

2. Anger is expressed overtly toward an object that elicits the anger.

3. Physical symptoms are described less frequently and are less extensive over time.

4. Loss of or separation from the loved object is worked through realistically.

5. Strengths and limits are realistically spoken of and accepted; statements indicate an increase in self-esteem.

6. Guilt feelings are resolved and are not described out of proportion to an event.

7. Activities are resumed, or new activities as an outlet for feelings and as a means of fun are learned.

8. Feelings are expressed verbally to professional staff, and their meanings are resolved.

9. Statements and behavior express hope and a desire to live.

You may think of other goals as you care for the depressed client. The nursing interventions for each of these nine goals will be discussed in the next section.

NURSING INTERVENTIONS RELATED TO CLIENT-CARE GOALS

Nurses can use a variety of approaches from different theorists. Use of Second and Third Force theories, (the dynamic and humanistic approaches), with their emphasis on feelings, uniqueness of the person, relationships, and individual life process, offers a framework that is pertinent to nursing practice and is useful for promoting recovery in the client.

Interpersonal care, acceptance, and concern make up a major portion of intervention with the depressed person. You must genuinely care, but you must remain objective enough so that you are not manipulated or controlled by the emotional pain as you guide the client toward healthy patterns of behavior. The depressed person needs to feel

that he/she is the center of your care but not the center of the universe. This is a difficult position to try to attain.

Crisis intervention principles apply to the suicidal person. Refer to Chapter 8 for further information.

Self-Awareness of Nurse as a Basis for Promoting Self-Awareness of Client

How do you feel about yourself when you are with the depressed person? How do you respond to someone who is obviously blue? How do you respond to someone who complains about many physical problems? How do you react to anger? Are you afraid of someone who is angry? Can you deal with your own anger in such a way that the depressed person will be able to accept his/her own anger and express it? Are you able to control your expression of elation and pleasure? Do you recognize that your optimism and cheerful statements can increase the client's depression? Do you attempt to define your goals for each interaction? Do you look forward to helping and listening? As you listen to the depressed person talk about loss, you may feel your own unresolved losses. Or you may feel sad about your own aging or the potential loss of loved ones. Look at yourself first. If you don't, you will have difficulty helping the depressed person look at him/herself.

Goals and Interventions

Goal I: Personal hygiene is managed without assistance.

Intervention

General hygiene will be maintained when the person begins to feel better about self and regains physical and emotional energy. Personal appearance becomes disheveled, and personal hygiene is omitted because of decreased interest in the body, lowered energy level, feelings of worthlessness, less interest in the reactions of others, agitation with hyperactivity, and decreased self-esteem. When the depression lifts, interest in appearance and hygiene will return, along with feelings of self-esteem and worth, which are related to appearance and cleanliness. To encourage a neat appearance seems to encourage the recovery process.

A severely depressed person will be unable to care for self and will need you to care for basic needs and make decisions. At first you may have to give oral hygiene, hair care, nail care, the bath, apply lotion to dry skin, and protect pressure areas. You may have to choose and assemble hygiene articles and clothing. Work through your feelings about caring physically for the dependent adult. Your approach must be nonpunitive; encourage self-directive, independent behaviors when the client is able to help himself/herself.

Goal 2: Anger is expressed overtly toward an object that elicits the anger.

Intervention

A primary element in the feelings of most depressed people is anger. Anger may be manifested in combative, defiant, teasing, sarcastic, obstructive, passive, withdrawn, agitated, or self-destructive behavior. Do not avoid this person and his/her anger. Encourage talking about angry feelings rather than having the person act them out behaviorally. You may first have to tell the person that you sense there is anger about something and that you would like to hear about it. The client's response may be to sneer, to make a sarcastic remark denying anger, to withdraw, or to curse. He/she may be unable to accept the anger. If you show acceptance of anger and of him/her and wait patiently, remain close, and continue to encourage talking, he/she will probably burst forth with angry statements. Since you invited expressions of anger, you must be prepared to hear it out, which can take time. Do not take anger personally, even if the person makes derogatory statements about you. Recognize the underlying causes and that the anger is turned against someone with whom the person feels safe. This is not an easy process because most of us were taught to suppress anger or to express it indirectly. Indirect expression, however, does not provide for self-understanding or for a full release of feelings, but rather promotes a deeper depression.

After the person has talked about angry feelings and what is considered to be the cause, be calm and supportive. Do not appear critical or distant toward the person because of what he/she has said, for if you do, he/she will probably no longer share with you, or perhaps with any other professional, in the future. Gently encourage the client to continue exploring causes for feelings until he/she can get back to the initial cause or loss. State that you understand the feelings, even if anger seems inappropriate in response. If the person is casting blame or making unrealistic statements, you can gradually clarify them. If mutual feelings of trust, respect, and caring exist between the two of you, the person will be able to listen as you present another viewpoint. You may gradually be able to help him/her understand how angry behavior has kept loved ones away, further adding to his/her problems. You may be able to suggest ways to reestablish relations with loved ones.

The principle of reinforcement of appropriate behavior can work over a period of time in this situation. You reinforce the person's expression of feelings by continuing to seek out, invite statements, and listen. As anger lessens, you can suggest other ways to get his/her needs met. You recognize verbally the attempts to change behavior and to look at self and others in a new way. Thus, you reinforce continued growth. But he/she is also reinforcing self. As responses to other people change, these others will change their responses to him/her in a positive direction. The person begins to feel better about self. Feelings of worthlessness and being bad or fears of aloneness diminish because others are showing care and affection. This circular process takes time and is completed to varying degrees, depending on how long and how severely the person has been depressed. If he/she has been a pessimistic person with depressive tendencies for a long time, change will be slow in coming. The person will also have to feel motivated to change behavior. Yet, people need people, and the depressed person is no exception. Your concern and assistance can motivate new behaviors, and with results and feeling better about self, the person will become motivated from within.

Some people may be unable to express anger and to go through the process described above, either because of personal beliefs forbidding such expression, aphasia, brain damage, or various physical, emotional, and social reasons. Here you can help express anger through constructive activities that can be physically managed, such as hammering, painting, squeezing play-dough or clay, walking, singing, working on a loom, scrubbing floors or walls, or digging in the garden. Activity provides some release, and your attitude of respect, acceptance, encouragement, and care helps the person feel better about self. In turn, he/she may respond less angrily toward others.

Sometimes the person can only talk about feelings indirectly. Thus anger will be expressed by complaining about the food, hospital, staff, relatives, or various world events. Your helpful response will be to follow the process in the above section.

Goal 3: Physical symptoms are described less frequently and are less extensive over time.

Intervention

Whether or not the depressed client's physical symptoms are directly related to the depression or are a manifestation of denial and masked depression, he/she is usually very disturbed and preoccupied with them. The pain or physical problems are real to him/her. Usually, the client does not understand the relationship between physical complaints and depression.

At first, listen to complaints fully and intently. This may help you establish rapport. Also help the person to be as comfortable physically as possible. Your attention to his/her needs conveys understanding and hope. Explain that the physical symptoms can be a manifestation of depression, that there is a good chance for improvement and that depression is a time-limited illness—it comes to an end. Say that by your both working together, many of the symptoms will disappear. Encourage the idea that you are an ally, a partner in care. Then the emotional emphasis related to the symptoms should begin to diminish.

A behavior modification approach may be used. The client's expression of feelings and interest in activities, people, and living is reinforced with positive responses. Preoccupation with self and bodily symptoms is given no response or only minimal matter-of-fact attention. Be careful that your responses are not phony or that you do not become mechanized in your reaction to the client. You will need to give treatment to some of the symptoms, but do not focus on them. Further, do not ask, "How are you?" as an opening remark because a question like this only encourages statements of physical complaints. Instead, try to direct the conversation to the emotional state, to important past experiences, or to involvement with present interests.

Your goal of emphasizing the emotional impact upon the person's life does not mean that the physical areas should be ignored. Expert care should be given to all areas of difficulty. The individual may be too depressed or too listless to eat or too agitated to take the time to eat, or he/she may refuse food in a suicidal attempt or gesture. Organic changes may result. Record the amount of intake, and determine whether there is any problem of malnutrition. Observe the ability to chew. Offer favorite foods in an attractive setting and sit while he/she eats. Often as you drink a beverage, the client will begin to eat as if imitating you. Encourage the person to set up a timetable around eating habits. Small, frequent meals may be helpful; a large quantity may not be appetizing. Give nutritional supplementary feedings. Encourage a well-balanced diet with plenty of fluids. Evaluate the need for natural laxatives (raw or bulk foods) since constipation is a common complaint. Encourage physical exercise and activity early in the day if possible. Also encourage certain chores or activities to increase appetite. To promote adequate nutrition, you must individualize the care according to the client's particular desires, needs, and activities.

Many depressed clients are preoccupied with defecation and bowel problems. They experience irregularity and constipation because of the slowed body processes. The lack of activity and minimal fluid intake increase the problem. Regression in some clients can cause soiling, incontinence, or retention. The manic or agitated depressive may be too active or preoccupied to take the time for elimination. Encourage a time for elimination. Keep a record.

Laxatives and enemas should be used only when necessary because of their habit-forming effect. Further, consider the meaning of the enema to the depressed person. Although the procedure may sometimes be seen as help from a concerned staff, it may also mean a well-deserved punishment, an invasion, a sexual attack, or a way of control. Enemas may become a part of a delusional system: ''My bowels are stone and closed; that tube will kill me.'' Feelings of fear and suspicion can be the result of a staff concerned only with the physical problem and the means to solve it. The more the client is made a partner in solving the problem, the more he/she will feel in control.

A common symptom of depression is sleep disturbance. The severely depressed person may have difficulty falling asleep or may wake up early; the agitated person may be too active to rest. Explore usual sleep patterns and sleep difficulties. Ask the patient what sleeping means to him/her. The person may fear falling asleep and having horrible dreams. Ask what he/she dreams about. If dreams are filled with fears and are laden with

emotion, perhaps talking about some of the fears will be helpful. Discuss ways to facilitate sleep. He/she may have to adjust the daily schedule to meet individual needs. The person should be sufficiently tired, but not too exhausted to sleep. A rest period during the day may be helpful. Light rather than strenuous activity in the evening may prevent exhaustion. If able, the person should adjust the environment to enhance rest and sleep: a quiet room, soft music, or a lighted or darkened room. You may help with muscle relaxation techniques. Or you might try a warm bath, milk, tea, soup, or whatever the person has used before. Talk softly to the person in a relaxing tone. Touch soothingly. A back rub is frequently very effective in promoting rest and sleep.

Sleep is important to restore energy. Sedatives and hypnotics may be given. However, at times giving barbiturates may distort dreaming, cause confusion, prolonged drowsiness, and deeper depression. Paradoxical stimulation may occur so that the person is awake and agitated all night. Other dangers include: (1) falls or incontinence because of the lethargic, confused state, (2) headache and irritability the following day, (3) fearfulness because of the nightmares that may occur with drugged sleep, (4) tolerance so that an increasing dosage is needed, (5) allergic reactions, and (6) dependency and addiction.

Some doctors recommend giving the full day's dosage of a tranquilizer or antidepressant at bedtime so that the person sleeps well, awakens refreshed, and remains tranquil during the following day. Table 15-4 summarizes the commonly used nonbarbiturate sedatives and related nursing responsibilities. Always be aware that any of these drugs may excite rather than quiet the person, however rarely you see that reaction.

Certainly nursing measures to induce sleep are preferable to the use of drugs.

Goal 4: Loss of or separation from the loved object is worked through realistically.

Intervention

Identification of the loss itself and its resolution comes with the person's response to your relationship, therapeutic communication, and time. Listen for negative feelings related to specific events or subjects. The person may have suffered

TABLE 15-4.   Nonbarbiturate Sedatives/Hypnotics

DRUG	DOSE	SIDE EFFECTS	NURSING RESPONSIBILITIES
Glutethimide (Doriden)	0.1–0.5 gm per os	Nausea. Nonpruritic skin rash. Headache. Dizziness. Stupor. Peripheral collapse rarely occurs.	Use nursing measures to prepare patient for sleep. May be given late at night because of short action and minimal hangover. Assist patient if he gets up after taking medication. Give judiciously; may be habit-forming. An overdose may cause deep sleep or coma lasting up to 72 hours. May not be suitable for suicidal patients.
Methaqualone (Quaalude)	150–300 mg orally	Mild and transient side effects. Headache. Dizziness. Nausea and epigastric distress. Dry mouth.	Prepare for sleep. Give only at bedtime. Limit activity after medication is taken; assist as necessary. May potentiate suicidal tendencies.
Ethchloroynal (Placidyl)	100–150 mg orally	Mild side effects. Bad dreams. Headaches. Ataxia. Dizziness. Nausea and vomiting. Unpleasant taste in mouth. Confusion.	Prepare for sleep. Store medication in dark, tight container. Give glass of fluids with drug to delay absorption and minimize dizziness or confusion. Discontinue drug slowly to prevent untoward effects.
Flurazepam hydro-chloride (Dalmane)	15–30 mg orally	Ataxia, vertigo, and falling, especially in the elderly.	Prepare for sleep. Observe for unsteadiness. Use safety precautions.

Source: **Murray, et al.** *Nursing Process in Later Maturity* (Prentice-Hall; © 1980), Table 21.2. Used with permission, Prentice-Hall, Inc., Englewood Cliffs, N.J.

loss or deprivation, then covered the feeling related to the loss and forgotten or repressed the precipitating event (16). Try to connect the present with past events. If anything significant is uncovered, talk with the client about the event when the time is appropriate. It is not enough for you to be aware of his/her loss; the client must also understand.

To learn that the client has lost a son, a home, or a spouse usually takes very little time. However, it may take much longer to prepare him/her to deal with the experience. Treat this suffering person tenderly. As you would not apply salt to a reddened infected wound, neither should you confront this wounded psyche with painful information too fast or without a caring attitude. The time for confronting the person about the meaning of loss depends on the closeness of your relationship, on the nurturing attitude of others in the environment, and on his/her personality strengths. There is probably no perfect time to talk about feelings, but your client must be able to attend. The person will not be shattered by what you say if your statement is gentle and conveys concern. Encourage the person to talk; a client often will repeat the same things everytime you meet with him/her. But resolution of feeling is not possible until one talks about them. Talking is difficult for this person, but eventually it provides a release.

For example, Mr. B. may know that his wife's death caused his depression, but he needs help in talking about what his wife meant to him, the role she had in his life, and how he feels about himself. He needs help in exploring new patterns of living so that he does not rigidly hold onto the depression.

Goal 5: Strengths and limits are realistically spoken of and accepted; statements indicate an increase in self-esteem.

Intervention

One of the most crucial areas is how the person feels about self (65). Usually the depressed person has damaged self-esteem and feels of no value. First of all, this destructive concept of self needs to be recognized by the person—if possible. You may think that the person recognizes these feelings. However, he/she may just *feel* all the depressive feelings and not have the slightest understanding that they apply to himself or herself. The person in the depths of depression has great difficulty seeing the unreality of his/her thoughts. Instead, he/she experiences feelings of being ugly, bad, homely, and hopeless, and undeserving of food, space, or life.

Remind the person that most of these feelings are caused by the depressive illness. Repeatedly state that the feelings do not represent his/her *true* self, and that he/she should work with you to overcome the illness and to feel better. You may say to your client, "I understand that it is hard to recognize these feelings as the result of the depression, but try to see that many of your ideas are unfounded."

Your acceptance of the person also conveys that the person is valued. Many times, however, the client will think that you are just being nice because it is your job. Yes, caring is your job. However, it is also your job to be honest and genuine and to do what is best for the person. You can help the

person to trust you, accept your humanness, and thus grow to accept self.

Insight comes when the person can appreciate you as a helping, unique person, not as a god or all-knowing supernurse, and when he/she can appreciate self as a worthwhile person, not a helpless, useless being. Such understanding comes gradually as you listen to physical complaints, provide needed physical care, convey your honest feelings, and spontaneously share a joke, a sunset, or a holiday. Through experiences of human warmth the person can be helped to accept his/her own human dignity and worth. In turn, he/she will learn to trust and respect others.

You do not help the client gain self-esteem by just putting your arms around him/her and saying you care. If you compliment too early, feelings of being overwhelmed occur. The client does not feel your warmth. He/she feels that you are not being honest. The repeated honest appraisal of strengths through the recognition of an activity done well helps improve feelings about self. Watch the person's reaction when you recognize strengths. The client may blush, frown, look away, or laugh. If he/she accepts your statement without rebuff, you will know that he/she is beginning to accept your feedback. Move ahead cautiously, always evaluating the effect of your interactions. After a while the answer may be, "If you think I'm OK, maybe I am." Eventually the person will feel positive about self even when no one is continually supporting him/her. At that point the person has recovered from the illness.

Goal 6: Guilt feelings are resolved and are not described out of proportion to an event.

Intervention

Guilt feelings are resolved slowly. Guilt is influenced by the standards and ideals of the person. Most people have been raised in an environment that promoted a strict conscience. Depressed people are notorious for having strict, unrelenting rules for themselves and their lives. Thus, the depressed person looks at self in a depreciating, accusatory manner, and blames himself for not living up to standards of perfection and for losses or problems. The person may feel that he/she is being punished for being bad or worthless and that the feelings surrounding depression are deserved. Anger arises when expectations about self are not kept, and ultimate feelings of guilt result.

There are times when talking about the person's feelings of anger and thoughts about self-expectations will alleviate the guilt. As the person talks, he/she will realize the futility of strict standards and that lowering self-expectations is acceptable. The goal is to see reality in a new perspective and to blame self less for events. Your listening and realistic feedback can help moderate expectations of self and others. Your acceptance of human weakness and failure may help him/her to accept personal limits. The following statements will be helpful: "You are awfully hard on yourself." "You deserve better treatment than that." "You seem to be blaming yourself for just being human." Your surprised expression upon hearing the client blame self, yet showing an understanding feeling, will be important. You may say, "I realize that it is difficult for you, but try not to hurt yourself for something over which you have little control." Never hesitate to give encouragement and praise for any efforts, including personal hygiene, feeding of self, or various activities.

Many times the person feels that God is blaming him/her for sins and errors. Convey empathy. Confront perfectionism. Speak of God's love if appropriate. Attend to spiritual needs yourself or seek the assistance of a clergyman. The depressed person often turns away from religious life as the depression increases. He/she may feel punished. The person may believe that God is a just, kind God, and that such a God would not punish; he/she therefore reasons that since he/she is depressed, there must not be a God. Or the depressed person who has always been a faithful churchgoer and led a religious life may now believe that he/she is being punished for being good; therefore, God is not just, and he/she either blames God or says that God does not exist. Many were taught by their religion to believe that man is a sinful creature, so suffering is what is deserved, and punishment for sins is appropriate. There may be varying degrees of added guilt caused by the recent turning away from a lifetime of religious beliefs. It is not your place to convert the person or to say what to believe, but you can help him/her find a comfortable and productive spiritual position. If you have an understanding of the person's religious beliefs, you may counsel him/her, or you can collaborate with a minister, priest, or rabbi who understands the ill-ness of depression and can convey love rather than judgment (100).

Goal 7: Activities are resumed, or new activities as an outlet for feelings and as a means of fun are learned.

Intervention

Interest in activities and other people is a sign of emotional health. Your client may be so caught up with self and personal sorrow that there is little energy left to be involved with others. Your relationship and activities with a client can stimulate his/her interest in others. However, do not become so involved in activity yourself that you forget that the project is only a means to an end. The activity is the means for the client to establish a relationship, to invest interest in someone other than self, and to increase self-esteem through a job well done. If your ultimate goal in activity with a client is to make a doll, play a game or take a walk, then nothing much is being accomplished.

Choose activities that reflect the individual's interest. If the person is severely depressed, has a short attention span, and is easily fatigued, the activities should be simple. Many times the person will want to make something for someone else, maybe a granddaughter or grandson. Some people become involved willingly in a menial task because it helps to displace anger and guilt. If the client is severely agitated, the activity should productively use restless energy, such as tearing rags to make a rug or making a flower garden for later bouquets. If the client is restless, the activity should not be stimulating or overwhelming, and it should have definite limits. In every activity, encourage the contact of others in order to counteract the loneliness so prevalent in the depressed person.

Goal 8: Feelings are expressed verbally to professional staff and their meanings are resolved.

Intervention

Through your humanistic approach, listening, caring, and the interventions described in relation to the other goals, you enable the client to increasingly describe rather than act out feelings. As he/she gains communication skill, relationships with others—at home, on the job, and in the community—are improved. As the person gains insight into the meaning behind behavior and feelings, and is encouraged to apply these insights to all of life, self-awareness and emotional health are enhanced.

Goal 9: Statements and behavior express hope and a desire to live.

Intervention

Goal 9 is both a short- and long-term goal. Prevention of suicide must be the immediate goal for the personnel if the client makes suicidal gestures or statements. But helping the person *feel* that life is worth living is the ultimate goal.

Find inner controls to prevent suicide. Your supportive, warm relationship to the person is a powerful deterrent to suicide. The more involved you can be with the client as a person, and the more you convey wanting to help, the less the chance that he/she will try to commit suicide.

Listen; try to see life as the person sees it. Hear the anger and give direct, structured support. Let the person know that you understand that he/she is suffering and that life seems so painful that it is no longer worth living. Say that you do not think that the person is bad because he/she is thinking of suicide. Tell him/her that you recognize these ideas as part of the illness. Convey the thought that you care, perceive strengths, want to help, and that together the two of you can work to improve the situation. You may need to make yourself available by phone as well as directly.

Consider any statement about suicide from the person as a cry for help. Give any gesture or statement serious consideration. Realize that while the person is overtly withdrawing from any help, at the same time he/she is hoping that someone will find the answers to his/her problems. Getting the person to say the words that have been kept hidden often brings relief. And these statements also give you a chance to convey your intention to help and to show your respect for the person. Often you can stimulate others in the environment to show more interest. You may also be able to secure practical help to overcome various economic, social, or health problems.

If the suicidal person tells you that he/she will contact you when he/she feels the impulse to end life and prior to carrying out any plan, you have a safeguard against any suicidal attempt. A study of 600 persons who indicated to medical professionals that they had decided not to carry through their suicide plans showed no fatalities over a five-year span (29).

Certainly safeguards need to be taken to decrease dangers in the person's environment. At the same time, do not dwell on or be obsessive about these dangers. It is impossible to have the surroundings completely free of objects with which to commit suicide. *Your best safeguard is your relationship with the person.* Your next safeguards are your observation and caring. You can also carry out unobtrusive measures. Make your rounds at different times, not just at predictable hours. Keep the person with someone or in the group whenever possible. Observe carefully that he/she swallows the medications. Many patients pretend to swallow pills but actually accumulate them in order to have them available for an overdose. Listen carefully for clues to intentions. Even though you are cautious and take necessary precautions, you must also convey that you trust him/her. Discuss feelings and thoughts with the person frankly and on a continuing basis.

People who live alone, are depressed, and have little contact with helping others are the ones who are more likely to commit suicide. A community service program can reduce suicide in the elderly. In an English community, a program was begun to give a variety of assistance to the suicide-prone senior. The suicide rate dropped over 60 percent (104). Certainly any depressed person who has been hospitalized needs follow-up services after discharge to maintain improvement.

Responsibility of the Nurse in Somatic Treatments

Part of your responsibility in care of the depressed person is to assist with somatic treatments, such as electroshock treatment. Convulsive therapy began in 1927 with the use of Metrazol given intravenously to produce a seizure. It was helpful, but many complications and dangers existed. In 1938 an electric current was found to produce the same results but with far fewer difficulties. Since that time, electroshock (EST) or electroconvulsive

(ECT) therapy has been a major procedure in treatment of depression. (It is also used to reduce delusional thinking, to reduce activity in catotonic excitement, and with manic behavior in a schizoaffective illness.) The treatment consists of applying a current of 110 volts (20 to 30 milliamperes) to the temperofrontal region of the brain until there is evidence of a grand mal seizure. A short-acting barbiturate, such as sodium pentothal or Brevital, and a muscle relaxant, usually Anectine, are given intravenously to reduce the severity of the muscular reaction. The nervous system reacts to the stimulation with both the tonic first stage and the clonic second stage of seizure. Usually, the first stage is noted by facial twitching or the curling of the toes. Little more than a tremor follows. The electric stimulus causes unconsciousness; however, the suffocating effect of the current-like medication, Anectine, can create great fear and anxiety; thus, sodium pentothal or Brevital is also given. A physician is usually present during this procedure. However, many times nurses are responsible for administering the treatment. Usually the nurse is specially prepared and has experience in emergency treatments. At first you may find it difficult to observe or assist with this procedure. Talk to your instructor or supervisor about your feelings.

The risks of ECT treatments to most patients are few; 1 in 25,000 has an untoward reaction. Age is not a contraindication. If the person is suicidal, severely depressed, or agitated, the physician may order this treatment. Cardiac symptoms, hypertension, phlebitis, aneurysm, and multiple sclerosis are contraindications. With increased intracranial pressure ECT is never done. The person must have a thorough physical examination, an electrocardiogram, and a chest X-ray prior to treatment.

Major complications of ECT are fractured bones and strained muscles. Fractures are usually caused by the strength and weight of the large muscles jerking the bone in the spasm of the seizure. Cardiac arrhythmias are another major area of difficulty, especially in people with a prior history of cardiac disease. The other complications are memory loss and confusion, depending on the amount and number of treatments. The closer the treatments, the greater the confusion. Confusion and some memory loss are always expected with ECT; therefore reassure the person and family that the confusion is temporary. Memory usually returns in a week or two after treatment; however, sometimes impairments last from six to twelve months. Some individuals complain of permanent loss and reduced learning capacity.

You must give supportive care before and after the treatment. The person may ask many questions about the treatment and why it is necessary. Give information generally about what to expect. However, no one really knows why depression lifts after ECT. Listen to fears and try to alleviate anxiety. Touch is reassuring to the person; he/she may request that you go along to the area where the treatment is given. Hold the person's hand and talk until he/she is asleep. An airway must be maintained during the treatment and until respiratory function returns spontaneously. The client sleeps for a short time after treatment. During this 15- to 30-minute period, pulse, respirations, and blood pressure are taken until the client is responding and breathing regularly. As the person awakens, he/she will feel hazy and confused; this regressed period is an ideal time for nurturing. Further emotional support is needed until the person is fully awake, relaxed, and feels more secure (16).

Drug Therapy

Medications are widely prescribed for depression. Table 15-5 lists the tricyclic derivatives, which are the drugs most commonly used. Side effects and the nursing responsibilities are also given in the table.

Lithium carbonate has been used effectively with people with bipolar depression alternating with hypomanic states. Blood levels should be carefully monitored since clients sometimes stop taking the drug when they feel better. Few adverse reactions occur when serum lithium levels are below 1.5 mEq/1 liter of blood. However, long-term use can be toxic to the kidneys, causing permanent damage. Take this complication seriously. Renal function tests, urinalysis, and serum creatinine and blood urea nitrogen tests should be done at periodic intervals. These patients should be taught to keep in touch with professionals and report symptoms. Any excessive thirst, voluminous urine output, edema of extremities, weight gain, cloudy urine, or reduction in urine output should be reported (74, 81, 101). Also refer to Chapter 19 for further information on lithium.

TABLE 15-5. Antidepressants: Tricyclic Derivatives

DRUG	DOSE	SIDE EFFECTS	NURSING RESPONSIBILITIES
Amitriptyline (Elavil)	25–50 mg orally 2 to 4 times daily	This classification of drugs may cause dry mouth, nausea, and vomiting, constipation, weight gain, urinary frequency, confusion, insomnia, dizziness, hypotension, tachycardia, arrhythmias, tremor, bone marrow depression, agranulocytosis, jaundice, and Parkinsonism.	Observe for changes in mood while drug takes effect. Note suicidal ideas during therapeutic lag. Teach client about side effects. Teach mouth care and use of mints, gum, or ice chips for dry mouth. Check bowel and bladder elimination. Weigh weekly. Record intake and output. Use safety precautions. Take vital signs daily. Observe for early signs of granulocytosis; sore throat, fever, and malaise. Take monthly blood counts. Observe for jaundice of sclera and skin. Check with physician if signs of bone marrow depression, liver damage, or Parkinsonism. Do not administer with monoamine oxidase inhibitors.
Desipramine hydrochloride (Norpramin)	25–300 mg; 150 mg average; onset in 3–5 days.		
Doxepin (Sinequan)	25–300 mg; 75 mg average		
Nortriptyline (Aventyl)	25–300 mg; 150 mg average		
Protriptyline (Vivactil)	5–60 mg; 30 mg average		
Imipramine (Tofranil)	25 mg orally 1 to 3 times daily		

Source: Murray, et al. *Nursing Process in Later Maturity* (Prentice-Hall; © 1980), Table 21.3. Used with permission, Prentice-Hall, Inc., Englewood Cliffs, N.J.

Working with the Family and Health Team

Previous chapters have discussed the importance of working with family members and how to include them in care. Such intervention is equally important for the depressed person. Help the family understand the needs and behavior of the depressed person, especially while he/she is regressed or confused as a result of ECT. Help them realize this behavior is temporary. Furthermore, no care plan is successful unless all members of the health team who have contact with the client, including home health-care personnel, can plan and work together. When staff members share their assessments and suggestions for intervention, the client, family, and each staff member benefit. The person is not distressed by inconsistency or an inappropriate referral. Staff members also have a better understanding of the person and what they are doing.

EVALUATION

Although you cannot presume to make up for the many losses experienced by the depressed person, in a symbolic and practical way you can fill in some of the gaps.

Evidence of your effectiveness is shown in various behaviors. If the client becomes increasingly interested in the relationship, he/she may ask questions about your life, partly from curiosity and partly from wanting to reach out. Answer these questions briefly and then redirect the conversation to him/her. The person will soon show renewed interest in surroundings and community events, personal appearance, group activity, and family life. Appearance will be less dejected and anxious, with fewer or no comments about physical symptoms. The individual will be alert and mentally active and will make fewer self-depreciating remarks; he/she will smile, laugh, and find humor in life.

However, you should expect the change to be gradual. The recovery and maturing will come in spurts, and relapses will occur. Evaluate your attitude as time passes. Accept the person, assist in the progress, and avoid giving excessive approval when progress is apparent. It is a heavy load for any client to carry when the helper's mood is dependent on the client's progress. You are to be *for* the person, without strings, to care, and to be *with* him/her as progression occurs, to the extent the individual is capable at the time.

REFERENCES

1. Abraham, Karl, *Selected Papers on Psychoanalysis.* London: Hogarth Press Ltd., 1948.

2. American Psychiatric Association, Committee on Nomenclature and Statistics, *Diagnostic and Statistical Manual of Mental Disorders-III.* Washington, D.C.: American Psychiatric Association, 1980.

3. Anthony, James, and Therese Benedek, eds., *Depression during the Life Cycle.* Boston: Little, Brown & Company, 1975.

4. Arieti, S., and J. R. Bemporad, "The Psychological Organization of Depression," *American Journal of Psychiatry,* 137, no. 11 (1980), 1360–65.

5. Banks, Susan, "Agitated Depression," *Nursing Times,* 69 (September 27, 1973), 1250–51.

6. Beck, Aaron, *Depression, Causes and Treatment.* Philadelphia: University of Pennsylvania Press, 1967.

7. Beck, A. T. et al., "Hopelessness and Suicidal Behavior," *Journal of American Medical Association,* 234 (December 15, 1975), 1146–49.

8. Benson, R., and D. Brodie, "Suicide by Overdoses of Medicine among the Aged," *Journal of American Geriatric Society,* 23 (July 1975), 304–8.

9. Berndt, D. J., T. P. Petzel, and S. M. Berndt, "Development and Initial Evaluation of a Multiscore Depression Inventory," *Journal of Personality Assessment,* 44, no. 4 (1980), 396–403.

10. Bishop, Susan, "Depression," *Nursing Times,* 71 (October 2, 1975), 1567–69.

11. Braden, W., and C. K. Ho, "Racing Thoughts in Psychiatric Inpatients," *Archives of General Psychiatry,* 38, no. 1 (1981), 71–75.

12. Brearley, Paul, "The Deprivation Syndrome," *Nursing Times,* 71 (November 27, 1975), 1914–15.

13. Breslow, R., J. Koesis, and B. Belkin, "Contribution of the Depressive Perspective to Memory Function in Depression," *American Journal of Psychiatry,* 138, no. 2 (1981), 227–30.

14. ——, "Memory Deficits in Depression: Evidence Utilizing the Wechsler Memory Scale," *Perceptual and Motor Skills,* 51, no. 2 (1980), 541–42.

15. Brown, C. W., T. Harris, and R. Copeland, "Depression and Loss," *British Journal of Psychiatry,* 130 (1977), 1–18.

16. Burgess, Ann, and Aaron Lazare, *Psychiatric Nursing in the Hospital and the Community.* Englewood Cliffs, N.J.: Prentice-Hall, Inc., 1976.

17. Burgess, Helen, "When a Patient on Lithium Is Pregnant," *American Journal of Nursing,* 79, no. 11 (1979), 1989–90.

18. Busse, Ewald, and Eric Pfeiffer, *Mental Illness in Later Life.* Washington, D.C.: American Psychiatric Association, 1973.

19. Cassidy, W. et al., "Clinical Observations in Manic-Depressive Disease," *Journal of American Medical Association,* 164 (1957), 1535–46.

20. Chenitz, W. C., "Primary Depression in Older Women," *Psychiatric Nursing,* 17, no. 8 (1979), 20–23.

21. Clough, Dorothy, and Anayis Derdiarian, "A Behavioral Checklist to Measure Dependence and Independence," *Nursing Research,* 29, no. 1 (1980), 55–58.

22. Cohen, M. A. et al., "An Intensive Study of Twelve Cases of Manic Depressive Psychosis," *Psychiatry,* 11 (1954), 103–37.

23. Coin, A. C., and I. Fast, "Childrens' Reactions to Parent Suicide," in *Survivors of Suicide,* ed. A. C. Coin, pp. 93–111. Springfield, Ill. Charles C Thomas, Publisher, 1972.

24. Commer, Leonard, *Up from Depression.* New York: Simon & Schuster, 1969.

25. "Coping with Depression," *Newsweek,* January 8, 1973, pp. 51-54.

26. Crary, Williams, and Gerald Crary, "Depression," *American Journal of Nursing,* 73, no. 3 (1973), 472-75.

27. "Dealing with Depression," *Emergency Medicine,* 11, no. 24 (1979), 9.

28. Doherty, G., "The Patient in Pain: Handling the Guilt Feelings," *Canadian Nurse,* 75, no. 2 (1979), 31.

29. Drye, R., R. Goulding, and M. Goulding, "No Suicide Decisions: Patient Monitoring of Suicidal Risk," *American Journal of Psychiatry,* 130 (1973), 171.

30. Eaton, J. W., and R. J. Weil, *Culture and Mental Disorder.* New York: The Free Press, 1955.

31. Eggland, E., "Dealing with Tragedy, the Aftermath of Suicide," *Journal of Nursing Care,* 11, no. 12 (1978), 14-15.

32. Escaber, Jovier, "Cytogenetic Study of Bipolar Affective Illness," *Comprehensive Psychiatry,* 19, no. 4 (1978), 331-35.

33. Farberow, Norman, *The Many Faces of Suicide.* New York: McGraw-Hill Book Company, 1980.

34. Farberow, N., and E. Schneidman, eds., *The Cry for Help.* New York: McGraw-Hill Book Company, 1965.

35. Floyd, Gloria Jo, "Nursing Management of the Suicidal Patient," *Journal of Psychiatric Nursing and Mental Health Services,* 13, no. 2 (1975), 23-26.

36. Flynn, Gertrude, "The Development of the Psychoanalytic Concept of Depression," *Journal of Psychiatric Nursing and Mental Health Services,* 6, no. 3 (1968), 138-49.

37. Freeman, Ramono, *1980 Year Book of Psychiatry and Applied Mental Health.* Chicago: Year Book Medical Publishers, Inc., 1980.

38. Freud, Sigmund, *Mourning and Melancholia,* vol. 4, pp. 152-70, in *Collected Papers.* London: Hogarth Press Ltd., 1946.

39. Frost, Monica, "Depression—the Mental Cold," *Nursing Mirror,* 137 (1973), 46-47.

40. Fulton, R., and G. Geis, *Death and Identity.* New York: John Wiley & Sons, Inc., 1965.

41. Gage, Frances, "Suicide in the Aged," *American Journal of Nursing,* 71, no. 11 (1971), 2153-55.

42. Goldberg, E. L., "Depression and Suicide Ideation in the Young Adult," *American Journal of Psychiatry,* 138, no. 1 (1981), 35-40.

43. Greenacre, Phyllis, *Affective Disorders.* New York: International Universities Press, 1953.

44. Hamilton, Max, "Rating Depressive Patients," *Journal of Clinical Psychiatry,* 41, no. 12 (1980), 21-24.

45. Harris, T., "Social Factors in Neurosis with Special References to Depression," *Research in Neurosis,* ed. H. M. Van Praag. New York: Medical and Scientific Books, 1978.

46. Haynal, A., "Some Reflections on Depressive Affect," *International Journal of Psychoanalysis,* 59, nos. 2-3 (1978), 165-71.

47. Hofling, Charles K., and Madeleine Leininger, *Basic Psychiatric Concepts in Nursing.* Philadelphia: J. B. Lippincott Company, 1960.

48. Jacobson, Edith, *Depression.* New York: International Universities Press, 1971.

49. Johnson, C. F. S., and M. M. Leeman, "Ancestral Secondary Cases on Paternal and Maternal Sides in Bipolar Affective Illness," *British Journal of Psychiatry,* 133, no. 7 (1978), 68-72.

50. Jones, H., and M. Ponsa, "Some Nonverbal Aspects of Depression and Schizophrenia Occurring during the Interview," *Journal of Nervous and Mental Disorders,* 167, no. 7 (1979), 402-49.

51. Kendell, R. E., "The Classification of Depressive Illness," *Institute of Psychiatry Maudsley Monograph.* London: Oxford University Press, 1968.

52. Kicey, Carolyn, "Catecholamines and Depression: A Physiological Theory of Depression," *American Journal of Nursing,* 74, no. 11 (1974), 2018-20.

53. Klein, Melanie, *The Psycho-analysis of Children.* London: Hogarth Press Ltd., 1937.

54. Kline, N., "Practical Management of Depression," *Journal of American Medical Association,* 190 (1964), 732-40.

55. Kovacs, M., "The Efficacy of Cognitive and Behavior Therapies for Depression," *American Journal of Psychiatry,* 137, no. 12 (1980), 1495-1501.

56. Kraepelin, Emil, *Manic-Depressive Insanity and Paranoia,* trans, R. Mark Barclay and George Robertson. Edinburgh: E. & S. Livingstone Ltd., 1921, reprint 1976.

57. Kramer, B. A., and J. L. Katz, "Circadian Temperature Variation and Depressive Illness," *Journal of Clinical Psychiatry,* 39, no. 5 (1978), 439-44.

58. Large, S., "Reactive Depression: A Problem of Personality," *Nursing Mirror,* 149 (July 5, 1979), 44-46.

59. Laughlin, Henry, *The Neuroses.* London: Butterworth Co., 1967.

60. Leonard, Calista V., "Treating the Suicidal Patient: A

Communication Approach," *Journal of Psychiatric Nursing,* 13, no. 2 (1975), 19-22.

61. Lewis, A., "Melancholia: A Historical Review," *The State of Psychiatry: Essays and Addresses.* New York: Science House, 1967.

62. Lipman, R., L. Covi, and A. K. Shapiro, "The Hopkins Symptom Checklist (HSCL)—Factors Derived from the HSCL-90," *Journal of Affective Disorders,* 1, no. 1 (1979), 9-24.

63. Luscomb, Richard et al., "Mediating Factors in the Relationship between Life Stress and Suicide Attempting," *The Journal of Nervous and Mental Disease,* 168, no. 11 (1980), 644-48.

64. Lyons, D. C., "Endogenous Depression," *Nursing Mirror,* 139 (October 17, 1974), 93-94.

65. Mackinnon, Roger, and Robert Michels, *The Psychiatric Interview in Clinical Practice.* Philadelphia: W. B. Saunders Company, 1971.

66. McHugh, P., and M. Falstein, *Psychopathology of Dementia in Congenital and Acquired Cognitive Disorders,* ed. P. Katzman. New York: Raven Press, 1979.

67. Mendels, Joseph, *Concepts of Depression.* New York: John Wiley & Sons, Inc., 1970.

68. Menninger, Karl, *Psychoanalytic Aspects of Depression.* Springfield, Ill.: Charles C Thomas, Publisher, 1960.

69. "Metabolites in Depression," *Medical News Report,* January 7, 1980, p. 12.

70. Mitchell, Ross, "Depression," *Nursing Times,* 20 (July 11, 1974), 1085-87.

71. Moss, L. M., and D. M. Hamilton, "The Psychotherapy of the Suicidal Patient," *American Journal of Psychiatry,* 112, no. 4 (1956), 814-20.

72. Murray, Ruth, M. Marilyn Huelskoetter, and Dorothy O'Driscoll, *The Nursing Process in Later Maturity.* Englewood Cliffs, N.J.: Prentice-Hall, Inc., 1980.

73. Nelson, J. C., and D. S. Charney, "The Symptoms of Major Depressive Illness," *American Journal of Psychiatry,* 138, no. 1 (1981), 1-13.

74. Neu, C., T. Manschreck, and J. Flacks, "Renal Damage Associated with Long-Term Use of Lithium Carbonate," *Journal of Clinical Psychiatry,* 40, no. 11 (1979), 460-63.

75. Neylan, Margaret, "The Depressed Patient," *The American Journal of Nursing,* 61, no. 7 (1971), 77-78.

76. Parker, S., "Eskimo Psychopathology in the Context of Eskimo Personality and Culture," *American Anthropologist,* 64 (1962), 76-96.

77. Pfeiffer, Eric, "What to Do about Mental Disorders of the Elderly," *Modern Hospitals,* 2 (August 1974), 57-61.

78. Pitt, Brice, *Psychogeriatrics, An Introduction to Psychiatry of Old Age.* Edinburgh: Churchhill Livingstone, 1974.

79. Pollock, G. H., "Process and Affect: Mourning and Grief," *International Journal of Psychoanalysis,* 59, nos. 2-3 (1978), 255-76.

80. *Psychology Encyclopedia,* p. 80. Guilford, Conn.: The Kushkin Publishing Group, Inc., 1973.

81. Reubin, Richard, "Spotting and Stopping the Suicide Patient," *Nursing 79,* 9, no. 4 (1979), 83-85.

82. Richman, A. et al., Minimal-Change Disease and the Nephrotic Syndrome Associated with Lithium Therapy," *Annals of Internal Medicine,* 92, no. 1 (1980), 70-72.

83. Rippere, V., "Some Historical Dimensions of Commonsense Knowledge about Depression and Antidepressive Behavior," *Behavioral Research and Therapy,* 18, no. 5 (1980), 373-85.

84. Ritchie, C. A., "Depression Following Childbirth," *Nurse Practitioner,* 2, no. 4 (1977), 14-17.

85. Robins, E. et al., "The Communication of Suicide Intent," *American Journal of Psychiatry,* 115 (1959), 724.

86. Rodman, Morton, and Dorothy Smith, *Clinical Pharmacology in Nursing.* Philadelphia: J. B. Lippincott Company, 1974.

87. Rosenbauer, A., "Suicide Prevention in the Emergency Room Nurse," *Heart-Lung,* 7, no. 1 (1978), 101-4.

88. Roy, Alec, "Early Parental Loss in Depressive Neurosis Compared with Other Neurosis," *Canadian Journal of Psychiatry,* 25 (1980), 503-5.

89. Ruggieri, V., C. Guiliano, and A. Fusco, "Relationship between Depression and Self-Contact," *Perceptual and Motor Skills,* 51, no. 1 (1980), 195-98.

90. Sacks, M., and S. Eth, "Pathological Identification as a Cause of Suicide on an Inpatient Unit," *Hospital and Community Psychiatry,* 32, no. 1 (1981), 36-40.

91. Savage, M., "Suicidal Survival," *Free Association,* 6, no. 4 (1979), 1-2.

92. Schapira, Kurt, "The Masks of Depression," *Nursing Mirror,* 140 (June 19, 1975), 46-48.

93. Schneidman, E. S., and N. L. Farberow, *Some Facts*

about Suicide. Washington, D.C.: U.S. Govt. Printing Office, 1961.

94. Schwartzman, Sylvia, "Anxiety and Depression in the Stroke Patient: A Nursing Challenge," *Journal of Psychiatric Nursing,* 14, no. 4 (1976), 13–17.

95. Smith, M. L., "Depression: You See It—But What Do You Do about It?" *Nursing,* 8, no. 9 (1978), 42–45.

96. Spitz, René, "Hospitalitism: An Inquiry into the Genesis of Psychiatric Conditions in Early Childhood," *The Psychoanalytic Study of the Child,* vol. 1, pp. 54–74. New York: International Universities Press, 1945.

97. Spry, W. B., "Prevention of Suicide," *Occupational Health,* 28, no. 7 (1976), 354–58.

98. Stafford, Linda, "Depression and Self-Destructive Behavior," *Journal of Psychiatric Nursing,* 14, no. 4 (1976), 37–40.

99. Stotsky, Bernard, *The Elderly Patient.* New York: Grune & Stratton, Inc., 1968.

100. "Suicide," *St. Louis Globe-Democrat,* Sunday, April 12–13, 1980, Sec. C, pp. 1–8.

101. Travelbee, Joyce, *Intervention in Psychiatric Nursing.* Philadelphia: F. A. Davis Company, 1969.

102. Tryrer, S. et al., "Lithium and the Kidney," *Lancet,* no. 1 (January 12, 1980), pp. 94–95.

103. Walk, D., "Suicide and Community Care," *British Journal of Psychiatry,* 113 (1967), 1381-91.

104. Ward, J. A., and J. Fox, "A Suicide Epidemic on an Indian Reserve," *Canadian Psychiatric Association Journal,* 22, no. 8 (1977), 423-36.

105. Weingartner, H. et al., "Cognitive Processes in Depression," *Archives of General Psychiatry,* 38, no. 1 (1981), 42–47.

106. Weissman, M. M., and J. K. Myers, "Rates and Risks of Depressive Symptoms in a United States Urban Community," *Acta Psychiatrica Scandinavica,* 57 (March 1978), 219-31.

107. Wendt, R. L., "Good Morning World, I'm Glad to Be Back," *American Journal of Nursing,* 79, no. 5 (1979), 949.

108. Wernstein, M. R., and M. D. Coldfield, "Cardiovascular Malformation with Lithium Use during Pregnancy," *American Journal of Psychiatry,* 132 (May 5, 1975), 529-31.

109. "What You Should Know about Mental Depression," *U. S. News and World Report,* September 9, 1974, pp. 37-40.

110. White, C. L., "Nurse Counseling with a Depressed Patient," *American Journal of Nursing,* 78, no. 3 (1978), 436-39.

111. Whitlock, F. A., and M. M. Siskind, "Depression as a Major Symptom of Multiple Sclerosis," *Journal of Neurological Neurosurgical Psychiatry,* 43, no. 10 (1980), 861-65.

112. Woodruff, Robert A., Donald Goodwin, and Samuel Guze, *Psychiatric Diagnosis.* New York: Oxford University Press, 1974.

16

The Withdrawn Person

Study of this chapter will help you to:

1. Discuss the continuum of withdrawal behavior and the many situations in which the person may experience withdrawal.

2. Explore the dynamics of withdrawal behavior.

3. Relate withdrawn behavior to the schizophrenic process.

4. Assess symptoms of extreme withdrawal.

5. Formulate client-care goals and a care plan for the withdrawn person, and individualize the care plan for the level of withdrawal and regression.

6. Adapt the principles of communication and relationship to meet the needs of the extremely withdrawn person.

7. Intervene, working with the person individually and as a team member, to change behavior to a higher developmental level and toward more integrated function.

8. Compare the effects of a supportive environment vs. a nonsupportive environment on the withdrawn person.

9. Assist, with supervision, the family to understand and work with the withdrawn member.

10. Evaluate the effectiveness of your care by determining the change in the person's behavior.

This chapter contributed by M. Marilyn Huelskoetter, R.N., M.S.N.

WITHDRAWAL: A CONTINUUM

Withdrawal is an adaptive or coping mechanism that involves physically pulling away from, or psychologically losing interest in, an anxiety-producing situation, person, or stressful environment. Examples of this behavior include the child who consistently plays alone instead of with a friend, the adolescent who becomes absorbed in reading instead of being involved with peers, the young adult who jogs to avoid personal contact with others, or the recluse who shuts windows and locks doors to close out the world. Everyone will at times seek solitude by going on a vacation or to the beach or by reading a book instead of seeking the company of others. But when this pattern is consistently used to distance or isolate self from people or from anxiety-provoking, stressful situations, the withdrawal behavior becomes unhealthy. Distancing and pulling away from other people may resolve an immediate problem, but such behavior eventually leaves the person bitter and alone. Withdrawn behavior is commonly found in unhappy people and in a variety of mental disturbances.

For example, the *chronically depressed* person discussed in Chapter 15 devalues and depreciates self, feels unworthy of others' affections, and withdraws from people. He/she may give up so many attachments that death is hastened. Suicide may result.

The *hypochondriacal* person withdraws from people and relates to self with constant preoccupation with the body and its functions. In this state of self-absorption, self-respect is lost, and regression into the helpless child position occurs. Suffering is apparent with a variety of infirmities. The person waits to be cared for by others, blaming failures and the deteriorating relations with others on his/her many physical illnesses. The behavior causes others to reciprocally withdraw as they become disinterested in the constant complaining and moaning. Friends and relatives pull back from involvement and allow the person to suffer alone.

The *narcissistic*, extremely self-centered, proud, and selfish person also uses the withdrawal pattern. This individual has probably always been self-centered, seeking recognition or approval from the external environment but giving little to it. Little energy is left to love or feel affection for anyone other than self. The cool, detached style is a cover-up for being easily hurt.

The maladaptive patterns of *neurosis* may be

manifested by a variety of symptoms; anxiety and withdrawal are common features. In all probability this withdrawal pattern has been a predominant feature in the individual's life for years. Through the years, more and more defensive mechanisms are used to save self-esteem and to cope with the stresses of living. Gradually, the person retreats into apathy, seclusiveness, or neurotic withdrawal. The neurotic retreats after minimal social contacts and waits for support from others. The neurotic is very aware of and uncomfortable about these symptoms; he/she longs for contact with others yet continues to live life in the same self-defeating manner.

A person suffering from *organic and intellectual decline* frequently withdraws from others in the face of frustration, embarrassment, and growing distress. Of course, the premorbid personality and characteristic defensive style determine coping behaviors, but a common behavior is that of withdrawal. The person stays home more, avoids contact with family members, and lives in secrecy.

At the farthest end of the withdrawal continuum is the isolated, disengaged individual who lives in a world of fantasy and autism. The person regresses or decompensates to an early phase of development, one that is comparable to the phase in which the child had difficulty perceiving the self as "me" and the outside environment as "not me." This autistic, daydreaming state can become the decompensated, regressed state of *schizophrenia.*

THE SCHIZOPHRENIC PROCESS

> . . . although living in a state of utter confusion, tried to recapture some understanding and to give organization to his fragmented universe. [5, p. 441]

What is Schizophrenia?

Schizophrenia is a severe psychotic illness that affects the mood, regulation of emotion, thought process, behavior, and total personality integrity (51). It is commonly thought of today as more than one illness—as one label covering a heterogeneous group of syndromes. Two major groupings can be seen: (1) the more fulminating, long-term, nonremitting illness with a poor prognosis is called *chronic schizophrenia, process schizophrenia, nuclear schizophrenia,* or *nonremitting schizophrenia,* and (2) the less severe or less chronic form of the illness is differentiated as *schizophreniform, schizoaffective, remitting acute schizophrenia,* or *reactive schizophrenia* (85, 118). There is a great diversity of symptoms, etiological factors, and treatment approaches.

Description, Dynamics, and Etiology

Schizophrenia was systematically described in 1896 by Emil Kraeplin. He called the behaviors and symptoms *dementia praecox,* meaning a deteriorated, hopeless condition with poor prognosis. He divided the behaviors and symptoms into four major disease types: simple, catatonic, hebephrenic, and paranoid (63).

The term *schizophrenia* was first used by E. Bleuler in 1911 to emphasize the schism or splitting off of the mind between the functions of feeling and thinking (16). Many people falsely think of schizophrenia as the splitting of the personality into two parts; the term actually was meant to describe the disorganization of the thinking and emotional processes (81).

Bleuler also set up criteria of primary and secondary symptoms, criteria that are still in use today for the diagnosis of schizophrenia. The primary symptoms are denoted by the four A's: (1) autism, (2) ambivalence, (3) affective disturbance, and (4) associational disturbance. Secondary symptoms include: (1) illusions, (2) delusions, (3) hallucinations, (4) symptoms related to muscular activity, (5) withdrawal, and (6) lack of touch with reality (16).

Primary process thinking develops before secondary process thinking; in schizophrenia, this primitive thinking process occurs with a narcissistic withdrawal and regression. The primary process thinking is unable to develop out of symbolic, autistic, cognitive processes into reality-based, logical thought forms. The regression occurs because of a weakened and fragmented ego function; it allows a break with, but also a protection from, reality. Freud believed primary process thinking originated in the id and archaic ego and was prominent early in the child's life, in dreams, and in schizophrenic conditions and other abnormal processes (36). See Table 2-3 in Chapter 2.

Both Freud and Kraeplin believed that schizophrenia had a poor prognosis because the person could not develop a relationship or transference phenomenon. Later therapists challenged their pessimism. After World War II, psychoanalytic therapists such as Sullivan, Fromm-Reichmann, Rosen, Lidz, and others worked with schizophrenic patients with commitment, optimism, and greater prognostic success.

Adolf Meyer conceptualized schizophrenia as a habit disorganization resulting from a progressive maladaptation. He saw this process as logical due to the person's life history and personal experiences (71). The individual would avoid difficulties by inefficient and faulty attempts to balance and reorganize (62). Meyer did not feel that this person had any organic structural changes but that the etiology was in some sense due to an inferior constitution and other physical conditions (62).

Sullivan worked with groups of young schizophrenic men at Sheppard and Enoch Pratt Hospital, and through these experiences and others, organized his Interpersonal Theory of personality. Sullivan hypothesized that when the child is first born, there is a period of "Not-Me," which gradually evolves into a recognition and experience of self (106). The organization of experiences marked by Not-Me is primitive, unelaborated, made up of parataxic symbols, and often attended by awe, horror, and dread. The Not-Me can be known by the adult in times of nightmares, and by the schizophrenic or severely mentally ill individual. Regression to Not-Me brings about extreme anxiety and other dissociated behaviors (106). (Refer to Chapter 2.)

The concepts of Kraeplin, Bleuler, Freud, Meyer, and Sullivan form a foundation of understanding, but they are not enough. Other important theorists have been John Rosen, Frieda Fromm-Reichmann, Karen Horney, and Edith Weigart.

Studies of twins in the last 50 years also give evidence of the existence of an inherited predisposition to the schizophrenic diseases. Franz Kallman found that if schizophrenia existed in one monozygotic twin, it occurred in the other 85.8 percent of the cases (62). Other past research with dizygotic twins, siblings, and adoptive children leads to similar findings. Yet the research methodology of some of those early studies is now being questioned as inadequate since many of the variables present were not taken into consideration. (Refer to Chapter 2, pp. 25–26, for further information.)

In the literature, every conceivable cause has been given for schizophrenia. The psychosocial and organic or biological theorists have all produced material to fortify their particular stands. Organic theory includes genetic predisposition, dopamine metabolism, and various other biochemical, endocrine, and neurological factors (105). (Refer to Chapter 2, pp. 26, 27, 28, for further information.) Psychodynamic theorists hypothesize the cause to be a psychic conflict, much like the conflict causing neurosis but more severe, or an ego or personality defect caused by organic, neurophysiological, neurobehavioral, or environmental factors. Between these two extremes are many other positions (115).

J. Bateson and D. Jackson were two early writers to claim disturbed patterns of communication in schizophrenic families (58). The thinking disturbances were said to come about because of *double-bind messages that were received from parents or family members during childhood, obligating the child to respond in a specific but often illogical way, either consciously or unconsciously.* For the double bind to work, honest responses to messages must be forbidden in the interaction. For example, a mother says, "Come here darling so I can hug you." The child knows from past experience that he will not be hugged but pushed away. If he disobeys his mother, he will be punished; if he obeys, he will be rejected and literally be pushed away. Either way he is unable to receive satisfaction. When dishonest communications and mixed messages are a pattern and the resulting confused feelings in the child continue over a period of years, the child grows up not trusting self or others, feeling bad and worthless, having a negative self-concept, unable to perceive or respond to people or events realistically, and experiencing identity diffusion. Consequently the person will have difficulty in all areas of life with interpersonal and social relations and with school and job performance. Eventually the person is labeled as mentally ill. Other writers on this process were Lidz, Laing, Esterson, Fleck, and Erikson (27, 30, 58). (Refer to Chapter 2, p. 71, for Laing's hypothesis.)

L. West and D. Finn integrate the various models of etiology. They feel that people who become schizophrenic are highly vulnerable to stress in the internal and external environments. Causes include ecological, developmental, learning, hereditary, and neurophysiological variables. (115).

Most authors agree that schizophrenia is a multifactor illness that involves an injury to the total personality, and that it may have a variety of causes. Genetic and neurotransmitter disturbances should be viewed in the framework of total personality disturbance. The child's perception of parenting and the parents' actual reaction to and disturbed nurturing of the child may trigger abnormal biochemical processes in the body, which in turn produce other emotional and personality maladaptations. The current research on organic and physiological changes must be interpreted in light of many years of case histories of family dynamics and communication processes with the person who eventually becomes schizophrenic. The complexity and unique combinations of the physical, emotional, cognitive, and social aspects of the person must be considered in determining etiology.

Schizophrenia: A Major Health Problem

Thirty years ago the mental hospitals were teeming with a large percentage of schizophrenic patients. For example, Michigan's Ypsilanti Regional Psychiatric Hospital designed to house 900 patients in 1931 had 3,400 inmates in the 1950s, many of whom were diagnosed as schizophrenic (75). Today, for every diagnosed schizophrenic in the hospitals of New York State, there are three living in the community (62). E. G. Mishler and N. A. Scotch state that three percent of the general population are suffering from schizophrenia (72). Schizophrenia continues to be a major health problem in terms of loss of manpower, disorganized family living, and individual disability.

ASSESSMENT OF THE WITHDRAWN PERSON

You will observe the basic pattern of recoiling or pulling back seen in any withdrawn person as well as in the person diagnosed as schizophrenic. Other behavioral symptoms are found in varying degrees and in individualized patterns. When these symptoms are extreme and combine, they form what is diagnosed as the *schizophrenic process.*

Thought Disorders

The person who is withdrawn and alienated from his/her fellow human beings will over time develop thought processes and ideas that are different from those of other people. The more withdrawn, the more evidence there is of thought disorder.

One of the common defining characteristics in schizophrenia is impairment in the areas of thinking and cognition. This includes *inability to perceive the whole pattern or unity and to think realistically* (51). The average person perceives a gestalt or the whole of anything, whether it be a tree, a bush, or a picture. The healthy person envisions the sum total of the subject or situation. But if you show the client a picture, it may not be seen or noticed in its wholeness, for example, that it is a picture of a baseball game or a park. The schizophrenic person will point out one small aspect and may talk in detail or at length about the bat of the third baseman or the bench in the park. The unity of the personality has been ruptured; in turn, the person has difficulty seeing unity in the environment.

Illogical, scattered, incoherent patterns of thinking are noted as you talk with your client and are a cardinal signal of schizophrenia (51). Normally in talking to another person, you will be aware of a sequence or pattern of ideas and thoughts. Words are normally associated by a common idea, and the sentences flow toward a goal. In talking to a person suffering from a schizophrenic illness, you hear a looseness, a disorganization of thinking in the person's conversation. The words do not hang together, and links to connect the ideas to form a logical ending are missing. The person may say his/her thoughts are racing or wandering. A young male stated to his nurse, "When you color me red, my knee jerks up, blast, summer is near, I will state too bad." These fragmented statements do have meaning, certainly on a symbolic level; but on first hearing them, you would wonder, "What is this all about?" Sometimes a client may speak more clearly and seem more lucid, and your only clue to the disorganization of the thinking person pattern is your sense of his/her confusion.

This person also has difficulty organizing the information perceived from reality, for example, in reading a book, watching television, or following a conversation. Part of the problem is the person's inability to block out irrelevant information and distracting thoughts; the very disorganized sense of self is unable to focus thoughts. Research findings substantiate schizophrenia as a perceptual disorder (79).

Other symptoms to look for would be: (1) ideas without logical connections, (2) words that sound alike spoken together, (3) concretization of words denoting specific objects, (4) circumstantial speech (moving indirectly towards a verbal and mental goal), (5) stereotyped or rigid thinking, (6) automatic knowing—feeling that others know the thoughts, (7) unclear referents—assuming that others know the object or person being spoken of, and (8) the splitting phenomenon, in which the thoughts, feelings, and actions are not consistent (66).

Unrealistic thinking, obvious fantasy, or symbolic thought is a major feature of the disease (51). Jung termed schizophrenia as the "waking dream." The person's thinking may sound like a dream. The psychological mechanisms of condensation, symbolism, displacement, and dissociation produce thoughts and mental pictures of people, objects, and places that are understood only by the person. Thus the thinking is autistic. Words are "coined" or made up, they have special meaning and significance only to the person. The words he/she uses do not have the same meaning to the listener, and the meaning may change from time to time. For example, rubbing the nose may represent a danger signal one time, but two hours later it may represent sending a message. This thinking is unrealistic. Unless the patient is grossly psychotic, his/her thinking will continually fluctuate between being realistic and clear at one time and fantasy-filled and disorganized at another. The world seems confusing to the schizophrenic person, and the schizophrenic is confusing to the world.

Childlike, primitive thinking occurs, except that the child's thinking is basically logical (51). The person thinks in specific, concrete, tangible terms. He/she is unable to think abstractly or conceptually. An object exists only if it can be seen. A proverb or a joke will not be understood. Primary, childlike thinking is also characterized by the absence of a sense of time; the person lives in the present, unable to wait, to imagine alternative modes of action, or to make specific decisions (109). To test for the lack of abstraction or con-

ceptualization, ask the client, "What is the same about a fork, a knife, and a spoon?" The obvious answer is that they are all eating utensils. The person with an impaired thinking disorder might tell you that his/her mother used to insist that everyone eat with a fork, or he/she might list the different foods that could be eaten with each utensil. Symptoms of disordered thinking occur in physical illness as well as in schizophrenic disorders, but the major difference is the symbolic nature of the thought content in the functional disorder. Assess this by exploring the person's thoughts and by getting to know the person better.

Affective Disorders

The withdrawn person may be perceived by others as cold, distant, a loner, unable to reciprocate feelings in an interpersonal situation. Developmentally, this person is infantile or childlike, lacking trust in others and self. His/her self-concept is often composed of negative characteristics, and the person may feel uncomfortable with self as well as with others.

The more withdrawn the person, the fewer are the harmonious emotional ties to others; and the more the dynamics of the schizophrenic process apply to the person, the more you will observe the manifestations of affective disorders, typical of schizophrenia, that are described in the following pages.

Major Emotional Manifestations

Since schizophrenia is considered primarily a thought disorder, emotional changes may be overlooked. Yet, they are of major importance. Disorders of affect or emotion are withdrawal, inability to show emotions or to respond appropriately, uncanny sensitivity, extreme anxiety, regression, emotional arrest, and accessory symptoms.

Emotional withdrawal, or the inability to express appropriate feelings in a situation, is a major and fundamental symptom of any form of withdrawal and schizophrenia. The person fears that he/she will be hurt emotionally by others and so pulls back from others to avoid rejection. The environment seems frightening, and he/she retreats to inner thoughts and fantasies. Fear of the external world, for whatever reason, may be greater than the fear of the personal world, even though the world of the schizophrenic seems chaotic and alien to us.

Emotional withdrawal can be seen in many ways. The family may tell you that the person no longer sees friends and remains alone at home. You may observe the person staring into space, watching television with a blank stare, or being unresponsive. You may feel as you talk that you are not in contact with the person. You may feel unresponsive and apathetic with little understanding for the pain and suffering that the person is experiencing. Your own feelings are an important clue to the client's feelings. Isolation of feelings is a prominent defense, and you may sense that you are relating to little of the real person. As the person withdraws, his/her thoughts and energies are directed inward, making an inner fantasy life that is usually confused, chaotic, and frightening.

Inability to externalize or show emotion is characteristic. You may note a flat, cold, indifferent expression; little feeling or emotion is evident. Your client may look at you without any warmth or recognition. It may be difficult to differentiate a flat affect from a deeply depressed, retarded affect. Look for other symptoms; never expect one symptom to give you a picture of a total behavior or illness. Many times you will feel depression yourself when you interview a depressed person, whereas you will feel little emotion, a distance, and detachment when you interview a withdrawn person.

Inability to respond appropriately with the proper emotion at the proper time is characteristic of the schizophrenic. The person may tell you that he came to the clinic because he lost his wife and then may laugh giddily. Seconds later he may cry when he looks at his hand or is given a piece of gum. This inappropriate response may also carry over into anger. He may submissively follow the rules and regulations of the institution and then defiantly resist an insignificant request.

Richard Corrodi studied facial expression as an indicator of the affect in both normal and schizophrenic people and set up four parameters for assessment (25), as shown in Table 16-1. As you interview your client and observe his/her face, you may notice that the person either avoids eye contact with you by looking everywhere except in your eyes, or directly gazes at the side of your face, never changing the gaze (101). Equally as common is the schizophrenic person who stares coldly and blankly into your eyes with the "schizophrenic stare" that some writers feel represents a wish for and fear of fusing. Milton Wexler described the schizophrenic as looking on a void, an inner emptiness (116). Thus schizophrenic behavior can be diagnosed at times by the style of eye contact.

Uncanny or extreme sensitivity to the feelings of others, or the ability to perceive any feeling or thought another person is having that might be threatening to self is a feature of schizophrenia and of few other mental illnesses. This person has an uncanny sensitivity to your feelings and your state of mind at one point in time; whereas later you may note his/her complete insensitivity to any feelings or to the overall reality situation. Many times the schizophrenic client is able to perceive feelings and attitudes of staff that are unspoken and covert and yet affect the entire attitude of the unit. Forty-eight hospitalized schizophrenics and 48 normal persons were given a set of emotion recognitions that included photographs depicting facial expressions. The normal people (of similar age, sex, and educational level to the schizophrenics) were significantly better than the schizophrenics at realistically identifying all of the emotions (111).

Extreme, overwhelming feelings of anxiety (akin to panic) are experienced by the schizophrenic because the weakened ego is unable to handle the internal or external stresses and organic changes. The anxiety may be observed overtly in tremors, perspiration, laughing, pacing, or wringing of hands. The anxiety also leads to regression, secondary symptoms, and sometimes to consumption of alcohol and drugs. It is cruel to suggest that this person should not be given medication for relief from the inner pain.

Arrested emotional development causes symptoms of emotional immaturity. According to Erikson's stages of development, the client is still emotionally in the first crisis period (30). Symptoms of lack of trust of self and of others and a fear of being rejected are readily seen upon meeting the person for the first time. The person is aloof and distant; he/she creates an emotional barrier so that secondary symptoms are unnoticed. Communication is limited; mutual contact is minimal. The infantile developmental level is a prominent feature in withdrawal and the schizophrenic process. Other characteristics of emotional immaturity include ambivalence, dependency, and lack of insight.

TABLE 16-1.   Comparison of Assessment Parameters for Normal, Withdrawn, and Schizophrenic Persons

PARAMETER	NORMAL	WITHDRAWN	SCHIZOPHRENIC
Range of affect	Capacity for expressing a wide range of emotion in interpersonal relations.	Capacity for expressing wide range of emotion is limited. Reserved and distant in interpersonal relations.	Constricted range; expresses few emotional extremes. Fixation at one end of emotional continuum; usually withdrawn and introvertive rather than extrovertive.
Mobility of affect	Orderly and spontaneous movement. Feelings conveyed by variety of behavioral clues. Smooth transition from one emotional state to another.	Limited movement of affect. Slow to express feeling state in a situation. Apathy, distance, seriousness, lack of reciprocation of spontaneous warmth.	Mood fluctuations abrupt; person lacks smooth transitions when expressing several feeling states. May move suddenly into extremes of potential range, i.e., sudden sadness, joy, rage, submission.
Appropriateness of affect	Congruity between ideas or content of the situation and affective responses.	Consistency between ideas and emotional response present at times. Unable to express warmth and positive feelings consistently in response to other's behavior.	Incongruity between ideas and manifested affect. Observer must know content of thinking to judge appropriateness of emotional response.
Communicability of affect	Ability to produce affective response in another.	Leaves others with cold, angry, or apathetic emotional response. Inconsistent in ability to convey emotion through nonverbal clues.	Inability to transmit emotion through facial and other clues.

Even though researchers are still struggling for additional facts about the etiology and development of the schizophrenic process and diseases, we know from current knowledge about the emotional experience of these people. Many articulate patients have described their experiences, and many therapists and psychiatric nurses working closely with their patients/clients have experienced with and described the feelings of these people. Many theorists and researchers have also studied and summarized consequences of this emotional state. The subjective experience of schizophrenia is one of loneliness, fear, dread, depression, rupture, and utter confusion. It then behooves you as an empathic, caring nurse to continue to strive to give emotional support and nurturing.

Accessory Symptoms

The major accessory symptoms are: (1) *delusions (false beliefs)*, (2) *hallucinations (false sensory perceptions without external stimuli)*, (3) *ideas of reference (thinking that situations around him/her refer to or are pertinent only to self)*, and (4) *ideas of influence (thinking one can influence or control in a supernatural way)*. All four symptoms are frequently present in autistic thinking; hallucinations are more common in the withdrawn schizophrenic and occur in about two-thirds of the clients.

J. F. Small et al. found that 38 out of 50 newly admitted schizophrenic patients hallucinated (103). *Hallucinations*, particularly visual hallucinations, may occur in a wide range of medical problems. Hallucinations that occur in organic states seem to have a greater degree of color, movement, and complexity (50). Some writers believe that purely visual hallucinations are likely to indicate organic disease (37).

Hallucinations often progress from comforting to frightening. In the assessment of schizophrenia, importance is attached to the nature and quantity of the hallucinations (26). In the psychodynamic view, functional hallucinations result from the projection of inner ideas or thoughts into the environment, and are perceived as real experiences. Signs of hallucinating include looking into space as if attending to some person or object. This person may answer back, cry out, laugh inappropriately, or say that the voices are giving commands. He/she may ask if you heard a sound or look at you to see how you are responding. The experiences are usually auditory, but they may be visual, tactile, or olfactory. The patient may see frightening animals or people, or may taste or smell something unusual. One male said, whenever he ate, "The food is horse dung." He actually perceived that everything he ate tasted like animal feces. While you assess the presence of accessory symptoms, also assess the meaning that the thoughts or hallucinations have to the patient. The patient who tasted horse dung was probably relating his feelings of worthlessness and attempting to organize his perception of the world by saying that he was worthless and therefore needed to eat horse dung.

Assess the client's reaction to the hallucinations. Does he/she feel suspicious of the motives of the perceived figure, or an absolute trust in or control by the perceived figure? If the voice or command is trusted, the client may be at greater risk of self-mutilation or injury (100).

Delusions and *ideas of reference* are also present in schizophrenia. The withdrawn patient's delusions are not as systematically organized as are those of the paranoid patient, and the content is more dissociated from or lacking in emotional input. Ideas of reference are related in the schizophrenic to his self-centered thinking in which almost anything in the environment pertains to self. The paranoid's ideas of reference are related to suspicion and fear.

Illusions (misperceptions of external stimuli) may also occur.

Identity Disorders

The withdrawn person may have an intact sense of identity even if the self-concept is negative. But the person with schizophrenia has a very tentative sense of identity. The sense of self is weak; the body boundary and the sense of "who I am" and "if I am" fluctuates. Many clients will not or cannot acknowledge a sense of self. They will not use personal pronouns such as "I" or "me" or call themselves by name, such as "Mary" or "John." They may refer to themselves in the third person, such as "we," or as an object, such as "it." One gentleman always referred to himself only as "one." When asking for anything, he would say, "May one have ____." As you talk to the person, notice how he/she addresses self. Loss of identity may also occur as he/she feels self merge with or become another person or object, as shown by the following examples:

One elderly hospitalized patient saw the nurse write his name in the chart on rounds one morning. The nurse had difficulty finding the patient for medication that afternoon, but when she did find him, he reminded her in all seriousness that she should have looked in the chart because he had been put there.

A group of people with chronic schizophrenia were occupied in painting one day. Each person had a sheet of paper. Each was busy painting and coloring. After a time the group leader took one large piece of paper and asked each member of the group to paint the same picture he had drawn on his own sheet of paper on the large sheet as a mural to decorate the wall. The members looked frightened. One began pacing. One became angry. Another sat down and refused to move. Two began to paint. The fourth never got anything on the paper, and the last drew a small painting in the far corner of the paper.

This is a dramatic yet symbolic example of how many patients fear merging and loss of their very identity. Schizophrenics may complain of feeling lost or engulfed when they are touched by another person.

The unstable ego state can also cause confusion of body image. As you watch the severely withdrawn person, you may notice a rigidity of movement or a difference in body coordination. The person may look at his/her legs to see if they are moving, or may place his/her feet down as if they were not connected to the rest of the body. Posture conveys unsureness of body structure and movement.

Surgery, an illness, or a temperature may give this person a feel of body contour that presents a feeling of identity. One patient was extremely lucid one day and said to the nurses on the division, "I am whole! I am whole!" He was later found to have an elevated temperature, which emphasized awareness of his body. The next day the temperature was gone, and so was the lucidity and perceived body boundaries. This phenomenon has been observed by nurses for years.

One way to get in touch with the person's sense of identity is to ask him/her to draw a stick figure of self. Ask the person to tell you about self. If the person is able to talk about his/her body, he/she may tell you about a diseased and rotting body, feelings of unrealness, merging with people or objects, and a changing and disorganized self. There are other tests to assess the concept of body image in relation to a wide range of phenomena: these include the Body Image Aberration Scale, Perceptual Aberration Scale, and Physical Anhedonia Scale (23).

Yet testing must be done with caution and insight and by a qualified person, as listed by the following example:

A female student nurse was working with a five-year old boy suffering from childhood schizophrenia. He had periods of psychosis but for the most part was lucid. The student wanted to talk about the child's identity and one day asked him to lie on a big paper. She drew his outline. The child thought the project was fun and quickly was involved. When the activity was finished, the child jumped up to view the outline and was overwhelmed by what he saw. The large outline of a boy was threatening to his sense of self and body image. He may have felt separated, torn, and unsure of who or where he was. The child became disorganized in thoughts and behavior; anxiety increased, and he began to hallucinate.

Communication Disorders

The withdrawn person usually communicates in a terse but adequate style for meeting basic needs. Words and ideas match and are considered appropriate to the situation. Communication may not be initiated, but response will reveal generally realistic thought processes.

In contrast, when you assess the schizophrenic person, you will be aware of disturbances in varying degrees. Thoughts may be from a special dream world with a private language and style. Sullivan thought that language use was magical in an effort to gain security (105). Sometimes the thoughts are too painful to say or too hurtful to share.

Words may be *autistic (having meaning only to self)*, or they may be jumbled by *neologism, words made up by the person that have very personal thoughts or meanings*. Words may be incoherent or mixed together incorrectly in a sentence. Some of the lack of communication may be a defensive distancing maneuver to keep people away. For example, if the person can speak only in a monotone or cannot be understood, he/she will be unable to become involved with other people. Some people in a regressed state will mumble, groan, or speak with a primitive-type language. Significant communication will be nonverbal because many times words are not trusted and the person wants to remain private. The communication will be seen in gestures, body motions, voice tone, expressions, and a variety of nonverbal forms.

Suicide Potential

Suicide in schizophrenia is not an uncommon problem (33). It may be the result of spontaneous acts (77) (in a flurry of depression from listening and acting on the direction of perceived voices and commands), or it may result after years of self-inflicted life-threatening behavior (2). Many times it occurs from motivation other than the intent to die.

Assess carefully the following areas to determine suicide risk in the withdrawn person (2):

Logic of thinking: Does the patient think in the strange logic of the schizophrenic person?

Content of thinking: What is the situation causing anxiety? What are the delusions and hallucinations? What are they saying?

Ego strengths and weaknesses: What supports are available? What emotional constraints are present?

Nonverbal communication: What does the person mean by his/her behavior? What is communicated unconsciously?

Ego control and reality testing: Is the person able to respond to the environment? Is the person able to delay gratification of impulses? Is the person impulsive?

Mood: Is the person depressed or confused? What is the general feeling tone?

NURSING DIAGNOSIS AND FORMULATION OF CLIENT-CARE GOALS

Nursing Diagnosis

Your *nursing diagnosis of withdrawn behavior* may include the following assessments of the person:

1. Shows a pattern of pulling back in a variety of ways when encountering anxiety-provoking, threatening situations.
2. Remains alone or engages in purposeless or little activity in order to maintain physical withdrawal.
3. Displays various degrees of emotional withdrawal, such as through daydreaming, fantasizing, or autistic communication.
4. Demonstrates self-centered preoccupation and has little interest in other people or activities.
5. Demonstrates a variety of primitive ego defense mechanisms to cope with anxiety.

Client-Care Goals

Long-term goals for the client may include the following:

1. Some degree of trust is established, as demonstrated in a satisfying relationship.
2. Appropriate speech and nonverbal behavior are used to express thoughts and feelings to others in an understandable way.
3. Interest in other activities is shown, which contributes toward more realistic behavior.
4. A feeling of security is developed about the self and environment to the fullest extent possible.
5. Constructive mechanisms to cope with feelings of anxiety are demonstrated to the greatest degree possible.

Short-term goals for the client may include the following:

1. Presence of another person is tolerated.
2. Interest in a brief activity shared with another is stated.
3. Some feelings are stated realistically to another person.
4. Sentences are progressively more understandable.
5. Different or more appropriate behaviors to handle anxiety are tried after encouragement.

You will think of other goals as you care for your clients.

NURSING INTERVENTIONS RELATED TO CLIENT-CARE GOALS

Self-Awareness of the Nurse as a Basis for Promoting Improvement in the Client

While planning for care and intervening with extremely withdrawn clients you need to constantly monitor your own feelings. The progress of the client is usually slow; achievement of your goals should be measured not by the time or by the amount of change but by the efforts that are extended. Until you have developed skill and self-knowledge, discouragement and frustrations will be common feelings as you work with the person. Over a period of time, you can help the person to achieve increasing ability to relate to others, further development of the personality, and the ability to live in the community as a contributing citizen (68).

Your own self-awareness aids you in being open to the client's needs, which is basic to implementing care in a Humanistic Framework.

Goals and Interventions

The five long-term goals (see p. 542) will be described here along with pertinent nursing interventions.

Goal 1: Some degree of trust is established, as demonstrated in a satisfying relationship.

Interventions

Begin with contact that is safe to the client. Even though this person conveys a desire for closeness and affection, he/she will maintain distance until the emotional barrier of lack of trust and fear of rejection can be broken. Your first task is to establish some contact with the person. This may be done symbolically by lighting a cigarette, giving a piece of candy, or bringing a book, any of which represents giving of yourself and being received by the person. Be sensitive to the person's fears and sense of vulnerability. If you are too enthusiastic and assertive in giving support, warmth, or gifts, the person may feel so anxious that he/she breaks off contact by leaving the immediate area or the agency or by asking for another nurse. Move slowly and with genuine concern in establishing emotional and physical closeness. Dependency behavior may be a call for help, yet the person may push you away as you offer guidance. On one hand, the infantile, unrealistic thinking may demand attention from you to the extent that you may feel overwhelmed and have difficulty maintaining interest. On the other hand, your client may be so cold and aloof that you feel that you are not getting anywhere and will want to quit. However, your own withdrawal will contribute to the client's withdrawal from a relationship with you, and thereby continued withdrawal from others (48). Or you may feel incorporated or engulfed by the client when you are with him/her, and you may

want to get away from this discomfort by discontinuing efforts at healthy movement into a relationship.

Establishing a feeling of mutual trust and a relationship occurs slowly and as a result of your attempts at contact. Read again Chapter 6 on the nurse-client relationship and apply the information with the withdrawn person. Establishing a relationship is difficult because the client expects you to cause pain. Thus, after moving a step closer, he/she pulls away. Just as you use the four A's in diagnosis (see page 534), use the following four A's as a guide to forming a relationship. Focus on: (1) acceptance—accept yourself and your shortcomings and the person's experience, (2) awareness—listen to verbal, nonverbal, and symbolic communication, (3) acknowledgment—recognize fears and communication, and (4) authenticity—show honest human-to-human contact (9). The key to helping the person is to develop trust. With your encouragement, he/she learns to feel good about being with you; and then gradually he/she learns to feel secure with others.

If the ability to trust remains underdeveloped, the person is flooded by disorganizing anxieties. To defend against the anxiety and loneliness, he/she freezes into "I-it" relations. The person tries not only to master the material world, but he/she also tries to manage others as objects in order to compensate for loneliness. But neither the highest managerial success nor the solitary perfection can meet the need for trust in others and self, that is, being accepted and understood by another. Trust is a basic human need; it *can* be rekindled in this person. Trust promotes personality integration, turns despair to hope, and permits acceptance of the limited freedom and responsibility of one's unique existence (114).

Encourage emotional involvement with you to develop a relationship. **Relatedness** *is the emotional, perceptual and cognitive capacity to become involved with another person* (105). The withdrawn individual must slowly but progressively become involved with life and must do this through another human being. Thus you must also slowly become involved with him/her. You represent the rejecting, fearful world, but you offer another experience with that world, one that is more comfortable. The person may have suffered many losses and may have been rejected too often. At first, the risk may be too great, and response is slow to your presence, conversation, and concern. If the impediments are not too great, anxiety can be overcome. The person may pull back several times and may manifest the symptoms discussed in the previous section. You must wait. Give distance and then seek the person out again. If people have caused too much hurt and if your own approach is too brusque, too fast, or too pushy, he/she may never move out at all. However, if you are perceptive of his/her feelings as you attempt to form a bond, and if you try over and over again, you will be given a chance to succeed. The bond, the involvement, will continue, depending on the time you both have and the ability of both of you to become emotionally close.

The nursing profession and the field of psychiatry may be moving to a more scientific approach to care. This may mean an emphasis on cognition to solve problems—on organic causes of mental illness that appear exact and defined. However, one very basic fact about humans is that caring and relatedness must be in feelings, not just words, to produce growth. Growth and recovery from extreme withdrawal or from other emotional disorders do not come about in many instances because the risk to move close is not shared by both the health worker and the client. The feeling level must be present as well as the knowledge and skill to have the bond succeed. The mother who is bonding with the newborn child may say all the right words and have the proper sound and method, but if she does not really care for or love the infant, or if fears and anxieties block the feelings of love, the infant will go without the close ties that are so important for the nurturing process to continue. Let us work and desire that nursing, as a caring profession, will continue not only to develop knowledge but that it will also continue to *care.*

Goal 2: Appropriate speech and nonverbal behavior express thoughts and feelings to others in an understandable way.

Interventions

Encourage communication that is less autistic and increasingly understood by others. In the early stages of a schizophrenic break, the major communication is nonverbal. The way to reach the person is by attempting to understand the primitive feeling and thinking level. Let the client know you

want to understand. Paraphrase, reflect feelings and thoughts, and clarify as indicated. Gradually, communication may be attempted at a higher, more cognitive level as the client feels safer with you.

Try to understand the person's words when he/she sounds illogical or incoherent. Look for topics, themes, and symbols. Ask the client to help you understand. Paraphrase what you think are thoughts or feelings; state the implied. Say the words that you think are being said. Encourage the person to say the words coherently, if at all possible. Never try to fool him/her by saying you understand when you do not. Trust is a very basic problem; be honest. If you do not understand, say so, or remain silent until you think you may have an idea. It may be helpful to say, "I hear you saying ——." "Tell me what you mean by ——." Always let the client know that you want to understand and that you appreciate his/her difficulty in talking about ideas and feelings. Try to be creative by allowing the person to find alternate ways of communicating. Some people can draw or make figures, whereas others are expressive in other nonverbal methods: gestures, mime, singing, or dance (20). The most important method of communication is the unidentifiable energy that moves between people that says, "I care about you."

Focus on tangible issues to strengthen communication skills. The withdrawn person is hard to live with. When the person is trying to solve a problem, especially in an area ridden with conflicts, he/she may tend to have difficulty in thinking. The person may become vague, increasingly disorganized, unsure of perceptions, and unable to focus on issues. He/she may say things that make no sense. Guide the client through the vagueness to solve problems and assist in giving a sense of past and future. As the person feels more secure and begins to identify with you, you can help him/her describe events in daily living that cause difficulty and determine how to handle these events. Carefully look for causes of the difficulty and reason for failure, withdrawal, regression, or secondary symptoms.

Hallucinations can also be handled as a tangible issue. The person can recognize hallucinations and can realize that they occur only in certain situations and that certain events can cause them. This is called the *listening attitude,* for he/she learns to anticipate and listen or watch for these experiences. The person may tell you about the hallucinations, for example, what the voices are saying. The hallucinatory voices may say never to trust anyone. Thus, only after some time in a relationship, after a deep trust has been established, will the client share information with you about the voices, people, or other hallucinations. As you discuss these experiences with your client, explore when he/she expects to hear the hallucination. Ask, "What happens right before the voice? What brings about the voice?" The following case illustrates this point:

> A student nurse visited Mrs. R., an elderly patient, in her home. During each visit she took Mrs. R. shopping. Each time they returned home, Mrs. R. would tell the student that the voices were saying Mrs. R. was dumb. As this information was examined, Mrs. R. was able to see that when she expected to hear the words, she would hear them. The words were based on her own feelings that she was a dumb person, on her own feelings of inadequacy and worthlessness. Much later, the voices in the store disappeared because Mrs. R. was able to recognize the precipitating cause and her feelings.

The person may or may not be able to gain this kind of insight. Such connections may be too anxiety-provoking or too abstract. However, other simple cause and effect relationships may be attained in lieu of this deeper insight.

In exploring any hallucinating experience, be aware of the client's anxiety or disturbed feelings. Listen to the manifest content (116). Listen to the underlying conflicts, needs, and wishes. Carefully present reality, as appropriate, by telling the client that you do not hear the voice or see the situation, but that you can understand how the experience is real. Do not go along with the hallucinations or encourage them in any way. Try to decrease the anxiety or underlying feelings. Over time, explore the precipitating feelings, events, or places so that the person can relinquish the hallucinations and meet needs in a more realistic way.

Goal 3: Interest in other activities is shown, which contributes toward more realistic behavior.

Intervention

The severely regressed, chronically ill schizophrenic client may be helped by reality orientation and remotivation sessions. Activity groups are also helpful to withdrawn clients, regardless of severity of illness, because the person feels safer at first doing an activity while having contact or an interaction with another person.

Activity groups have been found to alter the self-concept of the withdrawn person while at the same time increasing interaction. J. Lancaster chose twelve patients, six people from each of two wards, and established two activity groups. Twelve other patients, six from each ward, served as control subjects. The group members selected their activities—drawing, reading, looking at pictures, baking, and playing the piano. Sometimes discussion centered around activities, and sometimes it centered on thoughts and feelings. As a result of these sessions, there was a significant change on the Osgood Semantic Differential Score for Self-Concept within the experimental group but no significant difference within the control group (65). Review Chapter 11 for ideas on the kinds of groups that can be helpful to the withdrawn client.

Certainly before the withdrawn person can be comfortable in a group, he/she must first feel comfortable with you or with one or two other people. Gradually bring the client into increasingly larger groups.

Goal 4: A feeling of security is developed about the self and environment to the fullest extent possible.

Intervention

All of the previous interventions mentioned for Goals 1–3 contribute to a sense of security and the slowly emerging positive self-concept. In addition, *maintain a helpful environment* to foster personality development, trust, security, and positive self-concept. Review Chapter 4 for information on the therapeutic milieu. *Milieu therapy, using the environment as a treatment measure,* has proven successful. Within an institution, in the community, and in home settings, the environment should be considered as a means to produce comfort and alleviate anxiety. Thousands of withdrawn schizophrenic persons have been placed in nursing homes, apartments, or foster homes to rehabilitate them in the community so that they will not become dependent on an institution. Today the emphasis is to keep as many individuals as possible outside the hospital. They are encouraged to participate in community activities. It is preferable to have such people in the community where they can live independent lives, free from hospital rules and restraints.

The paradox is that since so many of these people are unable to be free in their own minds, they are as isolated in the community as they were in the hospital. Often they receive little treatment or are without the supportive environment necessary for healthy functioning. G. Serban studied the measurement of functioning and adjustment to the community of the discharged chronic schizophrenic person and found that the maintenance of low levels of stress, depression, and particularly anxiety plays a central role in preventing rehospitalization (98).

In another study, levels of experienced stress were studied in acute and chronic schizophrenia and in a normal control group. The chronically ill group reported the highest levels of stress in almost all areas of daily life. The acutely ill group reported significantly lower levels of stress. In this group, the stress was primarily evident in disturbed relationships with close ones. The normal group experienced the lowest levels of stress. The stress in this group appeared to be associated with the inability to reach and maintain high standards of behavior (98).

Maintain an environment that promotes trust and is as secure as possible. If not, the return into the family and community from treatment in the institution (or long-term institutionalization) may increase anxiety, stress, and symptom formation.

In the hospital setting you can maintain a safe, secure, attractive environment for the person. A team approach that provides consistent care and emphasizes gradual involvement with others is important. Continuity of such care in the home environment is more difficult but necessary. The public health nurse, social worker, vocational counselor, and psychiatrist must continue to plan together for the client's care. Home management goals would include securing support of family or friends and involvement of the client in social activities and in the pursuit of an occupation and hobbies. An excellent opportunity for a psychiatric nursing experience for student nurses would be working in community home-care facilities with withdrawn persons.

Goal 5: Constructive mechanisms to cope with feelings of anxiety are demonstrated to the greatest degree possible.

Intervention

Strengthen the identity of the client through your relationship with him/her. The confusion of identity can be strengthened by the person's identification with you, by his/her gaining a greater sense of self-worth through the relationship, by being treated as a unique person, and by having personal possessions. Always call the person by name. Allow adequate body and environmental space. Refer to possessions and handle them with care. Support unique qualities and show respect for the worthwhile individual that he/she is.

Personal hygiene is important for a whole body image and self-respect. Physical activity, such as walking, playing ball, or swimming, may be helpful. Activities using the five senses and touch may give more of a sense of self. Think of your client and some of the interests, symptoms, and difficulties; then plan activities with him/her.

Be careful to touch the person only if he/she responds comfortably to being touched. Touching can be a helpful contact to reinforce body boundaries. If you sense that the person is withdrawing or tightening, wait until he/she is responsive to physical closeness.

Promote understanding of dynamics. As you empathize with and get to know the client and his/her situation, begin to explore about patterns of behavior, defense mechanisms, the background for feelings and self-concept, the people who are important, and how he/she relates with others and with you. As you begin to make sense of the person's life and understand the underlying dynamics, help to clarify feelings and focus on the difficult life situations. Assist with decision making and foster success instead of failure. Gradually you can encourage understanding of self to some degree, the reasons behind behavior, and the effect of behavior on others. In turn, you can work with the client to develop healthier ways for relating to people and coping with stressful situations.

Be a role model for the client. As much as you can, become a companion to the person while also maintaining objectivity. As you talk, present reality. As you share your ideas and are supportive, he/she will learn to deal with life's realities, gradually gaining enough strength to return to independent activity and the community. To experience with the person may give him/her courage to become more involved in other relationships, social activities, and former interests, as is shown by the following case:

Miss J. was discharged from the state hospital to live with another former patient in an apartment. The other patient dominated Miss J. and Miss J. withdrew more and more into herself. She sat by the window and looked out hour after hour—bored, listless, and apathetic. She had always loved to cook but was fearful of doing so in this situation.

A nurse assigned to Miss J. began to visit, build a relationship, and talk about meaningful topics. She felt it was important to help Miss J. become more involved, so together they bought several cookie mixes. Two afternoons were spent together mixing and baking. The next time they baked cookies it was Miss J.'s suggestion, and cookies were made from a recipe. Miss J. had gained enough confidence from mutual experience to bake cookies from a recipe by herself.

Such encounters can lead the way to a fuller life. As you become more involved in a mutually trusting bond, you may cry, laugh, or express anger with the person and through this experience teach him/her how to live.

Working with the Family and Health Team

Working with the Family

The client becomes withdrawn or ill with schizophrenia within the family unit. There may be any one of many causes: (1) lack of parental care in childhood, (2) distorted communication patterns among family members, (3) scapegoating of the client, (4) identification with a withdrawn parent, (5) learning withdrawal or schizophrenic behaviors as a way to meet needs and obtain response from others, or (6) genetic predisposition to a perceptual distortion of communication and the environment or a biochemical abnormality.

Often the extreme identity disruption and the severe withdrawal and acute manifestations of schizophrenia develop gradually, so that interaction patterns within the family have become firmly entrenched. You and other team members need to work with the family unit concurrently with therapy for the client, for if the client returns to the same family environment, he/she will sooner or later evidence illness again. The client cannot maintain healthier behavior if the members of the family unit do not also change their behavior toward the client.

Review Chapter 10 for principles in working with the family unit. Establish rapport, a sense of trust, and if possible, a relationship with the family. Avoid judging or blaming the family unit or individual members for the client's behavior. Rather, help the members become aware of their feelings toward the client as well as how they interact and communicate with the client and among themselves. Explore ways for them to live more harmoniously with the client, if possible. Both the client and the family must become responsible for their own behavior and must consciously work at realistic communication and conveying acceptance of and caring for each other.

Sometimes the old hurts and hates are so deep that the client cannot return to live in the same family environment, but can maintain health only if he/she moves outside of the home situation. Your ability to listen, clarify, and offer alternatives can help the client and family arrive at this decision in a way that allows for ongoing personality development for all concerned.

Working with the Health Team

Because the client has identity, trust, and communication problems, it is extremely important that all health team members are consistent in implementing the treatment plan. Thus, the team members must confer among themselves so that the client does not receive opposing or distorted messages. Consensus among the team promotes achievement of the short- and long-term goals previously listed. Do not wait for team conferences and a team approach to happen. Initiate teamwork, if necessary.

Responsibility of the Nurse with Somatic Treatments

Use of Tranquilizers

Use of tranquilizers is a humane method to alleviate many of the accessory symptoms associated with the schizophrenic illness. You have an important function in giving the medication, helping the person understand the medication and why it is prescribed, and in achieving a dosage with maximum effect and the fewest possible side effects.

Monitoring of any drug given is essential since the person's tolerance for medication and susceptibility to toxic effects are individualized (10). Maintenance dosage is usually smaller in the elderly.

Major tranquilizers for the person include the phenothiazine derivatives as shown in Table 16-2.

Possible Side Effects

Table 16-3 summarizes the main side effects and related nursing measures for the phenothiazines listed in Table 16-2. Acute toxicity is very low (10).

Other complications below may occur besides those described in Table 16-3.

Water Intoxication

Water intoxication is an interesting phenomenon that can occur in schizophrenic clients receiving antipsychotic drugs but does not occur in normal individuals. Three types of water retention have been reported (10):

1. Water intoxication from unknown causes.
2. Water intoxication from abnormal secretion of antidiuretic hormone (A.D.H.).
3. Water intoxication precipitated by diurectic therapy.

The person begins to drink large amounts of water, saying he/she is thirsty from the medicines or wants to "wash out the worms," the "inside smell," or the "voices." The person may drink excessive fluid by standing in the shower to drink, or standing by the water fountain, or downing glass after glass of fluid. You may first notice a distended abdomen or aberrant drinking behavior. Next lethargy, disorientation, confusion, and grand

TABLE 16-2. Major Tranquilizers (Phenothiazine Derivatives)

GENERIC NAME	TRADE NAME	DOSAGE RANGE PER 24-HOUR PERIOD (mg)
Dimethylamine subgroup		
Chlorpromazine hydrochloride	Thorazine	30 to 1200
Triflupromizine	Vesprin	60 to 150
Piperidyl subgroup		
Thioridazine	Mellaril	30 to 800
Mepazine	Pacatal	50 to 400
Mesoridazine	Serentil	100 to 400
Piperazine subgroup		
Acetophenazine	Tindal	40 to 80
Fluphenazine	Permitil; Prolixin	1 to 20
Perphenazine	Trilafon	6 to 64
Prochlorperazine	Compazine	15 to 150
Thiopropazate	Dartal	15 to 100
Thiothixene	Navane	6 to 60
Trifluoperazine	Stelazine	2 to 20

TABLE 16-3. Summary of Phenothiazine Side Effects
and Related Nursing Implications

SIDE EFFECTS	NURSING IMPLICATIONS
Discomforts Drowsiness Dizziness Hypotension Blurred vision Faulty reflexes and faulty perceptions	Explain the value of the drug in spite of unpleasant effects. Ensure safety precautions. Encourage rising slowly or holding onto furniture. Assist person initially if necessary. Avoid slippery floors or clutter on floor. Warn that drug may interfere with driving, especially at beginning of therapy. Check blood pressure in prone and standing positions.
Dry mouth	Encourage sucking on mints or ice chips, chewing gum, holding fluids in mouth. Vaseline may be applied to lips.
Nasal stuffiness	At home, add humidity to room through steam. Use vaporizer.
Weight gain	Encourage low-calorie diet and exercise within limits.
Constipation	Encourage bulk and fluids in diet, exercise, regular times for elimination; may need mild laxative.
Libidinal changes	Teach person that this may occur but may also return to normal after a period of time.
Dermatological effects Photosensitivity Pruritis Skin discoloration (grayish-purple)	Warn to avoid exposure to sun because sunburn, rash, and discoloration are intensified in direct sunlight. Lotions relieve itching. Lowering dosage should decrease discoloration. Use sunscreen, sunglasses, protective clothing.
Blood dyscrasia Agranulocytosis (more common in women and after 40 years of age)	Teach person to report fever, sore throat, unusual malaise, any infection such as vaginitis, dermatitis, gastritis. Should have periodic complete white blood count and differential. Dosage decreased if dyscrasia occurs.
Jaundice, liver damage	Prolonged treatment of high dosage may cause decreased liver function. Teach family to observe for yellowish sclera or skin. Should have occasional liver function tests.

Neurological effects
Extrapyramidal reactions
  (Parkinsonism)
  Rigid limbs and face
  Drooling
  Tremors of hands and
    limbs
  Skin taut, waxy
  Gait and posture
    changes
	Occurs most commonly in people between 15 and 18 years, the elderly, and in women. Reduce dosage. Anti-Parkinson drugs usually ordered. Promote safety measures. Modify care and activities so that patient maintains self-esteem. May need assistance with eating, hygiene, grooming, and mobility.

Akinesia
  Weakness, fatigue
  Limbs may become
    painful
	Same as above.

TABLE 16-3.   Continued

SIDE EFFECTS	NURSING IMPLICATIONS

Tardive dyskinesia
  Involuntary movement of
    face, jaw, tongue
  Convulsions may occur
	Same as above.

Acute dystonia
  Increased muscle tone
  Oculogyric crisis
	Teach family to recognize signs: fixed stare, nystagmus, open mouth, protruding tongue, head back, facial expression of pain. Encourage to lie in darkened room with little stimulation.

Source: Murray, et al. *Nursing Process in Later Maturity* (Prentice-Hall; ©1980), Table 22.1. Used with permission, Prentice-Hall, Inc., Englewood Cliffs, N.J.

mal seizures occur. Coma and death result if excessive fluid intake is not terminated.

Tardive Dyskinesia

Tardive dyskinesia is a neuroleptic-induced complication of long-term phenothiazine use. The number of patients described in the literature is increasing. The cause is thought to be a development of dopamine receptor supersensitivity. Symptoms consist of slow, rhythmic, stereotyped movements in the buccolingual masticatory area. These may include puffing of cheeks, rolling tongue, and smacking of lips. These movements are increased by stress and activity and disappear during sleep. Eventually, brain damage may occur (55).

The symptoms may first appear when medication is changed. Withdrawal of the neuroleptic drug may increase symptoms temporarily, but symptoms may then subside. Anticholinergic and dopaminergic drugs are of no value.

Further research is needed on these complications, as well as on the total effects of long-term neuroleptic drug therapy.

Other Somatic Treatments

In addition to the use of tranquilizers, electroconvulsive therapy (ECT) and *psychosurgery (incising the frontal lobe of the cerebrum)* are occasionally used. The ECT is used with the person so that motor and accessory symptoms and mood may be improved. Psychosurgery is outdated, drastic, and may or may not be effective. The personality is changed, and behavior is less spontaneous. Regression may occur (74).

EVALUATION

You will observe an improvement in the client's behavior as you work closely with him/her over time. However, the importance of relationships is not just intuitively understood (74). Nursing interventions have been evaluated in a study by E. Gelperin on the motivation of withdrawn and regressed institutionalized, chronically ill elderly patients (40). The nursing intervention consisted of a one-to-one trust relationship in which interactions were held daily, averaging three hours a week for two months. The intervention included planning rehabilitative, therapeutic, and recreational activities, along with mutual reevaluation and modification of nursing plans. The result of the study showed significant behavioral changes; withdrawn and regressed behavior was decreased.

Nursing could do much more with therapeutic relationships. Relationships take time and effort, but the effort produces results. You may notice signs of renewed interest in surroundings and activities, an increased interest in clothing, food, or most significantly, in other people. Perhaps the best evaluation can be based on the person's capacity to respond to you. The person behaves in a less testing manner; he/she smiles as you approach and shows excitement about an activity you are planning together. You may become aware of a setback in the behavior when you miss a day of interaction with the person or take a vacation. Gradually, you will sense a bond developing between you. As this happens, usually the client extends the bond to others.

REFERENCES

1. Adelson, P. Y., "The Back Ward Dilemma," *American Journal of Nursing,* 80, no. 3 (1980), 422-25.

2. Anderson, Nancy, "Suicide in Schizophrenia," *Perspectives in Psychiatric Care,* 11, no. 3 (1973), 106-12.

3. Arieti, S., "From Schizophrenia to Creativity," *American Journal of Psychotherapy,* 33, no. 4 (1979), 490-505.

4. ___, "Individual Psychotherapy of Schizophrenia," *American Handbook of Psychiatry.* New York: Basic Books, Inc., 1959.

5. ___, "Man's Spirituality and Potential for Creativity as Revealed in Mental Illness," *Comprehensive Psychiatry,* 21, no. 6 (1980), 436-43.

6. ___, "Psychotherapy of Schizophrenia," *Treatment of Schizophrenia: Progress and Prospects,* eds., Louis West and Don Flinn. New York: Grune & Stratton, Inc., 1976.

7. ___, "Schizophrenia: The Psychodynamic Mechanisms and the Psychostructural Forms," *American Handbook of Psychiatry.* New York: Basic Books, Inc., 1959.

8. ___, "The Schizophrenic Patient in Office Treatment," *Psychotherapy of Schizophrenia—Symposium.* Basel, Switzerland: S. Karger, 1964.

9. Arnold, Helen, "Working with Schizophrenic Patients—Four A's: A Guide to One-to-One Relationships," *American Journal of Nursing,* 76, no. 6 (1976), 941-43.

10. Ayd, Frank, "The Major Tranquilizers," *American Journal of Nursing,* 65, no. 4 (1965), 70-78.

11. Beaumont, S., "Nursing Care Study: A New Life at 61," *Nursing Times,* 76, no. 20 (May 15, 1980), 863-65.

12. Beels, C. C., "Social Networks, the Family, and the Schizophrenic Patient: Introduction to the Issue," *Schizophrenic Bulletin,* 4, no. 4 (1978), 512-21.

13. Berner, P., "Modifications in the Psychopathologic Definition of Schizophrenia—Alterations during the Last Two Decades: Expectations for the Future," *Comprehensive Psychiatry,* 21, no. 6 (November-December 1980), 475-82.

14. Betz, B. J., "Curtain on Schizophrenia: A Twenty-Five-Year Clinical Follow-Up," *American Journal of Psychotherapy,* 34, no. 2 (1980), 252-60.

15. Billett, G., "Nursing Care Study: Sam—A Long-Term Psychiatric Patient," *Nursing Times,* 75, no. 7 (February 15, 1979), 277-79.

16. Bleuler, E., *Dementia Praecox of the Group of Schizophrenias.* New York: International Universities Press, 1911.

17. Boyajean, A., "Fighting Despair," *American Journal of Nursing,* 78, no. 1 (1978), 76-77.

18. Bull, A., "Nursing Care Study: Schizophrenia," *Nursing Times,* 74, no. 11 (March 16, 1978), 442-44.

19. Burgess, Ann, and Aaron Lazare, *Psychiatric Nursing in Hospital and Community.* Englewood Cliffs, N.J.: Prentice-Hall, Inc., 1976.

20. Burkett, Alice, "A Way to Communicate," *American Journal of Nursing,* 74, no. 12 (1974), 2185-87.

21. Carser, D., "The Defense Mechanism of Splitting," *Journal of Psychiatric Nursing and Mental Health Services,* 17, no. 3 (1979), 21-28.

22. Carson, V., and K. Huss, "Prayer—An Effective Therapeutic and Teaching Tool," *Journal of Psychiatric Nursing and Mental Health Services,* 17, no. 3 (1979), 34-37.

23. Chapman, L., J. Chapman, and M. Raulin, "Body-Image Aberration in Schizophrenia," *Journal of Abnormal Psychology,* 87, no. 4 (1978), 399-407.

24. Coburn, D. C., "The Experience of Schizophrenia," *Journal of Psychiatric Nursing and Mental Health Services,* 15, no. 12 (1977), 9-13.

25. Corrodi, Richard, "Clinical Assessment of Affect in Schizophrenia," *The Journal of Clinical Psychiatry,* 39, no. 6 (1978), 493-96.

26. Critchley, E. M., and C. J. Rossall, "Hallucinations," *British Journal of Hospital Medicine,* 19, no. 3 (1978), 264-70.

27. Davis, D. R., "The Family Processes in Schizophrenia," *British Journal of Hospital Medicine,* 20, no. 5 (1978), 524-31.

28. Delamothe, K. J., "Nursing Care Study: Schizophrenia or Not," *Nursing Times,* 75, no. 39 (September 27, 1979), 662-65.

29. Eaton, Merrill, Margaret Peterson, and James Davis, *Psychiatry,* 3rd ed. New York: Medical Examination Publishing Company, 1976.

30. Erikson, Erik, *Childhood and Society,* 2nd ed. New York: W. W. Norton & Co., Inc., 1963.

31. Famuyiwa, O. O. et al., "Tardive Dyskinesia and Dementia," *British Journal of Psychiatry,* 135 (December 1979), 500-504.

32. Fandetti, D. V., and D. E. Gelfand, "Attitudes towards Symptoms and Services in the Ethnic Family

and Neighborhood," *American Journal of Orthopsychiatry,* 48, no. 3 (1978), 477–86.

33. Farberow, Norman, et al., "Suicide among Schizophrenic Mental Hospital Patients," *The Cry for Help,* eds., Norman L. Farberow and Edwin S. Schneidman, pp. 78–109. New York: McGraw-Hill Book Company, 1965.

34. Forrest, D. V., "Nonsense and Sense in Schizophrenic Language," *Schizophrenia Bulletin,* 2, no. 2 (1976), 286–301.

35. Freeman, T., "On Freud's Theory of Schizophrenia," *International Journal of Psychoanalysis,* 58, no. 4 (1977), 383–88.

36. Freud, S., *The Interpretation of Dreams.* New York: Basic Books, Inc., 1960.

37. Frieske, D. D., and W. P. Wilson, *Psychopathology of Schizophrenia,* pp. 49–62. New York: Grune and Stratton, 1966.

38. Fromm-Reichmann, F., *Principles of Intensive Psychotherapy.* Chicago: University of Chicago Press, 1959.

39. ———, *Psychoanalysis and Psychotherapy.* Chicago: University of Chicago Press, 1959.

40. Gelperin, E., "Psychotherapeutic Intervention by Nurse Clinical Specialist," *Journal of Psychiatric Nursing and Mental Health Services,* 14, no. 2 (1976), 16–18.

41. Gendlin, E., "Therapeutic Procedures in Dealing with Schizophrenics," *The Therapeutic Relationship with Schizophrenics.* Madison, Wis.: University of Wisconsin Press, 1967.

42. Glazer, W. M., "Assessment of Social Adjustment in Chronic Ambulatory Schizophrenics," *Journal of Nervous and Mental Diseases,* 168, no. 8 (1980), 493–97.

43. Gottheil, E., R. Exline, and R. Winkelmayer, "Judging Emotions of Normal and Schizophrenic Subjects," *American Journal of Psychiatry,* 136, no. 8 (1979), 1049–54.

44. Gough, H., "Nursing Care Study. Schizophrenia: Silence Filled with Sound," *Nursing Mirror,* 151, no. 6 (August 1980), 42–46.

45. Green, D. E., "Schizophrenia: Some Problems for the Nurse," *Southern New Zealand Nursing Journal,* 73, no. 1 (January 1980), 11–13.

46. Grigg, W., "Nursing Care Study of Chronic Schizophrenia," *Nursing Times,* 75, no. 32 (August 1979), 1350–52.

47. Hafner, J. L., L. V. Corotto, and M. E. Fakouri, "Early Recollections of Schizophrenics," *Psychological Report,* 46, no. 2 (1980), 408–10.

48. Hall, Beverly, "Mutual Withdrawal: The Non-Participant in a Therapeutic Community," *Perspectives in Psychiatric Care,* 14, no. 2 (1976), 75–93.

49. Hardin, S. B., "Comparative Analysis of Nonverbal Interpersonal Communication of Schizophrenics and Normals," *Research in Nursing and Health,* 3, no. 2 (1980), 57–68.

50. Higaski, H., and K. Koshika, *Bulletin of the Osoka Medical School,* Suppl. 12 (1967), p. 155.

51. Hock, Paul, "Differential Diagnosis, in *Clinical Psychiatry,* eds. Margaret Strahl and Nolan Lewis, pp. 601–48. New York: Science House, 1972.

52. Hole, R., A. Rush, and A. Beck, "Cognitive Investigation of Schizophrenic Delusions," *Psychiatry,* 42, no. 4 (1979), 312–19.

53. Jameson, R., "Psychiatric Nursing for the Eighties: Into the Arms of the Big Wise World," *Nursing Times,* 76, no. 40 (October 1980), 1730–32.

54. Jeffries, J., "The Trauma of Being Psychotic," *Canadian Psychiatric Association Journal,* 22 (1977), 199–205.

55. Jeste, Dillip N., and Richard Jed Wyatt, "In Search of Treatment for Tardive Dyskinesia: Review of the Literature," *Schizophrenia Bulletin,* 5, no. 2 (1979), 251–93.

56. Johnson, J. J., "An Ambulatory Mental Health Clinic," *Nursing Clinics of North America,* 12, no. 4 (1977), 571–81.

57. Jones, I. H., and M. Pansa, "Some Nonverbal Aspects of Depression and Schizophrenia Occurring during the Interview," *Journal of Nervous Mental Disease,* 167, no. 7 (1979), 402–9.

58. Jones, S. L., "The Damned If You Do and Damned If You Don't Concept: The Double Bind as a Tested Theoretical Formulation," *Perspectives of Psychiatric Care,* 15, no. 4 (1977), 162–69.

59. Kay, D., and M. Roth, "Environmental and Hereditary Factors in the Schizophrenias of Old Age," *Journal of Mental Science,* 107 (1961), 649.

60. Kilgalen, R. K., "The Effective Use of Seclusion," *Journal of Psychiatric Nursing and Mental Health Services,* 15, no. 1 (1977), 22–25.

61. Klein, H. E. et al., "Transcultural Nursing Research with Schizophrenics," *International Journal of Nursing Studies,* 15, no. 3 (1978), 135–42.

62. Kolb, Lawrence, *Modern Clinical Psychiatry.* Philadelphia: W. B. Saunders Company, 1977.

63. Kraepelin, E., *Dementia Praecox and Paraphrenia.* Edinburgh: E. and S. Livingstone Ltd., 1919.

64. Lamb, H. R., "Schizophrenia through the Eyes of Families," *Hospital Community Psychiatry,* 29 (1978), 803–6.

65. Lancaster, Jeanette, "Schizophrenic Patients: Activity Groups as Therapy," *American Journal of Nursing,* 76, no. 6 (1976), 947–49.

66. Lawton, K., "Nursing Care Study. Schizophrenia: Laura Learns to Make Friends," *Nursing Mirror,* 148, no. 24 (June 1979), 32–33.

67. Manaser, Janice, and Anita Werner, *Instruments for Study of Nurse-Patient Interactions.* New York: Macmillan Publishing Co., Inc., 1964.

68. McArdle, Karen, "Dialogue in Thought," *American Journal of Nursing,* 74, no. 6 (1974), 1075–77.

69. Mellow, June, "The Experiential Order of Nursing Therapy in Acute Schizophrenia," *Perspectives in Psychiatric Care,* 6, no. 6 (1968), 249–55.

70. Melzer, M., "Group Treatment to Combat Loneliness and Mistrust in Chronic Schizophrenics," *Hospital and Community Psychiatry,* 30, no. 1 (1979), 18–20.

71. Meyer, A., "The Dynamic Interpretation of Dementia Praecox," *American Journal of Psychology,* 21 (1910), 385.

72. Mishler, E. G., and N. A. Scotch, "Sociocultural Factors in the Epidemiology of Schizophrenia," *Psychiatry,* 26 (1963), 315–51.

73. Morris, M. L., "Nursing Experience: Turnabout on the Locked Unit," *RN,* 42, no. 1 (1979), 77.

74. Murray, Ruth, M. Marilyn Huelskoetter, and Dorothy O'Driscoll, *The Nursing Process in Later Maturity.* Englewood Cliffs, N.J.: Prentice-Hall, Inc., 1980.

75. "Newsweek Medicine—Drugs and Psychiatry: A New Era," *Newsweek,* November 12, 1979, pp. 98–104.

76. Osler, M., and J. Singer, "Ethnic Differences in Behavior and Psychopathology: Italian and Irish," *International Journal of Social Psychiatry,* 2 (1956), 11–23.

77. Osmond, Humphrey, and Abram Hoffer, "Schizophrenia and Suicide," *Journal of Schizophrenia,* 1, no. 1 (1967), 54–64.

78. Ostendorf, Mary, "Dan Is Schizophrenic: Possible Causes, Probable Causes," *American Journal of Nursing,* 76, no. 6 (1976), 944–47.

79. Pao, P. N., "On the Formation of Schizophrenic Symptoms," *International Journal of Psychoanalysis,* 58, no. 4 (1977), 389–401.

80. Place, E. J., and G. C. Gilmore, "Perceptual Organization in Schizophrenia," *Journal of Abnormal Psychology,* 89, no. 3 (1980), 409–18.

81. *Psychology Encyclopedia,* p. 86. Guilford, Conn.: The Dushkin Publishing Group, 1973.

82. Putnam, M., "Nurse, Could you Care More?" *Nursing Times,* 76, no. 2 (January 1980), 56.

83. Pyke-Lees, P., "Care of the Schizophrenic at Home," *Midwife Health Visit Community Nurse,* 14, no. 9 (September 1978), 300–302.

84. Rawat, G. M., "Schizophrenia: Nursing Care Study," *Nursing Mirror,* 145, no. 22 (December 1977), 18.

85. Roberts, Sharon, "Territoriality: Space and the Schizophrenic Patient," *Perspectives in Psychiatric Care,* 7, no. 1 (1969), 28–33.

86. Robins, E., and S. B. Guze, "Establishment of Diagnostic Validity in Psychiatric Illness: Its Application to Schizophrenia," *American Journal of Psychiatry,* 126 (1970), 983–87.

87. Robinson, Alice, "Communicating with Schizophrenic Patients," *American Journal of Nursing,* 60, no. 8 (1960), 1120–23.

88. ——, "A Therapeutic Paradox—To Support Intimacy and Regression or Privacy and Autonomy," *Journal of Psychiatric Nursing and Mental Health Services,* 17, no. 5 (1979), 19–23.

89. Rodman, M. J., "Controlling Acute and Chronic Schizophrenia, Drug Therapy Today," *RN,* 41, no. 4 (1978), 75–83.

90. Rosser, R., "The Psychopathology of Feeling and Thinking in a Schizophrenic," *International Journal of Psychoanalysis,* 60, no. 2 (1979), 177–78.

91. Roth, M., "Interaction of Genetic and Environmental Factors in the Causation of Schizophrenia," in *Schizophrenia,* ed. K. Richter. Elmsford, N.Y.: Pergamon Press, Inc., 1957.

92. Rouslin, Sheila, "Relatedness in Group Psychotherapy," *Perspectives in Psychiatric Care,* 11, no. 4 (1973), 165–71.

93. Sawford, R., and S. Lee, "Nursing Care Study. Restoring Speech: The End of a Long Silence," *Nursing Mirror,* 148, no. 9 (March 1979), 34–35.

94. Schneider, K., *Clinical Psychopathology.* New York: Grune & Stratton, Inc., 1959.

95. Schroder, P. J., "Nursing Intervention with Patients with Thought Disorders," *Perspectives of Psychiatric Care,* 17, no. 9 (1979), 329.

96. Schwartz, D. M. et al., "Six Clinical Features of

Schizophrenia," *Journal of Nervous Mental Disease,* 166, no. 12 (1978), 831-38.

97. Seeman, M., and H. Cole, "The Effect of Increasing Personal Contact in Schizophrenia," *Comprehensive Psychiatry,* 18, no. 3 (1977), 283-93.

98. Serban, G., "Mental Status, Functioning and Stress in Chronic Schizophrenic Patients in Community Care," *American Journal of Psychiatry,* 136, no. 7 (1979), 948-51.

99. ____, "Social Stress and Functioning Inventory for Psychotic Disorders: Measurement and Prediction of Schizophrenics' Community Adjustment," *Comprehensive Psychiatry,* 19, no. 4 (1978), 337-47.

100. Shore, David, "Self-Mutilation and Schizophrenia," *Comprehensive Psychiatry,* 20, no. 4 (1979), 384-93.

101. Silk, Kenneth R., "The Schizophrenic Stare," *Bulletin of the Menninger Clinic,* 42, no. 1 (1978), 10-21.

102. Silverman, Julian, "Shamans and Acute Schizophrenia," in *Consciousness: The Brain, States of Awareness, and Alternate Realities,* eds. Daniel Coleman and Richard Davidson, pp. 120-25. New York: Irvington Publishers, 1978.

103. Small, J. F., J. G. Small, and J. M. Anderson, *Diseases of the Nervous System,* 27 (1966), 349.

104. Smith, W. O., and M. L. Clark, "Self-Induced Water Intoxication in Schizophrenic Patients," *American Journal of Psychiatry,* 137, no. 9 (1980), 1055-60.

105. Solomon, Phillip, *Handbook of Psychiatry.* Los Altos, Calif.: Lange Medical Publications, 1971.

106. Sullivan, H. S., "The Language of Schizophrenia," *Language and Thought in Schizophrenia.* Berkeley: University of California Press, 1964.

107. Stewart, Barbara, "Biochemical Aspects of Schizophrenia," *American Journal of Nursing,* 75, no. 12 (1975), 2176-79.

108. Toner, E., and P. Cabanban, "Schizophrenia: A Sense of Identity," *Nursing Mirror,* 147, no. 14 (October 1978), 35-37.

109. Verwoerdt, Adriaan, *Clinical Geropsychiatry.* Baltimore: The Williams & Wilkins Company, 1966.

110. Wadeson, H., and W. T. Carpenter, Jr., "Subjective Experience of Schizophrenia," *Schizophrenia Bulletin,* 2, no. 2 (1976), 302-16.

111. Walker, E., S. J. Marwit, and E. Emory," A Cross-Section Study of Emotion Recognition in Schizophrenics," *Journal of Abnormal Psychology,* 89, no. 3 (1980), 428-36.

112. Walsh, R., and L. Roche, "Precipitation of Acute Psychotic Episodes by Intensive Meditation in Individuals with a History of Schizophrenia," *American Journal of Psychiatry,* 136, no. 8 (1979), 1085-86.

113. Watson, C., K. Daly, and A. Zimmerman, "Effects of Patient Attitude and Staff Indulgence on Improvement in Schizophrenics," *Journal of Abnormal Psychology,* 88, no. 3 (1979), 338-40.

114. Weigert, Edith, *The Courage to Live.* New Haven, Conn.: Yale University Press, 1970.

115. West, Louis, and Don Flinn, *Treatment of Schizophrenia.* New York: Grune & Stratton, Inc., 1976.

116. Wexler, Milton, "Schizophrenia: Conflict and Deficiency," *Psychoanalytic Quarterly,* 40, no. 1 (1971), 83-99.

117. Wilson, Janet S., "Deciphering Psychotic Communication," *Perspectives in Psychiatric Care,* 17, no. 6 (1979), 254-56.

118. Woodruff, Robert, Donald Goodwin, and Samuel Guze, *Psychiatric Diagnosis.* New York: Oxford University Press, 1974.

119. Zerbin, Edith, and P. Ruedin, "Genetics," in *Modern Perspectives in the Psychiatry of Old Age,* ed. John C. Howells. New York: Brunner/Mazel, Inc., 1975.

17

The Suspicious Person

Study of this chapter will help you to:

1. Identify factors that contribute to suspicious thinking and behavioral patterns.

2. Describe the continuum of suspicion and the dynamics of the paranoid process.

3. Assess the paranoid process, either as the primary mental illness or as part of the symptomatology of another illness.

4. Formulate the nursing diagnosis, client-care goals, and a plan of care for the person who is manifesting the paranoid process.

5. Intervene with the client in such a manner that he/she does not have to adhere to the paranoid process.

6. Help family members to adapt to the behavior of the suspicious person.

7. Work with the health care team to maintain a consistent approach and secure environment for the client.

8. Evaluate changes in the person's behavior that indicate an effective approach.

This chapter contributed by M. Marilyn Huelskoetter, R.N., M.S.N.

The *suspicious or paranoid thinking process* is a reaction to anxiety and insecurity, whereby projection (attributing personal feelings and thoughts to others) is the basic defense mechanism used. Additionally, the person mistrusts and blames others, rationalizes behavior, is wary of and feels persecuted by others, and misinterprets others' behavior (60).

SUSPICION: A CONTINUUM

We have made little progress in curbing and eliminating discrimination, exploitation, violence, and war because of our refusal to recognize and acknowledge that all humans depend heavily upon paranoid processes throughout their lives (55).

We all feel mistrust at times, and the feelings may be protective. But if mistrust is persistent and occurs in most situations, it is maladaptive. The paranoid syndrome can be viewed on a continuum ranging from suspicion that is induced by family, society or the culture, or by extreme stressors, to temporary periods of extremely suspicious thinking, to paranoid states in mental illness and the psychotic delusional thinking in an extreme schizophrenic break.

The Greeks first used the term *paranoid* and called one another that name, as we do today. We use the term to describe nonpathological thinking as well as pathological thinking of suspicion, blaming, resentment, sensitivity, jealousy, and guardedness. Feelings of insecurity are transferred and blamed on many external causes, people, environments, or situations. Blaming can take the form of criticizing, attacking, belittling, ridiculing, accusing, and fighting. The object of the blaming can be political parties, religious groups, community agencies, and moral crusading groups. Or an individual can hide behind good causes such as religious groups, a police department, or a governmental department and can commit attacks and atrocities because of pathologically suspicious thinking. Blaming also occurs with stereotyping and prejudices, when hatred and anger are focused against men, women, Catholics, Jews, blacks, whites, or whomever. Paranoid thinking causes widespread distrust and suspicion.

Suspicious thinking is stimulated by many facets of our society and culture (60). The words may begin, "That guy took advantage of me. He doesn't like what I say or how I look, or what I do. He is out to get me, so I'll get him first." This reaction can disturb individual relationships as well as those involving family, spouse, siblings, peers, or employment. The suspicious attitude can spread into an attitude of one group against another or one organization against another. The so-called cold war psychology can be a paranoid attitude on a large scale (60). Labor and management conflicts that bring out suspicious thinking in both parties are another example. Even when there are no real hostilities, either or both parties may perceive them to be present.

Paranoid thinking brings about activity in a paranoid mode (19). The individual is hyperalert or hypervigilant to find the attacker, the potential enemy, the threat. Events are related to self and are scrutinized for the missing or hidden clues. Nothing can be left undone or unattended.

In contrast, reality thinking is the ability to view the environment as other realistic or healthy people view it and to be aware of self as a part of the environment; reality thinking occurs in the ordinary mode of human activity, when the individual lives in a matter-of-fact way, dealing with problems as they arise and at face value (19). The normal person lives with the flow of events, monitoring the environment only when necessary. This process also occurs in the group, family, and community. The security within the setting and with one another brings about a certain sense of trust that enables a freedom of activity. A person with an autonomous ego is able to adapt to threat; he/she may feel a sense of attack but does not always respond with distrust. E. Erikson described that trust implies not only that one has learned to rely on the sameness and continuity of other providers, but also that one may trust oneself and the capacity of one's own organs to cope with urges; and that one is able to consider oneself trustworthy so that the providers will not need to be on guard (24). Reality thinking, therefore, includes the ability to test the environment and decide when to trust and what situation or person should not be relied on. The person then may come to the conclusion that another is not trustworthy, based on fact, not paranoid thinking.

HISTORICAL NOTES AND THEORIES OF ETIOLOGY

The Greeks first coined the term *paranoia,* and it was used by Hippocrates to refer to delirium or disorganized thinking (44). The term then fell into disuse but was renewed in 1863 by Karl Kahbaum who believed that paranoia was a persistent delusional illness that remained unchanged throughout its course (47). E. Kraepelin in the early 1900s described paranoia as an insidious chronic illness characterized by a fixed delusional system, absence of hallucinations, and lack of deterioration of the personality (44). Bleuler recognized a paranoid form of schizophrenia, and Ernest Jones spoke of paranoia as a shrinking of self.

Freud used the now famous case of the German Judge Daniel Schreber to formulate his concept of paranoia. Schreber was a distinguished judge and had a well-known career in politics. He was hospitalized several times. After the last hospitalization he wrote about his experiences, his belief about the end of the world, and about his bizarre and elaborate delusions in a work called *Memoirs.* He then took legal action to be discharged from the hospital and was released. In 1903 his book was published. The book came to Freud's attention, and he published an analysis of the case in 1911 just after Schreber's death (28).

Freud's theory of paranoia centers on the idea that delusional thinking in both sexes comes from the projection and reaction formation of unacceptable homosexual wishes (28, 29). Freud's premise was that the repressed desire "I love him," is unacceptable; it is reacted against and emerges as "I do not love him, I hate him." This thought is unacceptable to the ego; therefore it undergoes projection and is perceived as "He hates me; therefore I must hate him (28)." These ideas result in persecutory delusions, based on "If he hates me and persecutes me, I must fear him." Thus the once loved object is turned into a persecutor, and the repressed love is transformed into a conscious hate (47). Freud's views have had great influence on modern concepts of the paranoid, particularly the concept of projection as a defense mechanism to explain suspicion and related symptoms. But the premise that the paranoid delusion results from repressed homosexual wishes has not proven acceptable. However, much research has concluded that there is a positive association in male psychotics between paranoid and homosexual tendencies (17). This correlation does not imply causation, although research gives massive evidence that the paranoid does have an intense level of manifest hostility, which when projected onto significant others, transforms into persecutory delusions (17).

H. S. Sullivan postulated that the paranoid person suffers from a deep sense of inferiority, insecurity, and feelings of rejection (64). These feelings keep the person from security and satisfaction and bring feelings of loneliness and unworthiness that are intolerable. Security is obtained by the projection of these feelings and by transfer of blame onto others. The self-system must continually draw into the projective system as the person attempts to disguise or exclude the underlying sense of inferiority (47, 64).

Melanie Klein believed the paranoid style of adjustment resulted from fixation at the oral and early anal sadistic phases of development. Klein saw the child projecting aggressive impulses onto the frustrating mother, who is incorporated as an internal persecutor. Klein also saw a close association between the early development of paranoid and depressive states (38, 47). Her other views have been controversial, but her views about aggressive impulses of the paranoid shifted thinking away from libido as the basis for aggressive behavior (47).

O. Fenichel discussed the role of the superego in paranoid delusions (25). A person with a strict or severe superego, with high standards and ideals, internalizes guilt, shame, and feelings of inadequacy; these feelings are then projected in the form of terrifying and sadistic delusions in order to maintain self-protection and defense (25, 47).

Since these early writers, others have described paranoia and masochism (the power operation in paranoia) and the relationship between depression and paranoia. J. Cameron described the paranoid pseudocommunity or community that has relevance and significance to the sensitive and vulnerable person. A person (or family) may believe that he (it) is the focus of a whole community and may become paranoid, believing that real, misidentified, or imagined persons are untrustworthy and may persecute him (it). (15). Such paranoid feelings develop as the person/family experiences blaming, unusual events, or actual persecution.

The studies on family dynamics, which are rich in interest about schizophrenia, seldom focus on the paranoid style of adaptation. H. Bonner described the strictness, harshness, and domination of the paranoid client's early pattern of family life (8). I. Sletten and S. Ballous studied the paranoid delusional system. They found when the father was the most feared parent, the subject had delusional ideas that concerned men only; when the mother was the most feared parent, the subject had delusions that involved both men and women (59).

Other researchers found that paranoid persons showed greater distortions of hypothetical people than did normal people; the paranoid persons tended to perceive faces as tense, suspicious, hostile, and threatening, and they overrated themselves (47). Friedman, with an 80-statement Q-sort test to characterize the hero in the Thematic Apperception Test, found that the paranoid person reflected greater degrees of feelings of inadequacy, dissatisfaction, and pessimism, as well as more stressful interpersonal relationships (47).

Biological and genetic studies have given little evidence to refute C. Miller's research on 400 psychotic persons with marked paranoid trends (50). He found clear evidence of dynamic causation: paranoid illness was found among the ancestors of only eight patients (50). Differences in innate makeup, early life experiences, and neuron sensitivity may later be linked with adult hypersensitivity. Some writers believe that the paranoid streak is a part of the nature of all people (43).

INCIDENCE AND CONTRIBUTING FACTORS

The incidence of paranoid thinking is considered by most to be high (15). Since the person is usually secretive, tends to be isolated, has an intact personality, and usually much self-control, he/she may live his/her life without disclosure. The illness may be found in a routine physical examination, emergency situation, legal situation, industrial or employment examination, nursing admission assessment, or by accidental personal encounter (15).

We live in a stressful age, and stress seems to predispose to suspicious thinking. The paranoid person seems very self-sufficient; but as stress increases, it takes greater energy and defense to hide the suspicion and maintain control. The paranoid process seems to occur more often in the mature adult or in late life than during the younger years. As life progresses, there are more stressors, responsibilities, and adjustments to disappointments, with decreasing opportunities and changes in energy and physical status. Stressors may include illness, sensory deprivation, loss, rejection, loneliness, and abuses.

In one study, a group of elderly rated their most severe problem to be physical illness (6). The paranoid aged were found to have a high incidence of physical disorders (68). Increased physical illness erodes trust in one's body, restricts social contact, and tends to diminish self-esteem.

A number of researchers have reported that the stress or sensory deprivation or defects leads to paranoid ideas (15, 23, 56). R. Houston and A. Royse demonstrated a higher proportion of paranoid symptoms among deaf psychotics than among psychotics with normal hearing (35). Suspicion may also be seen in deaf children. Blindness may contribute to suspicion but not to the same extent as deafness does. Many have noted acute paranoid reactions in patients with temporary deprivation of sight because of eye patching; recovery occurs when the bandage is removed (23). A. Eisendorfer and F. Wilkie also reported that blind persons have more primitive thought processes on Rorschach testing (23).

Loss, whether financial, social, emotional, physical, or intellectual, causes loss of self-esteem, a sense of emptiness, anxiety, and loneliness. Rejection and disappointment come to all in life but are especially noticed by the very sensitive or mistrusting person. The normal person can adjust to stressors more readily, whereas the mistrusting, rigid, isolated, angry, and fearful person may adjust poorly or not at all. Decreased social contact and increased isolation typical of the suspicious person bring further loneliness and increased dwelling on inner thoughts and dissatisfactions. This dwelling on fears, anxieties, and insecurities results in even higher anxiety and in the need for more defense in the form of the paranoid process.

DYNAMICS OF PARANOID THINKING

Figure 17-1 outlines the dynamics of the paranoid process as it progresses. The person with a paranoid thinking process suffers from insecurity and uncertainty, lacks self-confidence and ability to cope, and has feelings of low self-respect and low self-value, which is evidenced by the behavior and inner life of the person. The more threatened the person becomes and the greater the losses, the more that the self-esteem and sense of personal integrity suffer. Increased anxiety results. If the person has a tendency to handle problems in aggressive, compensating ways, and to use the paranoid process, he/she responds to anxious feelings with anger, mistrust, and increased sensitivity. These feelings are too painful for the individual to consciously acknowledge, so they are denied until the defensive mechanisms crumble. The blaming or accusing of others for the painful inner thoughts, feelings, attitudes, and experiences, relegated to the "not-me" portion of personality, becomes the basis for the process of projection (65). This process of externalizing feelings or projection is used by everyone at some time. For example, the young child blames the chair for a fall, or the student blames the teacher for a failing grade. The more difficulty the person experiences, the more negative feelings he/she attributes to others.

The paranoid person has greater ability to compensate, more intact mental functioning, and less personality disorganization than most mentally ill people. A high level of energy is used to maintain self-image, self-control, and pseudoextroversion in the face of inner fragility and fragmentation (47). Reaction formation is a mechanism used to enable this person to be more outgoing, independent, organized, in control, and self-assured. Although there are underlying feelings of powerlessness, weakness, and need for dependency, the paranoid appears independent, strong, and concerned with personal power and omnipotence. Many believe that they are gifted to influence, control, and persuade other people (47); their behavior is often ingratiating.

A *narcissism (self-love or investment in self)* brings the person to believe that everything in life, all events, center around him/her. It is very difficult to understand life and other people with such a focus of thinking. If stress increases and if denial, projection, and reaction formation are inadequate to help him/her feel secure, the person turns to other mechanisms to make sense of the confusing world. First, the person will support the projection by *rationalization, a logical sounding, acceptable reason for the suspicious response.* The use of

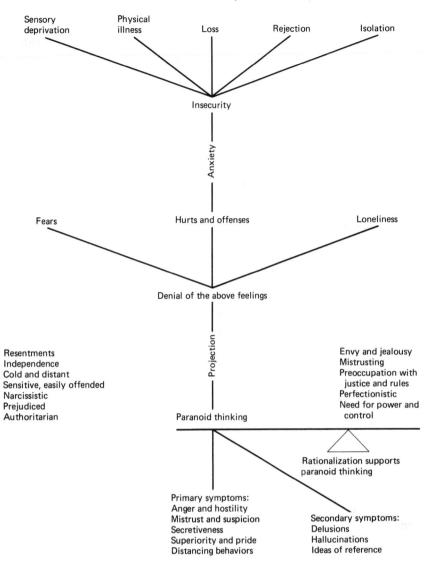

FIGURE 17-1   A model of the dynamics of paranoid thinking.

rationalization says to the person the he/she is right in the way of thinking because ———. This defense also helps to keep the real motives and feelings out of awareness. Rationalization combined with suspicious thinking and the self-assurance borne out of reaction formation reduces the chances for a realistic life view.

If stress and anxiety continue to increase, the person begins to fantasize and further rationalize circumstances. Ideas of reference develop as everything in the environment begins to have personal significance and actions of others are related to the self. These ideas of reference imply that there is a relationship between "me here" and "them over

there." For example, the person may hear a physician's name called on the loudspeaker and assume the doctor is calling him/her. Or the elderly man may see the mailman talking to several people in front of his house and assume that the mailman is saying something about him to other people.

Over time, the rationalizations, fantasies, and misinterpretations, combined with bits of truth, are developed into a delusion. The more organized and systematic the delusion becomes, the more logical and realistic it may seem to others. The organically confused person is unable to organize a logical, complex delusional statement; however, if the delusional person has little organic damage, he/

she may build upon the basic premise with such logic and precision that the delusion is difficult to detect. *As a delusion develops into an increasingly logical, organized network of beliefs, it is called a delusional system,* which is very difficult to change.

At times, delusions are *encapsulated* or *compartmentalized,* that is, *held apart from the rest of the person's life.* The individual may seem perfectly normal. One area of his/her life may be dominated by the delusion, whereas other areas of life are intact, integrated, and little influenced by the delusional idea.

The paranoid person may eventually come to a *"paranoid resolution"—the complete transfer of all insecurities and difficulties to the environment outside of self.* The person becomes totally secure in delusion, projection, and suspicious thinking. Anxiety is minimal; the person is calm and satisfied. He/she states beliefs in a matter-of-fact way; rationalizations are unnecessary. Prognosis becomes poor. When the person states with certainty that he/she is God, there has been in his/her own mind a resolution in which there is (in all probability) security.

DISORDERS DEMONSTRATING THE PARANOID PROCESS

The American Psychiatric Association has classified various paranoid diagnoses in the *Diagnostic and Statistical Manual,* 3rd ed. (2) (also see Appendix). Some of the common disorders will be discussed in the following pages.

The Paranoid Personality Disorder

The *paranoid personality is typically one who has a lifetime pattern of being suspicious, nontrusting, secretive, rigid, and proud.* Such a personality pattern often begins in earlier life and continues until death. The person may be able to live fairly successfully, but probably not as fully as if he/she had been more open to others. Some may maintain borderline stability; personality traits, such as being cantankerous, eccentric, and demanding, may cause real difficulty with others. He/she may be easily hurt and unforgiving, holding a grudge for a long time. The more insulted and alone he/she feels, the more seclusive, angry, alienated, and bitter he/she becomes.

The paranoid personality is relatively harmless to others; the real suffering is within the person as he/she becomes more isolated and alienated. Others may avoid relating with this individual. Many persons maintain a lifetime of unhappiness, even to their final years, alone without any support and friendships. Some remain in their homes isolated and avoided by all except delivery men or governmental employees, such as tax collectors or assistance workers. The following case is an example:

Mary Brown had been hypersensitive, rigid, blaming person all her life. She lived in a small Ohio town, never married, but supported herself as a salesperson in a local real estate office. She was a member of the Catholic Church and active on the board of a local children's home and adoption center. After retiring, she became increasingly more involved in gardening and reading, and less involved in any social life as her hearing impairment increased. Later, she developed a cardiac condition so that her gardening activities had to be curtailed. As she became more ill and isolated, she became suspicious of her neighbors; she thought they were talking about her and sending X-rays to attack her, change her, and poison her. Her thoughts caused her to become more frightened, and she shut herself in her home. She received no outside visitors. She did call occasionally to the police to check up on her neighbors, especially if they tried to initiate any contact. When she stopped picking up her mail, the neighbors became concerned and finally called authorities to check. She was found dead and had been dead for several weeks.

Often the paranoid person refuses help when it is offered by others, even when he/she desperately needs help. If there has been an unhappy experience with a health professional, which feeds into a delusion of persecution from health workers, all health professionals may be grouped together as "out to get me." The well-intentioned professional may have a hard time understanding this person's thinking process and may become resentful and rejecting, leaving him/her alone even when help is urgently needed. Yet, the person may accept help later if the worker is gentle and patient. If the person thinks you are going to help with some physical problem, he/she is more likely to let you stay.

Paranoid States

The person suffering considerable stress may regress to a *paranoid state, a condition of transitory psychotic, delusional behavior precipitated by stress.* Often a major, rapid loss causes this decompensation. The more the loss pertains to a conflicted or important area, such as the sense of manliness or femininity or separation or rejection from a loved one, the more likely the person will formulate a delusion to compensate the loss. Often, after the delusion is formulated, the person appears to adjust to the loss, returning to earlier behavior, especially if familiar activities intervene. The following case study is an example:

> Susan lived in a small apartment in a large metropolitan city. She was a successful accountant, organized in her life and occupation. She was married and had one child. When the child was diagnosed as leukemic, Susan had difficulty adjusting. She turned away from her husband and centered her life on her daughter. The child's progress was poor; she died after one year's illness. Shortly after the death, Susan seemed more alert, cautious, and irritable with her husband. One day she ran in after work and told her husband she was being followed. The husband took necessary precautions, but this repeatedly happened. Susan described the man as one who waited for her each night after work and the description was similar to the husband's appearance. This lasted for several weeks. Then Susan began working in an organization to help parents of dying children; shortly the delusion subsided.

Frequently after the delusion begins, the person either readjusts to the loss or else develops disturbed mood, behavior and thinking. Later the person returns to the former coping mechanisms present in the premorbid personality. For example, the person may use projection and respond aggressively against threats, or he/she may develop a rigid, obsessive personality, be fearful of change, and respond to a threat in a more primitive way.

Presence of Paranoid Process in Other Conditions

Cognitive Impairment

The person with reversible or irreversible cognitive impairment is often suspicious (57, 66). At first he/she may deny confusion and disorientation. As functioning is diminished, he/she explodes with indignation when confronted. Elaborate excuses are made for the behavior, and projection occurs as if others are to blame for the condition. Usually the people who are closest to the individual will get the most blame and will be worked into the delusion. However, the delusion is easily recognized for what it is since it is poorly organized, may change from day to day, is self-aggrandizing, and is obviously an unrealistic statement (56). Yet, mistrusting statements can be difficult to cope with.

Depression

The psychotic depressed person may also be suspicious of others, often accusing others of poisoning or persecuting him/her and maintaining these delusional beliefs in spite of reassurance to the contrary. The more worthless the person feels, the more likely the statements that everyone is out to get him/her. This mistrust of others prevents acceptance of helpful gestures from others.

Withdrawal

The withdrawn person may be diagnosed as having *paraphrenia, a late life schizophrenia with paranoid ideation.* This person is usually a female who lives alone, is partially deaf, is considered eccentric, and has few close relatives or associates. The person appears to have an intact personality but demonstrates an organized, strongly adhered-to delusion, with or without hallucinations. When hallucinations do occur, they are vivid, exciting, and threatening (37, 56, 58, 61). Often the person's response to the delusions and hallucinations is to run away. However, the thoughts and sensations continue to oppress the elderly person until he/she may commit suicide. If this person is treated successfully with phenothiazines, he/she still lacks insight into the illness, saying "The ——— is gone," rather than "I was sick and the medicine helped

(56)." The following case is an example of a paraphrenic senior:

> Mary Smith, at age 66, became suspicious of her minister. She saw the minister gesturing in the pulpit during a church service and said he was signaling for her to get away. She phoned the minister and told him that she had sent him a dollar and wondered when she would receive the return from it. He did not understand and asked her what she meant. She yelled at him, calling him a fool and a cheat. Then she became suspicious of her neighbors; she thought they were talking about her when she saw them talking to each other. Soon she began to hallucinate, and the voices were loud and rude, calling her dirty names. As time progressed, she became more isolated, for she believed a young teen-age neighbor was waiting to rape her. She closed her windows and blinds, locked her door, and had her groceries delivered. Gradually, she believed the teen-age neighbor had the key to her house and was waiting to come in. When this belief became fixed, she moved from her home where she had lived for 50 years.

Classical Paranoia

Classical paranoia is a relatively rare state in which a person holds to a well-organized rigid delusion that relates to only one area of life; otherwise the personality is well-integrated. The person frequently has been successful and relatively well-adjusted in earlier life, and the duration of delusional thinking is unknown. Often someone who has known the person well will recall that the delusional idea has existed for a long time. Only when the person experiences difficulties will the delusion become obvious, because the older person is less discrete in talking about it. Then others begin to recognize the belief as a delusion. Yet, the person with paranoia may continue to function adequately in other spheres of life. We do not know how many people have gone to their deaths with a systematized delusion so that even their relatives do not know how paranoid they really were.

Alcohol and Drug-Induced Paranoid Thinking

Paranoid thinking is a common occurrence during alcohol withdrawal or after a large ingestion of alcohol. C. Miller reported 1 percent of patients admitted to a state hospital with paranoid symptoms had alcohol-induced paranoid psychoses (50).

Paranoid behavior is frequently reported with marijuana and amphetamine use, chronic bromide intoxication, barbiturate abuse, and cocaine abuse. It is not an uncommon feature during withdrawal from barbiturates, minor tranquilizers, and hypnotics (45).

Shared Paranoid Disorders and Psychosis

A shared or mutual agreement in a delusion or system of thinking between two persons can be termed folie a deux and refers to the smallest paranoid group, a psychotic two-group. The two people may be friends, husband and wife, two relatives such as sisters, or one paranoid person and a suggestible person with weakened identity. The group can increase in size and become a paranoid community with religious, political, professional, or reform motives and beliefs. Usually the leader of the group is paranoid and takes vulnerable needy or young people and molds them into a system of belief with persecutory and hate feelings toward a common enemy (45). (Hitler is an example.)

Paranoid Schizophrenia

The person who is suffering from *paranoid schizophrenia has symptoms of schizophrenia along with paranoid characteristics.* According to recent investigators, paranoid schizophrenics can be differentiated from nonparanoid schizophrenics by several features: (1) a stronger family history of schizophrenia in nonparanoid schizophrenia, (2) more formal thought disorder, emotional incongruity, and catatonic traits in nonparanoid schizophrenics, and (3) more persecutory delusions in paranoid schizophrenics. Also paranoid schizophrenics are more likely to have held a job, have been married, have recovered, or have fewer symptoms (45). The paranoid person usually is diagnosed at a later age, normally after age 30 (45). This person tends to be more compensated, less disorganized, more outgoing, more aggressive, and have fewer hallucinations and more delusions. However, research findings are contradictory. Fowler et al. found no significant difference between the frequency of schizophrenia in families with paranoid schizophrenics than in families with no paranoid schizophrenics, but O. Kellman found lower risk of schizophrenia in families with paranoid schizophrenia (45).

ASSESSMENT OF THE SUSPICIOUS PERSON

Typical Statements

Assessment of the suspicious person or of the paranoid thinking process may be difficult because the illness is often hidden by an extrovertive or aggressive behavior. The person appears to be in firm control of self, and the personality appears intact.

However, if you listen closely, you will hear a pattern of denial, rationalization, and projection. The person will first deny the obvious. He/she might say, "No, I am not sick." "No, I do not need help." "I came here (to the hospital) for a rest." You may also hear denial of responsibility for personal behavior. For example: "Somebody keeps moving my glasses." "People keep taking my things." "Nobody remembers to tell me things." You might also hear denial of the defensiveness: "I'm not touchy; they are all prima donnas." "I'm not irritable." "I've always been easy to live with."

Then you become aware of how much is blamed on others. For example, the male says that he lacks certain things because: "My wife is so sloppy." "My kids are dumb." "You nurses aren't doing your job." Other significant statements, when part of the total suspicious pattern, might be: "They let me go at the plant because the bosses are no good." "Did you ever notice how everybody is starting fights these days?" "Nobody has time for a person without money."

If you regularly hear projections dispersed throughout the person's conversation, you can be sure of suspicion, even if you do not see any other evidence. Eventually you will see other signs of mistrust, anger, rationalization, and denial. Or you may notice first a number of rationalizations as if the person were hiding something. If the delusions and suspicious thoughts are firmly entrenched and if the person is sure of misgivings about other people, the rationalizations are operating within the paranoid process and may not be openly stated. If the paranoid process is wavering, or if he/she is cognitively or emotionally struggling to maintain adaptation, rationalization fosters feelings of adequacy. Then you will hear such statements as: "Nobody likes to listen to me because they are all jealous of my experience and knowledge." "People keep taking my things because I have collected invaluable items throughout the years." "Nobody likes to listen to me because they know I have the answers." "They won't let me back in the office to straighten things up; they're afraid of me."

Typical Behaviors

You may first be aware that the client is angry, hostile, openly aggressive, berating others for a variety of abuses, or demanding and expecting too much from others and attacking them for their inadequacies or weaknesses. Or he/she may be controlled so that anger is only expressed about unimportant issues or neutral topics.

Another prominent behavior is the ever-present suspiciousness or mistrust, manifested by glancing about furtively while entering the room, looking for flaws and minor details, and approaching you and others warily. He/she listens carefully and defensively to your words, looking for meanings as if to catch you in an act of harm and protecting self from imagined hurts. The person's body language may express suspicion: he/she carefully moves about, sits on the edge of the chair, or perhaps sits with arms folded as if closed to a "hostile world."

Usually the person is also secretive, wary, or sensitive about being seen, hiding self from you in order to feel safe, talking in a guarded manner, screening words, and protecting thoughts. He/she withholds, gives out information carefully, and evaluates your intentions before disclosing self. You may observe this secretive behavior as you watch how he/she holds any papers, states his/her health history, talks about money in the bank, or clutches the change in his/her hand.

In addition to the clusters of behavior described above, another cluster of behavior consists of the attitudes of superiority, pride, and aloofness. The person may discuss achievements and emphasize people he/she has known or places visited. The person may struggle to show superior knowledge and experience, or use words to impress you. He/she may try to control the conversation between the two of you, responding in a condescending manner. In the hospital he/she will have difficulty accepting and following the patient role; this may be shown by asking for a private room and expressing fears about sleeping with another person, stating a feeling of superiority to other patients in the hospital, or refusing to talk about any problem. The person may never be able to admit that there is no one to love, no one to care about him/her, or nothing worthwhile to do. In the home or apartment he/she will remain distant or even refuse to open the door rather than trust the assistance of a health professional.

Listen Carefully to the Client's History

As the person tells you about his/her life, listen to overt and hidden statements, observe defenses and behaviors used, and examine carefully the manner in which the story is told. Statements are circumstantial and hesitant; everything is explained in extreme detail without ever getting to the point, and conversational spaces are filled with information that seems to fit logically at first but later seems irrelevant. Careful listening can provide clues to delusions.

As the person tells the history, carefully listen to the content. Listen for ideas that do not seem to fit together or are not in tune with reality. Sometimes related ideas are jumbled together as a delusion is explained, so that you feel confused. For example, as you listen to such a conversation, you would feel uncertain about whether the person is losing the home to a greedy landlord, losing money to an unscrupulous caretaker, or being taken advantage of by an unloving daughter. Listen carefully for information that does not fit together or is of such a bizarre nature that you know the material is delusional.

Be Aware of Your Feelings

Be perceptive to your feelings as you talk with the suspicious person. Your own feelings about the person, especially if they validate the overt symptoms, can help you to make a nursing diagnosis. You may feel distance, notice lack of emotional contact between you, and feel "put down" as the person struggles to feel superior to you. The most diagnostic feeling you will have is that of being attacked, assaulted, belittled, stupid, or dumb, as the person is projecting and blaming you or others for his/her difficulties. Eventually the helping person—you—becomes the object of projection, blame, and delusions. Such behavior may cause an open confrontation between you and the client. When you feel yourself pulling back from the onslaught of his/her behavior, or if you feel a desire to retaliate, you have an important clue that the client is projecting and you are the recipient.

NURSING DIAGNOSIS AND FORMULATION OF CLIENT-CARE GOALS

Nursing Diagnosis

Your nursing diagnosis of *suspicious or paranoid ideation* may include assessment of the following behaviors:

1. Demonstrates behavior that is aggressive, abusive, angry, or hostile.
2. Demonstrates varying degrees of mistrust and secretiveness.
3. Responds to stress situations with statements that distort and indicate misunderstanding.
4. Blames other individuals or groups when he/she feels inadequate or uncomfortable.
5. Acts aloof or remains solitary in order to maintain feelings of superiority over others.
6. Makes statements that convey feelings of insecurity, jealousy, possessiveness, fearfulness, or distrust of others.

Client-Care Goals

Long-term goals for the client could include the following:

1. Feelings of trust toward family or close associates are described and demonstrated.
2. Stressful situations are handled without excessive or prolonged denial, projection, or blame.
3. Activities of daily living, work, and leisure are engaged in with others as appropriate to the life situation.
4. Life situations are more realistically appraised.

Short-term goals for the client could include the following:

1. Tolerates increasing physical and emotional closeness of yourself or other significant persons.

2. Engages in activities of daily living with others as appropriate.

3. States strengths and limits realistically.

4. Enters into activities with others for a limited period of time.

You will think of other goals as you work with suspicious persons.

NURSING INTERVENTIONS RELATED TO CLIENT-CARE GOALS

Goals and Interventions

The four long-term client-care goals are discussed here, along with pertinent nursing interventions.

*Goal 1: Feelings of trust toward
family or close associates
are described and demonstrated.*

Interventions

Develop a satisfying relationship. Trusting, caring contacts are difficult to establish but are essential for this person to overcome suspicious thinking (13, 54). Practice of the behaviors described in Chapter 6 and understanding of the dynamics of behavior just described will help you to develop a therapeutic relationship.

Convey to the person that you are aware of his/her feelings. Give an opening by saying, "You feel you have not been treated fairly," or "You seem upset about what is happening." Listen carefully to statements that subtly convey feelings and then validate that you heard the feelings. Do not defend that which is attacked verbally or try to reason away the feelings.

State that you respect his/her desire for privacy or distance. The suspicious person often has real difficulty in maintaining contacts with others unless he/she can keep emotional distance. To keep others away, paranoid people put up a "smoke screen," filibuster, become confused, lash out, or do anything they have to do to push people back. Allow the client to set the pace for closeness and involvement. Listen to the words carefully; there will be clues when you are moving in too fast and getting too close. For example, the person may be talking about the weather or the food, and will state that he/she is feeling closed in, attacked, or taken over. Remain matter-of-fact and somewhat passive in response. Do not move in, emotionally, too fast or be overly friendly or assertive.

Be *consistently reliable;* do what you say you plan to, and do not respond defensively to the anger or condescension. Appeal to the person's healthy behaviors. Let him/her know it is all right to ask for help. If you handle the person with care, you may become very significant to him/her. From you, he/she can learn that people can be trusted, are dependable, and give self a sense of value. As the relationship with you becomes closer, look for a family member or friend who will add to the individual's life.

Teach social skills so that he/she can expand contacts and activities. The person who has mistrusted for a long time will always remain cautious, but perhaps he/she can learn that people can be trustworthy and enjoyable to be with. Help the person to gradually extend self to others. This is important because you cannot always be present when needed, or when the person wants to talk about feelings, fears, or stresses. If the person is willing, have him/her write what would be said to you or another person if he/she is alone and wants to communicate thoughts. Also you have other people to care for and will eventually terminate the relationship. Reaffirm that memories of important relationships, including the relationship with you, can help sustain him/her when alone.

Be genuine and honest. Since the biggest problem this person has is trusting others, it is important to be as honest as possible. Be open, not secretive, so that you do not give the person reason to wonder about you. Be genuine, for this person is having a difficult time trying to evaluate what is and is not true. Protect your relationship. Explain misgivings or misunderstandings. This does not mean defending every word you say but rather responding truthfully, so that he/she at least hears your intention to help and protect. However, being honest and open does not mean being irritable when you are angry or telling him/her you are bored. Being honest also does not mean expressing yourself freely and fully to your clients. There is never any reason or excuse to be hostile toward or to belittle the person. In contrast, presenting a *facade* of compassion can be based upon your own needs, and will not be felt as genuine behavior by the client. You must solve your own problems and work through your own feelings before you try to help the client meet needs. Any suspicious person has a particular facility for finding your weaknesses. You will not fool the client. If your caring and affection are not genuine, he/she will know it.

Increase the client's self-esteem. Your lack of retaliation to the anger and abrasiveness can do more than anything to help the client accept self. Further, as you listen to feelings, complaints, and opinions, and act on them when indicated, you show that you value him/her as a person. Reinforce accomplishments and give praise and recognition when earned. Praise reliability. Encourage the person to make choices. Give opportunities for demonstrating abilities and skills. Promote acquisition of social skills by including him/her in activities, games, and social affairs. Have the person write an autobiography so that you better understand him/her; such an activity also stimulates identity formation and helps the person realize the worth of his/her life. As self-esteem improves, so will the person's ability to trust self—one of the major needs of the person with paranoid thinking (62).

Intervene in a consistent, matter-of-fact and objective manner. A consistent secure environment is important. Avoid creating suspicion. Avoid touching unless you have found it successful with this person. Speak clearly and concisely. Avoid laughing in groups near the person. Whenever you make changes, allow for the client's suspicious questioning: "Why did you move the chair over there?" "Why are we eating at 4?" or "Why are you coming to see me at 4 instead of 6?" Listen to the inquiries. Do not argue. Confront carefully about the suspicious nature of questioning; give the reason for any change in a calm manner. Because he/she mistrusts everything and everyone, he/she may even ask you to taste the food before it is eaten. Do so, and state matter-of-factly that it is not poisoned. The person may also refuse medications or secretively not take them. Observe carefully while administering oral medications and explain the importance of the medication. Answer any questions objectively. If the person wishes to check out the room allow him/her to do so. Explain in a calm, gentle manner about the reality of the situation and that you have nothing but helping in

mind. Be considerate of feelings; respond with kindness even when he/she is irritating to you.

Although the person's suspicious questioning and behavior may cause you to feel defensive, carry on your activities normally. Sometimes when you have someone checking your every move, you behave differently. Do not be maneuvered by questions or behavior. When he/she feels more comfortable with you, suspicion will decrease. You need patience to wait out the gradually increasing comfort.

*Goal 2: Stressful situations
are handled without excessive
or prolonged denial, projection,
or blame.*

Interventions

As you *implement measures just described for goal #1* to increase the client's self-esteem, and as you develop a close relationship, interacting in an honest therapeutic way to his/her behavior, you help the person to feel less hopeless and helpless. As the person feels more in control of self, he/she feels more able to handle stressful situations. Refer to Chapter 12 for specific ways to teach the client to manage stressors healthfully. Through your teaching and modeling of coping behavior, the client learns how to respond to stressors without excessive or prolonged use of defensive mechanisms.

Reduce stressors by working with the client, family, agency staff, employer, or others to maintain an accepting, supportive, consistent environment. Teach the siginificant persons in the client's life how to respond to his/her behavior, which will help to reduce insecurity in the client.

Certain aids may also be necessary to reduce stress. Eye glasses or a hearing aid help overcome sensory impairments. The illness should be treated so that there is energy to cope with other stresses. Safety hazards in the environment should be removed. Community resources should be used to obtain necessities, such as food or shelter, when indicated. Crisis intervention principles described in Chapter 8 can help him/her work through loss, rejection, or loneliness.

The physician may order phenothiazines as described in Chapter 16 to help alleviate anxiety. Drugs of choice include Thorazine, Mellaril, and Haldol (12). These drugs are best given in liquid form because it has been estimated that 70 percent of the pills given to paranoid clients are not taken. All of the phenothiazines come in liquid form.

Goal 3: Activities of daily living, work, and leisure are engaged in with others as appropriate to the life situation.

Interventions

Teach the client how to engage in the normal activities of life in a way that is satisfying to self and others. Your own response to his/her behavior is the first step.

At first the suspicious client, who is accustomed to being alone, may have to be separated from others to decrease the mutual irritability and anger that may result from his/her behavior. However, *avoid seclusion as punishment* since the person needs to learn to relate to others rather than gain satisfaction from being alone.

Avoid confrontation, although the suspicious person is often angry, hostile, and demanding, which interferes with relating and activities in all of life's spheres. Do not take this behavior personally nor retaliate with like behavior. Retaliation does not "teach him a lesson"; rather, it increases insecurity and acting-out behavior. Do not argue or try to give advice to the angry, suspicious client. Do not tease to attempt to humor him/her out of the feelings. Instead, try to understand what caused the explosive behavior and why the person is feeling threatened, rather than belittle what the person believes to be the difficulty. Remain calm, kind, and accepting. Let the person know you care but that you cannot allow behavior that is harmful to self or others. Discuss with the person the consequences and implications of the behavior so that he/she can understand why it cannot be permitted. However, this cannot be done early in the relationship. At first the person may not feel safe enough with you to hear the reality of the situation, but eventually he/she needs to hear in a nonpunitive way that anger only creates problems in living. Explore more acceptable ways of handling feelings. Help the person feel more sure of self and the immediate situation. Timing is crucial.

The suspicious person first needs experience with one person who can be trusted before he/she can dare to trust others. Initially he/she may be fearful in groups of people. Encourage involvement in group activities; however, let him/her set the pace of involvement. Avoid competitive, aggressive activities and those necessitating close bodily contact. Support will be needed. Remember this person is sensitive to little details, small remarks, and minor slights. Also remember that this person is lonely and frightened within the group even if the overt reaction is one of anger rather than fear. Help the client talk about feelings and reactions to the group.

Limit setting at times is important. You need to be firm but not authoritarian in stating restrictions in activity or rules to be followed. The paranoid person becomes threatened when he/she feels a loss of control. Allow the need for control to be expressed in healthy ways.

Activities may be helpful to an overtly angry person. A long walk, working with wood by sanding or hammering, pounding bread, or riding a bike may release energy to cope with angry feelings.

However, the most direct release of angry feelings is through talking. Sometimes it helps to discuss neutral topics where anger can be displayed and be channeled through a topic that the person feels he/she can handle. Also encourage talking about self and feelings, rather than about others and how they are behaving or feeling. Move very cautiously; the person's ego and self-concept are very fragile when he/she appears the most threatening or hostile. Support positive feelings so that the person feels safe enough to allow some degree of closeness.

Often the person is demanding of you and your time. Listen to requests. Be considerate. Do not feel that you must meet all of the requests, but if requests are reasonable, and you can meet them, do so. When you cannot, explain why. Evaluate the requests and try to understand the needs that he/she is trying to meet. If limits must be set, do so with kindness and consistency. If you can anticipate needs before the request or demand is made, you can reduce some of the demanding behavior. If you do not know what he/she wants, ask the person to help you by explaining. Be calm; avoid punitive measures. Try to help the person feel that you do want to help.

The person with some degree of inner control and personality integrity will frequently be in command of words and information. He/she may seem intellectual and use this to maintain a superior position with you. He/she may act very proud, belittle you, and behave in a condescending manner. Often he/she will refuse to go along with rules of an agency or hospital regulations because he/she does not want to admit illness or the need for help. Gently but firmly state the rules that the person must follow and that it is advantageous not to create a fuss. Recognize that the proud, superior, condescending manner is a defense, and do not try to top his/her stories or be superior. Avoid a power struggle by avoiding giving unnecessary demands. Rather, recognize any accomplishments and experiences—where he/she is realistically ahead of you. Give any opportunity to excel. When he/she feels accepted and secure, he/she will be less condescending.

Goal 4: Life situations are more realistically appraised.

Interventions

Explore reality. When the suspicious person begins to feel safe with you, explore alternatives to paranoid ideas. When he/she realizes that the spontaneous expression of feelings, especially hostility, causes difficulty with others, he/she may want to find another way of handling feelings. Discuss ways to control explosive or irritable behavior. Help the person discipline self to delay expression of feelings by intellectually looking at the facts before responding. Encourage putting limits on personal behavior, but realize that he/she will sometimes fail. Although the person can achieve some change, do not expect too much too fast. Even a small change is an accomplishment.

Accept that the delusional person is not realistic; he/she is misinterpreting the surroundings. Much of the literature says for you to present reality. However, it is unrealistic to assume that a paranoid person is capable of accepting our reality. This is true with any of the person's thinking as well as the delusions. To say to a suspicious person in either a harsh or a caring manner, "Those are crazy ideas," or "Those voices are just in your head" is a method of pushing the person away. First assess the level of the relationship. Second, listen carefully so that you can understand as much as possible what is being said.

If you say that something is not true or try to argue the person out of the delusion, he/she will become defensive and not disclose the innermost ideas. Asking questions to get further information does not encourage or agree with the delusion but helps you to know what he/she is thinking. Then you can create doubt about the delusion. The more

subtly you do this, the more successful will be the result. Say to the person, "Do you believe that the mailman has it in for you?" or "Is is possible that your daughter is out to get you?" Question with a doubting voice rather than challenge, oppose, or argue, or the person will feel that he/she must defend the delusion. If he/she asks, "You believe what I am saying, don't you?" respond to the feelings rather than the false belief. Reply, "I realize you *feel* the way you say, and that it is hard for you right now to see things another way." Or you may say, "I do not believe your daughter wants to hurt you, but I know you feel that she does. It is important for us to discuss your ideas because I know they cause you much pain." This gives you an opening for further discussion but you still are presenting reality.

The more you encourage the person to talk about feelings before, during, and after an incident, the more you can foster recognition of the falseness of the belief and the motive for it.

The delusion has meaning to the person. The content usually is organized around two main themes: wishes and fears. The person usually fears not living up to expected standards and being unable to maintain a personal level of perfection. When these fears lessen and he/she either obtains or dismisses the wishes, then the delusion can be given up (61).

The delusional material also has meaning for the listener. Listen for themes and connections. Certainly the man who said, "I am God" will not change his idea just because you tell him he is not, but you then understand how small and insignificant he must feel to have to believe that. The symbolic meaning of the delusional material will give you invaluable information for understanding your client better.

Notice what the delusion means, and what it accomplishes as the person discusses it. Delusional thinking is defensive and is a response to anxiety. It does not make good sense to strip a defense away from a client in times of anxiety. Instead, help the person to feel safe rather than anxious. When the relationship between you sustains the client, when he/she allows you to get close enough to understand and support, then the paranoid person can look at self and the world more realistically. In time it will be important for the person to know that the delusion keeps him/her from living a full life and from being constructive and useful.

WORK WITH THE FAMILY AND HEALTH TEAM

Teach the family ways of responding to the behavior, using the nursing approaches previously described in this chapter. However, the family members may have difficulty carrying out matter-of-fact or helpful responses; the memories of old harangues and the client's habitually aggravating responses keep intruding.

Often the suspicious person comes to your attention because the family can no longer handle him/her. The behavior is so intolerable to them that they wish to institutionalize the person. At times this is necessary, depending on the extent of suspicious behavior. Regardless of the arrangement for client care, the family will need your support and helpful suggestions. However, when you discuss family problems, the client should be present in the conversation. Whatever decisions are made, they will succeed only if the client feels it is his/her choice. The paranoid client struggles against authority, so unless it is contraindicated, and at times it is, allow decisions to be made by your client.

Engage the person in tasks that foster control and success.

Some paranoid persons present a real danger to the family and others. In this case, the family may need protection. Help them to accept and cope with this. In such a situation the person may need a structured life with specific limits and reduced stress.

If the suspicious person is counseled in the community crisis clinic, be cautious initially about the intensity of your relationship. Follow directions of your instructor or supervisor. You will become part of a paranoid person's delusional system if you get emotionally involved too quickly and without limits.

Anytime you care for a suspicious person, all health team workers who have contact with him/her must have a similar approach and be consistent in their behavior. Confer frequently with the other health workers who are involved in the client's care, and keep the client as informed as possible.

EVALUATION

Observe changes in behavior toward you and other people. As the suspicious person improves, you may also note that you feel differently toward him/her. You will feel warmth from and feel warmth toward the client. As the person gains security, he/she will be more comfortable with others, act less angry, or attack others less.

Can you expect changes in the paranoid person? The prognosis is guarded, although a slowly built relationship and the phenothiazine drugs can help. Prognosis is most guarded in the severely suspicious, withdrawn person (39). In the treatment of 93 patients over 60 years of age, for one year,

Post found that 6 became employed and 29 were able to carry out domestic duties effectively. Yet, he felt the results were mostly unfavorable since their way of looking at life did not change very much. Results in this study were highly dependent on adequate drug treatment (56).

Favorable prognostic signs are an immediate behavioral response to phenothiazines, married status, a high social status, and good family relationships (56). Certainly a long-term therapeutic relationship with a caring professional will also improve the prognosis.

REFERENCES

1. Aaronson, Luren, "Paranoia as a Behavior of Alienation," *Perspectives of Psychiatric Care,* 15, no. 1 (1977), 27–31.

2. American Psychiatric Association, Committee on Nomenclature and Statistics, *Diagnostic and Statistical Manual of Mental Disorders,* 3rd ed. *(DSM-III).* Washington, D.C.: American Psychiatric Association, 1980.

3. Barber, R., "Nursing Care Study: Psychopathic Personality with Paranoid Traits," *Nursing Mirror,* 146, no. 19 (1978), 26–27.

4. Berger, K. S., and S. H. Zarit, "Late-Life Paranoid States: Assessment and Treatment," *American Journal of Orthopsychiatry,* 48, no. 3 (1978), 528–37.

5. Berner, P., E. Gabriel, and H. Schanda, "Nonschizo-

phrenic Paranoid Syndromes," *Schizophrenic Bulletin,* 6, no. 4 (1980), 627-32.

6. Beverly, Virginia, "Beginnings of Wisdom about Aging," *Geriatrics,* 30 (1975), 116-28.

7. Blum, H. P., "Paranoia and Beating Fantasy: An Inquiry into the Psychoanalytic Theory of Paranoia," *Journal of American Psychoanalytic Association,* 28, no. 2 (1980), 331-61.

8. Bonner, H., "Sociological Aspects of Paranoia," *American Journal of Sociology,* 56 (1950), 255-62.

9. Bridge, T. P., and R. J. Wyatt, "Paraphrenia: Paranoid States of Late Life. Part I. European Research," *Journal of American Geriatric Society,* 28, no. 5 (1980), 193-200.

10. _____, "Paraphrenia: Paranoid States of Late Life. II. American Research," *Journal of American Geriatric Society,* 28, no. 5 (1980), 201-5.

11. Brink, T. L. et al., "Hypochondriasis and Paranoia: Similar Delusional Systems in an Institutionalized Geriatric Population," *Journal of Nervous Mental Disease,* 167, no. 4 (1979), 224-28.

12. Burnside, Irene, "Recognizing and Reducing Emotional Problems in the Aged," *Nursing 77,* 7, no. 3 (1977), 56-59.

13. Busse, Edward, and Eric Pfeiffer, *Mental Illness in Later Life.* Washington, D.C.: American Psychiatric Association, 1973.

14. Butler, Robert, and Myra Lewis, *Aging and Mental Health.* St. Louis: The C. V. Mosby Company, 1977.

15. Cameron, J., "Paranoid Conditions and Paranoia," in *American Handbook of Psychiatry,* ed. S. Arieti, pp. 475-84. New York: Basic Books, Inc., 1959.

16. Carson, V., and K. Huss, "Prayer—An Effective Therapeutic and Teaching Tool," *Journal Psychiatric Nursing,* 17, no. 3 (1979), 34-37.

17. Chalus, Gary Anton, "An Evaluation of the Validity of the Freudian Theory of Paranoia," *Journal of Homosexuality,* 3, no. 2 (1977), 171-86.

18. Coburn, D., "The Experience of Schizophrenia," *Journal of Psychiatric Nursing,* 15, no. 12 (1977), 9-13.

19. Colby, Kenneth, *Artificial Paranoia: Common General Psychology Series,* pp. 1-9. Los Angeles: University of California, 1975.

20. Corrodi, R. B., "Clinical Assessment of Affect in Schizophrenia," *Journal Clinical Psychiatry,* 39, no. 6 (1978), 493-96.

21. Day, D. W. K., and M. Roth, "Physical Accompaniments of Mental Disorder in Old Age," *Lancet,* 2 (1955), 740.

22. Di Bella, G. A., "Educating Staff to Manage Threatening Paranoid Patients," *American Journal of Psychiatry,* 136, no. 3 (1979), 333-35.

23. Eisendorfer, A., and F. Wilkie, "Auditory Changes in the Aged," *Journal of American Geriatric Society,* 8 (1972), 377-82.

24. Erikson, E. H., *Childhood and Society,* 2nd ed. New York: W. W. Norton & Co., Inc., 1963.

25. Fenichel, O., *The Psychoanalytic Theory of Neurosis.* New York: W. W. Norton & Co., Inc., 1945.

26. Fish, F. J., "Senile Paranoid States," *Gerontology Clinics,* 1 (1959), 127-31.

27. Freeman, A. M., and F. T. Melges, "Temporal Disorganization, Depersonalization, and Persecutory Ideation in Acute Mental Illness," *American Journal of Psychiatry,* 135, no. 1 (1978), 123-24.

28. Freud, S., *Psychoanalytic Notes on an Autobiographic Account of a Case of Paranoia Dementia Paranoides,* standard ed., vol. 12, pp. 1-82. London: Hogarth Press Ltd., 1958.

29. _____, *The Complete Psychological Works of Sigmund Freud,* vol. 14, pp. 82-91. London: Hogarth Press Ltd., 1959.

30. Fry, W. F., Jr., "Paranoid Episodes in Manic-Depressive Psychoses," *American Journal of Psychiatry,* 135, no. 8 (1978), 974-76.

31. Gollicker, Jacqueline, "A New Life at 77," *Nursing Mirror,* 137 (July 13, 1973), 34-37.

32. Green, D. E., "Schizophrenia: Some Problems for the Nurse," *New Zealand Nursing Journal,* 73, no. 1 (1980), 11-13.

33. Henker, F. O., "Acute Brain Syndromes," *Journal Clinical Psychiatry,* 40, no. 3 (1979), 17-20.

34. Hinton, John, "Portrait of a Recluse," *Nursing Times,* 71 (October 30, 1975), 175.

35. Houston, R., and A. Royse, "Relationship between Deafness and Psychotic Illness," *Journal of Mental Science,* 100 (1954), 990-93.

36. Hunter, R. C., "Forgiveness, Retaliation and Paranoid Reactions," *Canadian Psychiatric Association Journal,* 23, no. 3 (1978), 167-73.

37. Kay, D. W. K., and M. Roth, "Environment and Hereditary Factors in the Schizophrenics of Old Age and Their Bearing on the General Problem of Causation of Schizophrenia," *Journal of Mental Science,* 107 (1961), 649.

38. Klein, Melanie, *The Psycho-Analysis of Children.* New York: Grove Press, Inc., 1960.

39. Langley, G., "Functional Psychoses," in *Modern Perspectives in the Psychiatry of Old Age*, ed. John Howells, pp. 326–55. New York: Brunner/Mazel, Inc., 1975.

40. Limentani, A., "The Differential Diagnosis of Homosexuality," *British Journal of Medical Psychology*, 50 no. 3 (1977), 209–16.

41. Lipscomb, W., "Acute Paranoia," *Emergency Medicine*, 1 (1969), 17–23.

42. MacKinnon, Roger, and Robert Michels, *The Psychiatric Interview in Clinical Practice*, pp. 259–94. Philadelphia: W. B. Saunders Company, 1971.

43. MacLean, Paul, "The Paranoid Streak in Man," *Consciousness: The Brain, States of Awareness, and Alternate Realities*, eds. Daniel Goleman and Richard Davidson, pp. 24–26. New York: Irvington Publishers, Inc., 1979.

44. Manschreck, T. C., "The Assessment of Paranoid Features," *Comprehensive Psychiatry*, 20, no. 4 (1979), 370–77.

45. Manschreck, T. C., and M. Petri, "The Paranoid Syndrome," *Lancet*, 2 (July 27, 1978), 251–53.

46. Martin, Ian, "The Intruders," *Nursing Times*, 73 (February 17, 1977), 244–45.

47. Meissner, W. W., *The Paranoid Process*. New York: Jason Aronson, Inc., 1978.

48. ___, "Addiction and Paranoid Process: Psychoanalytic Perspectives," *International Journal of Psychoanalysis Psychotherapy*, 8 (1980–81), 273–310.

49. ___, "The Wolf-Man and the Paranoid Process," *Psychoanalytical Review*, 66, no. 2 (1979), 155–71.

50. Miller, C., "The Paranoid Syndrome," *Archives of Neurology and Psychiatry*, 49 (1941), 953.

51. Modly, D. M., "Paranoid States," *Journal Psychiatric Nursing*, 16, no. 5 (1978), 35–37.

52. Murray, Ruth, M. Marilyn Huelskoetter, and Dorothy O'Driscoll, *The Nursing Process in Later Maturity*. Englewood Cliffs, N.J.: Prentice-Hall, Inc., 1980.

53. Neadley, A. W., "Nursing Care Study: Paranoid Depression," *Nursing Times*, 73, no. 41 (October 13, 1977), 1590–92.

54. Pfeiffer, Eric, "Psychotherapy with Elderly Patients," in *Geriatric Psychiatry*, eds. Leopold Bellak and Taksoz Karasu, pp. 191–205. New York: Grune & Stratton, Inc., 1976.

55. Pinderhughes, C. A., "The Universal Resolution of Ambivalence by Paranoia with an Example in Black and White," *American Journal of Psychotherapy*, 24 (1970), 597–610.

56. Pitt, Brice, *Psychogeriatrics*. London: Churchill Livingstone Publishers, 1974.

57. Relterstal, N., *Prognosis in Paranoid Psychoses*. Springfield, Ill.: Charles C Thomas, Publisher, 1970.

58. Roth, M., "The Natural History of Mental Disorders in Old Age," *Journal of Mental Science*, 101 (1955), 201–301.

59. Sletten, I., and S. Ballous, "The Selection of Delusional Persecutors," *Canadian Psychiatric Association Journal*, 12 (1967), 327–31.

60. Solomon, Philip, and Vernon Patch, *Handbook of Psychiatry*. Los Altos, Calif.: Lange Medical Publications, 1971.

61. Spanton, John, "Paraphrenic," *Nursing Times*, 71 (December 25, 1975), 2053–54.

62. Stankiewicz, B., "Guides to Nursing Intervention in the Projection Pattern of Suspicious Patients," *Perspectives of Psychiatric Care*, 2, no. 1 (1964), 39–47.

63. Storr, A., "Sadism and Paranoia. Cruelty as Collective and Individual Response," *Journal of Child Psychological Psychiatry Book Supplement, vol. I*, pp. 1–11. 1978.

64. Sullivan, Harry S., *Clinical Studies in Psychiatry*. New York: W. W. Norton & Co., Inc., 1956.

65. ___, *Conceptions of Modern Psychiatry*. New York: W. W. Norton & Co., Inc., 1953.

66. Travelbee, Joyce, *Intervention in Psychiatric Nursing*, pp. 177–211. Philadelphia: F. A. Davis Company, 1969.

67. Verwoerdt, Adrian, *Clinical Geropsychiatry*. Baltimore: The William & Wilkins Company, 1976.

68. Whitehead, J., *Psychiatric Disorders in Old Age*. New York: Springer Publishing Co., Inc., 1974.

69. Wicks, Robert, *Counseling Strategies and Intervention Techniques for the Human Services*. Philadelphia: J. B. Lippincott Company, 1977.

70. Winokur, G., "Delusional Disorder (Paranoia)," *Comprehensive Psychiatry*, 18 no. 6 (1977), 511–21.

71. Wurmser, L., "Phobic Core in the Addictions and the Paranoid Process," *International Journal Psychoanalytical Psychotherapy*, 8 (1980–81), 311–35.

18

The Cognitively Impaired Person

Study of this chapter will enable you to:

1. Discuss personal feelings about the loss of cognitive functions and the value of the deteriorating person.

2. Describe general etiology and manifestations of reversible (acute) and nonreversible (chronic) cognitive impairment.

3. Contrast abilities and limitations of the person with impaired cognitive function with those of the cognitively unimpaired person.

4. Discuss how to generally differentiate between the person with functional illness and one with an organic brain disorder.

5. Use an effective assessment tool to determine a nursing diagnosis of cognitive impairment.

6. Formulate client-care objectives and a care plan for a person with a reversible brain disorder and one with a nonreversible brain disorder.

7. Adapt nursing intervention to the needs of the client with cognitive impairment related to etiology, signs, symptoms, and behavior.

8. Work with other health team members to initiate or continue a reality-orientation program.

9. Evaluate the effectiveness of your care by looking at your feelings and approach, and patient's response.

This chapter contributed by M. Marilyn Huelskoetter, R.N., M.S.N.

SCOPE OF THE PROBLEM

The twentieth century has changed the population configuration of the United States from that of a large population of young people to an increasing number of elderly people (11). Today, one in every nine Americans is over 65 years of age, and it is estimated that in 50 years, one in every five people will be over 65 (67). More people are living longer, and many are remaining healthy to enjoy their later years. However, some are not remaining healthy. Approximately 25 to 50 percent of those over 75 years are disabled with a variety of illnesses and infirmities (11). One problem among the aged is cognitive impairment; 4 to 6 percent of the aged suffer from neuronal degeneration arising from cerebrocirculatory problems or unknown causes (44).

Although only 2 or 3 percent of persons over 65 years are institutionalized as a result of cognitive deterioration or psychiatric illness, three out of every ten patients in mental institutions are over 65 years of age, and 94 percent of these elderly have been diagnosed as suffering from chronic brain disease or cerebral multi-infarct disease.

Not only is life extending for a longer period, but the difficulties found during the years of later maturity are also expanding. The presenile or degenerative illnesses occurring before 65 years are not new, but they are becoming a broader problem. Some authors estimate that Alzheimer's Disease, a presenile brain disease, is the fourth or fifth commonest cause of death in the United States today (12, 43).

You will be working with the elderly not only in the psychiatric setting but also in the acute care, extended care, community, emergency, and home settings. You may be caring for elderly persons within your own family. You will probably encounter the cognitively impaired, either in a fleeting period or during an extended illness. Therefore you need to understand as fully as possible what cognitive impairment is and what can be done to improve the lives of the elderly suffering from it as well as the lives of their loved ones.

DEFINITIONS

Cognitive impairment is caused by a variety of conditions associated with brain tissue dysfunction and is seen in any age group (5). This chapter will focus on impairment in the adult. Chapter 21 discusses impairment in the child/adolescent. Many terms are used to explain or classify this impairment, and they can be confusing. First, the terms *organic* and *functional* relate to causation. The term **organic** *refers to cognitive impairment resulting from brain tissue changes.* Agents of causation include: (1) genetic or congenital defects, (2) intracranial and systemic infections, (3) drugs, poisons, and systemic intoxication, (4) brain trauma, either at birth or later in life, (5) epilepsy, (6) disturbance of metabolism, growth, or nutrition, (7) intracranial neoplasms, and (8) degenerative disease of the central nervous system. The term **functional** *is used if there is no discernible or identifiable cause,* such as in psychosis or neurosis (27).

In early times, *dementia* was the term used to denote madness; however, later it meant organic loss of intellectual ability. Today the term is used much less, and some condemn the usage entirely (51). As people began living longer and evidencing more cognitive difficulty, senile dementia was separated in the literature from arteriosclerotic disease. Functional problems began to be differentiated according to symptoms, such as depression, delusional thinking, and paranoia. M. Roth later classified all disorders of later life into affective, senile, and arteriosclerotic psychoses (62). In the *Diagnostic and Statistical Manual-II* by the American Psychiatric Association, acute and chronic brain disorders were classified into psychotic, neurotic, and behavioral reactions. As if this were not confusing enough, in *DSM-II*, the classifications were changed to psychotic and nonpsychotic disorders (5). The *nonpsychotic conditions are those in which the person, though troubled, can test reality and can handle basic daily habits of living without the presence of gross perceptual distortions,* such as hallucinations and delusions. The *psychotic reactions are those in which the person has impaired reality testing and gross interference in the ability to meet the demands of life because of deficits of language, memory, or perception* (68).

In the *DSM-III*, published in 1980 (see Appendix), the organic brain syndromes were classified as Delirium, Dementia, Amnestic Syndrome, Organic Delusion Syndrome, Organic Hallucinosis, Organic Affective Syndrome, Organic Personality Syndrome, Intoxification, Withdrawal, and Atypical (6).

Under a second category are the dementias arising in the senium and presenium. The major type of presenium disease, Alzheimer's Disease, is now believed to be the major dementia in late life and is called Alzheimer Disease Senile Dementia Complex by some medical researchers. J. C. Brocklehurst states that the future of geriatric care will hinge on fundamental research into senile dementia and cerebrovascular disease (11).

GENERAL ASSESSMENT

The Interview

When you first meet the person in the assessment interview, rely on your observations and listening skills. Although you may observe obvious data about failing cognition as the person walks into the room, you will probably have to look for subtle changes such as clues in conversation, memory, judgment, affect, and orientation. If the person is interviewed with family members, their perception can be exceedingly important. They may openly state such symptoms as, "Mom wanders around the house at night," or "She laughs and cries all in a matter of minutes." Or they may say no more than, "Mom is failing." Follow these clues until you have a clear understanding of the symptoms. As the interview begins, you may observe that the person's anxiety is increasing, which in turn increases his/her confusion. Perhaps you will notice that the family members discuss the person as if he/she were not present, and they speak of him/her negatively. Determine how to progress with the interview. Perhaps you may want to talk to the family or the client alone. Or you may want to make a first-level assessment of the person quickly and then continue further assessment later in several short sessions.

The first interview usually produces fear in the person. Even in the best situation, such as at home, the person is struggling to think and to hold on to failing mental capabilities. With the added stress of new people, ideas, or an unfamiliar setting, the client experiences greater difficulty. Feelings of uneasiness, vulnerability, fear, and confusion are frequently experienced.

Adjust the interview to the person you are meeting. Patience and gentleness can help to promote a sense of safety in the setting. If you try to create a safe, comfortable setting, you will usually be rewarded with enough information to make an early assessment. Do not feel that you must ask every question on the interview tool. Do not rush the client. Allow time and space for the client to tell his/her story. If pushed, anxiety and disorganization will result, and your purpose may be defeated (72). While the interview is progressing, carefully notice the level of functioning. You may want to apply more stress by challenging a point that the person has made or questioning a date given in order to observe the reaction. You may want to provide more structure to assess whether or not he/she can function within a more defined framework. Never press the client more than is necessary. Whenever possible, respond in a helpful manner. You can support with an empathic statement, or you can give a reassuring smile to convey the impression that the person is in good hands. At times, you may be able to make a sound assessment in one interview; in other cases, it will take longer. Now is the time to begin the nurse-client relationship, which may be the most helpful tool in the assessment process.

No typical person complaining of confusion and suffering cognitive impairment, with either acute or chronic organic syndrome, exists. A wide range of behaviors is seen from client to client. Behaviors may change. And severity changes. Complications are as varied as are the personalities of the individuals concerned. Furthermore, the type and severity of the behavior are not always related to the extent of brain damage. The person with little neuropathology sometimes shows severe behavioral change. And those with profound pathology may have only mild symptoms. In some instances, even normal-behaving people may have

brain changes as marked as others with senile or arteriosclerotic disorders (22, 41).

The wide range of symptoms or behaviors manifested by cognitively impaired people is caused by a variety of factors: long-term personality patterns; the crisis of loss; death of loved ones; complications of neurotic, psychotic, and behavioral disorders; stressful social and economic environments; lack of religious or family support; or pathology located in different areas of the brain.

Common Symptoms: Comparison between Cognitive Impairment and Functional Illness

The basic features of cognitive impairment are found in the acronym JOMAC (*J*udgment, *O*rientation, *M*emory, *A*ffect, *C*ognitive) (27). They include: (1) faulty judgment; (2) sensorium impairment, such as impaired orientation, loss of memory, and disordered intellectual functioning; and (3) lability of affect (27). As indicated by the following discussion, assessment of these areas aids differential diagnosis between reversible (acute) or nonreversible (chronic) cognitive impairment and functional illness.

Faulty Judgment

Judgment is the ability to perceive and distinguish relationships or alternatives, with the capacity to make reasonable decisions. When you are assessing the person's ability to make judgments, you will be looking at the form, speed, and content of expressed thought. For example, you may ask the person to explain a fable or old saying. During the interview you may notice a lack of sequence of thought, or the inability to make and act on a decision, or unrealistic thinking. If you observe illogical thinking, you have reason to question the person's ability to judge and decide. As judgment deteriorates, so does the ability to think in the abstract. Frequently the most difficult problems encountered by the person struggling with impaired judgment center around situations in everyday living. The family may tell you about unwise investments, permissive sexual activity, or family embarrassments from behavioral indiscretions. Wills may have been changed or money given away. Friends may comment about "change in living habits'' or "going back to childhood." You may observe inappropriate dress, excessive makeup or perfume, or an unkempt, dirty appearance. The client with severe functional problems, such as schizophrenia or mania, will also have difficulty in judgment, which can cause difficulty in diagnosis differentiation (27).

Impaired Orientation

Orientation is the ability to locate self in one's environment as to person, place, or thing. Loss of orientation is fairly easy to assess (31). Disorientation for time, day, hour, month, or year occurs first, and can readily be determined by questioning. Disorientation about location or place seems to occur next. To determine place disorientation, ask the following questions: "Where are you? What city do you live in? What state do you live in? What country do you live in?" Next, the person tends to lose the identity of the people around him/her. Finally, knowledge of self is lost. Ask the person who he/she is, what his/her name is, or whom he/she sees in the mirror. Disorientation may be first noted at night when sensory stimulation is lower, as the person wanders around, gets lost, or does not answer to his/her name. Major difficulties in orientation usually accompany advanced brain disease.

In the person diagnosed with reversible (acute) brain syndrome, the disorientation may fluctuate from hour to hour; whereas a person with nonreversible (chronic) brain syndrome may have longer periods of disorientation, then become oriented for a time, and then return again to disorientation. In comparison, clients with functional illnesses often lose sense of identity first, and then they lose their orientation for time, place, and person.

Secondary Symptoms

Secondary symptoms such as hallucinations, illusions, and delusions may also interfere with the person's orientation. Hallucinations occur without sensory stimuli or impairment, whereas illusions may occur because of hearing, vision, or tactile impairment. Delusions may be unrelated to current life experiences, for example, a suspicious, frightened patient may refuse food because he/she believes that it is poisoned. Or he/she may hide in a room because of a belief that the nurses are going to steal his/her money. The schizophrenic or manic patient may also have sensory perceptions that promote disorientation, but in this case the hallucinations or illusions are much more bizarre and symbolic. Often the delusions are extremely autistic and are poorly understood by others because they are responses to personal fears and fantasies.

Memory Loss

Memory is the retention of material over a period of time and involves differing forms of response. You may tell the person several items at the beginning of the interview and later ask what information he/she was given in order to check recent memory loss. *Immediate memory, reproduction, recognition, or recall within a period of not more than five seconds,* may be tested by showing a picture, then removing it and asking the person to tell you about the picture. *Recent memory, reproduction, recognition, or recall after 10 seconds or longer,* may be tested by reading a story or showing a list of words and asking the person to repeat them to you (27). This type of assessment must be done carefully and sensitively; you must wait for the person's reaction. In some cases, the person may think that it is a game or a fun situation and may not respond accurately; or he/she may feel used, especially if the assessment can be done in other ways, or vulnerable and frightened. Such assessment might be perceived as exploitation or ridicule.

Assessing memory of the person is not easy. When the person is able to compensate, detection may come only with time or detailed questioning. In the early stages of memory loss, the person may have difficulty recalling names and may use phrases for places and events. He/she may be *circumstantial, talking around the topic,* or may *confabulate, filling in gaps of conversation with fantasy.* When the person is trying to hide the loss from others and self, his/her communication may include pleasantries and banter. Some people are consciously aware of the initial loss. Others may show signs of anxiety about the condition without wanting to share it with you. Note these emotional clues; then make further inquiries. For example, during an interview a client hesitates, searches for words, flushes, and begins to tremble when asked what day it is. He states that the day is Tuesday, the 4th, even though he was told earlier in the day it is Monday, the 24th. With increasing memory loss, the deficit will be noticed more frequently in situations involving people. The person may forget names of close family members, relatives, or neighbors. He/she may call out, "Oh Mary, I haven't seen you in years. How I remember the good times we had together." In reality, the two people are strangers.

The last memory deficit to be noted is that of the self. In the interview the person may also complain of fatigue or exhaustion because of the amount of energy needed to maintain integrity and to cope with failing memory and intellectual ability.

A common belief is that people, especially the elderly, suffering from advanced brain disorders have well-preserved remote memory. In actual fact, their remote memory is significantly inferior to that of normal persons of comparable age and education. However, even the person suffering from greater deterioration will retain longer the events that have made an impact and have been repeated many times; in this case, the remote memory is better than the recent memory (51).

Contrary to general belief, recent memory loss does occur with many elderly people. In cases in which they view it as a feared mental illness, the problem may be exaggerated. Memory loss frequently occurs in conjunction with depression and anxiety. However, with a functional illness there will be little difference between recent and remote memory loss.

Lability of Affect

Affect refers to the emotional expression, reaction, or stability of the person. Definite emotional changes occur in brain disease, but most normal people show more pronounced personality characteristics and manner of response as age progresses. A common feature is *lability of affect, rapid fluctuation in emotional response.* The person reacts excessively and inappropriately, laughing one minute and crying the next. He/she may mimic your emotions, acting angry if you appear angry. He/she may look sad, cry, and say, "I don't know why I am crying; I don't feel that bad." A later characteristic is the emotional outburst called *emotional incontinence, inability to control aggressive*

or sexual impulses (18). The elderly person will be particularly unable to hold back or defend against unacceptable feelings and loosened inhibitions and may become very angry, irritable, or depressed. As the disease progresses, a leveling of affect takes place. Spontaneity, range of response, and appropriateness are lost. Response becomes more apathetic, dull, and monotonous.

Throughout the illness the person may suffer from added stress and may experience symptoms of psychotic, neurotic, and behavioral disorders. These disorders may in turn present emotional symptoms that will cloud the picture. Depression, for example, may result from a changing neurological picture or it may be a reaction to severe cognitive impairment.

Disordered Intellectual Functioning

Cognition involves the ability to know, think clearly, concentrate, and function intellectually. This area, as well as the other areas just described, varies in degree of impairment and may be classified from mild to severe. Clinical observation and neuropsychological testing help to determine general intelligence, reasoning, problem solving, speed and flexibility of response, attention and concentration, language performance, and extent of deterioration (32). Assess levels of education, manner of speech, topics of conversation, comprehension, flow of thought progression, and manner of communication. You need information about previous performance in order to make an accurate comparison; consider prior occupation and organizational involvements. (Do not assume that the ditchdigger was less intellectually bright or less complex than the traveling salesman, for example.) Look for impoverishment of ideas, reduced flow of thoughts and ideas, and inability to abstract (18).

Assessment Tools

Assessing cognitive function is a subjective area. The interview and the use of JOMAC as a guide are essential. The assessment tools in Chapter 4 may also be helpful. You may find simple ways to assess cognitive function, such as using pictures or having the person copy simple drawings (a circle or square). Various psychological tests can be used. You may find Goldfarb's 10-point scale helpful for assessing the extent of the impairment (35). The questions to ask are:

1. Where are we now? (place orientation)
2. Where is this place located? (place orientation)
3. What month is it? (time orientation)
4. What day of the month is it? (time)
5. What year is it? (time)
6. How old are you? (memory)
7. When is your birthday? (memory)
8. Where were you born? (memory)
9. Who is the president of the United States? (general information and memory)
10. Who was the president before him? (general information and memory)

The evaluation is done by counting up the number of incorrect answers (35):

0–2   No impairment to mild impairment.
3–8   Moderately impaired.
9–10 Severely impaired.

Another scale used to assess deterioration in the spheres of orientation, emotional control, motor ability, and communication was developed by a team at Kingston Psychiatric Hospital in Canada. Content and scoring of the scale are described in detail in J. Lawson, M. Rodenburg, and J. Dykes (50).

Remember that test results can be influenced by many factors, including response to the test and the tester. Do not be hasty in your conclusions about the past and present functioning.

COMPARATIVE ASSESSMENT OF REVERSIBLE (ACUTE) AND NONREVERSIBLE (CHRONIC) COGNITIVE IMPAIRMENT (BRAIN DISORDERS)

The previous discussion on assessment relates generally to anyone with cognitive impairment. However, it is useful to know the different manifestations of reversible (acute) and nonreversible (chronic) brain disorders. The following discussion and Table 18-1 will help to clarify the differences. Usually cognitive impairment, both reversible and nonreversible, has multiple causation (45, 51).

Reversible Cognitive Impairment

Reversible (acute) brain disorder is a confusional state in a severe, fulminating form and produces symptoms related to the functions of the brain area involved. For example, subdural hematoma or epidural bleeding in the temporal lobe might cause olfactory hallucinations; bleeding in the occipital lobe would cause visual hallucinations.

Frequently, however, the total brain reacts in a diffuse manner. You may observe clouding of consciousness, disorientation, fluctuation of confusion, and reduced attention span. Perceptual disturbances usually occur in severe cases. The client may complain of various perceptions when awake or upon awakening, or may experience them as nightmares during sleep. Hallucinations are common, vivid, and frightening. Illusions are also

common; the person may misinterpret common objects in the environment to be animals, insects, or frightening people. Often the perceptions produce fear and anxiety. Many clients with acute brain syndrome are also delusional. Frequently the delusions are persecutory in nature, and the client may feel trapped or endangered by someone or something.

You should note not only the various physical and behavioral symptoms but also the duration, fluctuations in severity, and possible precipitating causes. Such observations can help determine the diagnosis.

Just as a child may react to an elevated temperature with a seizure, so the adult may react to elevated temperature, immobility, fecal impaction, stress, pain, and the other etiologic factors given in Table 18-1, with resulting confusion or a variety of other symptoms of impaired cognition (64).

Often, diminished cognition is a presenting sign of other problems, although the person cannot label symptoms clearly or recognize any abnormalities. Or he/she may indirectly tell you about being ill by complaining about food, mobility, and relatives, or by restating past complaints. Emotional lability, confusion, disorientation, or poor judgment frequently precede myocardial infarction,

TABLE 18-1. Comparison of Reversible and Nonreversible Cognitive Impairment

CHARACTERISTIC	REVERSIBLE (ACUTE)	NONREVERSIBLE (CHRONIC)		
		Impairment from Neuronal Degeneration in Pre-senium	Impairment from Neuronal Degeneration in Senium	Impairment from Hypertensive Cerebral Vascular Disease or Multi-infarct Senile Dementia
Onset	Sudden	Slow, insidious.	Slow, insidious.	Slow, insidious.
Etiology	Temporary, diffuse disturbance of brain function, which results from a toxic process. Examples include cerebral hypoxia; intracranial tumor or abscess; head trauma; infection; altered cellular content; dehydration; electrolyte imbalance; malnutrition; metabolic disorder such as uremia or diabetes; intoxication by poisons, drugs, or alcohol; seizure disorders; sensory deprivation; liver dysfunction; hemorrhage, anemia; psychological abuse.	Major atrophy in fronto-temporal region of cerebral cortex. Pick's Disease: atrophy of brain cells. Alzheimer's Disease: eurofibrillary changes and nerve cell loss, especially in cerebral cortex and white matter. Abundance of senile plaques. Degeneration from Huntington's Chorea and Jakob-Crentzfield Disease, which is caused by a viral agent, has a rapid onset with deterioration in 4 to 8 months.	Alzheimer's Disease. Senile Dementia causes changes in nerve cells with senile plaques and abnormal cortical cells, as well as atrophy of of brain substance. Ventricular enlargement. Most common of non-reversible confusion in senium.	Arteriosclerotic changes in vessels, causing decreased blood supply to brain cells. Small cortical scars from multiple widespread emboli may cause cerebral dysfunction. Tissue softens and discolors.
Age of onset	Any age, depending on etiology.	Any time after age 40. Most common in 50s and early 60s.	Age 65 to 70 years, or later.	Age 50 to 65 years. May not occur until later.
Sex	Either male of female.		Females more frequently.	Males more frequently.
Physical symptoms	Related to etiology. Any organ system may be affected. Delirium, stupor, coma.	Restlessness. Ataxia. Increased appetite. Muscle twitching and seizures in final stage.	Fatigue; nocturnal restlessness; deterioration of self-care habits; disturbed sexual behavior; incontinence.	Dizziness; headaches; hypertension in 50 percent of cases; fatigue; drowsiness; syncope; marked physical deterioration; stiff and shaky voluntary muscles; ataxia; poor coordination. Often symptoms of a small stroke.
Speech pattern	May or may not be abnormal.	Speech and understanding of communication impaired.	Dysphasia—impaired ability to speak and perhaps to comprehend.	Dysphasia and slurred speech.
Mental symptoms	Rapid impairment of orientation, memory, intellectual function, and judgment. Confused.	Progressive memory loss. Disoriented as to time and place. Confused. Impaired judgment, especially in personal habits.	Disoriented; confused; impaired abstract thinking, memory, and judgment.	Poor concentration and judgment; memory loss.
Emotional symptoms	Impaired affect; may have psychotic or neurotic reaction.	Irritability with temper outbursts. Distractible. Personality change. Loss of spontaneity. Flat affect.	Anger and irritability; emotional lability; use of rationalization, denial, or projection; increased dependency; helplessness; possibility of suicide or accidents.	Personality degeneration; may have insight into difficulty up until the last stages which causes depression, anger, suspicion, delusions.

TABLE 18-1.   Continued

CHARACTERISTIC	REVERSIBLE (ACUTE)	NONREVERSIBLE (CHRONIC)		
		Impairment from Neuronal Degeneration in Pre-senium	Impairment from Neuronal Degeneration in Senium	Impairment from Hypertensive Cerebral Vascular Disease or Multi-infarct Senile Dementia
Clinical course	Brief. Recovery unless there are physical complications that do not respond to treatment.	Three stages: (1) Death from diseases closely related to cerebral degeneration. (2) Wasting away process. (3) Reduced life expectancy.	Intellectual and physical deterioration progressing for years, ending in death; reduced life expectancy.	Death from cerebral vascular accident.

Source: Murray, et al. *Nursing Process in Later Maturity* (Prentice-Hall; © 1980), Table 20.1. Used with permission, Prentice-Hall, Inc., Englewood Cliffs, N. J.

cerebrovascular accident, congestive heart failure, or cardiac arrhythmias (76).

The acute physical adaptive process itself may cause further difficulty. Toxins from tissue damage are circulated to all body cells, cutting off adequate oxygen supply, and with it, nutrients and fluids, thus upsetting the body chemistry. In the end this causes more confusion (57).

Many times the well-functioning person temporarily reacts to a change of environment or stress with complaints of not knowing where he/she is, misinterpreting people, or forgetting what has just been going on. Although the younger person who has suffered a toxic state or a head injury may return to normal functioning rapidly, the older person is not so likely to do so. Even without a history of degeneration, the elderly person has a greater chance of nonreversible cognitive impairment because deterioration is begun or accelerated by the acute assault. It seems that since the elderly person has moved to a more precarious mental position, any one of a number of factors may cause disorganization of mental abilities and brain functioning.

Nonreversible Cognitive Impairment

Assessment of *nonreversible (chronic) cognitive impairment (chronic brain disorder)* may be easier and more accurate in the home than in the clinic or doctor's office. During visits to a family, you can check the client for beginning signs of mental difficulty: amnesia, misidentification, disorienta-

tion, confusion, defective judgment, and poor impulse control. Your assessment in the home will be more accurate than in an institution since the person functions at the highest level in familiar surroundings. Further, you can also assist the family to understand and deal with behaviors they are noticing for the first time, and to intervene in the early stages. If the client is elderly and is diagnosed with chronic (nonreversible) brain syndrome, you must also assess for various physical problems. Common problems could be cardiac decompensation, cardiac attacks, transient ischemic attacks, cerebral hemorrhage, fractures, decubitus, peripheral circulatory problems, anemia, uremia, infection, and pulmonary complications. (All these conditions could also cause reversible cognitive impairment.) Further, observe for signs of depression, suicidal ideation, withdrawal, alienation, loneliness, and disengagement. While working with this client, you must be attuned to many nursing specialties.

Case Studies

The following are three different examples of people who are suffering from cognitive impairment or chronic nonreversible brain disease:

Mr. S. is a well-known lawyer and an active member of a small town community. He graduated from the state college and came back home to begin his law practice. He worked long, hard hours and soon had an established business. He joined clubs, ran for office, and served in politics. He married and raised four sons. In his late fifties he began to complain of headaches, dizziness, and periods of forgetfulness. He went to his family practice physician and discovered he was suffering from high blood pressure and related arteriosclerotic problems. He was given medication and soon felt better. Several years later he began to have symptoms of inability to concentrate, disorientation, loss of memory, and confusion.

Miss Sarah B., the third-grade teacher at the town school, had never married and had been occupied in education and related activities all her life. She lived alone in a small house on the edge of town. She was a quiet person, very responsible, and dedicated. People admired her, but she had few friends. At 65, she retired, and people soon realized they were seeing her less. Rumors about her activities included seeing her peeking out of her windows and yelling at the delivery man. A distant cousin came to the area to visit and went to see Miss Sarah. She let him into the house, which was covered with feces and foul-smelling food. She seemed disoriented and disorganized; she could not remember him or the family. She was disheveled in appearance. When he asked her to go with him to the physician in the community, she refused.

Mrs. M. was the wife of the city chief of police. She had three daughters and was a conscientious mother and homemaker. As the daughters grew and married, several crises came into the family life and Mrs. M. had difficulty adjusting. Friends said she was never the same. At age 53, she began to wear heavy makeup, unmatched clothes, and inappropriate outer garments, such as coats or sweaters in the summer. Her husband said she did not bathe, although she wore a lot of powder. She became progressively confused and began to have trouble stating her sentences. At times she did not comprehend what was said to her. Her body movement was disorganized; at times she walked with a scissorlike gait.

Diagnostic Procedures

Brain disorders are usually discovered by: (1) careful observation and interview, (2) JOMAC assessment by the nurse, (3) a history showing abnormalities in physical, neurological, and psychological examinations, or (4) an electroencephalogram or brain scan. Skull X-rays, lumbar puncture, arteriography, air studies, CT, and PET Scan may also be done.

Diagnostic measures should be directed toward the whole person. The physician may only look for the precipitating cause of the acute state and its physical complications. In the hospital, the client may be diagnosed with diabetes, heart disease, or any number of chronic illnesses, and no one notes the acute brain syndrome the person is suffering. If the acute brain syndrome is not diagnosed, further complications may occur.

A variety of diagnostic studies is the best way to determine if the symptoms result from a temporary condition, age deterioration, or vascular problems. Very specific body chemistry tests and X-rays can help to diagnose a physical disease that is causing an acute confusional state. In multi-infarct dementia, small brain vessel accidents will produce infarcts or dead tissue and coagulated blood which causes brain changes. Often there has been a history of hypertension and cerebrovascular accidents. If the client has generalized vessel disease, he/she may be having cardiac, kidney, lung, and vascular complications as well. Neurological symptoms are common. In senile dementia, various skull X-rays may show diffuse cerebral atrophy or shrinking with dilatation and enlargement of the ventricles and widening of the cortical sulci, but senile dementia cannot be conclusively and effectively diagnosed (32). Senile dementia may be positively confirmed at autopsy when a higher than normal density of senile plaques are found on the brain.

Some elderly people who function adequately have been found at autopsy to have advanced brain pathology. Clients diagnosed with either Alzheimer's disease or multi-infarct senile disease may have atrophy, tangles, plaques, and softening of the brain. The extent of brain changes may influence behavior as well as the emotional aspects of the personality. Many times depression will cause some of the same symptoms as chronic (nonreversible) brain disorder; therefore differential diagnosis is difficult.

The physician may diagnose cerebral vascular disorder from an assessment of the symptoms and signs. It can be much more difficult to diagnose senile or presenile dementia. A person with senile dementia is characteristically over 65, may also have arteriosclerotic changes, and would reveal, on autopsy, cerebral plaques and abnormal cortical cells (74). A person with presenile Alzheimer's disease is characteristically under 65 and does not have cerebral vascular changes nor the typical history of symptoms of *aphasia (disturbance in speech or communication), apraxia (disturbance in movement), agnosia (disturbance in comprehension through senses),* and changes in activity (74). The autopsy would provide a characteristic picture with an abundance of plaques, neurofibrillary changes, and nerve cell loss. The person with Pick's disease, a rare presenile disease, is usually under 65 years of age and has behavioral changes of reduced spontaneity, lack of insight into his/her behavior, and changes in moral personality. An autopsy would reveal atrophy with a Pick cell, but without the number of plaque cells (74).

A group of researchers reported a follow-up study of 51 patients in whom presenile dementia was diagnosed from 1963–1972 (61). This diagnosis was made in individuals under age 65. In 1977, 18 of these patients were still alive; 32 patients had died, and 1 patient was not followed (61). In a retrospective study, 7 appeared to have a functional illness, primarily depression; 25 appeared to have a presenile dementia, and 16 appeared to be normal. Thus it was concluded that presenile dementia was incorrectly diagnosed in a high proportion of the population (61).

FORMULATION OF NURSING DIAGNOSIS AND CLIENT-CARE GOALS

Nursing Diagnosis

Your *nursing diagnosis of impaired cognitive function* (reversible or nonreversible) may include the following assessments of the person:

1. Demonstrates varying degrees of impaired alertness, orientation, and rationality.
2. Demonstrates various amounts of inaccuracy when responding to directions.
3. Is unable in varying degrees to recall data appropriate to the situation.
4. Displays varying inability to think through situations; encounters difficulty in making decisions; judgments are not based on data.
5. Shows pattern of involving self in hazardous situations or in situations that will somehow jeopardize him/her in varying ways.
6. Responds apathetically or inappropriately to stimuli that might otherwise be expected to elicit interest and curiosity.

Client-Care Goals

The long-term goal for the person with reversible (acute) cognitive impairment is to regain mental abilities and prevent recurrence.

The long-term care goals for the person with nonreversible (chronic) cognitive impairment could include the following:

1. Tasks related to all spheres of daily living are accomplished to the fullest degree possible, considering limitations. Strengths are utilized.
2. Information that is essential to daily living is retained or learned to the fullest possible degree, considering limitations.

3. Cognitive impairment is realistically accepted to the degree possible, and adequate feelings of self-esteem and hope are retained.

Short-term goals for the client with reversible (acute) cognitive impairment include:

1. Physical status stabilizes and improves.
2. Sensory perception, cognitive competencies, and ability to relate are regained. Reality situation is comprehended.
3. Adequate rest is maintained in a safe environment.
4. Self-esteem and positive self-concept are maintained or regained, as demonstrated by statements and behavior.

Short-term goals for the client with irreversible (chronic) cognitive impairment include:

1. Physical health and sense of security are maintained to the degree possible.
2. Reality contact is maintained.
3. Communication and problem-solving abilities are related to the activities of daily living and to the expression of feelings to the extent possible.
4. Interaction with other individuals and in a group setting is maintained.
5. Physical care is maintained by self to the degree possible; assistance is accepted when necessary.

Both sets of short-term goals along with recommended nursing interventions will be discussed in the next section.

CLIENT-CARE GOALS AND RELATED NURSING INTERVENTIONS

Be sincere, respectful, and responsive to the person when you work with the confused or cognitively impaired client. If you can be empathic, your interventions will have meaning. Recognize the client as a unique person and feel compassion for the suffering, and he/she will in turn be touched and respond with as much growth as possible. If you believe that this person, who may be unable to remember the time of day or your name, is less than human, you do little for him/her. In fact, you may be disturbing.

Most nurses have real empathy for someone suffering from a malignancy or chronic emphysema, but they may have little understanding of the realness of the experience and the suffering and fear that confusion, disorientation, failing memory, and hallucinations produce. The pain of terror for this client is as great as the pain of physical suffering.

Care is similar in many ways, although the following discussion differentiates intervention for reversible and nonreversible cognitive impairment. In either case, the person needs excellent physical care; a helpful, trusting relationship, empathic communication appropriate for his/her condition; touch; adequate sensory and emotional stimulation; protection from injury; social interaction from loved ones or a peer group, depending on the specific condition; and spiritual care based on beliefs. This person is not just a diagnosis. This person is not just senile. In fact, striking the word *senile* from the medical vocabulary would probably do a great service for many elderly persons. The word clouds our vision and creativity; it causes us to feel hopeless and to consider only custodial care.

Reversible (Acute) Cognitive Impairment

Goal 1: Physical status stabilizes and improves.

Interventions

Immediate treatment and intervention must be related to the stressor, precipitating cause, and degree of impairment of the acute state. For example, if the client has pneumonia, the immediate care must relate to the bacteria or virus. Anti-biotics must be given regularly. Oxygenation must be maintained. Fluid and electrolyte balance, nutrition, and elimination require careful monitoring. Rest is essential. Safety precautions are necessary. All prescribed treatments must be done. Nursing intervention must also relate to the specific mental and emotional problems the client is having.

Nutrition, fluid and electrolyte balance, and state of mind are closely related. The well-adjusted person living at home may suffer confusion from an inadequate intake or a slightly elevated temperature. An elderly person in a nursing care unit who is malnourished or dehydrated may begin to show subtle signs of confusion. A newly admitted client suffering from severe infection and dehydration or a chronic illness such as arthritis may have a serious electrolyte imbalance and consequently an acute brain syndrome. When the imbalance has been discovered and treated, a rapid return to equilibrium usually occurs.

Adequate nutrition is essential to provide nutrients and energy. Intake and output must be accurately recorded. Daily infusions of intravenous fluids, usually with vitamins and minerals, are given if the person is unable to take fluids by mouth. Carefully observe the speed and amount of fluids given parenterally; always observe for cardiac overload. Daily intake should usually be about 2 liters (8 glasses) of fluids. Adequate protein in the diet is encouraged with supplementary feedings. Always consider the person's preferences; serving something that he/she will not eat is pointless.

Goal 2: Sensory perception, cognitive competencies, and ability to relate are regained. Reality situation is comprehended.

Interventions

Communication to provide for sensory stimulation, cognitive motivation, and emotional closeness is essential. If the client is showing signs of confusion, disorientation, delirium, stupor, or coma, he/she has probably reached an isolated, nonadaptive state. To continue to reach out, provide human contact, and maintain a stimulating environment, you must provide continual verbal and nonverbal communication. Listen carefully to anything said, no matter how brief or difficult it is to hear. Speak in a slow, gentle manner to this person. A familiar face, voice tone, and language are important. Kindly and concisely give directions: for example, "Open your eyes, Mr. Brown," or "Raise your arm." Use orienting conversation, such as, "You are in St. Christopher's hospital, Mrs. Baron." Make supportive comments, such as, "You are progressing; your temperature is nearer normal today." Long sentences confuse the client. Avoid negative, condescending, and joking conversation, or the person may wonder how interested you are in caring and may feel frightened. Instead of beginning with a question, talk about something of interest to the person. Do not threaten, bribe, or demand. Never assume that understanding is absent. Often clients will have partial amnesia after an acute episode, but they will remember threatening or anxiety-provoking experiences (27, 52, 65, 72).

Establishing trust is basic because it allows the client in this very vulnerable position to feel secure and to depend on you. However, the person who is forced to be dependent for complete care may feel that he/she will not be cared for properly, and he/she may become suspicious, guarded, and delusional. This can trigger further problems of agitation and panic. Everything about the helping relationship applies to this person, even if he/she appears stuporous or delirious at the time.

The person may benefit by being in a room with another client or in a room close to the nurses' station. Or ask the family to remain with the person if possible. Visual and auditory devices are important if the individual is able to wear them. Glasses and hearing aids as well as dentures provide environmental contact and maintain a sense of identity and body image.

Communication may be nonreciprocal; that is, you may have to continue without much response from your client. However, you may find that without any feedback your communication suffers. You continue to care for the person's physical needs, but you perceive him/her as less than human. Watch for your feelings of anxiety, boredom, irritation, hopelessness, and discouragement. Such feelings may reinforce the client's anxieties if he/she is conscious, and they may trigger insecure and worthless feelings. Or the client may be conscious, but the family may sense your feelings and be concerned that their loved one will not get adequate care. Explore your feelings with another person to determine why you feel the way you do. Fully expressing these feelings may neutralize them and free you to respond to your client more positively through your care, your touch, and your spirit.

Goal 3: Adequate rest is maintained in a safe environment.

Intervention

A safe, protected, restful environment is essential for the maintenance of the client's abilities and to achieve any improvement in his/her condition. Treatments and care routines should be organized and timed so that they do not interfere with rest or sleep. Often sleep deprivation adds to the symptoms of brain disorder.

Measures of protection will depend on the severity of illness. If treatment such as infusions are necessary, assess the client's ability to understand and cooperate with the treatment. For example, some clients can keep their arm relatively immobile for an infusion; others cannot. One person may be able to tolerate a gastric tube in daylight hours but will become agitated by it at night. Treatment measures can be modified, depending on response.

Your calm, understanding approach or the presence of a family member will probably be the best protective measure. Do not underestimate the power of purposeful communication and previously established feelings of trust in quieting the person who is agitated, fearful, or potentially self-destructive.

Verbal reassurance is usually enough to orient the person to reality and to calm him/her. If communication does not work over a period of time, sedative drugs or physical restraints may be necessary if the person is dangerous to self or others (34). Yet, these protective measures can create other problems. All drugs that have depressant effects on the central nervous system may cause confusion, even if given in small doses. Also drowsiness caused by drugs may interfere with perception and reality testing, causing further confusion. Since individuals respond differently to drugs, you must observe the reaction in each case. A hot drink or glass of wine can sometimes do more than a tranquilizer (78).

In some cases, you may feel that a waist restraint, posey belt, or full restraints are necessary. However, physical restraints should be considered only as a last resort; they threaten self-esteem and add to anger. A client wandering about may fall and injure self, but a physically restrained client may have skin damage, become more confused and distraught, or suffer other complications such as pneumonia, decubitus, or constipation. If restraints are needed, additional nursing measures are imperative. First of all, frequently tell the client the reason for the use of the restraint. This is necessary even if it seems to be useless or to cause further agitation. Also examine the skin frequently for tears, cuts, and abrasions. Provide skin care by turning and massage; give range-of-motion exercises to maintain circulation, joint mobility, and muscle tone. Offer fluids frequently. Provide communication and sensory stimulation by frequently stopping at the bedside.

Evaluate which method of restraint works best, such as the presence of people, the use of drugs, or physical restraints, but do not threaten the person. The immediate result of a quiet client should never have priority over the long-term loss of the sense of integrity. *Be certain that use of drugs or a physical restraint is an intervention for the client's well-being and not just a time-saving measure for you.* Also evaluate your approach while you are restraining the person. Many times a severely agitated client may be provoking and irritating, and even the most accepting nurse might feel satisfaction in restraining him/her. But remember that the client is the first to pick up feelings of anger, resentment, and punishment in your nonverbal expressions.

Goal 4: Self-esteem and positive self-concept are maintained or regained, as demonstrated by statements and behavior.

Interventions

Support to the fearful, confused person is essential. The client in coma or delirium may not be aware of his/her mental functioning; however, many persons suffering acute brain syndrome are very aware of confusing feelings and thoughts. For example, Mr. S. G., a 75-year-old single man, was admitted to the hospital suffering with acute hepatitis. After being taken to his room, he asked frequently where he was and appeared to receive no reassurance. The disorientation seemed to be more upsetting than the physical symptoms, for he repeatedly asked, "What is the matter with me?" I just don't know what is happening."

Symptoms of cognitive impairment are usually a new and bewildering experience to clients. Their response is influenced by present fears and past experiences with confused people, if those past experiences were traumatic. The person may fear deterioration, becoming insane, or losing his/her mind. The person may have known a neighbor or grandparent who committed suicide or was admitted to a custodial institution. Whatever the degree of organic impairment, it is usually increased by fear and anxiety. Added to the concern about changed mental functioning are fears of strange surroundings, discomfort of physical illness, loneliness, and boredom. Self-esteem and self-concept may be drastically damaged. The client feels overpowered by vulnerability and weakness. Regression and shame become prominent. The person may feel very old, worn out, and hopeless.

As a nurse, you come into close touch with the human condition—not only your client's but also your own. If you have insight into the frailty of the human being, in a holistic sense, and know how fragile a hold any person has on the reality of life, you can be considerably changed. Such insight can help you accept and care for the person without fear and with the resolution that "Yes, life is hard, it is momentary, but there is hope, and there can be more life ahead." Your nonverbal support and how you feel about the meaning of life, illness, and death may be the most comforting intervention you bring to the person. You can encourage life and promote solutions to current problems. Give necessary information repeatedly. Be available as needed.

Nonreversible (Chronic) Cognitive Impairment

Assess your feelings concerning the future, value, and progress of your client. You must deal with feelings of pessimism and discouragement as you face mental deterioration, emotional deprivation, suffering, and multiple physical complications and problems. Because you may fear your own death, you may hold yourself back from your client. You may not want to become involved because you know that in the end, loss is inevitable. You may find the lack of intellectual ability or dependency repulsive to you, and may feel no empathy and warmth for the client. You may want to see progress and feel defeated if you only see degeneration. Many times nurses find it difficult to admit such feelings to themselves, but all of us have these feelings at times. Certainly, at the same time, there are feelings of concern, desire for excellent nursing care, and compassion for another human being. But the negative feelings should be acknowledged because they prevent aspirations for quality care from being fulfilled.

> Goal 1: Physical health
> and sense of security are
> maintained to the degree
> possible.

Interventions

Intervention relating specifically to the client with nonreversible (chronic) brain syndrome presents multiple, complex problems that may be present for a long time. *Drug therapy* has produced little or no results, although a recent study indicated that Naftidrofuge (Praxilene) has improved reaction time and short-term memory in persons with mild nonreversible brain syndrome. Many clinical studies have been done with vasodilators and senile dementia; but results are still uncertain (80). Therefore, *nursing care is the crucial factor* for this person. This client needs communication, particularly nonverbal, as well as support, sensory stimulation, adequate diet, fluids, rest, and protection from injury or other illness, just as the client with reversible (acute) brain disorder does (9). He/she needs privacy and a place for possessions—a territory. Modesty must be respected during routine care and during diagnostic and treatment measures. Special preferences, such as in food, drink, an activity, or wearing apparel, should be granted whenever possible so that personal integrity is maintained.

Management and care should begin with careful observations. The diagnostic label of "nonreversible" or "chronic" often precludes further observation or planning of care. Mistakes in interaction, treatment, and use of resources can be avoided if you do not allow labels to interfere with your commitment to quality care. Early, careful,

and continued assessment helps you to assist the client and family to adjust to many practical problems. Clients' families might be spared much of the guilt they later carry if they were given early information and counseling.

> Goal 2: Reality contact
> is maintained.

Interventions

Supportive measures will help the person to maintain his/her remaining abilities. Also, emphasizing the person's strengths, rather than his/her impairments, will help you to avoid a pessimistic outlook and to maintain a philosophy of rehabilitation.

Environmental aids for reality orientation are helpful to the confused, cognitively impaired client, and they should be consistently used. Be creative about developing new ways of letting the person know about reality. Reinforce realistic behavior. Provide a dependable schedule. Adjust the environment to fit failing senses and decreased motor coordination: use brighter colors, better illumination, well-marked exits, color-coded doors and rooms, clocks, calendars, family pictures, and treasured objects to help the client remain oriented. Flowers, a fish tank, a bird, or having a small pet makes the environment more homelike. Set limits for the client's protection since he/she cannot rely on personal reality testing. Convey rules clearly and consistently to increase a sense of security (8, 20, 28, 39, 40).

> Goal 3: Communication
> and problem-solving abilities
> are related to activities of daily
> living and to the expression of
> feelings to the extent possible.

Interventions

Communication is a major avenue of intervention. You need to be as skillful as possible in the techniques and methods of communication discussed in Chapter 5. You should know the person you are working with and his/her style of communication, manner of response, and any sensory impairments. There are many reasons for inappropriate response from the client. Often the cause is not confusion, disorientation, or senility, but perhaps a hearing impairment or lack of understanding of the language used by professionals. Even though the person appears confused, realize that what he/she is talking about may be based on a real experience, on an event much earlier in life that you do not know about. Listen carefully and ask related questions to help clarify the story. Show respect. Stimulate further rational conversation and promote life review. Your lack of understanding of the conversation may add to your confusion, but should not add to his or hers! Pick out meaningful comments and continue talking.

Watch for emotional and nonverbal cues for evidence of how the person perceives your communication. The client's perception of your communication is far more influential on his/her behavior than what you actually say. Avoid injuring a relationship by making a careless remark about his/her behavior. Through maintenance of communication skills you can help the client use whatever memory, judgment, or problem-solving ability remains.

In order to maintain and stimulate communication and cognitive abilities, do everything possible to *minimize communication barriers*. A major communication barrier is anxiety, which may come from within the client, from yourself, or from the environment. For example, the elderly person, with or without sensory and perceptual disabilities, frequently is suffering from a damaged self-concept and body image. Cultural influences and expectations, family goals, personal ideals and aspirations, and many other influences impinge upon him/her. The person may feel that he/she is losing a life style, friends, his/her place in society, and a sense of hope; or the person may feel insecure and that he/she is not worth the time and effort it takes for the care or that he/she has little to say that you would be interested in knowing; or the person may think that you have some hidden motive for wanting to talk. Factors in the environment that may increase anxiety are: threatening or hostile staff members, routines that evoke hopelessness and dependency, little contact with the community, or offensive surroundings. Your level of anxiety may also influence the person's feelings (46).

Another barrier to communication might be the person's withdrawal, whether it is the physical withdrawal of lying in bed or staying in his/her room, or an emotional withdrawal with its apathy,

isolation, bizarre reactions, or unresponsiveness. The more active, aggressive client usually receives more attention from the staff than does the withdrawn client. Frequently staff members respond to the withdrawn person with a withdrawn response— a distancing behavior to cope with their own anxieties and fears (34). The soundest approach in treating an apathetic or withdrawn client is to try to establish some rapport and contact. Get to know him/her so that trust can develop and so that he/she can know and respond to your approach.

Other barriers to communication with confused persons are staff unresponsiveness; stereotyping, joking, demanding, or demeaning statements; and talking over the client as if he/she did not exist. Such behaviors will discourage the client from expressing his/her feelings and ideas and may injure the nurse-client relationship.

Goal 4: Interactions with other individuals and in a group setting is maintained.

Interventions

Social interaction needs to be considered and can begin with reality orientation and remotivation therapy groups and then progress to more complex activities or group experiences as described in Chapter 11. Family visits, group activities, parties, trips, and shopping tours are important if the person is able to participate. Encourage friendships between clients and responsibility one for another. It may be helpful if one person is assigned to take another person for a walk. One benefits from the socialization, and the other benefits from the responsibility. Both of them receive satisfaction from the adventure. Or you might ask several clients to decorate the unit or a living room; you can give them some assistance and support. Music therapy, listening to records, playing an instrument, or singing solo or in a group can promote reality contact, reminiscing, a release of feelings, renewed interaction with others, and a sense of joy. Working with various handicraft projects in occupational therapy can also promote social interaction and helps meet personal needs. Physical exercise, activity groups, reminiscing groups, and any type of stimulation are important in keeping the person as active and alert as possible and in helping maintain a sense of identity (64).

Socialization may be a problem for the elderly person if he/she is reluctant to join groups because of such problems as urinary frequency or urgency, poor sphincter tone, poor manual dexterity for eating or for various routine tasks, ataxia, or poor memory. Wearing protective apparel can help avoid embarrassment about elimination, or the use of special forks or spoons may prevent spilling or dropping food. Unobtrusive guidance on your part may also help coping with ataxia or poor memory.

Goal 5: Physical care is maintained by self to the degree possible; assistance is accepted when necessary.

Interventions

As time passes, the person will be able to engage in activities of daily living less and less. Complete physical care becomes inevitable if the person lives long enough (8). Thus, assistance with physical care is also important as habits and abilities deteriorate. The person may have to be reminded of such activities as brushing teeth and combing hair. A list of activities can be made and checked off as they are accomplished. Encourage the client to write any information that must be remembered—if the client is able to do so. However, sometimes this causes anxiety and thus defeats the purpose. You may have to give the client total routine care after a period of time.

EVALUATION

Over the years the authors have had many experiences with cognitively impaired persons in a variety of settings—including the community, acute care setting, client home setting, and nursing homes. Evaluation of care includes looking at relationships and recalling memories of happy and sad human experiences while working with these persons. Tears were sometimes shed as relationships ended or as a client recalled memories of his/her life and better times. Sometimes the person's subtle sense of humor brightened the day. There were discouraging times as well, such as when a family forgot to visit or a healed decubitus broke down.

An unforgettable experience involved an elderly man confined to a wheelchair. He was disoriented and apparently recognized only his own name and his own person. He had snow-white hair and a kind smile, and he always wore pajama bottoms, a shirt, and a bow tie. One student nurse had been assigned to him for a long-term experience and to learn basic physical care. She had worked with this man for four months, and termination of the relationship had been dealt with. On her last day she reminded him that this would be their last visit together. Just as every other day, there was no response—not a word, not a grunt, not a twinkle in his eye. She had always talked to him and had tried to form a relationship with him, but she had received very little feedback. In fact, she had told her instructor that it seemed inappropriate

to discuss termination because she was not sure that he even knew she was there. As she said goodbye and turned to leave, he said, "Wait." He then pulled her face to his and kissed her on the cheek. The inferences to be made from this experience are that a cognitively impaired person may perceive more of your feelings and care than he/she overtly indicates and that working with the cognitively impaired elderly can be a rewarding experience.

Evaluation of care should be in terms of the person's ability to maintain or regain some cognitive functions, accept limitations, work with assets, and gain satisfaction from personal and group activities. Recovery from the disease that causes reversible (acute) brain disorder can be evaluated by various tests. Evaluation of the person's cognitive function and feelings and of your nursing approach is more subjective, but it is just as essential. Sometimes the only time you can evaluate the client's feelings is when an incident occurs similar to the one mentioned above.

Eventually the client may become totally regressed or unable to respond. But you will know you are effective if you prevent further complications, if family members or other observers recognize that you are maintaining the dignity of the person, if the family feels comforted by your information and counsel, and if you do unto the client as you would want done unto you.

REFERENCES

1. Adams, M. et al., "The Confused Patient: Psychological Responses in Critical Care Units," *American Journal of Nursing*, 78, no. 9 (1978), 1504–12.

2. Alfano, Genrose, "There Are No Routine Patients," *American Journal of Nursing*, 75, no. 10 (1975), 1804–7.

3. Amburgey, Pauline, "Environmental Aids for the Aged Patient," *American Journal of Nursing*, 66, no. 9 (1966), 2017–18.

4. American Psychiatric Association, *Diagnostic and Statistical Manual of Mental Disorders*. Washington, D.C.: American Psychiatric Association, 1952.

5. ____, *Diagnostic and Statistical Manual of Mental Disorders*, 2nd ed. (DSM-II). Washington, D.C.: American Psychiatric Association, 1968.

6. ____, *Diagnostic and Statistical Manual of Mental Disorders*, 3rd ed. (DSM-III). Washington D.C.: American Psychiatric Association, 1980.

7. Armstrong, Priscilla, "Comment: More Thoughts on Senility," *The Gerontologist*, 18, no. 3 (1978), 315–16.

8. Baines, J., "Effects of Reality Orientation Classroom on Memory Loss, Confusion, and Disorientation in Geriatric Patients," *The Gerontologist*, 14 (1974), 38–42.

9. Bartol, M. A., "Dialogue with Dementia: Nonverbal Communication in Patients with Alzheimer's Disease," *Journal of Gerontological Nursing*, 5, no. 4 (1979), 21–31.

10. Branconnier, R., and J. Cole, "The Impairment Index as a Symptom-Independent Parameter of Drug Efficacy in Geriatric Psychopharmacology," *Journal of Gerontology*, 33, no. 2 (1978), 217–23.

11. Brocklehurst, J. C., "Evaluation of Geriatric Medicine," *Journal of American Geriatric Society*, 26 (October 1978), 433–39.

12. Burnside, Irene, "Alzheimer's Disease: An Overview," *Journal of Gerontological Nursing*, 5, no. 4 (1979), 14–20.

13. ____, "Clocks and Calendars," *American Journal of Nursing*, 70, no. 1 (1970), 117–19.

14. ____, "You Have Been Here Before," *Journal of Gerontogical Nursing*, 6, no. 1 (1980), 377–79.

15. Burnside, Irene, and B. A. Moehrlin, "Health Care of the Confused Elderly at Home," *Nursing Clinics of North America*, 15, no. 2 (1980), 389–402.

16. Busse, E., and E. Pfeiffer, eds., *Behavior and Adaptation in Late Life*, 2nd ed. Boston: Little, Brown & Company, 1977.

17. Butler, Robert, D. Dastur, and S. Perlin, "Relationship of Senile Manifestations and Chronic Brain Syndrome to Cerebral Circulation and Metabolism," *Journal of Psychological Research*, 3 (1965), 229–38.

18. Butler, Robert, and Myrna Lewis, *Aging and Mental Health*. St. Louis: The C. V. Mosby Company, 1977.

19. Chivers, T., and J. Westwater, "Hospital Care of Confused Elderly People," *Nursing*, 10, no. 1 (1980), 393–96.

20. Citrin, Richard, and David Dixon, "Reality Orientation —A Milieu Therapy Used in an Institution for the Aged," *The Gerontologist*, 17, no. 1 (1977), 39–43.

21. Cohen, Gene, "Comment: Organic Brain Syndrome," *The Gerontologist*, 18, no. 3 (1978), 313–14.

22. Corsellis, J., *Mental Illness and Aging*. London: Oxford University Press, 1962.

23. Cybyk, M. E., "Alzheimer's Disease," *Nursing Times*, 76, no. 7 (February 14, 1980), 280–82.

24. Davidson R., "The Elderly Disturbed Patient," *Nursing Mirror*, 246, no. 14 (April 1978), 23–24.

25. Davies, Peter, ed., *American Heritage Dictionary*. New York: Dell Publishing Co., Inc., 1973.

26. Davies V., "Social Care: Finding the Best Home for the Confused Elderly," *Nursing Mirror*, 147, no. 17 (1978), 51–53.

27. Eaton, Merrill, Margaret H. Peterson, and James A. Davis, *Psychiatry*, 3rd ed., pp. 253–67. New York: Medical Examination Publishing Company, Inc., 1976.

28. Folsom, James, "Reality Orientation for the Elderly Mental Patient," *Geriatric Psychiatry*, Spring 1968, pp. 291–307.

29. Folsom, James, and Geneva Folsom, "Team Method of Treating Senility," *Nursing Care*, 6 (December 1973), 17–23.

30. Fovall, P. et al., "Choline Bitartrate Treatment of Alzheimer-Type Dementias," *Community Psychopharmacology*, 4, no. 2 (1980), 141–45.

31. Fowler, Roy, and Wilbert Fordyce, "Adapting Care for the Brain-Damaged Patient," *American Journal of Nursing*, 72, no. 11 (1972), 2056–59.

32. Friedman, A. M., I. H. Kaplan, and B. J. Sadack, "Organic Brain Syndrome," *Modern Synopsis of Comprehensive Textbook of Psychiatry*, pp. 268–311. Baltimore: Williams & Wilkins Company, 1972.

33. Friedman, F. B., "It Isn't Senility: The Nurse's Role in Alzheimer's Disease," *Journal of Practical Nursing*, 31, no. 2 (1981), 17-19.

34. Gerdes, Lenore, "The Confused or Delirious Patient," *The American Journal of Nursing*, 68, no. 6 (1968), 1228-33.

35. Goldfarb, A. I., "Psychiatric Disorders of the Aged: Symptomatology, Diagnosis, and Treatment," *Journal of the American Geriatric Society*, 8 (1960), 680.

36. Gottschalk, L. A. et al., "A Cognitive Impairment Scale Applicable to Verbal Samples and Its Possible Use in Clinical Trials in Patients with Dementia Proceedings," *Psychopharmacological Bulletin*, 16, no. 4 (1980), 25-27.

37. Guralnik, David, ed., *Webster's New World Dictionary*, 2nd college ed. New York: World Publishing Co., Inc., 1972.

38. Hall, Beverly A., "Mutual Withdrawal: The Non-Participant in a Therapeutic Community," *Perspectives in Psychiatric Care*, 14, no. 2 (1976), 75-77.

39. Harris, Clarke, and Peter Ivory, "An Outcome Evaluation of Reality Orientation Therapy with Geriatric Patients in a State Mental Hospital," *The Gerontologist*, 16, no. 6 (1976), 496-503.

40. Hirchfield, Miriam, "The Cognitively Impaired Older Adult," *American Journal of Nursing*, 76, no. 12 (1976), 1981-84.

41. Jarvik, L., C. Eisendorfer, and J. Blum, eds., *Intellectual Functioning in Adults*. New York: Springer Publishing Co., Inc., 1973.

42. Kahn, R. L. et al., "Brief Objective Measures for the Determination of Mental Status in the Aged," *American Journal of Psychiatry*, 111 (1960), 326-28.

43. Katzman, R., and R. B. Korasu, "Differential Diagnosis of Dementia," in *Neurological and Sensory Disorders in the Elderly*, ed. W. S. Fields. New York: Stratton Intercontinental Medical Books Corp., 1975.

44. Kay, D., "Epidemiological Aspects of Organic Brain Disease in the Aged," in *Aging in the Brain*, ed. C. M. Gaitz, pp. 15-26. New York: Plenum Publishing Corporation, 1972.

45. Kay, D., and Alexander Walk, "Classification and Etiology in Mental Disorders of Old Age: Some Recent Developments," *Recent Development in Psychogeriatrics: A Symposium*, pp. 1-17. Ashford, Kent, England: Headley Brothers Ltd., 1971.

46. Kazmiarczak, Frances, Dorothy Moser, and Mary Russo, "Communication Problems Encountered When Caring for the Elderly Individual," *Journal of Gerontological Nursing*, 1, no. 2 (1975), 21-27.

47. Kral, V. A., "Confusional States, Description and Management," *Modern Perspectives in the Psychiatry of Old Age*, ed. John G. Howells, pp. 356-62. New York: Brunner/Mazel, Inc., 1975.

48. Kroner K., "Dealing with the Confused Patient," *Nursing*, 9, no. 11 (1979), 71-78.

49. La Vorgna, D., "Group Treatment for Wives of Patients with Alzheimer's Disease," *Social Work Health Care*, 5, no. 2 (1979), 219-21.

50. Lawson, James, M. Rodenburg, and J. Dykes, "A Demential Rating Scale for Use with Psychogeriatric Patients," *Journal of Gerontology*, 32, no. 2 (1977), 153-59.

51. Lillie, Douglas, "Attitudes in Geriatrics," *Nursing Times*, 72 (July 15, 1976), IIIff, Supplement.

52. MacKinnon, Roger, and Robert Michels, *The Psychiatric Interview in Clinical Practice*, pp. 339-60. Philadelphia: W. B. Saunders Company, 1971.

53. Murray, Ruth, M. Marilyn Huelskoetter, and Dorothy O'Driscoll, *The Nursing Process in Later Maturity*. Englewood Cliffs, N.J.: Prentice-Hall, Inc., 1980.

54. Nowakski, L., "Disorientation—Signal or Diagnosis," *Journal of Gerontological Nursing*, 6 (1980), 197-202.

55. Patrick, Maxine Lambrecht, "Care of the Confused Elderly Patient," *American Journal of Nursing*, 67, no. 12 (1967), 2536-39.

56. Perez, F. I. "Behavioral Studies of Dementia: Methods of Investigation and Analysis," *Proceedings of Annual Meeting of American Psychopathology Association*, 69 (1980), 81-95.

57. Pitt, Brice, *Psychogeriatrics*, pp. 24-45. Edinburgh: Churchill Livingstone Publishers, 1974.

58. Preston, Tonie, "When Words Fail," *American Journal of Nursing*, 73, no. 12 (1973), 2064-66.

59. Roberts, Rosemary, "Senile Dementia and Depression," *Nursing Times*, 71 (December 4, 1975), 1931-33.

60. Robinson, C. W., "The Toxic Delirious Reactions of Old Age," in *Mental Disorders in Later Life*, ed. I. Kaplan. Stanford, Calif.: Stanford University Press, 1972.

61. Ron, M. A. et al., "Diagnostic Accuracy in Presenile Dementia," *British Journal of Psychiatry*, 134 (February 1979), 161-68.

62. Roth, M., "The Natural History of Mental Disorders in Old Age," *Journal of Mental Science*, 101 (1955), 281-301.

63. Roth, M., B. Tomlinson, and G. Glisted, "Correlation between Scores for Dementia and Counts of Senile Plaques in Cerebral Gray Matter of Elderly Patients," *Nature*, 209 (1966), 109-10.

64. Savage, B., "Rethinking Psychogeriatric Nursing," *Nursing Times*, 70 (February 1974), 282–84.

65. Schwab, Sister Marilyn, "Caring for the Aged," *American Journal of Nursing*, 73, no. 12 (1973), 2049–53.

66. "Senile Psychoses May Be Psychologic, Not Organic," *Geriatric Focus*, 8, no. 9 (1969), 1ff.

67. Sloan, R. Bruce, "Psychiatric Problems of the Aged," *Continuing Education*, 9 (November 1978), 42–50.

68. Solomon, Philip, and Vernon Patch, *Handbook of Psychiatry*, pp. 201–9. Los Altos, Calif.: Lange Medical Publications, 1971.

69. Stedeford A., "Understanding Confusional States," *British Journal of Hospital Medicine*, 20, no. 6 (1978), 694–98, 703–4.

70. Steven, Carolyn, "Breaking through the Cobwebs of Confusion," *Nursing*, 74, no. 8 (1974), 41–48.

71. Stotsky, Bernard A., *The Elderly Patient*, pp. 108–12. New York: Grune & Stratton, Inc., 1968.

72. Szanto, Stephen, "Dementia in the Elderly," *Nursing Mirror*, 140 (June 19, 1975), 64–65.

73. Trimble M., "Altered Consciousness," *Nursing*, 8, no. 12 (1979), 344–47.

74. Turisha, I., "Circumscribed Cerebral Atrophy in Alzheimer's Disease: A Pathological Study," *Alzheimer's Disease*. Symposium on Alzheimer's Disease, Summit, N.J.: The Ciba Foundation, November 11–13, 1969.

75. Voelkel, D., "A Study of Reality Orientation and Resocialization Groups with Confused Elderly," *Journal of Gerontological Nursing*, 4, no. 3 (1978), 13–18.

76. Wahl, Patricia, "Psychosocial Implications of Disorientation in the Elderly," *Nursing Clinics of North America*, 11, no. 1 (1976), 145–56.

77. Wang, H., "Organic Brain Syndromes, in *Behavior and Adaptation in Late Life*, eds. Ewald Busse and Eric Pfeiffer, pp. 263–88. Boston: Little, Brown & Company, 1969.

78. Whitehead, J. A., "Helping Old People with Mental Illness," *Nursing Mirror*, 138 (March 22, 1974), 76–77.

79. Worth, D., "Community Nursing: Not in Their Perfect Mind," *Nursing Mirror*, 147, no. 18 (1978), 50–52.

80. Yesavage, Jerome et al., "Vasodilators in Senile Dementias: Review of the Literature," *Archives of General Psychiatry*, 36, no. 2 (1979), 170–76.

19

The Person
Whose
Behavior Is Abusive

Study of this chapter will assist you to:

1. Compare and contrast medical and nursing diagnoses for clients whose behavior includes aggressive or emotional/physical abuse of others.

2. Distinguish these behaviors on a continuum from normal to pathological.

3. Identify behaviors that are characteristic of the pathological states for each selected nursing diagnosis.

4. Explore the psychodynamics related to each selected nursing diagnosis.

5. State goals for client care and describe the related nursing interventions.

6. Assess and intervene with these clients, with supervision and increasing skill.

7. Discuss effectiveness of care as well as available community services with other team members.

This chapter contributed by Virginia Luetje, R.N., M.S.N. Portions of this chapter also provided by Ruth Murray, R.N., M.S.N.

Nurses not only experience the joy of caring for delightful, lovable clients, but they also experience the distress of trying to maintain their own health in caring for clients who are unnerving, insulting, intrusive, crabby, offensive, and perhaps assaultive and violent. We are then challenged by three overriding goals:

1. The abusive client needs assistance in adopting and using nonhurtful patterns of relating to others.
2. Other clients need protection from the abusive client.
3. Staff and self need to function in a reasonably safe milieu.

We accept a goal of helping abusive clients become less abusive because we are the product of a period of time and a culture that believes in the premise that people who hurt other people have something wrong with them that should be fixed. Many have answered the call to find out what is wrong and how to fix it, including clergymen, philosophers, faith healers, sociologists, psychiatrists, biologists, psychologists, ethnologists, anthropologists, and parents. Fortunately, nurses are not averse to absorbing the good ideas from any of these professions if they provide a lead to giving better client care. As a result, you will find ideas from several disciplines underlying the intervention suggestions in this chapter.

PSYCHIATRIC DIAGNOSES RELATED TO ABUSIVE BEHAVIOR

Abusive behaviors may occur in clients with almost any psychiatric diagnosis or in persons with no clear psychiatric disorder. In this chapter, the author arbitrarily selected those diagnoses where the essential symptoms are such that you might anticipate some form of behavior potentially injurious to self or others. Any diagnosis primarily addressed in other chapters is omitted except for a brief summary.

The following paragraphs are an alphabetized list of diagnoses related to abusive behavior, summarizing the key symptoms of each disorder. In order to study psychiatric diagnoses in more depth, refer to the current American Psychiatric Association's *DSM-III* (2). (See Appendix.)

Affective Disorder, Manic: A diagnosis for clients manifesting tireless overactivity and excitement, plus extreme verbosity and push of speech, along with an affect that is generally euphoric or elated. Underneath the euphoria are anger and hostility, which are being directed outwardly. These clients often are busily, but somewhat randomly, making grandiose plans and boasting of their marvelous abilities. They are highly distractible even by internal stimuli; they show flight of ideas and impulsivity and have difficulty sleeping or taking time to eat. (One individual put it this way: "I feel like I am a 33-rpm record that has been turned up to a 78-rpm speed.") Judgment is limited or inappropriate. These clients seek attention, often do considerable clowning, joking, or punning, (unfortunately, staff may laugh at them) and may be sexually casual or exhibitionistic. They are over-responsive to external stimuli and may quickly become hostile or even combative if they feel thwarted or psychologically threatened.

Antisocial Personality: A personality disorder most commonly diagnosed in young adult males, and to a lesser extent in females, who have a lifelong history of disregard for others. These clients can state moral principles but do not abide by them unless it is personally convenient. The lack of an effective social conscience results in a history of multiple social infractions and/or lawbreaking. These clients consistently strive to maintain their own satisfaction rather than sometimes setting personal desires aside out of regard or loyalty to others. They have been variously described as narcissistic, egocentric, selfish, impulsive, manipulative, exploitive, ruthless, and irresponsible. Often they are charming con artists who will rationalize and project all responsibility for their behavior onto others. Formerly described in psychiatric literature as *sociopaths* or *psychopaths*, these individuals sooner or later wreak havoc in the lives of self, family, or those who offer love and friendship. To live with such a person is emotionally abusing and may involve physical abuse as well.

Attention Deficit Disorder with Hyperactivity: A disorder most usually described in children and variously also referred to as hyperkinesis or minimal brain dysfunction. The develop-

goal-directed but rather results from impulsive responses to stimuli as well as from an impaired concentration ability. The degree of symptoms often varies with the situation, but group settings such as the classroom are often particularly difficult for these children. During the toddler and preschool years, these children have excessive gross motor activity, such as running, climbing, and dismantling toys and machines. Older children may be restless and constantly disruptive. Problematic behaviors include a low frustration tolerance, temper outbursts, mood lability, and negativism. It is difficult to find ways to effectively discipline these youngsters. The person who cares for such a child may feel emotionally and physically abused. An *Attention Deficit Disorder without Hyperactivity describes an illness where inattention and impulsivity prevail, but hyperactivity does not* (2).

Borderline Personality Disorder: A category characterized by clients with persistent patterned behaviors of impulsivity, instability, unpredictability, and emotional lability. Their behaviors are often self-damaging, such as intensely and repetitively seeking demeaning relationships with other unstable individuals. Suicidal behaviors are frequent, along with affective instability and a low frustration tolerance. Deficient in their sense of self-identity, these clients experience chronic feelings of emptiness as well as an intolerance for being alone. To live with this person may leave one feeling emotionally abused as a result of the unstable behavior.

Conduct, Disorder, Socialized Aggressive: The manifest behaviors of this disorder are very similar to Conduct Disorder, Undersocialized Aggressive, but dynamically there is a striking difference. These youths experience guilt and anxiety in relation to the values of their own subculture; thus they have peer friendships. There are also parental or adult figures whom they love and emulate. However, values regarding right and wrong are deviant from the values of the larger society. Earlier texts sometimes classified these behaviors as *dyssocial sociopathologic*. These people may be abusive to those people who do not hold the same value system.

Conduct Disorder, Undersocialized Aggressive: A descriptive diagnosis for a child or adolescent with repetitive, persistent problem behaviors such as hostility, fighting, rebelliousness, theft, and truancy. Whether it is a lack of consistent discipline or an inability to benefit from discipline, these youngsters seem unable to relate with emotional depth to peers, parents, or authority. Evidence of experienced guilt or anxiety in relation to their behavior is minimal or nonexistent.

Dependent Personality Disorder: Clients with this disorder have a habitual pattern of relating to others in an overly dependent fashion. They display helplessness, passivity, and indecisiveness. Subordinating their own needs, they want others to make all major decisions. In a sense they abuse others with their constant clinging helplessness. These clients also may tolerate being the victim in a chronically abusive situation because they do not view themselves as having the power or ability to get out of the situation.

Explosive Disorders: These disorders are subcategorized. *Isolated Explosive Disorder is used to refer to a single episode of impulsive loss of control and consequent injurious assault on others or significant property destruction. The aggression is obviously out of proportion to any precipitating stressor.* These clients are genuinely regretful and distressed after the outburst. *Intermittent Explosive Disorder is a category used to refer to clients who have had periodic episodes of explosive outbursts followed by remorse. Some texts will describe a repetitive outburst syndrome as an Explosive Personality.* Sometimes there are clinical findings suggesting related organic pathology in clients with Explosive Disorders pathology such as epilepsy (rarely) or other brain disease.

Oppositional Disorder: A diagnostic term often utilized in child psychiatry for habitual behavior patterns of disobedience, negativism, stubbornness, and provocative insubordination. These youngsters do not violate major societal norms but are distressing to parents and authority figures because of constant argumentativeness and uncooperativeness.

Organic Mental Disorders: A broad general category used here to summarize a whole group of disorders with organic etiology, such as drug reactions or withdrawal; drug, alcohol or other poison intoxications; systemic infections; cranial infections; endocrine, metabolic, or nutritional disturbances; intracranial tumors; and cerebrovascular disease. Cognitive and personality changes, impulsive behaviors, paranoid attitudes, affective lability, and decreased control over sexual and aggressive impulses. Refer to Chapter 18 for more information. These persons may wreak more emotional than physical abuse.

Passive-Aggressive Personality: This term describes clients who express a general hostility through indirectly resisting demands made on them. On the surface they are generally pleasant and agreeable, yet they perpetually procrastinate, "forget" the promises they made, are purposely inefficient, and sabotage the plans with which they have agreed, all of which leaves those they live with feeling emotionally abused.

Sexual Deviations: The terms used here define behaviors that individuals may manifest as a preferred or exclusive method for achieving sexual excitement. Exhibitionism: The intentional exposure of the genitals under innappropriate conditions to persons of the opposite sex. It is rare for any further sexual activity to be attempted along with the self-exposure or for any physical assault to also occur. Usually the shocked reaction of the unexpecting viewer is necessary for the sexual excitement of the exhibitionist. *Masochism: Achieving sexual pleasure through suffering pain or humiliation.* It may involve self-mutilation or the seeking out of others who will inflict pain, harm, or be abusive. *Pedophilia: An adolescent or adult engaging in genital fondling or other clearly sexually seductive activity with prepubertal children. Sadism: Repeatedly and intentionally inflicting psychological or physical suffering on another consenting or nonconsenting partner to achieve sexual excitement. Voyeurism: Sexual excitement is achieved via viewing unsuspecting people who are disrobing, naked, or engaged in sex.*

NURSING DIAGNOSES RELATED TO ABUSIVE BEHAVIORS

Early psychiatric nursing texts made a commendable effort to derive nursing interventions directly from the patient's psychiatric diagnosis. This approach worked to a degree. In addition, this approach insured that nurse and physician could communicate with each other in terms that had mutually validated meaning, an advantage that we risk losing as we develop our own communication system via nursing diagnoses.

By the early 1960s, nurses were becoming increasingly aware that psychiatric diagnoses did not of themselves point directly toward specific nursing interventions. Texts were written with chapter headings like: "Nursing Care of Patients with Socially Aggressive Patterns (34)," "Patients Whose Behavior is Characterized by Antisocial Attitudes (38)," or "The Patient with Feelings of Distrust (8)." This changing approach was useful for developing a theory of independent nursing intervention. An example will help illustrate. In the psychiatric diagnoses summarized in the previous section, the behavior "impulsivity" is mentioned in six categories and perhaps implied in several more. Thus it appears that there are certain independent actions that nurses can take to assist impulsive clients, regardless of their specific psychiatric diagnosis.

The National Conference for Nursing Diagnosis has been engaged since the early 1970s in developing and clinically testing proposed nursing diagnoses to see if they are valid and useful to practicing nurses (12). Until this group formulates a set of clinically tested classifications, the author is presenting a *temporary* set of diagnoses related to abusive behaviors, based on clinical observations, for you to utilize and test.

The following classification schema will use the word *state* or *mode* as the final term in each label category. *State will be used to mean the current behavior. State further indicates a temporary set of behaviors highly susceptible to the influence of environmental factors and/or internal organic factors.* Nursing diagnoses identified as states of behavior are: Rational Anger State, Aggressive Response State, Impulse-Dominated State, and Self-Exalted State.

Mode will be used to mean the characteristic or usual manner of acting or doing. Mode implies an enduring but not necessarily permanent pattern of behavior. Innate determinants or interaction styles learned early in childhood are likely to be important factors in abusive modes. Nursing diagnoses identified as modes of behavior are: Aggressive Coping Mode, Impulsive Coping Mode, Manipulative Coping Mode, Subtle Obstructive Mode, and Dependent Coping Mode. Note that two of the state diagnoses have corollary mode diagnoses (see Table 19-1).

A total of nine diagnostic categories relative to abusive behaviors are defined in the following list:

1. **Rational Anger State**: *A temporary condition in which the person is angry for understandable, valid reasons, and the expression of the anger is direct, yet socially and morally acceptable.* Others are not abused by this behavior except in the sense that it is often anxiety-provoking to be confronted by another's anger.

2. **Aggressive Response State**: *A temporary condition in which the individual is hostile, argumentative, or assaultive out of proportion to the provocation or in a socially or morally objectionable manner.* Other people may be verbally or physically injured (even killed) as a result.

3. **Aggressive Coping Mode**: *A patterned and repetitive style of responding to interpersonal stress by using hostility, argument, or assault, including physical and psychological abuse, to control or overpower others.* In its extreme manifestation, fatalities or serious injuries may occur to the victim.

4. **Impulse-Dominated State**: *A temporary condition in which the behavior is highly unpredictable. Actions are sudden, heedless, unwise.* Behavior is not mediated by self-control, forethought, or discriminating social judgment. Other's needs are not sufficiently considered, and thus abuse may occur.

5. **Impulsive Coping Mode**: *A patterned and repetitive style of reacting to life events without the intervening processes of forethought and realistic consideration of consequences.* Others' rights or needs may be violated in the process.

6. **Self-Exalted State**: *A temporary condition in*

which the individual self-aggrandizes and giddily presents self as having unrealistic superior abilities and qualities. Others are abused by being considered lesser beings unworthy of consideration.

7. **Manipulative Coping Mode:** *A patterned and repetitive style of influencing, persuading, or managing others to suit one's own self-interests.* The free choice of others is taken advantage of and is disregarded.

8. **Subtle Obstructive Mode:** *A patterned, repetitive style of resisting the demands and expectations of others with noncompliance and passive sabotage.* The person is not fully aware of the motivation of his/her behavior or its alienating consequences. Others are constantly angered and frustrated by this client.

9. **Dependent Coping Mode:** *A patterned, repetitive style of relating to others through helplessness.* The other person is relied on to make all significant decisions and choices. Others are abused by being used as an extension of self.

More than one diagnosis may be made simultaneously for a given client. Figure 19-1 shows the diagnoses that could occur simultaneously. When more than one diagnosis is indicated, select relevant goals and interventions from every chapter section that relates to caring for your client.

All of the mode categories do not have a corresponding state diagnosis. For example, manipulation, subtle obstructiveness, and dependency are

TABLE 19-1.   Nursing Diagnoses Relevant to Abusive Behaviors

STATES	MODES
Rational Anger	—
Aggressive Response	Aggressive Coping
Impulse-Dominated	Impulsive Coping
Self-Exalted	—
—	Manipulative Coping
—	Subtle Obstructive
—	Dependent Coping

passing, temporary behaviors; these can be resolved with effective communication and do not entail a detailed intervention plan. (See also the Dynamic Considerations paragraphs for each of these modes in the section on nursing assessment and intervention.) Theoretically, a person in an extreme situation, such as a political hostage, might experience Rational Anger in a modal fashion, although this is unlikely.

These nursing diagnoses are not just a rewriting and rewording of the psychiatric diagnoses presented earlier, but you will see some relationships between the two. For example, the nursing diagnosis, Subtle Obstructive Mode, and the psychiatric diagnosis, Passive-Aggressive Personality, appear similar. Therefore, consider what you can do independently if your client is in the outpatient medical

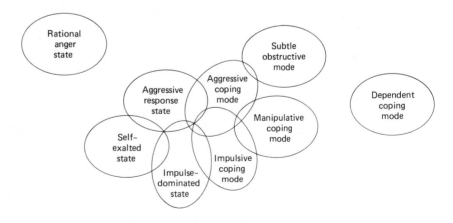

FIGURE 19-1   Diagram of various nursing diagnoses that could occur simultaneously.

clinic, yet resists complying with most treatment efforts. Will referral to a psychiatrist, based on the diagnosis of Passive-Aggressive Personality, be your first nursing action? Probably not, because you know the result would be noncompliance. Rather, start with a nursing diagnosis that points toward appropriate *initial* nursing actions.

Furthermore, a nursing diagnosis may be applicable to more than one psychiatric classification. Impulsive behavior is an example. The manic person may be impulsive because he/she is too emotionally high to be concerned with consequences. The hyperactive child is too energy-driven to slow down and think. The antisocial person wants immediate gratification. The person with borderline personality disorder does not know what he/she really wants. The explosive client is impulsive for unknown reasons. The person with organic brain disease may be impulsive because the brain cells are trying to cope with the effects of a toxin. The sexually deviant client may be impulsive because stimuli have created urges that are experienced as uncontrollable. Yet, as soon as you have data to assess Impulse-Dominated State and/or Impulse Coping Mode, you can institute therapeutic nursing actions even if you have no immediate knowledge of precise causation or psychiatric diagnosis. How these nursing diagnoses can be utilized and combined should become increasingly clear as you proceed through the rest of this chapter.

FACTORS CONTRIBUTING TO VIOLENCE PRONENESS

Probably our greatest fear is that "crazy people" might maim or even kill us. But how do we tell what people are potentially violent? Unfortunately, predictions of this sort cannot be made with certainty (19). Violent individuals are violent only some of the time (32), and then only under the circumstances that are violence-inducing for that particular client. J. Rappeport, G. Lassen, and N. Hay cite a number of studies, some dating back more than fifty years, that indicate that discharged psychiatric patients were not more dangerous than the population as a whole (44). However, in recent years, some studies are finding that discharged clients are more likely to commit crimes against persons than people in the general population (see Chapter 23). As a nurse, you are probably safer in psychiatric care settings where personnel are skilled in anticipating and minimizing the effects of violence than you are in many other places where you routinely go. For example, the only knife pointed toward this author was wielded not by a psychiatric patient but by an enfeebled aging man hospitalized for congestive heart failure.

It is essential to your personal safety to realize that nursing role behaviors appropriate to the planned care in a treatment setting may be inappropriate or dangerous in encounters with violent or potentially violent strangers. If someone approaches you on the street or in your home with physically threatening behaviors, that individual is an assailant, not a client. Respond with self-defense and/or survival strategies. Your goals might be to distract and escape, scream for help, fight back, submit and wait your chance, or use verbal trickery. But above all, do not assume that if you cooperate, show empathy, and use therapeutic communication that an assailant will do you no harm!

History of Violence

A history of violent behavior is the most reliable predictor of future violent behavior (32, 60). Interviewers will need to ask specific questions (like those listed below) about many factors commonly documented in the violence-prone (26, 31, 45, 52, 60):

1. Is the individual having homicidal thoughts, wishes, or fantasies about a specific intended victim or type of victim, such as an ethnic group or a particular group of females?
2. Is the individual a person of action who shows the capacity to effectively carry out threats?
3. What is the individual's access to weapons, especially guns? The lethality of the weapon in hand may be the determining factor between homicide and assault, and of more importance than either is the intent or motivation of the aggressor. [See J. Godwin (19).]
4. Is there a potential victim continually provoking the potentially dangerous person?
5. What is the extent of the use or abuse of drugs, such as alcohol, amphetamines, and hallucinogens?
6. What has been the usual past behavior during intoxicated states?

7. Is there a history of spouse abuse, child abuse, sexual assault, or rape?

8. Is there a childhood history of the behavioral triad of fire-setting, cruelty to animals, and enuresis?

9. Was the individual physically abused as a child?

10. Is the individual part of a family or subculture that honors violence or teaches physical aggression as a response to frustration?

11. Was there a particular or unusual set of events or circumstances that preceded any previous violent acts?

12. Does the individual demonstrate an inability to be sensitive and empathic to the needs and feelings of others?

13. Is there a history of many traffic violations or auto accidents related to aggressive driving behaviors?

14. Is a psychotic and volatile individual who has managed to function with the aid of psychotropic drugs now refusing to continue following the medication program?

A positive history on any one of the above questions may be the only predictive factor you have. Yet these questions do have a somewhat additive effect in that a positive history on several variables probably indicates very high violence potential.

However, a single act of extreme and perhaps murderous violence may not be anticipated by any of the above questions. E. I. Megargee describes the "overcontrolled" person who for years tolerates frustration and perhaps seethes inwardly but is viewed by outsiders as a conforming, gentle, and a nice neighbor. Then one day he/she may explode in an unexpected and shocking violent act (36). You may never anticipate the violence potential of this client unless you are a nurse who inspires sufficient trust that the client discloses plans or fantasies of violence, which you should treat with seriousness.

Spouse Abuse

Refer to Chapter 8 for discussion of one kind of violence—sexual assault/rape. Some of the dynamics and care pertinent to the rape victim are also applicable to the abused or battered spouse. Violence frequently occurs in the home (19). Signs and symptoms of an abused adult are similar to those described in Chapter 21 for child/adolescent abuse. The dynamics also have similarities. The abuser may have been abused as a child. Or the abuser may not have learned constructive ways of releasing anger and frustration. Being frequently beaten, often with no provocation or for different reasons at different times, causes feelings of fear, passivity, humiliation, low self-esteem, helplessness, hopelessness, and guilt at being the cause for the attacks. These feelings contribute to being too ashamed or afraid to admit the situation or to ask for help, and they may contribute to the abused (frequently the woman) standing by passively while one or more of the children are also beaten. The woman may stay in the battering relationship for other reasons, including: love for the batterer, remorse of the batterer and promises that it will not happen again, lack of means to get away (battered women's shelters are a recent development), society's view that husbands own wives and can treat them as they wish, threats of worse harm if she leaves, and lack of a support system or resources if she does leave. In one study, when asked how the wife could prevent the violence, the answers referred to being passive: by keeping quiet, giving in, grinning and shuffling, letting the husband do what he wants.

Sometimes the wife or husband does not leave, but the provocation becomes so great that she/he carefully plans how to kill the partner so that there can be a final release for self (and children). Godwin cites material Dr. George Bach gathered in interviewing 74 spouse-slayers (3, 19). Bach found these slayings occurred when there was a sharp disparity in marital power, with an aggressive mate insatiably demanding "giving" behaviors on the part of the spouse. A crisis point came when the passive, giving partner finally rebelled. The domineering partner tried to block the rebellion. It was then most often the "blocking mate" who ended up as the victim. This description of a passive partner becoming a rebelling slayer seems to correspond to Megargee's description of the "overcontrolled" personality discussed earlier (36).

Violence, hostility, and dominance are primary factors in many offenses of rape or sexual assault as well as in spouse abuse. The question is often raised as to what extent such events are victim-precipitated. Erich Fromm's theory describes masochistic persons as having difficulty in initiating excitation or in reacting readily to normal stimuli. Instead, they react when the stimulus overpowers them; when they can give themselves up to the excitement forced upon them. Sadists have a "passion" to absolutely and completely control another person. Masochistic people admire, love, and submit to those who have power, whereas sadists despise and want to control those who are powerless and cannot fight back. The sadist needs a victim. Fromm says both the sadist and the masochist seek a symbiotic relationship because neither has his/her center in self (17). However, given the power orientation of the sadist, the sadist will be the one who is active and skillful in seeking out vulnerable individuals without regard for whether there are significant masochistic tendencies in the victim. Do not assume that the victim wanted to be hurt or provoked or deserved the attack. No matter how much provocation there is, short of physical violence, violence is not justified as a response to anger, frustration, tension, or deprivation of needs.

Child Abuse

Child abuse may be perpetrated by anyone involved in a caretaking role with a child (57). The incidence of psychosis in child abusers is about the same as the incidence of psychosis in the general population. Drugs, alcohol, sociopathy, and sadism each may be the most pertinent factor in explaining certain cases of child abuse. However, most abusers are not generally violent, but rather blend in with the surrounding community as indistinct except in the aggression manifested within the confines of the home. Refer to Chapter 21 for a detailed discussion of assessment, intervention, and advocacy in child abuse.

Parent-child incest or other forms of sexual abuse may occur simultaneously with child abuse but this is certainly not always the situation. Frequently the incestuous family appears normal to the outside observer and there is no history of social deviance. Referring to these families as *endogamous families*, Alvin Rosenfeld writes of an immature,

dependent father unable to cope with adult women, a needful mother with low self-esteem, and an ambivalent child who may find the sexual attention to be pleasurable as well as coming from the more supportive and nurturant parent, but also anxiety-provoking if the child recognizes that the incestuous activities are furtive and at odds with social norms. Jailing the father or removing the child from the family may be more psychologically destructive to the child than the incest has been. The most helpful response will usually be therapy for the family as a unit (48).

Influence of Milieu and Staff Behaviors

Milieu factors and staff behaviors can provoke violent reactions in generally manageable clients. This means we need to recognize and respond to a tense ward climate caused by unresolved conflicts among staff or the treatment team. Inconsistent and conflicting responses to the client from various staff may precipitate power struggles between the client and others, which can escalate to violent acting out (28).

We must also ask ourselves uncomfortable questions as to how we personally may be contributing to a client's violence-proneness. Is our inexperience with assaultive persons so obvious that the client senses we will be unable to institute any firm controls? Are we somewhat immobilized by our own intrapersonal conflict regarding the aggressive or sexual impulses we experience in confrontive situations? Is a physical fear of being injured inhibiting us from relating to the client? Is our perception of the client distorted because of physical size, reputed strength, sex, or ethnicity? Are we verbally or nonverbally communicating to the client that assaultive behavior is the expected behavior (28, 53)? "Yes" answers to these questions may point us to problem-solving behaviors for ourselves.

NURSING ASSESSMENT, CLIENT-CARE GOALS, AND NURSING INTERVENTIONS

Care of the Person Who Is Rationally Angry

Assessment of Rational Anger State

The diagnosis of Rational Anger State is established when the client directly communicates

anger appropriate to a situation. Behavior is goal-directed. The thought processes are alert, oriented, and organized. Usually the person has an angry, tense facial expression and will readily verbalize frustration. Enduring hostile attitudes, physical assault, or environmental destructiveness as well as impulsive actions are behaviors that are incompatible with this nursing diagnosis. Rational Anger

State is a nursing diagnosis to use when a person is upset for valid, understandable reasons and is expressing the anger in a socially acceptable manner.

Dynamic Considerations

We have experienced rational anger throughout our lives. Perhaps one of our early experiences with rational anger occurred when a nurturing person offered us cereal mixed in milk. Our infantile response was that plain milk found its way down our throat much more comfortably. We reacted with spit, sputter, and fuss. Thus, we began to experience that everybody was not always going to treat us in precisely the way we desired to be treated.

Does our lifelong experience with rational anger enable us to be anxiety-free and comfortable with the reasonable anger of ourselves and our clients? No, we prefer to pretend that Perfect Nurse and Perfect Client do not experience anger, although we may intellectually acknowledge anger as an emotion basic to survival (42). Carl Rogers tells us that we may have an inner self that fears destruction by the client's anger (47). Betty Cuthbert reminds us that often we learn at a very early age how the expression of strong emotion is to be avoided. This past experience conditions us to protectively become defensive against experiencing direct emotion or being open to the client's emotion (15).

There are many valid reasons why clients experience Rational Anger States. Anger is a normal response to physical or psychological discomfort. Anger is also a predictable consequence of being forced to depend on others or conversely of feeling pushed into independence. Anger may occur when the person perceives the nurse is pressuring for too much self-disclosure of very personal data, or when the nurse is presuming a trustful, helping relationship that does not exist in the client's mind (59). Clients may be righteously angry about an unwieldy health care system and related dehumanization, angered by other clients who share the facilities, angered by the insensitivities of any health care giver, or angered by the actions of significant others and beloved ones. A typical case study is given below:

> Mrs. A., age 46, has been hospitalized for several weeks with an admitting psychiatric diagnosis of Bipolar Disorder, Depressed. She approaches the nurse with a swift step and says tersely, "Is Dr. B. here at the hospital yet?" The nurse answers that she does not know. Mrs. A. frowns and continues,

> "She said she would be by to see me before 9:30. It's almost 10 o'clock. I'm supposed to be at the lawyer's office by 10:30 to talk with him about my pending divorce. My friend who is going with me is here waiting and I need to leave. I'd like to know where Dr. B. is and why she isn't here like she said she would be."

Although Mrs. A. may have been admitted for the treatment of depression, that is not what the nurse assesses at this point. Instead, the nurse wants to ascertain whether Mrs. A. is experiencing a Rational Anger State, and if so, to consider appropriate nursing responses for this particular patient.

Goal 1: The client validates anger state with the nurse and develops appropriate avenues for expressing anger and a plan of action.

Interventions

The therapeutic communication skills described in Chapter 5 are essential to help the person express and resolve anger. Use active listening skills and ask clarifying questions to ascertain the breadth and depth of the anger. Validate when anger is an understandable reaction of the client. Apologize with concern and sincerity if you are at fault in creating or contributing to the client's rational anger. Do not feel responsible for defending the behavior of other health care givers, but you can explain your view of other health care givers' behavior if this aids in problem resolution. Consider and plan with the client any actions that can be taken in response to aggravating situations. For example, you can guide the person in thinking through how he/she can approach another who is triggering the anger. You can assist the client in planning what to say in a way that promotes resolution of anger rather than increased frustration.

Goal 2: Client states that discomfort due to anger state has been alleviated.

Interventions

Validate whether client feels less angry. If not, be active and creative in implementing the interventions of the previous goal. Explore how the person could more effectively cope with rational anger in future situations.

The Rational Anger State is the only "healthy" diagnosis this chapter will discuss. The other eight categories all describe behaviors that are pathological to at least some extent. Aggressive and impulsive modes and states describe behaviors that we have learned to fear.

Care of the Person in an Aggressive Response State

Assessment of Aggressive Response State

The diagnosis of an Aggressive Response State is established when the client appears hostile, tense, unduly agitated, and possibly argumentative. Reality testing and judgment are impaired. The person perceives a goal conflicting or goal blockage, but his/her insight about self as contributing to the conflict is limited. It is contradictory to this category for the client to be behaving in a fully rational manner.

A client who is potentially assaultive or combative may be maintaining a tense "ready to spring" posture or else pacing in an agitated, restless manner. He/she may be expressing distorted perceptions of the environment along with fear and defensiveness. There may be verbal threats to others to "leave me alone" or "keep away." Ventilation of hostility leads to increasing signs of physical tension rather than to increased self-control. Offers of therapeutic assistance, such as talking about the problem or accepting a P.R.N. medication, are rejected.

Dynamic Considerations

Unless you have gone through life without ever poking, biting, hitting, kicking, or screaming, you have experienced some degree of aggressive coping state as part of the pathology of everyday living. The labeling of these behaviors as "pathologic" will depend on the definition given earlier: that the aggression is beyond what is reasonable for the situation. "Beyond what is reasonable" is often not easily determined and depends on the values of a given culture. There is even considerable variance in different psychiatric settings as to what behavior is tolerated and what is not.

Aggressive Response behavior may result when the individual manifests a flight reaction to fear, such as fears related to hospitalization or to invasions of space and territorial needs. Many defensive maneuvers result in aggressiveness. Examples of this include *displacing* anger felt toward one person and taking it out on a safer person; or *overcompensating* for feelings of inadequacy or inferiority by intrusive interactions.

Often aggressive acts are attributed to *acting out.* In acting out the individual is thought to be experiencing an unconscious conflict about impulses that seem forbidden or dangerous. To relieve anxiety accompanying any impinging awareness of the conflict, the person will permit expression of the desire, i.e., act out or show conflicts or feelings he/she is experiencing (1, 13, 30). For example, an adolescent who feels mistreated by a teacher may vandalize the schoolroom. The conflict may revolve around the student's actually liking and respecting the teacher but feeling unachievable expectations are being set for him/her. Therefore, to vent his/her anxiety, the schoolroom, (especially the teacher's own materials) may be destroyed.

Sometimes staff members unwittingly encourage a client to act out. They may get vicarious satisfaction out of seeing one client punch another client they themselves have found troublesome. They refrain from intervening before the punch is thrown. After it happens, they rationalize that they could not have stopped it, and that the client got what he deserved. Staff may also set themselves up as such parental or authority figures that clients are triggered into acting out as unruly children.

One popular theory regarding aggressiveness is that it occurs in response to frustration incurred when attainment of a desired goal is blocked. K. Scherer, R. Abeles, and C. Fischer present a revised Frustration-Aggression Theory (52). They postulate that environmental frustrations lead to emotional arousal, which in turn energizes aggressive behaviors. The forces that arouse, sustain, and direct aggression are reactions to the blocked goals in the environment. In addition, general, nonspecific arousal feelings may sensitize a person to aggressive cues, and thus make an aggressive response more likely, and may also increase the strength of aggressive behavior (52).

Many factors are potentially etiologic to aggression, not only psychological factors. Physiological factors such as hormonal and biochemical alterations, temporal lobe and anterior hypothalamic pathology, hypoglycemia, allergic food reactions (40), and untoward reactions to medication may trigger aggression. For example, aggressive responses in the manic or hyperkinetic child may be influenced both by environmental frustration and a general state of high physiologic arousal related to biochemical alterations. Your observation and clear description of circumstances preceding an aggressive outburst will aid the psychiatric and medical diagnosticians.

Goal 1: The client shows recognition that the nurse is acting to assist him/her in effecting better self-control.

Interventions

A client who is highly agitated and verbally threatening should not be psychologically cornered. Do not imply that you are treating the agitation lightly or disrespectfully. Instead, acknowledge the intensity of the feeling state and reinforce any remaining self-control (43). For example, imagine that Mrs. W. has a shampoo bottle in her upraised hand aimed toward you. Maintain eye contact and say calmly, "In spite of how upset you feel, you are able to think before you act. Set the bottle down. Let's see what we can accomplish by talking." In this example, feelings are acknowledged, any capacities for self-control are affirmed, a simple direction is given, and a constructive response has been suggested as a mutual task.

Mrs. W. may well respond by lowering her arm only slightly and saying, "Where do you get off thinking you can order everybody around? I'm getting out of here and the devil himself isn't going to stop me!" Noting the increased signs of self-control shown by the lowered arm and verbalizing, you might then say, "You feel the best action you can take now is getting out of here. I would like to know what happened that made you feel leaving is the best choice you have." Be prepared to listen and allow ventilation as long as the ventilation is productive rather than generating further loss of control. You probably will not be able to influence the client's reasoning much at this point. Defensiveness impairs listening (61). Consider whether the basis of the client's fear or anger is rational, even if the behavior is not. Later you may be able to guide the client in naming and planning more adequate and acceptable choices of behavior. If the basis for the agitation is misperception or overreaction, you may be able to provide feedback of information on how you view the client's behavior as long as you can do so in a matter-of-fact, sensitive manner that does not impair the client's self-esteem.

Goal 2: The client shows realization that staff members have an obligation to intervene to prevent physical harm to client or others.

Interventions

Unfortunately there will be a few occasions where all the relationship and communication skills available to you will not be sufficient to enable you to maintain a safety priority. In such cases, you will have to consider chemical or physical restraint, or both. Administering either form of restraint is a dependent nursing function that necessitates a physician's orders. The only exception to this is temporary emergency physical restraint exercised as a nursing judgment to prevent immediate injury. The physician is then notified immediately, and an order for continued restraint is requested if indicated. In all decision making regarding the use of medicinal or physical restraint, you must consider legal rights of clients as well as institutional policies and procedures, which need to be clearly stated in writing (see Chapter 22).

Approaching a potentially or actively assaultive client to do bodily restraint requires a team of staff that is emotionally and procedurally prepared (29, 41, 58). S. DiFabio and E. J. Ackerhalt observe that nurses are often educationally unprepared to bodily restrain clients because educational programs and nursing texts have failed to present such material. These authors suggest structured role-play as a tool in such learning and describe their role-playing seminars (16).

Clients in any care setting can become combative. All of an institution's nursing personnel should attend regularly scheduled training sessions on restraining, just as most institutions now provide training for other emergencies, such as cardiopulmonary resuscitation (C.P.R.). You should have an opportunity to be physically restrained yourself. It will increase your empathy with the client to expose yourself to some of the same fears that the client experiences. You will also be more apt to believe that physical restraints should be used as a last resort!

Anyone locked in seclusion or restrained to a bed needs almost continuous care and observation in regard to safety, vital signs, fluids, nourishment, toileting, safe restraint and body positioning, and prevention of skin breakdown. Frequent verbal reassurances and reality orientation interventions are essential.

Chemical restraint is often the preferred choice of client, physician, and nurse. A prescribed medication given early enough may eliminate the need for any physical immobilization and may enable the client to better maintain a sense of self-esteem and self-control. Medications prescribed P.R.N. for agitation may include phenothiazines, diazepam, and barbiturates. However, these drugs may have hazardous side effects as well as interact with or potentiate the effects of each other or alcohol. Also too much chemical restraint can be a problem instead of a solution. Staff members or the client may become too reliant on medicinal control, and consequently they may neglect to utilize the full range of milieu and interpersonal interventions.

Overmedication can be a problem, too, especially for the elderly. Confusion, disorientation, and agitation in the evening and nighttime are common, especially in patients on psychoactive drugs with hypotensive side effects (50). Respiratory and total central nervous system depression are also common in the elderly as the result of psychotropic medications.

Goal 3:   The client utilizes opportunities to discuss and integrate an aggressive response state.

Interventions

Too often we neglect to intervene in the calm that follows the storm. The client may feel shame, humiliation, and puzzlement following an aggressive outburst, even if these feelings are masked by distancing or defensive maneuvers. Approach the person with acceptance. Initiate opportunities for him/her to discuss what happened, to reflect on factors involved, to learn from the experience, and to accept himself or herself. Other clients who have witnessed a violent incident also need opportunities to discuss their feelings and reactions. The same is true for staff members who have been involved.

Care of the Person with an Aggressive Coping Mode

Assessment of Aggressive Coping Mode

For the nursing diagnosis of Aggressive Coping Mode to be established, there must be a positive history of repeated assaultiveness, fighting, and destruction of property, with the intention of getting personal needs met through the use of force. This client appears tense, sullen, and resentful when questioned about past behavior. Perceptual distortion is evident in the client's world view; i.e., the client believes that he/she is a superior person struggling to assert himself or herself in a hostile world. Responsibility for actions is rationalized or projected. This client is often limited in verbally discussing anger and resentful feelings.

Dynamic Considerations

Social Learning Theory is useful in understanding individuals whose coping style relies persistently on aggressive responses. Albert Bandura hypothesizes that we learn from others how to be aggressive and we continue to be aggressive because of reinforcement (5, 6). We learn aggression responses to stimuli from parental models as well as from our subculture, from the symbolic modeling we observe in television programs or movies, and from our own trial-and-error experiences. We may become aggressive to forestall events we foresee will be threatening or painful. Or we may hurt others because we anticipate positive consequences will result or because we have experienced some success in controlling people through force.

According to the concepts of Social Learning Theory, the reinforcement of aggression may occur in a number of ways: (1) There may be *direct external reinforcement,* such as tangible rewards, status rewards, alleviation of mistreatment by defensively aggressing, or much more rarely, reinforcement by the pleasure of causing pain, as occurs in the sadist. (2) There may be *vicarious reinforcement* of aggression; i.e., we tend to do what we see others get reinforced for doing, and we avoid behaviors that we see bring punishment to others. An exception to this is that reactive aggressive behavior may increase if we see the other as being unjustly punished. (3) Finally there may be *self-reinforcement.* We may minimize our own conduct by pointing our finger to the greater aggression of someone else, make noble rationalizations, displace or diffuse our own responsibility, or dehumanize the victim into labels and stereotypes. As we convince ourselves that our aggression occurs only in righteous circumstances, we become progressively and somewhat unwittingly desensitized to our own aggressiveness (5, 6).

Thus far the discussion has dynamically presented the Aggressive Coping Mode in terms of "we," "us," and "our." This is because as you are probably aware, our aggressive, competitive American society has developed certain aggressive inclinations in most, if not all, of us. The pathology of the behavior depends on the degree and circumstances of the aggressiveness.

In an empathic discussion of clients who repetitively act out aggressively, F. Carney discusses four specific inabilities these clients have (11):

1. The inability to trust, with perhaps an incapacity to believe that other human beings can be sincere.
2. The inability to experience feelings (they may unconsciously refuse to acknowledge feelings).
3. The inability to fantasize and empathize.
4. The inability to learn, i.e., to transfer learning from past experience to a sense of the future, with the idea that actions have consequences.

In light of Carney's identification of such major inabilities, you can see that therapeutic care for these individuals is no small challenge. In fact, most institutional settings do not try to change the behavior of those operating in an aggressive mode. They simply try to contain and control the behavior until they can release the client. Changing the behavior requires months or years of intensive and sophisticated intervention followed by regular aftercare with a therapist with whom there is a trusting relationship.

Some clients will faithfully follow a medication regime of major tranquilizers and thus have sufficient control of behavior. For others, major tranquilizers may be used simultaneously with therapy to teach the client new behaviors.

Goal 1: The client describes awareness of the experience of a milieu that controls and contains major aggressive actions.

Interventions

The treatment setting should be well staffed with calm, nonthreatening personnel who are capable of warmth and a trusting relationship. These personnel should be highly visible, yet not impinge unnecessarily on the territorial distance that a tense,

sullen client needs. The environment should be free of objects that can serve readily as weapons. Necessary limits should be firmly and fairly identified for the client. Any consequences that the client faces for rule violations should be clear and reasonable, and the client should be fully cognizant that the staff has the capacity to enforce any needed measures to control aggression. Therefore, do not be provoked into making threats you cannot fairly enforce. Also staff members must try to avoid a punitive or judgmental approach. Punitive treatment furnishes aggressive examples to the client and may reinforce the belief that aggressiveness is the best way to solve problems. High aggressors may become even more aggressive when a punitive approach is used (5). Shaming or belittling should be avoided as this also may provoke further aggression (23). It has been common in psychiatric facilities to believe that aggressive patients benefit from catharsis. Objects such as punching bags were readily available and were encouraged for use to "drain off" aggressive energy. Learning Theory suggests this may be momentarily true; however, in the long run, catharsis may result in reinforcing aggressive habits (52). Rather, what the aggressive client needs is a full, busy, and active day.

Guidelines for intervening in the Aggressive Response State (see pages 609–610) may be applicable for clients in the Aggressive Coping Mode. Sister Kiening suggests that some patients, especially those with strong authoritarian traits, respond to limit setting much more readily than they do to discussion and ventilation. Their anxiety is lessened when they feel that the caretakers show no signs of weakness, seem to be in firm control, and can be depended on to help them preserve their self-respect (24). You may find Kiening's suggestions particularly applicable early in treatment for an aggressive client who is testing limits and security.

Goal 2: The client changes behavior in a positive direction, indicating experience with corrective emotional experiences.

Interventions

Repeated caring from considerate, empathic staff in response to inappropriate aggression can provide corrective emotional experiences to clients (27), as illustrated by the following case study of a hospitalized patient:

M. O., although only ten years of age, was described in the morning report by the night nurse as a new patient who was tough, unsocialized, and had pretty much raised himself on the inner city streets of St. Louis.

After listening to the report about patients, the nurse G. M. makes an initial approach to introduce herself when she sees M. O. standing alone in the hallway near the locked exit door. G. M. is still 6 to 8 feet away and about to speak when M. O. glares at her and states belligerantly, "Stay away from me, you bitch!"

G. M. stops in her tracks. But she meets M. O.'s stare and responds, "That's smart of you not to trust strangers. Never mind calling me 'bitch' though, because that word could mean a lot of things besides me. Call me 'G.' Now pick out two chairs for us to sit in so we can learn more about whether or not to trust each other."

M. O. hesitates only a surprised moment before rather meekly selecting two chairs. He sits in one after scooting them a few inches further apart.

The nurse was also surprised by the chain of events. She had not anticipated being greeted as "bitch." However, she knew how to apply the principles: (1) give M. O. space, (2) state her observations as to what his behavior might mean in an esteeming way, (3) state a limit with an explanation, (4) offer the client the control of choice of chairs, and (5) state an expectation that some goal in respect to trusting would be broached. Pleased that her response worked, G. M. relaxed a bit and smiled to herself as M. O. selected the two chairs.

M. Wolfgang offers the following principles based on evidence from all the healing arts and behavioral sciences (62):

1. Give the infant, child, adolescent, and adult family member affection, recognition, and reward for being alive and unharming to others.
2. Give freedom from excessive restraints.
3. Provide pleasures for the body as well as a broad repertoire of verbal ways to respond to stimuli in any social interaction.

In the past we have been reluctant to use comfort touching with the aggressive client because of several pertinent dynamic concerns. We do not want to induce pathological anxiety in a person who might not be able to tolerate physical or emotional closeness. We are also cautious about highly distorted transference and countertransference responses developing. Yet, new learning regarding human contact seems central to permanent change for the habitually aggressive. Perhaps clinical nursing research could address this issue of when and how to use comfort touching and begin to develop guidelines.

Goal 3: The client demonstrates socially acceptable measures for meeting needs.

Interventions

Consider how often role-play, rehearsal, and discussion of problematic situations are used in effecting learning for nurses. These techniques are equally useful for aggressive clients, either individually or in a group. For the child, play therapy may achieve these same aims. Remember these people have inexperience and difficulty with verbalizing, so use supportive techniques to help them frame verbal responses to situations where their rights are being challenged. Teach the difference between assertiveness and aggressiveness.

Goal 4: The client responds constructively to frustration.

Interventions

Consider using behavior modification principles along with a nurse-client relationship to achieve this goal. This involves first developing a clear understanding of the conditions under which behaviors are reinforced or extinguished. Have the staff agree upon a behavior modification program so that all involved with the client are applying the principles consistently. Determine what is truly rewarding and reinforcing for the individual. Perhaps it is something you would not ordinarily consider, such as an undisturbed hour of listening to the radio, or an opportunity to strum a guitar. Reward positive behaviors with verbal comment, privileges, and increasing freedom. Refer to Chapter 2 for further discussion of behavior modification theory and therapy.

You may not have the opportunity to see much progress with clients in an Aggressive Coping Mode because such progress may not happen. But if you do see the slow changes of personality transformation, it will be one of your most satisfying experiences as a nurse.

Care of the Person
in an Impulse-Dominated State

Assessment of Impulse-Dominated State

The diagnosis of an Impulse-Dominated State is made when the client demonstrates impulsive behavior and is restless, excitable, and somewhat unpredictable. Ability to concentrate is impaired. He/she may be aware of reality, but actions are often more influenced by internal factors than external considerations. Insight is very limited. The client often later expresses bafflement and dismay over his/her actions. Anxiety is not overtly obvious prior to the impulsive action, but he/she may express anxiety and guilt after the fact.

Dynamic Considerations

One way to get in touch with what the impulse-dominated client experiences is to recall occasions when your own behavior baffled you. Perhaps it was giggling inappropriately or saying something you didn't intend to say. Many of us have experienced sufficient states of stress that we tried to explain away what we viewed as our own strange behavior with comments such as, "I was so tired that I didn't know what I was doing."

Instinct or drive theories of behavior hold that certain urges, especially aggression and sexuality, are inborn and are driven by an innate energy to seek expression. Psychoanalytic Theory adds that through socialization we develop ego controls that aid us in containing or directing innate drives and in channeling their expression into acceptable activities. An impulsive act would be the result of an innate urge slipping through the retaining wall of ego control and manifesting itself in an insufficiently socialized way. For some impulse-dominated clients, organic impairment may be such that reality is not perceived accurately. Often, however, the client is perceiving reality but is not in possession of sufficient ego control to respond wisely to reality.

From the standpoint of pathology, impulsivity can wear many hats. In addition to addressing causative factors, there are interventions we can use to assist the client in immediate functioning without knowing causation, such as discussed below under goals.

Goal 1: The client experiences a milieu that is nonthreatening, low in stimulation, and safe.

Interventions

Communicate firm, fair limits in a simple, direct, matter-of-fact manner. Avoid power struggles. Insure that basic physical needs, often neglected by the client, are being met. Is the client getting sufficient fluids, nourishment, rest, and sleep? Are bowel habits and personal hygiene measures being maintained?

The disturbed person is particularly vulnerable to the emotional contagion of a chaotic milieu. Remove him/her to more subdued surroundings when indicated and provide activities that are interesting and can be engaged in successfully.

Goal 2: The client considers choices and exerts self-control consistent with current functioning.

Interventions

Self-control is developed over time. Present the client with feedback on the results of impulsive acts. Suppose Mr. Y. suddenly turns off a television program that others are watching. You might say, "Mr. Y., the others were irritated to have the T.V. turned off while they were watching. If the T.V. is bothering you, let's work out some solution besides turning it off." Limit choices to that which is safe and appropriate to the situation. Assist the client to make plans, set realistic goals, and work toward these goals for the day, week or month. Reinforce success in small delays of gratification. Reflect with the person about consequences of unplanned actions and unattained goals. As he/she progresses, you may be able to apply interactions suggested under the Impulsive Coping Mode, which is discussed in the following pages.

Care of the Person with an Impulsive Coping Mode

Assessment of Impulsive Coping Mode

As in other diagnoses designated as modes, the assessment of Impulsive Coping Mode is based to a great extent on history of past behavior. There is a history of hasty, ill-considered actions. Often these clients have been considered disciplinary problems, e.g., youngsters "who just don't listen but do as they please." Their overall activity level has been above the norm since at least early childhood. Affect is labile and is influenced almost entirely by circumstances of the moment. Frustration is poorly tolerated and often precipitates an impulsive response. Social judgment is impaired. Close and mutually meaningful friendships are not established. Family members indicate anger and emotional exhaustion from so frequently being called on to bail the impulsive client out of situations. There is often a history of sexual, aggressive, and self-destructive acting out. In the adult, there is a history of sudden school and job changes, geographic moves, and multiple erratic romantic liaisons.

Dynamic Considerations

In addition to factors discussed under the Impulse-Dominated State, these clients may be afflicted with perceptual and/or learning disabilities, even though specific neurologic pathology cannot be demonstrated. In recent years there has been considerable interest in the role of nutritional imbalance or food allergies (in particular, sugar) in explaining some impulsive and overactive behavior.

Parenting styles that are overpermissive, overindulgent, or inconsistent have been associated with the impulsive client (13). A "difficult baby" who is irritable and overreactive to stimuli may invoke parental confusion, inconsistency, and overindulgence in an effort to try anything to keep harmony within the home. Eventually it may become a "peace at any price" issue, and the family events will revolve around a center point of reacting to the behaviors of the impulsive child.

The first two goals and their interventions for the Impulse-Dominated State (see page 613) are applicable to the Impulsive Coping Mode.

> *Goal 3: The client states understanding of relationship of rewards and consistent environmental consequences with his/her actions and increasingly demonstrates self-control and responsible self-direction.*

Interventions

The client needs to become aware that coping with stress by permitting release of impulsive energies is the cause of much of his/her misery. This can happen if he/she is allowed to experience cause-and-effect events, with opportunities to discuss how *A* (action) produced *R* (result). Magical thinking should be confronted and identified as such. Esteem and reward the person for postponing gratifications. Involve him/her regularly in playing commercial games where winning depends on planning, patience, and strategy more than on impulse and chance. (For example, play Mastermind rather than Monopoly, or Gin Rummy rather than Blackjack.) Verbalize the strategic thinking you do to model how planning has its payoffs.

As with any modal diagnosis, treatment is a long-term proposition. You will need to cope with your irritation and anger at the client's gross impulsive action just when you thought that some progress had been made. Pay attention to your own needs for humor and a moderate blood pressure!

Care of the Person in a Self-Exalted State

Assessment of Self-Exalted State

Psychiatry refers to clients experiencing the extreme end of the Self-Exalted State as *manic* or *grandiose*. This nursing diagnosis is established when a client expresses ideas of being a supremely important person or of possessing untold wealth, power, magnetism, sexual prowess, or attractiveness. If these ideas extend to a frankly delusional level, the person may claim to be such personages as Napoleon, Jesus Christ, or "the President's Personal Emissary sent to Evaluate Sexual Behaviors of Psychiatric Staff," or some similar title. Insight, judgment, and reality testing are all impaired. Behaviors described under Affective Disorder, Manic (page 600) are observed.

Dynamic Considerations

There is research indicating that genetic and biochemical alterations are determining factors in the occurrence of manic affective disorders (see Chapter 2, pages 26, 27, 28.)

Psychologically, we can feel understanding for persons exhibiting self-aggrandizing or manic behavior by recalling the thrills of days when we felt on top of everything, able to overcome any obstacle and conquer any foe. The accompanying emotional high was exhilarating. However, we are brought "down to earth" when confronted with a stubborn problem or after a night of sleep subdues our former slap-happy state.

It is often helpful to view self-exhalted states from the other side—the feeling of being unworthy. A sense of self-failure might be overwhelming, were it to be acknowledged. Thus, the person defensively does a turnabout, claiming superiority. *Fears* of not being equal to a loss, or to a loss-potential situation, *are denied.* In addition the person *overcompensates* and presents self as all-powerful, all-competent, and all-knowing. This is a highly vulnerable position to maintain. Challenges from reality are constant. In response to these intentional or accidental challenges the client may become irritated and hostile.

Healing involves aiding the person to come to love and accept self with the assets and limits that exist; without need for gross reality distortion. The nurse who is able to *feel* esteem for the self-exalting person aids immeasurably in the healing process.

Goal: The client's statements regarding own abilities will become increasingly congruent with reality.

Interventions

Avoid laughter, smirks, or argument in response to self-exalted ideas. Commend the person for actual abilities, strengths, and skills that you observe. Avoid the reinforcement of self-exaltation that occurs if you pay more attention to grandiose statements than you do to reality-oriented statements. State your perception of reality when the client misinterprets or is delusional or when you note that his/her self-aggrandizing statements are a source of interpersonal difficulties. However, do not argue or insist that your perception be accepted. Encourage all activities where the individual is likely to experience successful participation. Assist the person in setting goals and in realistically evaluating successes or failures. Avoid threatening or opposing his/her defensive system so much that you increase hostility and/or exacerbate symptoms. Convey to the client that your esteem for him/her derives from assessments apart from the area of self-exaltation.

This discussion of the Self-Exalted State concludes with a case study that illustrates a number of the intervention principles just presented:

Mrs. T. was hospitalized yesterday afternoon with a psychiatric diagnosis of Manic-Depressive Disease, Manic Phase. Her nurse renews an intervention process begun earlier that morning after she observes the following interchange between Mrs. T. and another patient, Miss U:

Mrs. T. (loudly): "Did you notice how your doctor avoided me? The doctors all know my powers go on for hours. Seductive eyes that hypnotize. They fall at my feet. You're jealous." Miss U. looks at Mrs. T. wide-eyed. Without verbally responding, she walks away to join a group of patients.

Nurse: "Mrs. T., I noticed Miss U. didn't answer you but rather walked away."

Mrs. T.: "She's jealous. You're jealous too. Doctors and nurses and T.V., I know what goes on."

Nurse: "Dr. J. seemed to me to be focusing his interest on the patients he has admitted."

Mrs. T.: "He's afraid of my husband. They all are. Whoop-de-do. Scaredy cat too!"

Nurse: "Am I correct that you've been married twenty years? You must have solved many a problem in that length of time."

Mrs. T.: "Yes, I can solve anything. Solver, Savior, oh woe is me."

Nurse: "Do you mean that a very difficult problem is troubling you now?"

Mrs. T.: "Right dearie, its getting you out of my hair!" (glares at nurse)

Nurse: "You are telling me to back off. OK. But I do want to spend time with you. I read in your chart that you were a cook for many years in one of our downtown restaurants. Could you share a few trade secrets?"

Mrs. T.: "Maybe there's hope for you yet, dearie. I've been wondering if there was anybody around here who could appreciate me."

The nurse in this sequence begins by describing an observed effect of Mrs. T.'s behavior on another patient. Next, rather than challenging Mrs. T.'s thoughts, the nurse offers her personal perception of events. The nurse chooses not to directly explore the statement about other men fearing Mrs. T.'s husband because she does not want to overattend to what may be contributing to Mrs. T.'s grandiosity. Instead the nurse alludes to the client's capacities to problem solve. In response, there is indication of a momentary lapse in Mrs. T.'s defense system. The nurse offers an opportunity for her to continue in this vein. At this, Mrs. T. feels threatened and becomes annoyed. The nurse understands and will use this insight later when appropriate. As the immediate goal is to foster rapport and help the person maintain control and self-esteem, the nurse now shifts the focus into an area that Mrs. T. can discuss successfully.

Care of the Person with a Manipulative Coping Mode

Assessment of Manipulative Coping Mode

Because the word *manipulation* is itself an abused term in nursing and psychiatry, Ben Bursten's criteria will be used to restrict the meaning of the term. Bursten suggests we look for four components to behavior before concluding it is manipulative (10).

1. There must be a *perceived* conflict of goals. (The client might be mistaken or inaccurate about there being a goal conflict, but he/she *believes* that personal wants are in conflict with what another individual wants.)
2. The client must *consciously intend* to influence the other person.
3. There must be *conscious deception and insincerity.*
4. There must be a *feeling of exhilaration, having put something over* on the other person.

As with each modal diagnosis, you will find a history of repeated attempts by the client to handle or cope with stressful events by consciously trying to influence and deceive another person, feeling pleased with him/herself for being so artfully tricky. (However, avoid the common pitfall of labeling all people who are more than routinely troublesome as manipulative.)

Dynamic Considerations

In the client's mind, the end justifies the means. And there may be many ends that the client desires. He/she may want to test personal power believing that a direct approach will be thwarted, rejected, or ignored. Or there may be a struggle to assert autonomy and/or mastery in a

distorted fashion. Depending on prior experience with parental/authority relationships, the client generally manifests a learned style of how he/she got what was wanted in early relationships.

Nurses don't like to be manipulated by clients. As H. Jensen and G. Tillotson noted, the nurse who is, or appears to be, unable to control the situation loses status with colleagues (22). The following example shows how a patient attempts to ridicule a young nurse.

> Mrs. B.H., a former registered nurse, is now a very charming and extroverted client. She holds other patients as well as some staff spellbound with graphic stories about her escapades—stories of sex in the linen closet and vodka in the orange juice.
> One early afternoon, a newly employed, 21-year-old nurse observes Mrs. B. H. talking very quietly to another female patient. The nurse approaches and asks to join them. Mrs. B. H. smiles as she responds, "Yes, of course. I was just giving Sharon some suggestions for an ideal suicide."
> The nurse, at a loss as to how to react, utters a reflexive, "Oh?"
> Mrs. B. H. is ready with a response, "On a fine spring day like today, a nice slow intravenous drip of pentathol would be ideal—over in the park across from the hospital. You know, you could lay under a tree, hang the bottle on a limb, and just drift off."
> Later the two clients explode with laughter. It was "all a game" they say; "a bit of fun," says Mrs. B. H., because the new nurse takes her work much too seriously.

Unless you are Perfect Nurse, accept that you may be manipulated on occasion. It may happen because a particular client is so artful, beguiling, and flattering that you do not feel "used" until later. Sometimes you may "go along" even when you sense that this is what is happening. Try to remain alert to the process and objective in response. A mesmerizing manipulator might be suspected when: (1) the previously harmonic staff or treatment team are in uproar over their treatment plan for the client; (2) clients are acting out and are being played "against" each other; (3) family members are giving you mixed and ambivalent messages about the client; (4) special privileges are convincingly pleaded for, (5) you are hearing bargaining statements such as, "If you will only do this, then I'll . . . ," (6) approaches begin with flattery; e.g., "You're the only nurse who can understand why I need to . . . ," or (7) the client is an expert in taking advantage of weak or vulnerable aspects of individual staff members.

Goal 1: The client decreases manipulative behavior in a milieu that consistently avoids reinforcing manipulations.

Interventions

The manipulative client can effectively change behavior when assigned to a well-integrated, secure, caring nurse on a one-to-one basis. *All* requests even for things so simple as a deck of cards or a pencil are then to be made to that staff member. This limits the successful manipulations that can be achieved by playing staff members against each other. Avoid unenforceable rules, but stick to the limits that are enforceable. Tell the client (and follow through) that his/her progress will be evaluated on the basis of actions you see rather than words you hear. Avoid long interactions when the client is engaged in manipulation. Spend time with the client when manipulation is not occurring.

Goal 2: The client directly communicates needs and demonstrates nonmanipulative approaches to stress; concern is shown for others.

Interventions

The client's behavior will change very slowly; consistent rewards for nonmanipulative behavior are necessary. Role-playing of alternative behaviors may be useful, as mentioned under the Aggressive Coping Mode. Share with your client your feelings when you sense manipulation and say what approach would feel more fair and honest to you.

M. Meldman, G. McFarland, and E. Johnson present an extensive list of interventions that may be selected to utilize for a particular manipulative client (37). B. Bursten points out that the manipulator needs to be able to identify with the therapist for engagement to occur and that this may involve "being more clever" than the client, i.e., achieving respect and admiration as a basis for identification (10). It is easy to mistakenly trust the manipulator too soon, as he/she may "act" new behaviors as just one more manipulation. Treatment is an extremely long-term proposition. You may make significant strides if you are able to confront with sincere empathy. Take the following example:

Imagine a hypothetical situation where J. N. has once again manipulated the staff. You might open with: "Jonah, it looks like you have backed staff members into a corner again. If you get by with this, you'll believe that we are fools whom you have tricked. If we enforce the rules, you'll convince yourself that we're up-tight bad guys. You are clever! Let's explore why backing people into corners is the way you frequently want to operate."

You have challenged J. N. You may well get a wordy response that is angry, defensive, and rationalizing.

Respond: "Hmmm, I'm not sure how much truth I heard in all that. Your actions will show me in time. Meanwhile, I'll play the heavy. The rule still stands. You know, you are so good at figuring angles that you will be a terrific guy when you put that together with caring about people. I guess I'm saying that I feel disappointed but not hopeless about you. I'll be back as soon as I check on a couple of matters. See you in about ten minutes." Walk away.

Care of the Person with a Subtle Obstructive Mode

Assessment of Subtle Obstructive Mode

Clients with the diagnosis of a Subtle Obstructive Mode are not ordinarily seeking treatment for their obstructive patterns, as they are not insightful as to how these patterns are contributing to their interpersonal difficulties. Their problems generally come to the attention of the nurse in the context of treating them for some other illness. Or in trying to cope with them as a co-worker, these people irritate you in constant subtle ways that are difficult to define and to respond to in a direct manner. They do such things as sit quietly and agreeably through a long committee meeting and then begin nit-picking just as the committee is resolving a matter and getting ready to adjourn. These people (1) procrastinate, (2) are habitually late, (3) "don't recall having heard" a point they may have agreed to earlier, (4) neglect to do jobs for which they are responsible—but always offer "reasons" for why not, (5) botch an assignment they didn't really want to do, or (6) pester and provoke you with comments and questions while doing the task. Two case studies are given below:

Maria is a seven-year-old pediatric patient hospitalized for minor surgery. She has been incessantly demanding staff attention. When staff become counterresistive, Maria spills her juice, gags on her medication, loses her possessions, and falls and scrapes her knees.

C. R., a clinical specialist in medical outpatient care, is not really surprised that Mr. A. S., age 45, is late again. She anticipates that he will again have reasons for not being able to come on time, follow his diet, and refill his prescription. If Mrs. A. S. is along, she will be nagging Mr. A. S. Soon Mr. A. S. will be sitting like a sullen, silent lump in the waiting area.

Dynamic Considerations

These clients have learned to handle autonomy, authority, and dependency conflicts through indirect measures. Perhaps such behavior has been survival-adaptive, such as in asserting personal identity in a struggle with an excessively controlling parent, teacher, or spouse. In a situation where direct expression of feelings was perceived as hazardous, the person's feelings were suppressed or repressed. Through identification with a role model, cleverness, or trial and error, the client finds that some satisfaction can be gained by subtle obstructionism.

Passive-resistance techniques have been repeatedly presented in the news as strategy for inducing social change. Chances are that you also have at some point subtly avoided doing something you were expected to do but did not really want to do. Recalling such actions on our own part helps us empathize with a client's subtle obstructiveness and consider whether we want to alter some of our own indirect measures of expressing feelings.

Goal 1: The client's behavior changes in a positive direction in response to a direct, nonhostile message as to how the nurse views the client's actions.

Interventions

Using descriptive statements, tell the client what you have observed. Offer speculations as to

why this may be occurring. Tell the person you would like to work with him/her in gaining sufficient control and security in this situation. An adult client, such as Mr. A. S. in the above example, might react with anxiety and defensiveness. Restate what you said, emphasizing that you have spoken because you care and want to be involved with him in achieving better health. Emphasize his freedom of choice and your respect for that freedom.

With a young client such as the seven-year-old Maria, you might say,

Maria, in the past hour you have spilled your juice on the bed, asked us to help you find your lost doll, gagged on your medication, and scratched both knees in a fall. Are you trying to tell us you want us to stay close by? If that's it, we have got to come up with a better plan. What do you think?

You may need to repeat these interventions in many future contacts with the client since change is not produced with ease.

Goal 2: The client develops a sense of control and freedom and becomes involved in his/her own treatment process.

Interventions

Convey to the client that you feel he/she is competent to develop with you an individualized approach to treatment of the behavior and illness. Get the person involved in learning about his/her health and physical state as well as any current disease. Becoming more knowledgeable increases one's sense of control and self-esteem.

Goal 3: The client decreases subtle obstruction behavior.

Interventions

Be as objective and matter-of-fact as possible. Try not to react emotionally to subtle obstructive behaviors. This is not easy because the person may react by trying even harder to irritate you. If the client indicates distress or anxiety regarding interpersonal difficulties, validate his/her difficulties and talk with him/her about referral possibilities for insightful therapies.

Care of the Person with a Dependent Coping Mode

Assessment of a Dependent Coping Mode

The diagnosis of a Dependent Coping Mode is not directed toward clients whose dependent behaviors increase temporarily and expectedly in coping with the stress of illness, injury, or pain. For this normal dependent client, acceptance and concerned response to the dependent behaviors will allow healthy independence to emerge. An example of functional dependence is the client who wants your presence and reassurance the first few times trying a new self-care procedure, but then confidently says he/she feels ready to manage alone.

In contrast, clients operating in a Dependent Coping Mode demonstrate such resistance to assuming responsibility for self-care that you may find yourself feeling angered by their determination to prove how helpless and incapable they are. The dependent coping client wants your presence. Strategies to keep you near may vary from overly sweet requests and chatter that invokes guilt feelings in you because of your desire to escape and continue with your work, to tearful, clinging requests that you not leave. Anxiety will surface if you pressure this client to make a choice or decision or to assume responsibility. Dependency needs will increase if you begin ignoring or avoiding this client. Somatic reactions may also develop. Desperate bids for attention, including self-injury or self-neglect, may result. Dependent clients abuse others by using them too much.

Dynamic Considerations

A domineering, overcontrolling parent may let a child know from the very beginning that life will occur on the parent's terms only and that the child is not competent to make decisions. An overprotective parent may fear to let the youngster make decisions on his/her own. A smothering parent may receive so much gratification from parenting that the natural separation maneuvers of the child are thwarted. S. Rouslin speaks of a mother who anticipated a client's needs so completely that in later life the client expected that others would know and respond to his needs without any necessity of his verbally declaring his wishes (49). Parents who don't wish to be bothered with devoting the extra time it takes to assist a child develop independent skills or learn through trial and error may rear dependent offspring. Or children who feel pushed prematurely into self-sufficiency may cope with stress by regression to extreme dependence. Similarly, people who have led a very self-sufficient life maintained by a counterdependent defense may lose the ability to maintain this defense in illness or other crisis and as a result behave with excessive dependence (20).

Considerable repressed anger often underlies the Dependent Coping Mode, anger that the client fears acknowledging or expressing. If you try to directly restrict the dependent actions, anxiety results over the anger you provoke. This increased anxiety may lead to even greater dependence or panic. Or the anxiety may result in the client becoming extremely compliant to your expectations. In other words, the client anxiously resorts to pleasing you in order not to lose you. What you create then is a bidirectional master-slave relationship, with you as master in telling the client how he must act in order to receive your ministrations *and* you as slave trapped into accepting the client's dependency as long as he/she is good. Functional care might appear easier that way, but the energy being consumed to control your mounting frustration is appreciable! Meanwhile the client is learning nothing new about how to live successfully.

Nurses need to consider how they respond to dependency needs. They may abuse dependency because care seems easier that way; or they may foster it to meet personal needs; or they may reject and avoid the dependent client (14). The need to reject or punish the client's dependency needs may mean the nurse has not worked through and accepted her/his personal dependency needs (27).

*Goal 1: The client explores
how dependency alienates
others and limits self, and gains
increasing independence
within the context of an
accepting relationship.*

Interventions

At first, give the attention and care needed by the person. Then gradually encourage the person to do some care tasks for self and to make some decisions about daily routine. The client must first feel your acceptance of dependent behaviors in order to feel trust of you and of self. Often the person will respond to your caring but encouraging behavior by becoming more independent. If not, when trust is established sufficiently, you can gently confront the person about his/her behavior. As rapport and trust develop, try a caring but bantering confrontation, such as, "Miss D., it's a good thing you're such a worthwhile person. If you weren't, I might start to get grumbly about doing so much for you." If this evokes an anxious response, rephrase, the idea, "I'm just trying to let you know two things. One, I like you. Two, your requests for assistance are more frequent than I find easy to handle. I guess I'm curious about whether you see this as a problem area in your life." Before closing an interaction of this type, assure the client of your continuing acceptance.

Continue to encourage independent behavior and decisions about daily routine, always commenting on the client's ability to make the appropriate choice. At a later time, you may again need to de-scriptively confront, e.g., "Miss D., you have asked three different staff members what you should do about this. I'm wondering if you don't trust your own judgment or are afraid of hurting someone's feelings?"

Validate when you observe the client in situations where anger or uncertainty is an appropriate response. Give opportunities to role-play, rehearse, or practice with you in making descriptively angry or assertive statements. Explore the client's awareness of how his/her behaviors drive others away and result in the opposite of what is wanted. Assist the person in realizing that he/she will not be destroyed by another's anger or displeasure. Verbally support and reinforce actions of initiative and self-sufficiency. Do not prematurely withdraw support as the client moves toward independence since this will indicate to the client that independence means loss of relationship. Ask the person to tell you when he/she feels ready to take action independent of your assistance.

EVALUATION

Because of the dynamics and learning involved, abusive, aggressive, or acting-out behavior is not quickly changed. You may feel very frustrated and angry as you care for the clients described in this chapter. You may not see your goals met during the time the person is admitted for hospitalization. It is useful to discuss your perceptions and feelings with your instructor, supervisor, and other team members so that you can gain a viewpoint about the person's changing behavior that extends over a period of time. Equally important, remain open to even the most subtle behavioral changes. Be ready to respond with warmth and encouragement at the moment when the person feels motivated (often because of the relationship with you) to try a different approach to people and problems. Then you may be a significant force toward change for this person and his/her family.

SOMATIC THERAPIES

In addition to the interventions described in this chapter and throughout the text, you will also care for the client by administering or assisting with *somatic therapies, those treatments that have as their purpose physiological or physical change of the person, with apparent consequent behavioral change.* These therapies are also discussed in other chapters as appropriate.

Convulsive Therapy

Because convulsive therapy is generally most effec-tive in conditions of fairly recent and sudden onset, it is of little or no use in treating most of the pathology described in this chapter. However, convulsive therapy may reduce the hyperexcited, agitated behavior of mania and thus may be useful if psychotropic drugs are not an appropriate alternative (27, 54). With an acutely psychotic, highly assaultive client, more than one treatment can be given in a day to achieve rapid behavioral control. The most appropriate use of convulsive therapy is in treating certain types of depression (see Chapter 15).

Psychosurgery

The use of psychosurgery, in particular amygadolotomy, has been reported to reduce aggressiveness (26, 31, 54). Such surgery is accompanied by risk, potential complications, negative side effects, and much ethical controversy. Thus it is generally not considered except for the rare patient where all other means of control for intractable assaultiveness have been tried. It is also more apt to bring relief when the aggressive outbursts are related to demonstrable organic abnormality. From a humanistic viewpoint, this treatment is unacceptable.

Chemotherapy

Lithium carbonate is a compound form of lithium, an element of the alkali metal group. Current brand names for the 300 mg. tablets or capsules include Eskalith, Lithane, Lithonate, and Lithotabs. A syrup form of lithium citrate, Lithonate-S, is also available (4). The use of lithium to treat acute mania was introduced by the Australian psychiatrist John Cade in the late 1940s. It came into use in American psychiatry in the early 1960s.

The specific action of lithium is unknown. It is generally considered clinically specific to manic phases of an affective disorder (pp. 600, 614–615). Over a period of one to two weeks, lithium frequently normalizes the behavior of a mania-affected person without causing the feeling of "being drugged" that often occurs when taking major tranquilizers. In addition, lithium appears to be of prophylactic value, i.e., when taken regularly in maintenance doses, it seems to prevent or diminish the occurrence of further manic attacks. For clients subject to cyclic mania and depression, lithium seems to have a mild antidepressant effect. At the same time, some clients on prophylactic lithium may develop an acute depression. An evaluation then needs to be made as to whether the lithium is contributing to the depression and should be discontinued by the physician, or whether maintenance lithium is still indicated in addition to the physician prescribing antidepressants (54).

In addition to the treatment of mania there are some reports of lithium being useful to: (1) relieve mood swings in clients with a borderline unstable labile personality (54), (2) decrease violent acts in some maximally reacting, impulsive, violence-prone clients (54), and (3) decrease aggression in severely disturbed children when the aggression is associated with excitability and explosiveness (54).

The daily dosage range for adults is usually between 1 to 3 grams, given in divided doses, over 24 hours. Toxic levels of lithium are often close to effective level. This necessitates superior levels of nursing observation and monitoring as well as an informed client/family.

One key to safe, effective lithium therapy is the frequent surveillance of serum lithium levels. These blood samples should be drawn 12 hours after the last dose. During initiation of therapy, the serum lithium concentrations should be in the range of 0.8–1.8 mEq/liter and should be checked every three to four days. The usual serum levels for the client on maintenance lithium are between 0.6 and 1.2 mEq/liter. Serum lithium levels greater than 2.0 mEq/liter are toxic!

Early signs of lithium intoxication include excessive thirst, fine muscle tremors or weakness, impaired coordination, drowsiness, nausea, vomiting, and diarrhea. These signs should be immediately reported to the physician. Advanced signs of toxicity include muscle twitching and/or rigidity, ataxia, polyuria, slurred speech, blurred vision, confusion, seizures, and coma. There is no specific antidote for lithium poisoning. Treatment for overdose may involve lavage, correction of fluid and electrolyte imbalance, and regulation of kidney function (4, 54).

Lithium is not metabolized by the human body and is excreted unchanged by the kidney (54). Lithium alters sodium dynamics in the body, and a diet or pathology that creates either sodium overload or depletion will affect the toxic response. Diuretics, sodium-restricted diets, dehydration, excessive sweating, diarrhea, and febrile infections may reduce lithium tolerance. Lithium is contraindicated for the extremely debilitated and those with siginificant renal or cardiovascular disease, or organic brain damage (4, 54).

Laboratory information that should be obtained before and during lithium therapy includes white blood count, differential cell count, hematocrit, blood urea nitrogen, urinalysis, thyroxine iodine level, free thyroxine level, and electrocardiograph (54).

Lithium crosses the placenta and exposes the fetus to the same concentrations as the mother; thus any lithium therapy during pregnancy needs very skillful supervision. Clients contemplating pregnancy need expert information and counseling regarding whether to discontinue the lithium. Lithium is also present in breast milk, and breast feeding is strongly discouraged for lithium mothers (9). There are lithium birth registries in the United States.

The amphetamines (Benzedrine, Dexedrine) are central nervous system stimulants when used for adults. Assaultiveness and psychotic behaviors are among the symptoms of abuse and overdosage. Yet, for children over age three, the amphetamines may help reduce hyperactivity and impulsiveness of Attention-Deficit Disorders, enabling these youngsters to maintain better self-control and concentration. Side effects may include assorted gastrointestinal disturbances, such as anorexia and nausea, or central nervous system effects, such as headaches, irritability, tremors, and insomnia (4).

Methylphenidate (Ritalin) may be used in children over age six with Minimal Brain Dysfunction for the same symptoms as are helped by the amphetamines described above. However, there is some evidence that the convulsive threshold may be lowered by Ritalin. Just as with the amphetamines, Ritalin is contraindicated for agitated adults (4). Blood pressure and pulse should be monitored in clients receiving amphetamines or methylphenidate.

Many of the major tranquilizers (antipsychotics) are useful in alleviating aggressiveness, some impulsiveness, and psychotic delusions such as grandiosity. In fact their appearance on the treatment scene in the 1950s paved the way for nursing to focus on verbal and milieu interventions rather than spend all day with procedures such as hydrotherapy and wet sheet packs or care for patients oversedated with barbiturates. The phenothiazines in particular may alleviate agitation and excitement. Chlorprothixine, thiothixene, and haloperidol may be particularly helpful when delusional ideas are the source of the agitation. All major tranquilizers have extensive potential adverse effects (see Chapter 16).

FAMILY, COMMUNITY, AND RECREATION

As previously discussed, your responsibility is never limited to just the individual client. Family members need your expertise to at least some degree. Your knowledge of the community is always an asset to the person and family who need additional services. You may also be active in some of the community organizations as a volunteer, using your nursing knowledge.

The Family

M. Guttmacher comments that families of psychotic patients should realize their responsibilities to the community (21). Once sensitized to the problems that families of abusive clients face, you might be inclined to add: "The community, and health professionals in particular, should be made to realize their responsibilities to the family!"

Families are often expected to take their relatives home on pass or discharge with little or no preparation or skill in knowing *which* behaviors of the client are indications of a need for prompt professional attention; *why* it makes any difference if medication is taken at the correct time in the correct dosage; or *how* they can specifically help their loved one. Nurses are making great progress in understanding the family as a treatment unit.

You must be bold in ensuring that no client who is dependent on family for total function and care leaves with an uninformed and unsupported family.

The Community

Check your community services. What resources exist for clients discussed in this chapter? Child abuse groups to provide support for abusive parents? Services for victims? Resources for parents of the learning disabled and/or hyperkinetic? Rehabilitation programs for criminals? Support groups for clients and families? Crisis services for families? Shelters for abused women and children?

What group can you help get organized? You might suggest a family discussion group for the relatives of clients on your unit. If a needed resource doesn't exist, today is the earliest opportunity you have for planning its beginning!

Recreation

What activities can you encourage for your clients that will be renewing for them? For example, scheduled listening to subdued music might be calming for some agitated clients. A hobby that gradually develops compulsiveness and planning skills might benefit the impulsive client. An interest that demands choices and decisions can help the dependent, as long as it is not too anxiety-provoking. Which of your clients can benefit from relaxation exercises or from activities that develop body awareness? Encourage healthy defenses and new sources of self-esteem. And last—because it is really first—facilitate the client's spiritual growth and recreation as a human being! Facilitate your own!

REFERENCES

1. American Psychiatric Association, *A Psychiatric Glossary*, 5th ed. Washington, D.C.: American Psychiatric Association, 1980.

2. ———, *Diagnostic and Statistical Manual of Mental Disorders*, 3rd ed. (DSM-III). Washington , D.C.: American Psychiatric Association, 1980.

3. Bach, George, *Creative Aggression*. New York: Ballantine Books, Inc., as cited in John Godwin, *Murder USA*, pp. 20–21. New York: Ballantine Books, Inc., 1978.

4. Baker, Charles, Jr., ed., *Physicians Desk Reference*. Oradell, N. J.: Medical Economics Co., A Litton Division, 1979.

5. Bandura, Albert, *Aggression: A Social Learning Analysis*. Englewood Cliffs, N.J.: Prentice-Hall, Inc., 1973.

6. ———, "Learning and Behavioral Theories of Aggression," in *Violence: Perspectives on Murder and Aggression*, Irwin Kutash et al., eds. San Francisco, Calif.: Jossey-Bass, Inc., Publishers, 1978.

7. Brooks, Beatrice, "Aggression," *American Journal of Nursing*, 67, no. 12 (1967), 2519–22.

8. Brown, Martha, and Grace Fowler, *Psychodynamic Nursing*, 3rd ed., Chap. 14. Philadelphia: W. B. Saunders Company, 1966.

9. Burgess, Helen, "When a Patient on Lithium Is Pregnant," *American Journal of Nursing*, 79, no. 11 (1979), 1989–90.

10. Bursten, Ben, *The Manipulator: A Psychoanalytic View*. New Haven: Yale University Press, 1973.

11. Carney, Francis, "Treatment of the Aggressive Patient," in *Rage, Hate, Assault and Other Forms of Violence*, eds. Denis Madden and John Lion, pp. 223–48. Jamaica, N. Y.: Spectrum Publications, Inc., 1976.

12. Clearing House, National Group for Classification of Nursing Diagnoses, St. Louis University Department of Nursing, 3525 Caroline St., St. Louis, Mo. (Contact for list and/or publication regarding most current listing of accepted nursing diagnoses.)

13. Coleman, James C., and William Broen, Jr., *Abnormal Psychology and Modern Life*, 4th ed., Chaps. 6, 9, 10, 11, 13, 15, 17. Glenview, Ill.: Scott, Foresman & Company, 1972.

14. Committee on Therapeutic Care, Group for the Advancement of Psychiatry, *Toward Therapeutic Care*, 2nd ed., vol. 7, no. 77 (1970).

15. Cuthbert, Betty, "Switch Off, Tune In, Turn On," *American Journal of Nursing*, 69, no. 6 (1969), 1206–11.

16. DiFabio, Susan, and E. Judith Ackerhalt, "Teaching the Use of Restraint through Role Play," *Perspectives in Psychiatric Care*, 16, nos. 5–6 (1978), 218–22.

17. Fromm, Erich, *The Anatomy of Human Destructiveness*, pp. 280–324. New York: Holt, Rinehart and Winston, 1973.

18. Galdston, R., "Observations on Children Who Have Been Physically Abused and Their Parents," *American Journal of Psychiatry*, 122 (1965), 440–43.

19. Godwin, John, *Murder USA*. New York: Ballantine Books, Inc., 1978.

20. Gruber, Karen, and Henry Schniewind, "Letting Anger Work for You," *American Journal of Nursing*, 76, no. 9 (1976), 1450–52.

21. Guttmacher, Manfred, "A Review of Cases Seen by a Court Psychiatrist," in *The Clinical Evaluation of the Dangerousness of the Mentally Ill*, ed. Jonas Rappeport, Chap. 3. Springfield, Ill.: Charles C Thomas, Publisher, 1967.

22. Jensen, Hellene, and Gene Tillotson, "Dependency in Nurse-Patient Relationships," in *Psychiatric Nursing*, 2nd ed., vol. 1, ed. Dorothy Mereness, pp. 100–107. Dubuque, Iowa: William C. Brown Co., Publishers, 1971.

23. Karshner, Judith, "The Application of Social Learning Theory of Agression," *Perspectives in Psychiatric Care*, 16, nos. 5–6 (1978), 223–27.

24. Kiening, Sister Mary Martha, "Hostility," in *Behavioral Concepts and Nursing Intervention*, ed. Carolyn E. Carlson, pp. 187–205. Philadelphia: J. B. Lippincott Company, 1970.

25. Kolb, Lawrence, *Modern Clinical Psychiatry*. Philadelphia: W. B. Saunders Company, 1977.

26. Kutash, Irwin et al., eds., *Violence: Perspectives on Murder and Aggression*. San Francisco, Calif.: Jossey-Bass, Inc., Publishers, 1978.

27. Kyes, Joan, and Charles Hofling, *Basic Psychiatric Concepts in Nursing*, 3rd ed. Philadelphia: J. B. Lippincott Company, 1974.

28. Lathrop, Vallory, "Aggression as a Response," *Perspectives in Psychiatric Care*, 16, nos. 5-6 (1978), 202-5.

29. Lenefaky, Barbara, Theo dePalma, and Dominick Locicero, "Management of Violent Behaviors," *Perspectives in Psychiatric Care*, 16, nos. 5-6 (1978), 212-17.

30. Loomis, Maxine, "Nursing Management of Acting-Out Behavior," *Perspectives in Psychiatric Care*, 8, no. 4 (1970), 168-73.

31. Madden, Denis J., and John Lion, *Rage, Hate, Assault and Other Forms of Violence*. Jamaica, N. Y.: Spectrum Publications, Inc., 1976.

32. ____, "Treating the Violent Offender," in *Violence: Perspectives on Murder and Aggression*, eds. Irwin Kutash et al., Chap. 21. San Francisco, Calif.: Jossey-Bass, Inc., Publishers, 1978.

33. Madow, Leo, *Anger*. New York: Charles Scribner's Sons, 1972.

34. Matheney, Ruth, and Mary Topalis, *Psychiatric Nursing*, 4th ed., Chap. 15. St. Louis: The C. V. Mosby Company, 1965.

35. McGreevey, Abigail, and Judy Van Heukelm, "Crying: The Neglected Dimension," *Nursing Digest*, Spring 1977, pp. 61-63.

36. Megargee, E. I., "Undercontrolled and Overcontrolled Personality Types in Extreme and Social Aggression," *Psychological Monographs*, vol. 80, no. 1 (1966).

37. Meldman, Monte, Gertrude McFarland, and Edith Johnson, *The Problem-Oriented Psychiatric Index and Treatment Plan*. St. Louis: The C. V. Mosby Company, 1976.

38. Mereness, Dorothy, and Louis Karnash, *Essentials of Psychiatric Nursing*, 7th ed., Chap. 16. St. Louis: The C. V. Mosby Company, 1966.

39. Moritz, Derry Ann, "Understanding Anger," *American Journal of Nursing*, 78, no. 1 (1978), 81-83.

40. Moyer, K. E., "The Physiology of Aggression and the Implications for Aggression Control," in *The Control of Aggression and Violence*, ed. Jerome Singer, Chap. 3. New York: Academic Press, Inc., 1971.

41. Penningroth, Philip, "Control of Violence in a Mental Health Setting," *American Journal of Nursing*, 75, no. 4 (1975), 606-9.

42. Plutchik, Robert, "A Language for the Emotions," *Psychology Today*, February 1980, pp. 68, 78.

43. Pribula, Sister Irene, "Disarming the Agitated, Combative, or Destructive Patient," *Free Association*, 4, no. 1 (1977), 1-3.

44. Rappeport, Jonas, ed., *The Clinical Evaluation of the Dangerousness of the Mentally Ill*. Springfield, Ill.: Charles C Thomas, Publisher, 1967.

45. Rappeport, Jonas, George Lassen, and Nancy Hay, "A Review of the Literature on the Dangerousness of the Mentally Ill," in *The Clinical Evaluation of the Dangerousness of the Mentally Ill*, ed. Jonas Rappeport, Chap. 9. Springfield, Ill.: Charles C Thomas, Publisher, 1967.

46. Revitch, Eugene, and Louis Schlesinger, "Murder: Evaluation, Classification, and Prediction," in *Violence: Perspectives on Murder and Aggression*, eds. Irwin Kutash et al., Chap. 6. San Francisco, Calif.: Jossey-Bass, Inc., Publishers, 1978.

47. Rogers, Carl, "Characteristics of a Helping Relationship," *Canada's Mental Health*, 27 (March 1962), 1-18 (Supplement).

48. Rosenfeld, Alvin, "Treating the 'Emotional Orphans' of Incest," *Medical News*, January 7, 1980, p. 15.

49. Rouslin, Sheila, "Developmental Aggression and Its Consequences," *Perspectives in Psychiatric Care*, 8, no. 4 (1975), 170-75.

50. Salzman, Carl, Bessel van der Kolk, and Richard Shader, "Psychopharmacology and the Geriatric Patient," in *Manual of Psychiatric Therapeutics*, ed. Richard Shader, Chap. 10. Boston: Little, Brown & Company, 1975.

51. Sarles, Richard M., "Child Abuse," in *Rage, Hate, Assault, and Other Forms of Violence*, eds. Denis Madden and John Lion, pp. 1-16. Jamaica, N. Y.: Spectrum Publications, Inc., 1976.

52. Scherer, Klaus, Ronald Abeles, and Claude Fischer, *Human Aggression and Conflict*. Englewood Cliffs, N.J.: Prentice-Hall, Inc., 1975.

53. Schwartz, Morris, and Emmy Shockley, *The Nurse and the Mental Patient*, pp. 21-71. New York: Russell Sage Foundation, 1956.

54. Shader, Richard, ed., *Manual of Psychiatric Therapeutics*. Boston: Little, Brown & Company, 1975.

55. Singer, Jerome, ed., *The Control of Aggression and Violence*. New York: Academic Press, Inc., 1971.

56. Stanton, Alfred, "Personality Disorders," in *Harvard Guide to Modern Psychiatry*, ed. Armand Nicholi, Jr., Chap. 14. Cambridge, Mass.: Belknap Press of Harvard University Press, 1978.

57. Steele, Brandt, "The Child Abuser," in *Violence: Perspectives on Murder and Aggression*, eds. Irwin Kutash et al., Chap. 15. San Francisco, Calif.: Jossey-Bass, Inc., Publishers, 1978.

58. Stewart, Allen, "Handling the Aggressive Patient,"

Perspectives in Psychiatric Care, 16, nos. 5–6 (1978), 228–32.

59. Sundeen, Sandra, et al., *Nurse-Client Interaction: Implementing the Nursing Process*. St. Louis: The C. V. Mosby Company, 1976.

60. Tupin, Joe, "Management of Violent Patients," in *Manual of Psychiatric Therapeutics*, ed. Richard Shader, Chap. 7. Boston: Little, Brown & Company, 1975.

61. Veninga, Robert, "Defensive Behavior: Causes, Effects, and Cures," *Nursing Digest* (May–June 1975), pp. 58–59.

62. Wolfgang, Marvin, "Violence in the Family," in *Violence: Perspectives on Murder and Aggression*, eds. Irwin Kutash et al. San Francisco, Calif.: Jossey-Bass, Inc., Publishers, 1978.

20

The Person
Who Has
Sexual Role Conflicts

Study of this chapter will assist you to:

1. Define terms that relate to the concept of sexual role conflict.

2. Compare and contrast biological, psychoanalytic, social learning, and cognitive developmental theories of sexual development.

3. Relate socialization of the child to dependency, passivity-aggressivity, self-esteem, and achievement feelings and behavior patterns.

4. Distinguish traditional from current trends in life styles and the implications for health and nursing.

5. Assess behaviors that may indicate sexual role conflict as a single nursing diagnosis or in combination with other nursing diagnoses.

6. Formulate goals pertinent to care of the client who may feel sexual role conflict.

7. Describe ways to help the client resolve conflicts and gain a stronger sense of identity.

8. Confer with other team members to determine the effectiveness of your contribution toward the care of this person.

This chapter contributed by Marcea Kjervik, R.N., M.S.

CHANGING SOCIETAL ROLES

Nurses, like other people in health care, need to learn about trends in the public interest. Sex-role conflict is an area of study that has only recently been given some attention in nursing texts, despite its significance for the client as well as the nurse.

In Western society, as elsewhere, sex is a major societal determinant. Men and women are channeled into particular roles that in turn influence their interactions with others. Until a few decades ago, women were generally restricted to a single major societal role of homemaker, whereas men occupied two roles—household head and worker. Thus, men had two major sources of gratification—family and work, whereas women had only one source of gratification—the family. Unsatisfied men could psychologically abandon one role in favor of another. Women, however, could not easily abandon the homemaker role in favor of other roles.

Strict division of roles still exists today for some people in the United States, but society is increasingly more open. More than half of the women in the United States now combine home and career roles. Men are also increasingly involved with child care and homemaking tasks. Some men,

as well as women, constitute single-parent families, having responsibility for child care and home-making as well as a job.

Where societal restrictions exist, women may become frustrated with their status and major role of homemaker. However, in seeking roles outside of the home, low-paying jobs with little prestige may be all that is available. These roles are often unstructured and all but invisible, even though they are essential to the maintenance of society. Women who are aware of such role restrictions may become distressed, which further adds to the discomfort involved in certain roles. Refer to Chapter 12 for studies on stress levels of working men and women (married and unmarried) compared to homemakers. Married working women experience more stress than working men, in that the woman must be much more flexible in combining career, homemaker, and mother roles. In her multiple roles, the woman works more hours totally per day than the man (28).

The difficulty encountered by males and females in the United States is that there is no one ideal model of behavior pattern to follow. The task, then, is to discover what will meet individual needs at a particular time. Each person has many roles made up of demands, expectations, and responsibilities. Other people also impose pressures on the person in any given role. Each person has his/her own perceptions of what ought to be done in a specific role, and these perceptions influence behavior. Behavior is further shaped by demands and expectations of self and of others relative to each role.

In order to cope with sex-role conflict, men and women need to manage these competing sets of expectations as well as their own behavior. There are three ways to cope:

1. Attempt to change others' expectations (redefine roles of men and women).

2. Change personal expectations about behaviors of men and women.

3. Accept the various demands placed on men and women and find a way to meet all of them.

The first two methods of coping involve redefining roles of men and women. The third involves an attempt to comply with all roles as currently defined. This may lead to one of the basic types of overt conflicts—the clash of roles. Without clear role definitions and a shared sense of priorities, men and women may experience crossed signals, different motivations, a lack of support and, more often than not, sheer overload. Managing multiple life roles, for instance, in a two-career family, is a frequent source of stress (31).

DEFINITIONS

In order to adequately understand the meaning of sex-role conflict as used within the confines of this chapter, it is necessary to define the following terms:

Sex will be defined according to gender.

Gender refers to the psychological connotations of maleness or femaleness, to the sense of masculinity or femininity.

Gender identity refers to the awareness of belonging to one of the two sexes.

Role refers to both a personal and societal set of expectations, values, attitudes, and behaviors associated with a position in the functional units of the social structure, including the family, formal and informal groups, and society generally.

Sex or gender roles are the activities or overt behaviors that society reserves for males and females. Social standards serve as guides to individuals and groups as to what is ideally desirable, not what is actually possible (41).

Role stress is a social structure condition in which role obligations are vague, irritating, difficult, conflicting, or impossible to meet, which results in a subjective sense of role strain or feelings of distress.

Role conflict is a condition in which existing role expectations are contradictory or mutually exclusive.

Sex-role conflict is a condition in which existing gender role expectations are contradictory or mutually exclusive.

THEORIES OF SEXUAL DEVELOPMENT

The emergence of humans into sex roles can be explained in a number of ways. Four theories of sexual development will be explored: biological, psychoanalytic, social learning, and cognitive.

Biological Theory

Biology tends to direct a chain of events that begins with conception and continues throughout the prenatal period. Socialization related to the sex of the child then contributes to the acquisition of masculine and feminine behaviors.

Genetic Inheritance

Genetic inheritance is the first major factor in establishing the sex of the person. The woman provides the ovum with an X chromosome; the man provides the sperm cells with the X or Y chromosomes. When the ovum and sperm join, the XX chromosomes produce a girl, and the XY chromosomes produce a boy. Chromosomal sex is thus determined by the father, contrary to the belief held in many cultures that the woman is responsible for the sex of the newborn child (15).

Influence of Hormones

Hormones, after the chromosomes, are the most potent biological factors in developing sex differences (71). The hormones influence differentiation of the internal system and external genitalia (86). Until the sixth or seventh week of maturation, the human fetus contains neither testes nor ovaries, only prefunctory gonads. There are two systems of primitive ducts that exist in the fetus: (1) the Mullerian system—which gives rise to the oviducts, uterus, and upper vagina, and (2) the Wolffian system—which gives rise to the epididymis, vas deferens, and seminal vesicles. The genotype decides the direction of the development of the primitive gonads. An unidentified fetal morphogenic testicular substance prompts the masculine development of the Wolffian duct system and inhibits the development of the Mullerian duct system. However, there is no specific substance that prompts the feminine development of the Mullerian duct system and the regression of the Wolffian ducts. Rather, these reactions occur as the result of either the presence or absence of a fetal testicular substance. A similar process occurs on the external genitalia (71), although the physical appearance of genitalia may be ambiguous in some infants.

Physiological Processes

Physiological processes are the third factor that establishes the differences between males and females. These differences increase with maturation. For instance, at birth, male and female Apgar scores are similar, but proportionately, girls have less muscle and more fat than boys from birth on. They also generally weigh less and are shorter than boys. However, females are more skeletally mature for the first six weeks of life. From early on, girls generally are slower and less well coordinated than boys, with the exception of fine hand movement. Boy babies are less sedentary, sleep less, are more irritable, and cry more (15). In adults, when looking at body size and activity level, women have a lower metabolism than men in the normal state. There is a more conspicuous physiological reaction to stress, however, and a more rapid recovery in women (71). These female differences appear to be adaptive for the reproduction and survival of the species.

There are apparently sex differences in the hypothalamus; thus sex differences could also occur in the central nervous system (6). The critical period in humans in regard to the central nervous system is one week before or after birth. The presence or absence of sex hormones in the fetus/neonate provokes permanent changes in the psychophysiological processes. The hormones that are found in the fetus/neonate decide which hormones the brain centers react to. For instance, in a study of rats, all were female but were masculinized by the presence of testosterone. If the baby rat was castrated but given testosterone within the critical period (one week), it would develop into a male rat. Therefore, the critical factor was the presence or absence of testosterone during the critical stage (6).

In general, newborns differ in terms of their vulnerability and mortality. Males are more vulnerable than females for the first year of life; they also are more frequently aborted, and they die more often of birth trauma, injuries, congenital malformations, and infectious diseases. Susceptibility to disease is controlled by a gene that is carried on the X chromosome.

The ratio of the sexes conceived and born is 120–150 males to 100 females (15).

Assigned Sex through Socialization: Biological Fact and Fiction

Assigned sex through socialization is the last major factor to influence gender (15). When looking at the biological background for socialization over life's course of events, the various meanings of sexuality for men and women need to be understood. Fear of pregnancy has been used for years as a practical restraint to female sexuality. Now, more reliable birth control methods are available, but the internalized attitudes and values of people in society still prevent women from making a free choice regarding their sexuality. Women still remain the responsible persons for birth control (84).

A popular myth is that there is a stronger male sex drive. According to M. Sherfey's investigations, the female sexual drive is actually stronger because of the possibility of multiple orgasms. Repressive measures such as clitoridectomy, seclusion, and severe punishment for adultery were historically used to change females' sexuality (72).

The male orgasm (and consequent pleasure in the sexual act) is required for reproductive success, but it is not necessary for females. Visual materials, female adornment, and pornography are aimed at motivating the male for copulation.

The physical difference in the accessibility of the sexual organs is at least partially responsible for the supposed greater male sex drive. The external presence of the penis seems to make it an inborn object of pleasure to the boy. The clitoris, on the other hand, is less accessible and less likely to be eroticized by the girl (6).

During childhood, both sexes secrete small amounts of both estrogen and androgen. The girl's androgen and the boys' estrogen come chiefly from the adrenal cortex. When puberty begins, the amounts of the secretion of these hormones sharply increase (86).

Puberty is the developmental time period that occurs between childhood and maturation and involves emotional and social as well as physical changes. The timing of puberty is a function of the hypothalamus, which stimulates the pituitary gland to secrete hormones that regulate the functions of the ovaries and the testes. In general, girls develop secondary sex characteristics and enter puberty one or two years earlier than boys. The average age for this maturation is eleven years in girls; the average for boys is thirteen to fifteen years.

The biological as well as the social impact of the menstrual cycle is very involved. The general cultural tone is usually negative. The avoidance of talking about the menstrual cycle is a covert message to girls of the private nature of the experience. Unfortunately, without prior learning about the upcoming menstrual experience, fears of hideous injury, impending death, or sexual misconduct are common. These apprehensions may influence the individual girl's later outlook about her entire sexual functioning, not only her feelings about menstruation. Even if girls are given some information about their changing body, boys are usually not given much information about menstruation. Myths proliferate and contaminate attitudes about women and their sexuality (84). Therefore women's learned expectations and ascriptions about the effects of menstruation may have a greater effect on their behavior than do the actual cyclic changes (48).

Some sexually mature women undergo changes in feelings and emotional states, changes that occur simultaneously with menstrual cycle change. For example, premenstrual tension is experienced by some women and frequently includes symptoms of depression and irritability (6). When estrogen increases at the beginning of the cycle, emotions are usually outward, active, object-directed, and heterosexual—but may also be homosexual in direction. At the time of ovulation, the active sexual tendency blends with the passive-receptive tendency, which biologically and emotionally prepares the woman for conception. When ovulation is completed, tension is relieved and there is a sense of relaxation and well-being. During the menstrual flow itself, some women report symptoms such as anger, excitability, fatigue, crankiness, and crying spells (6).

It is possible that men may also experience physiological cycles that cause emotional changes. Unfortunately, little research has been done in this regard. Some evidence shows a great variability among men in their mood and physical symptoms. Men may also be at a disadvantage because of their lack of knowledge of actually having cycles, whereas women at least are aware of their cycle (48).

During pregnancy, the estrogen and progesterone levels are high in the woman. T. Benedek found that when progesterone is high there is an intensification of receptive-retentive tendencies that prepare women for pregnancy as well as maintain the patience and nurturance of the healthy, mature woman. Therefore, the increase in nurturance depends both on the hormone level and on the personality characteristics of the women (10). However, other factors may also contribute to personality changes in pregnancy, including fatigue and other physical discomforts that occur with pregnancy, reaction to the changing body image, anxiety about new responsibilities, and possible resentment of an unwanted child (48).

S. E. Taylor and T. J. Langer found that people in our culture, especially men, respond to pregnant women with avoidance and staring. Pregnant women in our society are expected to withdraw from social and job-related activities (although this is less true now than formerly). Therefore, women receive a double message: the mother-to-be is glorified and yet stigmatized because of her unusual and delicate condition (75). Our culture, like all cultures, teaches how pregnant women are supposed to feel and act.

Climacterium applies to both women and men. In the female, less estrogen and progesterone are produced; breasts and genital tissues undergo atrophy; and the menstrual period stops (menopause). The decrease of testosterone in the male varies with the individual, and effects become more apparent in the fifties although a very gradual decrease may occur from age 30 onward. In response to the approaching menopause, women may experience physical symptoms such as hot flashes and headaches, as well as emotional symptoms such as depression and irritability. Yet most women do not have disabling symptoms with menopause. The physical symptoms in men are not clearly obvious, but the emotional symptoms of depression and lowered feelings of self-worth are seen in mid-life. Culturally, women are taught to expect some change; men are not (48). In spite of myths, the middle-aged and older person has sexual desires and remains sexually active. Sexual satisfaction is important to the self-concept and to the sex-role image of the person.

Psychosexual Abnormalities

Psychosexual abnormalities shed light on the sex-role development of children. Three will be briefly discussed here: adrenogenital syndrome, hermaphroditism, and transsexualism.

Children who have features of the *androgenital syndrome* (AGS) have malfunctioning adrenal glands that release large amounts of androgen rather than cortisol during the critical period of sexual differentiation before birth. Males with AGS need cortisone treatment to prevent early puberty, but they have no abnormalities in the genitalia. Females with AGS need to be placed on cortisone before the critical period, or else masculination occurs. Tomboyish behavior plus higher intelligence levels have been found in these females. For the *hermaphrodite*, socialization can usually overcome the hormonally imposed direction if during the period of eighteen months to three years consistent support is received from the parents and other people in the child's environment. *Transsexualism* is marked by a primary feeling on the part of a person that she/he was born into the

wrong sex. The biological inputs are unknown because not enough research has been done in this area (84). For more information on these conditions, refer to S. Weitz (84).

Psychodynamic Theories

In all psychodynamic theories, the concept of identification is addressed. How identification occurs varies from theory to theory, and these differences will be explored in this section.

Identification is the process whereby a person receives approval by patterning after an important individual in his/her environment. The individual:

Relates with an important person in the environment.

Admires traits, thoughts, feelings, or actions of the important person.

Unconsciously patterns self after the important person.

Receives approval from the important person.

Assimilates the admired trait, so that it becomes an element of the individual's self.

The three primary psychodynamic theories discussed in this chapter are Psychoanalytic, Social Learning, and Cognitive-Development Theories. Differing views on identification will be examined for each theory.

Psychoanalytic Theory

Freud

Psychoanalytic Theory has become society's most authoritative theory of human behavior. Freud, whose formulations about women reflect values that emanated in the Victorian era in which he lived, believed that people are motivated by forces buried in their minds. The world during Freud's time was dominated by men; thus he held the phallocentric viewpoint that emphasized the penis as a source of power (6).

Freud's psychosexual theory of development assumes that the sexuality or pleasurable experience of children is centered in various zones of the body at different ages. The first year, an oral stage, has erotogenic responses centered around the mouth. The second year, an anal stage, focuses on bowel functioning. Differences between the sexes arise in the third or phallic stage of development (71).

According to Freud, identification for males is first with the mother and then must be reversed in order to achieve sex-role identity with the father. The son is then motivated to acquire masculine values and traits as well as norms and prohibitions, particularly in regard to sexual repression. The son identifies with his father, the aggressor, because of the fear of castration after the original love link with his mother (84).

The process in female development is more complex. The daughter's original love object is the mother, but the daughter is no threat to the father. Two problems exist in the Freudian view of female sex-role identity. These are: (1) the transfer of affection from the mother to the father, and (2) the acquiring of the mother as the primary identification figure. The daughter is seen as coveting the missing organ (penis), which results in penis envy; she then experiences the castration complex and the feeling of being castrated, which influences her interactions with others. Upon discovering that her mother also does not possess a penis, she blames her mother and then rejects her as a love object while turning to her father as her mother's replacement. The daughter's identity is realized because of the inability to have her father for herself and the fear of the loss of the mother's affection as a consequence. Thus the mother is then taken as the daughter's identification figure (84).

The Freudian concept of identification involves three factors: (1) a *motive* or wish of a child to become more like the parents, (2) the *process* or mechanism by which the child comes to imitate the model, and (3) the actual *behavior* similar to that of the parent. The child internalizes parental and societal standards for appropriate sex-role behavior and moral conduct and incorporates many of the attributes and characteristics of the parents, especially of the same-sex parent (14).

Freud sought a common pattern of development that could come only from a common cultural pattern. However, there are no universal patterns of family life. Thus, Freud underestimated the importance of the child's immediate environment and overrated the uniformity of family patterns (70).

Helen Deutsch

Helen Deutsch was schooled in the Freudian tradition. She did, however, revise the two concepts of penis envy and resolution of the Oedipal conflict. She interpreted envy as being common for both boys and girls in their need for love and attention. The girl's abandonment of the mother as a love-object in favor of the father is never fully accomplished according to Deutsch, whereas Freud believed that the Oedipal conflict was resolved in early childhood (19).

Deutsch seemed unimpressed with cultural factors as sources of change in the feminine psyche, despite her observing the transition of women's behavior during World War II. She felt different male characteristics, such as competitiveness, might change the facade, but the feminine core would remain (19).

Deutsch's interest was in the development of the child's ego and the growth of the self, which she felt were guided by emotional and intellectual aspects of the personality rather than by Freud's psychosexual stages per se. She believed that the ego wanted to master the environment through adjustments and resolving conflict. Thus, the child's relationship would be independent of the sexual instincts (19).

Deutsch also believed that sex differences existed from birth that were psychologically significant in the phallic phase. The inhibited sexual activity in the female undergoes a transformation into passivity, which would be the normal path to femininity. The female's sexual energy is manifested in receptive readiness rather than active aggressiveness as seen in the male. Thus she believed that the female's sexual activity is dependent on the physiologically based man's activity and leads to feminine passivity (19, 84, 86).

Narcissism, passivity, and masochism were central personality traits used to describe women, and Deutsch defined them as follows: *Narcissism is loving and valuing oneself.* In *passivity, the women is supposed to be receptive, expectant, and willing to wait for the male. Masochism is the seeking out of suffering and pain.* All are normal conditions for women, according to Deutsch. To her, the healthy woman will accept pain associated with her traditional functions because of the underlying pleasure (6, 19, 86).

The normative base that Deutsch worked from was that women were biologically equipped to become mothers and most did. The active-aggressive components of girlhood were transformed into the service of femininity. Therefore women driven to achieve intellectual and competitive goals had personalities that were always in conflict because this masculine element prevented them from accepting their role as women (19, 86).

Karen Horney

Karen Horney was also a member of Freud's early group as well as the head of the American Institute of Psychoanalysis. She was one of the first persons who took issue with Freud's theory of psychosexual development (48).

Horney believed that from the male's viewpoint, the penis played too major a role. She learned through her clinical work that males were envious of the female's reproductive role. She suggested that the degree of men's desire to create and achieve was related to an overcompensation for their unconscious sense of inferiority in not being able to produce their own child. Men might depreciate women because of this envy rather than because women do not have a penis (48, 73, 84).

Horney suggested that a girl's psychosexual development centered around her own anatomy rather than around the male's. Further, Horney gave credance to a connection between the cultural and inner dynamics in forming the personality since society generally encourages rejection of the feminine role because of the traditional belief that women are inadequate and inferior (48, 73, 84).

The girl is exposed from birth to the concept that she is inferior. To envy the male and his role would seem logical since she receives none of the power he automatically has been given. According to Horney, it is difficult for the woman to compensate for this. Therefore, women, because of their supposed position of weakness, adopt male values and then suppress their true selves. Thus diverging from the norm set by men, women apply others' values and pretensions to self that are biologically foreign. The result is that the individual woman then feels inadequate, and the cycle renews itself when a daughter is born to the woman. Motherhood is often felt as a burden or a handicap. Since women occupy few positions in the masculine world, they seem barred from accomplishment. These factors only increase women's sense of inferiority (6, 86).

Clara Thompson

Clara Thompson was influenced by her analyst, Sandor Ferenczi, as well as by Karen Horney and Harry Stack Sullivan. Thompson had a different perspective on personality development, based on an interpersonal view. She felt that the basic human drive was the need to grow and master one's environment. People are influenced not so much by libidinal urges or instincts as by interactions with significant persons and social forces around them. Childhood development was directed toward the formation of self and the emergence of an identity separate from the mother. Varying and increasingly mature ways of interacting with others occur as the child goes through the stages of development.

Thompson disagreed with Freud's view of female personality being the inevitable result of her original biological inferiority. Jealousy, feelings of inferiority, weak superego, prematurely arrested development, rigidity, and other characteristics of penis envy were accounted for by Thompson's theory of cultural causation, which explained how women in Western society have had to adapt to society's values. Thompson believed that women view the penis as a symbol of privilege. Jealousy and envy occur in competitive societies in which one person has to lose. Women's feelings of inferiority are a reflection of their actual position in society and not a biological lack, as Freud postulated. In many cases, women's security depends on the approval of powerful people around them, which accounts for the lack of their own internalized standards (48, 78, 86).

Thompson objected, as did Horney, to Freud's masculine viewpoint of female development; she noted that Freud observed women only in his patriarchal society, where it was assumed that women were inferior to men. Thompson also rejected that woman (her body and her functions) was inferior. She believed that opportunity to pursue various experiences, a lack of restriction on achievement of developmental tasks, a secure attitude toward the sexual nature, and social and economic independency will assist women's development of a sense of worth and equality.

When women choose to move out of their traditional roles, they have no models other than men. The conflict returns as to whether to accept male values and behavior in order to be able to achieve any significance in the world outside of the home. The race for success does not enrich the lives of those trapped in it, whether they are male or female (6, 48, 78, 86).

Erik Erikson

Erik Erikson agreed with Freud that biology as well as the unconscious has an impact on experience and behavior. He focused on the female and male anatomies. Regarding women, he spoke about the "inner space," which included the uterus and reproductive system. To him, these organs had an unconscious meaning of being productive, safe, and life-giving. Erikson felt that the different body experiences of women and men predisposed them toward different approaches to life. Men are more interested in "outer space"—caring, nurturing, and creating a stable environment. He did not add that each sex is capable of learning the other's style, therefore, the predispositions are not restrictive (6, 22, 23).

Erikson also denies the importance of penis envy but suggests that women envy men's greater social importance. He feels that the Oedipus complex is less common in women than in men. Erikson also denies the importance of masochism but concedes that the acceptance of pain is important. Erikson was less concerned with intrapsychic events and more concerned with the customs of society as a means of identification (6, 22, 23).

Social Learning Theory

In Social Learning Theory, *identification is defined as the occurrence of similarity between the behavior of the model and the child, where the model's behavior serves as the stimulus for matching responses* (4).

The social process precedes the individual because everyone is born into a social environment. As a result of interaction with the social environment, the biological organism is greatly modified. The infant's biologic impulses, instincts, and emotions are modified and channeled through interactions with others (48). The Social Learning theorists relied on learning principles to explain the acquisition of a sex role. Reinforcement, observation, and limitation were the most important Social Learning principles (15).

Albert Bandura proposed that the sex-role identity did not need to be formulated through a relationship with a same-sex parent. Internalizing parental standards and personality characteristics was not necessary because the child only had to *act* like his/her same-sex parent. Bandura claims that the original sex-role identity was caused by the varied reinforcement histories of the two sexes but is eliminated by reward. Therefore, learning by modeling is determined by observational and cognitive processes and can occur without any direct reinforcement (3, 4, 5).

There are two kinds of processes by which children acquire attitudes, values, and patterns of social behavior. The first occurs when parents or other socialization agents are explicit about what they want the child to learn and then attempt to shape his/her behavior through punishment and reward consequences. The second process involves the acquisition of personality patterns by the child's active imitation of parental attitudes and behaviors, most of which are never directly taught by the parent (4). All models in a family affect the sex-role learning of the child; therefore, the child's social behavior is not just a child-sized version of that exhibited by the same-sex parent. Bandura believes that children do not exclusively rely on their parents as models (4). However, studies do indicate a greater tendency to imitate the same-sex parent.

Cognitive-Development Theory

Cognitive-Development Theory provides a background for a cohesive concept of sex role that helps to organize the child's perceptions of and attachments to the world and, in particular, to parental figures and activities. Such a theory does *not* eliminate the information of Social Learning Theory. The Cognitive-Development Theory of the sex-role concept development for females has not been fully supported. This theory favors a "uni-sex" course with no sexual peculiarities, and it attempts to base female sex roles and positive sensations on a male-based size and strength evaluation.

Jean Piaget

Jean Piaget's observations led him to define several stages of imitation during infancy. In the first two stages of infancy, imitation did not involve novel responses and was labeled "pseudo-imitation" (66). The third stage, between 7 and 10 months of age, brings about imitation of new models, for example, matching a visually perceived mouth movement of an adult. Between 10 and 18 months, the child imitates conceptually perceived new movements of parts of the body not actually visible to him/her. Finally, after 18 months, the child imitates a new action when the model is no longer present. The child will play at being an absent person in the sense of deliberately enacting a set of behaviors characterizing another person. This is the first developmental approximation of identificationlike behavior (66).

Early in the period between two and five years of age, the child first fantasizes, enacting roles other than his/her own. Then gradually a firm sense of the limits of his/her own identity is learned during selective modeling of a person similar in identity (66).

Identification, as a cognitive process, is closely related to the mental capacity of visualizing another model in relation to one's self (51). Play, involving language and imitation, leads to communication with an outside world and to a gradual process of socialization. Successful identification depends on the intellectual capacity to differentiate and on the affective incentive to imitate (66).

Lawrence Kohlberg

Lawrence Kohlberg believed that as intellectual growth goes, so goes the development of a sex-role identity. He theorized three stages in sex-role acquisition. First, children initially learn that the world is divided into two groups, male and female, and that they belong to one of the two groups. The second stage involves the process of *sex-role acquisition, which is the attachment of value to people and attitudes and behaviors of the same sex.* Imitation of same-sex individuals is *not* due to a previous reinforcement history but to the recognition of same-sex persons as comparable to self and, thus,

valued. Finally, after the children learn to value same-sex people and their activities, they learn to identify with their same-sex parent (15).

The process of identification originates from the development of gender identity and then learning to value one's maleness or femaleness, rather than from the fear of love or retaliation as Freud states. According to the Cognitive-Development Theory, identification depicts a positive, internal process motivated by the child's striving to understand and master his/her world (15).

Jerome Kagan

Jerome Kagan created a model of sex-role development that seems to combine social learning and cognitive-developmental formulations. He believes the *sex-role standard is a learned association between the person's attributes, behavior, and attitudes, and perceptions of maleness and femaleness* (39, 84). The child learns to differentiate between males and females by the assistance of parents and other socialization agents. Once discrimination between the sexes is learned, sex-typed responses are also learned. The child uses social learning as well as a desire to obtain the goals of the models (84). Appropriate behaviors come from the consistent example of parents and socialization agents. The child acts to conform to a previously acquired standard (40). Behavior in consistent ways is self-reinforcing. Kagan adds a cognitive and affective scope to the social learning model, and reinforcement is seen as a prime factor in behavior (84).

In order to summarize the similarities and differences of the Psychosexual, Social Learning, and Cognitive-Development theories, the identification concepts of Freud, Bandura, and Piaget are compared in Table 20-1.

TABLE 20-1.   Comparison of Three Theorists' Concepts of Identification

CHARACTERISTIC	FREUD	BANDURA	PIAGET
Importance of identification for development of person.	Identification with same-sex parent essential for development.	Environmental and social reactions to maleness or femaleness define differences chosen by boys or girls.	Cognitive development is asexual.

TABLE 20-1.   Continued

CHARACTERISTIC	FREUD	BANDURA	PIAGET
Source of motivation for identification.	Internal fears are externalized in order to keep lost or feared object choice. Identification inborn or hereditary.	Behavior is modified in response to external stimuli. Identification depends on all social influences.	Intellectual development results in gradual stages of identification development. Assimilation of environment for identification.
Influence on identification.	Mother and then father direct identification; family provides only object choices for sex-role identification.	Anyone can be a model. Child imitates whatever is available and continues behavior that is reinforced.	Child learns from self and then from parents.

SOCIALIZATION

Socialization refers to individuals learning the needed skills, developing the knowledge, and internalizing values and attitudes of a particular social system in order to play a specific role in the system (32). Socialization continues over the life span.

The infant is born into a rich social world and interacts with mother, father, extended family members, siblings, peers, and other people. Even though these relationships vary in intensity, all have an impact on the infant's perception of the world. Each society has its own set of beliefs about sex differences and appropriate sex roles. Apparently all societies prefer male children (15).

The family is the initial and most influential intermediary of the child's sex-role acquisition. Later, school-age children experience pressure from external sources, like teachers and other children. Finally, the adolescent has to face independence from the family, assimilation of the peer culture, and pursuit of a career, lover, and mate (15).

Boys are described as independent, aggressive, competitive, leadership-oriented, task-oriented, outward-oriented, assertive, innovative, self-disciplined, stoic, active, objective, analytical, courageous, unsentimental, confident, and emotionally under control (15).

Girls are described as dependent, passive, frag-ile, nonaggressive, noncompetitive, inner-oriented, interpersonally oriented, empathetic, sensitive, nurturant, subjective, intuitive, yielding, receptive, unable to risk, supportive, emotional, and as having a low pain tolerance (77).

Yet, according to E. Macoby and C. Jacklin, many of the popular beliefs about psychological characteristics of the sexes have little basis in fact (50). Perhaps as the boundaries between the feminine and masculine roles become less fixed, the concept that both men and women have the same feelings and needs and similar characteristics will be better understood by our society, as well as by other societies. Factors that contribute to life satisfaction can then be viewed as similar rather than different for the two sexes. Women may come to learn that personal competence and work satisfaction are compatible expectations with both femininity and masculinity (53, 56).

It is important to explore several special areas of socialization of boys and girls in more depth. These areas are dependency, passivity-aggression, self-esteem, and achievement/competition.

Dependency

Dependency is defined as lacking self-reliance

(21), the inability to make decisions, and the impulse to lean on others for advice, guidance, and support (34). Excessive independence may lead to poor adaptation in relating to people. Excessive dependency may lead to hypersensitivity to other people's reactions (6), and difficulty in relationships as well.

Society expects many more dependent behaviors in girls than boys. Girls are seen as adaptive and normal when they are dependent. If boys are dependent, they are considered maladjusted, insecure in their masculinity, and immature (6).

Research suggests that females are more dependent, passive, and conforming than males. However, white middle-class Americans were the subjects of this research, so comparisons to other groups cannot be made. Greater dependency was found in girls over six years of age; apparently this increase in dependency is a function of pressure to behave in the socially expected way (71).

It needs to be emphasized that infant studies of dependency behaviors have only used proximity with the mother, touching, and clinging as variables. Studies with older children have dealt with a greater variety of behaviors and are usually observational in nature (86). In reviewing eight observational studies of children's dependency behavior with people outside the family, five showed *no* sex differences and the rest were *inconsistent!* (50).

Parents respond to dependent behavior in boys and girls differently. In most cultures, close behaviors (dependence) are expected of their daughters and distant behaviors (independence) are expected of their sons. Yet the best predictor of dependency is not the sex of the child but rather the culture in which the child is raised (15).

Parents of independent sons and daughters demonstrated different behavior. Consistent discipline, high demands for maturity, reassurance about their having independent lives especially in relating to others, reasoning with them in order to comply, and not being overly coercive or restrictive—all create an atmosphere for children to learn to be independent (6).

Dependency was a stable measure for females but not for males in a longitudinal study of 44 males and 45 females over a 25-year period. In other words, when girls were dependent as children, they grew up being viewed that way, whereas dependent boys did not grow up to be dependent men. Therefore, the assumption can be made that

societal pressures teach children how they are to behave and continue behaving into adulthood (40).

Although our society focuses on independence, especially for males, healthy dependence may mean a sensitivity to the needs of significant persons. It is important to learn that depending is not negative; asking for assistance at a time of need may lead to a development of an interdependent relationship. Being able to be both dependent and independent is healthy—for both women and men.

Passivity-Aggressivity

Biological differences in aggressivity exist, according to J. Williams, in all societies, and sex differences in aggressivity supposedly appear at about two years of age (86). Similar sex differences are found in some animal studies. Apparently, levels of sex hormones change the degree of aggressiveness (86).

Most societies have the norm of passivity for females and aggressivity for males. Deutsch defines **passivity** *as activity that is inwardly directed and is perceived as vital to life* (19). Traditionally, passivity is referred to as *the lack of activity or aggressiveness of a person.* A very passive person may seem infantile, dependent on others for self-esteem, fearful of rejection, and indirectly aggressive. Unfortunately, the picture of the passive girl is oftentimes overstated. Girls tend to withdraw from direct physical aggression because of being prohibited by society or because they believe that they are physically weaker, not because they are passive. Thus women, using withdrawal of friendship, verbal slams, and other behavior, may really be using these as a means of handling their aggressiveness. It is true that girls are not as likely to hit, bite, kick, and wrestle as boys. Girls, who traditionally have had better verbal skills, use verbal aggression instead. Therefore, differences in the form of expression do not negate the fact that the motives may be similar (6).

Aggression may be viewed as a way to hurt or control another person (50). In Maccoby and Jacklin's review of the literature, males were found to be more aggressive than females. Such behavioral sex differences can be found in various cultures.

No consistent evidence has been found to indicate that parents are more overtly tolerant of aggression in boys than in girls, although the payoff for aggressive behavior is different for boys than for girls. Operant Conditioning Theory illustrates how aggression is learned. Severe reprimands are used by fathers for their son's aggressive behaviors, whereas fathers are more permissive with their daughters. In contrast, mothers are more lenient with their sons' aggressiveness than with their daughters' aggression (86). Perhaps mothers discourage their daughters' aggressiveness because of their own ambivalence about aggression. If the child is seeking approval of the opposite-sexed parent, and imitating and then identifying with the same sexed parent, as Psychoanalytic Theory suggests, the child soon learns how to act and with whom.

Classical Conditioning Theory assumes that aggression is an involuntary response to environmental stimuli (25). I. Frodi, J. Macauley, and P. Thome have suggested that differences in aggression anxiety between males and females are partially responsible for sex differences in aggression. This argument is supported by another source that said women reported more guilt and anxiety about aggression and were more self-punitive after being aggressive than men (48).

The Social Learning Theory emphasizes modeling, imitative learning, or vicarious learning via observation. D. Hicks found that girls learn from observation as well as boys, but girls recall fewer destructive actions against toys than boys can recall (33). Power seems to be an important factor of modeling of either sex, and power needs seem related to aggressive behavior (48). Original sex differences are caused by different reinforcement histories for boys and girls (3). A. Bandura and R. Walters found increased aggressiveness in boys related to parental and social pressure for this behavior. Therefore, social reinforcement and modeling processes are held to contribute to sex differences in aggressiveness (5).

Identification seems to be the significant variable in determining aggression. It is difficult to say whether parental identification or sex-role identification affects boys' and girls' aggressiveness differently (48). Girls are less likely to use physical aggression than boys, possibly because of temperament. Verbal and interpersonal skills are better in girls, which helps them to cope with frustration without being aggressive. Even though they have physically aggressive fathers, girls usually receive support and warmth from them. Their mothers, on the other hand, are the primary frustration or discipline agents. Mothers frequently use verbal forms of discipline or aggressiveness, so daughters imitate or model verbal behavior as an expression of aggression. All in all, girls have learned not to use direct, overt, physical forms of aggressiveness (6).

In summary, from early childhood, boys exhibit a higher level of aggressive behavior than girls. Hormonal and physical characteristics contribute toward boys responding aggressively, but the socialization process has great impact in terms of aggressive behavior in both the male and female.

Self-Esteem

When the child of about two years of age begins to refer to self as "I," the self as a separate entity is developing. Even though the sense of self becomes fixed early in life, subidentities can be acquired later as a result of societal expectations for various roles. Role subidentities are a function of sex and age. Some say the traditional role for women may not encourage self-actualization, and low self-esteem may result (17). In specific, as well as in general, situations, women experience more role conflict than men, and this contributes to lower self-esteem. The conflict is between their existence as autonomous persons and as objects to please others. Since women are taught the latter, being passive objects is rewarded and therefore autonomy is renounced.

When men and women were asked to rate themselves on personal characteristics, they had the same number of positive and negative self-esteem items (50). But there were also differences. Men expect to do well when approaching problem-solving tasks, and they judge their performance favorably after completing the work. Women, on the contrary, function differently and seem to be more hesitant about boasting. Women are generally more accepting of others, as well as of themselves, than are men. Women apply high standards to intellectual or academic pursuits but do not expect to excel in their personal lives. Women also seem to feel less in control of their own fate. In Rotter's locus of control studies, there is a trend in women, during college years, to have an external locus of control and to rely on external forces for reward (67). Therefore, women hesitate to take responsibility or praise for their accomplishments. The feeling of low dominance and power may also affect self-confidence in engaging in a task (50). Women's sense of self-achievement often comes later in life than for men (84).

Positive correlations were found between femininity in females and high anxiety, low self-esteem, and low social acceptance (3). Yet there is an unclear picture as to how the sexes differ in their self-satisfaction over the life span. Other areas that need to be investigated further are early developmental talents, quality of marriage, kinds of adult occupations, and societal changes as these relate to self-satisfaction and self-esteem.

Achievement/Competition

People with achievement motivation have a stable personality and strive for success in all situations where criteria of excellence are applicable. The Thematic Apperception Test (TAT) has been utilized to measure performance in competitive situations as well as career performance. Data from female subjects were difficult to explain. Females tended not to respond to "achievement-involving" task instructions and in general did not appear to achieve as much as males when tested. D. McClelland and his colleagues concluded that there are sex differences in achievement motivation (52).

However, since more females have been researched, the achievement motive has been found to be more complex. Perhaps different forms of arousal are needed for females. Females tend to utilize the affiliation motive (need to be liked or accepted) and external support, whereas males use the achievement motive (task completion) and internal motivation as the basis for achievement. Thus, women are more threatened by future success, and men are more threatened with the thought of failure (48). Males are supposed to be competitive and economically oriented, whereas females are supposed to be expressive and domestic. Perhaps males achieve because they feel they have to (84).

Horner found that females who scored high in fear of success actually did more poorly in competitive tasks than in noncompetitive situations. Those who were low in the fear of success did better in competitive situations (36). Fear of success is aroused when women have some reason to fear that negative consequences, such as loss of femininity and social approval, will result from success. When males fear success, they are punished more severely because they are told to ignore their feelings and be persistent despite their fears (48).

J. Veroff found that females in our culture emphasize process rather than impact; therefore they would be less aware of the social ramifications of achievement and less persistent in achievement than males (80). Luck rather than skill is how females seem to account for their success (84).

Sex discrimination in society is factual, but one reason for females' lower productivity is their hesitancy to take on a long-term career commitment. The key is commitment to effort, performance, and the desire to excel (6). Ability to achieve in the female is fostered when the child has opportunity to develop independence, has experiences with mastery of stress in childhood and adolescence, is accepted by others as an achiever, and has a good role model. Females who feel independent, have high self-esteem, and defer an early marriage to initiate their vocational life will be more likely to meet self-actualized needs (6).

In contrast, males show less hesitancy in pursuing goals. They have learned in childhood to compete directly in sports instead of indirectly in school. They have also been rewarded for being aggressive to obtain what they want. They defend their positions whether they are right or wrong. Males are not so concerned about receiving love and approval from others. They are taught to be independent, and when they hesitate, they receive negative sanctions from society. Anxiety and avoidance do not occur unless males are socialized to be feminine (86).

Outwardly, it appears that families, universities, businesses, and other institutions have been programmed to support male rather than female achievement patterns. The dual-career couple finds that society is hesitant to make adjustments. Females are paid less than males because of the careers open to them, and even in the same career. Male nurses not infrequently earn more than female nurses in the same position slot. If women are competing with men for the same positions, they find that promotions are less frequent, especially as they move up the career ladder. Raising a family complicates the picture. But a single female is also at a disadvantage in upward career mobility because she is not likely to receive the support that males obtain simply by being married.

LIFE STYLES

Traditional

Early socialization affects personality development and coping mechanisms of males and females throughout their lifetime and impacts on their life style and occupational choice.

The female is reinforced for conformity to traditional feminine behavior. Women conform by their inaction, emotionality, and unhappiness. Therefore, women have been limited in pursuit of goal-directed activities, in an effort to win society's approval. Males are expected to conform too, but to action, problem solving, and pleasure pursuits.

Men are described in terms of their occupational roles; women are seen in terms of their sex roles (29). But both may be motivated toward self-development. When people are forced to stay at a single level, they become bored with what was initially interesting. They want to learn and grow and, if allowed to, may become self-actualized; if not, they may become fixated or regressive. Internal motivation pushes people toward growth and fulfillment. Men have been socialized to be internally motivated and therefore have a self-development advantage over women who have been taught to be motivated by external supportive rewards.

Men are motivated to achieve primarily because they were taught from childhood to be growth-oriented and outward-reaching. They were not taught to conform, to be passive, or to allow others to control their lives. Because women are rewarded for being less competent than men, they are also more often rewarded for irrelevant behaviors (29). The professional woman in American society experiences stress from conflictual role demands, minority group status, and negative societal sanctions (76).

Developmentally, then, a lesser view of self is learned by girls. They are prepared for a life of inequality where their power, autonomy, self-directedness, energy, and productivity are discouraged. The care and support of others become the focus of the girl's energy. Boys, on the other hand, learn to accept emotional support but may not be taught how to be supportive. Consequently, when a woman marries, she may find that her need for nurturing, as well as the opportunity to be independent, is not as easily fulfilled. The girl is taught to accept being second and that being non-assertive is safer (63). This contributes to the tendency for women to be more ambivalent about role change (87).

The status of men in American society continues overall to be superior to that of women. Men and masculine characteristics are more highly valued. Even as young children, boys as well as girls prefer to be boys (49). Behaviors that fit the feminine stereotype seem to be incompatible with behaviors appropriate to being equal (9). There is great societal pressure on women to conform to the norm because when differences in values and beliefs arise, conflict results.

Hindrances creating achievement problems for women are the inflexible structure of many professions, the isolation of the nuclear family, and the still prominent social view that masculinity is superior (35). The price of a traditional life style for women may include less autonomy, less opportunity for education, and subordination to males. Benefits are economic and emotional security, the cult of beauty, possible nurturance, and lack of pressure to achieve. However, these same hindrances cost men less (41). Men have a great deal of autonomy and can continue to explore the environment outside the home for growth; some men are even sent through school by their spouses. Economically, married men earn more money than single men, and they receive the added benefits of emotional security and nurturances that women have been socialized to give. A major cost of a traditional life style for men is probably the pressure to achieve since they are task-oriented persons.

As people, especially women, learn to utilize conflict productively, they will develop their own standards to meet personal needs instead of accepting society's standards. They will learn how to identify external and internal expectations of relationships, and they will pursue collegial or cooperative bonds. They will learn to accept that productive conflict involves change, expansion, and happiness, as well as pain (54).

New Ways

In the process of self-actualization, a person creates a self-image of what he/she is and a self-ideal of what he/she would like to be. Hopefully, the two roles are congruent with the life style. If identity can be maintained despite societal demands, old roles can be unlearned and new roles accepted (29).

In selecting roles, a person needs to find those that are compatible with self. In a study by M. O'Neill, it was found that women who were not in role conflict thought that women's primary fulfillment was homemaking and children but that women ought to be free to choose whether to work after marriage, especially if there are no children, if their children are in school, or if the children have left home. Most felt women should be in the home when their children are preschoolers (61). For the woman, the role choice is either a traditional relationship with a man or a career, or trying to accomplish both. In order to work through this conflict, a sense of trust, parting from traditional values, working through social stereotypes and personal ambiguity, and resocializing of the family are necessary.

The process of establishing a professional as well as a personal identity is more intricate and problematic for women than for men because independent goals and risk taking may not be considered "feminine." Fears of loss of approval and rejection come from being viewed as aggressive or competitive (58). D. Nevill and S. Damico found that stress levels in employed women were highest with respect to time management and expectations of self. Children were an added stressor, especially immediately after birth or if the woman has a large number of children (59).

Several workplace problems hamper women. Women do not seem to fit the image of competence in American society (29). Organizational mentors, who are usually men, tend to allow only males to risk climbing the ladder. N. Kogan and K. Dorros found male subjects pinpointing highly achieving women as more exceptional than their male counterparts, in addition to being risk-takers (45). Another problem is the societal expectation that persons have to be single-minded in pursuing a career. This casts doubt on women since they have the capability at any time of exercising the homemaker option. Finally, mobility may be an additional requirement for advancement (35).

If sexual equality is to be promoted and reinforced, the two-career family needs to work to eliminate some of the obstacles discussed above. Flexible work schedules, negotiating to work part time without losing major benefits and professional status, and sharing one position are possible solutions for the two-career family (35).

Provided this direction continues, men will profit the most because masculinity has been very restrictive. Women can use masculine as well as feminine traits with more ease than men can do the reverse (63).

The aim needs to be a clarification of options so that everyone, including married persons, can find the standard that is satisfactory to their needs. What is problematic is that the dual-career couple does not have a role model. Therefore, each couple must discover what works out best in their relationship. Allowing the other person to complete and make mistakes at tasks in his or her own way builds trust (31). Learning to work together is of the utmost importance. Areas needing attention include: (1) limiting the number of obligations taken on at any one time, (2) saying no when appropriate, (3) scheduling of routine activities by each partner to minimize conflict, (4) reviewing and committing to realistic goals and expectations, (5) examining demands and delegating responsibility, (6) reducing uncertainty by establishing customary tasks under one's control, (7) discussing life and career plans to decrease stress, and finally, (8) managing the changes in life (31).

Despite the increase in formal rights that women are obtaining educationally and economically, there has not yet been a dramatic change in the status of women. Since women still have the traditional sex role, that is, responsibility for child care, change may be slow in coming. Goals of the feminist movement are to increase the prestige and economic lives of women and to enable women to develop their own values and guidelines. One method to achieve this is to obtain status and rewards for work done by women. This may be done by placing a monetary value, possibly for tax purposes, on child care and other duties usually performed by women.

Age, educational level, and employment impact on choice of life style within sex roles. Sex-role differences have been found to first increase and then decrease with age (50). Orientation toward traditional life styles decreases with higher educational level (50). Some older working mothers are less traditional than new working mothers in their attitudes toward sex roles. Therefore, since aging is unavoidable and trends toward higher educational level and increased female employment exist, it appears that *new ways* will gradually supplant traditional life styles. According to a recent study, sex-role stereotyping is undergoing some changes, although many stereotypes about typical female and male behavior still exist (26).

Implications for Nurses

The issue of changing societal roles has relevance for nurses, especially female nurses. You will work with clients, men and women, who are experiencing role dissatisfaction and conflict. But conflicts simultaneously related to sexuality and role will probably be seen more frequently in women. You may also experience sex-role conflict, either as a female who is combining marriage, child rearing, and a profession, or as a male who is working in a predominately female profession. That the medical profession is primarily male will impact on both female and male nurses, but the response to each sex is likely to be different, although possibly just as demeaning and anger-provoking. The competent female nurse is often perceived as aggressive or castrating by other male health professionals. And the nurturing male nurse is often perceived as feminine or as a homosexual.

Nurses need to be leaders in trying to break down social stereotypes about what is male and female behavior and in reducing barriers to achievement. You can help to change ideas as you teach and counsel pregnant women and their partners, as you talk to families about their developing children, as you encourage autonomous behavior, a healthy identity, and a positive self-concept in people of any age, and as you involve yourself as a citizen in legislative and economic decision making and policy formulation.

But before you can engage in this, you must face and resolve your own sex-role conflicts. If necessary, seek a counselor who can help you feel good about yourself—man or woman, who can help you balance the expectations of self and others and make a decision about the roles you wish to pursue.

THE NURSING PROCESS

Assessment

The positive aspects of mental health include feelings of self-worth, satisfaction with life roles, and ability to establish positive relationships with others. For the person to be mentally healthy, he/she needs to be able to function well in a variety of situations, to relate positively with others, and to be reasonably healthy and content.

Having role options is a source of freedom, but this freedom adds to role conflict. Therefore, life style choices are not without pain (6). It may be discovered that women will suffer the same health problems as men when allowed to reach executive status. Women who choose to seek executive status find themselves in the position of having to constantly prove themselves, working harder than men, and receiving little support from others, except perhaps from a supportive significant other. Once men are allowed into the executive suite, they become part of the "old boy network" and do not necessarily have to prove themselves to the same extent as women do. There is automatic support from their peers and presumably from their significant others. The question is whether either men or women are happy and content and able to adjust and remain healthy with the demands placed on them by upward occupational mobility and by the changes in our fast-paced society.

The health threat related to occupation and role behaviors needs to be investigated when assessing individuals, families, or groups presenting themselves for treatment. It must be determined whether or not the person has been able to cope with such stresses in the past and what means were utilized to do so. The client's perception of psychological, physical, familial, occupational, social, and cultural situations may give you some cues as to the resources, including any insight and judgment that the client may have.

Case Study

Mary, a 26-year-old married Caucasian woman was self-referred to the mental health clinic. She gave the initial impression of being a somewhat sensitive, retiring, and vulnerable person. There were no immediate signs of acute distress manifested during the initial interview. Her main complaint was, "I have been terribly depressed lately." She stated she had been previously depressed but was concerned because she could no longer cope with her feelings by herself. She experienced limited ability to concentrate, fear of the unknown, and frequent and easily provoked crying about which she stated, "I seem to have no control over my emotions." When her husband went to the store, she was afraid to be alone, became "panicky," and was likely to cry because she felt deserted and helpless. She scolded herself for being too dependent on her husband. Finally she would regain her composure.

Mary's depression was manifested by both a mild insomnia and a loss of appetite. She acknowledged a moderately diminished sexual drive. Her ability to concentrate at work as a college-level professor was greatly reduced, and she was concerned whether others had noticed her change in performance. She believed that her long-term depression had always impaired her efficiency. She recalled a fear of success after graduating from high school, even though she was able to complete a doctorate in education and be employed as a professor.

Mary remembered having had panicky feelings for many years when in groups of people that she did not know well. She had never suffered anxiety in one-to-one relationships, although she characterized herself as shy, reserved, and submissive. Being depressed was not new, but not being in control of her feelings was very upsetting to her and she tended to dwell on this. Mary had many thoughts about how life should be and talked at length about her frustration over the fact that life was not as she thought it should be.

Mary attributed the severity of her symptoms to her marriage of four months to a 28-year-old process engineer. She knew him for about one year prior to their marriage and came to like him because he was "sensitive" and "very possessive." Since their marriage he had become less possessive, sought out the company of others at parties, been flirtatious with women, and as a result, paid less attention to her. At these times she felt defenseless and panicky, and she cried. She was fearful that her marriage would terminate. Mary claimed that she had confronted her husband but was unable in therapy to role-play their interactions.

Before her marriage, Mary dated a fairly large number of men. All these relationships were casual with neither emotional nor physical intimacy. She was very selective and always found something wrong with the men she dated. Her major attraction was that of being a "nice girl," and she only fantasized about being the center of attention.

Mary's parents were divorced when she was three-years old. She saw little of her father afterwards and there was no closeness between them. Her mother remarried when she was five, and she feared her stepfather who was an alcoholic. When her mother and stepfather had marital discord, her role was to care for her younger siblings. She felt neglected but never complained.

Mary was viewed by the treatment team as a

responsible young woman with a dependency problem that she expected her husband to accommodate. She was fearful of desertion. Chronic over-ideation, shyness, and low self-esteem were noted. Her tendency to self-punishment and lack of decisiveness sabotaged any movement in treatment (8). She avoided therapy by not showing up after two sessions, claiming that she felt guilty complaining about her husband.

Formulation of Nursing Diagnosis and Client-Care Goals

The nursing diagnosis of the above care study client was long-standing depression related to fear of another desertion and to unmet, dependency needs, resulting in conflict between personal identity, self-concept, and role performance. Mary was caught between being a successful career woman and traditional wife. Her performance as homemaker and sexual partner was diminished, and performance in her career could become compromised in the future. In this case, few somatic and no suicidal thoughts were elicited.

Your nursing diagnosis of sexual role conflict in regard to Mary may include the following assessment (73):

1. Statements that reflect the following:
   a. Change in perception of roles.
   b. Denial of roles.
   c. Change in others' perception of role behavior.
   d. Conflict in roles.
   e. Change in the physical capacity to resume roles.
   f. Lack of knowledge of roles.
   g. Change in the usual patterns of responsibility.
2. Behaviors of avoidance, withdrawal, and ambiguity.
3. Depression associated with feelings of uselessness and futility with the current roles and an inability to see alternatives that could lead to greater satisfaction.
4. Fears of being seen as emotionally distant or cold, of being regarded by others as powerful, competitive, or competent.
5. Somatic complaints and frigidity in sexual relationships.

Ambiguity about roles causes dissatisfaction, brings to light unfulfilled expectations, and produces much strain on women's attitudes toward work inside or outside the home. Conflicts may emerge at each stage of development but seem to occur more frequently during periods of transition (82). People can tolerate a great deal of inconsistency as long as it does not conflict with their self-interest and self-concept. In men, role strain may be manifested in condescending intellectual relationships with women friends and negative attitudes toward working wives.

Although Mary did not remain in therapy long enough to accomplish all the desired goals, the following long-term client-care goals would be appropriate to help her work through sexual role conflict:

1. Explore feelings about current and past life situations, and the impact of these feelings on behavior.
2. Describe realistic ideas about strengths and limitations.
3. Increase positive feelings and statements about self and decrease self-defeating feelings.
4. Practice assertive communication skills in seeking need-fulfillment with partner and colleagues.
5. Determine role behaviors appropriate to marriage and profession and alternate ways to carry out these behaviors.

Nursing Interventions

The previous chapters have described interventions appropriate to the goals that have been listed that relate to improving negative self-concept and depression. The following discussion will relate to interventions for behaviors related to sexual role conflict, the primary nursing diagnosis in this study.

The selection of a therapist is crucial for the care of the person with sexual role conflict. In 1970, I. Broverman and associates found that views of mental health were affected by sex-role stereotypes (16). Mentally healthy adults were ascribed masculine characteristics, and unhealthy persons were ascribed feminine characteristics by mental health professionals. Nurse therapists were not included in this study. In another study, nurse therapists were found to be more accepting of men and women having both masculine and feminine characteristics (43). Certainly a therapist imposing values on clients is not conducive to their mental health. Personality characteristics and values shared between therapist and client may be more important than the techniques used in therapy. Sometimes a shared gender can enhance the therapeutic process. All in all, empathy on the part of the nurse therapist leads to development of insight in the client.

It is necessary to teach clients like Mary to learn to observe behaviors in interactions with others, to become more astute about automatic thoughts before, during, and after each interaction, and to learn which feelings follow the process. All of this needs to be recorded by the nurse therapist. Assertiveness training, consciousness-raising groups, behavioral modification, and interpersonal techniques are all interventions that could be utilized in the course of treatment in addition to insight-oriented therapy.

According to H. Peplau's process and concept of learning, eight steps of behavior are required of the client in the therapeutic process to promote insight and mature development (64):

1. Observation of what went on or goes on in interactions with others.
2. Description of these events in specific terms.
3. Analysis of assessment information with the therapist.
4. Interpretation and making connections based on the analysis.
5. Consensual validation to check inferences and formulations with the therapist.
6. Practice of new behavior patterns.
7. Integration of new behaviors with previously acquired usable behaviors.
8. Utilization of what was learned in this process in other situations.

Be sensitive to the problems created by conflicts between demands of professional adaptation and internalized contradictory expectations received from developmental experiences. A look at symptom formation and how it relates to real life events, as well as to intrapsychic conflicts, is warranted in working with individuals, couples, families, or group members (58). Help the client explore the following issues:

Sense of self-esteem and worth as a woman.

Role choices related to traditional sexual stereotypes.

Expression of anger.

Pleasing others to one's own detriment.

Risks involved in changing life patterns.

Exploring ideas about the behaviors, thoughts, feelings, and goals that a person holds on a conscious level may lead to an understanding of his/her unconscious needs, conflicts, and goals. Help men focus on coping with their feelings of weakness, vulnerability, helplessness, and other unresolved issues. Help women to discover their real potential for cooperativeness and creativity. Detaching ideas and feelings from their related symptoms may be a long-term process.

Alternative methods of reacting to stress and/or anxiety need to be investigated (see Chapter 12). The client needs to be taught to distinguish between attainable and unattainable goals and how to alter behavior in order to meet attainable goals (12).

As you work with clients, realization of how you have prevented or worked through sexual role conflict is important. Your acceptance of and empathy and support for the person can be enhanced as you share some of the feelings you have experienced in managing home and career. You may also be able to share practical suggestions for balancing the workload required in each role.

Through exploration of feelings, teaching, and your encouragement, the client can learn to make use of conflict in a constructive way. By understanding the concept of conflict as an inevitable fact of life and by learning new ways to handle conflict, fear will lessen, and the client can problem-solve at a more abstract level (71).

One tool that can be utilized in helping the person communicate needs and feelings and gain a sense of autonomy is assertiveness training. Expressive abilities as well as feeling and being competent in specific roles may enhance interpersonal effectiveness (1). The person will need help in differentiating between assertive and aggressive behaviors.

Behavioral techniques are powerful in that overt change can be seen quickly. Trying out a new behavior may initially feel uncomfortable, but once the person is over the hurdle of beginning a change, the process will proceed quickly. As the person feels new energy, there can be more in-depth exploration if he/she wants to understand under-lying conflicts. For example, keeping records of moods may assist in the discovery of the relationship between these states and their expectations of reinforcers (24).

Consciousness raising usually occurs in homogenous groups (all men or women). Here, contact with people in similar circumstances may allow them to learn that they have commonalities, which can make them feel less "crazy" and less "alone" with their conflicts. These groups are effective in developing an awareness in persons of culturally accepted roles. The group members can then critically evaluate sex roles and the behaviors and attitudes that perpetuate stereotyped roles. This supportive atmosphere leads to change (42).

Helping the client with constructive and creative conflict resolution is of primary concern as you teach the client about changing behavior in various roles. Constructive conflict resolution results in more effective communication and insights about life with others (29). A collaborative relationship between you and the client and between the client and others is an important aspect of conflict resolution, particularly if change is to be a growth-producing experience. People need to relate to both sexes as different but equal because then it is possible to draw support from shared experiences. A free choice as to roles is a necessity for personal fulfillment and becomes possible with resolution of conflicts related to sexual roles.

When the client learns to love self, she/he also learns to accept and value self, and success in life is more likely. Conflict can act as a catalyst for maturing and also as an opportunity to improve social conditions. If spouses can learn to view both male and female characteristics as being essential for a full range of human emotional expression, and to communicate this feeling to others, then the archaic cultural prejudices about restrictive roles can be eliminated. Your work with clients can facilitate such a change.

Evaluation

Each action that the nurse therapist uses should be evaluated for the purposes of examining the client's progress and decide which behavior works best for him/her, which problems have been resolved or unresolved, and what new problems the client chooses to work through.

Outcome criteria specific for the client can be

formulated from the goals. For example, based on the specific case of Mary and the long-term goals that were formulated (see p. 646), the following criteria could be used to evaluate success of the therapy:

1. Described feelings about her marriage and work demands and how these feelings relate to earlier experiences.
2. Analyzed how her feelings contributed to distancing behavior between herself and her husband.
3. Identified four strengths that could help to build a solid marital relationship; these strengths were validated by the spouse.
4. Identified five limits that contributed to poor communication with spouse and which were validated by the husband.
5. Recorded one event daily that contributed to a positive self-concept.
6. Role-played assertive communication techniques in therapy and recorded in a log one interaction daily where she had been assertive rather than nonassertive.
7. Set aside one hour weekly to talk with husband about their role behaviors appropriate to marriage and profession and ways to improve their marriage.
8. Reported that after three weeks of therapy, appetite and sleep patterns improved.
9. Reported that after two months of therapy she no longer cried or felt deserted or panicky when her husband left her.
10. Reported greater energy level, increased libido, and better concentration at work after four months of therapy.
11. Requested ongoing therapy to maintain progress in overcoming dependency behavior and to work through deep-seated emotional problems.

Although all the above criteria may not be met, at least the majority of them would be applicable. You can formulate similar criteria of evaluation for clients that you work with.

REFERENCES

1. Adams, Kathleen, "Assertiveness Training, Androgyny, and Professional Women," *Dissertation Abstracts International*, 37, no. 12-B (June 1977), 6311.

2. Alpert, Judith, and Mary Richardson, "Conflict, Outcome and Perception of Women's Roles," *Educational Gerontology*, 3, no. 1 (1978), 79–87.

3. Bandura, Albert, "Influences of Models; Reinforcement Contingencies on the Acquisition of Imitative Response," *Journal of Personality and Social Psychology*, 1, no. 6 (1965), 589–95.

4. ——, "Social Learning Theory of Identificatory Processes," in *Handbook of Socialization Theory and Research*, ed. D. A. Goslen, pp. 215–17. Chicago: Rand McNally College Publishing Company, 1969.

5. Bandura, Albert, and Richard Walters, "Aggression," in *Child Psychology*, ed. Harold Stevenson, pp. 364–415. Chicago: University of Chicago Press, 1963.

6. Bardwick, Judith, *Psychology of Women: A Study of Bio-Cultural Conflicts*. New York: Harper & Row, Publishers, Inc., 1971.

7. ——, "The New Women and Mental Health." Paper presented at the Meeting of Human Development Seminars, Minneapolis, March 13, 1981.

8. Beaulieu, Dean, "MMPI Profiles of General Hospital Psychiatric Patients." Unpublished manuscript.

9. Bem, S. L., W. Martyna, and C. Watson, "Sex-Typing and Androgyny: Further Explorations of the Expressive Domain," *Journal of Personality and Social Psychology*, 34, no. 5 (1976), 1016–23.

10. Benedek, Therese, "Sexual Functions in Women and Their Disturbance," in *The American Handbook of Psychiatry*, ed. S. Arieti, pp. 727–48. New York: Basic Books, Inc., 1959.

11. Bernard, Jessie, *The Future of Marriage*. New York: Bantam Books, Inc., 1972.

12. ——, *The Future of Motherhood*. New York: Penguin Books, 1974.

13. Brinkman, June, "The Relationship between Marital Integration and the Working Wife-Mother," *Dissertation Abstracts International*, 37, no. 3-A (September 1976), 1826–27.

14. Bronfenbrenner, Urie, "Freudian Theories of Identification and Their Derivatives," *Child Development*, 31, no. 3 (1960), 15–40.

15. Brooks-Gunn, Jeanne, and Wendy Schempp-Matthews, *He and She: How Children Develop Their Sex-Role*

Identity. Englewood Cliffs, N.J.: Prentice-Hall, Inc. 1979.

16. Broverman, I. K. et al., "Sex-Role Stereotypes and Clinical Judgments of Mental Health," *Journal of Consulting and Clinical Psychology,* 34 no. 1 (1970), 1–7.

17. Bush, Mary Ann, and Diane Kjervik, "The Nurse's Self-Image," in *Women in Stress—A Nursing Perspective*, eds. Diane Kjervik and Ida Martinson. New York: Appleton-Century-Crofts, 1979.

18. Chesler, Phyllis, "Are We a Threat to Each Other?" *MS,* 1, no. 4 (1972), 89.

19. Deutsch, Helene, *The Psychology of Women.* New York: Bantam Books, Inc., 1944.

20. Dohrenwend, D. P., and B. S. Dohrenwend, "Social and Cultural Influences on Psychopathology," *Annual Review of Psychology*, 25 (1974), 417–52.

21. English, Horace, and Ava English, *A Comprehensive Dictionary of Psychological and Psychoanalytic Terms.* New York: David McKay Co., Inc., 1958.

22. Erickson, Erik, *Childhood and Society* (2nd ed.). New York: W. W. Norton & Co., Inc., 1963.

23. ——, "Womanhood and Inner Spaces, in *Women and Analysis*, ed. J. Strouse. New York: Dell Publishing Co., 1974.

24. Fodor, Iris, "Sex-Role Conflict and Symptom Formation in Women: Can Behavior Therapy Help?" *Psychotherapy: Theory, Research and Practice*, 11, no. 1 (1974), 22–29.

25. Frodi, A., J. Macaulay, and P. R. Thome, "Are Women Always Less Aggressive than Men?" *Psychological Bulletin*, 84, no. 4 (1977), 634–60.

26. Gilbert, L., C. Deutsch, and R. Strahan, "Feminine and Masculine Dimensions of the Typical, Desirable and Ideal Woman and Man," *Sex Roles*, 4 (1978), 767–78.

27. Goldman, Noreen, and Renee Ravid, "Community Surveys: Sex Differences in Mental Illness," in *The Mental Health of Women*, eds. Marcia Guttentag, Susan Salasia, and Deborah Belle, pp. 33–55. New York: Academic Press, Inc., 1980.

28. Gove, Walter, and Jeanette Tudor, "Adult Sex Roles and Mental Illness," *American Journal of Sociology*, 78, no. 4 (1973), 50–73.

29. Grissum, Marlene, and Carol Spengler, *Womanpower and Health Care.* Boston. Little, Brown & Company, 1976.

30. Hall, Douglas, and Francine Gordon, "Career Choices of Married Women: Effects on Conflict Role to Behavior, and Satisfaction," *Journal of Applied Psychology*, 58, no. 1 (1973), 42–48.

31. Hall, Francine, and Douglas Hall, *The Two-Career Couple.* Reading, Mass.: Addison-Wesley Publishing Co., Inc., 1978.

32. Hardy, Margaret, and Mary Conway, *Role Theory. Perspectives for Health Professionals.* New York: Appleton-Century-Crofts, 1978.

33. Hicks, D. J., "Imitation and Retention of Film-Mediated Aggressive Peer and Adult Models," *Journal of Personality and Social Psychology*, 2, no. 1 (1965), 97–100.

34. Hinsie, Leland, and Robert Campbell, *Psychiatric Dictionary.* New York: Oxford University Press, 1974.

35. Holmstrom, Lynda, *The Two-Career Family.* Cambridge, Mass.: Schenkman Publishing Co., Inc., 1972.

36. Horner, M., "Sex Differences in Achievement Motivation and Performance in Competitive and Non-Competitive Situations." Unpublished Ph.D. dissertation.

37. Horney, Karen, *Feminine Psychology,* New York: W. W. Norton & Co., Inc., 1967.

38. ——, "The Flight from Womanhood," in *Psychoanalysis and Women*, ed. J. B. Miller, pp. 5–20. Baltimore, Md.: Penguin Books, 1973.

39. Kagan, Jerome, "Acquisition and Significance of Sex Typing and Sex Role Identity," in *Review of Child Development Research*, eds. M. L. Hoffman and L. W. Hoffman, vol. 1; New York: pp. 137–67, Russell Sage Foundation.

40. Kagan, Jerome, and A. Moss, *Birth to Maturity: A Study in Psychological Development*, pp. 49–84. New York: John Wiley & Sons, Inc., 1962.

41. Keller, Suzanne, "The Female Role: Constants and Changes," in *Women in Therapy—New Psychotherapies for a Changing Society*, eds. Violet Franks and Vasanti Burtler, pp. 416–30. New York: Brunner/Mazel, Inc., 1974.

42. Kirsh, Barbara, "Consciousness-Raising Groups as Therapy for Women," in *Women in Therapy—New Psychotherapies for a Changing Society*, eds. Violet Franks and Vasanti Burtler, p. 350. New York: Brunner/Mazel, Inc., 1974.

43. Kjervik, Diane, "The Stress of Sexism on the Mental Health of Women," in *Women in Stress—A Nursing Perspective*, eds. Diane Kjervik and Ida Martinson. New York: Appleton-Century-Crofts, 1979.

44. Kjervik-Doremus, Marcea, "The Identification Concepts of Freud, Piaget, and Bandura." Unpublished manuscript, Spring 1975. Hennepin County Medical Health Center, Minneapolis, Minn.

45. Kogan, Nathan, and Karen Dorros, "Sex Differences

in Risk Taking and its Attributions," *Sex Roles*, 4, no. 5 (1978), 755–66.

46. Komarovsky, Mirra, "Cultural Contradictions and Sex Roles: The Masculine Case," *American Journal of Sociology*, 78, no. 4 (1973), 873–84.

47. Krutien, Dean, "The Declining Status of Women: Popular Myths and the Failure of Functionalist Thought," *Social Forces*, 48, no. 2 (1969), 183–93.

48. Lips, Hilary, and Nina Colwill, *The Psychology of Sex Differences*. Englewood Cliffs, N.J.: Prentice-Hall, Inc., 1978.

49. Lynn, David B., "The Process of Learning Parental and Sex-Role Identity," *Journal of Marriage and the Family*, 28, no. 4 (1966), 466–70.

50. Maccoby, Eleanor, and Carol Jacklin, *The Psychology of Sex Differences*. Stanford, Calif.: Stanford University Press, 1974.

51. Maier, William, *Three Theories of Child Development*. New York: Harper & Row, Publishers, Inc., 1969.

52. McClelland, D. A. et al., *The Achievement Motive*. New York: Appleton-Century-Crofts, 1953.

53. Menikheim, Marie, "Communication Patterns of Women and Nurses," in *Women in Stress—A Nursing Perspective*, eds. Diane K. Kjervik and Ida Martinson. New York: Appleton-Century-Crofts, 1979.

54. Miller, Jean Baker, *Toward a New Psychology of Women*. Boston, Mass.: Beacon Press, 1976.

55. Minnigerode, Fred, and Judith Lee, "Young Adults' Perceptions of Social Sex Roles across the Life Span," *Sex Roles*, 4, no. 4 (1978), 563–69.

56. Morgan, Carolyn, "Female and Male Attitudes toward Life: Implications for Theories of Mental Health," *Sex Roles*, 6, no. 3 (1980), 367–80.

57. Moulton, Ruth, "Women with Double Lives," *Contemporary Psychoanalysis*, 13, no. 1 (1977), 64–84.

58. Nadelson, Carol et al., "Success and Failure: Psycho-Therapeutic Considerations for Women in Conflict," *American Journal of Psychiatry*, 135, no. 9 (1978), 1092.

59. Nevill, Dorothy, and Sandra Damico, "Family Size and Role Conflict in Women," *Journal of Psychology*, 84, no. 3 (1975), 267–70.

60. ——, "Role Conflict in Women as a Function of Marital Status," *Human Relations*, 28, no. 5 (1975), 487–89.

61. O'Neill, Maureen, "An Investigation of Women's Sex-Role Conflict and the Predictability of Modes of Conflict Resolution," *Dissertation Abstracts International*, 35, no. 2-B (August 1974), 1058–59.

62. O'Neill, Nina, and George O'Neill, *Open Marriage*. New York: Avon Books, 1972.

63. Orbach, Susie, *Fat Is a Feminist Issue*. New York: Berkley Publishing Corporation, 1978.

64. Peplau, Hildegarde, "Process and Concept of Learning," in *Some Clinical Approaches to Psychiatric Nursing*, eds. Shirley Burd and Margaret Marshall, pp. 333–36. New York: Macmillan Publishing Co., Inc., 1963.

65. Phillips, D., and B. Segal, "Sexual Status and Psychiatric Symptoms," *American Sociological Review*, 34, no. 1 (1969), 58–72.

66. Piaget, Jean, *Play, Dreams and Imitation in Childhood*. New York: W. W. Norton & Co., Inc., 1962.

67. Rotter, J. B. and R. C. Mulry, "Internal Versus External Locus of Reinforcement and Decision Time," *Journal of Personality and Social Psychology*, 2 (1965), 598–604.

68. Salwen, Laura, "Few Conflicts for the New Woman," *Psychotherapy: Theory, Research, and Practice*, 12, no. 4 (1975), 429–32.

69. Sears, Robert, *Survey of Objective Studies of Psychoanalytic Concepts*, pp. 136–37. New York: Social Science Research Council, 1942.

70. ——, "Dependency Motivation," in *Nebraska Symposium on Motivation*, ed. M. R. Jones, pp. 25-64. Lincoln, Nebr.: University of Nebraska Press, 1963.

71. Seiden, Anne, "Overview: Research on the Psychology of Women: Women in Working Families, and Psychotherapy," *American Journal of Psychiatry*, 133, no. 10 (1976), 1111–34.

72. Sherfey, Mary, *The Nature and Evolution of Female Sexuality*. New York: Random House, Inc., 1972.

73. Sherman, Julia, *On the Psychology of Women: A Survey of Empirical Studies*. Springfield, Ill.: Charles C Thomas, Publisher, 1971.

74. Sinnott, Jan, "Sex-Role Inconsistency, Biology, and Successful Aging," *The Gerontologist*, 17, no. 5 (1977), 459–63.

75. Taylor, S. E., and E. J. Langer, "Pregnancy: A Social Stigma?" *Sex Roles*, 3, no. 1 (1977), 27–35.

76. Teulner, Patricia, "Women in the Professions: A Social-Psychological Study," *Dissertation Abstracts International*, 34, no. 8-A (February 1974), 5309.

77. Thagaard, Tove, "Academic Values and Intellectual Attitudes: Sex Differentiation or Similarity?" *Acta Sociologica*, 18, no. 1 (1975), 36–48.

78. Thompson, C., "Cultural Pressures in the Psychology of Women," in *Interpersonal Psychoanalysis: The*

Selected Papers of Clara Thompson, ed. M. R. Green. New York: Basic Books, Inc., 1964.

79. *U.S. Women and Their Changing Status*. Michigan State University, Ann Arbor, Mich., May 1976.

80. Veroff, J., "Process versus Impact in Men's and Women's Achievement Motivation," *Psychology of Women Quarterly*, 1, no. 3 (1977), 283–93.

81. Weissman, Myrna, and G. Klerman, "Sex Differences and the Epidemiology of Depression," *Archives of General Psychiatry*, 34, no. 3 (1977), 98–111.

82. Weissman, Myrna, and Eugene Paykel, *The Depressed Woman: A Study of Relationships*. Chicago: The University of Chicago Press, 1974.

83. Weisstein, Naomi, "Psychologic Constructs in the Female," in *Woman in Sexist Society: Studies in Power and Powerlessness*, eds. V. Goeniah and B. Moran, p. 221. New York: Basic Books, Inc., 1971.

84. Weitz, Shirley, *Sex Roles: Biological, Psychological, and Social Foundations*. New York: Oxford University Press, 1977.

85. Williams, Elizabeth, *Notes of a Feminist Therapist*. New York: Dell Publishing Co., Inc., 1976.

86. Williams, Juanita, *Psychology of Women: Behavior in a Bio-Social Context*. New York: W. W. Norton & Co., Inc., 1977.

87. Young, Rosalie, "Current Sex-Role Attitudes of Male and Female Students," *Social Issues*, 10, no. 3 (1977), 309–23.

SUPPLEMENTARY READING LIST

Allison, Janet, "Infertility and Role Conflict: A Phenomenological Study of Women," *Dissertation Abstracts International*, 37, no. 9-B (March 1977), 4660.

Bales, R. F., and P. E. Slater, "Role Differentiation in Small Decision-Making Groups," in *Family, Socialization, and Interaction Processes,* eds. T. Parsons and R. F. Bales, Chap. 5. New York: The Free Press, 1955.

Bardwick, Judith, *In Transition*. New York: Holt, Rinehart and Winston, 1979.

Brownmiller, Susan, *Against Our Will*. New York: Bantam Books, Inc., 1975.

Chesler, Phyllis, *Women and Madness*. New York: Avon Books, 1972.

Coopersmith, Stanley, *The Antecedents of Self-Esteem*. San Francisco: Freeman Company, 1967.

deBeauvoir, Simone, *The Second Sex*. New York: Vintage Books, 1974.

Denkmeyer, Don, *Child Development: The Emerging Self*. Englewood Cliffs, N.J.: Prentice-Hall, Inc., 1965.

DeRosis, Helen, *Women and Anxiety*. New York: Delacorte Press, 1979.

____, and Victoria Pellegrino, *The Book of Hope*. New York: Bantam Books, Inc., 1976.

Farrell, Warren, *The Liberated Man*. New York: Bantam Books, Inc., 1974.

Fogarty, Michael, R. Rapoport, and N. Robert, *Sex, Career, and Family*. Beverly Hills, Calif.: Sage Publishing Co., 1971.

Frances, Susan, "Sex Differences in Nonverbal Behavior," *Sex Roles*, 5, no. 4 (1979), 519–35.

Frisemer, David, "Success Avoidance and Gender Role," *Dissertation Abstracts International*, 35, no. 8-B (February 1975), 4263.

Goldberg, Herb, *The Hazards of Being Male*. New York: The New American Library, Inc., 1976.

____, *The New Male*. New York: The New American Library, Inc., 1979.

Gordon, Francine, and Douglas Hall, "Self-Image and Stereotypes of Femininity, Their Relationship to Women's Role Conflicts and Coping," *Journal of Applied Psychology*, 59, no. 2 (1974) 241–43.

Gornich, Vivian, and Barbara Moran, eds., *Women in a Sexist Society*. New York: The New American Library, Inc., 1971.

Guttentag, Marcia, Susan Salasin, and Deborah Belle, *The Mental Health of Women*. New York: Academic Press, Inc., 1980.

Horney, Karen, *Feminine Psychology*. New York: W. W. Norton & Co., Inc., 1967.

Janeway, Elizabeth, *Man's World, Woman's Place: A Study in Social Mythology*. New York: Dell Publishing Co., Inc., 1971.

____, *Between Myth and Morning: Women Awakening*. New York: William Morrow & Co., Inc., 1975.

Kanter, Rosabeth, *Men and Women of the Corporation*. New York: Basic Books, Inc., Publishers, 1977.

Klein, Elizabeth Ann, "Role Conflict in Feminist and Non-Feminist Women," *Dissertation Abstracts International*, 36, no. 3-B (September 1975), 1410.

Klein, Marjorie H., "Feminist Concepts of Therapy Outcome," *Psychotherapy, Theory, Research and Practice*, 3, no. 1 (1976), 89–95.

Konopka, Gisela, *The Adolescent Girl in Conflict.* Englewood Cliffs, N.J.: Prentice-Hall, Inc., 1966.

Krovetz, Diane, "Sex Role Concepts of Women," *Journal of Consulting and Clinical Psychology,* 44, no. 3 (1976), 437–43.

Laws, Judith, "Work Aspiration of Women: False Leads and New Starts," *Signs,* 3, no. 2 (1976), 33–49.

Marine, Margaret, "Sex Differences in the Determination of Adolescent Aspirations: A Review of Research," *Sex Roles,* 4, no. 5 (1978), 723–54.

Maslow, Abraham, *Toward a Psychology of Being.* New York: Van Nostrand Reinhold Company, 1968.

Meeker, B. F., and P. A. Weitzel-O'Neill, "Sex Roles and Interpersonal Behavior in Task-Oriented Groups," *American Sociological Review,* 42, no. 1 (1977), 91–105.

Michalson, Evelyn, and Walter Goldschmidt, "Female Roles and Male Dominance Among Peasants," *Southwestern Journal of Anthropology,* 27, no. 4 (1971), 330–52.

Mill, John, *The Subjection of Women.* Cambridge, Mass.: The M.I.T. Press, 1970.

Mitchell, Juliet, *Psychoanalysis and Feminism.* New York: Vintage Books, 1974.

Orlofsky, Jacob, and Michael Windle, "Sex-Role Orientation, Behavioral Adaptability, and Personal Adjustment," *Sex Roles,* 4, no. 6 (1978), 801–12.

Powell, Barbara, and Marvin Reznikoff, "Role Conflict and Symptoms of Psychological Distress in College-Educated Women," *Journal of Consulting and Clinical Psychology,* 44, no. 3 (1976), 473–79.

Rapoport, Rhona, Robert Rapoport, and Janice M. Bumstead, eds., *Working Couples.* New York: Harper & Row, Publishers, Inc., 1978.

Rich, Adrienne, *Of Woman Born.* New York: Bantam Books, Inc., 1976.

Richardson, Deborah, Anne Vinzel, and Stuart Taylor, "Female Aggression as a Function of Attitudes Toward Women," *Sex Roles,* 6, no. 2 (1980), 265–71.

Romer, Nancy, and Debra Cherry, "Ethnic and Social Class Differences in Children's Sex-Role Concepts," *Sex Roles,* 6, no. 2 (1980), 245–63.

Rubin, Richard, "Antecedents of Sex-Role Conflict in Gang Delinquents," *Dissertation Abstracts International,* Part 2, 34, no. 8-A, (February 1974), 5342.

Safilios-Rothschild, Constantina, *Love, Sex, and Sex Roles.* Englewood Cliffs, N.J.: Prentice-Hall, Inc., 1977.

Shepard, Winifred, "Mothers and Fathers, Sons and Daughters: Perceptions of Young Adults," *Sex Roles,* 6, no. 3 (1980), 421–34.

Sherman, J., "Social Values, Femininity and the Development of a Female Competence," *Journal of Social Issues,* 32, no. 3 (1976), 181–95.

Terman, L. M., and L. E. Tayler, "Psychological Sex Differences," in *Manual of Child Psychology,* 2nd ed., ed. L. Carmichael. New York: John Wiley & Sons, Inc., 1954.

Vellenga, Dorothy, "Changing Sex Roles and Social Tensions in Ghana: The Law as Measure and Mediator of Family Conflicts," *Dissertation Abstracts International,* 36, no. 3-A (September 1975), 1847–48.

Weis, Kurt, and Sandra Borges, "Victimology and Rape: The Case of the Legitimate Victim," *Issues in Criminology,* 8, no. 2 (1975), 71–115.

Welch, Mary, *Networking.* New York: Harcourt Brace Jovanovich, Inc., 1980.

Zaro, Joan, "An Experimental Study of Role Conflict in Women," *Dissertation Abstracts International,* 33, no. 6-B (December 1972), 2828.

Zuckerberg, Joan, "An Exploration into Feminine Role Conflict and Body Symptomotology in Pregnancy," *Dissertation Abstracts International,* 34, no. 8-B (February 1974), 4066.

21

The Child and Adolescent with Emotional Problems

Study of this chapter will help you to:

1. Relate vulnerability risk factors and their effects to the emotional health status of the child and adolescent.

2. Define selected emotional health problems of the child/adolescent and describe the etiologic factors of psychosis, learning disability, mental retardation, school phobia (separation anxiety disorder), and anorexia nervosa.

3. Define child abuse and describe the factors that contribute toward parental abuse of offspring.

4. Describe psychodynamic aspects in the family system when psychosis, school phobia, anorexia nervosa, or child abuse is present.

5. Assess and differentiate behaviors, signs, and symptoms of psychosis; of learning disability; and of mental retardation in the child/adolescent and the effects of these conditions on the family.

6. Assess behaviors in the family system and in the offspring that indicate school phobia or abuse.

7. Assess and differentiate anorexia nervosa from other physical illnesses of the adolescent.

8. Formulate nursing diagnoses based on assessment of the child/adolescent and family system.

9. Plan care with goals based on needs of the child/adolescent and of the family unit.

10. Intervene to assist the child/adolescent and family in meeting physical, emotional, cognitive, and social needs related to the specific health impairment and its effects.

11. Evaluate the effectiveness of your nursing intervention and of your collaboration with other health team members, recognizing that small increments of progress may be all that is possible.

This chapter contributed by Sandra Blaesing, R.N., M.S.N. and Patricia Kaufmann, R.N., M.S.N. Also a portion of the section on anorexia nervosa was contributed by Phillis Jacobs, R.N., M.S.N.

The preliminary report of the President's Commission on Mental Health has indicated a great need for mental health services for children. This commission reported in 1977 that 8.1 (15 percent) of the 54 million children and youth of school age need help for psychological disorders (51).

The kinds of services needed depend on etiological factors as well as on characteristics of the emotional and mental disorders found in this population. In 1970, the Joint Commission on Mental Health of Children identified five categories of problems believed to play a role in the origin of these disorders (33):

1. Faulty training and faulty life experiences.
2. Surface conflicts between children and parents that arise from adjustment tasks related to siblings and school, and social and sexual development.
3. Deeper conflicts within the child (the neuroses).
4. Difficulties associated with physical handicaps and disorders.
5. Difficulties associated with severe mental disorders such as psychoses.

It is estimated that 80 percent of emotional problems are related to the first two categories; 10 percent to the third; and 10 percent to the fourth and fifth (33).

Various combinations of etiological factors may contribute to the emotional disorders that may be manifested by a child in any phase of development. In this chapter selected problems that impair the health of the child and adolescent will be explored, with emphasis on use of the nursing process. The condition described here are those that affect the development of the child and adolescent and are distinctly different from conditions encountered in adulthood.

Although child psychiatric nursing is a specialty role that requires graduate education, nurse generalists who work with children and their families in any setting can make a valuable contribution to the field of child mental health. For example, if you work with children in any setting, your ability to assess behaviors that differ from the general norms can assist in case finding of illness and early treatment. You can also share with families general knowledge about the behavioral problems discussed in this chapter and can refer them to in-depth psychological help when such problems arise. Further, you can teach parents the importance of proper prenatal care and nurturing in childhood as a means to help prevent these behavioral problems. Along with the various nursing modalities recommended here for intervention with the child/adolescent and family, keep in mind the importance of using a Humansitic Framework as you plan and give care to the individual and as you work with the family system.

VULNERABILITY—RISK FACTORS IN CHILD MENTAL HEALTH

Assessment of vulnerability is extremely important for effective primary and secondary prevention. Those that work in the field of child mental health have observed the recurring paradox of some children raised in psychologically and mentally enriched environments who succumb to what appears to be minor stresses; whereas conversely, some children suffering from effects of poverty and prejudice seem invulnerable to influences that leave others incapable of coping. Recent studies have investigated these aspects of vulnerability in children.

E. J. Anthony developed a vulnerable-invulnerable continuum (1). According to this author, constitutional and environmental factors interact to cause children to be placed at either end of the continuum. A vulnerable state results from such factors as: (1) genetic loading (or familial schizophrenia), (2) constitutional factors (temperament type), (3) reproductive factors (prematurity), (4) parental pathology or loss (death, divorce, or separation during the child's first two years), and (5) disadvantaged environment. Children with high constitutional vulnerability are more prone to disturbed behavior when also exposed to high environmental risks (1).

A. Thomas, S. Chess, and H. Birch have established nine categories by which to study temperament, and they suggest that there are definite relationships between temperament and childhood behavior disorders (59). Their categories of temperamental reactivity are: (1) activity level, (2) rhyth-micity, (3) approach-withdrawal, (4) adaptability, (5) quality of mood, (6) threshold of responsiveness, (7) intensity of reaction, (8) distractibility, and (9) attention span or persistence. From these nine categories three temperamental clusters are developed: (1) difficult, (2) slow to warm up, and (3) easy. Each of these three clusters reflects a characteristic style of relating to life situations. Of special note is the "difficult temperamental type." These children demonstrate irregularity in bodily functions, negative withdrawal responses to new stimuli, high-intensity reactions, slow adaptability to changes in the environment, and negative mood. In these studies, 70 percent of the children with the "difficult" termperamental cluster later developed behavior problems, in contrast to 18 percent of the "easy to handle" children. These findings suggest that useful predictions can be made about vulnerability based on early temperamental behaviors that are difficult for parents to handle (59).

Norman Garmezy relates vulnerability in children to levels of competence. *Competence is viewed as the ability to adapt and master situations.* The assumption is that the higher the level of competence, the greater the resistance to stress (21).

You, as a nurse, are in an excellent position to identify vulnerable children and their families and to assist them in healthy adaptation. Information in this chapter will present a general background for such a role.

THE NURSING PROCESS WITH CHILDREN EXHIBITING SEVERE BEHAVIOR DISORDERS (CHILDHOOD PSYCHOSIS)

Childhood psychosis represents a profound and dramatic disorder; etiology, classification, and treatment are not fully known in spite of a substantial body of research. The incidence is also not precisely known because various diagnostic criteria are used; estimates are that less than 1 percent of this youthful population are affected (63).

Criteria, as listed below, were originally formulated by M. Creak and were supported by the Group for the Advancement of Psychiatry; these have been factors widely accepted by professionals as a general description of childhood psychosis (12):

1. Severe and continued impairment of emotional relationships with others.
2. Tendency toward preoccupation with inanimate objects.
3. Loss of speech or failure in its development.
4. Disturbances in sensory perception.
5. Bizarre or stereotyped behavior and movement patterns.
6. Marked resistance to environmental change.
7. Outbursts of intense and unpredictable panic.
8. Absence of a sense of personal identity.
9. Blunted, uneven, or fragmented intellectual development.

Assessment

In this chapter, the term *childhood psychosis* is used in a broad sense, encompassing early infantile autism, symbiotic infantile psychosis, and childhood schizophrenia. There is considerable confusion as to the identification of differential diagnostic criteria as well as the question whether these are indeed separate and distinguishable conditions (18, 39). Table 21-1 summarizes the primary characteristics of the clinical picture for the childhood psychoses (39). Early infantile autism is differentiated from childhood schizophrenia on the basis of age of onset, autistic aloneness, and insistence on sameness in the environment. Symbiotic psychosis is differentiated by the child's inability to separate from the mother. As the symbiotic psychosis progresses, it becomes indistinguishable from autism.

Etiological Theories

There are multiple etiological theories. The controversy centers around psychogenic (environmental) theories versus biological (inborn) theories. Psychogenic theory sees early childhood psychosis as the child's response to severe stress and anxiety in the environment. The psychosis is a fortress erected by the child to shut out the world. Parents are viewed as the primary pathological agents. Biological theories, conversely, point to alterations in physiological arousal or central disorders in perception or cognition as the cause for childhood psychosis.

Current research data strongly suggest that the primary etiological factor is a neurological defect, although the specific nature of the impairment is speculative (18, 39). Psychogenic considerations, however, are extremely important because the nature of the interaction between the child and family sets the parameters for the child's subsequent adjustment/maladjustment.

Apparently, the newborn who manifests a temperament that is difficult for the mother to respond to causes interference with the normal development of attachment and nurturing. The mother's anxiety and rejection may reinforce rather than overcome any innate impairments and apparently contribute to anxiety and withdrawal in the infant. A vicious circle may be established in a matter of weeks. As the mother's anticipation of a baby to love changes to feelings of anxiety, passivity, despair, and conscious or unconscious rejection, she touches, talks to, and cuddles the baby less. The baby, in turn, becomes unresponsive to whatever overtures are made. The infant must be touched, stroked, talked to, cuddled, and loved for certain brain structures and functions to develop. Thus, innate physiological impairments may become fixated. This process of impaired maternal attachment is made worse when the baby is unwanted or the mother does not receive loving support or help from a partner, her parents and friends, or health professionals. What may begin as a physiological problem in the baby is heightened through interaction processes. Or if perceptual or neurological problems were not present at birth, they may soon develop if attachment between mother and baby does not occur and a loving relationship does not develop (5, 6, 42, 49, 57).

Characteristic Symptoms/ Behaviors

A cardinal symptom of the severely disturbed child is disturbance of affect. Attempts to cuddle or show affection to the child result in a total lack of response and a profound inability to relate to other people develops. The child does not seem to know or care whether or not he/she is alone or with others. E. Ritvo et al. summarize an array of behaviors reflecting disturbances of relating: poor or deviant eye contact, lack of anticipatory response to being picked up, aversion to physical contact, reacting to only a part of another person, and absent or overreactive stranger anxiety (53). The child operates from a personal reality.

Another major symptom characteristic of the severely disturbed child is the inability to commu-

TABLE 21-1. Summary of the Clinical Picture for the Three Childhood Psychoses

CLINICAL PICTURE	CHILDHOOD SCHIZOPHRENIA	EARLY INFANTILE AUTISM	SYMBIOTIC INFANTILE PSYCHOSES
Onset	Gradual between age two to eleven after period of normal development.	Gradual from birth.	Between two and one-half to five years after normal development.
Social and Interpersonal	Decreased interest in external world, withdrawal, loss of contact, impaired relations with others.	Failure to show anticipatory postural movements; extreme aloneness; insistence on sameness.	Unable to tolerate briefest separation from mother; clinging and incapable of delineating self.
Intellectual and Cognitive	Thought disturbance; perceptual problems; distorted time and space orientation; below average I.Q.	High spatial ability; good memory; low I.Q. but good intellectual potential.	Bizarre ideation; loss of contact; thought disturbance.
Language	Disturbances in speech; mutism, and if speech is present, it is not used for communication.	Disturbances in speech; mutism, and if speech is present it is not used for communication. Very literal; delayed echolalia; pronoun reversal; I and Yes are absent till age six.	
Affect	Defect in emotional responsiveness and rapport; decreased, distorted, and/or inappropriate affect.	Inaccessible and emotionally unresponsive to humans.	Severe anxiety and panic over separation from mother; low frustration tolerance; withdrawn and seclusive as psychosis persists.
Motor	Bizarre body movements; repetitive and stereotyped motions; motor awkwardness; distortion in mobility.	Head banging and body rocking; remarkable agility and dexterity; preoccupied with mechanical objects.	
Physical and Developmental Patterns	Unevenness of somatic growth; disturbances of normal rhythmic patterns; abnormal EEG.	Peculiar eating habits and food preferences; normal EEG.	Disturbed normal rhythmic patterns.
Family	High incidence of mental illness.	Aloof, obsessive, and emotionally cold; high intelligence and educational and occupational levels; low divorce rate and incidence of mental illness.	Pathological mother who fosters the symbosis.

Source: Table from Knopf (39, p. 259). Used with permission.

nicate. Some children remain mute several years after speech is normally acquired. When speech is present, it is seldom used as a form of verbal communication. *Echolalia, repetition of last words heard*, is a frequent response. This lack of speech or communication interferes with the development of the child's self-image, which is necessary for reality testing. Typically, personal pronouns either are not used at all or they are misused. T. Shapiro, I. Chariandini, and B. Fish note that speech patterns are rigid and stereotyped with no ability to symbolize. They conclude that the severely disturbed child's speech represents a central cognitive disorder with disturbances of association and conceptualization (56).

Sameness in the environment is essential. If a piece of furniture is moved or a routine is changed, the child becomes quite upset and frightened. Thus he/she uses a rigid compulsiveness to maintain some sense of control. One of the most striking behaviors demonstrated by the severely disturbed child is a repetitive, self-stimulating activity, such as rocking the body, twirling, flapping hands, and spinning objects for long periods of time in an incessant manner. This type of behavior seems to block responsiveness to external stimuli.

Temper tantrums and self-mutilating behaviors are also frequently seen. These destructive rages are directed against self or others. The child may scream, kick, bite, or bang his/her head against walls so forcefully that it causes tissue damage. These rages can be brought on by a minor restriction, an environmental change, or for no apparent reason.

Some of these children appear to have sensory deficits. Parents may incorrectly suspect the child of being blind or deaf. There are extreme variabilities in attentional behavior. A child may not react to an immediate loud noise, but may indicate awareness of a distant, barely audible sound. Many also seem insensitive to pain and show no awareness of physical injury.

In addition to these behavioral problems, the severely disturbed child tends to develop few self-care skills, such as feeding, dressing, and toileting, and shows little understanding of common dangers.

Stress on the Family System

Family assessment includes information about current stressors and problems as well as about resources. The intense stress on the family system

of the severely disturbed child must be assessed as a critical factor. Often after a long and expensive search for someone to tell them what is wrong with their child, the parents are given a diagnosis that leaves them confused and with little hope. The parents of a severely disturbed child often experience guilt. Until recently the most common theory of autism placed the blame on the parents, and some health professionals still adhere solely to this theory. However, personal experience of this author suggests that the dysfunctional parent-child relationships often reported are reciprocal rather than etiological. As parents grow more perplexed and discouraged in trying to meet the needs of their disturbed child, their responses become less effective and less rational.

Because the severely disturbed child's behavior is bizarre and causes disruption and embarrassment, he/she is often kept at home. The result may be social isolation for the whole family. The family does not eat in restaurants because the disturbed child may scream and throw food. Even a drive in the family car involves some risk. Babysitters usually cannot handle these children; therefore, getting away for even a brief vacation becomes nearly impossible. Thus the family of a severely disturbed child often revolves around the needs and demands of that child. This has significant implications for all other relationships within that family system.

Formulation of Nursing Diagnoses

Some of the nursing diagnoses that are pertinent to the severely disturbed child are:

1. *Affective isolation* related to *inability to interact with others.*
2. *Impaired communication* related to *language confusion and/or distortion.*
3. *Ineffective individual coping* related to *need for sameness in environment.*
4. *Stereotyped, repetitive behaviors* related to *need for sensory stimulation by own body.*
5. *Tantrum behavior* related to *low frustration tolerance.*
6. *Potential for self-injury* related to *self-mutilating behaviors and sensory deficits.*
7. *Self-care deficits in activities of daily-living* related to *cognitive and affectional impairments.*

8. *Compromised family coping* related to *increased stress*.

Client-Care Goals and Related Nursing Interventions

Based on your nursing diagnoses, you are now able to formulate goals and to plan appropriate interventions.

Goals

1. *Child's self-stimulating and self-mutilating behaviors diminish.*
2. *Child begins to appropriately communicate feelings and thoughts verbally and nonverbally.*
3. *Child recognizes and responds as appropriate to own physiological needs.*
4. *Child develops appropriate play and self-care skills.*
5. *Child forms a satisfying relationship with one significant adult and begins to form attachments to others.*
6. *Child begins to engage in peer interaction.*

Interventions

Almost every form of treatment has been tried with these children, including behavior therapy, milieu therapy, psychotherapy, and chemotherapy. Behavior modification is currently the major therapeutic approach, although it is not a panacea (18, 39, 45). Reinforcement techniques are used to reduce disruptive behaviors and to teach more appropriate behaviors, with emphasis on teaching the skills of interpersonal relations.

Because of the inverse relationship between self-stimulating motor behavior and appropriate social, affective, and intellectual behavior, self-stimulating behaviors should be actively suppressed. This can be done by anticipating and intervening with alternative motor activities or patterns.

Various studies have demonstrated that the self-mutilation behavior demonstrated by severely disturbed children is a learned social behavior that disappears when ignored (45). Therefore, you should *cautiously* ignore this type of behavior, remembering that the safety of the child should never be jeopardized.

Establishing meaningful attending skills is a critical step in communication. One way of achieving this is to hold the child's hands and look straight into his/her eyes saying, "Look at me." When the child begins to attend, he/she is taught nonverbal behaviors (touching body parts, facial expressions, and gestures) and then verbal behaviors through imitation. Various discriminations are developed through reinforcement of responses.

When the disruptive behaviors are reduced and the child has a beginning repertoire of general imitative responses, all the normal behaviors that these children do not typically display—such as self-help skills, appropriate play with toys, and peer play—are taught. The process is the same as general behavior modification: specific target behavior is broken down and more normal behavior is shaped and reinforced. Throughout, the child needs a structured, secure environment; a sense of sameness contributes to more flexibility in behavior in the long run because a sense of trust and self-confidence is established.

Although there are few well-designed studies comparing drug therapy to other treatments, clinical experience has demonstrated that drugs can be a valuable adjunct in the total treatment plan of the severely disturbed child (9). Tranquilizers and antidepressants are used to improve the child's accessibility by reducing anxiety and disruptive behavior patterns.

Although shaping and reinforcement of behavior and use of medications can be effective in changing behavior, the child learns to emotionally relate to first one person and then to other people *only* if someone invests consistent caring attention, patience, affection, and love in the child. External behavior may change, but a positive change in feelings about self and other people does not come about from automatic or mechanized techniques. The child learns to be human (or a social being) through prolonged and intense emotional contact with another human. As a nurse, you may be the first caring, patient, attentive person that reaches the child on a feeling level as well as on a perceptual and behavioral level. Your use of the Humanistic Framework for nursing care must be combined with whatever other treatment techniques are used.

Goals

7. *Family develops affective coping skills to deal with increased stress.*
8. *Family utilizes appropriate support systems.*

Interventions

The most important interventions you can provide for the family of a seriously disturbed child are empathy, support, use of principles of therapeutic communication, and a helping relationship, discussed in Chapters 5 and 6. Listen empathetically, reduce guilt, and assist parents in clarifying and resolving their ambivalent feelings. Help them see any positive aspects in the child's behavior. Assist them to reinforce appropriate behavior and solve problems in areas they identify in order to better meet the needs of all family members. Assess dysfunctional parent-child dynamics and make appropriate referral for treatment. You are also in an excellent position to serve as a role model for effective communication with the child and family system.

Provide resource information to parents about respite homes that take care of severely disturbed children for a short period of time so parents can have occasional relief. Introduce them to parent groups such as the National Society for Autistic Children. Assist the family in finding suitable educational programs and explore with them the possibility of residential treatment when appropriate.

THE NURSING PROCESS WITH THE LEARNING DISABLED (LD) CHILD

Learning disability (LD) is a condition that makes the child and family vulnerable to additional problems. The term learning disability is often interchanged by professionals with multiple other labels such as "minimal brain dysfunction," "hyperactivity," and "learning dysfunction;" there is much disagreement about its definition. *Learning disability will be defined here as a significant discrepancy between expected and actual academic achievement in children who are not handicapped regarding general intelligence* (average, near average, or above average intelligence is present), *sensory processes, emotional stability, or the opportunity for learning*

When doing long-range planning with the family of a severely disturbed child an equation evolves. On one side is the strain that such a child puts on the family, and on the other side are the resources to cope with that strain. When the strain is greater than the resources, the equation must be rebalanced either by changing the child's behavior or by increasing resources. You as a nurse have much to offer on both sides.

Evaluation

Our understanding of childhood psychosis is still quite limited. A *combination* of behavior modification, chemotherapy, psychotherapy, and environmental structuring seems to be the preferred treatment, and nurses may be responsible for any of these modalities. Although even the most comprehensive treatment programs have produced few "cures," there does seem to be evidence that early therapeutic interventions, before maladaptive patterns are firmly established, are the most effective.

Evaluation needs to be systematic and programmed into your nursing care. When interventions do not achieve expected outcomes, reassess and/or alter interventions. Make allowances for the normal maturation process as well as for those deficits that cannot be corrected.

For a poignant account of the impact of a seriously disturbed child on his family we recommend the book *A Child Called Noah* (25).

(39). The academic skills referred to primarily include the basic skills of reading, writing, arithmetic, and spelling.

Learning disability is often due to a developmental delay in the area of receptive and expressive language (18). The diagnosis of learning disability is based on results of individually administered intelligence and achievement tests. This definition excludes the mentally retarded child, the emotionally disturbed child, the child with hearing and vision loss, and the environmentally deprived child.

Assessment

A conservative estimate is that 4 to 10 percent of the children in the United States are learning disabled (LD) (60).

Etiological Theories

The etiology responsible for learning disabilities is not proven. A diagnosis of LD is made only when there is no evidence of gross neurological impairment. The majority of the professionals in this field attribute learning disability to a minimal cerebral dysfunction, based on a group of behaviors often seen in the LD child (39). Experts have associated LD with a variety of prenatal, perinatal, postnatal, and psychological factors, including severe illness, injury, nutritional deficiencies, and quality of parent-child interactions. The electroencephalogram findings in LD children show an inconsistent increase in slow wave activity, and there are numerous soft neurological signs involving fine and gross motor deficits inconsistently present in LD children (60).

Characteristic Symptoms/ Behaviors

The LD child exhibits characteristics that are identifiable during the different stages of childhood (18, 36). The infant often exhibits restlessness, colic, sleep disturbances, a frequent high-pitched cry, disturbance in normal reflexes, and difficulty responding to the parent (36, 60). During the preschool and school years, the child may exhibit impaired coordination, especially with fine motor activities, such as printing, drawing, and cutting with a scissors (60). The preschooler may also be unable to inhibit activities and may react with a forced responsiveness at a point in time when he/she should have developed some internal controls and have differentiated between right and wrong (60).

Although the majority of authors in this field agree that a learning disability cannot be classified as a syndrome or a single pattern, they agree that LD children do exhibit very similar characteristics or behaviors, which are highly correlated (39, 60). These characteristics can be divided into five major areas: (1) lack of impulse control, (2) deficiency in cognitive processes, (3) motor dysfunctions, (4) poor interpersonal relationships, and (5) abnormal emotional reactivity (39, 55, 60).

Lack of impulse control

Lack of impulse control is the central aspect of a learning disability. The LD child is unable to inhibit a response and has a very low frustration tolerance level (60). These characteristics are also typical of the mentally retarded child so a differential diagnosis must be made. The LD child is unable to delay gratification and displays poor planning and a lack of foresight expected for the chronological age. Lack of attention to detail results in ineffective organizing of the environment, especially if structure is imposed by others. The LD child is usually very messy but becomes angry if someone else tries to organize or straighten the immediate environment, such as his/her room or possessions.

Difficulty in impulse control also results in antisocial behavior and destructiveness, an early sign of LD. He/she may frequently fight with others, break or destroy objects, lie, or steal. The motivation and quality of destructive behavior differ from that of the emotionally disturbed child because the LD child is not acting intentionally or with malice. Actions simply cannot be controlled. Lack of judgment and coordination problems may precipitate damage to objects and may involve fights with others. Stealing is not done for personal gain, and the stolen objects are not hidden. For example, the child may take pencils or erasers from the teacher's desk, where they are very visible and accessible, and not make any effort to hide them. Then he may lie to save face when accused of stealing or when questioned relentlessly about the objects. Fire-setting is another frequent behavior of this child, often occurring as a result of recklessness, clumsiness, and poor spatial concept, which may result, understandably, in overprotection on the part of the parents.

Deficiency in cognitive processes

Another major aspect of LD is a deficiency in cognitive processes manifested by high distractibility, inability to control or delay incoming environmental stimuli, and a very brief attention span (18, 39, 60). He/she depends on others to reduce environmental distractions and generally functions better in a structured environment.

The Stanford Binet Intelligence Test is utilized to diagnose LD in a child under six years of age, and the Wechsler Intelligence Test for Children (WISC) is utilized for older children. The LD child demonstrates excessive variation in abilities, and the verbal scale intelligence scores (I.Q.) on the Stanford Binet or WISC tend to be lower than the performance scale I.Q. scores (18, 60). These results correspond with the increased frequency of receptive and expressive language delays in LD children. Subtest scores on intelligence tests can be utilized to evaluate a child's strengths and weaknesses. However, test results may not be valid. This child is hard to test because of the short attention span and difficulty with sitting still during the tests.

Reading disability (dyslexia) is one of the most common forms of a learning disability, and perceptual-visual problems and short-term memory problems are also frequent (18, 39). Tests frequently utilized to assess visual perception include the Frostig Test, the Bender-Gestalt Test, and the Memory for Designs Test. The Berry is a visual motor test often utilized, which requires the child to duplicate various symbols, such as +, -, =, o, x, and 1. The Leiter Test, requiring no verbal instructions or responses, is most helpful in evaluating children with language dysfunctions. Instructions are demonstrated manually, and motor responses, such as arranging blocks in a certain pattern, are required. Auditory perception tests should also be done. If a learning disability is suspected, vision and hearing losses should first be ruled out (18, 39).

The mentally retarded child differs from the LD child regarding the variation of abilities. The mentally retarded child has a consistently low score on the I.Q. subtests in various skills, and a general I.Q. score of below 70. The LD child has a general I.Q. above 70, and a wide scattering of abilities. The mentally retarded child also has a significant impairment of daily living skills, such as feeding or dressing, assessed primarily through interview or by utilization of a scale such as the Vineland Social Maturity Scale.

Motor dysfunctions

Motor dysfunctions form a third problem area for the LD child. Much difficulty with gross motor coordination, such as walking or climbing, may exist. Fine motor incoordination is even more common, such as difficulty in cutting with a scissors, printing, fastening buttons, and tying shoelaces (39). Many of these children have left and right hand confusion. Also the LD child's general activity level is often either deficient or excessive. If the activity level is consistently excessive, especially during difficult tasks, and if he/she cannot inhibit motion or constantly shifts activities and fails to complete tasks, the child is described as *hyperactive* (39, 60). Internal body states such as fatigue, hunger, or a full bladder often precipitate a hyperactive response.

Poor interpersonal relationships

A fourth area of concern for the LD child is poor interpersonal relationships (39, 60). Friendships may be made easily, but temper outbursts cause loss of friends. The child tends to be controlling and bossy, prefers to play with younger children, and may be a loner, unconcerned about being separated from the parents even as a young toddler. Or he/she may be excessively dependent and clinging. He/she is often described as stubborn because of resistance to social demands. The child does not seem to learn from mistakes; punishment and reasoning do not have a noticeable effect. A low self-concept and a sense of inferiority develop as he/she perceives rejection by others (36, 39, 60).

Abnormal emotional reactivity

Abnormal emotional reactivity, either an inappropriate deficient or an excessively emotional response, is the fifth characteristic. Parents often report that their child has frequent mood swings and is very unpredictable or labile (20, 60). Characteristic feelings are excessive anxiety, being preoccupied with death or impending injury to self, complaints of not feeling well, appearing depressed, or having a decreased reaction to pain (60).

The multiple problems experienced by the LD child and his family are evident in the following case study:

Jeff is an eight-year-old boy with a diagnosis of LD who currently presents problems both at home and at school. At school he fails to complete tasks, exhibits a short attention span, and is restless. He is easily distracted by other children when he is doing schoolwork. He frequently leaves his seat and fidgets with papers and pencils, rather than working on the assigned tasks. His general intelligence level score is 95; his language skills are lower than his motor skills. Reading is his most difficult subject. He has no close friends, and often fights with other children at home and at school. He has been accused of stealing small items, such as erasers, from his peers. He makes no attempt to hide the items. His parents describe him as very moody or labile, and they complain that reasoning with him and punishing him are ineffective. Following a thorough psychological evaluation and testing, a recommendation was made to enroll Jeff in a class for LD children and to initiate family counseling.

Formulation of Nursing Diagnoses

Some of the nursing diagnoses that are pertinent to the learning disabled child are:

1. *Impaired verbal communication* related to *both expressive and receptive language delays.*
2. *Ineffective individual coping* related to *poor impulse control.*
3. *Potential for injury* related to *motor incoordination, distractibility, and hyperactivity.*
4. *Noncompliance with parental rules and with educational programs* related to *distractibility, attentional deficits, and forced responsiveness.*
5. *Disturbance in self-concept* related to *a sense of inferiority.*
6. *Social isolation* related to *frequent temper outbursts.*
7. *Compromised family coping* related to *increased stress of behavior and social problems of LD child.*
8. *Sensory perceptual alterations* related to *a possible cerbral dysfunction.*

Client-Care Goals and Related Nursing Interventions

Once the nursing diagnoses have been made on the basis of the nursing assessment, client-care goals should be identified. Nursing interventions are then planned in order to attain these goals. You may formulate other goals related to the child's specific behaviors and needs and to the family's concerns.

Goals

1. *Child's thoughts and needs are communicated either verbally or nonverbally.*
2. *Child's behavior and verbal expression indicate understanding of others' communication.*
3. *Planned health program is followed.*

Interventions

When a diagnosis of LD is suspected on the basis of language delays, you may be involved in both the hearing and vision screening as part of primary prevention and identification. Or you may be involved in the planning for or care of an LD child when he/she is hospitalized for further evaluation and testing or because of an illness. You may also be a member of a community or school diagnostic team, consisting of many professional disciplines, that evaluates developmentally delayed children.

Approach the child at the level of current functioning and not at the chronological age level. Demonstrations, diagrams, and visual aides will be helpful when teaching the LD child about health care. Directions should be simple and direct, and they may need to be repeated. Any health care teaching should be initiated in a setting with a minimum of distractions, isolated from the activities of others. The teaching sessions should be brief because of the child's short attention span. A return demonstration, utilizing appropriate medical equipment or teaching aides, and repeat of instructions by the child will clarify understanding and retention of the material presented.

Play therapy is another means of communicating with the child and facilitating his/her communication with you. Through play the child expresses feelings and ideas that cannot be stated directly because of language delays (16). Play therapy also provides a sense of control for the child and a means of working through anxiety about various interpersonal situations, illnesses, or other life conditions. You, as the child's nurse, may initiate play therapy on the basis of your frequent close contact and your nursing assessment of his/her needs. Provide an unstructured setting for play with a minimum of distraction, either in the child's room, or in another pleasant, nonthreatening location. Provide material to work with, such as dolls, puppets, models of hospital equipment, paper, crayons, pencils, paints, water, or cornmeal. Liquid or flexible media such as water and cornmeal, provide a form of mobility and the child feels that he/she is in control. Cups, straws, and sponges can be used for moving water or cornmeal and expressing feelings. The child may utilize the puppets, dolls, or drawings to act out perceptions of scenes or events from daily life (58). Explain to the child that he/she has freedom to play with the material as desired and that you will participate only as an observer unless your participation is invited. V. Axline is an excellent reference for additional information about play therapy (2). If the child is given the opportunity to express feelings about the treatment program, and if the program is presented in a manner that he/she understands, following through with the program is more likely to occur.

Goals

4. *Child's behavior and social contacts demonstrate ability to control some impulses and aggression through the use of effective coping mechanisms.*
5. *Child remains free from injury.*
6. *Child's behavior and statements reveal a positive self-concept.*
7. *Family demonstrates through verbalization and behaviors an acceptance of the LD child, including a realistic awareness of both his/her strengths and weaknesses.*
8. *Behavior and verbal expressions by family and child reflect a realization of the child's individual maximum potential for achievement.*

Interventions

The three primary methods of treatment for the LD child are drug therapy, behavior modification techniques, and educational specialization (39, 60).

Drug therapy

There is much disagreement about the benefit of drugs, and there is a variety of choices, ranging from stimulants, such as ritalin, to depressants, such as thorazine. Ritalin and other stimulants are frequently found to have a positive effect on the LD child, resulting in a generalized quieting, increased attention span, decreased distractibility, and improved self-control and social interactions (60). This should result in a decreased frequency of injuries as well as in better interpersonal relationships. You can instruct the family about expected positive effects and side effects associated with the specific medication and about any specific requirements for the administration of individual medications: for example, whether the drug should be

administered with or without foods, the duration of action, and the time of administration. If prescribed drugs do not appear to be giving the expected results, encourage the family to call the physician and persist until an effective medication routine is established.

Behavior modification

Operant conditioning is one of the behavior modification routines frequently utilized with positive results in LD children, and it is combined with special education techniques. By helping the family to assess the child's strengths as well as weaknesses, you may assist them in planning a program of positive reinforcement for their child's appropriate behavior. (See Chapter 2 for additional details.) This approach should result in fewer temper tantrums, improved social contacts, and a more positive feeling toward the child, so that his/her self-concept becomes more positive. The family should view the child as an individual, and positive reinforcers should be planned according to the individual's specific situation. You may act as a role model to demonstrate conditioning methods for behavior modification. You may also refer the family for counseling.

Additional guidelines that should be helpful to the family include the need for immediate rather than delayed reinforcement because of the child's low frustration tolerance. If a child takes belongings from others, direct parents, siblings, or teachers to remove tempting items from view. If the child does take something, do not ask, "Did you take it?" when that fact is already known. Avoid forcing the child to lie to save face. Established routines for daily living will be helpful in controlling anxiety related to a poor self-concept and poor self-control.

Educational specialization

Educational placement in a structured class for LD children is recommended because these children are unable to control environmental stimuli themselves. Individual educational plans (IEPs) and precise individual goals are necessary for each child, and success is measured by observed changes. The child benefits from the interaction with a teacher especially educated to work with this problem. Further, until the LD child is able to control behavior in a socially acceptable direction, the child benefits from not having to endure the taunts and rejection from healthy children in a regular classroom.

Throughout your contact with the LD child and family, your empathy and relationship are important. The parents and siblings experience much frustration and disappointment with this type of child; often family life is disrupted by the child's behavior. It takes more than medications to help the child live in a socially acceptable way. Listen to and help the family members work through their feelings. Reaffirm that they are doing the best possible with the child. Avoid criticism. Acknowledge any behavior or characteristics of the child that are positive and lovable. Reaffirm ways that the family members can remain patient and consistent in their guidance and care of the child. If you remain as a supportive person, the family members can in turn be more supportive to the child and to each other.

THE NURSING PROCESS WITH THE MENTALLY RETARDED (MR) CHILD AND ADOLESCENT

Mental retardation is defined by the American Association on Mental Deficiency (AAMD) *as significantly subaverage general intellectual functioning that exists along with deficits in adaptive and developmental behavior* (39). I.Q. is measured by standardized individual intelligence tests, such as the Stanford Binet or the Wechsler. An intelligence score (I.Q.) of below 70 is not enough to diagnose mental retardation. The child/adolescent under eighteen years of age must also be below normal in interpersonal skills and self-help skills, compared to peers. These adaptive skills are often assessed by means of interviewing the child's caretaker and by using a scale, such as the Vineland Social Maturity Scale or the AAMD Adaptive Behavior Scale, which evaluate the child's usual behavioral level skills. The intellectual and adaptive behavior levels usually correlate well with each other.

Assessment

Three percent of all Americans are estimated to be mentally retarded (39). The causes of mental re-

Evaluation

The entire family of an LD child is affected by his/her behavior and reactions. Therefore involve both the child and family in evaluation of the effectiveness of the plan in order to meet needs and in determining if behavior is improved. The family's feedback can help you and other team members decide if maximum individual potential for achievement and self-satisfaction has been reached. If the child's behavior is considered more appropriate in most situations than previously, intervention can be considered effective. The goals will not be accomplished quickly; time and repetition will be needed to accomplish them.

Although the same interventions may accomplish several goals, realize that you may accomplish only one or two goals at a time and then later you may accomplish additional goals with persistent use of the same nursing interventions or with the family's continued love and consistent care to the child.

tardation are many and varied, including genetic, prenatal, perinatal, and postnatal physical factors, such as chromosomal disorders; malnutrition; viral and bacterial infections; anorexia; lead poisoning; and head injuries. Thus frequently physical/congenital anomalies exist concurrently with mental retardation. Environmental and psychological factors that also have an important causative effect on mental retardation include sensory deprivation and frequent variable changes in environmental stimulation (18). The sensory deprivation may be related to impaired hearing or vision or to decreased environmental stimulation (36). However, all children who have impaired hearing or vision are not mentally retarded.

I.Q. scores resulting from standardized intelligence tests form the basis for the AAMD four classification levels for mental retardation. Mental retardation (MR) is diagnosed when the score is more than two standard deviations below the average I.Q. score of 100. Table 21-2 classified these four levels according to the 1973 AAMD.

Approximately 90 percent of all MR children fall in the mild retardation category (39). They are

TABLE 21-2.   Levels of Retardation

LEVELS OF RETARDATION	INTELLIGENCE (I.Q.) SCORE		PROJECTED MENTAL AGE AS ADULTS
	Stanford Binet or Cattel	*Wechsler*	
Mild	68–52	69–55	6–10 years
Moderate	51–36	54–40	2– 6 years
Severe	35–20	39–25	2– 6 years
Profound	19 and below	24 and below	0– 2 years

usually not diagnosed until they are of school age, and they achieve the optimal functioning level of the six- to ten-year-old. They are classified as "educable," and their special education classes focus on basic learning skills of reading, writing, and arithmetic. They often marry, function independently as adults, and hold unskilled labor jobs.

The moderately retarded or trainable child has more difficulty with basic school subjects than the mildly retarded. Therefore, special education classes focus on learning self-help skills rather than academic skills. This child may have more motor coordination problems and more physical abnormalities than the mildly retarded.

Some of the children in the severe range of retardation may also be considered trainable. Others may learn only minimal self-help skills. The profoundly retarded child often requires constant supervision or institutionalization and may be unable to ambulate without assistance due to sensory, motor, or central nervous system disabilities. The care of the moderately, severely, and profoundly retarded child continues through the lifetime of the person. With better medical care today, even the profoundly retarded live into adulthood.

The MR child may have behavior and personality characteristics similar to the normal child of the same chronological age. However, he/she appears to be at an increased risk for developing personality and emotional instability as a result of the interaction between intellectual limitations and input from social interactions (44, 65).

The child's basic central nervous system disorder frequently precipitates behaviors such as irritability, hypersensitivity to environmental stimulation, motor hyperactivity, short attention span, poor impulse control, and frequent acting out or temper tantrums (65). Problems in making and maintaining friends may result from reduced cognitive functioning. Rejection by others or a perception of disappointing others may cause a low self-esteem and excessive dependency (44). Self-concept is dependent on interaction with others, which may be impaired by disabilities in areas of sensory, motor, or integrative functioning, resulting in poor reality perception or increased fantasizing.

Because parents are the child's primary social contact, their reaction to and influence on the child are vital to development. Parents may react to the initial diagnosis of a MR child with shame, a sense of failure, guilt, anger, frustration, depression, denial, or fear (40, 44, 65). If the parent rejects the child and gives inadequate nurturing, the child's development is affected. Also if the parent reacts by overprotecting the child or by placing excessive demands on siblings for the care of the child, the child may be unable to develop to an optimal level of independence, and further stress is placed on the family system. The MR child who develops psychopathology demonstrates a typical personality profile: autism, passivity, inflexibility, immaturity, and deficiency in ego function (65). Parents may express anger and a sense of being overwhelmed when they realize that the child's condition will never change appreciably. Parents may be able to enjoy the educable child, but the child who becomes an adolescent and adult only in chronological years continues to present social, health care, and financial challenges and concerns to the parents. The emotional stresses involved for parents and siblings can be lifelong, and they need ongoing support from you and other significant people.

See Chapter 12 for additional information about the reactions to and care of a person with a chronic condition.

The multiple problems facing the MR child and his/her family are characterized in the following case study:

> Cathy is an eight-year-old girl with a diagnosis of Down's Syndrome. Her general I.Q. on the Stanford Binet is 40, which places her in the moderate range of retardation. The subtests were consistently below normal. Cathy requires assistance with daily living skills, such as dressing, fastening clothing, and cutting food with a knife. She was toilet-trained at age four, and her developmental milestones of sitting, crawling, walking, and language development were delayed. She is generally a friendly child, but she requires parental assistance with controlling frequent temper outbursts caused by a low frustration tolerance. She is enrolled in a public special education class for the mentally retarded. The outlook is that she will always require assistance with activities of daily living and supervision to maintain basic social skills.

Formulation of Nursing Diagnoses

Some of the nursing diagnoses that relate to the MR child are:

1. *Impaired verbal communication* related to *general intelligence deficiency.*
2. *Ineffective individual coping* related to *low frustration tolerance.*
3. *Compromised family coping* related to *both physical disabilities and behavioral dysfunctions.*
4. *Impaired physical mobility* related to *physical disabilities (frequently present in the severely and profoundly retarded child and may be found in all levels of retardation).*
5. *Self-care deficit in activities of daily living* related to *developmental motor delays and excessive dependency.*
6. *Disturbance in self-concept* related to *low self-esteem and frequent sense of failure.*
7. *Potential for injury* related to *motor coordination problems.*
8. *Social isolation* related to *rejection by peers.*

These nursing diagnoses are often compounded by a knowledge deficit in the public about etiological risk factors for MR.

Client-Care Goals and Related Nursing Interventions

Every child should have the opportunity to develop to his/her maximum potential; thus developmental delays should be identified early. You can assist with primary prevention, early case finding, and home management (36). As a community health nurse, obstetric nurse, or pediatric nurse, you have numerous opportunities to educate the public about the necessity and purpose of routine prenatal and pediatric follow-up, the importance of adequate prenatal nutrition, and the dangers of specific illness, such as rubella during pregnancy and lead poisoning during childhood, which can cause MR in the child. As the pediatric nurse or community health nurse, you also have excellent opportunities to detect delayed development in young children and to refer them for intervention to prevent further damage. Developmental screening tests and evaluation of developmental milestones may be utilized to facilitate early detection of delayed development. Thorough nursing histories and assessments may help identify conditions such as phenylketonuria, hypothyroidism, hearing and language delays, and mobility problems. Early referrals for diagnosis and treatment can minimize developmental delays. The first three years of life are most important for optimal development, but mental retardation is often not detected until school age (36). Further, the person who is mentally retarded may also be mentally ill, so he/she needs care for the illness. Often differential diagnosis is difficult, but depression or withdrawal, for example, is not part of mild or moderate retardation. The person who is less retarded can relate to others in a harmonious way. Explore with parents how to adjust the home environment and schedule to meet the developmental needs of the child as well as the needs of other family members.

After identification of nursing diagnoses, client-care goals and interventions can be planned as discussed below. You may formulate other goals for specific children in your care.

Goals

1. *Child's behavior and expressions reveal a positive self-esteem.*
2. *Family's priorities, decisions, and behavior indicate that it considers both the needs of the MR child and of other family members.*

Interventions

Home management as a nursing role can begin when the child is born. You are in a position to support the family and assist them in expressing and working through feelings about a diagnosis of MR. Accept the initial denial that may be expressed. Remain realistic about the diagnosis, which will help the parents come to accept it. Refer them to supportive agencies, such as Down's Syndrome Association or the local chapter of the Association for Retarded Children. Most parents react to the birth of the MR child by first grieving over the loss of the anticipated normal child. If the parents continues to reject the child, this results in a poor self-concept in the child as well as a sense of shame in the family. Help the family through the grieving process. Provide opportunities for members to ventilate their feelings. Evaluate and work through your own feelings about the MR child. Your acceptance of the child as a person of worth is conveyed to the child and parents. Patience, support, and being realistic are important in working with the child and family (36, 64).

Goals

3. *Child's behavior and verbal expressions indicate realization of the individual maximum potential for achievement.*
4. *Parents' behavior and statements demonstrate realistic, appropriate expectations for the child's capacity to learn or achieve.*
5. *Child's behavior and daily living activities reveal that he/she is functioning as independently as possible within individual limits.*
6. *Child's daily activity schedule demonstrates participation in normal society to the extent possible.*
7. *Child's aggressive, hostile impulses are controlled, and effective coping mechanisms are demonstrated.*

Interventions

Help parents work with the other children in the family and with each other to meet needs of all members of the family rather than focusing only on the retarded child. The potential of normal offspring should not be compromised for that of the retarded child, just as the retarded child should not

be neglected. Support from friends, relatives, teachers in special education, and health care professionals can help the family remain a close working unit that develops the potential of each member.

Work with the family in realistically determining the child's strengths and weaknesses and in creating an environment that will reinforce independence, aid in impulse control, and enable the child to socialize with others. A loving environment, behavior modification methods, and some structuring of the physical setting may aid in developing impulse control and in controlling temper tantrums. Help the family members work through feelings about societal reactions to, and expectations about, the child's and their own behavior. You can be a model for providing stimulation and in utilizing appropriate control measures to handle behavior problems. Assist the family in teaching activities of daily living, such as feeding, dressing, and toileting skills, to the retarded child. Encourage the family members to avoid making the child overdependent on them when he/she is capable of doing the task.

Other health professionals are often involved in working with the families of MR children, including the speech therapist; occupational, vocational, recreational, and physical therapists; and the special education teacher. You, as the community mental health nurse, may act as a coordinator of care among these various professionals.

Goal

8. *Child communicates verbally or nonverbally and demonstrates some understanding of other's communication.*

Intervention

You may utilize play therapy to aid in encouraging self-expression because language delays often predominate. See the section on learning disabilities (pp. 664–665) for further information on play therapy as a tool to facilitate communication.

Evaluation

Evidence of change is often slow and requires much patience in the parents, siblings, other relatives, and health professionals involved. The efforts of daily teaching often result in frustration. The family continues to require much support and patience from the nurse. All health team members and family members who are involved in the care of the child must perceive and reinforce the small steps in developmental progress so that achievements are maintained over time.

The moderately, severely, or profoundly retarded child may be placed in an institution by the family who is unable to provide care. Do not feel your intervention was unsuccessful. Do not be judgmental. Rather, your assistance in helping the family clarify their needs, values, and goals can result in the best plan for all concerned. Your ongoing support may enable the family to remain in contact with the institutionalized child. Some institutions have foster grandparent programs that can be very supportive to and successful with the children.

THE NURSING PROCESS WITH THE CHILD WITH SCHOOL PHOBIA

School phobia, the fearful avoidance of school attendance, is a common problem among school-age children and involves dynamics that are deeper than that child wanting to miss a day of school.

Assessment

Some children show an extreme reluctance to go to school because of severe anxiety and an expressed dread of some aspect of the school situation. Frequently these children are afraid of separation from home rather than fearful of school itself. The parent-child relationship often reveals an intense bond with a fear of separation on both sides. L. Eisenberg's classic analogy, the umbilical cord pulls at both ends (13), describes the intense, mutual dependency between parent and child. The school-phobic child gets mixed messages: "I want you to go to school, but if you do not feel well you can come home. You know I am lonely, but you should go to school." The usual reasons for keeping the child home from school are somatic complaints, including headache, abdominal pain, tiredness, joint pain, vomiting, and diarrhea. A complete physical assessment to rule out organic cause should be done as soon as a pattern of these complaints, accompanied by frequent absences from school, is detected.

Some children express school anxiety because of particular situational problems at school. For these children, resolution of the particular situation will usually solve the problem.

Nursing Diagnoses

Some of the nursing diagnoses that are pertinent to the child with a school phobia are:

1. *Anxiety reaction* related to *fear of separation from home.*
2. *Disturbed self-concept* related to *overdependence on parents.*
3. *Impaired parent-child relationship* related to *ambivalent feelings about child's dependency.*

Client-Care Goals and Related Nursing Interventions

Based on your nursing diagnoses, you are able to formulate nursing goals and to plan interventions. Other goals may be pertinent to specific children and family situations.

Goals

1. *Child returns to school.*
2. *Child demonstrates a gradual reduction in manifest anxiety.*
3. *Parents demonstrate a reduction in ambivalent behaviors regarding separation.*

Interventions

P. Nadar (50) and D. Gelfand (22) have shown that the most effective treatment for school phobia is forced school attendance in conjunction with family counseling, although not all experts agree with forced school attendance. If the child is allowed to stay home, the dread of going to school is usually increased. Prepare the child for going to school one day at a time. Empathy, but firmness, should be conveyed. The parent can say, "I know it is hard, but you can go to school." It is important that parents reinforce this message by recognizing physical complaints while they simultaneously take the child to school. Give both the child and parent positive reinforcement for school attendance rather than staying home.

Working with the family system is of critical importance. You will often find that it is less difficult for the child to go to school than it is for the parent to let him/her go to school. Assist parents in recognizing and exploring their own feelings. You can say, "It is frightening for you to have him (her) go off to school. You feel lonely without the child." Explore anxiety about the child's safety and other problems. Help the mother cope with immediate separation by encouraging her to use available support systems, for example, phoning a friend after the child leaves for school. Make a referral for continued counseling when appropriate.

School authorities and the teacher must be involved in the treatment plan from beginning to end or it will not be effective. Conflicting expectations between home and school must be resolved. Include the school nurse in the treatment plan. School phobia is best treated while the child is young and before school absence has become prolonged. As a nurse oriented towards health and who understands the dynamics of mutual dependency, you are the ideal person to help the child and family. You serve as a visible bridge between home and the teacher and school administration and as a support to both the parent and child.

Evaluation

Your support, counseling, and reinforcement to parents and child have been effective when the child can attend school regularly, without physical complaints, and when he/she interacts with peers and teacher in ways to ensure school success. Also, you can evaluate that the parents no longer give the child a double message of "stay at home and go to school," and that they have overcome anxiety about the separation and are able to anticipate future separations as part of the developmental tasks for themselves and the child.

THE NURSING PROCESS WITH THE CHILD OR ADOLESCENT WITH ANOREXIA NERVOSA

Anorexia nervosa is a disorder of eating precipitated by mother-daughter conflicts, problems in self-image, separation from home, or traumatic events such as sexual encounters. The condition affects adolescent females. The client sees herself as being obese or as unworthy of food and decreases the intake of food until there is a profound weight loss with accompanying physical symptoms. At times the decreased eating is a way to gain attention or to control others. The disordered eating often continues on into adulthood, although weight may be stabilized. Many types of treatment ranging from psychotherapy to behavior modification have been used with the anorexia nervosa client with varying degrees of success. The disorder has been known for many years, although at present its incidence seems to be increasing. Up to 15 percent of all cases die of malnutrition, and some are suicidal (65).

Assessment

Anorexia nervosa is considered a psychosomatic illness, and it can be fatal, usually because of infection. In this client there is no known medical illness that accounts for the anorexia or weight loss. Thyroid function and adrenal cortical function are normal. Usually there is no other psychiatric illness. The criteria often used for diagnosis include the following (52):

1. Under 25 years of age.
2. Anorexia with weight loss of 20-25 percent or more of total body weight or a weight 20-25 percent below average for age-appropriate height.
3. Distorted attitude toward eating, food, or weight that overrides hunger and reason, including denial of pleasure, increased pleasure in losing weight, a desired body image of thinness, and unusual hoarding or handling of food.
4. At least two of the following signs or symptoms are present:
   a. Bulimia (increase in the sensation of hunger), often accompanied by feeling of fullness after a small intake of food.
   b. Lanugo (fine, downy hair covering the body).

c. Amenorrhea and sexual organ atrophy.
d. Periods of overactivity.
e. Bradycardia (pulse less than 60 per minute).
f. Vomiting (after eating).
g. Use of large amounts of laxatives.

The client is most often a teen-age girl who is usually a good student but has lost interest in attending school. Since the illness is often long-term, it can have serious physical, emotional, and educational ramifications during this crucial developmental period. Dieting usually begins spontaneously, but weight loss goes far beyond expectations. There is often obsessive thoughts about food and its preparation. Although the client may weigh well below 100 pounds and look emaciated, she does not see herself as appearing particularly thin. About 50 percent of all anorexics are liable to overestimate both their own body size and the size of others (26).

The client eats only a very small amount of food daily and feels "full" after only a few bites. The diet may include only a small selection of food, and fluids may be limited. Binge eating may occur occasionally wherein large amounts are eaten. Then vomiting is induced, as the client feels guilty for eating. Self-induced vomiting may become a regular practice and allows the client to eat at the urging of others, especially parents, yet not gain weight.

Physical symptoms that may occur as a result of the weight loss include muscular weakness as the body breaks down stored proteins for energy and changes in sleep patterns such as early morning awakening. There may be changes in blood composition, including anemia, feelings of being cold, cyanosis, dry hands and feet, lanugo, constipation, and hypotension (26). Typical lab values show leukopenia, anemia, hypoglycemia, hypercholesterolemia, lowered basal metabolic rate, and reduced gonadotropins (65). An increase in activity may be a means of increasing weight loss. A vigorous exercise routine may be initiated and strictly adhered to, although the exercise is usually done in isolation.

The client often withdraws from previous social contact, rejecting friendships, becoming withdrawn, and losing interest in hobbies or other activities.

Psychodynamics reveal that this condition involves more than its physical manifestations. Often a sense of trust has not been firmly established. The marriage relationship in the family of a client with anorexia nervosa is often not satisfying. The parents may involve the daugher in this conflictual relationship as a way of avoiding or suppressing their own dissatisfactions. By focusing on the daughter's anorexia, emphasis is removed from the marriage relationship. The adolescent involved in the family conflict does not want to achieve womanhood with the potential of becoming embroiled in the same kind of relationship her parents have. As the onset of menstruation and the development of body contours signal the development of womanhood, dieting is begun. In order to control personal sexual desires and interests and sexual responses from others, the client maintains control over her body. There is an identity struggle. Dieting becomes an area over which the client has control and therefore feels she has an identity.

In the client with anorexia nervosa, three areas of disordered psychological function are often found. The first area is a disturbance of delusional proportions in the body image and body concept. The emaciated appearance is viewed as being normal, and the person strives to maintain it. A change in this body image must occur in order to achieve long-term progress in stabilizing weight at a safe level. A second disturbance is in the accuracy of the perception of stimuli arising in the body, particularly the stimuli of hunger. Hunger is denied, yet there are constant thoughts of food. The client "feels" full after only a few bites or feels once she starts eating she will be unable to stop. When gorging occurs, followed by self-induced vomiting, there is a feeling of total lack of control, which further threatens identity. The third area of psychological maladaptation is the client's feeling of ineffectiveness or of acting only in response to others instead of doing what she wants to do. The stubbornness often seen can be a camouflage for the sense of helplessness that is felt. Clients with anorexia nervosa often have been very obedient children, and the onset of adolescence with its development of independence seems to generate overwhelming fears of losing control (8).

Formulation of Nursing Diagnoses

Nursing diagnoses based on your assessment, which are relevant to the client with anorexia nervosa, are:

1. *Ineffective individual coping* related to *a loss of self-control.*

2. *Nutritional deficiencies* related to *inadequate intake of food.*

3. *Disturbance in self-concept* related to *inaccurate perception of self as obese.*

4. *Potential for self-injury* related to *excessive weight loss.*

5. *Sexual dysfunction of amenorrhea* related to *excessive weight loss.*

6. *Decreased cardiac output* related to *excessive weight loss.*

7. *Potential for fluid volume deficit and electrolyte imbalance* related to *vomiting and excessive weight loss.*

8. *Sleep pattern disturbance* related to *anxiety over weight status.*

9. *Impairment of muscular strength* related to *excessive weight loss.*

10. *Potential for impairment of skin integrity* related to *dry skin and lanugo.*

11. *Alteration in bowel elimination (constipation)* caused by *deficient food and fluid intake.*

12. *Social isolation and fear of sexuality* related to *poor self-image.*

13. *Compromised family coping* related to *marital discord.*

14. *Client's perceptual alterations* related to *body states, especially that of hunger.*

Client-Care Goals and Related Nursing Interventions

Based on your nursing diagnoses, you are now able to plan client goals and interventions. You may formulate additional goals specific to your client.

Goals

1. *Client's behavior and verbalizations express ability to form trusting relationships with others.*

Intervention

Of major importance is the development of a trusting relationship between the client and the nurse who will be consistently caring for the client. You can achieve this goal by being honest and dependable when working with the client. Development of trust requires time and patience on your part and a genuine concern for the client's welfare. Refer to Chapter 6 for further information on the helping relationship and on promoting trust and emotional development in the client.

Goals

2. *Client's weight is stabilized within normal limits.*

3. *Client's behavior and statements indicate sense of self-control.*

4. *Client's perceptions regarding body stimuli, such as hunger, are accurate or appropriate, as revealed by appropriate eating patterns and behavior.*

Interventions

Treatment for the client with anorexia nervosa ranges from psychoanalytically oriented therapy to a stringent behavior modification program, which is usually most effective when initiated in a hospital setting (65). Although the goal is to gain weight, the inappropriate eating habits that have been learned and that have been a major source of intrinsic reward must be altered. The program is initiated with the client having no privileges; privileges are gained as weight is gained, thereby indirectly rewarding appropriate eating habits. Privileges are lost as weight is lost. Thus the client maintains some control over the food eaten and the privileges gained. The feeling of being in control is very important to the client. Within the framework of a trusting relationship, you can deal with such factors as the client's anxiety over weight gain and necessary supervision of the client during and after meals or when the client is suspected of hoarding food.

In a behavior modification program, you have a major role in planning and implementation. Remain firm in carrying out the necessary supervision. The anorexic client develops multiple and varied methods to avoid food intake. She dawdles at mealtime, eating very slowly, or she attempts to maneuver staff by talking or crying, thereby removing the focus from her eating habits. Duration of the meal should be limited to prevent dawdling, and the client should eat alone. Check to see that the diet is appropriate, nutritious, and pleasing in appearance. Supervise her on a one-to-one basis during meals. She may hide food to avoid eating, or she may hoard food in order to gorge herself later and then induce vomiting (65). Her food choices are often inappropriate, and she may try to over-exercise to burn up excess calories. Supervise her on a one-to-one basis for at least 30 minutes follow-ing meals, checking to see that food is not hidden or given away to others, and that vomiting is not induced. Restrict bathroom privileges and oppor-tunity for exercise after meals. Chart her activity level frequently and weigh her at least once weekly at the same time of the day and with the same clothing. Do not attempt to use logic to convince her to eat. She is not ready to voluntarily change her eating habits at this time.

Other programs allow the client more control within reasonable limits (32), especially when the client is treated in the home. These programs advo-cate ignoring the client when she sneaks food, re-fuses meals, or vomits. Food intake is not charted daily, and activity limits are not set.

Goals

5. *Client's behavior and statements demonstrate a realistic, positive self-concept and body image.*
6. *Client's social relationships with peers indicate normal behavioral development.*
7. *Family members demonstrate appropriate cop-ing mechanisms by their behavior and verbali-zations.*

Interventions

Family therapy may be initiated on the basis of a nursing referral to help the family members deal with their problems concerning the client as well as to help the parents develop a more normal marriage relationship (see Chapter 10). Some com-munities have anorexia nervosa societies that serve as support groups for clients and families. This also provides an opportunity for peer relationship development. The address of the national society is:

Anorexia Nervosa and Associated Disorders
Suite 2020
550 Frontage Road
Northfield, Illinois 60093

When working with the anorexic client in the hospital, assist the parents in working through overwhelming guilt feelings about their child's debilitated condition. Teach them how to appro-priately show their caring and how to reinforce their daughter's appropriate behavior.

You also have a major role in helping the client to develop appropriate coping mechanisms and in developing a positive self-image. The hospitalized client often becomes angry over her loss of auton-omy over food, and she is ambivalent much of the time. You need to clearly present the treatment plan to her; remain consistent and firm and avoid arguing over the fairness or the rules of the plan once it has been presented (32, 65).

Provide positive reinforcement for the client and ample opportunity for peer relationships through activities, such as recreational or occupa-tional therapy to promote a positive self-image and social and emotional coping skills (64).

Acknowledge the client's defense mechanisms of denying that any problem exists and of placing her entire focus on eating. Deemphasize the focus on eating, thereby minimizing the gains that she receives from fasting. Convey an interest in her as an individual, unrelated to food, and concentrate on the present and the reality of daily activities, rather than theorizing with her about the psycho-logical meaning of her behavior (65). You can do this by approaching her with positive activities based on her own interests rather than nagging her to get out of bed or to get involved. This approach will facilitate the development of a posi-tive self-image. The anorexic client is often distant, superficial, and manipulative (65). This client needs a primary nurse, that is, the same nursing care-taker over a period of time, as well as open staff communication in order to avoid staff manipula-tion by the client (32). The care approach must be consistently implemented by all health team mem-bers involved with this person.

Goal

8. *Client demonstrates improved physical condi-tion and appearance.*

Intervention

The client suffering from anorexia nervosa often has dry skin and dry hair, skin breakdown, and unstable vital signs. Safety practices are neces-sary if hypotension is severe. Monitor vital signs regularly while she is hospitalized. Discourage daily baths and hair washing, and instruct her to massage skin with lanolin, particularly over bony prominences (65). Adequate food and fluid intake will correct physical problems.

Evaluation

Just because a safe level of weight has been obtained does not mean a long-term cure has been secured. The client may still have disordered eating patterns, particularly gorging and then induced vomiting. The client may have gained weight in order to please you or the parents, but the problems that engendered the eating habits may still be present. Evaluation of the effectiveness of your nursing interventions is based on achievement of the identified goals. A continuing trust relationship, behavior modification program, and counseling are vital to the achievement and maintenance of these goals for the child with anorexia nervosa and for her family.

THE NURSING PROCESS WITH THE ABUSED CHILD AND ADOLESCENT

Child abuse is defined by the Federal Child Abuse Prevention and Treatment Act (Public Law 93-247), which states, *"Child abuse and neglect mean the physical or mental injury, sexual abuse, negligent treatment or maltreatment of the child, under the age of eighteen years, by a person who is responsible for the child's welfare under circumstances which indicate that the child's health or welfare is harmed or threatened thereby."*

Assessment

Remember that not only young children are abused. The schoolchild and adolescent may also be victims of abuse, and the abuse may have started in infancy. Child abuse is currently regarded as the greatest single contributor to childhood deaths (43). Child abuse crosses all economic, racial, and class barriers. The distinguishing feature in child abuse is the abuser's attitude toward discipline and child rearing (30). The abuser was often abused as a child. He/she did not receive mothering and was not provided with a good parental model. Thus the same harsh forms of discipline are used on his/her children that were received from his/her parents. (An example of identification with the aggressor.) Expectations for the child's behavior, appropriate to the ego, are often unrealistic; the child is supposed to act like an adult. The disciplinary measures are usually inconsistent in mode and in relation to the degree of the behavioral offense. A typical example of an unrealistic expectation is a parent who is attempting to toilet-train a one-year-old child. The child is not physically or mentally prepared for this task, but the parent views the child as being stubborn, bad, or deliberately malicious when he/she fails to comply with the toilet training and so is punished for the lack of compliance. Further, the child is seen as existing primarily to please and meet the demands of the parents.

There are three components necessary for child abuse to occur: the potential abuser, the potential child, and the stress or crisis (37). Eighty-seven percent of the abusers are parents or parent substitutes (23). There is a high proportion of abuse in one-parent families, often in female-headed households, and less than 10 percent of the parental abusers are psychotic (37). The majority of the parents wanted the children prior to birth, but they wanted them for the wrong reasons, such as satisfying their own unmet needs for love. The potential abuser usually has a low self-esteem, is immature, self-centered, and impulsive. There is often a poor relationship between the child's parents, which contributes to an inadequate support system and a sense of isolation. These parents are very vulnerable to criticism due to their low self-esteem, and they often feel threatened by outside agencies. Therefore they have much difficulty in seeking help, which increases their isolation. Misuse of alcohol or of drugs is often a characteristic of child abusers.

The abused child (usually only one in a family is singled out) often reminds the parent of him/herself as he/she sees self reflected in the child's personal faults. The parent may also endow the child with the spouse's shortcomings, and the child then becomes a scapegoat for the angry feelings directed toward the spouse. The child may be perceived and described as "different" or "bad." The abused child often appears fearful, wary of physical contact, and apprehensive when other children cry. The child has not learned to trust because needs have not been met by others. In fact, the child may appear overprotective and comforting toward the parents because he/she has been expected to meet their needs rather than receiving comfort from them. The abused child may be well-fed and clothed or may be undernourished and inadequately dressed. An example of this is a child found in an unheated building in freezing weather, wearing only a diaper, and hungrily crying because he/she has not been fed that day. The abused child may cry often and hopelessly, increasing the parent's sense of inadequacy regarding his/her personal ability to satisfy the child's needs.

Premature infants, ill newborns, and mentally retarded, handicapped, and hyperactive children are at an increased risk of being abused because of the increased demands on the parents and the elevated stress level. Even the gifted child may be abused because he/she is a threat to the parents. Abused children also have an increased incidence of delays in motor and language development due to their initial inability to complete the task of developing trust. The abused child is often aggressive, unresponsive, or negativistic, and exhibits low self-esteem and self-destructive behavior because he/she has identified with the aggressor, the parent (24).

When a child is brought to a hospital or to a physician for treatment for an injury, the parent may blame someone else, such as sibling or even the injured child, explaining that the child is clumsy. However, there is often a discrepancy between the history given of how the injury occurred and the actual clinical findings, for example, a toddler falling from a couch and fracturing a femur. It is very important to compare the child's age and developmental level with the size, shape, and location of bruises, burns, and wounds, and with the type of fracture or injury. The following injuries are typical evidence of abuse in young children:

1. Bilateral facial bruises or hand prints.
2. Finger-tip bruises around the elbows or knees where the child was grasped or shaken.
3. Cuts, scratches, bruises, and puncture wounds in different stages of healing.
4. Evidence of numerous scars, poor hygiene, and general neglect.
5. Teeth marks.
6. Cigarette burns.

7. Bilateral scaldings of lower limbs below the buttocks as a result of immersion.
8. Tears of the upper lip resulting from forcing a bottle or striking the child's mouth.
9. Subdural hematoma resulting from shaking an infant.
10. Bilateral skull fracture in an infant under one year of age.
11. Spiral fracture of the long bones in infants under six months of age.
12. Avulsion fracture.
13. More than one fracture in different stages of healing.
14. Posterior rib fractures that are unaccounted for, with no history of a car accident or other obvious cause.
15. Fractures simultaneously existing in siblings of the injured child.
16. History of failure to thrive or repeated attempts of poison ingestion in the same child.

Physical abuse of the older schoolchild and adolescent may include some of the above signs and symptoms. But instead of fractures, the main signs may be extreme underweight, lethargy, and persistent fatigue and drowsiness related to lack of sleep, muscular tremors or tics, nightmares, flinching from physical contact, or a pregnancy that results from incest. The abused child/adolescent may seek relief through use of alcohol or drugs or staying away from home as much as possible.

Emotional and sexual abuse of the school-age child and adolescent are more difficult to detect unless there is gross psychopathology or pregnancy. Thus it is often the subtle signs that are significant: the general mistrust of people; the withdrawal from peers and adults; preoccupation with self, a pet, or some object; and/or lack of involvement in school or other age-appropriate activities. School truancy problems may be present, although sometimes this person excels in school by overcompensating for the home situation. This young person may attempt, or be successful, in running away from home. Or in an attempt to find love and security, this adolescent may marry early or live with another; these relationships usually fail also. Adult psychopathology may be the result.

The parent may delay in reporting the child's injuries, or may completely fail to report injuries or behavioral changes. A humanogram, an overall

X-ray of the body, is utilized to detect previously unreported fractures in various stages of healing. Parents who repeatedly bring the child to the emergency room for no apparent reason, seeking assistance for minor ailments, should be regarded as sending out a plea for help.

The crisis or stress in the family that precipitates the child abuse may be major, such as a divorce or separation, unemployment, illness, or a death in the family. It may appear to be an insignificant problem to others, such as a broken television, an argument, or the adolescent asking for additional privileges, but for that particular parent at that point in time, it represents a crisis! The stress usually contributes to the parent's sense of isolation, and displacement of feelings into abuse of the child (24).

The following case study illustrates some of the factors involved in child abuse:

> Brian C. is a ten-month-old boy admitted to a pediatric hospital unit with a fractured femur. His father and mother are nineteen years old, and his father recently lost his job. They have no close family members or friends in this city. Mr. C. reported that Brian bumped into a stereo set and injured himself. Mrs. C. reported that Brian fell from a couch, but she later admitted that Mr. C. had physically abused Brian while he had been drinking heavily. Brian had a previous hospital admission at three months of age because of a skull fracture, and his parents had reported at that time that he fell from his bed. His general hygiene and nutritional status are good, but he appears to be a solemn child, seldom smiling, and fearful when other children cry. His development indicates slight delays: he sat alone at age nine months, began crawling recently, and does minimal babbling. Brian is being treated with traction in the hospital. Family Services is following this family.

Formulation of Nursing Diagnoses

Some of the nursing diagnoses, based on your assessment, that are pertinent to the abused child are:

1. *Child's pain* related to *injuries inflicted by parents.*
2. *Compromised family coping* related to *poor support system and elevated stress level.*
3. *Child's fear* related to *past history of abuse.*
4. *Potential for injury to the child* related to *a history of child abuse.*

5. *Impaired home management and maintenance* related to *elevated stress and isolation of parents.*
6. *Unrealistic expectations of child* related to *parental knowledge deficit about growth and development and age-appropriate tasks.*
7. *Parental noncompliance with recommended treatment or health care for child* related to *intimidation by health care system.*
8. *Potential for less than adequate nutritional requirements* related to *parental neglect.*
9. *Alterations in parenting* related to *inappropriate expectations of child behavior and parental immaturity.*
10. *Disturbance in self-concept of child* related to *identification with the aggressor (parent) and a sense of inferiority.*
11. *Social isolation of parent* related to *inadequate support system and poor self-concept.*
12. *Ineffective individual coping skills of child* related to *developmental delays.*

Client-Care Goals and Related Nursing Interventions

Based on your nursing diagnoses, you are now able to formulate nursing goals and to plan interventions for the abused child and the family. Goals always have to be specific for the specific injuries or problems of the child.

Goals

1. *Child remains free from injury.*
2. *Family remains intact whenever possible.*
3. *Parental statements and behavior demonstrates understanding of child development and of positive parenting skills.*
4. *Child's verbalizations and behavior reflect an achievement of maximum potential for development.*

Interventions

Nurses play a vital role in the prevention and treatment of child abuse. You identify families at risk for abuse, and you act as advocator, educator, counselor, and coordinator (34). You assume a major role in primary prevention of child abuse by identifying high-risk families and by referring them to appropriate resources for counseling or follow-up. In the nursing assessment you will identify the areas of concern previously discussed regarding the family characteristics and the potential for crisis or stress. As the obstetric nurse, postpartum nurse, pediatric nurse, mental health nurse, or the nurse teaching parent education classes, you have an excellent opportunity to explore with parents their reasons for having children, their expectations for the child's behavior, and their knowledge of growth and development. You can assess the family's support system, provide accurate information about growth and development, and explore guidelines for positive parenting with the families. You may teach courses on family life in high school or initiate a support group for single parents. You can make referrals for home follow-up through the community health nurse at these times.

You also have a legal responsibility to report all suspected incidences of child abuse. All fifty states now have mandatory reporting laws regarding child abuse and give immunity to professionals who make such reports in honesty and good faith. All persons with responsibility for the care of the children, such as nurses, physicians, teachers, and day-care workers, are obligated by law to report any suspicion of child abuse or neglect. You are guilty of a misdemeanor and you may be fined $1,000 or be imprisoned for up to one year if you don't report child abuse. Any reporter of abuse is immune from liability. Although all of the states in the United States now have mandatory abuse laws, the laws are not uniform because they vary regarding the age of the child and the agency to which you report. This agency, often a state family service division, will promptly investigate all reports received through the state's telephone hot line. The individual state's central registry maintains a cross-reference file on all abuse reports to prevent families from hiding the abuse by obtaining medical care from multiple agencies.

When a problem of abuse has already been identified, you may work with the family, making home visits at frequent intervals. As a community health nurse, you act as an educator by assessing and increasing the parental knowledge of a child's growth and development, along with approved practices of child rearing. You provide a positive role model for parenting skills, such as developmental stimulation and discipline. These parents may have had a negative role model in their own

parents, or they may just be too immature to be parents.

Goals

5. *Parent's behavior demonstrates ability to form trusting relationships with others. Frustration is expressed openly and verbally.*
6. *Child's behavior demonstrates ability to form trusting relationships with others.*
7. *Parental statements and behavior demonstrate increase in parental self-esteem and a positive self-image.*
8. *Child's statements and behavior demonstrate increase in self-esteem and a positive self-image.*

Interventions

You must first examine your own feelings regarding child abuse, and you must view child abuse as a family dysfunction, regarding the family as worthy of help. You need to develop a trusting relationship with the family which can be facilitated if you are honest, dependable, and are viewed by the family as being helpful to them (34). As a result of this positive relationship and support to the parents, their self-esteem will be enhanced. Areas in which the nurse is viewed as helpful may include assisting the family in obtaining food stamps, assisting with toilet training or discipline, or helping to find someone to relieve the mother from the constant burden of parenting by taking the children for a few hours each week.

Goal

9. *Parental behavior demonstrates ability to seek and utilize help from others when necessary.*

Intervention

Due to the abuser's low self-esteem, he/she is often intimidated by the health care system and needs assistance in working with the system. You can be the parent's advocate by assisting with making and keeping health care appointments, and by working with the family and other personnel to plan realistic treatment regimes for the child and family. The parent(s) should eventually function independently in obtaining health care.

Goal

10. *Constructive coping mechanisms to deal with stress are developed by the parents to the greatest degree possible. This will initially be apparent by the parent's attempts to utilize new coping mechanisms with the nurse's assistance and guidance.*

Interventions

You act as a counselor by exploring the parent's feelings and expectations with them, and by referring them to appropriate agencies for further help when their own support system is inadequate. Self-help groups, such as Parents Anonymous and Mother's Hotline, in addition to homemaker services, parent aides, and crisis nurseries, may provide additional support systems for these families. Parent aides are supervised volunteers who are parents themselves; they attempt to meet some of the parents' needs and provide positive role models. Crisis nurseries care for children and allow parents free time when their stress level is high. Homemaker services and 24-hour mother's hotlines or parent's groups strive to reduce the parent's feelings of stress, give practical suggestions, and promote effective coping mechanisms. Unfortunately, often there is an insufficient number of such services available. Being a parent can be another disappointment in a long series of disappointments for these parents because their children are not able to satisfy their needs for love and dependency. When several agencies are involved with the same family, the nurse may act as a coordinator to ensure mutual goals, avoid role duplication, and prevent overwhelming of the family with conflicting directions from the various involved agencies.

Evaluation

Working with abusive families is both a stressful experience and a challenge for you. You must continually examine and resolve your own feelings concerning abuse. Progress may be slow, but evidence of successful intervention should be seen in the parent's ability to form trusting relationships, initially with the nurse, and subsequently with others. The parents' behavior and statements will indicate some insight into their own stresses and coping mechanisms. They will establish new coping mechanisms and attempt alternate methods of child rearing. As they progress, their dependency on you will decrease, and they will ultimately make appropriate, independent decisions regarding their own needs and those of their children. Over time, the physical and emotional status of the offspring should show some improvement as abusive behavior decreases, although long-term effects of abuse, in spite of your care, may be difficult to determine.

REFERENCES

1. Anthony, E. James, "The Syndrome of the Psychologically Invulnerable Child," in *The Child in His Family*, vol. 3, eds. E. James Anthony and Cyrille Koupernik, pp. 529–44. New York: John Wiley & Sons, Inc., 1974.

2. Axline, Virginia, *Play Therapy*. Boston: Houghton Mifflin Company, 1947.

3. Barnard, Martha Underwood, "Early Detection of Child Abuse," in *Family Health Care*, eds. Debra P. Hymovich and Martha Underwood Barnard, pp. 365–76. New York: McGraw-Hill Book Company, 1976.

4. Barnard, Martha Underwood, and Lorraine Wolf, "Psychosocial Failure to Thrive," *Nursing Clinics of North America*, 8, no. 3 (1973), 557–65.

5. Barnett, Kathryn, "A Theoretical Construct of the Concepts of Touch as They Relate to Nursing," *Nursing Research*, 21, no. 2 (1972), 102–9.

6. Bowlby, John, "Disruption of Affectional Bonds and Its Effect on Behavior," *Canada's Mental Health: Supplement*, no. 59 (January-February 1969), 2–12.

7. Brown, Catherine, "It Changed My Life," *Psychology Today*, November 1976, 47–112.

8. Bruch, Hilde, *Eating Disorders: Obesity, Anorexia Nervosa, and the Person Within*. New York: Basic Books, Inc., 1973.

9. Campbell, Magda, and Arthur Small, "Chemotherapy," in *Handbook of Treatment of Mental Disorders in Childhood and Adolescence*, eds. Benjamin Wolman, James Egan, and Alan Ross, pp. 9–27. Englewood Cliffs, N.J.: Prentice-Hall, Inc., 1978.

10. Ciseaux, A., "Anorexia Nervosa: A View from the Mirror," *American Journal of Nursing*, 80, no. 8 (1980), 1468–70.

11. Claggett, M., "Anorexia Nervosa: A Behavioral Approach," *American Journal of Nursing*, 80, no. 8 (1980), 1471-72.

12. Creak, M., "Schizophrenic Syndrome in Childhood: Report of a Working Party," *British Medical Journal*, 2 (1961), 889-90.

13. Eisenberg, L., "School Phobia: A Study in the Communication of Anxiety," *American Journal of Psychiatry*, 114 (1958), 712-18.

14. Erickson, Florence, "The Toddler during Illness," *Hospital Topics*, 42, no. 9 (1964), 95-97.

15. ____, "When 6 to 12 Year Olds Are Ill," *Nursing Outlook*, 13, no. 7 (1965), 48-50.

16. ____, "Helping the Sick Child Maintain Behavioral Control," *Nursing Clinics of North America*, 2, no. 4 (1967), 695-703.

17. ____, "Nursing Care Based on Nursing Assessment," in *Current Concepts in Clinical Nursing*, ed. Betty Bergersen, pp. 171-77. St. Louis: The C. V. Mosby Company, 1969.

18. Erickson, Marilyn, *Child Psychopathology*. Englewood Cliffs, N.J.: Prentice-Hall, Inc., 1978.

19. Fagin, Claire, *Readings in Child and Adolescent Psychiatric Nursing*. St. Louis: The C. V. Mosby Company, 1974.

20. Freeman, Stephen, "Learning Disabilities and the School Health Worker," *The Journal of School Health*, 43, no. 8 (1973), 521-22.

21. Garmezy, Norman, "The Study of Competence in Children at Risk for Severe Psychopathology," in *The Child in His Family, vol. 3*, eds. F. James Anthony and Cyrille Koupernik, pp. 77-97. New York: John Wiley & Sons, Inc., 1974.

22. Gelfand, Donna, "Social Withdrawal and Negative Emotional States: Behavior Therapy," in *Handbook of Treatment of Mental Disorders in Childhood Adolescence*, eds. Benjamin Wolman, James Egan, and Alan Ross, pp. 330-53. Englewood Cliffs, N.J.: Prentice-Hall, Inc., 1978.

23. Gil, David, *Violence against Children*. Cambridge, Mass.: Harvard University Press, 1970.

24. Green, Arthur H., "Child Abuse" in *Handbook of Treatment of Mental Disorders in Childhood and Adolescence*, eds. Benjamin Wolman, James Egan, and Alan Ross, pp. 430-55. Englewood Cliffs, N.J.: Prentice-Hall, Inc., 1978.

25. Greenfield, Josh, *A Child Called Noah*. New York: Holt, Rinehart and Winston, 1972.

26. Grossniklaus, D., "Nursing Interventions in Anorexia Nervosa," *Perspectives in Psychiatric Care*, 18, no. 1 (1980), 11-15.

27. Haber, Judith et al., *Comprehensive Psychiatric Nursing*. New York: McGraw-Hill Book Company, 1978.

28. Hagamen, Mary, "Childhood Psychosis: Residential Treatment and Its Alternatives," in *Handbook of Treatment of Mental Disorders in Childhood and Adolescence*, eds. Benjamin Wolman, James Egan, and Alan Ross, pp. 421-29. Englewood Cliffs, N.J.: Prentice-Hall, Inc., 1978.

29. Harris, Merril, "Understanding the Autistic Child," *American Journal of Nursing*, 78, no. 10 (1978), 1682-85.

30. Hopkins, Joan, "The Nurse and the Abused Child," *Nursing Clinics of North America*, 5, no. 4 (1970), 589-98.

31. James, Muriel, and Dorothy Jongeward, *Born to Win: Transactional Analysis with Gestalt Experiments*. Reading, Mass.: Addison-Wesley Publishing Co., Inc., 1973.

32. Johnson, B. S., and V. Ritchie, "Milieu Management of the Patient with Anorexia Nervosa," in *Current Perspectives in Psychiatric Nursing: Issues and Trends*, vol. 2, eds. C. R. Kneisl and H. S. Wilson, pp. 34-43. St. Louis: The C. V. Mosby Company, 1978.

33. Joint Commission on Mental Health of Children, *Crisis in Child Mental Health: Challenge for the 1970's*. New York: Harper & Row, Publishers, Inc., 1970.

34. Josten, Lavohn, "Out-of-Hospital Care for a Pervasive Family Problem—Child Abuse," *American Journal of Maternal-Child Nursing*, 3, no. 2 (1978), 111-16.

35. Juenker, Donna, "The Child's Perception of His Illness," in *Nursing Care of the Child with Long-Term Illness*, ed. Shirley Steele, pp. 133-71. New York: Appleton-Century-Crofts, Inc., 1971.

36. Kalkmann, Marion, "Mental Retardation," in *New Dimensions in Mental Health-Psychiatric Nursing*, eds. Marion Kalkmann and Anne Davis, pp. 178-201. New York: McGraw-Hill Book Company, 1980.

37. Kempe, C. Henry, and Ray Helfer, *The Battered Child*. Chicago: The University of Chicago Press, 1980.

38. Kestenbaum, Clarice, "Childhood Psychosis: Psychotherapy," in *Handbook of Treatment of Mental Disorders in Childhood and Adolescence*, eds. Benjamin Wolman, James Egan, and Alan Ross, pp. 354-84. Englewood Cliffs, N.J.: Prentice-Hall, Inc., 1978.

39. Knopf, Irwin, *Childhood Psychopathology*. Englewood Cliffs, N.J.: Prentice-Hall, Inc., 1979.

40. Kolb, Lawrence, *Modern Clinical Psychiatry*. Philadelphia: W. B. Saunders Company, 1977.

41. Kramer, Marlene et al., "Extra Tactile Stimulation of the Premature Infant," *Nursing Research*, 24, no. 5 (1975), 324–34.

42. Kunzman, Lucy, "Some Factors Influencing a Young Child's Mastery of Hospitalization," *Nursing Clinics of North America*, 7, no. 1 (1972), 12–26.

43. Lancaster, Jeanette, and I. Wade Lancaster, "Psychiatric Nurse's Role in Community Mental Health," in *Principles and Practice of Psychiatric Nursing*, eds. Gail Stuart and Sandra J. Sundeen, pp. 533–59. St. Louis: The C. V. Mosby Company, 1979.

44. La Vietes, Ruth, "Mental Retardation: Psychological Treatment," in *Handbook of Treatment of Mental Disorders in Childhood and Adolescence*, eds. Benjamin Wolman, James Egan, and Alan Ross, pp. 354–84. Englewood Cliffs, N.J.: Prentice-Hall, Inc., 1978.

45. Lovaas, O. Ivan, Douglas Young, and Crighton Newsome, "Childhood Psychosis: Behavioral Treatment," in *Handbook of Treatment of Mental Disorders in Childhood and Adolescence*, eds. Benjamin Wolman, James Egan, and Alan Ross, pp. 385–420. Englewood Cliffs, N.J.: Prentice-Hall, Inc., 1978.

46. McDiarmind, Norma et al., *Loving and Learning*. New York: Harcourt Brace Jovanovich, Inc., 1975.

47 Milman, D., "When Thin Is Not Beautiful: Anorexia Nervosa," *Resident and Staff Physician*, 27, no. 1 (1981), 47–54.

48. Misil, I., "Dr. Evans, Obsessed with Food, Was Starving Himself," *Nursing 80*, 10, no. 3 (1980), 54–56.

49. Montagu, Ashley, *Touching: The Human Significance of the Skin*. New York: Columbia University Press, 1971.

50. Nadar, P., "School Phobia," in *Principles of Pediatrics: Health Care of the Young*, ed. R. A. Hoekelman, pp. 558–60. New York: McGraw-Hill Book Company, 1978.

51. President's Commission on Mental Health, *Preliminary Report to the President*. Washington, D.C.: U.S. Government Printing Office, 1977.

52. Richardson T., "Anorexia Nervosa: An Overview," *American Journal of Nursing*, 80, no. 8 (1980), 1470–71.

53. Ritvo, E. et al., eds., *Autism: Diagnosis, Current Research, and Management*. Jamaica, N.Y.: Spectrum Publications, Inc., 1976.

54. Savino, Anne, and R. Wyman Sanders, "Working with Abusive Parents," *American Journal of Nursing*, 73, no. 3 (1973), 482–84.

55. Schroeder, Carolyn, Stephen Schroeder, and Melvyn Davine, "Learning Disabilities: Assessment and Management of Reading Problems," in *Handbook of Treatment of Mental Disorders in Childhood and Adolescence*, eds. Benjamin Wolman, James Egan, and Alan Ross, pp. 212–37. Englewood Cliffs, N.J.: Prentice-Hall, Inc., 1978.

56. Shapiro, T., I. Chariandini, and B. Fish, "30 Severely Disturbed Children: Evaluation of Their Language Development for Classification and Prognosis," *Archives of General Psychiatry*, 30 (1974), 819–25.

57. Spitz, Rene, and K. M. Wolf, "Anaclitic Depression: An Inquiry into the Genesis of Psychiatric Conditions in Early Childhood," in *The Psychoanalytic Study of the Child*, vol. 2, pp. 313–42. New York: International Universities Press, 1946.

58. Stone, L. Joseph, and Joseph Church, *Childhood and Adolescence*. New York: Random House, Inc., 1973.

59. Thomas, Alexander, Stella Chess, and Herbert Birch, "The Origin of Personality," *Scientific American*, 223 (1970), 102–9.

60. Thompson, Robert, Jr., and Aglai O'Quinn, *Developmental Disabilities*. New York: Oxford University Press, 1979.

61. Vigersky, R., ed., *Anorexia Nervosa*. New York: Raven Press, 1977.

62. Watson, L. S., *Child Behavior Modification: A Manual for Teachers, Nurses, and Parents*. New York: Pergamon Press, Inc., 1973.

63. Werry, J. S., "Childhood Psychosis," in *Psychopathological Disorders of Childhood*, eds. H. C. Quay and J. S. Werry, pp. 173–233. New York: John Wiley & Sons, Inc., 1972.

64. Wieczorek, Rita, and Janet Natapoff, *A Conceptual Approach to the Nursing of Children: Health Care from Birth to Adolescence*. Philadelphia: J. B. Lippincott Company, 1981.

65. Wilson, Holly, and Carol Ren Kneisl, *Psychiatric Nursing*. Reading, Mass.: Addison-Wesley Publishing Co., Inc., 1979.

V

Realities in Comprehensive Mental Health Nursing

22

Law and the Mental Health Client: An Overview

Study of this chapter will assist you to:

1. Define terms that pertain to legal actions in health care.

2. Discuss legal trends and the implication for your practice.

3. Compare and contrast voluntary admission and involuntary commitment, and the meaning of each of these to the person and to your nursing practice.

4. Explore patient's rights that are protected by law and the consequences of neglecting these rights.

5. Compare and contrast rights of adults and children.

6. Explore the implications of caring for the person when criminal actions have been committed prior to hospital admission.

7. Determine ways that negligence could occur in psychiatric care, ways to prevent negligence, and consequences of legal negligence.

8. Identify potential examples, with guidance, of battery, assault, imprisonment, intentional infliction of emotional distress, defamation of character, and invasion of privacy, and describe ways to prevent these situations from occurring.

This chapter contributed by Dorothy O'Driscoll, R.N., M.S.N., J.D.

LEGAL TRENDS

The care and treatment of people who are mentally ill have changed dramatically since Philippe Pinel first crusaded to gain humane conditions for them (see Chapter 4). Today, the mental health professional is confronted by legislation and court decisions outlining methods and procedures all focused on protecting the rights of mentally ill clients. Right to treatment, informed consent, right-to-refuse treatment, due process requirements and standard of proof for commitment and continued hospitalization, freedom of information, and right to privacy are all legal principles now being utilized to secure and protect clients (in this chapter referred to as *patients* to differentiate from other legal clients) from infringement of the rights guaranteed to them by the Bill of Rights and the civil rights amendments. This is making the practitioner's job more difficult because of the necessity for understanding and then respecting and protecting these rights.

Everyday issues involving the care and treatment of patients are considered and decided in courts and legislatures all across this country. Legislation outlining the methods of commitment are being reviewed, written, adopted, and implemented in an attempt to guarantee the patient's due process rights. Likewise, existing laws are continuously being challenged in courts of law on the basis of being unconstitutional as a result of failure to provide due process.

From this discussion it should be evident that this is an extremely dynamic and complex topic. State laws vary as to commitment, guardianship, and other issues that might affect care and treatment of mentally ill patients. Therefore the discussion that follows will attempt to focus on majority positions, modern trends, and model legislation. However, be aware of what the law is in the states where you practice. Also, stay attuned to pending legislation and recent court decisions in your state.

LEGAL IMPLICATIONS OF HOSPITALIZATION

Voluntary Admission

Persons hospitalized in a psychiatric facility may be there voluntarily or involuntarily. One state legislature defines the *voluntary patient as a person over sixteen years of age who applies to the facility for admission because of symptoms of mental disorder. Mental disorder is defined as any organic, mental, or emotional impairment including those induced by alcoholism or drug abuse, which has substantial adverse effects on his cognitive, volitional, or emotional functioning.* The mentally ill minor may be voluntarily admitted when application is made by his/her parent or guardian. A guardian of an incompetent adult may also have his/her ward admitted voluntarily upon securing an order authorizing admission from the court (§ 202.123 R. S. Mo.).

If a voluntary, competent adult patient wishes to be discharged, or if the guardian or parent wishes the discharge of the voluntarily admitted ward or child, the patient is discharged immediately in some states. In other states, the patient may be detained for a brief period (varies from state to state) if the physician or director of the mental health facility does not concur in the patient's release. At this point, involuntary commitment proceedings are initiated (§ 202.123 R. S. Mo.). You should be familiar with the mental health code of your state. In addition to remedies outlined in the code, common law recognizes the right of a person held against his/her wishes to sue for false imprisonment. Any nurse confronted with a patient who has not been declared incompetent and who is demanding to be released from the hospital should immediately contact that person's physician, the nursing supervisor, and the administrator. Hospitals should establish policies to deal with such situations. These policies should be reviewed periodically by legal council for the institution to determine if such policies are in compliance with the state's statutes and court decisions.

Involuntary Commitment

Involuntary admission, once the usual route into psychiatric hospitals, has become the less frequently used method of admission (33). This is due in large part to the growing acceptance of mental health care as just another type of health care and the destigmatizing of mental disease.

Protecting the person's due process rights has made involuntary hospitalization a complex procedure, which has contributed to its less frequent use. *Involuntary admission means that the request for hospitalization does not originate with the patient, and he/she may or may not be resistive to the idea* (33). State laws in this area differ considerably, with some states having very modern statutes and others still having outmoded, probably unconstitutional, procedures for involuntary commitment. A typical modern statute establishes criteria for involuntary admission, outlines the procedure that must be followed to protect the person's rights, identifies a right to treatment, and outlines the individual's rights generally. For involuntary commitment, there usually must be proof that the person is suffering from a mental disorder that presents a likelihood of serious physical harm to self or to others and is in need of treatment. The physical harm to self includes failure or inability to provide for essential human needs. Recent court cases would suggest that the standard or burden of proof for the above is by "clear and convincing evidence" and requires that the proof must be greater than the preponderance of the evidence standard applicable to other categories of civil cases (*Addington v. Texas*, 441 U.S. 418 [1979]).

From this discussion, it becomes obvious that merely showing that a person is mentally ill and in need of treatment is not sufficient for involuntary admission. It must be shown by clear and convincing evidence that the individual represents an actual danger to self or others.

The due process right of the individual is protected by providing adequate notice and judicial hearings along with the assurance of legal representation at the hearing. Hearings and new commitment orders are required from time to time after admission to guarantee that the person, once committed, will not be forgotten in some back ward, as could have occurred in earlier times. You, as a health professional, must be aware of the time and procedural requirements involved in an involuntary admission. If these are not strictly followed, an action for false imprisonment may be brought. A judgment in favor of the person bringing the action could result in monetary damages being awarded. Also, the person could allege state action and could sue for his/her freedom as well as for damages, based on a denial of constitutionally guaranteed due process. By following the procedures outlined for involuntary admission and by adhering to time limitations for reviews and evaluations, the health professional protects self and the patient. For the health professional, court actions, even if successful, are time-consuming, unnerving, costly, and often demoralizing. The patient suffers also because the care and treatment that he/she needs are often interrupted and sometimes terminated, with the outcome not always in the person's best interests.

PROTECTING PATIENT'S RIGHTS

Effects of Commitment

In modern mental health statutes, persons committed to psychiatric facilities retain their civil rights, whereas the person involuntarily committed under some older state statutes is considered to be incompetent. With legal incompetency, civil rights such as the right to vote, hold public office, drive, be issued a driver's license, marry, divorce, be a juror, enter into contracts, or obtain a professional license are lost.

Incompetency Procedures

Usually *incompetency is determined in a court hearing in which an adult will be declared not to possess the mental ability to carry out personal affairs.* The reason for seeking to have someone adjudged incompetent is so that a guardian, conservator, or committee may be appointed to take care of his/her estate and/or person. This procedure arises as a result of society's desire to safeguard the person's assets and to provide for care if the person cannot care for self. To have legal competency restored requires another court hearing to reverse the previous ruling. In states where the commitment carries with it an adjudication of incompetency, mere discharge from the hospital may not be enough to restore personal rights; a court hearing may also be required. The state probate code and mental health code will reveal what the procedure is for incompetency determinations and commitment procedures, and their implications.

Modern statutes also outline the rights of patients and usually include a right to humane care and treatment, freedom from verbal and physical abuse, and medical care and treatment in accordance with the highest standards in available facilities and circumstances (§ 202.205 R. S. Mo.)

You should be aware that incompetent persons cannot sign for themselves. Therefore, when permits need to be signed, the guardian must sign for the ward. This does not apply to persons who have not been declared legally incompetent. This person, if possible, must sign for self. If he/she cannot, then it is probably necessary to initially get a court order, and then seek to have the person declared incompetent.

Habeas Corpus

Any person who is detained involuntarily also has a right to apply for a *writ of habeas corpus.* This writ *is intended to secure the speedy release of any individual who claims he/she is being deprived of liberty by being illegally detained* (24). A person committed may file this writ at any time on the basis that he/she is sane and should be released. The writ is heard in a court of law where a jury may or may not be present. If the person is found to be sane, the order is issued that he/she be released immediately from the hospital.

Informed Consent

In the absence of an emergency situation, a therapist is under an obligation to engage in *informed consent, explaining procedures to the patient, the risks involved, alternative treatments, and other information necessary for the patient to make an intelligent and informed choice.* A minor or patient declared legally incompetent cannot give consent for self, and the parent or guardian's consent must be secured.

The amount of disclosure required varies among states. When informed consent is challenged in court, the majority position requires expert testimony as to what a reasonable medical practitioner would have disclosed under the same or similar circumstances.

An evolving trend, however, holds that the community standard rule is an unnecessary delegation to the medical profession of the responsibility as well as an abrogation of the individual patient's right to make an informed choice. The court in *Canterbury* v. *Spence* (464 F2d 772 [D.C. Cir., 1972]) intimated that the individual's right to make choices in the light of his/her own individual value judgment is the very essence of freedom of choice and should not be left entirely to the medical profession to determine what the patient should be told. Therefore, in a court action where informed consent becomes a question, the jury should be able to make a ruling on the question as to whether a particular piece of information should have been disclosed to the patient.

Because informed consent is so important in avoiding actions for assault and battery as well as negligence, you must be constantly alert for the manner in which consent is secured and the understanding demonstrated by the patient. Any patient who withdraws consent or who has questions regarding a procedure, which show that he/she has little understanding of an impending procedure, must be treated cautiously. The patient's physician and the administration of the institution should be contacted. Careful documentation as to information conveyed and patient understanding is important. Action taken when a patient withdraws consent or seems to lack understanding should be documented. It is also important that the patient be able to give informed consent when it is sought. Therefore, it must be secured when he/she is not under the influence of sedative drugs or alcohol or in such an emotional state as to preclude free choice. Therefore, threats, coercion, and bribes must never be used in securing consent.

Right to Refuse Treatment

Because of the necessity for informed consent, patients have a right to refuse treatment. Electroshock and other treatment modalities may be specifically identified in some state statutes.

Written consent that is informed and voluntary is usually required. A court order may be required for involuntary electroshock treatment (§ 202.207 R.S.Mo.).

A New Jersey court recently held that mental hospitals must disclose the risk of drugs, in writing, to patients and must attempt to get the patient's informed consent. Without this consent, the court held that the hospitals would be required to meet additional conditions before forcing patients to take drugs against their will. Decisions to forcibly medicate must be reviewed by an independent psychiatrist. Forced medication is allowed only in carefully defined circumstances involving emergencies, legally incompetent patients, and functionally incompetent patients. When the hospital wishes to administer medication to nonconsenting patients who are not in these three categories, the patient must be given a hearing before an independent psychiatrist (*Rennie* v. *Klein*, No. 77-2625 [D.N.J. Sept. 14, 1979]). This New Jersey court relied on a Supreme Court decision *Parham* v. *J. R.* (99 S.Ct. 2493 [1979]) and *Secretary of Public Welfare* v. *Institutionalized Juveniles* (99 S.Ct. 2523 [1979]) to conclude that involuntary patients have privacy and due process rights and that voluntary patients have privacy rights and an absolute right to refuse medication.

A Massachusetts court held that mental hospitals cannot forcibly seclude or medicate patients, voluntary or involuntary, without the consent of the patient or the consent of his/her guardian except when there is a substantial likelihood of, or as a result of, extreme violence, personal injury, or attempted suicide. This court held that the practice of forcibly medicating patients in nonemergencies is "an affront to basic concepts of human dignity" (*Rogers* v. *Orkin*, No. 75-1610-T [D. Mass., filed Dec. 29, 1979]). The U.S. Court of Appeals for the First Circuit further considered the question of forced medication presented in the *Rogers* case. This additional decision requires physicians to balance the pros and cons involved in emergency medication and demands determination of incapacity before a patient is forcibly medicated for treatment purposes. For emergencies, this court ruling requires an individualized estimation of the possibility and types of violence, the likely effects of particular drugs on the individual, and an appraisal of less restrictive courses of action. For treatment purposes, the ruling says that prior to the use of antipsychotic drugs, the individual must be incapable of making a competent decision concerning treatment (*Rogers* v. *Orkin*, 49 USLW 1097 [Dec. 23, 1980]).

The area of informed consent is a rapidly evolving area. Therefore, you must be aware of the statutes and court decisions relative to informed consent when you are doing mental health therapy.

Other Rights

Other rights of patients may be spelled out in the statutes. These rights can be restricted, if necessary, for the medical welfare of the patient, but restriction must be documented in the medical record. One state lists the following patient's rights in its Mental Health Code:

1. To wear his/her own clothes and keep personal possessions.
2. To keep and be allowed to spend a reasonable sum of his/her own money.
3. To communicate by sealed mail, or otherwise, with persons outside.
4. To receive visitors of his/her own choosing at reasonable hours.
5. To have reasonable access to a telephone to make and receive confidential calls.
6. To receive a nourishing, well-balanced, and varied diet.
7. To have opportunities for physical exercise and outdoor recreation.
8. To have reasonable, prompt access to current newspapers, magazines, and radio and television programming.

Every patient has an absolute right to receive visits from his/her attorney, physician, or clergyman in private, at reasonable times, and to communicate by sealed mail with the court and mental health department. These rights are outlined in writing, along with the procedure for requesting discharge, and are given to the person at admission (§ 202.215 R.S.Mo.).

Respecting these rights while providing for the patient's safety, treatment, and well-being may seem to be a very difficult task. You should remember that these rights can be restricted if it is for the patient's medical welfare. However, it is absolutely necessary to document restrictions and the reasons for their imposition. Absolute rights cannot be impinged, but they can be regulated so that they are met in a reasonable manner and do not infringe on the rights of others.

Right to Privacy and Confidentiality

Confidentiality is spelled out in modern statutes that usually stipulate that records may be disclosed only with the patient's written consent. However, under the law, records usually can: (1) follow a patient to another facility, (2) be disclosed for insurance claims and other types of aid, (3) go to an administering court, (4) be used for research while maintaining the anonymity of the patient, (5) be used by law enforcement officers when necessary for the responsibilities of their office, and (6) be released to the patient's attorney (4).

As a mental health professional, you must be aware of your obligation to safeguard the confidentiality of records and other disclosures made by the patient. Even revealing the name of the patient or taking his/her picture without permission and showing it indiscriminately could be very detrimental to the patient. Computerization and data banks may threaten a person's right to privacy. Because of this, all mental health practitioners must be extremely cautious about when and to whom information is released. Information should be given only with the patient's knowledge and with his/her signed consent.

A physician-client privilege may exist in a specific state. This means that in certain situations where a special relationship exists, the persons cannot testify against each other. For example, in the physician-patient privilege, if a physician is called to testify against the patient in a court of law, he/she cannot reveal the information told by the patient unless the patient gives permission (4). This condition only exists where specifically established by statute. A very small number of states recognize a nurse-patient privilege as well.

A patient's hospital record can be subpoenaed for a legal action and can be used as evidence. Therefore, it is very important that it be accurate, written carefully, and complete. Only those persons involved in the patient's care should be allowed to read the chart.

Compulsory disclosure of medical information may be required outside the courtroom by statutes that have been enacted to safeguard the public welfare. The areas usually requiring disclosure are communicable disease, child abuse, drug use, birth, death, and knife and gunshot wounds (4). In these situations, state legislatures have determined that societal interests outweigh individual interests in nondisclosure. A recent court decision spoke to this problem and chose the interests of the community in regulating drugs over the confidentiality interests of the individual patient. This decision further observed that many necessary invasions of privacy are associated with health care and that disclosures to doctors, hospitals, insurance companies, and public health agencies are essential to modern medical practice (*Whalen* v. *Roe*, 97 S.Ct. 869, 878 [1977]). The physician may also have a duty to reveal the patient's secrets without his/her consent when a competing interest involving life, safety, well-being, or other important interest is in jeopardy (*Berry* v. *Moench*, 331 P.2d 814 [Utah, 1958]).

As a therapist, you may encounter problems when the patient reveals intentions to do harmful or dangerous acts. There is a duty imposed on the therapist to initiate steps to protect the patient, and there may also be a duty to protect or warn third parties. In *Tarasoff* v. *Regents of University of California* (551 P.2d 334 [Cal. 1976]), the California Supreme Court required a psychotherapist who determines that a patient presents a danger to a third party to warn that third party. The court held that the relationship of psychotherapist to patient is sufficient to create a duty of care to all persons who are foreseeably endangered by the patient's acts. This decision requires that confidential communication be disclosed where the risk to be prevented is the danger of violent assault and not where the risk of harm is self-directed or property damage. Also the U.S. District Court for the Middle District of Pennsylvania, in applying *Tarasoff*, has held that the group to be protected must be readily identifiable (*Leedy* v. *Hartnett*, 49 USLW, 1167 [Mar. 24, 1981]). The therapist's duty to protect the patient's privacy may be safeguarded in these situations: by (1) requiring a second opinion before disclosure, (2) waiting until the danger

is imminent, (3) intervening and disclosing only to the degree necessary to prevent the danger, and (4) warning the patient that the therapist may be required to disclose some confidential communications, and thereby gaining informed consent (4).

An institution should draft policies outlining actions to be taken regarding the release of information. Safeguarding confidentiality while providing for the patient's safety or the safety of another must be carefully considered and weighed. Actions to be taken in situations where a patient reveals self-destructive thoughts or threats of violence to another must be worked out in advance. The therapist must know what these policies are and then must follow them. If the therapist acts contrary to these policies, or if there are no policies and the therapist does not institute appropriate measures to safeguard the patient or another, a lawsuit for negligence becomes a definite possibility.

Right to Treatment

A right to treatment is an evolving concept frequently litigated today. The right to treatment was first recognized in the 1960s (7). In *Rouse* v. *Cameron* (373 F.2d 451 [D.C. Cir. 1966]), the court held that patients committed by criminal courts had the right to adequate treatment and that confinement without treatment transformed the hospital into a penitentiary. This court held that the purpose of commitment was treatment and not punishment, and if treatment was not provided, the person could be transferred, released, and/or even awarded damages.

In the early 1970s, in the case of *Wyatt* v. *Stickney* (325 F. Supp. 781 [M.D. Ala. 1971]), the judge observed, "To deprive any citizen of his or her liberty upon the altruistic theory that the confinement is for humane therapeutic reasons and then fail to provide adequate treatment violates the very fundamentals of due process." The consent order in this case identified with great specificity standards for the mental hospitals involved. The order called for treatment plans that are continuously reviewed by a qualified mental health professional and modified if necessary. It further ordered that at least every 90 days, each patient should receive a mental examination and the treatment plan should be reviewed by a qualified mental health professional other than the professional responsible for supervising and implementing the plan.

Other aspects of the plan were to include: (1) a statement of patient problems and needs, (2) a statement of the least restrictive treatment conditions necessary, (3) intermediate and long-range goals and a timetable, (4) a statement of rationale for the plan, (5) a description of proposed staff involvement, (6) criteria for release to a less restrictive environment and discharge, and (7) notation of therapeutic tasks to be performed by the patient.

In the mid-1970s, in the case of *O'Connor* v. *Donaldson* (95 S.Ct. 2486, [1975]), the Supreme Court stated,

> Now the purpose of involuntary hospitalization is treatment and not mere custodial care or punishment if the patient is not a danger to himself or others. Without such treatment, there is no justification from a constitutional standpoint for continued confinement unless you should also find that he was dangerous either to himself or others.

In this case, the plaintiff was awarded damages, both actual and punitive.

The concept of right to treatment in the least restrictive setting is also spelled out in some state statutes. Lawsuits have been brought in states where the least restrictive setting was not specified in the state statutes, as well as in states where it was specified and it was not being complied with. In addition to this type of suit, there is also the type of action that arises when the patients are placed in less restrictive settings but with little or no treatment. Such placements are also being challenged in the courts on the basis that the patient's liberty right is still being infringed, even if he/she is in a less restrictive environment, when proper care and follow-up are not provided.

When the patient is released to a less restrictive environment, periodic evaluations of progress and adequate documentation are necessary for a defense when right to treatment is challenged. Discharge planning and referrals must be documented in patients' records. Again, policies and procedures worked out in advance can help avoid lawsuits.

Other Legal Protections

Other laws have been utilized by patients bringing actions against mental health institutions. For example, it would appear from a recent decision relative to the Fair Labor Standards Act (29 U.S.C. § 201 *et seq.*) that patients, even when committed to mental institutions, enjoy the protection of other federal and state legislation. In *Sander* v. *Brennan* (367 F. Supp. 808 [D.D.C. 1973]), the minimum wage provisions of the Fair Labor Standards Act were made applicable to patients at state and county institutions for the mentally ill who engage in voluntary and therapeutic work programs.

Other laws that may be used to challenge the actions of hospital officials and others responsible for the care and treatment of mental patients are: (1) Rehabilitation Act of 1973, (2) Social Security Act, (3) Special Health Revenue Sharing Act, (4) Community Health Center Amendments, and the (5) Developmentally Disabled Assistance and Bill of Rights Act.

In 1980, Public Law 96-247 became effective. This law, entitled "Civil Rights of Institutionalized Persons Act," grants authority to the U.S. Attorney General to initiate actions in federal courts against a state, a political subdivision of a state, or a person acting on behalf of persons who are residing in or confined to any institution and are subjected to egregious or flagrant conditions that deprive them of rights protected by the Constitution or other U.S. laws. This law applies to institutions for mentally ill or handicapped persons. It applies to jails, prisons, and other correctional and pretrial facilities. Facilities for juveniles and institutions providing skilled nursing, intermediate or long-term care, or custodial or residential care are also covered by the act.

Additionally, patients can bring actions against the hospitals, physicians, or other health care workers if they feel that they have a complaint due to a tort perpetuated against them or their property or if a contract has been breached. More will be said about tort liability later in this chapter. Patients also have defenses that can be used if a hospital, physician, or other person sues them. For example, in a hospital collection suit in Georgia, a voluntary psychiatric patient who was held in a hospital against her will in violation of state law was not liable for any charges during the period that she was involuntarily held (*Fulton*

DeKalb Hospital Authority v. *Fletcher*, No. 718524 [Dec. 13, 1979]).

RIGHTS OF CHILDREN

The rights of children are becoming more important as courts decide sensitive issues relating to a child's constitutional rights. Until the 1970s, children were not considered to have constitutional rights apart from their parents (3). In the 1970s, many court decisions and state laws have brought about a widening recognition of the rights that children enjoy under the constitution.

The Supreme Court has recently decided several cases in which the constitutional rights of children were under consideration. In the case of *In re Gault* (387 U.S. 1 [1967]), the Court observed that neither the Fourteenth Amendment nor the Bill of Rights is for adults alone. The Court also identified a minor's right to freedom of speech and expression under the First Amendment in *Tinker* v. *Des Moines School District* (393 U.S. 503 [1969]). The procedural safeguards against self-incrimination established by the 6th Amendment were recognized in *In re Winship*, and in the case of *Wisconsin* v. *Yoder* (406 U.S. 243 [1971]), the Court reviewed these decisions and observed that recent cases have clearly held that children have constitutionally protectable interests.

Although, as was stated earlier, state mental health codes allow parents to voluntarily commit their minor children or children under sixteen to mental institutions, it is becoming questionable whether this can be done without some safeguarding of the child's due process rights. The California Supreme Court, in *In re Roger S.* (No. 19558 [Cal. Sup. Ct., July 18, 1977]), held that a fourteen-year-old boy had a right to a precommitment hearing before a neutral fact-finder in order to guarantee his due process rights. It further observed that minors fourteen years of age or older possess rights that may not be waived by parents or guardians. These minors have federal and state constitutional rights to procedural due process in determining whether or not the minor is mentally ill or disordered, or dangerous to self or others as a result of mental illness, and whether

or not the admission sought is likely to benefit him/her.

The case of *Morales* v. *Turman* (383 F. Supp. 53 [E.D. Tex., 1974]) found a right to treatment for juvenile offenders. This case attacked the entire juvenile correctional system of Texas and resulted in the closure of several institutions along with sweeping reforms relative to mail censorship, visitation privileges, and discipline procedures. The court found that the state has a duty to create and foster alternatives such as home placement, day-care programs, halfway houses, and group homes. The court ordered the state to create a system of community-based treatment alternatives adequate to serve the needs of juveniles for whom the state institution is not appropriate.

A right to refuse treatment has been recognized in the IJA-ABA Standards Relating to Juvenile Delinquency and Sanctions. These standards recommend that children may voluntarily refuse services except in three cases: (1) services juveniles are legally obliged to accept (school attendance), (2) services required to prevent clear harm to physical health, and (3) helpful services mandated by the court as a condition to a non-residential placement (17).

Children also have certain rights to privacy. In most states, the parent or guardian may have access to all information in the minor's medical record (4). However, most states have statutes that enable minors to be treated directly by a physician without parental consent for venereal disease, family planning, alcohol and drug abuse, and mental health. Because of this, records and information relative to these areas should not be made available to anyone, not even to parents, without the child's permission.

The Family Educational Rights and Privacy Act (20 U.S.C. § 1232) applies to all school-children. This law provides for inspection and review of school records, and compliance is a precondition to the availability of federal funds to the institution involved. This act spells out what information must be made available to the individual, the procedures to afford access to the records, hearings that must be held, and when corrections or deletions must be made. When medical records are a part of the school record, they are also covered by the Act (4).

The area of informed consent also has been recognized for children. As was stated earlier, children have a right to consent for themselves for medical treatment of venereal disease, family planning, drug or alcohol abuse, and mental health (4). For all other medical and surgical treatments, the parent or guardian must give consent.

Abortion laws requiring parental consent for an unmarried minor's abortion have been held unconstitutional in *Planned Parenthood of Central Missouri v. Danforth* (96 S.Ct. 2831 [1976]). The Missouri Supreme Court held that to impose blanket parental consent requirements was unconstitutional and that the abortion decision must be left to the medical judgment of the pregnant woman's attending physician. It also said that constitutional rights do not mature and that minors as well as adults are protected by the Constitution. However, state abortion statutes calling for notification of parents prior to an abortion are constitutional, at least as

applied to immature and unemancipated minors dependent on their parents (*H. L. v. Matheson*, 49 USLW 1145 March 24, [1981]).

Parents who challenged a state-supported family planning clinic's distribution of birth control information and contraceptives to their unemancipated minor children without their consent on the basis that the parent's Fourteenth Amendment liberty interest in relation to the care and custody of their children was being violated were not successful in a case in the Sixth Circuit—*Doe v. Irwin* (48 USLW 2588 [3/11/80]). In this case, the rights of the parents, the rights of the children, and the interests of the state were all considered. The court upheld the privacy right of the child and stated that the rights of the parents were not really being impinged upon.

In summary, the constitutional rights of children have been recognized. As a health professional, you must be aware that whenever the child is the client, these rights must be respected. State statutes regarding age of majority and age for giving consent for medical and surgical treatment should be known. The minor being admitted by the parents to an institution for mental care should have due process rights safeguarded. Adequate notice, a hearing, and appointment of someone to represent the child's interests should be considered even if not called for by statute.

CRIMINAL ACTIONS

Persons accused of a crime may utilize several defenses that may result in their acquittal or avoidance of trial. The insanity defense results in acquittal by reason of insanity and prevents the accused from being retried. Incompetency to stand trial is a bar to trial since it alleges that the accused is presently in no mental condition to stand trial (19). He/she can at a later date be tried if competency is regained. The accused also can be hospitalized, but civil commitment must be secured to permit an extended period of confinement.

The insanity defense involves the establishment of certain proof. According to the traditional M'Naghten Rule used in some states, it must be proved that the accused at the time of the crime suffered from a mental illness that

caused a defect of reason, and because of this, he/she lacked the ability to either know the wrongfulness of the actions or understand their nature and quality (19).

There is a trend among courts to use the Model Penal Code Test in which it must be proved that the accused suffered from a mental illness or defect and as a result lacked substantial capacity to either appreciate the criminal nature of his/her action or to conform his/her conduct to the law's requirements.

Proof of insanity is established through the use of psychiatric examinations and the testimony of psychiatrists at the trial. Remember that the term *insanity* is strictly a legal one and relates to the criteria stated above.

GENERAL LEGAL PRINCIPLES

The following legal principles are important to you as a nurse. Nurses and other health personnel may find themselves in situations where a *legal wrong is committed against the person or property of another. This is referred to as a **tort**.* The law allows the injured party to bring a civil action against the wrongdoer, usually to recover a sum of money referred to as "damages."

Negligence

Torts may be either intentional or unintentional. Negligence is an unintentional tort. Every person is responsible for behaving in a reasonably prudent manner. *When the person fails to act in a reasonable and prudent way and harm befalls another due to his/her action, then the person may be legally negligent.*

A professional who fails to meet the required standard of care in the practice of his/her profession and causes another to be injured may be sued for malpractice. The standard that the professional's conduct is measured against is that of other reasonably prudent members of the same profession in the same or similar circumstances. Many jurisdictions have eliminated this "locality rule," and some do not hold the practitioner to a standard of reasonably careful or prudent care but only that such care was employed by other members of his/her profession (16). However, a specialist will be required to exercise that degree of skill and knowledge that is ordinarily possessed by similar specialists. A student nurse will usually be held to the standard of care required of the professional when performing duties customarily performed only by the professional (32).

Federal and state regulations, accreditation standards, and a facility's own bylaws may be admissible as evidence in court concerning certain responsibilities that hospital authorities, other health professionals, and state officials who license health facilities deemed appropriate for hospitals to assume. Such standards and regulations have been successfully invoked to find liability on the part of health care facilities (*Darling* v. *Charleston Community Hospital,* 211 N.E. 2d 253 ([Ill. S.Ct., 1965], *cert. denied,*

383 U.S. 946 [1966]). Therefore, administrators and health professionals in a facility that is licensed by an accrediting agency, participating in a federal or state funding program, or operating under bylaws outlining standards or quality assurance measures must be constantly vigilant in order to assure that specified laws, regulations, and standards are known, adhered to, and monitored to assure compliance. Violation of such standards has been found to be evidence of negligence (*Mikel* v. *Flatbush Convalescent Hospital,* 370 N.W.S. 2d 162 [N.Y.S.Ct. 1975]), or could be negligence per se if a statutory violation is involved.

The ***doctrine of respondeat superior*** *is a legal concept that holds an employer liable for the negligent acts of an employee when carrying out the employer's orders or otherwise serving the employer's interests.* This doctrine applies only when there is an employee-employer relationship and only when the negligent act committed is within the scope of employment (32). This doctrine does not relieve the negligent employee of liability, but it does provide the injured person another party to sue (11). Thus, an employer, even if blameless except for the negligence of his employee, can be found liable because of this doctrine. The employer can in turn sue his negligent employee to recover whatever loss he sustained (11).

When a practitioner does not possess the skills needed to carry out an assigned function, the concept of "acting with reasonable care" requires the employee to refuse to perform the function, even at the risk of appearing insubordinate.

If a *patient fails to exercise reasonable care and thus contributes to an injury initially caused by the practitioner's negligence, the patient will be said to be **contributorily negligent*** and will not be permitted to recover damages (16). Since this is a rather harsh doctrine, there is a *trend for courts to weigh degrees of negligence and apportion recovery accordingly. This doctrine is referred to as that of **comparative negligence*** (11).

In a malpractice case, the plaintiff has the burden of proving the defendant's liability by the preponderance of the evidence. This means that there is enough evidence to persuade the court that the allegations are more probably true than not. The plaintiff is required to introduce expert witnesses to prove the standard of care and whether the professional conformed to that standard. Expert testimony is not required to prove negligent conduct involving something within the knowledge or experience of most laymen (16).

The doctrine of *res ipsa loquitur* can be used when a plaintiff sustains an injury under circumstances that make it difficult or impossible for him to prove how the injury was sustained or who was liable (30). In a case such as this, the jury is permitted to infer that the defendant was negligent without the need for any expert testimony. This doctrine can only be applied when: (1) the injury is of a type that ordinarily does not occur unless someone has been negligent, and (2) the conduct causing the injury was under the exclusive control of the defendant (11).

Intentional Torts

Professionals may encounter situations where they may become liable for intentional torts. For example, assault and battery may be alleged when procedures are undertaken without the patient's consent. A *battery is defined as an unconsented to, intentionally harmful or offensive contact to the plaintiff's person.* An *assault is an intentional causing of apprehension or immediate, harmful or offensive contact to the plaintiff's person.*

If a patient refused treatment or withdraws his/her consent for treatment, he/she should not be forced to submit, threatened, or coerced (16). The physician and nursing supervisor should be contacted. Or the patient's guardian should be contacted if he/she is incompetent. Or the court should be contacted if he/she is involuntarily committed. These contacts are made to secure permission for treatment. The voluntary patient should not be subjected to treatment unless informed consent has been given. All refusals and actions pursued should be documented in the patient's record.

False imprisonment is another intentional tort that may be alleged against the health professional. *Imprisonment is defined as the intentional confining or restraining of the plaintiff to a bounded area* (11). There must be physical barriers, force, or the direct threat of force to the plaintiff's person or property. Any competent voluntary patient who demands to be released should not be kept in the hospital against his/her wishes beyond that period that the state statute provides for the institution to begin involuntary commitment procedures.

Intentional infliction of emotional distress is a tort that involves intentional outrageous conduct causing the plaintiff severe emotional distress (22). Courts are reluctant to recognize this tort (11) and often limit recovery to the plaintiff who is "sensitive" and thus susceptible to emotional distress. Thus this tort is often only available to certain groups such as children, pregnant women, and elderly people. It is conceivable that a patient who is in a weakened condition could allege that he/she fits into this category of sensitive individuals and could sue for severe emotional distress.

Defamation may be a writing that is called libel or may be an oral communication that is referred to as slander. Defamation involves the use of defamatory language concerning the plaintiff, revealed by the defendant to a third party, and resulting in injury to the plaintiff's reputation (22). Defamatory language tends to adversely affect one's reputation because of inferences of dishonesty, lack of integrity or virtue, or insanity.

Invasion of privacy is another tort that is *based on the right of the individual to be protected from unreasonable interferences with solitude.* Areas covered by this tort are: (1) appropriation by the defendant of the plaintiff's picture or name for the defendant's commercial advantage, (2) intrusion by the defendant into the affairs or seclusion of the plaintiff, (3) publication by the defendant of facts that place the plaintiff in a false light, and (4) public disclosures of private facts about the plaintiff by the defendant.

Defamation and invasion of privacy overlap and in certain areas are similar. It is important for you to be constantly on guard to protect the privacy of patients and to avoid revealing any information about them except when permission has been given or when the state mental health code covers the information involved.

SUMMARY

You must be aware of the laws governing mental health clients. Check your state mental health code, the guardianship provisions, and the state probate code for the procedures governing commitment and guardianship. Be aware of recent court decisions relative to mental health clients.

Children present special problems and their rights under the Constitution make up a rapidly developing area of the law. Careful policy making on the part of the institution caring for children is a must. Legal input should be available during the drafting of these policies, and all policies should also be checked and updated frequently.

As a nurse, you can become involved in tort actions. Following the highest standards of care and establishing good professional-client relationships are the major defenses against involvement in tort allegations and actions.

You always have a dual responsibility for the client: one involves his/her health state and care, and the other involves protection of his/her legal rights. Humanistic nursing involves caring for the person in such a way that legal rights will be ensured and negligence or intentional torts will be avoided.

REFERENCES

1. Barron, John O., "Incompetency Proceedings: Standard of Proof—Delany Revisited," *Journal of the Missouri Bar*, 35, no. 6 (1969), 395–97.

2. Brooks, Ruth, "Behind the Heavy Metal Door," *American Journal of Nursing*, 79, no. 9 (1979), 1547–50.

3. Burgdorf, Marcia, "Legal Rights of Children," *Nursing Clinics of North America*, 14, no. 3 (1979), 405–15.

4. Cooper, Almeta, "The Physician's Dilemma: Protection of the Patient's Right to Privacy," *St. Louis University Law Journal*, 22, no. 3 (1978), 397–432.

5. Creighton, Helen, *Law Every Nurse Should Know*, 3rd ed. Philadelphia: W. B. Saunders Company, 1975.

6. Dunn, Lee, "Legal Aspects of Nursing and Medicine," in *Family Health Care*, 2nd ed., eds. Debra Hymovich and Martha Barnard, vol. 1, pp. 373–81. New York: McGraw-Hill Book Company, 1979.

7. Ennis, Bruce, and Loren Siegel, *The Rights of Mental Patients—The Basic ACLU Guide to a Mental Patient's Rights*. New York: Avon Books, 1973.

8. Fenner, Kathleen, *Ethics and Law in Nursing*. New York: Van Nostrand Reinhold Company, 1980.

9. Haber, Judith et al., *Comprehensive Psychiatric Nursing*, p. 26. New York: McGraw-Hill Book Company, 1979.

10. Hatton, Corrine, "The Evolving Health Clinical Nurse Specialist in Private Practice," in *The Law and the Expanding Nurse Role*, Bonnie Bullough, ed. New York: Appleton-Century-Crofts, 1980.

11. Hemelt, Mary, and Mary Ellen Mackert, *Dynamics of Law in Nursing and Health Care*. Reston, Va.: Reston Publishing Company, 1978.

12. ——, "Your Legal Guide to Nursing Practice—Part I," *Nursing '79*, 9, no. 10 (1979), 57–64.

13. ——, "Your Legal Guide to Nursing Practice—Part II," *Nursing '79*, 9, no. 11 (1979), 57–64.

14. ——, "Your Legal Guide to Nursing Practice—Part III," *Nursing '79*, 9, no. 12 (1979), 57–64.

15. ——, "Your Legal Guide to Nursing Practice—Part IV," *Nursing '79*, 10, no. 1 (1980), 57–67.

16. Hullverson, Thomas, "Medical Malpractice Law in Missouri," *St. Louis Bar Journal* 25, (1978), pp. 8–15.

17. Joint Juvenile Justice Standards Project of the Institute of Judicial Administration and the American Bar Association Standards (1977), tentative drafts. Cambridge, Mass.: Ballinger Publishing Co., 1978.

18. Juvenile Rights Litigation Project, "Voluntary Commitment to State Mental Institutions: Juveniles' Due Process and Equal Protection Rights," *Clearinghouse Review*, 11, no. 5 (1977), 465.

19. Kolb, Lawrence, *Modern Clinical Psychiatry*. Philadelphia: W. B. Saunders Company, 1977.

20. Levy, D. Allan, "The Legal Rights of the Psychiatric Patient," in Lois Dunlap, ed., *Mental Health Concepts Applied to Nursing*. New York: Wiley Medical Publication, 1978.

21. Litwick, Lawrence, Janice Litwick, and Mary Ballou, *Health Counseling*, pp. 214–35. New York: Appleton-Century-Crofts, 1980.

22. Logue, Karen, "Legal Rights and Obligations," in *Basic Psychiatric Concepts in Nursing*, 4th ed., eds. Joan Keyes and Charles Hofling, pp. 667–97. Philadelphia: J. B. Lippincott Company, 1980.

23. Maebius, Jed, "Law and the Family, in *Family Health Care*, 2nd ed., eds. Debra Hymovich and Martha Barnard, vol. 1, pp. 109–21. New York: McGraw-Hill Book Company, 1979.

24. Manfreda, Marguerite, and Diane Sydney, *Psychiatric Nursing*. Philadelphia: F. A. Davis Company, 1977.

25. Mental Health Law Project, "Mental Health Development," *Clearinghouse Review*, 14, no. 2 (1980), 129–31.

26. National Center for Youth Law, "Bellotti v. Baird: A Minor's Right to Consent to Abortion," *Clearinghouse Review*, 14, no. 10 (1980), 763–64.

27. Padberg, Joan, "Nursing and Forensic Psychiatry," *Perspectives in Psychiatric Care*, 10, no. 4 (1972), 163–67.

28. Rogers, Yolande, "The Involuntary Drugging of Juveniles in State Institutions," *Clearinghouse Review* 11, no. 7 (1977), 623–28.

29. Rothman, Daniel A., and Nancy Lloyd Rothman, *The Professional Nurse and the Law*. Boston: Little, Brown and Company, 1977.

30. Shapiro, E. Donald, "Medical Malpractice: History, Diagnosis and Prognosis," *St. Louis University Law Journal*, 22, no. 3 (1978), 469–84.

31. Stachyra, Marcia, "Nurses, Psychotherapy, and the Law," *Perspectives in Psychiatric Care*, 7, no. 5 (1969), 200–213.

32. Streift, Charles J., *Nursing and the Law*, 2nd ed. Rockville, Md.: The Health Law Center, Aspen Systems, 1975.

33. Stuart, Gail, and Sandra Sundeen, *Principles and Practice of Psychiatric Nursing*. St. Louis: The C. V. Mosby Company, 1979.

34. Swanger, Harry, "Juvenile Institutional Litigation," *Clearinghouse Review*, 11, no. 3 (1977), 219–21.

35. Willig, Sidney, *The Nurse's Guide to the Law*. New York: McGraw-Hill Book Company, 1970.

36. Wilson, Holly, and Carol Kneisl, *Psychiatric Nursing*, Chap. 25. Reading, Mass.: Addison-Wesley Publishing Co., Inc., 1979.

23

Nursing Advocacy
in
Mental Health Settings

Study of this chapter will assist you to:

1. Review the historical development related to the need for a client advocacy movement.

2. Define advocacy and describe its meaning for nursing practices.

3. Explore moral, ethical, and legal aspects of client advocacy.

4. Relate advocacy to the steps of the nursing process.

5. Assess your potential strengths and limits as an advocate.

6. Describe instances when the nurse can intervene as a client advocate.

7. Examine ways to effectively communicate so that advocacy actions will be helpful to the client.

This chapter contributed by Virginia Luetje, R.N., M.S.N.

THE DECADES OF DEINSTITUTIONALIZATION

Community Mental Health: The Vision

In 1950 the hospitalization rate (number of days in the hospital per 1,000 of population) for state, county, and private mental hospitals was approximately 1,700. Twenty-five years later that rate had decreased to about 500. But although the length of hospitalization was decreasing, the admission rate was increasing by 129 percent. Nearly two-thirds of these admissions were readmissions within a year of discharge (8). A look at events and factors affecting what A. Slavinsky and J. Krauss term recycled patients (54) will help you comprehend the entreaty for nursing advocacy that comes later in this chapter.

Congress in 1955 established a Joint Commission on Mental Illness and Health, which, among other directives, was charged with developing a national plan for meeting mental health needs. Partially in response to the Joint Commission's findings, as well as to John Kennedy's presidential request for a "bold new approach" to mental illness, Congress legislated the Mental Retardation Facilities and Community Mental Health Centers Construction Act of 1963. This, in addition to other federal funding grants to assist in staffing these community centers, was to be an impetus for providing nationwide availability of a complete array of neighborhood-located mental health services. The provision of five services was essential to qualify for federal monies as a community health center: (1) inpatient care, (2) outpatient care, (3) emergency treatment, (4) partial hospitalization, and (5) consultation and education. Yet twenty-five years later, the President's Commission Report of 1978, published during Carter's presidency, concluded that the effects of deinstitutionalizing patients and the system of community aftercare were far short of what had been envisioned.

Several hundred thousand chronically mentally ill clients eat and sleep between readmissions in poorly organized or perhaps even nonexistent after-care programs. Originally, mental health planners envisioned a very comprehensive network of coordinated after-care services that would include day care or night care (partial hospitalization), foster care for the chronically mentally ill, halfway houses, group homes, supervised apartment living, home visiting mental health teams, 24-hour crisis services, vocational and social programs, and sheltered workshops. In addition, this array of services was to occur in the midst of an involved community, with everyone from bartender to clergy, hair stylist to educator, and homemaker to entrepreneur participating in the prevention and rehabilitation for mental illness. Planners in the midst of the 1960s social and civil rights outcries also argued for community control and direction for these comprehensive health care systems, based on the theory that a given community system would reflect the needs and priorities perceived by the community rather than have services defined and directed by outsiders.

Community Mental Health: The Reality

With few exceptions, the vision has had little semblance to reality. For example, in Missouri a recent study found that although nursing homes were the most widely used alternative to mental hospitals, 56 percent of the mental health patients in those homes should be elsewhere (57). In fact, throughout the nation, most chronic patients discharged from state hospitals are in privately owned nursing or boarding homes. Many others drift through the streets of urban areas. As E. Bassuk and S. Gerson word it, these discharged patients form a new kind of ghetto subpopulation, a captive market for unscrupulous landlords (8).

The stigma for this discharged population is even greater now than it was, a stigma now fed by real social and financial problems (8). As just one example of the reality stigma, M. Greenblatt reports a study on increased homicides and higher arrest rates for crimes against persons by discharged mentally ill patients in the last ten years (30). There are a number of reasons why the reality has fallen short of the dream.

1. *The planning did not necessarily incorporate what the institutionalized client wanted or needed.* H. Lamb, in commenting on his study of 101 residents of a board-and-care home in California, reminds us to be realistic (37). We do not have the answers to make life happy, anxiety-free, and meaningful for persons in board-and-care homes, just as we do not have those answers for

persons in society generally. He reports 42 percent of the residents saying they were content or reasonably content. He speaks of this board-and-care environment as an "asylum from life's stresses" where the resident's can come to adaptation by decompression (37).

One who remembers the open chronic wards of the state hospitals in the early sixties has feelings of *déjà vu* in reading Lamb's descriptions of board-and-care homes. In fact, Slavinsky and Krauss claim that deinstitutionalization has changed the location, but not the conditions, of the chronically mentally ill (54).

2. *The deinstitutionalization movement was often politically and economically problematic.* State legislators were understandably eager to see state hospital patients discharged and reclassified under a status where they could be supported by federal assistance such as Supplemental Security Income, rather than continuing to drain state treasuries as state hospital inpatients. The possible reduction in expenditures looks good to a state senator—unless of course it means putting out of work several hundred state hospital employees residing in that senator's district. Situations occurred where a state hospital "overnight" became retitled a "community mental health center" and thus eligible to apply for federal funding. In other cases, private hospitals quickly added a community mental health center to their existing array of services. However, their intention was not so much to meet the comprehensive mental health needs of all potential clients in their geographic area as to continue serving the same paying or well-insured clients that they were already serving and to refer difficult or chronic patients to the state system of care.

3. *The needs and problems of today's patients in state hospitals are being neglected.* In the sixties there were many relatively functional patients in state hospitals who could be better served by less restrictive settings. These patients may have been helpful to less functional patients and in addition were often utilized by staff in various jobs and roles. Although we can rejoice that this

servitudinal use of patients has greatly diminished, we need to be aware that their absence creates a care vacuum that paid workers should be employed to fill. Nearly 100 percent of today's state hospital inpatients are manifesting acute or severe behavioral problems and have generally been underresponsive to current psychiatric treatment approaches. Where there were once a number of wards with no particularly violent or suicidal patients, there are now a significant number of actively suicidal or violent or actively psychotic patients on nearly every unit. Therefore, a state legislator's understandable assumption that less patients should mean less staff and less money is in error, given the nature of the patient.

4. *In most communities there is no organized systematic after-care program that has defined what good after-care involves and then makes such care available on a 24-hour, seven-day a week basis.* Day or night, workday or holiday, clients in the community may need temporary: (1) protection from self or others in a crisis, (2) intervention and perhaps removal from a distressed family or group situation, (3) practical assistance with the decisions and activities of daily living and health maintenance, (4) appropriate social and occupational services, and (5) a dependable counselor to assist the client in resolving emotional or interactional problems. Often there is nothing and no one consistently available to respond to these needs.

These are but a few of the problems facing those who advocate for better mental health care. Fortunately there are some programs that implement community care for the discharged institutionalized person. M. Bayer describes a "sustaining care" program that cut rehospitalization rates and reduced the stay for those who had to be readmitted. The nurses rendering the "caring and advocacy" in this rural program looked at the problems from broad perspectives. They asked: (1) Who is the client and what are his/her needs for successful deinstitutionalization? (2) What are the learning needs of state hospital staff and the potential caretakers (foster and boarding home proprietors, family, etc.)? (3) What resources are in the community and how can these be both supported and utilized? With priorities established and the nursing process as the means of approach, the nurses in this program were so successful in implementing specific improvements that statewide visibility had administrators asking why this "sustaining care" role should be filled by a nurse rather than by someone from another mental health discipline. The nurses' response was to present documented cases where their knowledge of normal physical conditions and development as well as their ability to quickly detect deviations had been important in crisis intervention (9).

All nurses will probably find that they too must be increasingly involved in developing and documenting theory, roles, and methods for meeting mental health needs on a coordinated spectrum basis.

ADVOCACY: DEFINITIONS AND CONNOTATIONS

You have probably been informed that one of your nursing roles is client advocacy. However, if you ever have tried to ascertain just what behaviors are expected of you as a client advocate, you will have had good reason to become confused. We have no consensus within either the health care system or nursing as to how advocacy should be demonstrated in behavior.

The noun *advocate is the first of all a term to denote*: (1) *the person who pleads, argues, or defends on behalf of another*, (2) *the person who supports and pleads the cause of another in a court of law*, and (3) *a synonym for lawyer*. Over the past several decades, we have seen this

term taken from its traditional legal context. Now we use the word, *advocate, in the context of consumer advocate or civil rights advocate, and meaning not only an attorney but all who argue for or uphold a given cause.* Simultaneously with other advocacy movements, various health professionals began promoting the idea that health professionals *should* be client advocates. Nurses began claiming that they needed to take action not only to protect clients from health care system abuses but also to enable clients to get a fuller measure of informed and high quality care.

As nurses began making advocacy statements it became obvious that quite differing connotations were being associated with this concept. S. Kosik in a 1972 article equates patient advocacy with "fighting the system" and writes that patient advocacy is seeing that the patient knows what to expect and what his/her rights are, and then displaying the willingness and courage to see that our system does not prevent the person from getting them (36). Kosik believes that nursing needs nurses to become patient advocates (36).

In an article published a year later, W. Nations, a nurse-lawyer, differs from Kosik. She describes her role in a Veterans Administration Hospital as an "ombudsman-plus" who educates staff, serves as the patients' relations officer, is a legal interpreter, and counsels patients regarding legal action and representation. It is not clear whether Nations sees her only advocacy responsibility as being toward the client. She relates that when a group of patients inquired as to whether the therapy team was violating the patients' rights via token economy therapy, she responded by explaining that token economy therapy was a medically approved, widely accepted mode of treatment (43). This response does not seem to directly address the issue of whether rights of patients were being violated.

Perhaps examples such as that above from Nations help us understand why Attorney George Annas cautions patients not to let a hospital representative tell you he is your representative! The most important thing about a patient advocate, regardless of title, is that *he/she must actually represent the patient* since the goal is to enhance the patient's position in making decisions concerning health care (1).

Annas points out that many hospital administrations have employed patient representatives whose goal is to smooth over patient complaints and improve the hospital's image; these are public relations programs, *not* patient advocate programs (1).

F. Schontz suggests that the term *advocate* may not be the best term because it implies that patient-hospital interaction is an adversary procedure. As an alternative, Schontz offers the term *liaison agent* to describe *an individual who works for the benefit of both client and institution to ensure communication and mutual understanding.* Schontz acknowledges that the liaison agent role

is difficult since this individual will be caught between economic identification with the agency and personal identification with the patient. Schoentz sees the liaison agent in the role of diplomat or statesman rather than champion or adversary (52).

This liaison role involves loyalties to both client and employer and is one that many nurses have tried to fulfill for generations. It is not a role to be slighted since diplomacy can prevent not only wars but lawsuits! However, the needs of the clients and the needs of the institution may be oppositional. It is not difficult to think of examples. Clients may need the reduced stimulation of a private room, whereas the institution presses for the more economical choice of a shared room. The client might need one-to-one nursing care, whereas the hospital is short-staffed. Mental health clients may need opportunities to test new behaviors that involve taking risks whereas the hospital is short-staffed. Mental health clients may need opportunities to test new behaviors that involve taking risks, whereas the agency overseeing the treatment is validly concerned about the legal redress that may occur if the client or others are injured as a result of risk. These are but a few areas of potential conflict. Related moral and legal issues will be discussed shortly.

M. Whitley and L. Madden seem in substantial agreement with Schontz as they describe a family advocate as an intercessor, not champion of a cause (60). Their discussion speaks of advocacy in terms of guiding, clarifying, and assisting a client to understand how an agency functions.

S. Archer and R. Fleshman take a considerably stronger approach in their text. They write of assisting a client to obtain what he/she is entitled to from the system, and propose that it is an essential nursing responsibility to pressure the agency into modifying policies. These authors conceive of an advocate as speaking up for something and being different from an ombudsman who mediates and intentionally does not take sides. One of their examples of what client advocacy might include was that of testifying in court on behalf of clients (2).

Emergent nursing seems to be most closely adhering to the *advocacy interventions* of the type that Archer and Fleshman espouse, i.e., *speaking up for principles of respect, justice, equality, and rights when you assess that a client cannot adequately represent or advocate for self* (2).

M. Burgdorf, in an article regarding children's legal rights, separates advocacy into two types: formal and informal advocacy (17). *Formal advocacy refers to legal interventions by the nurse, such as testifying in court on a client's behalf, researching and developing data to be utilized by attorneys, and perhaps even initiating court cases on behalf of clients.*

Nurses are increasingly being utilized in the courts as **expert witnesses,** *persons who by education and experience possess knowledge that others do not have* (49). The expert witness, in addition to giving facts, may give opinions that are based on knowledge and experience. This witness should honestly believe in the point of view that he/she will be called upon to support, although S. Perry maintains that this belief should not extend to emotional involvement or advocacy (48). It is not clear how Perry defines advocacy, or how, if one gives an opinion that he/she sincerely believes is based on professional knowledge and experience, this is not in some sense advocating.

Expert nurse witnesses may be utilized in testifying in nursing malpractice; on the value of nursing services; or on standards of nursing care, education, and administration (45). It is beyond the scope of this text to prepare you to be an expert nurse witness. However, several states have developed guidelines or services to aid expert nurse witnesses. Nurse-authors such as C. Northrop (41) and S. Perry (44), who have expertise in this area, are active in trying to disseminate information and in encouraging nurses to be informed about this role.

Informal advocacy refers to actions taken to see that clients' rights are respected, that clients are well-informed, that cover-ups of information to which client and public are entitled do not occur (17), *and that strategies are developed to impel improvements in settings rendering unsafe and/or inhumane care.*

Before we can consider principles that the nurse can follow in both formal and informal advocacy dilemmas, we need to realize that advocacy events are in their very nature always surrounded by ethical and/or legal implications.

MORAL STANDARDS, ETHICS, AND LEGAL PARAMETERS

If our advocacy actions are to be more than knee-jerk responses, we first need to understand the legal parameters of nursing practice; and second, we need to examine how advocacy actions are either consciously or reflexively undergirded by our moral standards and to a varying degree by our ethical level of development. T. Szasz states that therapeutic action in the mental health field always involves moral values and constitutional rights (58).

Several terms need to be defined before proceeding. *Law refers to man-made rules that regulate human social conduct in a formally prescribed and legally binding manner.* Law may be made in the form of **statutes,** *formal enactments by a legislative body,* or **common law,** *rulings developed through judicial decisions that interpret legal issues* (12). *Legal rights are claims considered valid by the legal system* (56). (See also Chapter 22.)

L. Churchill differentiates ethics from morals. He defines **morality** *as behavior in accordance with custom and tradition,* and says that *to be **ethical** the person must take the additional step of exercising critical, rational judgment to assess courses of action in terms of principles* (19). This leads us to considering the interplay of advocacy with morality, ethics, and law. M. Bayles expresses the dilemma with a question: To what extent should a nurse be a patient's advocate and to what extent should a nurse's own standard of the value of life be the basis of action (10)?

M. Kohnke suggests that her advocacy standard is one of informing a client of choices and rights and then supporting the decision the client makes. The decision a client makes is his/her own, even if, in your opinion, it is not the best decision. He/she has the right to make decisions freely and without pressure. This is advocacy in the best sense of the word. Kohnke's ethical statement about what advocacy *ought* to be (ideal ethical rights) seems to derive from a concern that nurses not fall blindly into the rescuer role or a "we know best" attitude (35).

A different ethical viewpoint is to assert that if a client's decision is not the best decision in our professional viewpoint, then we have an obligation to try and influence that decision and in selected situations to try and prevent the implementation of that decision by using legal manuevers. In addition, many would insist that you have an ethical responsibility to yourself not to compromise your personal standards to the extent that you impair your own physical, emotional, or spiritual health.

Law, morality, and ethics are all constructs that are bound by time and culture and in a dynamic society are constantly in process. Morality usually lags behind the ethics of ethical leaders in society. Laws usually are not enacted by statute until they represent the moral development of a substantial segment of society. Once legislated, statutory laws may linger on the books long beyond their moral acceptance by a plurality. Contrary to what happens with statutory law, judicially interpreted or common law is sometimes contrary to the wishes of significant numbers of citizens. The point here is that advocate-nurses may very likely experience dilemmas where their own moral standards or ethical sense is either contrary to statutory law or unsupported by recent decisions in judicial findings. (See also Chapter 22.)

One assertion you will find in researching advocacy literature is that the nurse's primary ethical responsibility is to the client (20, 56). Dilemmas occur then for the nurse employed in an agency since this nurse: (1) has legal obligations both to the agency and to the clients, (2) works with physicians who are considered to have the ultimate accountability for patient care, and (3) is limited by institutional policies that circumscribe the nurse's authority to act (56).

There is light at the end of this moral-ethical-legal tunnel. Many advocacy dilemmas can be significantly alleviated by continual effort to sharpen two skills: (1) moral-ethical self-awareness, and (2) communication that is assertive, nonthreatening, and nondefensive.

Moral-Ethical Self-Awareness

As a challenge to sharpening ethical awareness,

you can look at the following strong advocacy statement and articulate the ethic espoused by B. Ennis and R. Emery:

> Psychiatric diagnoses are not always reliable or agreed upon by two or more experts. Experts have not always been able to predict dangerous behavior, including suicide. Therefore mental health professionals should refuse to make the legal, ethical, and social judgments for involuntary confinement (25).

Curiously and ironically, one ethic being expressed in the foregoing is that it is *unethical* to make *ethical* judgments for involuntary confinement! Recognizing an ethical-based statement such as the one above is a way to begin thinking about your own ethical standards—questioning and analyzing the culturally developed morals that you may have accepted as truth since childhood. Statements that directly assert or clearly imply how people *ought to behave* are statements deriving from a *moral standard or ethical principle* Noticing this can lead to challenging yourself to more conscious levels of awareness and growth in your own ethical principles. You can then help clients make more ego-syntonic decisions because you can help them enunciate and weigh what values, ethics, and morals are central to them in making a *"peace-full"* decision.

Communication That Is Assertive, Nonthreatening, and Nondefensive

In reading statements below about the second skill of using assertive, nonthreatening, nondefensive communication, you will probably now be attuned to looking for ethic-based statements.

1. *In deciding to advocate on behalf of a primary client, the nurse owes the sufficiently energized and rational client (or the family/guardian of the seriously impaired client), physician, and employer, precise nondefensive, noncritical information regarding the nurse's advocacy decisions.*

   In one general hospital, nurses said they were not allowed by the physicians to give the local crisis hot-line telephone number to clients as an additional resource after these clients were hospitalized for a suicide attempt. One nurse decided that advocacy was vital in this situation. She very calmly but firmly explained to the physician and nursing supervisor why she felt professionally obliged to offer the crisis phone number to potentially suicidal clients. The physician complained to the Director of Nursing, who called the nurse in to be counseled about insubordination. She explained to her director that she viewed her own actions as consistent with the state nursing practice act that defined one of her responsibilities as *that of preventing illness*. This approach was successful and the physicians' unwritten policy was changed as a result.

2. *When personal limitations are affecting professional counseling abilities, the nurse-advocate owes clients this information.*

   Mr. Z. was a "natural" at nursing. From childhood through adolescence he took care of an alcoholic mother. Throughout several years of student nursing experience he considered himself lucky in not being assigned clients with health problems directly attributed to alcohol consumption. But the day came when he was to render primary care to an alcoholic homemaker. Mr. Z found he could not feel at all comfortable with this patient. He talked to his nursing instructor who felt he should contine to try to relate more therapeutically with the patient. Finally Mr. Z. made the only decision with which he could be comfortable at that point. He said to the client, "Mrs. F., due to some of my own past experiences, I really am not able to help you consider your problems in depth. But you certainly deserve someone who is. Let's explore how we can assure that you find someone to help you work through your problems."

   Nurses often do not have the feeedom to choose their clients on the basis of whom they feel they can help effectively. Surely then they are entitled to tell the client that they feel personally limited, but that they do feel they can help the client find alternative significant counseling relationships.

3. *The customer is not always right! Neither is the client when viewed in terms of the nurse's own values.* The nurse's professional judgment in a given situation may be that the interests of the family, institution, physician, or society supersede the nurse's obligation to a particular client. In other words, the nurse's ethic in this situation will prevent effectively advocating for the client in terms of what the client says he/she wants. The nurse should communicate this to the client and should assist the client in obtaining fair advocacy from someone who does not feel as he/she does.

ADVOCACY AND THE NURSING PROCESS

Experience with the nursing process makes you aware of how cyclic the process is. Beginning with initial assessment, you then form your first nursing diagnosis. Based on that, you begin planning intervention. Advocacy is one kind of intervention. Sometimes an initial nursing assessment and diagnosis will indicate advocacy needs, for example, when an abuse victim's self-perception is that of being powerless, helpless, and dependent.

However, much of the time your awareness of advocacy needs comes later in the process of client care. For example, suppose you have assessed and made a nursing diagnosis of Dysfunctional Grieving. As you begin your interventions, you are also continuing to assess and thus you observe that the client's apathy is immobilizing him from self-assertion in response to a roommate's intrusiveness. You ask the client if he would prefer a different roommate. He says yes, but he is sure what he wants is of no consequence in such a huge medical complex. When you investigate a room change, you are told there are no other beds available. Thus the client becomes increasingly convinced that he can have no influence over external circumstances. At this point, you intervene by telling the client that he has had the power to influence your behavior. You then convince the admitting office that a room change request is not just a whim for this client but a component of providing him quality care. You can use this to help the client see that he can influence the world around him. It is a stepping-stone to a later intervention of assisting him to be autonomously self-assertive.

Advocacy, then, is not a diagnosis but rather an intervention. However, you do assess whether advocacy is an indicated intervention and whether you are the appropriate intervener.

Assessing the Need for Advocacy

Various tools and resources can be used to assess advocacy needs. For example, does the patient care in the setting under question meet the American Nurses' Association Standards of Psychiatric and Mental Health Nursing Practice? Does it comply with licensing regulations and mental health codes of the particular state? Manuals or references that put forth standards that have been widely accepted by the nursing profession are appropriate to use in validating a need for advocacy in a given situation.

D. Wineman and A. James, in entreating social work educators to respond more appropriately to advocacy needs, present a list of many of the forms of dehumanization that occur too often in mental "health" settings. Their list, which is enumerated below, serves nurses well in sensitizing them to events where they need to advocate. Hopefully you are witnessing a high enough level of care that you will be shocked at the items on the list. Yet there are an uncounted number of both private and public facilities where the types of care described below are not even rare events. The list of nine categories of dehumanization include (61):

1. *Physical brutalization*: Restraining a client to meet staff needs rather than responding appropriately to the client's need is brutality. Isolation procedures by their nature create sensory deprivation and need to be accompanied by regulating external stimuli at individual therapeutic levels. Unrestrictive settings and understaffing are brutal to clients who are actively suicidal, self-mutilating, and/or highly impulsive.

2. *Psychic humiliation*: Frustrated ineffective staff may use shaming such as, "John, you know better than that!" Clients who are harrassing or exploiting other clients may be tolerated or ignored. The use of authority may be routine, arbitrary, and demeaning. Offensive terms such as "old codger," "big baby," etc., may be directed to clients or used in verbal interchanges to describe the client.

3. *Sexual traumatization*: In settings that are insufficiently supervised, weaker residents can be victimized by sexual intimidation, assault, or rape. Reports of such victimiz-

ation may be essentially ignored because "after all, she/he is crazy."

4. *Condoned use of feared indigenous leaders for behavioral management*: Where staff are in short supply or perhaps just insecure, they are apt to covertly encourage stronger residents to maintain order even at the expense of other residents.

5. *Chronic exposure to programless boredom*: Much of the regression, withdrawal, and acting out for which clients are supposedly being treated is in fact being induced by enforced inactivity in inadequate custodial settings.

6. *Unclean grouping*: Wineman and James point out that individuals may be forced to live together who are clinically incompatible and thus cannot avoid symptom and trait clashes that increase their problems.

7. *Symptom-squeezing forms of punishment*: Wineman and James pinch the professional's conscience with examples such as: restricting home visiting for one who needs his/her family; isolating a person who is fearful of being left alone; restricting food in an attempt to shape the behavior of the severely regressed; or punishing a masochist. Settings that utilize Behavior Modification Therapy should first examine which reinforcements and aversive approaches are dehumanizing.

8. *Enforced work routines in the guise of vocational training!* Even the courts have intervened in this area to rule that involuntary servitude is not treatment. Jobs and the vocational rehabilitation of clients are to be appropriately designed and individualized as a response to the particular client's vocational and social needs.

9. *Violation of privacy*: Here, too, the courts have intervened to issue directives about clients' rights for sufficient quarters, personal property, and freedom from unauthorized searches of persons and property. Yet staff in many settings still assume that privacy considerations can be sacrificed for security and efficiency. Hospital records used inappropriately violate privacy, as does interview data obtained to merely satisfy personal curiousity. Clients also are entitled to protection from the violation of their privacy by other clients.

Finally, there are some general questions to explore in determining if advocacy is indicated. For example: What is the basic advocacy issue? (Does it have to do with quality of care, access to care, fully informed care, or choices and alternatives in care?) What are the legal rights and responsibilities of the client? What is being risked as far as the client is concerned if advocacy does/does not occur? Why does the client need an advocate? (Why is the client not totally able to represent self?)

If you have determined a client's need for advocacy, there is a second equally important question to be assessed: Are you the individual who should do the advocating? Table 23-1 below lists questions you can ask to assess yourself as advocate.

TABLE 23-1.   Assessing Self as Advocate

1. Are you aware of your legal rights and responsibilities?
2. What can you foresee that you might be risking?
3. What will happen if you take a position in conflict with existing institutional policy?
4. Is there another issue or hidden agenda motivating your urge to advocate?
5. How can you be sure that you are not just displacing your own anger or acting-out your own identification or transference issues?
6. What do you foresee will be the results of successful advocacy?
7. What might the ripple effect be? What further events may occur due to throwing an advocacy-rock into a calm body of water?
8. What resources can you utilize, such as public opinion, legal opinion, community support?
9. Why should it be *you* to advocate in a given situation?
10. Should it be a group advocacy action?
11. Who needs the advocacy—an individual in a unique situation, or a whole group or class of clients experiencing similar distress or powerlessness?
12. What is the current status of both your physical and emotional energy level?
13. Can you handle the related anxiety and perhaps lonesomeness?
14. Who will support you if the going gets rough?
15. How will you deal with the phenomena that advocacy often facilitates the client's dependency on you?
16. What data-gathering and documentation do you need to do before arriving at a decision on advocacy?

Principles of Advocacy Intervention

The primary skill of advocacy intervention seems to revolve around the appropriate use of power. B. Brown, K. Gebbie, and J. Moore define *power* as *the ability and willingness to affect others' behavior to bring about change* (14).

Nurse-power

Use nurse-power appropriately. In health care systems, the power struggles regarding client care are continual. Dr. Brown gives the example of a patient who is scheduled to go to physical or perhaps respiratory therapy, whereas your nursing assessment is that the client cannot tolerate these treatments at this time. It is nursing's prerogative to intervene and decide that such therapy be postponed. If we do not exercise our prerogative as client advocates and control the massive subsystems of organizations operating in our hospitals, we deserve to lose the rightful role of nursing (14).

To affirm and utilize nurse-power, we must

be willing to make decisions with awareness of our accountability and risk-taking (14). We too often confuse medical expertise with nursing expertise and rely on the physician to make nursing decisions. For example, suppose the physician writes an order that the client must attend all sessions of occupational therapy (O.T.). Does that mean you are required to have the physician's altered order before you can hold that client out of a given O.T. session? No, it means that when you have a nursing-based rationale for not following the order, you assume professional accountability for your decision. You also communicate your decision and rationale to the physician and to the O.T. staff.

In more complex advocacy dilemmas there are many questions to explore. Let's take an illustrative dilemma of a physician recommending electroconvulsive therapy (ECT), whereas you believe this to be against the client's best interest. What are your advocacy responsibilities then? What is appropriate use of power? This is not an easy dilemma, and if you randomly researched this in a population of both nurses and physicians, you would get varied answers. However, there are questions that can help you decide what you want to do—questions that you can apply to many other situations by substituting other adjectives and nouns for the abbreviation ECT, as noted below:

1. What do you think you know about ECT, based on your balanced research of the literature and your own nursing observations?
2. Are you totally against ECT under all circumstances, or just against ECT for this specific treatment for this client?
3. What nursing theory or evidence is your opinion against ECT based on?
4. Are you able to pull out the subjective components of your objection? (When one "doesn't like" something there are usually subjective and sometimes even unconscious reactions involved. It is important to identify and examine the values and ethical positions so that you can consider how they are affecting your perceptions.)
5. What is the client's power in this situation?
6. Is the client or client's guardian fully informed as to the effectiveness of ECT compared to other alternatives, the cost, the anticipated outcome, all risks and/or adverse effects?
7. What does the client want?
8. Has an independent second opinion from another psychiatrist been obtained?
9. If the client has been adjudged mentally incompetent, what are his/her rights in regard to refusing ECT?
10. What discussion have you had with the physician to understand the physician's point of view?
11. What do your peers, co-workers, faculty, and/or supervisor say when you discuss the situation with them?

You may reach agreement with the physician through exploring some or all of the above questions. If you do not reach agreement, then the alternatives you have (once you are a *licensed professional*) involve decidedly increased risk-taking: (1) You can nondefensively ask the physician to reconsider, based on your data and reasons for your objection, in which case you are risking the physician's reaction. (2) You can ask the client and family to consider your point of view. In this case, you risk upsetting the client, family, nursing supervisor, and physician, and possibly even risk being sued. (3) You can refuse to participate in the care of that client. Now you risk promotion, job, and further opportunities to be of help to that client. (4) You do nothing, choosing loyalty to the physician as your higher value or convincing yourself that authority knows best. With the last two alternatives (3) and (4), you risk losing your nursing perspective and your self-esteem.

M. Donahue states that in order to fully realize our potential as patient advocates, we must first become nurse advocates and proponents of nurses' rights (22).

Have you considered what your rights are as a nurse? Our legal professional rights are the subject of each state nursing practice act (statute) and may be known to you. However, a large number of states have so recently updated their nurse practice acts that related common law judicial interpretations have not yet been made. There are practice acts in such states as New York and Missouri which identify nursing functions, such as nursing diagnoses, health teaching, counseling, and prevention. But nurses have yet to implement these functions so visibly and assertively that the public reacts with legal processes of their own which will clarify the parameters of nurses' legal rights. The abortion controversy helped define the right of nurses *not to do* nursing actions that were contrary to their beliefs. There is no similar precedent for defining what you have a legal right *to do* (4,5,15,26).

We have much professional growth to achieve in organizing in accord with the "safety in numbers" truism so we can clarify our rights. We can collaborate in interpreting our practice acts and the professional standards issued by the American Nurses' Association. We can influence both agency and individual practice nursing so that burgeoning role definitions become traditional functions at a pace consistent with our knowledge and competence. Earning the public's trust is as simple as demonstrating and documenting that we have the skills to promote, maintain, and restore health in a humane, cost-efficient manner. The following case is a good example of successful advocacy:

B.W., a medical nurse, called L.V., a psychiatric nurse, for consultation. Mrs. T., a retired, widowed client in the medical clinic where B.W. practiced, had been told by a psychiatrist in private practice that he could be of no further help to her unless she agreed to hospitalization for a series of ECT treatments. Mrs. T. did not want ECT. She sought the opinion of B.W.

Through data that B.W. had collected, L.V. learned that Mrs. T. lived alone at home with involved family nearby whom Mrs. T. visited frequently. Mrs. T. had lost interest in all her usual activities but was continuing to accomplish the basic functional activities of living at a diminished level. Mrs. T. had significant symptoms of depression in emotional and physical spheres. However, her spiritual functioning remained a source of strength and meant that active suicidal behaviors were out of the question.

Based on this data, L.V. supported B.W. in a decision to assist Mrs. T. in obtaining a second opinion. Mrs. T. insisted that the referral be to a psychiatrist rather than to a non-physician, and one with an office near her home. B.W. made inquiries, with the additional requirement that the referral be to someone particularly attuned to the problems of senior citizens. Mrs. T. then chose from a couple of referral possibilities. The new physician used a cognitive and stress-reducing approach. After her first visit to him, Mrs. T. told B.W. that the doctor had given her "homework" that she was dubious about but was going to try to do. Mrs. T. was even marginally eager to see what future visits to this physician could accomplish. B.W. was an advocate!

Nurse-advocacy

Nurse-advocacy may be indicated in judicial incompetency and guardianship proceedings as well as in reversing an incompetency ruling (see Chapter 22). This might occur through court testimony as well as through careful and precisely recorded nursing observations that describe the client's capacities and incapacities. An article by D. Hyland considering the pros and cons of judicial incompetency rulings notes that clients may react to such a serious legal step with fear, frustration, anger, depression, withdrawal, uncooperativeness, and regression. Yet, guardianship may promote feelings of security for the debilitated individual because the guardian may be the only caring person in his/her world (34).

An incompetency ruling may be so horrendous for one individual that a successful, sudden, and impulsive suicide occurs. For another the ruling may be acknowledged with equanimity. A third individual might be motivated to see the ruling as a challenge and for the first time might cooperatively engage in therapy. The following is an example:

The family of B.F., who is 35 years of age, asked a clinical specialist in psychiatric nursing to accompany them to a lawyer to discuss incompetency proceedings for B.F. The nurse, who had been familiar with the problems of B.F. and her family over a period of several years, agreed. The lawyer asked the nurse to testify regarding her experiences with B.F. The nurse talked this over with B.F. and the family. The nurse's professional opinion was that an incompetency ruling would be health-promoting for both B.F. and family, and she agreed to give testimony. The incompetency hearing took most of the day. The state hospital psychiatrist, psychologist, and social worker presented data and testimony that they believed indicated B.F. should retain her competent legal status. A private psychiatrist employed by B.F.'s family testified and presented data that he believed indicated incompetence, as did B.F.'s mother and the nurse. B.F. also testified in her own behalf; in fact, she was insistent on doing so against the counsel of her attorney. The judge's ruling was for incompetence.

B.F. was highly ambivalent about the ruling. One year later she still vacillated between "demanding" to have her rights restored and relief over the protectiveness and leverage the guardianship offered. Her ambivalence was similar in its manifestations to early adolescent struggles with dependence and independence.

A revealing sidenote occurred at lunchtime on the day of the hearing when B.F., B.F.'s family, the social worker, and the nurse found themselves left standing together in a cluster as the others left to eat. As this group began walking to a nearby cafeteria, B.F. challenged the nurse and social worker as to how they could both claim to care about her and yet hold divergent opinions. They each tried to honestly answer. Perhaps what B.F. witnessed at that point was advocacy operating both at its peak and within its limitations.

Nurses are becoming quite alert to the need for advocacy in child abuse situations. Chapter 21 identifies several signs, symptoms, or injuries that may indicate abuse. R. Olson developed a weighted index that can be used in assessing for potential abuse. In the tool, he weights the factors of attitude towards staff, family structure, family problems, religious affiliation, labor and delivery, and cultural factors (47). Refer to Chapter 21, pp. 677–679, for information on how you can be an advocate for the abused child and his/her family.

J. Holter notes that about 70–75 percent of identified abusive parents are believed to desire professional assistance in changing their child-rearing practices and will respond to planned intervention that meets their individual needs (33). One of the difficulties in reaching the abusive parent before irreparable injury or death occurs is the same problem that occurs in reaching the violence-prone in general. (See Chapter 19.) Holter helps us by identifying some categories of parents that are generally less responsive to help:

1. Parents who are severely depressed and/or psychotic.
2. Parents with severe character disorders or antisocial personalities.
3. Parents suffering severe alcohol and/or drug addiction.
4. Parents with severe mental retardation.
5. Parents living a violent subcultural life style.
6. Parents whose religious values affirm cruel punishment or medical neglect.

If one or more of these categories are indicated, you may need to consider whether the child should be at least temporarily removed from the home.

Adults may also be abuse victims, particularly a spouse, the intellectually or emotionally vulnerable, and the elderly. Perhaps it is surprising that the same observations that help you recognize abused/neglected children will also help you recognize abused/neglected adults. A number of states are in the process of writing or updating abuse laws to respond to the protection needs of adults (40).

Emily Eckel and Joseph Nagy were advocates. As former nursing aides working in a nursing home, they, along with social worker Mary Lewin, published a 100-page report, *Kane Hospital, A Place to Die*, a documentation of abuse and neglect in the Pittsburgh, Pennsylvania, institution. They did not stop with a report; they also formed committees and coalitions, involved the community, and confronted politicians and bureaucracy. These well-organized efforts were successful to the tune of millions of dollars in economic resources and hundreds of new staff positions for the hospital (51).

Organized advocacy efforts are often a very effective way to generate reforms. A recent edition of the *Encyclopedia of Associations* listed 1,336 health and medical organizations and 879 social welfare organizations (62). Many of these groups either identify advocacy as a primary function or imply that it is one of their functions. Space allows for only a few of these organizations to be listed here (62).

> Parents Anonymous, a self-help group for abusive parents, has about 880 local chapters. It estimates that physical or emotional abuse injures 5 million children a year.
>
> The Mental Health Association claims 850 local groups. The National Association for Retarded Citizens claims 275,000 members in their 1800 local groups.
>
> The American Schizophrenia Association, sometimes referred to as the Huxley Institute, advocates for its viewpoint on the cause and treatment of schizophrenia. It conceives schizophrenia to be the expression of a probably inherited physical disorder rather than a "psychosociological" condition that can be treated only by "psychiatric means." In relation to its causality position, this group maintains a library on orthomolecular treatment. There are local chapters of this organization in some metropolitan areas.
>
> The American Association of Homes for the Aging, the Association for Humanistic Gerontology, the Gray Panthers, and the Interna-

tional Federation on Aging are some of the groups that advocate for health and welfare interests of the senior citizen.

There are also advocacy groups that express themselves in voluntary and direct one-to-one relationships. Citizen Advocacy, which recently reported some 200 local chapters, is one example. Volunteers offer not only advocacy but friendship and problem-solving support to enable the mildly retarded to function more independently. Inquiries about this group can be made to the National Association for Retarded Citizens or their local chapter (38).

Some hospitals or institutions will motivate an advocacy group to form and lobby for improved care and facilities in one specific facility. Or relatives and friends may organize for the purpose of fund raising and developing alternatives of care, such as temporary housing, that are not currently available in a community. Both of these types of groups may benefit from the assistance of the nurse who wishes to work with them, who will listen to *their* perception of their needs, and who will *collaborate* rather than dictate in striving for mutual goals.

The telephone book, the community service directory of your own or a nearby locale, and reference library resources will help you discover whether you are alone or among talented company when a particular advocacy cause arises.

It is difficult, if not fanciful, to single out principles that apply uniquely to advocacy; but Table 23-2 identifies selected principles that have served nurses well in guiding their advocacy actions.

TABLE 23-2.   Principles of Advocacy Intervention

1. Do not do for the client what the client can do for self.
2. Validate with the client and/or the guardian as well as your support system regarding your plans and any results of your actions.
3. Seek out the knowledge, expertise, and support of individuals or organizations with goals similar to yours.
4. Minimize the use of abstract terms and generalizations in presenting your data.
5. Be thorough and inclusive of all pertinent examples in presenting documentary evidence.
6. Use nurse-power appropriately—as an efficient energy-source, rather than as an incendiary that flames out to burn anything and everything.
7. Patience and persistence are often required and may be more productive than an agitated clamor that soon dies, leaving the basic advocacy goals unachieved.
8. Advocacy does not always involve activity. At times, observation and communication about a problem will be sufficient to improve conditions for a client.

Advocacy and the New Professional

The question of what advocacy actions are reasonable expectations for the student or beginning professional is an intricate question. This chapter has amplified a position that advocacy decisions are arduous and accompanied by risk-taking. Should a new practitioner bombarded with reality shock also shoulder a burden of feeling a failure if there is no energy remaining for advocacy? Our answer is no!

How heavy a cloak of advocacy should we wear? The answer will change as we manifest professional growth. Stuart Chase tells a story of William Penn that somehow seems analogous:

> Penn, who was a gentleman by breeding, wore a sword as part of the traditional dress of the gentlemen of his day. Penn was subsequently converted to the Quaker faith and was much influenced in this conversion by George Fox. The pacifism that is central to Quaker faith put Penn in conflict between his value of a sword as the symbol of gentlemen's attire and his new commitment to Quaker values. He sought out the opinion of Fox about whether he should continue to wear the sword. Mr. Fox's insightful, challenging response was, "Wear it as long as thou canst (18)."

As new nurses, we may not need swords but rather figurative eye blinders and ear plugs as part of our attire. For us to face the advocacy implications of all what we hear and see could be literally overwhelming. Yet if we use self-protection as a permanent rationalization, we will sacrifice our self-esteem and our professional integrity. As we mature, the blinders and ear plugs will feel increasingly restrictive. We can wear them no longer. The cloak of silence becomes heavier than the cloak of advocacy. When that occurs, we look, we listen, we appreciate the support and validation of a colleague; for finally we know we are ready to speak and act.

REFERENCES

1. Annas, George, *The Rights of Hospital Patients* (the basic American Civil Liberties Union guide to a hospital patient's rights). New York: Avon Books, 1975.

2. Archer, Sarah, and Ruth Fleshman, *Community Health Nursing*. North Scituate, Mass.: Duxbury Press, 1975.

3. Aroskar, Mila, "Anatomy of an Ethical Dilemma: The Theory . . . and the Practice," *American Journal of Nursing*, 80, no. 4 (1980), 658-63.

4. Bandman, Bertram, "Do Nurses Have Rights? No," *American Journal of Nursing*, 78, no. 1 (1978), 84-86.

5. Bandman, Elsie, "Do Nurses Have Rights? Yes," *American Journal of Nursing*, 78, no. 1 (1978), 84-86.

6. Barnard, Kathryn, "Child Advocates Must Help Parents Too," *The American Nurse*, 3, no. 8 (September 20, 1979), 4.

7. Barry, Anne, *Bellevue Is a State of Mind*. New York: Harcourt Brace Jovanovich, Inc., 1971.

8. Bassuk, Ellen, and Samuel Gerson, "Deinstitutionalization and Mental Health Services," *Scientific American*, 238, no. 2 (1978), 46-53.

9. Bayer, Mary, "Easing Mental Patient's Return to Their Communities," *American Journal of Nursing*, 76, no. 3 (1976), 406-8.

10. Bayles, Michael, "The Value of Life . . . By What Standard?" *American Journal of Nursing*, 80, no. 12 (1980), 2226-30.

11. Bernhard, Robert, "The Dehumanized Hospital Hurts You and Your Patients," *Nursing Digest*, 5, no. 1 (1977), 39-41.

12. Bernzweig, Eli, *Nurse's Liability for Malpractice*. New York: McGraw-Hill Book Company, 1969.

13. Brill, Norman, "Overview: Individual and Societal Discontents," *The Bulletin of the American Association for Social Psychiatry*, 1, no. 4 (1980), 3-5.

14. Brown, Barbara, Kristine Gebbie, and Joan Moore, "Effecting Nursing Goals in Health Care," *Nursing Administration Quarterly*, 2, no. 3 (1978), 17-31.

15. Bruce, Joan and Marie Snyder, "The Right and Responsibility to Diagnose," *American Journal of Nursing*, 82, no. 4 (1982), 645-46.

16. Budson, Richard, "Sheltered Housing for the Mentally Ill: An Overview," *McLean Hospital Journal*, 4, no. 3 (1979), 140-57.

17. Burgdorf, Marcia, "Legal Rights of Children," *Nursing Clinics of North America*, 14, no. 3 (1979), 405-16.

18. Chase, Stuart, *Roads to Agreement*. New York: Harper & Row, Publishers, Inc., 1951.

19. Churchill, Larry, "Ethical Issues of a Profession in Transition," *American Journal of Nursing*, 77, no. 5 (1977), 873-74.

20. Curtain, Leah, "Is There a Right to Health Care?" *American Journal of Nursing*, 80, no. 3 (1980), 462-65.

21. Davis, Anne, "Pain q 3h," *American Journal of Nursing*, 80, no. 5 (1980), 974.

22. Donahue, M. Patricia, "The Nurse a Patient Advocate?'. *Nursing Forum*, 17, no. 2 (1978), 143-151.

23. Donaldson, Kenneth, *Insanity Inside Out*. New York: Crown Publishers, Inc., 1976.

24. Duran, Fernando, and Gerald Errion, "Perpetuation of Chronicity in Mental Illness," *American Journal of Nursing*, 70, no. 8 (1970), 1707-9.

25. Ennis, Bruce, and Richard Emery, *The Rights of Mental Patients* (an American Civil Liberties Union handbook), p. 6. New York: Avon Books, 1978. As cited in *New York Civil Liberties Newsletter*, 26, no. 7 (September-October 1978), 5.

26. Fagin, Claire, "Nurses' Rights," *American Journal of Nursing*, 75, no. 1 (1975), 82-85.

27. Friedberg, John, *Shock Treatment Is Not Good for Your Brain*. San Francisco: Glide Publications, 1976.

28. Galton, Lawrence, "A Serious Threat to the Elderly," *Parade*, November 4, 1979, pp. 6,9,12.

29. Gotkin, Janet, and Paul Gotkin, *Too Much Anger, Too Many Tears: A Personal Triumph over Psychiatry*. New

York: Quadrangle/The New York Times Book Co., Inc., 1975.

30. Greenblatt, Milton, "Violence and the Rights and Responsibilities of Patients and Staff," *The Bulletin of the American Association for Social Psychiatry*, 1, no. 4 (1980), 9–12.

31. Health Services Administration, U.S. Dept. of Health, Education and Welfare, *Background Papers: National Symposium on Patients' Rights in Health Care*, May 17-18, 1976.

32. ___, *Proceedings: National Symposium on Patients' Rights in Health Care*, May 17-18, 1976. DHEW Pub. No. (HSA) 76-7002.

33. Holter, Joanne C., "Child Abuse," *Nursing Clinics of North America*, 14, no. 3 (1979), 417–27.

34. Hyland, Dale, "Incompetence and Guardianship," *American Journal of Nursing*, 80, no. 10 (1980), 1863–64.

35. Kohnke, Mary F., "The Nurse as Advocate," *American Journal of Nursing*, 80, no. 11 (1980), 2038–40.

36. Kosik, Sandra, "Patient Advocacy or Fighting the System," *American Journal of Nursing*, 72, no. 4 (1972), 694–98.

37. Lamb, H. Richard, "The New Asylums in the Community," *Archives of General Psychiatry*, 36, no. 21 (1979), 129–34.

38. Lampe, David, "Just Being a Friend Can Work Wonders," *Parade*, November 30, 1980, pp. 6–9.

39. Leaman, Karen, "Recognizing and Helping the Abused Child," *Nursing 79*, 9, no. 2 (1979), 64–66.

40. Mancini, Marguerite, "Adult Abuse Laws," *American Journal of Nursing*, 80, no. 4 (1980), 739–40.

41. Munhall, Patricia, "Moral Reasoning Levels of Nursing Students and Faculty in a Baccalaureate Nursing Program," *Image*, 12, no. 3 (1980), 57–61.

42. Murray, Jacquelyn, "Failure of the Community Mental Health Movement," *American Journal of Nursing*, 75, no. 11 (1975), 2034–36.

43. Nations, Wanda, "Nurse-Lawyer Is Patient Advocate," *American Journal of Nursing*, 73, no. 6 (1973), 1039–41.

44. *New York Civil Liberties Newsletter*, vol. 26, no. 7 (1978).

45. Northrop, Cynthia, "The Expert Nurse Witness Service," *The Maryland Nurse*, August 1979, pp. 27–29.

46. Numerof, Rita, "Assertiveness Training," *American Journal of Nursing*, 80, no. 10 (1980), 1796–99.

47. Olson, Robert J., "Index of Suspicion: Screening for Child Abusers," *American Journal of Nursing*, 76, no. 1 (1976), 108–10.

48. Perry, Shannon, "If You're Called as an Expert Witness," *American Journal of Nursing*, 77, no. 3 (1977), 458–60.

49. ___, *The Nurse as an Expert Witness*. A self-instructional module prepared for the Arizona Nurses' Association, Phoenix, Ariz., 1977.

50. Quinn, Nancy, and Anne R. Somers, "The Patient's Bill of Rights," *Nursing Outlook*, 22, no. 4 (1974), 240–44.

51. Robb, Susanne, Mark Peterson, and Joseph W. Nagy, Jr., "Advocacy for the Aged," *American Journal of Nursing*, 79, no. 10 (1979), 1737–38.

52. Schontz, Franklin, *The Psychological Aspects of Physical Illness and Disability*. New York: Macmillan Publishing Co., Inc., 1975.

53. Schorr, Thelma, "Focus on the Nurse Shortage," *American Journal of Nursing*, 80, no. 9 (1980), 1587.

54. Slavinsky, Ann, and Judith Krauss, "Mutual Withdrawal . . . or Gwen Tudor Revisited," *Perspectives in Psychiatric Care*, 18, no. 5 (1980), 194–203.

55. Smith, Carol, "A Decade of Patient Advocacy," *The Heart and Lung Journal*, 8, no. 5 (1979), 926–28.

56. Smith, Sharon, and Anne Davis, "Ethical Dilemmas: Conflicts among Rights, Duties, and Obligations," *American Journal of Nursing*, 80, no. 8 (1980), 1463–66.

57. *St. Louis Post Dispatch*, February 13, 1981, Sec. A, p. 7.

58. Szasz, Thomas, *Law, Liberty, and Psychiatry*. New York: Macmillan Publishing Co., Inc., 1963.

59. ___, *The Myth of Mental Illness*. New York: Harper & Row, Publishers, Inc., 1974.

60. Whitley, Marilyn, and L. (Sissy) Madden, "Encountering Dysfunction in the Family System," in *Clinical Practice in Psychosocial Nursing: Assessment and Intervention*, eds. Diane Longo and Reg Williams, pp. 253–54. New York: Appleton-Century-Crofts, 1978.

61. Wineman, David, and Adrienne James, "The Advocacy Challenge to Schools of Social Work," in *Community Mental Health*, eds. Bruce Denner and Richard Price, Chap. 15. New York: Holt, Rinehart and Winston, 1973.

62. Yakes, Nancy, and Denise Akey, eds. *National Organizations of the U.S.*, 14 ed. Detroit, Mich.: Gayle Research Co., 1980.

24

Feelings and Adjustment of the Nurse in the Health Care Setting

Study of this chapter will assist you to:

1. Examine concerns and conflicts encountered by new graduates and experienced nurses in the work setting.

2. Identify behaviors that facilitate transition into the professional work situation.

3. Formulate your unique criteria for choosing a work setting and making job choices.

4. Consider alternatives for coping with frustrations that will occur within the work group and work setting.

5. Explore the unsuccessful job experience and ways to cope with the experience.

6. Review the rewards and maturing aspects that evolve from commitment to your profession.

7. Develop internal and external resources that will enable you to remain in nursing and to enhance your professional growth.

This chapter contributed by Margaret Ederer, R.N., M.S.N.

SOCIALIZATION INTO THE PROFESSION

Enter the Work Setting:
The World of Reality

This chapter deals mainly with the kinds of realities, struggles, and conflict you might encounter when you enter any new work setting. Conflict is inevitable. Without it, we would be unable to identify problems, seek solutions, and make progress. No matter how ideal a situation may appear, when people are seriously practicing their professions, exercising their options, behaving creatively, and making decisions, conflict will occur. The task is not to avoid conflict but to learn how to resolve it constructively.

Despite all the emphasis on rewards that nurses derive from working with clients, job satisfaction seems more closely related to how nurses get along with other nurses than to how they get along with clients. The nurse-client relationship is transient. You may develop very meaningful relationships with clients and their significant others, but you realize throughout the experience that the relationship will end. In fact, you plan for termination as part of your professional practice. This is not to negate the very real rewards that nurses and clients receive from working together. Still, the nurse-client relationship is temporary. Relationships within work groups, on the other hand, tend to be more permanent. Few nurses resign from positions because of clients when all other factors in the situation are ideal. Nurses can tolerate all kinds of frustrations and difficulties when they have a warm, dependable work group on which to rely.

Awareness of this phenomenon has implications for socialization into the work setting. Ideally there should be no problems with embracing the values of a new work group because the values of all "good" nurses would appear to be the same. In reality, conflicts arise because values differ, as do performance standards and interpretation of the essentials of nursing practice. You may be pulled one way by your desire to practice according to your own professional standards and in the opposite direction by your need to be accepted by the group, since both facets contribute to your job satisfaction and self-esteem.

The need for affiliation is a very basic one. Yet, attempts to have this need met in a work group whose values seem to differ from yours can present difficulties. Your need to belong may initially outweigh professional considerations. "Going along to get along" can result in guilt feelings and depression. Insisting on doing things "the right way," despite indications that your co-workers disapprove, can lead to rejection by the group and to feelings of isolation. M. Kramer and C. Schmalenberg discuss these conflicts in depth in *Paths to Biculturalism* and suggest useful methods for resolution (1). You will find this a valuable resource in dealing with specific work adjustment problems.

General Guidelines

The following are general considerations to keep in mind as you enter a new situation.

Establishing your nursing competence to the satisfaction of your co-workers, superiors, and self is your first objective. You need the power of your proficiency before you can have any constructive impact on the situation. During this time you may witness incidents in which co-workers perform in a less than ideal manner. Remember that your initial task is to learn, not to teach. Not only is it advisable to withhold comments while you are getting acquainted, sometimes it is essential for professional survival. Take comfort in the fact that this situation is temporary. When you have earned the authority to speak, others will listen. You are not ignoring or accepting the unacceptable; rather you are gathering and analyzing data in preparation for presenting it in the most effective way.

A certain amount of testing occurs when a new member enters a group. You have been subjected to testing, formal or informal, at various times and will continue to be throughout life. Work is no exception. Often the nature of the test will not be explained to you. It may be as simple as how long you stay at coffee break or as complex as whether or not you carry out a prescribed treatment on time. When you find yourself going along with the group in some situations, you will benefit more if you make a conscious decision to accept the group norms rather than feeling acted upon and out of control. Decide for yourself which battles you want to fight. Maintain your integrity in those things that really make a difference to you, but do so quietly. Let go of the things that really do not matter.

Be slow to criticize the performance of others. When you are in the process of establishing yourself, it is counterproductive to come on as an ex-

pert who will enlighten and meet the need of others. Take some time to figure out what is really occurring. For example, you may observe that your new co-workers are reluctant to spend time interacting with clients. You feel that is not good! That's not how it should be! Before pointing out the staff's apparent inadequacy and demanding improvement, observe and ask a few nonthreatening questions. Maybe the staff is recovering from a high-intensity client situation that occurred before you arrived. Maybe there have been significant changes in personnel, and people need time to readjust. Although withdrawing from clients is not a therapeutic behavior, there can be any number of possible reasons for it. It is a disservice to your co-workers and to yourself if you immediately assume people do not care. The same is true when you overhear co-workers discussing a client in very negative terms. Your education as well as your inclination point up the destructiveness of this behavior. Yet, as a newcomer, you have no idea of the co-workers' history with this client, of what hurts others might have experienced, or even the co-workers' usual patterns of communication. Caution is indicated. Watch as well as listen. Some people need to get rid of their frustrations verbally. This enables them to prepare again to approach the client therapeutically.

Learning the communication cues and behavior patterns of your co-workers is one of your important tasks. Listen to, but do not rely too heavily on, information volunteered by "helpful" others. Get to know your co-workers in your own way and time. Remember that different people have different things to offer clients. Look for the unique talents that are present and developing in the staff, with an eye to how your unique characteristics will fit in.

Some work groups socialize a great deal outside of work. You have choices about the extent of your participation. At first it may seem almost mandatory for you to be present. Although it might be one way to get to know your co-workers, you have the right to decline invitations that you are uncomfortable accepting. Some people find it difficult to "keep up" physically, financially, or emotionally with the social activities of co-workers. Others prefer to keep work and personal life separate to avoid potential complications. Whatever your choice, you have the right to decide for yourself. To "go along" in an effort to fit in without really wanting to will result in feelings of anger, resentment, or depression. You don't have to do what everyone else does. Your co-workers will respect your position regarding outside socialization if you show your willingness to cooperate and share at work. You will be accepted for your own uniqueness to the degree that you are able to accept others for theirs.

If you decide to participate in social activities with co-workers, remember there may be some overlap. Things that happen outside of work can cause positive or negative feelings that may carry over into work relationships. Be prepared also for having some after-work experiences being alluded to on the job. This can be surprising and, in some instances, embarrassing. Accept comments as part of the process and do not allow yourself to become too upset.

Unfortunately, the socialization process can sometimes involve hurtful feelings. Trial and error is often the method by which we get to know people. You may make some wrong decisions about whom to trust. Everybody does. You may hear gossip and be involved in some of it yourself. The potential for problems is present in any group. You do not have to become entrapped. Keeping your perspective, knowing what to expect, and being alert to signals can prevent some adjustment trauma.

Transition into the Work Group

The following are some suggestions you can follow to smooth your own transition with your work colleagues:

1. *Identify cliques.* You may be fortunate to discover no well-defined cliques in your work setting. It is more common, however, to find subgroups. Membership criteria can be varied and difficult to determine. Work subgroups can form on the basis of age, marital status, outside interests, amount of informal power in the system, attitudes about the job, or any other criteria imaginable. Some groups may openly compete for your membership. Others may make a point of discouraging your attempts to join.

   Initially it is wise to get to know everyone, to look at how people relate to each other, and to make choices. In some settings, choosing to belong to a subgroup is an "either/or" proposition. Belonging to one means you will automatically be excluded from others. Therefore, it is useful to observe the situation before you commit yourself. Sometimes, too, it is easier to get in a group than to get out, so take your time.

2. *Look at the informal power structure.* When you begin a new job, you will be shown organizational charts for the facility and for your area. Charts indicate the formal leaders and the chain of command within the organization. Do not assume that the organizational chart shows who is really in charge. Notice who leads and who follows, who speaks out on what issues, and how the power and work are distributed. Understanding the work setting is impossible without understanding the informal power structure. You may be invited to take sides on various issues. Be aware that you may be enmeshed in an ongoing power struggle before you realize what is really happening. It takes careful observation and thought to determine who really makes things happen in the situation and what the real lines of communication are. Informal power is fluid. Keep up with changes in your setting.

3. *Observe communication patterns with special attention to outcomes.* Does the "squeaky wheel" really get the "grease"? Do people ask directly for what they want, or do they rely on subtle hints and intimations? Do people become defensive when confronted in a straightforward manner? Learn *how* as well as to *whom* to speak to improve communication.

4. *Be cautious about confiding.* Gather information but use restraint in sharing it with co-workers. It is uncomfortable to make a derogatory remark about the head nurse, only to discover later that your listener is the head nurse's best friend. It is risky to do general grumbling about work at first. People develop a sense of ownership about their settings similar to those seen in a family. For example, I can complain loudly about the behavior of my child but I will not tolerate someone else doing the same thing. What you may see as simply joining in, others might interpret as disloyalty. If you do decide to share your opinions with a co-worker, do not be surprised if your words get around. Since you are unknown, people will be interested in sharing their impressions of you. If this happens, con-

sider it a learning experience and go on with the knowledge that you are important to the people around you. Feelings can be hurt and friendships ended before they really get started if you engage in negative communication. Instead of discussing your co-workers with another, write down your impressions and feelings. You will learn about yourself and about your perceptions. Review your observations in three months and again in six months. By that time you may know people well enough to be able to share your first impressions with those involved.

5. *Be yourself.* Do the best you can. Maintain your sense of humor. In due time you will not only be accepted into the work group; you will be helping to socialize others.

Transition Into the Work Setting

In addition to the variety of people you will encounter in your new job, you will also have to cope with the setting itself. Every work setting has its own personal history and emotional life, which will become apparent to you as you get acquainted. That "personality" was formed, just as your personality was formed, through a series of individual and group experiences. Often, explanations for some of the unusual reactions that a new nurse experiences can be found in the history of the setting. For example, you make a very rational, nonthreatening remark about an innocuous policy, and co-workers either laugh aloud or give you cold stares and walk away. Chances are the history, how that policy came into being, and what steps have been taken to adjust to it or modify it, would explain their reaction. If you do not seek additional information from people who know, you might conclude either that your co-workers dislike you or that there is something very wrong with them. Both conclusions can be hurtful and can interfere with future interpersonal relationships.

When you feel there is an inconsistency between what is actually happening and the feelings surrounding the incident, ask for background information. If someone responds to your suggestions with, "We tried that once and it doesn't work," ask for details or contact someone more willing to talk about it. Sometimes what appears to be resistance to change is actually very appropriate behavior when the history is considered. This is not to say you should stop trying to effect change. Rather, approach it from a different direction or at a more opportune time.

Pay attention during "remember when" sessions. Often these occur informally as situations similar to past events arise. You will learn much from them about the development of your setting. It is possible to have more formal group meetings when "old-timers" introduce newcomers to the setting by recounting significant events.

Another aspect of an area's unique personality is its informal norm system. Often you are not aware of norms until you violate them. Sitting in the "wrong" chair at a meeting and using an item "reserved" for the leader are examples of violating informal norms. Again, request more information. If you are told, "That's just the way it is," and if the issue really is not that important, conform to the norm. You will learn the informal norms just as you learn many important relationship skills—by trial and error. Be prepared to make mistakes and to learn from them.

Results of Socialization Efforts

As you can see, socialization into the work group and setting is no easy task. In addition to the high-visibility nursing skills necessary to succeed in your job, you will have to deal with politics, informal power and leadership structures, a diversity of co-workers, others' impressions of your behavior away from as well as during work, the history of your work setting, and informal norms.

Part of your learning about the informal group norms and structure will result from conflict encountered when following formal dictates. There is no way to avoid this; learn from each mistake. You will become very aware of the power some of your co-workers wield when you inadvertently displease or disagree with them. When this occurs, view it as an opportunity to gather information. Review the situation and evaluate the issues involved. Usually you will be able to determine when there is potential for a power struggle. If the other person is willing, discuss the situation in terms of the apparent issues, not in the context of power. This should be enough to help you determine what went wrong and what to avoid in the future.

An error that some newcomers make is insisting on debating the obvious issues and ignoring the dynamics involved. Thus, you may win for the moment but lose in the long term. It is difficult to maintain a seemingly passive or submissive stance when you are filled with enthusiasm and eager to make a good impression, but it will benefit you until you discover exactly how the informal system works. Remember, your task initially is to gather about the organization and the people with whom you work while demonstrating to them your competence and willingness to join them in working toward agreed upon goals.

During this data-collection stage, you may be exposed to situations that distress or trouble you. The informal leaders may engage in actions that you feel you cannot accept. Standards of care may not be maintained. Power struggles may be usurping energy and time that could be spent much more productively in improving care. Formal leaders may be bypassed consistently and to the degree that their real power is nonexistent. You have to observe and experience these situations before you can take any effective steps toward changing them. Stating your ideas too soon or too strongly can stop your ideas before you can begin to make change. Instead, remain quiet, observe, analyze, and then formulate an action plan.

Although this process of socialization into the profession and entry into the work world looks like an overwhelming task, you can accomplish it by being aware of your own feelings and behaviors and being sensitive to those around you. Remember that most things of value take time to accomplish. You cannot rush your acceptance into the group. Errors are inevitable. You will learn from them. The job of getting to know your co-workers, work setting, and organization is well worth the effort. Your reward is the ability to work competently, comfortably, and creatively in the area you have chosen.

In summary, the maxim for a newcomer is: Do not just do something; stand there until you really know what's going on.

CRITERIA FOR CHOOSING WHERE YOU WORK

Before making any job choice, it is essential that you honestly assess your needs, goals, and limitations. Take time to consider your strengths and weaknesses, what you would like to do now and in the future and what you do well as well as what you like to do.

Ask yourself the following questions before choosing a work setting:

1. Do I prefer to work with acute or chronic care patients?
2. Would I be more comfortable in a traditional setting or in one where more innovative therapies are practiced?
3. Do I want general psychiatric nursing experience or am I ready to specialize?
4. Will a hospital- or a community-focused facility best meet my needs?
5. What are the advantages and disadvantages of public versus private psychiatric facilities?
6. Where do I want to live? Would I be willing to relocate for the right job?
7. What are my basic salary and benefit requirements?
8. Does working a permanent shift work best for me, or can I rotate shifts with no problem?
9. What other factors need to be considered, for example, life style, leisure time activities, child-care arrangements?

After answering these questions and others that come to mind, arrange them in priority order. Writing your answers will help to clarify your thinking. Identify the essential items and those you are willing to negotiate or give up for the present.

The question and answer exercise is valuable whether you are a new graduate, or thinking of a new job, or because you feel ready to make a change, or because circumstances make a move necessary. The exercise promotes self-awareness and helps to clarify values. Even if on the basis of your answers you decide to stay where you are, you are ahead. You will know more about yourself, which is always useful.

In addition to discovering where you are now, think about where you want to be in one year, five years, and ten years from now. If your long-range goals are hazy at the moment, do not panic. They will come; do not wait for a decision about long-term goals before seeking employment. Work with what you have. Many new graduates might say, "At the end of a year I just want to know where to report to work, feel my performance is acceptable, and be able to pay my bills. I don't want to think past that." If that is your feeling, move from there, keeping in mind that formulating long-range goals will be necessary in the future. If you do not know where you are going, you will probably end up somewhere other than where you want. Therefore, gathering necessary information about yourself is essential.

Once your long-range goals are clear, you can work toward achieving them. For example, experience as a staff nurse, including floating and shift rotation, is useful for someone planning to go into nursing service administration. It not only provides an opportunity to develop nursing skills but also allows for observing management techniques from a subordinate perspective and lends credibility to future performance. Some experiences are good to have had even though they are not that appealing to live through. Having long-range goals makes such situations more tolerable. Sometimes being open to new situations provides valuable information that you did not know you wanted.

Considerations
for the New Graduate
and the Experienced Nurse

For the new graduate consider the advantages and disadvantages of working in the setting where you had clinical practice. One advantage is that you are already familiar with the physical set-up, policies, procedures, schedules, and some personnel. This frees you to expend more time and energy developing your nursing skills. However, one disadvantage is that those around you may continue to see you as a student and may fail to recognize your progress and increasing skill. This can interfere with your development of decision making, competence, and accountability.

For the experienced nurse considering a change in location, remember:

The same bureaucratic problems are everywhere, although the degree to which they

impact on you personally may be somewhat different depending on the setting.

Politics and power plays happen everywhere. If you are looking for a situation where you do not have to be involved, it does not exist.

Personal problems do not disappear just because you change environments. When problems arise between you and the world around you, it is important to begin solving those problems. Wait to relocate until you are feeling better about yourself and your ability to cope.

You can be hurried into an ill-advised change by negative circumstances that are temporary. An argument with a co-worker, being refused a promotion, or simply realizing how slowly changes occur in the system are not, in themselves, valid reasons for relocating. Give yourself some time, ask the questions pertinent to a job change (previously stated), and regain your perspective.

If after examining your needs, goals, and reasons, you decide you are moving toward rather than away from something, relocation is probably for you.

The next step then is to investigate, to discover what is available:

Obtain written information from various facilities and compare what each has to offer with your personal list of negotiable and non-negotiable issues.

Reduce the possibilities to a manageable number.

Contact the various facilities to inquire about available positions and hiring procedures. Some facilities have orientation classes only at certain times; other agencies individualize orientation. Ask about pre-employment physical examinations since sometimes waiting for results delays hiring.

Choose the better possibilities and schedule your interviews according to the established procedure. Some facilities depend on the personnel department to answer pre-employment questions. In such situations you will have to make an interview appointment with the appropriate person in the nursing department. You do deserve to have contact with both nursing and personnel before you make a decision. Divide your questions accordingly.

Investigate the Agency: Its Philosophy, Program, Policies, and Employment Practices

Get a copy of the nursing philosophy and discuss it. How are the concepts operationalized? (As a point of interest, if your contact has trouble finding a copy of the philosophy, it probably is not used to guide day-to-day behavior.) Is there a conceptual framework guiding care? Do goals and objectives flow naturally from the philosophy? How do these fit with your own personal goals, objectives, and philosophy? Do the nursing administrators, personnel director, and others you talk to convey a sense of caring for patients/clients as well as for staff?

If you are toured through the agency, notice how people react to each other. Is there an atmosphere of respect? Can you get a feel of caring and commitment from staff? What is the overall condition of the client/patient?

Get a copy of the job description. Is it consistent with the philosophy? Does it include responsibilities, expectations, and skills necessary to perform adequately? Are there different job descriptions for specialty areas?

Get a copy of the performance appraisal. Does it reflect the requirements in the job description? Is it specific enough to be helpful in planning professional growth? Who has input into the performance appraisal? How often are appraisals given? Are they tied to salary increases?

Ask questions about the orientation program. Obtain an outline if possible. How long is it? Does it include supervised clinical practice as well as interpretation of nursing policies and procedures? Will you be oriented to all three shifts? Is there a difference in orientation for new graduates and experienced nurses? Is there separate or additional orientation to specialty areas? Is there a probationary period after orientation? How long is it?

Provision for continuing education is another important consideration. Does the organization offer State Nurse Association-approved educational programs? How often? Are they offered on all shifts? Who may attend? Is it possible to attend during work time? If so, how is coverage arranged? Does the organization pay for attendance at off-site workshops or conventions? How is this arranged?

Ask questions about any other issues that concern you. Some common concerns include: (1) the type of charting and reporting systems used, (2) methods for evaluating quality of patient care, (3) committee involvement, (4) policies regarding being temporarily assigned to other areas, (5) procedures for transferring to another area for another shift, and (6) professional liability insurance.

Obviously it is impossible to include all the questions that might be of interest to you personally. Decide, before the interview, what you want to know about and make your own list. Take it with you. You probably will not remember to ask everything the first time. However, you should have the chance to get additional information before you make your final decision. As you ask your questions, be sensitive to the interviewer. Note which topics are dealt with comfortably and which seem to cause discomfort. You may want to explore the problematic issues more carefully.

Questions about opportunities for advancement can be directed to the nursing representative, the personnel representative, or both. You will probably want to know if the organization has a system for clinical or managerial advancement and the requirements. What are the policies and procedures for tuition payment or reimbursement if you attend advanced education during employment at the agency?

The personnel representative will be able to answer your questions about salary and fringe benefits. Ask about your salary; how often you will be paid; how salary increases are achieved and how often; how cost of living increases are handled; and if differential salaries are paid for educational preparation, shifts other than days, weekends, or holidays, and on-call status.

Information about medical and dental insurance, sick pay, paid holidays, and other benefits are usually presented to prospective employees in written form. Study this material so that you can ask pertinent questions. Again, making a list is recommended. It is much better to examine the information carefully than thinking six months later, "If I'd only known. . . ." Before you decide to become an employee in an agency, talk to people in the community. What is the reputation of the agency? Talk to someone who has received care in the agency? What was his/her impression?

The agency with the brightest ads and greatest promises may not be the best place for *you* to work.

THE "UNSUCCESSFUL" JOB ATTEMPT

Each person has his or her own unique criteria for success and failure. Society also teaches us what to view as positive and negative. Usually by the time you have finished school and acquired a job, you are quite familiar with success. You have set and achieved many goals and have developed some confidence in your ability to meet expectations. However, you should remember that people who have a history of succeeding have more difficulty coping with failure than those who have had previous experience with defeat.

You approach a new job or a change in job responsibilities with positive feelings based on previous successes in new situations. Even though you are realistic in your appreciation of problems, you face them with well-founded faith that you will overcome them. Therefore, when things start to go wrong, you may become anxious. Your usual coping skills may not work. You try to intensify your previously effective behaviors. Things get worse. Obviously, there is a potential for crisis when you encounter serious on-the-job problems.

Determining Ineffective Performance

In some instances, you may not be aware that the problems you are having are serious enough to jeopardize your position. Even after a supervisor has discussed your inadequate performance with you or co-workers have given you negative feedback, it is still difficult to grasp the idea that those in power view you as unacceptable.

Initially, you may minimize or dismiss negative evaluations. It is much easier to say, "My supervisor is impossible," or "She can't evaluate me because she really doesn't know what I'm doing," than to seriously consider making changes. This rationalization is an attempt to make the situation tolerable by distorting reality, but it may also be related to the way the negative information was presented. Any time you are told your per-

formance is lacking, you have a right to know specifically what will make it acceptable. Rather than attempting to explain or justify particular problems, focus on what changes are necessary for the future. You and your supervisor together have to determine specific behaviors that, when practiced, will indicate improvement. Without previously agreed upon goals, you may work very hard to change behaviors that are not seen as problematic and may ignore those behaviors that your supervisor finds unacceptable.

Again, it is easy to become defensive and rationalize that "the supervisor is wrong." The clash between what you have learned is good nursing practice and what is expected in the real situation can be very frustrating. Use effective communication methods to try to resolve the frustrations. The supervisor represents the philosophy, standards, and goals of the institution and profession as well as those of her/himself. Reality is that the supervisor has the power in the situation. This does not mean that you are powerless, but if you are to practice successfully, you must deal with reality rather than with how things "should" be. Maybe if you can learn from the situation, you can grow emotionally rather than just give in and give up.

Coping with the Situation

When you find yourself in serious conflict with your supervisor, first deal with your feelings of hurt, anger, self-doubt, or whatever you are experiencing. Although you may be admonished not to take criticism personally, it is almost impossible not to. After all, you are the person who has been found wanting. It is all right to express feelings about the unfairness or stupidity of the criticism as long as you go past this phase to a serious consideration of the problem. It may be true that no one understands you, but that does not mean that you can sit around until others see the light. You have a responsibility to make yourself understood. You can spend a lot of time and energy deciding what others should know, should understand, and should do, but there's no way you can make that happen. You can only change yourself.

Often it is tempting to involve others in your dissatisfaction. All of us have indulged in gripe sessions, even knowing that these accomplish little more than temporary relief. There is nothing wrong with temporary relief, but it is not a solution. You will usually be able to find others who will agree with your negative views of supervision or administration. Sometimes they agree because it is easier than telling the truth. Sometimes they would like to use you to voice criticism that they are unable to on their own. Sometimes it is exciting to see someone else really upset, so the behavior is supported rather than dealt with.

Although some co-workers may wholeheartedly agree that you are right and the supervisor is wrong and even urge you to confront authority figures, do not count on them to take steps in your behalf. Also, do not assume that because a group seems to agree with you, you have permission to speak for that group. If there is a consensus in the group that significant problems exist and action is necessary, each member must take responsibility and participate in problem solving. Too often one person assumes the role of group spokesman, only to find other group members are unable to take the risks necessary to effect change. As one nurse related:

> We all agreed on what the problems were. They all said they were behind me when I went to talk to the supervisor. What I didn't know was that they were so far behind me that I didn't see or hear from them again. I've never felt so alone, so angry, or so betrayed.

To avoid similar disappointments, take responsibility for yourself and allow others to do the same.

After dealing with your own negative feelings, go to someone who will help you sort out what is and is not real. If you have developed an open, honest relationship with one of your experienced co-workers, use this resource. Remember, though, you need tough reality orientation, not the false reassurance of sympathy. An experienced person who cares enough to tell you the truth can share insights about survival in the system, the politics, and power issues involved. You might want to see a counselor who can help you evaluate the total situation and can help you develop problem-solving skills as well as support your sagging self-esteem. Your organization may have someone who provides this service. If not, you may have to find an outside source. Consider the cost of counseling as an investment. Counseling at this time solves immediate problems, enables you to know yourself and your capabilities, assists you to improve adaptive capacities, and thus avoid problems in the future.

Self Assessment: A Step toward Resolution

The next step is to seriously consider the content of the criticism. Ask yourself the following questions:

1. Am I insisting that things be ideal?
2. Am I refusing to accept the realities of the situation?
3. Have I gotten into a power struggle with the supervisor and lost sight of the professional issues involved?
4. Am I spending more time criticizing others than in attempting to improve my own performance?
5. Have I been given specific plans for improvement?
6. Am I acting on those plans?
7. Have I asked for help or decided to go through this alone?
8. Am I being asked to do things that conflict with my basic values?
9. Have I discovered that this area of nursing is not for me but am reluctant to admit it?
10. Are there other things in my life requiring attention to the point that I am not willing to give necessary time and energy toward improving my performance?
11. Have I honestly looked at what it would take to change my behavior and decided it isn't worth the effort?
12. Have so many unpleasant or hurtful things happened that even if I become perfect overnight, the situation wouldn't really change?

Do not avoid answering the hard questions

because they're painful. You are in a position where you can use conflict to stimulate growth. Ignoring the opportunity is a disservice to yourself. Basically you need to consider if you know what is expected of you and if you are willing and able to meet those expectations. If the answer is no, you probably should consider working somewhere else. Making a conscious decision based on adequate information enables you to feel in control and purposeful rather than inadequate and a failure.

An Action Plan

Begin Looking for Another Job

When you decide it is time for you to leave, begin looking for another job. Sometimes this activity in itself helps to identify the positive factors in your present situation. Use the criteria presented earlier in this chapter. Try not to allow your negative feelings to come through when you interview for other positions. Avoid discussing in detail the problems in your present position with prospective employers. Remember, you have the same things to offer that enabled you to get a job in the past. In addition, now you have had the experience of discovering problems, identifying limitations (yours and the organization's), and attempting solutions. That experience can increase your value to your prospective employer; you are better prepared to utilize new skills and avoid pitfalls that others may not even recognize.

Consider Transferring

You may consider transferring to another area within the organization rather than terminating employment. Weigh the advantages and disadvantages. Review the reasons you chose your present facility in the first place. If the deciding factors included proximity to home, fringe benefits, provision for child care, i.e., overall organizational assets, and your expectations have been met, transfer might be the answer for you. (If you have been disappointed, working in another area will not change that.) Also, in transferring, you will usually retain your accumulated benefits and thus avoid the necessity of learning a whole new organizational system.

If you decide to transfer, talk openly with your supervisor about the implications of problems that you have had previously. State what you experienced and your plans for avoiding or overcoming similar problems in the future. Discuss what role the supervisor might play in your plans and ask for a commitment. Make arrangements for regularly scheduled feedback sessions and participate in them. Acknowledge the difficulties you have had but do not dwell on them. Instead, focus on what is necessary for your progress.

Your new co-workers will probably have heard about you through the grapevine prior to your transfer. Some may be eager to hear about your previous experiences. Refrain from giving negative accounts of your situation. You can briefly state why you transferred but do not elaborate. Although others might seem to enjoy your "horror stories" about another area, they will soon become uncomfortable with the idea that you may tell similar stories about them. Involve co-workers to whatever extent they are willing to be involved in your plans for growth, but do not subject them or yourself to nonproductive review of the past.

Some co-workers may have used grapevine information to make negative judgments about you prior to your arrival. It may not be fair or kind, but it does happen sometimes. Usually time and a little bit of distance will take care of the problem. There is really no way you can hurry the process. Trying to justify yourself often just makes people more resistant. The burden of proof is on you. Demonstrate your competence and your willingness to be part of the group. If problems continue after you feel you have shown that those preconceived opinions are false, or if some co-workers attitudes are so negative that they will interfere with your daily functioning, more active measures are in order. Approach the person in private, describe what you see happening and your feelings about it, and ask for help in finding a solution. If your attempts at conflict resolution do not work, be pleasant, maintain your distance except when contact is necessary to get the job done, and do not dwell on the situation.

You May Be Fired

You may be terminated (fired) when your job problems are such that the agency does not want to give the option for resignation or transfer. If this happens, give yourself some time to recover from the shock and then review the situation. This is a crisis point. Use it to foster maturity. Reread your supervisor's documentation and evaluation of your performance. This would have been reviewed with you in counseling sessions prior to termination unless you were dismissed for a single very serious incident. In either case, you can review the reports in the light of new events. You have a right to copies of all documentation in your personnel file. Ask about your organization's procedure and use it to obtain the records you want. Use them for learning, to look for patterns, to understand what really went wrong. Also familiarize yourself with the organization's policies and procedures concerning termination for cause, resignation, severance pay, and disposition of benefits. Do not make any rash statements or any decisions immediately. You need time to gather information before you determine steps to minimize the trauma of termination for you. Be sure to seek out reliable support people and get necessary help. Again, a counselor will be useful to help you turn a painful experience into an opportunity for personal and professional development.

COPING WITH STRESSES ON THE JOB

Developing Inner Resources

Recognizing when stress begins to interfere with rather than stimulate action is an important step in coping with stress. Self-awareness—tuning into your own unique responses to stress—is a learned skill and develops with time and effort. The headache that you get when you are driving to work and goes away when you are driving home is not a coincidence. It is a signal! Becoming angry at minor things at home, looking in the "help wanted" section of the newspaper, feeling irritated with your co-workers without apparent cause, and wondering how many sick days you have accumulated can also be symptoms of stress. Feelings are signals about how you and the world are getting along. When you discover, through awareness and interpretation of feelings, that work stress is causing discomfort, you can begin to do something about it.

Much stress is caused simply by the way people think about things. If you go into a situation "knowing" the way it should be, you will be stressed to the degree that your expectations

Exit Interview

You will be asked to participate in an exit interview in most organizations, whether you resign or are terminated. It may be verbal, written, or both. You have a professional responsibility to be honest about your reasons for leaving your position. You may feel so relieved at getting away from the problems that you have little energy to expend, but your input could help those who come after you. Do not assume no one cares or that it will not help. Describe situations and events as you experienced them and were affected by them. Be honest without being destructive. Avoid personal attacks but relate all the facts. If you kept written accounts of your difficulties, offer copies. Include suggestions you have for improving the situation. This interview should reflect your professional identity and concerns. When done in this manner, it will help you with closure to a difficult episode in your life and prepare you for more positive situations ahead.

differ from the real situation. You set yourself up for disappointment when you expect to have the "perfect day" at work since anything that happens to make the day less than perfect (and it always does) will create stress. Expecting the worst is just as self-defeating as expecting the best. The fact is when you enter a new situation, you just do not know how it will be. Control of stress is possible when you accept the uncertainty of the situation, resolve to take things as they come, and do your best.

Whenever you begin to think situations must be the way you would like them to be or even the way they should be, you are preparing yourself to experience stress. Events are the way they are. Of course, you should work to the best of your ability to change the things you can change. However, using time and energy to complain about how awful "things" are is a waste. Accept reality. While gathering information and formulating plans to solve problems, be realistic in order to decrease stress.

Another pattern of thinking that causes stress at work is the idea that people will change because they should, or because you want them to. However, you cannot change anyone but yourself. There is no point thinking that your supervisor should be fair, that your co-workers should care, that people in other departments should understand your problems, or that clients should be satisfied and appreciative. That is just not the way work always is. If you sit around waiting for everyone else to change, your stress response will rise. Rather, you can accept other people's limitations and get on with what you have to do.

Dwelling on past inadequacies or failures is another way you can stress yourself. For example, you plan to accomplish fifteen tasks at work one day but only complete twelve. You can berate yourself for the three tasks you did not do and ignore the twelve you finished; or you can realistically review your day, determine if your goal was attainable, decide what changes need to be made for success in the future, and enjoy the fact that you accomplished twelve tasks. The choice is yours. Why not choose the method that results in stress reduction? You have probably been warned against "resting on your laurels" and been encouraged to constantly strive for perfection. However, following this advice too earnestly can cause problems. You're entitled to your positive as well as negative strokes. And if no one else gives them to you, you have to give them to yourself.

Recognizing and changing ideas that are destructive develops inner resources, but is not a simple matter. It takes practice, and in some cases help, in identifying the thoughts that are causing stress. Getting such help is well worth the effort. With all you have to cope with, you do not need to stress yourself unnecessarily by thinking destructive thoughts.

There are other techniques you can use to reduce stress in addition to examining the way you think and discarding the irrational ideas that get in your way. Physical exercise can be beneficial, but be sure you select an activity that you really enjoy, in a location that is convenient, and engage in it with a compatible group or alone. Otherwise, it will be just one more thing you "have to do" and will not serve its purpose. Various types of meditation, relaxation techniques, imagery, and biofeedback can be learned in a relatively short period of time and practiced to meet the needs of your individual situation.

Refer to Chapter 12 for a description of methods of stress management.

You can also reduce stress and develop your inner resources by deepening your spiritual being and resources. Contact your spiritual advisor (minister, priest, rabbi), the Chaplain at your workplace, or a friend or relative who has deep spiritual maturity. Discuss your work problems with them, seek their counsel, and through their counsel and your worship gain new insights, strength, and courage. You may not be a member of a religious faith; however, you are a spiritual person. Some problems are best solved when you approach them on a spiritual, as well as an intellectual or emotional level. As you open new avenues to yourself, you will mature. In turn, you will become a more effective person, including on the job.

Developing Support Systems at Work

Certainly support systems are essential in reducing job stress. Developing effective support systems takes time, sensitivity, and a great deal of hard work. If you already know someone in the organization, that person will probably be your first support, helping you to learn your way around and explaining some of the subtleties of the situation. This can be useful initially to decrease the anxiety of knowing nothing about everything. Yet it is important to recognize when to move away from this resource and make your own way. Looking at the organization through someone else's eyes may make it more manageable at the beginning, but in time you will want to process information in your own unique way and make your own judgments. Continued dependence limits your ability to use new experiences for growth.

You and a friend might decide to change jobs together. This provides a preestablished support system. Even though both of you are new to the organization, you can support each other by sharing feelings, validating observations, and encouraging each other to take appropriate action. Again, there is a time when this kind of relationship is profitable and a time to be on your own.

An orientation group is another resource for initial support. Getting to know people who are at the same stage of adjusting to the organization is helpful. Although each of you might be going to a different area, you can benefit from sharing concerns and being united in common experiences. Getting together with your orientation group at regular intervals after you have been permanently assigned is a way to keep informed, to discuss common problems and solutions, and to gain support.

Staying too close to one outside person or group can be restrictive when it prevents you from developing support resources in your own area. The people who work with you on a daily basis have tremendous potential for assisting you. And you have much to offer them. There is no substitute for discussing mutual problems and accomplishments with co-workers who know the circumstances and people involved.

As you become acquainted with your co-workers, be aware of what you might need from support people. Different people have different gifts to offer. When the situation has been very demanding, you might want to spend time with a co-worker who has a talent for playing, or for using humor to relieve tension. When things are chaotic, find the calm, complacent co-worker who doesn't seem to react to anything. When you are feeling absolutely worthless and incompetent, go to a warm, caring co-worker or friend who is able to nurture and love others. And when you need guidance and direction, seek out the person who will analyze, think critically, and offer you an honest, though sometimes painful, evaluation of your performance, so you can begin planning for change.

On very rare occasions you might find one person who is able to do all these things for you: help you laugh when you are taking events too seriously; calm you when you are uptight; love you when you feel unlovable; require you to realize your potential when you do not feel like trying. If you do find such a person, value the relationship the way you would any extraordinary gift because that is indeed what you have. It is uncommon to find all these attributes in one person. Therefore your task is a little more complicated but not impossible. Seek out people who can provide what you need in a given situation. Reject "help" that is not helpful. People who cope best are those who keep looking until they find appropriate assistance and do not settle for what others say "should" satisfy them.

This process is another one that is guided by trial and error. At first you will go to people who are unable to give you what you require. This is part of the learning that helps you develop personally and professionally. When support is not forthcoming, it is advantageous to keep your perspective. Remember that not getting what you want does not mean your request is not valid or that you are not worthy of having your needs met. Neither does it mean the other person is withholding or uncaring. Accept that the person you contacted simply does not have what you need. That is inconvenient but understandable. (If you were asking for money rather than support, you would have little difficulty realizing that although you desperately need $1,000 and would use it wisely, few people will be able to give it to you.)

An important aspect in obtaining support is being involved and willing to enter into two-way relationships. Although it may not seem that you have much to offer those already established in the organization, you do. By looking at another person's performance without a history or preconceived ideas, you can make observations lost to someone in the midst of things. Do not withhold positive comments because you doubt others would value them. No one is immune to the benefits of a sincere compliment. This does not mean to compliment in order to manipulate. Be sincere and honest in your sharing. You will find admirable qualities in all your co-workers—if you look for them. Observe and acknowledge the positive things. Often people do not believe what they do is extraordinary because it is so routine to them. Your affirming comments will help them to appreciate themselves more.

Administration as a Resource

The administration can also be a support and an aid in stress reduction. Time really is money, and nurses have a responsibility to make clear to administration their need for time to deal with stress. Problem-solving and communication groups, assertiveness training, and programs on conflict resolution and stress reduction are ways that the administration can demonstrate its awareness of staff needs. Implementation of such activities is expensive but not nearly as expensive as the cost of stressed personnel.

It is the responsibility of professional nurses to inform the administration not only what is necessary but how it might be accomplished and evaluated. A thoroughly researched, written proposal sent through proper channels is the way to begin. After that it is necessary to organize proponents of your suggestions, engage in some political maneuvers, and negotiate. It is not easy, but it can be done.

When stress begins to interfere rather than motivate, take steps to reduce it. Fortunately, the people and techniques for stress reduction are readily available to those who are willing to discover, develop, and utilize them.

REFERENCES

Kramer, Marlene, and C. Schmalenberg, *Paths to Biculturalism*. Wakefield, Mass.: Contemporary Publishing, Inc., 1977.

25

Application of Mental Health Principles: Prevention Opportunities

Study of this chapter will assist you to:

1. Define primary, secondary, and tertiary prevention and contrast the services under each category of prevention.

2. Explore the traditional and emerging roles of the nurse in primary prevention.

3. Describe factors that must be considered in planning primary prevention programs.

4. Describe examples of primary prevention programs that are being implemented in your community.

5. Participate, either by teaching or counseling, with other nurses or health team workers in primary prevention.

6. Initiate primary preventive care in combination with other nursing intervention.

7. Describe secondary and tertiary prevention programs in your community and their benefit to clients.

This chapter contributed by Phyllis Jacobs, R.N., M.S.N.

DEFINITIONS

Gerald Caplan's definitions of primary, secondary, and tertiary prevention have been used extensively (11), even though some authorities argue that secondary and tertiary prevention are treatment of mental illness rather than prevention. The focus of this chapter is on primary prevention, but all three levels of prevention will be discussed.

Caplan defines *primary prevention as reduction of incidence of new cases of mental disorder in the population by combating harmful forces that operate in the community and by strengthening the capacity of people to withstand stress* (11). Thus there is a two-pronged approach. One prong refers to improving community conditions in physical, psychological, and sociological areas so that the individual can be strengthened. Physical resources that can be improved include lack of adequate food, shelter, or clothing, and unsafe living conditions. Stimulation of intellectual and emotional development will improve psychological resources. Strengthening the client's beliefs and values is in the sociocultural realm. The second prong is strengthening the capacity of people to withstand stress through crisis intervention strategies and support to at-risk populations. Incidence of mental illness in a community should be lowered if harmful factors can be eradicated. The influence of factors that cannot be eradicated must be coped with by the residents. Essentially the attempt is to decrease hazards and to provide safeguards so that exposed people can better cope. This two-pronged approach involves health promotion and protection from disease—in other words, primary prevention.

Secondary prevention is defined as reduction of the duration of mental disorders. By shortening the duration of existing cases, the prevalence of mental disorder is reduced (11). Early case finding and prompt intervention are emphasized. Reliable and sensitive instruments for detecting emotional illness must be developed and utilized, and priorities must be established for providing services. Other people, in addition to mental health professionals, must participate in case finding to reach the goal of early diagnosis and treatment.

Tertiary prevention is defined as reduction of the rate of residual defects that are sequel to mental disorder in the affected population. Tertiary prevention seeks to ensure that people who have recovered from mental disorders will be hampered as little as possible by their past illness in returning to full participation in the occupational and social life of the community (11).

Tertiary prevention includes treatment and rehabilitation services for those with mental disorders so that the client is rehabilitated to the optimal level of function.

COMMITMENT TO THE PROMOTION OF MENTAL HEALTH

Lip service has been paid to the term *primary prevention of mental illness* for many years. Primary prevention appears to be a laudable yet impossible goal. The lack of emphasis on primary prevention is apparent from the distribution of money spent for health care. In recent years, 40 cents of each health care dollar was spent for hospitalization; 3 cents of each dollar was spent for illness prevention; and less than one-half cent was spent for health education (22). There is a clear need for a reversal of priorities from an economic standpoint *and* from the standpoint of human welfare and quality of life.

Declared Need

The Joint Commission on Mental Illness and Health was convened by President John F. Kennedy for the purpose of determining the nation's mental health needs. The final report of the commission, *Action for Mental Health*, published in 1961, proposed a concerted attack on mental illness, in large part via delivery of psychiatric services in the community (35). This report proposed a massive program of preventive services.

President Jimmy Carter convened a commission for the same purpose. The commission's findings, titled *The Report of the President's Commission on Mental Health*, published in 1978, also emphasized the still prevalent need for primary prevention. The report specifically highlighted children as a vulnerable population whose needs for primary prevention are not being met (45).

Mental health professionals seem to agree on the need for prevention programs, but agreement on development and delivery of programs is difficult. Since results of a preventive mental health program are difficult to assess, funding frequently goes to programs whose results are more tangible. Some say the cause of mental illness needs to be delineated before attempts

at prevention are possible. We are ingrained with the medical-disease model, which is based on a linear cause-and-effect relationship (7). But the effect of divorce, physical illness, or poverty cannot be quantified as a precursor of mental illness. Although no direct cause-and-effect relationship may be found between some of the specific problems of society and some forms of psychological malfunctioning, an indirect relationship certainly exists.

Declared Goals

Many programs that have been implemented have been criticized, usually on the grounds that they are based on a one-to-one clinical ideology. Primary prevention must be grounded on: (1) ascertaining the at-risk population, and (2) providing services to strengthen coping resources of these groups to prevent development of symptoms (38). The individual is not discounted, but *the major focus in primary prevention is on groups of people.* Some mental health professionals are so accustomed to the individual client in the clinical setting that they are not able to adapt to working with a larger group where they may not have the same degree of influence on the client. Not all mental health workers feel comfortable in this somewhat fluid setting. Individual workers must decide what areas they are best suited for.

Criticism of some prevention programs that have been developed may stem from disagreement over goals or from global and interchangeable use of terms. The first priority is to establish what the goals of prevention are. The main goals must be: (1) a decrease in suffering from disease and (2) an enhancement of the capacity to cope with stress, rather than total elimination of stress and disease. The second priority is to define the terms relative to prevention, as these may differ in meaning depending on which definition is used. There is a need for a conceptual base upon which programs can be developed, but lack of agreement about terms and conceptual framework should not preclude the development of programs to meet the needs of people.

The Nurse's Role

Nursing has a role in primary prevention, and as a nurse you must seek to continue to develop this role, using your unique capabilities for promoting mental health. Community health nurses, occupational nurses, and school nurses have been engaged in primary prevention for many years. Nursing education is incorporating the principles of health maintenance into the general curricula. Some schools of nursing are teaching a course focusing on prevention as an introductory nursing course. Thus the nursing student develops a concept of the well client in the community setting, a concept that focuses attention on health maintenance and serves as a basis for caring for hospitalized patients. She/he gains awareness of the effect of the client's sociocultural background on illness, treatment, and hospitalization. Assessment of the client's physical, psychological, and sociocultural background requires the nurse to function in primary care as a generalist, reversing the specialist trend that has been occurring in other areas of nursing. The nursing profession today emphasizes improving the health status of the person and of the entire community.

No matter where you work and live, you will be a part of a system interacting with others. Prevention principles are practical in interactions with your own family, neighbors, friends and co-workers, as well as with clients. Teaching prevention principles does not need to be done in a formal setting with a prescribed curriculum. Prevention principles can be taught to the neighbor who is expecting her first child, to a co-worker who becomes very frustrated with superiors, to fellow committee members in every organization in which you are a member. Prevention should occur in every encounter you have, both personally and professionally.

SYSTEMS THEORY AND PREVENTIVE SERVICES

In attempting to provide preventive mental health services to groups of clients, the clients' social systems must be incorporated into your planning. You must understand the system the client functions within, the system of the agency within which you are involved, the social systems or institutions that are available in the community, and the general health care system. For many years the patient was seen solely as an individual; health professionals often did not take into account the systems within which the person functioned. Patients were discharged from psychiatric institutions without apparent concern about the interpersonal environment to which the person was returning. Employers threatened to fire long-time productive employees without concern about the reason for the employee's sudden decline in job productivity. The doctor prescribed a fairly complicated diet without inquiring about the patient's cooking skills, economic status, availability of prescribed foods, or knowledge of nutrition. Some of this behavior may have stemmed from a previously prevalent outlook that a person should be able to solve his/her own problems without relying on others, i.e., the patient's problem was a personal one to solve.

When Systems Theory is used in preventive mental health, emphasis is placed on the situation within which the person functions, and it is acknowledged that there are problems beyond the individual's capability to solve. A person should not be accused of not wanting to change a situation when change is outside of his/her control. The nurse's role is not that of the control person who will bring about change, but that of an enabler who can offer resources and a relationship to foster growth.

The recipient of health care services is no longer a passive patient but more frequently a person who initiates action on his/her own behalf. The client is an integral part of the health care system and must be involved in planning and treatment. The communication and relationships within the delivery of health care services must be analyzed so that humanistic care can be given. Formerly, a person sought health care when there was an ailment. So health care was in large measure set up as a complaint-response system. As the trend shifts from a curative to a preventive philosophy of health care, more emphasis will be placed on the client's life style and living patterns (34). The systems responsible for human services have in some instances become so bureaucratic that they are no longer capable of change, problem solving, or individualized care (5). The system of delivery of health care service must change as the philosophy of health care changes. As a nurse, you can utilize the principles of change discussed in Chapter 7 to foster changes in the health care system that will allow for humanistic care of the client.

THE COMMUNITY AS A PREVENTIVE MENTAL HEALTH DELIVERY SYSTEM

Defining and Assessing the Community

Developing a prevention program in a community must be defined. Then, community assessment is imperative before programs can be planned.

D. Klein has defined the *community as a set of patterned interactions where safety, security, support, and sense of self and significance are derived* (36). There are social, ethnic, occupational, religious, and political communities to which a person can belong, in addition to the geographic area of residence (19). If you are working in a community health setting, you may be concerned, as far as possible, with all that occurs within a specific geographic area. If you are in an occupational setting, you may focus on the workers and management in a particular department or plant, their families, and any recently retired employees from that department. In assessing mental health needs in a school setting, a realistic approach may be to focus on one grade, such as the kindergarten children and their families. A community may also be members of a church who are attempting to provide some mental health services for their own members or others.

In assessing the defined community, consider the following:

1. Geographical area, including distribution of residences, industry, or service facilities.
2. Income stratification and the amount of interaction between various income levels.
3. Educational levels and occupations of the population.
4. Cultural background of the community and its residents.
5. Age, sex, and family-size distribution of the population.
6. Service people in the community, such as police, clergy, social-welfare workers, and their utilization by the population.
7. Designated and informal community leaders and their roles.
8. Means of communication in the community, such as face-to-face interchange, directives, and nonverbal messages, as well as the formal communication systems.
9. The decision-making process and enforcement of decisions in the community.
10. Acceptance and integration of new residents into the community.
11. Level of trust in the community between residents, between leaders and residents, and between leaders and service providers.
12. Changes that have occurred in the last several years, as well as rapidity of change, cause of change, and acceptance of change by the community.
13. Degree of cohesion in the community.
14. Acceptance of members who do not conform to the cultural norm.
15. History of the community.

Change and its effect on a community are of major importance. The nurse, or anyone attempting to implement preventive concepts, must assess what effect change will have on the population. Will the community see changes as increasing the quality of life, or is it only the nurse who sees this potential? What does the individual see as the most relevant need? Most mental health workers come from a middle-class background (27). They have been accused of attempting to mold their clients to what the professional considers positive mental health. What the mental health worker sees as positive life goals, such as self-fulfillment and emotional security, may be construed as being manipulated into conforming by clients in a community.

A way to avoid inflicting your own values on the client and community is to study the community's values and customs and the sociocultural aspects of the client's life style. Accept the life style of the client and of the community as valid, even though it may be far different from your own. Your role is not to determine a life style for others but to help them gain the greatest physical and psychosocial well-being within their selected or prior-determined life style. You must determine who needs help as well as who wants help. Groups may be very skeptical of any professional, and you must take time to know the residents of a community. Be available where people tend to congregate: on a street corner, or in a tavern, store, laundromat, park, church, or community center. Any mental health services, to be accepted, must be easily available and must be seen by the recipients as meeting their own perceived needs.

Effect of Culture on Need for Mental Health Services

The rapid cultural changes in the United States may be one reason for certain groups being at greater risk to develop emotional problems and therefore in need of preventive services. In most stable cultures, the basic physical and psychosocial provisions for mental health may be considered adequate even if they are not consistent with our middle-class values. In unstable cultures, such as communities in transition due to immigration or emigration, or communities in the midst of change because of urbanization or industrialization, there may be confusion about values and traditions. Values may be in conflict. Traditional values may seem inadequate or out-of-date to cope with current problems (3). In a mobile society such as ours, patterns of living that were acceptable in a former community may not be acceptable in a new community. Close friends and family may not be available to help a new member assimilate the community's accepted patterns of behavior.

The delivery of mental health services is highly disproportionate to clients in different economic levels, ethnic and racial groups, levels of education, and geographical residence (17). Mental health professionals, including nurses, must take responsibility for the unbalanced manner in which mental health services have been delivered. You have a responsibility to evaluate your own biases and values and should become familiar with the culture within which you are working.

SUPPORT SYSTEMS WITHIN A COMMUNITY

Natural Support Systems: The Family and Lay Leaders or Groups

In each community you can assess some *natural support systems, those that are outside of the professional human services that function in the community* and that were functioning long before the intervention of mental health professionals. These natural systems provide material aid, knowledge of where further help can be obtained, and psychological support (6). Often a family member is designated the wise and helpful one for the rest of the relatives. Or one person in the neighborhood is always sought for help and listening. Bartenders, waitresses, barbers, and beauticians are examples of people in service occupations with whom clients tend to talk through their problems. For example, a significant amount of time may be spent with one's hairdresser, yet the relationship is neutral to the point that the hairdresser does not feel responsible for solving the client's problem, and there is enough anonymity in the relationship that the client does not fear repercussion regarding what has been disclosed. Often the service person has an astute awareness of the community and can be a source of information about the community for the mental health professional. This person can also be a source of information to the client about where help can be obtained if he/she (the service person) has been given this information.

In each community, whether the system is a hotel for older residents, a neighborhood, or an inpatient psychiatric service, natural leaders tend to emerge. Mental health professionals have attempted to utilize these lay leaders to provide a link between available professional services and residents who may be skeptical about professionals or anyone connected with a mental hospital. This approach has been successful to a degree. However, after training has been provided for these leaders, some have become so aligned with the professionals that they are no longer accepted as a part of the community. Some agencies have become caught up in how to fit the lay leader into the bureaucratic structure of the agency, and clients have become frustrated with the hassle. Also in some agencies, there has been a lack of follow-up assistance after the leaders were given training.

Groups of people who share a common disease or characteristic also form a natural support group, such as mothers of twins or parents of terminally ill children. Many of these kinds of groups have developed into structured organizations in recent years. These groups provide mutual support and understanding about the stigma of the disease that may occur in the community. Members of these groups feel there is a real understanding of their mutual problems by other members. Since these groups reach a large number of people at-risk, you can be helpful as a preventive caregiver: providing health care knowledge if needed and giving support and recommending resources.

You may initially become a member of such a group because of a shared problem with others in the group. You are looked to as an example; your handling of certain personal or family health problems may be used as a norm by others. As a nurse, usually you will be perceived as a knowledgeable person who can be trusted. In the neighborhood where you live there are many opportunities to do health teaching on an informal basis without making anyone feel guilty about his/her lack of knowledge or inability to handle a stressful situation.

If you are employed in a health care agency, you also have a responsibility to be concerned about the health care needs of colleagues and staff members working with you or for you. If personnel policies in psychiatric institutions were evaluated in terms of providing preventive mental health services to their employees, such preventive care would often be found to be non-existent. The employee who is depressed is not given support by fellow mental health workers but is faced with a "you need to snap out of it"

attitude. Thus we need to meet the mental health needs of those who are expected to *provide* support as an initial means of preventive care.

You must also look at your own degree of mental adjustment and honestly assess how you deal with stressful situations, both personally and professionally. As we administer to others by helping them simplify their lives, confront situations, or learn relaxation techniques, we must look at how these methods are useful in our own lives. We cannot provide preventive services to others if we do not use them ourselves.

Professional Support Systems

In addition to the various natural support systems in any community, *professional support systems exist in the form of professional or para-professional individuals and agencies.*

There are many members of the health team who may be supportive with clients and clients' families in individual or group practice. Table 25-1 shows some of the main categories of health workers who have specific educational training in their field and can contribute to primary prevention in mental as well as physical health. Some of these workers will be better prepared than others for such a task, although any individual in any discipline may intuitively be supportive and promote emotional growth.

Professional agencies or settings that may provide a support system to people in the community are numerous and varied and may include the following:

1. Physician's offices, including individual or group practice, such as Health Maintenance Organizations.
2. Schools—public, private, or special education centers for any age.
3. Occupational health centers in industries, stores, or wherever people are employed.
4. Neighborhood health centers or storefront clinics.
5. Health department—city, county, or state.
6. Home health services, such as Visiting Nurses Associations, that give care to people in their homes.
7. Hospitals—private, public, or governmental;

TABLE 25-1.   Categories of Health Workers

1. Administration of health services.	20. Osteopathy.
2. Anthropology and sociology.	21. Midwifery.
3. Automatic data processing in the health fields.	22. Nursing and related services.
4. Basic sciences in the health fields.	23. Occupational therapy.
5. Biomedical engineering.	24. Optometry and opticianry.
6. Chiropractic services.	25. Orthotic and prosthetic technology.
7. Clinical laboratory services.	26. Pharmacological and other services.
8. Dentistry and allied services.	27. Physical therapy.
9. Dietetic and nutritional services.	28. Podiatry.
10. Economic research in health fields.	29. Psychology.
11. Environmental control.	30. Radiologic technology.
12. Food and drug protective services.	31. Secretarial and office services in health fields.
13. Health and vital statistics.	32. Social work.
14. Health education.	33. Specialized rehabilitation services.
15. Health information and communication.	34. Speech pathology and audiology.
16. Library services in health fields.	35. Veterinary medicine.
17. Medical records.	36. Vocational rehabilitation counseling.
18. Medicine.	37. Miscellaneous health services (such as inhalation therapy technician).
19. Naturopathy.	

Source: Table from R. Murray and J. Zentner (p. 37, 51). Used with permission.

general or specialized; and including emergency and outpatient departments.

8. Long-term care facilities—extended care and rehabilitative institutions, geriatric day-care centers, or nursing homes.

9. Other social or welfare agencies or services, such as Crisis Hotline Centers, drug abuse crisis centers, telephone referral services, halfway houses, Salvation Army centers, Traveler's Aid.

Some of these places where health care is delivered may purposefully and systematically include primary prevention for mental health in the services rendered. In other places, primary prevention happens incidentally because of the skill or intuitive helpfulness of certain individuals who work there. Unfortunately, in still other places, primary prevention for either mental or physical health may be overlooked completely as a purpose or program.

GUIDELINES FOR ASSESSING MENTAL HEALTH

In addition to the lack of agreement on the etiology of mental illness, there is disagreement on what is mental health. (Some have defined health as loosely as "the absence of disease.") The Preamble of the Constitution of the World Health Organization defines health as "a state of complete physical, mental, and social well-being and not merely the absence of disease or infirmity." In all of us there are varying degrees of this state of well-being (21). Psychiatry says there is no such thing as a completely normal person because the same phenomena seen in the mentally ill may be present in anyone.

The following guidelines can be used in

assessing your own and the client's mental health as well as providing indications for primary prevention:

1. The person is a social being with autonomy needs who functions in the context of a group.
2. Stress is a precursor of disease. Stressors cause both physiological and psychological effects; behavior and function are influenced by how stressors are managed and by the intensity and duration of the stress-causing factors.
3. High levels of anxiety interfere with interpersonal relationships and decrease ability to function in daily living.
4. Emotionally healthy people feel good about themselves or have reasonably high self-esteem.
5. A holistic approach should be used in prevention and in health maintenance.

As a mental health nurse, you incorporate these guidelines into your interactions with clients. A supportive approach, which includes decreasing the client's anxiety as well as increasing the client's self-esteem, is an important nursing intervention. The five guidelines listed above can be applied to strengthen the function of those who may be vulnerable.

The Person Is a Social Being with Autonomy Needs Who Functions in the Context of a Group

The most immediate group is the family, who serves as a means of psychological support, although this function does not occur in some families. The nurse plays a preventive role in teaching families how to give psychological support. The nurse can help families to communicate therapeutically by learning to listen, to give positive feedback, and to explore feelings. Assertive training can also be utilized by families to strengthen skills in interacting in a helpful way with its members.

Mentally healthy people are capable of becoming intimate with other people. They are not afraid of disclosing information, personal feelings, and their own values. The school nurse has an opportunity to teach principles important in developing an open relationship with another when teaching classes on preparation for marriage and parenting.

Mentally healthy people have a securely developed identity and realize that their feelings and values will often differ from others in their group. Because they know who they are and what they believe, they can maintain a sense of self, yet interact closely with others. They can choose between when to follow the crowd and when to function independently of outside influences. The nurse teaching values clarification is fostering primary prevention by helping develop decision-making resources.

Some people are lonely because of anxiety about interactions with others, because they have never learned how to establish relationships, or because they will not take initiative in establishing relationships. Others live in relative isolation because of external circumstances. The nurse can establish a relationship with the client as well as refer the person to appropriate support groups, such as clubs for elderly people or groups sharing a common problem or characteristic such as parents of autistic children.

Stress Is a Precursor of Disease

Stress and its relationship to disease and illness were described in Chapter 12. Stressors that interfere with mental health and primary prevention are myriad. For example, environmental causes include lack of food, inadequate housing, or unsafe conditions, such as combat, flood, or other disasters, from which the person cannot escape. Rapid change of any kind is stressful. *Role conflict, when the role an individual assumes is different from that which society has stereotyped for that individual,* is a source of stress. The mother who returns to work when her extended family disapproves and the adolescent whose behavior differs from what the parents feel is appropriate are examples of role conflict.

As a nurse, you have a prevention role in helping clients learn to deal with stress. Review Chapter 12 for methods you may use to help the client eliminate specific sources of stress, decrease the intensity of stress when it cannot be eliminated, or cope more effectively.

High Levels of Anxiety Can Decrease One's Ability to Function

Review the effects of anxiety in Chapter 12. Helping people gain adaptive mechanisms to handle anxiety is a major prevention activity of the nurse. Learning which situations trigger high anxiety and the consequent behavior, such as anger, withdrawal, or physical illness, is necessary. Classes about decreasing anxiety, such as relaxation and desensitization techniques, can be taught in all settings. The nurse in an elementary or secondary school or in a college student health service can conduct groups focused on reducing anxiety that inhibits learning. Groups whose purpose is to help participants reduce anxiety are being conducted in some schools of nursing. Classes are also conducted in the hospital setting for those adjusting to a change in their lives, such as the amputee or the new diabetic, in order to help reduce anxiety and provide group support. Education about anxiety related to child care and ways to manage it should be incorporated into prenatal classes. Every nurse must be alert to symptoms of anxiety in clients and should attempt to decrease the anxiety.

Emotionally Healthy People Have Reasonably High Self-Esteem

Self-concept refers to the total way a person sees self; self-esteem is the perceived sense of value and worth. If people have a basic sense of liking self and are realistically aware of their limitations, attributes, and potential, they have a sense of self-esteem. Self-esteem varies according to circumstances but remains fairly constant throughout life.

The development of self-concept begins within the family and continues to be molded during the school years. A mother with low self-esteem may engender this same attitude in her child through the care she gives the child. The person with a low self-esteem will expect failure and may not attempt to do things or try to grow because of fear of failure. A person who is unsure of self cannot reach out to others in intimate re-lationships. Marriage problems or job dissatisfaction may result. The person may fail to live up to personal standards or may feel other people judge him/her as inadequate. If the person feels inadequate, he/she tends to feel judged that way by others. The inadequacy role is then fulfilled if the person's behavior becomes less competent. Dissatisfaction with life and fear of death in old age often result from long-standing low self-esteem.

Promotion of positive mental health must emphasize increasing the person's self-esteem. This is a major task usually accomplished through contact with people, for example, in prenatal and parenting classes, hot lines to give support to mothers of young children, teaching psychosocial concepts in the required curriculum for teachers, junior high and senior high school classes on preparation for marriage, emphasis on increasing job satisfaction in industry, and increased psychosocial support for the aged.

A Holistic Approach Should Be Used in Prevention and in Health Maintenance

Health professionals are realizing that there are many ways to foster health maintenance. Emphasis is being placed on the effect of emotional factors on physical disease to the extent that some feel that most disease is caused by stress. *Holism means accepting the ability of the human body to be fully potentiated in maintaining health and overcoming disease* (16). Proponents of the holistic health movement emphasize that assessments and diagnosis should include listening to the person and family, and that intervention should include the cultural beliefs and remedies, human contact, touch, and emotional warmth and support. As the public is increasingly knowledgeable and sophisticated about health matters, health professions have a responsibility to include the client in making decisions about his/her care. Health workers must be informed and must maintain an open mind about new developments in health care and must be prepared to incorporate these developments into their program of care. Care of the whole person has long been a part of the philosophy of nursing and must be continually expanded. As a nurse, you can incorporate methods of the holistic health movement since you were taught these as a part of your basic education.

PRIMARY PREVENTIVE CARE TO HIGHER-RISK GROUPS

Since no one always functions at the optimum level, everyone can benefit from preventive mental health care. However, there are those that tend to be a higher risk than others to develop a psychiatric illness. *Populations at risk are those that have a large number of individuals who have undergone stresses sufficient to interrupt their emotional equilibrium* (38). Finding the at-risk population without bias is difficult. The problem may be that the criteria used are developed by the middle-class mental health worker. The test instrument may be skewed toward predicting high rate of illness in a lower economic level population if the instrument focuses on status, value, and life style. What must be considered in addition are other elements such as money and power. Lack of money is a stressor and contributes to the incidence of emotional disorders. Lack of money may result in poor and crowded housing, nutritional deficiencies, medical neglect, and unemployment. These factors have been found rather regularly to correlate with emotional disorder. Certain kinds of stressful events, such as minor illness, may be merely inconvenient for the rich but often are disastrous for the poor (21).

When any population is studied to determine those who are at higher risk to develop an emotional disorder, measurement along several dimensions is needed to give the best prediction. This could involve use of psychological tests, peer ratings, and judgments by those in care-giving roles. For example, studies by T. Bower have shown school personnel to be reliable in predicting subsequent psychiatric illness of students (60). These same studies report that a majority of individuals hospitalized in state hospitals are not served by any agency during the three years prior to hospitalization. Thus, there is a need for accurate instruments to be developed for predicting vulnerable people and also for care services to be offered before hospitalization is required. How much better to prevent the hospitalization through an active program of support in an effort to attempt to prevent illness from developing.

One instrument that has had widespread use in determining magnitudes of stress is the Holmes and Rahe Social Readjustment Rating Scale (30). (See also Chapter 8.) This scale attempts to measure the magnitude of the stressful situations a person has encountered during the previous ten years. The authors feel that all events, both untoward and desirable events, that occur in a person's life cause stress and therefore require a significant change in the ongoing life pattern of the individual. Frequent changes in life pattern due to a large number of significant events occurring in close proximity tend to decrease a person's ability to deal with stress, and physical illness may be the result. Studies using the Social Readjustment Rating Scale have found that people who have experienced a high rate of life change events have had a higher rate of heart disease, tuberculosis, accidental injury, skin disease, hernia, and even pregnancy than those experiencing a lesser amount of life change events (30). Using an instrument such as the Social Readjustment Rating Scale will assess the degree of change that has occurred in a person's life. Prevention programs can provide intervention to groups of people when they are undergoing major social stress or crises, such as moving to a new community, getting a divorce, or seeking a new job. There are also developmental crises such as the birth of a baby or entry into a nursing home. During these crises the nurse can provide preventive care because of her close interaction with the person or family.

Developmental Crises

The Expanding Family

When a baby is born, this time of physiological, psychological, and family stress represents a prime opportunity for preventive intervention. Pregnancy is initially disruptive, whether planned or not, and may impair ability to cope with stress for a period of time. A. Clark and D. Affonso identify four tasks of pregnancy: (1) pregnancy validation, (2) fetal embodiment (incorporation of the fetus into the body image), (3) fetal distinction (viewing the fetus as an individual being), and (4) role transition (13). All of these tasks may be stressful and require adaptation.

The time spent waiting in a prenatal clinic is a good opportunity for the nurse to convene a group of pregnant women to help them prepare for the psychological changes that occur before and after the baby is born. Prenatal classes for mothers and fathers should emphasize the changes that will be occurring and help the expectant parents adapt to them.

The birth of a baby can be disruptive to the couple's relationship. Stressful factors that may occur in the new mother are interrupted sleep, chronic tiredness and exhaustion, a sense of being tied down, decrease in social activities, loss of adult companionship, resentment of the husband's unequal participation in the care of the baby, and guilt feelings about having these feelings.

The father's stress regarding the new baby may center around economic problems, lack of quiet, a wife who is irritable and wants to go out, and wanting to see the baby while the wife would like the baby in bed. Discussion of these issues in prenatal classes will help the new family to know these are normal feelings. One or several home visits by the nurse in the early period following delivery also may prevent future crises.

The expanded family needs continued support to manage stress; supportive services include a mothers' crisis line, mothers in the LaLeche League (a group dedicated to good mothering through breastfeeding), and babysitting services. Helping parents recognize their positive reactions to the baby is also necessary.

The single parent, the mother who must return to work shortly after her child is born, the family with multiple births, an unplanned pregnancy, and having a very active baby are all situations in which the parents are more vulnerable during the postpartum period. These parents may respond very positively to preventive intervention.

The Preschool Child

The preschool child, particularly one who attends a day-care center, may be a candidate for preventive services. Over 50 percent of children under six years of age are now cared for by others while their parents work, and much of this care takes place in day-care centers. With the rapid rate of physical and psychological growth that occurs during the preschool years, health problems that have only a minor effect during the adult years may cause lifetime deviations from normal when they occur during the preschool years (46). The nurse should teach communication and psychosocial development to preschool teachers and teachers' aides in addition to doing mental health assessments on the children. With the increased mobility of families and the consequent decline of an extended family to provide psychological support, parents of preschoolers often need outside help. Convening parents of preschool children for discussions on all aspects of parenting may help fulfill this need. Classes must be scheduled so mothers (and fathers) can conveniently attend, and provisions should be made for child care during meetings.

The Schoolchild

Beginning school may be a crisis because this is a time of change for both the parents and child. Periods when the child is most vulnerable to stress, regarding school, are entry into kindergarten or high school or a transfer to a different school. For the beginning schoolchild, the school experience may transmit a very different message about values and behavior than has been learned at home. For some children this may result in a positive change in behavior, but the child must still adapt to this learning. The teacher's acceptance of the child is a factor in the child's acceptance of the school experience.

An interview by the school nurse with the parents of a child entering kindergarten, or with a new family who has moved into the district, provides an initial neutral contact with the family and an opportunity to make at least a general mental health assessment. This may initiate a positive feeling between family and school instead of the parents feeling the school only contacts them when there is a problem with their child.

Health education for adolescents can be applied to prevent both immediate and long-term problems. Problems with immediate effects are, for example, sexually transmitted diseases, high-risk pregnancy in early adolescence, and motor vehicle accidents. Other problems are the long-term risks for cancer, cardiovascular disease, mental illness, maladaptive dietary patterns, heavy alcohol use, and maladaptive human relationships. Before health-damaging patterns are firmly established, there is a crucial opportunity for preventive intervention.

One effort to prevent disease and protect health throughout the life span is a peer counseling program. In this type of program, the credibility of peers is used as a strength. Programs usually focus on clarifying tasks of this phase of the life cycle, giving information on the processes of interpersonal relationships and providing continuing supervision to the student counselors (29).

The school is a natural area for preventive programs because it is one of the few places where large numbers of children can be reached. Few children who need services should be missed in a comprehensive school mental health program. Programs need to be focused in the lower grades since later school achievement problems can often be traced to difficulties in the earlier grades (28). However, continued preventive programs throughout the school years are necessary.

Schools are a logical place for the dissemination of preventive mental health care. In recent years, school administrators and teachers have realized that they must deal with the whole child instead of only teaching academics. There is strong evidence that emotional factors hinder learning. Schools must realize what an impact they have on the child since about 30 hours a week are spent at school. The administrators and teachers at school do not have a choice about being agents that can affect psychological growth. They simply are.

The school nurse may find some obstacles in trying to initiate a school-based program of preventive care. At present, schools are vulnerable to accusations of fomenting a variety of problems, such as poor academic achievement, school violence, and drug and alcohol abuse. Also school administrators may feel initiating new programs will call attention from parents and the media to school problems. They may want to preserve an "all is well" image. If straightforward meetings with school administrators fail to convince them of the need for a program, the nurse can meet with school board members, parents, and teachers.

School administrators may try to justify the lack of preventive programs because of financial constraints. Thus there may be advantages in having a school nurse implement preventive programs. The prepared school nurse is in the unique position of being an established member of the school staff, which eliminates the need to hire outside mental health staff. Also the teachers will not feel competition from outside staff coming in to direct a program. When outside staff are brought in for an hour a week to conduct a mental health teaching program with students, the teachers may relinquish responsibility for teaching in this area and may not want to work with them.

Another obstacle to prevention programs is the tendency of schools to intervene only *after* learning or behavioral problems emerge. Thus the nurse may need to sell a preventive mental health role to an administrator who comes from this tradition. Presently there is an emphasis on basic subjects in schools, and the schools are concentrating on fundamental academics to the exclusion of programs focusing on the child's affective development. However, the ability to resolve conflicts, to cope with everyday stressors, to set realistic goals, and to cooperate with others constitute "the basics" in their own right. Studies have shown that building adaptive strengths in young people can lead to improved scholastic achievements (56).

A preventive program (initiated by the nurse) needs to have a two-pronged focus: (1) altering systems and social environments detrimental to individuals, and (2) helping the individual develop life skills to better deal with the environment. The nurse in the school system must analyze the school's social environment. Policies of the school, such as posting grades instead of giving them out privately, or disciplining a child in front of peers or in a manner that is deameaning may serve to decrease a child's self-esteem. The nurse can work with the school administrator and teachers by assessing school policies and making concrete suggestions about methods that will increase children's self-esteem. Authority figures are more willing to accept something new when a specific plan is offered. Therefore you should avoid a tirade of fault-finding with present policies which may result in no change.

The nurse may find in assessing the classroom situation that it is the teacher's attitude, outlook, and relationship with students that are detrimental factors in the environment. There is certainly evidence to suggest that the teacher's mental health is very important in fostering the mental health of pupils (19). The teacher may be under considerable stress because of a variety of factors. For example parents sometimes have very high expectations of what the teacher ought to accomplish with their child. Also juvenile delinquency, school dropouts, and sexual promiscuity are sometimes blamed on the teacher. Or the teacher may feel the need to be the perfect behavioral example to students.

The nurse's counseling of teachers may be made more acceptable if conducted in an informal manner. Small group meetings are helpful to provide teachers a discussion forum for expressing their frustrations that occur in or out of the classroom. The nurse may also conduct programs for other staff, including cooks and custodians, to help sensitize them to children's mental health needs.

The nurse can be very active in direct care to students as well. Value education is often taught at the junior and senior high school level and may be taught by the school nurse. Value education provides a framework on which students can base sound decisions. Including information on mental health in health classes, personal and health and teaching relaxation exercises to students with test anxiety are other examples of ways to help the individual develop better coping skills for life.

Certain groups of school children can be classified in an at-risk category. These include children with some disability, such as retardation, speech impairment, or a sensory defect. If these children are placed in schools with normal children, reactions from other children may put such a strain on the disabled child that self-esteem is diminished. Such a child has a higher risk of developing mental illness. This child may need an individually designed curriculum to meet individual needs, modification of the schoolroom milieu, such as a small classroom setting, and support from the nurse by frequent informal interactions.

Other children who are at risk include those who may have a particular life crisis that makes them more susceptible to mental illness, such as divorced parents, death or chronic illness in their immediate family, or a recent move to a new community. These children may need additional support through: (1) individual counseling, (2) convening of small groups of children with similar needs to develop increased self-awareness, (3) parent conferences, or (4) home visits.

Potential school dropouts are a prime group for the nurse to work with. The nurse may convene small groups of students to help them look at present stressors, reactions, and consequences of decisions, and to provide a place for exchange of opinions.

The Adult Years: Preventive Intervention in Occupational Health

As the schoolchild spends a large proportion of time at school, likewise the adult spends a large proportion of time at work. Formerly companies did not consider an employee's mental health to be a company concern. This attitude began to change when industry realized how much work output was lost and how many accidents were related to alcoholism and drug abuse, even among long-time, productive employees. Thus, instead of employees being fired, programs were developed to help the employee overcome the addiction. Employers are now realizing that non-work problems have an effect on the employee's productivity. Up to 15 percent of the national work force struggles with personal problems that adversely affect their work performance (6).

Workers who have a relatively high degree of job satisfaction show either a high or moderately high level of mental health. Individuals who cannot appreciably satisfy their psychological needs in their work environment have either a low or, at best, a moderate level of mental health (32). Stress related to the job situation is particularly prevalent between 35 and 45 years of age. Data confirm that the most important changes in a job, such as promotion, demotion, or transfer to lower status jobs or less challenging assignments, occur in this age range (6).

Companies are now expanding employee benefits to include free professional counseling for workers and their dependents. Approximately 10 million workers are now covered by Employee Assistance Programs (EAP). These programs are usually in the form of an in-house counseling staff or a private, off-site, counseling firm that employees can contact. Confidentiality is a major factor in these programs. The employee's supervisor in most cases does not know assistance is being sought for a personal or work problem, so the employee's performance evaluation will not be affected. In other cases, employees are asked to make use of the counseling service as a condition of continued employment. Such far-ranging problems as marital discord, child adoption, over-eating, child care for a working mother, and legal services are handled by EAP.

The occupational health nurse is changing her role in that increased emphasis is being placed on preventive programs. Health education and disease detection programs are being offered to employees by nurses. The occupational health nurse is also placing increased emphasis on employees' mental health. Since the majority of companies do not participate in an Employee Assistance Program, the nurse can often fulfill this role. The prepared nurse can do counseling and can give assistance with environmental manipulation either on the job site or outside of the work situation. Making home visits to assess a situation and to provide support is within the role of the occupational health nurse.

Programs must be developed according to the workers' needs, rather than according to the nurse's perception of the workers' needs. The total worker population the nurse is responsible for must be assessed to determine what problems may be common to a large group of employees. Such areas as determining whether workers are socially and culturally disadvantaged, how many female workers support families, the logistics of child care, and hazardous materials in the work situation must be assessed. The nurse can develop a comprehensive family, social, health, and occupational history on individual employees. With these records, the nurse can ascertain what the general needs are and can then develop plans for health education (37). The nurse must assess the employees' ability to handle stress. In addition to the role of developing programs to prevent mental illness in groups at risk, the nurse also has a responsibility to interpret these problems to management to get appropriate support and action.

There are many groups of employees to whom the occupational health nurse can provide personalized preventive mental health services. For example, the new employee, particularly one who has recently moved to the area, may need information about the community as well as support in adapting to a new job. The employee's family may need the same type of help. Or the employee who is geographically mobile may start a new job frustrated and guilt-ridden because his/her family has opposed the move. The young worker who is just entering the work force may have concerns about his/her role and others'

expectations. Also the executive may feel under a lot of stress to succeed and may feel there is no one with whom these feelings can be shared without jeopardizing future advancement. The female executive is increasingly a significant percentage of the managerial staff in many companies. Although the numbers of female executives are increasing, there are still many male executives who will not accept them, and thus a woman executive may feel isolated. Such behavior toward her may make her question her abilities. Support for her, particularly in a beginning managerial position, is important, and the nurse may be the only other female in the area able to provide this support.

As more women are entering the work force, the nurse must be aware of the special needs of the female worker. A woman may have worries about working, particularly if working is something she feels compelled to do. Whether or not the marital partner agrees on the wife's working is an area of potential discord. The nurse may be active in assisting the mother to find adequate care for children and in helping develop child-care facilities at the employment site.

Many workers are exposed to noxious substances, such as air, noise, and water pollution at the work site, or they may have direct contact with harmful substances because of their type of work. Families may also be affected by particles carried home on workers' hair, skin, and clothing. The nurse working in this environment must be active in monitoring these substances, interpreting to management the potential health problems, and working to improve job conditions, which in turn enhance emotional health.

Psychogenic illnesses may develop among workers because of anxiety and stress. (See Chapter 12.) This can be a devasting experience for the individual worker, for the economy of the plant, and for future jobs for the workers. Research has found psychogenic illnesses that spread among workers are most often found where there are any of the following: (1) a predominantly female work force, (2) work that is boring, repetitive, or requires fast pacing such as assembly line work or where production quotas are set, (3) an unusually heavy workload, or (4) ambiguous or hostile relations with management (37). The nurse must be aware of this potential and must work with management to change working conditions before problems develop. Conducting groups on relaxation methods during the workday can increase ability to cope with stress. (See also Chapter 12.)

The person planning to retire also needs preventive services. The person whose retirement will be occurring in a period of months often has a decline in work output because he/she no longer feels a part of the work situation. Retirement may make the worker feel unneeded and unwanted. The nurse can conduct group meetings of those planning to retire to help workers know that they are not alone with these feelings. Individual counseling with the worker, and also with the spouse, can prevent some frustrations of retirement. The worker with a particular skill may be helped to find ways to pass along the knowledge to younger workers so others can derive the benefits of his/her experience, and the retiree's self-esteem is increased during a vulnerable period. Sometimes the worker wants to retire early to get away from an unpleasant work situation. This person also needs assistance in planning for retirement.

Preventive Intervention with the Elderly

The elderly as a group are more vulnerable to mental health problems than are other age groups. One reason is the number of losses that the elderly experience, involving sensory decline, health, productive work opportunities, possessions, income, death of spouse, and death or movement of other relatives and friends. Loss creates a stress response that predisposes any person to a breakdown of mental health. How much more devastating this is for older people who have to adapt to changes resulting from these losses at a time when their capacity for adapting to change is decreasing. Each loss causes worry, which produces a further stress response. Loss of physical health is of prime significance. Physical health has been reported to have a stronger correlation with life satisfaction than the variables of income, internal control, having a confidant, education, or sexual relations (38).

The role the elderly person is to assume is often very nebulous, particularly because the roles of spouse, parent, or worker are now over. The opportunities for choice decline for the elderly. Thus an older person may assume a sick role even if he/she is not sick. At least this *is* a role that can be assumed and may be preferred to having no role or the role of nonbeing that society may ascribe to the elderly. Society by its treatment of the elderly often says, "You are useless and incompetent." As a result, the aged often have a decline in self-esteem. Even if the person feels competent to handle situations, he/she may stop attempting to because of others' reactions. The nursing home staff, the apartment manager, or the children and grandchildren may demonstrate that they consider elderly people to be incompetent by making decisions for them.

The nurse can help the elderly person retain decision making and explore role alternatives, particularly those emanating from past accomplishments or hobbies that may not have previously been considered as useful (38). Previous experiences can be developed into useful activities. The nurse can encourage younger people to seek a variety of roles so there are still choices available when other roles are completed in old age.

Nurses can practice prevention principles for the elderly in a variety of settings: the nurse in a nursing home or residence for the elderly, the public health nurse who has elderly clients in his/her caseload, the nurse who has contact with senior citizens groups, the office nurse in a private physician's practice, the nurse in independent practice whose clientele includes senior citizens, and any nurse who interacts with elderly people in the community. A high percentage of senior citizens belong to voluntary organizations, which are excellent places for the nurse to establish contact with them and provide preventive care.

The nurse can also attempt to mobilize the client's support system. Three types of support systems that can be used are: (1) informal, such as family and friends, (2) nonprofessional, such as the American Association of Retired Persons and senior citizens groups, telephone services that call elderly people daily, and (3) health care professionals.

Prevention programs should focus on management of the environment to increase and retain the independence of the elderly. Such programs should include emphasis on teaching proper physical care to prevent illness and should provide rehabilitation services for physical illness. In general, nutritional problems and physical health rank higher as causative factors of mental illness in elderly than in younger people. The nurse can teach proper diet and easy meal preparation to groups and individuals. Individuals who eat alone sometimes do not prepare adequate meals because of loneliness or feeling it is not worth the effort. Encouraging the elderly to eat one meal a day at a neighborhood nutrition site can reduce the sense of loneliness and at the same time enhance nutritional status. Also, since the elderly often have much free time, the nurse may have a role in helping them find satisfying ways to spend this time. Continued participation in activities can promote intellectual stimulation and physical and psychological health. Loneliness can be overcome through social activities, and the support system can be expanded by making new friends.

Groups have been developed in institutions for the elderly for the purpose of reminiscing. It was found that talking about and sharing earlier experiences was positively correlated with a lower rate of depression (23). Cohesiveness and support were also gained from the groups as members began to feel comfortable about sharing present problems. The nurse can use reminiscing therapy with the elderly, individually or in groups, if there is a willingness to listen. (Refer to Chapter 11.) The nurse can also assist families to see the positive benefits of carrying on the family heritage and to explore ways to increase self-esteem in the elderly by incorporating the person into family living experiences.

Stressful Social Crises

In addition to naturally occurring stressful periods of life, certain circumstances such as geographic mobility, job changes, or financial problems, can create social crises. If these crises are not resolved on a short-term basis, they may cause life-long changes. The nurse oriented toward prevention must be aware of clients undergoing this type of stress. If the nurse does not have the opportunity or skills to intervene directly, these clients should be referred to agencies where help can be obtained.

Some examples of social crises, as mentioned earlier, involve children of single-parent families and children from geographically mobile families who have just entered the school system. The school nurse can be helpful to these children. Also college freshmen who are away from home for the first time may feel embarrassed about expressing feelings of loneliness to fellow students and may avail themselves of supportive programs

at the student health service. The community that has migrant workers among its numbers may include a high proportion of at-risk people who will not avail themselves of programs by going to the mental health center. In this case, the nurse must go to them. Other people who need help are single people who have finished their education and are working or looking for a job. They may be very lonely because they are no longer in the school system that provided a means of bringing peers together. Groups that have special needs are those who are addicted to drugs, including the alcoholic or the habitual user of prescribed or street drugs.

The abused also need special help. The magnitude of child abuse, spouse abuse, and abuse of parents in this country is just becoming known. A high percentage of child abusers are found to have been abused as children, so both the parents and children constitute an at-risk population. The nurse in any setting has a responsibility to pursue any perception of abuse of another human being and intervene directly or indirectly. Attempts should be made to prevent abuse through encouraging participation in programs for at-risk clients. Refer to Chapter 19 for additional information.

Institutionally Created Stress Situations

An institution has the responsibility to provide its clients with the opportunity for normal personality development, or at least to prevent damage to their personality development. An example is the hospitalized child and the possible long-term effects of hospitalization. In recent years, pediatric nurses have been very active in preparing children for hospitalization in order to minimize stress. Long-term care institutions for retarded, disabled, or emotionally ill children must also work to prevent further problems that would reduce the quality of these children's lives. Foster children who may be moved from institutions to foster homes, or between foster homes, need preventive mental health services including a continuity of experience and attention paid to the importance of their individual possessions. The individual in the welfare institution also suffers stresses related to stigma and the loss of privacy and possessions. The nurse must be particularly cognizant of increasing self-esteem in these clients and should maximize therapeutic communication between the client and health care institutions.

The nurse who works in a penal institution must also provide preventive health care services. In addition to physical assessment, a psychological assessment is necessary. Helping clients maintain contact with their families and helping the individual client and family prepare for the person's return to the community can be part of the nurse's role. Also assisting the community to understand and accept a member returning from a penal institution is necessary.

THE NURSE AS CONSULTANT

In addition to interacting directly with clients, in providing preventive mental health care services, the nurse meets with other professionals and groups as a consultant. Caplan defines *consultation as the interaction between two professional persons in regard to a current work problem with which the consultee is having difficulty and which he/she has decided is within the consultant's area of competence* (11). *Mental health consultation can be defined as the application of the consultative process by a mental specialist in interaction with a consultee, a health care provider or agency, with the end goal of preventing mental illness and promoting mental health both in the care-giver and in his/her clients* (20). The mental health nurse as consultant tries to help the consultee either with individual clients, with systems of clients, or with environmental problems. Consultation is directed toward either helping plan a program for a particular group or helping the consultee work through experiences with that group. The mental health nurse may in turn seek the help of another consultant, for example, a social scientist, in order to learn how to interact with clients from a particular culture.

The consultee should realize that consultation is not psychotherapy. The mental health consultant does not decide what will be done in a situation but only suggests, clarifies, and presents alternatives (11). The responsibility for carrying out any agreed upon action remains with the consultee. The consultee retains the right to modify the information or reject its use entirely.

As consultants deal with individual client problems, a need for change within the system may be apparent. Thus, the consultant may be viewed as a change agent. If the consultee feels that attempts at change within the system are a viable option, the consultant may become involved with the consultee in some of the following change activities (28):

1. Development of a plan showing the need for change.

2. Establishment of a change relationship between consultant and the consultee or the system.

3. Clarification or diagnosis of the client's system problems.

4. Examination of alternative goals and intentions for action.

5. Transformation of intentions into actual change efforts.

6. Generalization and stabilization of change.

7. Achievement of a terminal relationship.

The change that occurs as a result of consultation proceeds in an orderly way through these steps: (1) study and fact finding, (2) evaluation of the facts, (3) diagnosis, (4) formulation and implementation of a plan of action, and (5) evaluation of the outcome.

There are three steps in the process of consultation: trust building, problem solving, and ending. If trust is to develop, the consultee must feel confident that the consultant is concerned about him/her, is competent to help, and is interested not only in problem resolution but also in the consultee's own professional growth (20). The consultant will need an in-depth knowledge of the community or group with which the consultee is working in addition to sound communication skills and sensitive understanding of interpersonal relationships.

There are many pitfalls in mental health consultation. One is the consultant considering self as expert and moving in to solve problems. Trust must be developed with the consultee. Above all, the impression that the consultee is being criticized must be avoided.

Depending on the capacity of the nurse consultant, consultation may be done with a wide variety of groups. Schools and churches are two major areas that use consultants. The teacher may seek help with problem students, and the clergyman may need additional expertise in dealing with members who seek his help. Many ministers are trained to counsel parishioners and see this as one of their major functions. Consultation with clergymen and conducting educational programs to increase their expertise in preventing mental illness are within the role of the mental health nurse. Also, law enforcement officials are aware of their need for mental health training in dealing with people. Prevention occurs when a policeman intervenes in a therapeutic manner to defuse a volatile situation. Nurses working individually with policemen or providing educational programs for groups of law enforcement officers are engaged in prevention. Probation officers, prison guards, and staffs of juvenile detention centers can benefit from nursing consultation services. Often these groups will first need a good listener who attempts to understand some of the frustrations inherent in the nature of the job.

People living in rural areas have problems not encountered by those in urban and suburban areas. The stress encountered by the farmer may be totally foreign to the city person, but it can be just as devastating. Acceptance of professional services and views on mental illness seem to differ in rural areas. Delivery of services will also be quite different. The county agricultural worker, clergyman, teacher, pharmacist, bartender, beautician, and shopowner—with a knowledge of the area and its people—may be the most likely people to provide preventive services. The support of the mental health nurse as consultant can help these people do more effective prevention work. The nurse must see the importance of educating others in preventive principles so that there is a multiplier effect. The nurse who helps to train policemen, clergymen, community health nurses, teachers, and others, and emphasizes that these people in turn train others, is expanding the cause of mental health.

SECONDARY PREVENTION

If the person becomes emotionally ill, there are many care settings and treatment programs where he or she may receive care. The purpose and function of *secondary prevention are to provide early diagnosis and quick, effective treatment to improve the effectiveness of the client's social functioning at home, at work, and in the community.* Secondary prevention applies to the individual and family, or groups of which he/she is a member, and the community within which the person lives and works. Early diagnosis and treatment are essential to ensure that the psychiatric illness does not become fixed into a long-term behavioral pattern that interferes with individual life style or social functioning.

The first line of treatment is usually the family physician, or individual or group psychotherapy, as well as drug therapy by a private psychotherapist or in a clinic setting. Hospitalization may be needed to give the client relief when environmental stress is overwhelming and when the additional structure of the hospital setting would be the best intervention, or when the client is suicidal.

Secondary care settings may be limited in services or may be comprehensive and provide complete, semiprotected, or minimum protection for the client. General hospitals with locked and open psychiatric units often offer a variety of, if not comprehensive, psychotherapies and adjunct therapies. Psychiatric hospitals usually offer comprehensive services.

Milieu therapy is usually practiced in these care settings. *Milieu is a French word translated in English to mean environment. Milieu therapy emphasizes the total experience of the client as being significant for improvement.* Each contact with the client should promote recovery; a therapeutic milieu is a health-promoting environment over the entire 24-hour day. The physical aspects of the unit, including colors, furnishings, and architecture, are contributing factors, but more important are the attitudes and behaviors of personnel and the activities provided on the unit. Characteristics of a therapeutic environment are that it: (1) encourages a client to participate in his/her own plan of care, (2) helps the client gain new insights about self, (3) allows the client to test new patterns of behavior, (4) is accepting, (5) is democratic, and (6) provides adequate protection. Elements of a therapeutic milieu include open communication between clients and staff and among staff, individualization of treatment programs, and often some form of ward government led by clients. The self-government system implies that the clients will have some degree of input into planning daily activities, setting policies, orienting newly admitted clients, and in some cases, making decisions about fellow clients, such as appropriateness of a weekend pass or time of discharge.

Most inpatient settings include *adjunct therapies* as a part of the treatment regime. For example, *occupational and recreational therapy* have long been used to provide: (1) experience in a group situation, (2) practice in social skills, (3) opportunity for expression of regressive and aggressive tendencies in a socially acceptable manner, (4) relaxation, and (5) new areas of interest that can be important leisure-time activities during hospitalization and after discharge. *Educational therapy* usually is a somewhat formalized school setting seen primarily in children and adolescent psychiatric units. *Other therapies,* such as poetry, music, psychodrama, dance, art, and bibliotherapy, are important aspects of a comprehensive treatment center. Each is used as a tool that contributes to the increased functioning of the client but is not a sole means of treatment. The types that are available depend on the type of population a care setting serves, the conditions available in the setting, and whether there are personnel on the staff who are well trained in a particular therapy. Which clients would benefit from which types of therapy depends on the clients' interests and needs.

Poetry therapy is the use of poetry in a group setting, both writing it and reading it, to enable clients to work together and to gain insights into their behavior. Poetry may help the client get in touch with feelings through expression or through seeing parallels in the writings of others.

Participation in *music therapy* offers the challenge of expansion of knowledge; provides the discipline of orderly activity; promotes improvement in concentration, attention span, and memory; and provides pride of achievement (2). The coming together in a group experience, such as a singing group or a small band, provides opportunities for working together toward a common goal.

Dance therapy is defined by the American Dance Therapy Association as the psychotherapeutic use of movement as a process which enhances emotional and physical integration of the individual (55). The focus is on developing individual body awareness, group interaction, and cooperation, and sharing of feelings in movement.

Frequently clients can better express themselves through art than through verbal communication; an objective of *art therapy* is to foster this expression. The client, through drawing, painting, print work, or sculpture, often finds a media of expression for past experiences, feelings, and future plans.

In *bibliotherapy* the client is assisted to broaden experiences, see parallels with personal life, and perhaps assimilate values from books into his/her own life, in addition to providing a medium for discussion with others.

All of these adjunct therapies introduce nonthreatening media to the client and provide the opportunity to decrease inhibitions, share values at a feeling level, and allow vicarious experience of a variety of life experiences.

Partial hospitalization is another treatment alternative. Clients may participate in partial hospitalization as a substitute for 24-hour hospital care or may gradually progress from full hospitalization to partial hospitalization. Among the advantages of partial hospitalization over inpatient care are less separation from families, more family involvement in the treatment program, and a lessening of the client's preoccupation with the illness, which may be intensified by full hospitalization. In partial hospitalization, the client is involved in the treatment program and retains a high degree of independence, but without the full burden of independent living. The *day hospital* may be independent or may function as a part of a 24-hour psychiatric treatment center. Services are usually more or less comprehensive in psychotherapies and adjunct therapies. The *evening hospital* is designed to give sustaining help five evenings or less a week for the client who can continue to work at a job and live at home. The *night hospital* is for clients who can handle their jobs during the day but may be unable to deal with home and family situations during the evening and night hours. The night hospital also can serve as a transition between full hospitalization and becoming established again in independent living. Clients who have a job may use the inpatient hospital setting in this manner as they go to their job during the day and return to the hospital at night. The *weekend care center* is another form of partial hospitalization wherein clients may devote weekdays to their usual pursuits and obtain intensive treatment on Saturday and Sunday. This program is particularly useful for clients who do not require inpatient care but who live too far from a treatment center to obtain day care.

Various other types of treatment centers are a part of secondary prevention. For example, there are *small, homelike residential centers*, whether a camp, farm, or urban home, for adults or for children and adolescents who can not cope with the stresses and demands of home, school, the law, or community; these residences offer strict to minimum protection, depending on the needs of the residents. Usually residential centers of this kind provide group therapy and some adjunct therapies. In addition, behavior modification programs are often used, along with the residential environment and therapies, to alter behavior through reward, support, and limits so that the person learns adaptive behavior.

The *halfway house,* which offers a variety of therapies, facilitates transition between the hospital and independent living where the person is without the benefit of therapy except for weekly counseling sessions or maintenance drug therapy. Often the halfway house is a small, homelike place where the client resides 24 hours daily, or during evenings and weekends if the client is employed. The semiprotected environment helps the resident develop personal strengths and coping mechanisms before facing the demands of the real world.

Many psychiatric clients do not require live-in situations but are treated in the hundreds of *outpatient clinics* across the country. Timely assistance in a convenient outpatient service may prevent prolonged illness. The service may be one of the comprehensive services of a community mental health center, with the backup services of inpatient care available, or may be a separate facility. Other types of services that provide emotional care for clients on a nonhospital basis are 24-hour *walk-in services* staffed by psychiatric personnel in the *emergency room* of a general hospital, and 24-hour *telephone service* located in a general hospital and dealing specifically with calls for psychiatric help. *Home visits* may be made by a community mental health nurse either on an emergency basis or to nonemergency clients who require treatment at home because of physical illnesses, lack of transportation, or certain psychiatric illnesses that preclude the individual coming to the hospital or clinic. Innovative means must be found to provide accessible services to clients so there is effective treatment before an illness becomes long-term.

TERTIARY PREVENTION

If the person is not successfully treated in a relatively short duration of time or if the inappropriate behavior is of a chronic or longstanding nature, *rehabilitative services and agencies* exist to help the person return to a higher level of health. The same treatment methods are used in tertiary prevention as in secondary prevention with the same emphasis on returning clients to their optimal level of function. In *tertiary prevention, emphasis is placed on reducing disability resulting from the illness.* Tertiary prevention often means long-term care.

Disability may result from years of hospitalization, and nurses must make every effort to preserve the hospitalized client's identity and self-esteem. For many people, being hospitalized for a psychiatric illness connotes the end of a productive lifestyle and the beginning of long-term care. Even though much progress has been made, being labeled a "mental patient" is still very detrimental. The client may feel alienated from society. The family is disrupted when a member is hospitalized, and the longer the hospital stay, the more likely the family is to reassign the other members' roles and exclude this member. When the client is first admitted to a long-term care institution, you have a responsibility to begin planning for discharge through attempting to maintain the client's self-esteem and his/her contact with reality and social skills.

Many clients who need psychiatric care for a lengthy period are hospitalized in *public mental hospitals.* Others are hospitalized in *nursing homes.* Populations of state mental hospitals have decreased markedly, due in some measure to transferring clients to nursing homes. This may provide a less restrictive environment for the client, but some nursing homes are not equipped to provide the services available in a large hospital, such as vocational rehabilitation, music therapy, planned group outings, or even occupational and recreational therapies. Also some clients may be placed in a *geriatric day-care center* or a *halfway house,* or these facilities are used for clients to return to for periods of time when more structure is needed, instead of returning to the psychiatric hospital.

It is important that clients who have been hospitalized for long periods not be discharged without preparation for a return to society and assistance after discharge. One step toward rehabilitation is *reality orientation groups and remotivation groups during hospitalization.* Another step is the client *going out into the community,* initially accompanied by staff and later alone or with other clients. These clients may ride the bus, go to a restaurant, or buy something at a store for the purposes of gaining experience in interacting with strangers again and participating in aspects of daily living.

Most clients from long-term care institutions return to their families at discharge. However, in some cases the family will not allow the client to return, or the family unit is no longer functioning. Therefore, some clients may be discharged to a *group home, day-care center, halfway house, or a foster family.* Others may *live in an apartment* alone or shared with other discharged clients. The rent is often paid by the hospital, and the landlord may provide assistance with aspects of daily living. *Centers* are often set up either on the hospital grounds or on separate facilities supported by the hospital where clients go for social activities, to receive medications, get health care, take courses, and get assistance with finances or employment in a sheltered workshop. It is imperative that visits from hospital personnel to the home situation continue on a regular basis and that clients know where to go if assistance is needed.

Problems that former state mental hospital clients living in community residential facilities often face are: (1) reduced social competence, (2) alienation from significant others, (3) loss of supportive systems in society due to their absence from society, and (4) extrusion or rejection by the community (8). *Social linkability is defined as the act of joining a human being with other human beings, agencies, or community resources with the aim of reintegrating and maintaining him/her in the society or community* (8). Social linkability attempts to give the former mental hospital client a sense of belonging and involvement and a means of satisfying the need for respect, identity, and status. Too many former mental hospital patients live in the community but are not a part of it. By itself, placement in the community will not reintegrate the client into that community. We have a responsibility to take an active role in reintegration of discharged patients.

Because of the emphasis on community mental health services, custodial care has been deemphasized. However, unfortunately some people may receive only *custodial care, care that maintains the physical being but does not contribute to emotional or social care nor return the client to a higher level of function in these spheres.* Wards of state psychiatric hospitals or nursing homes still exist where the residents are considered regressed and demented, incapable of learning new behavior or changing their responses and unworthy of rehabilitative efforts. Social attitudes, employment of uneducated and unskilled workers in these institutions, and funding patterns from the public or private sectors foster this type of custodial care. As a nurse and citizen, you have a responsibility to work toward primary, secondary, and rehabilitative care in any or all settings, and to eliminate custodial care as an attitude and program.

REFERENCES

1. Adelson, Pearl, "The Back Ward Dilemma," *American Journal of Nursing,* 80, no. 3 (1980), 422–25.

2. Beavers, Stacie, "Music Therapy," *American Journal of Nursing,* 69, no. 1 (1969), 89–92.

3. Bellak, Leopold, *Handbook of Community Psychiatry and Community Mental Health.* New York: Grune & Stratton, Inc., 1964.

4. Bennett, Douglas, et al., "Towards a Family Approach in a Psychiatric Day Hospital," *British Journal of Psychiatry,* 129 (1976), 73–81.

5. Brill, Naomi, *Working with People: The Helping Process*. Philadelphia: J. B. Lippincott Company, 1973.

6. Brocher, Tobias, "Understanding Variables in Occupational Stress," *Occupational Health and Safety*, 48, no. 2 (1979), 26–31.

7. Broskowski, Anthony, and Frank Baker, "Professional Organizational and Social Barriers to Primary Prevention," *American Journal of Orthopsychiatry*, 44, no. 5 (1974), 707–19.

8. Brown, Frances Gold, "Social Linkability," *American Journal of Nursing*, 71, no. 3 (1971), 516–22.

9. Budson, Richard, "Sheltered Housing for the Mentally Ill," *McLean Hospital Journal*, 4, no. 3 (1979), 140–57.

10. Burgess, Ann, and Aaron Lazare, *Psychiatric Nursing in the Hospital and the Community*. Englewood Cliffs, N.J.: Prentice-Hall, Inc., 1976.

11. Caplan, Gerald, *Principles of Preventive Psychiatry*. New York: Basic Books, Inc., 1964.

12. ——, *Support Systems and Community Mental Health*. New York: Behavioral Publications, 1974.

13. Clark, A. L., and D. D. Affonso, *Childbearing: A Nursing Perspective*. Philadelphia: F. A. Davis Company, 1976.

14. Clark, Carolyn, *Mental Health Aspects of Community Health Nursing*. New York: McGraw-Hill Book Company, 1978.

15. "Community Mental Health Nursing," *American Journal of Nursing*, 70, no. 5 (1970), 1019–21.

16. Cousins, Norman, "The Holistic Health Explosion," *Saturday Review*, March 31, 1979, pp. 17–20.

17. Cowen, Emory, Elmer Gardner, and Melvin Zax, *Emergent Approaches to Mental Health Problems*. New York: Appleton-Century-Crofts, 1967.

18. Crejic, Helen, and Anne Smith, "The Evaluation of a School-Based Mental Health Program Using a Nurse as a Mental Health Consultant," *The Journal of School Health*, 49, no. 1 (1979), 36–39.

19. David, Henry, ed., *International Trends in Mental Health*. New York: McGraw-Hill Book Company, 1966.

20. Deloughery, Grace, Kristine Gebbie, and Betty Neuman, *Consultation and Community Organization in Community Mental Health Nursing*. Baltimore: The Williams & Wilkins Company, 1971.

21. Denner, Bruce, and Richard Price, eds., *Community Mental Health: Social Action and Reaction*. New York: Holt, Rinehart and Winston, 1973.

22. Dunton, Sabrina, "Prevention Today: Better Health Tomorrow," *Journal of Practical Nursing*, 28, no. 8 (1978), 12–14.

23. Ebersole, Priscilla, "From Despair to Integrity through Group Reminiscing with the Aged," *1974 ANA Clinical Sessions*. New York: Appleton-Century-Crofts, 1975.

24. Evans, Frances, *The Role of the Nurse in Community Mental Health*. New York: The Macmillan Publishing Co., Inc., 1968.

25. Freeman, Hugh, "The Environment and Human Satisfaction," *International Journal of Mental Health*, vol. 4, no. 3 (1975).

26. Gammonley, Judith, "New Directions for Mental Health Education," *Journal of Psychiatric Nursing and Mental Health Services*, 16, no. 12 (1978), 40–44.

27. Goldman, Elaine, ed., *Community Mental Health Nursing: The Practitioner's Point of View*. New York: Appleton-Century-Crofts, 1972.

28. Grunebaum, Henry, ed., *The Practice of Community Mental Health*. Boston: Little, Brown & Company, 1970.

29. Hamburg, David, "Disease Prevention: The Challenge of the Future," *American Journal of Public Health*, 69, no. 10 (1979), 1026–33.

30. Holmes, Thomas, and Richard Rahe, "The Social Readjustment Scale," *Journal of Psychosomatic Research*, 11, no. 2 (1967), 213–18.

31. Jacobs, Phyllis, "Stress and Respiratory Disease," Master's thesis, Washington University, 1967.

32. Jamal, Muhammad, and Vance Mitchell, "Work, Nonwork and Mental Health: A Model and a Test," *Industrial Relations*, 19, no. 1 (1980), 88–93.

33. Janzen, Sharon, "Psychiatric Day Care in a Rural Area," *American Journal of Nursing*, 74, no. 12 (1974), 2216–17.

34. Johnston, Maxene, "Ambulatory Health Care in the 80's," *American Journal of Nursing*, 80, no. 1 (1980), 76–79.

35. Joint Commission on Mental Illness and Health, *Action for Mental Health*. New York: Basic Books, Inc., 1961.

36. Klein, D., *Community Dynamics and Mental Health*. New York: John Wiley & Sons, Inc., 1968.

37. Kuchinski, Bernadine, and Michael Colligan, "Psychogenic Illness in Industry and the Role of the Occupational Health Nurse," *Occupational Health Nursing*, 27, no. 7 (1979), 7–17.

38. Lancaster, Jeanette, *Community Mental Health Nurs-*

ing: An Ecological Perspective. St. Louis: The C. V. Mosby Company, 1980.

39. Landsberg, Gerald, "The State of Prevention in Mental Health," *Perspectives in Psychiatric Care*, 15, no. 1 (1977), 15–17.

40. Lewis, Edith, and Mary Browning, eds., *The Nurse in Community Mental Health*. New York: The American Journal of Nursing Company, 1972.

41. Lewis, Howard, "Nurse Practitioners in Prevention and Health Education," *Hospital Progress*, 59, no. 1 (1978), 80–83.

42. Longo, Dianne, and Reg Williams, eds., *Clinical Practice in Psychosocial Nursing: Assessment and Intervention*. New York: Appleton-Century-Crofts, 1978.

43. Macht, Lee, "Beyond the Mental Health Center: Planning for a Community of Neighborhoods," *Psychiatric Annals*, 5, no. 7 (1975), 56–69.

44. McCarthy, Nancy, and Denise Brett, "Learning Primary Preventive Intervention in the Day Care Center," *Nurse Educator*, 4, no. 3 (1979), 12–14.

45. *MH-MR Report: A Morris Associates Report from Washington*, 15 (May 5, 1978), 1–8.

46. Miller, A. C., "Health Care of Children and Youth in America," *American Journal of Public Health*, 65, no. 4 (1975), 353–58.

47. Miller, Dean, and Jan Wiltse, "Mental Health and the Teacher," *The Journal of School Health*, 49, no. 7 (1979), 374–77.

48. Moore, Jean, "Community Mental Health Consultation in Police Courts," *Perspectives in Psychiatric Care*, 18, no. 5 (1980), 204–9.

49. Morgan, Arthur, and M. D. Morgan, *Manual of Primary Health Care*. Philadelphia: J. B. Lippincott Company, 1980.

50. Murray, Ruth, M. Marilyn Huelskoetter, and Dorothy O'Driscoll, *The Nursing Process in Later Maturity*. Englewood Cliffs, N.J.: Prentice-Hall, Inc., 1980.

51. Murray, Ruth, and Judith Zentner, *Nursing Concepts for Health Promotion*, 2nd ed. Englewood Cliffs, N.J.: Prentice-Hall, Inc., 1979.

52. Puetz, Belinda, "Occupational Health Nursing: Employee Mental Health," *Occupational Health Nursing*, 28, no. 9 (1980), 7ff.

53. Quick, James, and Jonathan Quick, "Reducing Stress through Preventive Management," *Human Resource Management* (Fall 1979), pp. 15–22.

54. Rapaport, L., ed., *Consultation in Social Work Practice*. New York: National Association of Social Workers, 1963.

55. Sandel, Susan, "Integrating Dance Therapy into Treatment," *Hospital and Community Psychiatry*, 26, no. 7 (1975), 439–41.

56. Schwartz, Sandy, "Obstacles to Implementing School-Based Prevention Program." Paper presented to the National Youth Workers Alliance, San Francisco, June 1979.

57. Shamansky, Sherry, and Cherie Clausen, "Levels of Prevention: Examination of the Concept," *Nursing Outlook*, 28, no. 2 (1980), 104–8.

58. Smith, Selwyn, "The Prevention of Child Abuse," *Canadian Journal of Public Health*, 70, no. 2 (1979), 108–10.

59. Vicary, Judith, "The Affective Domain as Prevention," *Health Education*, 10, no. 1 (1979), 11–12.

60. Whittington, Horace, *Psychiatry in the American Community*. New York: International Universities Press, 1966.

Appendix

DSM-III Classification: Axes I and II Categories and Codes

All official DSM-III codes and terms are included in ICD-9-CM. However, in order to differentiate those DSM-III categories that use the same ICD-9-CM codes, unofficial non-ICD-9-CM codes are pro- *vided in parentheses for use when greater specificity is necessary.*
The long dashes indicate the need for a fifth-digit subtype or other qualifying term.

DISORDERS USUALLY FIRST EVIDENT IN INFANCY, CHILDHOOD OR ADOLESCENCE

Mental Retardation

(Code in fifth digit: 1 = with other behavioral symptoms [requiring attention or treatment and that are not part of another disorder] , 0 = without other behavioral symptoms.)

317.0(x) Mild mental retardation, ___
318.0(x) Moderate mental retardation, ___
318.1(x) Severe mental retardation, ___
318.2(x) Profound mental retardation, ___
319.0(x) Unspecified mental retardation, ___

Attention Deficit Disorder

314.01 with hyperactivity
314.00 without hyperactivity
314.80 residual type

Conduct Disorder

312.00 undersocialized, aggressive
312.10 undersocialized, nonaggressive
312.23 socialized, aggressive
312.21 socialized, nonaggressive
312.90 atypical

Anxiety Disorders of Childhood or Adolescence

309.21 Separation anxiety disorder
313.21 Avoidant disorder of childhood or adolescence
313.00 Overanxious disorder

Other Disorders of Infancy, Childhood or Adolescence

313.89 Reactive attachment disorder of infancy
313.22 Schizoid disorder of childhood or adolescence
313.23 Elective mutism
313.81 Oppositional disorder
313.82 Identity disorder

Eating Disorders

307.10 Anorexia nervosa
307.51 Bulimia
307.52 Pica
307.53 Rumination disorder of infancy
307.50 Atypical eating disorder

Stereotyped Movement Disorders

307.21 Transient tic disorders
307.22 Chronic motor tic disorder
307.23 Tourette's disorder
307.20 Atypical tic disorder
307.30 Atypical stereotyped movement disorder

Other Disorders with Physical Manifestations

307.00 Stuttering
307.60 Functional enuresis
307.70 Functional encopresis
307.46 Sleepwalking disorder
307.46 Sleep terror disorder (307.49)

Pervasive Development Disorders

Code in fifth digit: 0 = full syndrome present, 1 = residual state.

299.0x Infantile autism, ____
299.9x Childhood onset pervasive developmental disorder, ____
299.8x Atypical, ____

Specific Developmental Disorders
Note: These Are Coded on Axis II.

315.00 Developmental reading disorder
315.10 Developmental arithmetic disorder
315.31 Developmental language disorder
315.39 Developmental articulation disorder
315.50 Mixed specific developmental disorder
315.90 Atypical specific developmental disorder

ORGANIC MENTAL DISORDERS

Section 1. Organic mental disorders whose etiology or pathophysiological process is listed below (taken from the mental disorders section of ICD-9-CM).

Dementias Arising in the Senium and Presenium

Primary Degenerative Dementia, Senile Onset

290.30 with delirium
290.20 with delusions
290.21 with depression
290.00 uncomplicated

Code in fifth digit: 1 = with delirium, 2 = with delusions, 3 = with depression, 0 = uncomplicated.

290.1x Primary degenerative dementia, presenile onset, ____
290.4x Multi-infarct dementia, ____

Substance-Induced

Alcohol

303.00 intoxication
291.40 idiosyncratic intoxication
291.80 withdrawal
291.00 withdrawal delirium
291.30 hallucinosis
291.10 amnestic disorder

Code severity of dementia in fifth digit: 1 = mild, 2 = moderate, 3 = severe, 0 = unspecified.

291.2x Dementia associated with alcoholism, ———

Barbiturate or Similarly Acting Sedative or Hypnotic

305.40 intoxication (327.00)
292.00 withdrawal (327.01)
292.00 withdrawal delirium (327.02)
292.83 amnestic disorder (327.04)

Opioid

305.50 intoxication (327.10)
292.00 withdrawal (327.11)

Cocaine

305.60 intoxication (327.20)

Amphetamine or Similarly Acting Sympathomimetic

305.70 intoxication (327.30)
292.81 delirium (327.32)
292.11 delusional disorder (327.35)
292.00 withdrawal (327.31)

Phencyclidine (PCP) or Similarly Acting Arylcyclohexylamine

305.90 intoxication (327.40)
292.81 delirium (327.42)
292.90 mixed organic mental disorder (327.49)

Hallucinogen

305.30 hallucinosis (327.56)
292.11 delusional disorder (327.55)
292.84 affective disorder (327.57)

Cannabis

305.20 intoxication (327.60)
292.11 delusional disorder (327.65)

Tobacco

292.00 withdrawal (327.71)

Caffeine

305.90 intoxication (327.80)

Other or Unspecified Substance

305.90 intoxication (327.90)
292.00 withdrawal (327.91)
292.81 delirium (327.92)
292.82 dementia (327.93)
292.83 amnestic disorder (327.94)
292.11 delusional disorder (327.95)
292.12 hallucinosis (327.96)
292.84 affective disorder (327.97)
292.89 personality disorder (327.98)
292.90 atypical or mixed organic mental disorder (327.99)

Section 2. Organic brain syndromes whose etiology or pathophysiological process is either noted as an additional diagnosis from outside the mental disorders section of ICD-9-CM or is unknown.

293.00 Delirium
294.10 Dementia
294.00 Amnestic syndrome
293.81 Organic delusional syndrome
293.82 Organic hallucinosis
293.83 Organic affective syndrome
310.10 Organic personality syndrome
294.80 Atypical or mixed organic brain syndrome

SUBSTANCE USE DISORDERS

Code in fifth digit: 1 = continuous, 2 = episodic, 3 = in remission, 0 = unspecified.

305.0x Alcohol abuse, ———
303.9x Alcohol dependence (Alcoholism), ———
305.4x Barbiturate or similarly acting sedative or hypnotic abuse, ———

304.1x Barbiturate or similarly acting sedative or hypnotic dependence, ——

305.5x Opioid abuse, ——

304.0x Opioid dependence, ——

305.6x Cocaine abuse, ——

305.7x Amphetamine or similarly acting sympathomimetic abuse, ——

304.4x Amphetamine or similarly acting sympathomimetic dependence, ——

305.9x Phencyclidine (PCP) or similarly acting arylcyclohexylamine abuse, —— (328.4x)

305.3x Hallucinogen abuse ——

305.2x Cannabis abuse ——

304.3x Cannabis dependence, ——

305.1x Tobacco dependence, ——

305.9x Other, mixed or unspecified substance abuse, ——

304.6x Other specified substance dependence, ——

304.9x Unspecified substance dependence, ——

304.7x Dependence on combination of opioid and other nonalcoholic substance, ——

304.8x Dependence on combinations of substances, excluding opioids and alcohol, ——

SCHIZOPHRENIC DISORDERS

Code in fifth digit: 1 = subchronic, 2 = chronic, 3 = subchronic with acute exacerbation, 4 = chronic with acute exacerbation, 5 = in remission, 0 = unspecified.

Schizophrenia

295.1x disorganized, ——

295.2x catatonic, ——

295.3x paranoid, ——

295.9x undifferentiated, ——

295.6x residual, ——

PARANOID DISORDERS

297.10 Paranoia

297.30 Shared paranoid disorder

298.30 Acute paranoid disorder

297.90 Atypical paranoid disorder

PSYCHOTIC DISORDERS NOT ELSEWHERE CLASSIFIED

295.40 Schizophreniform disorder

298.80 Brief reactive psychosis

295.70 Schizoaffective disorder

298.90 Atypical psychosis

NEUROTIC DISORDERS

These are included in Affective, Anxiety, Somatoform, Dissociative, and Psychosexual Disorders. In order to facilitate the identification of the categories that in DSM-II were grouped together in the class of Neuroses, the DSM-II terms are included separately in parentheses after the corresponding categories. These DSM-II terms are included in ICD-9-CM and therefore are acceptable as alternatives to the recommended DSM-III terms that precede them.

AFFECTIVE DISORDERS

Major Affective Disorders

Code major depressive episode in fifth digit: 6 = in remission, 4 = with psychotic features (the unofficial non-ICD-9-CM fifth digit 7 may be used instead to indicate that the psychotic features are mood-incongruent), 3 = with melancholia, 2 = without melancholia, 0 = unspecified.

Code manic episode in fifth digit: 6 = in remission, 4 = with psychotic features (the unofficial non-ICD-9-CM fifth digit 7 may be used instead to indicate that the psychotic features are mood incongruent), 2 = without psychotic features, 0 = unspecified.

Bipolar Disorder

296.6x mixed, ____
296.4x manic, ____
296.5x depressed ____

Major Depression

296.2x single episode, ____
296.3x recurrent, ____

Other Specific Affective Disorders

301.13 Cyclothymic disorder
300.40 Dysthymic disorder (or Depressive neurosis)

Atypical Affective Disorders

296.70 Atypical bipolar disorder
296.82 Atypical depression

ANXIETY DISORDERS

Phobic Disorders (or Phobic Neuroses)

300.21 Agoraphobia with panic attacks
300.22 Agoraphobia without panic attacks
300.23 Social phobia
300.29 Simple phobia

Anxiety States (or Anxiety Neuroses)

300.01 Panic disorder
300.02 Generalized anxiety disorder
300.30 Obsessive compulsive disorder (or Obsessive compulsive neurosis)

Post-Traumatic Stress Disorder

308.30 acute
309.81 chronic or delayed
300.00 Atypical anxiety disorder

SOMATOFORM DISORDERS

300.81 Somatization disorder
300.11 Conversion disorder (or Hysterical neurosis, conversion type)
307.80 Psychogenic pain disorder
307.70 Hypochondriasis (or Hypochondriacal neurosis)
300.70 Atypical somatoform disorder (300.71)

DISSOCIATIVE DISORDERS (OR HYSTERICAL NEUROSES, DISSOCIATIVE TYPE)

300.12 Psychogenic amnesia
300.13 Psychogenic fugue
300.14 Multiple personality
300.60 Depersonalization disorder (or Depersonalization neurosis)
300.15 Atypical dissociative disorder

PSYCHOSEXUAL DISORDERS

Gender Identity Disorders

Indicate sexual history in the fifth digit of Transsexualism code: 1 = asexual, 2 = homosexual, 3 = heterosexual, 0 = unspecified.

302.5x Transsexualism, ____
302.60 Gender identity disorder of childhood
302.85 Atypical gender identity disorder

Paraphilias

302.81 Fetishism
302.30 Transvestism
302.10 Zoophilia
302.20 Pedophilia
302.40 Exhibitionism
302.82 Voyeurism
302.83 Sexual masochism
302.84 Sexual sadism
302.90 Atypical paraphilia

Psychosexual Dysfunctions

302.71 Inhibited sexual desire
302.72 Inhibited sexual excitement
302.73 Inhibited female orgasm
302.74 Inhibited male orgasm
302.75 Premature ejaculation
302.76 Functional dyspareunia
306.51 Functional vaginismus
302.70 Atypical psychosexual dysfunction

Other Psychosexual Disorders

302.00 Ego-dystonic homosexuality
302.89 Psychosexual disorder not elsewhere classified

FACTITIOUS DISORDERS

300.16 Factitious disorder with psychological symptoms
301.51 Chronic factitious disorder with physical symptoms
300.19 Atypical factitious disorder with physical symptoms

DISORDERS OF IMPULSE CONTROL NOT ELSEWHERE CLASSIFIED

312.31 Pathological gambling
312.32 Kleptomania
312.33 Pyromania
312.34 Intermittent explosive disorder
312.35 Isolated explosive disorder
312.39 Atypical impulse control disorder

ADJUSTMENT DISORDER

309.00 with depressed mood
309.24 with anxious mood
309.28 with mixed emotional features
309.30 with disturbance of conduct
309.40 with mixed disturbance of emotions and conduct
309.23 with work (or academic) inhibition
309.83 with withdrawal
309.90 with atypical features

PSYCHOLOGICAL FACTORS AFFECTING PHYSICAL CONDITION

Specify physical condition on Axis III.

316.00 Psychological factors affecting physical condition

PERSONALITY DISORDERS
Note: These are Coded on Axis II.

301.00 Paranoid
301.20 Schizoid
301.22 Schizotypal
301.50 Histrionic
301.81 Narcissistic
301.70 Antisocial
301.83 Borderline
301.82 Avoidant
301.60 Dependent
301.40 Compulsive
301.84 Passive-Aggressive
301.89 Atypical, mixed or other personality disorder

V CODES FOR CONDITIONS NOT ATTRIBUTABLE TO A MENTAL DISORDER THAT ARE A FOCUS OF ATTENTION OR TREATMENT

V65.20 Malingering
V62.89 Borderline intellectual functioning (V62.88)
V71.01 Adult antisocial behavior
V71.02 Childhood or adolescent antisocial behavior
V62.30 Academic problem
V62.20 Occupational problem
V62.82 Uncomplicated bereavement

V15.81 Noncompliance with medical treatment

V62.89 Phase of life problem or other life circumstance problem

V61.10 Marital problem

V61.20 Parent-child problem

V61.80 Other specified family circumstances

V61.81 Other interpersonal problem

ADDITIONAL CODES

300.90 Unspecified mental disorder (nonpsychotic)

V71.09 No diagnosis or condition on Axis I

799.90 Diagnosis or condition deferred on Axis I

V71.09 No diagnosis on Axis II

799.90 Diagnosis deferred on Axis II

Source: Diagnosis and Statistical Manual of Mental Disorders, 3rd ed., Washington, D.C.: APA.

Copyright ©American Psychiatric Association 1980.

Index

Mental retardation, 253–54, 663, 666–70
Meprobate, 456
Mesmer, Anton, 22
Messick, J., 262
Methyphenidate (Ritalin), 622, 665
Metrazol, 524
Mexican-Americans, 276–79, 283, 284
Meyer, Adolf, 385, 388, 437, 535
Michels, Robert, 167
Middleton, Joan, 70
Mikel v. Flatbush Convalescent Hospital
    (1975), 696
Milieu therapy, 545, 754
Miller, C., 559, 564
Miller, David, 445
Miller, Lynn, 161
Miller, Neal, 30, 32
Mind body relationship, concept of,
    384–85
Mineralocorticoids, 376
Minimal Brain Dysfunction, 622
Minnesota Multiphasic Personality Inven-
    tory (MMPI), 120
Mishler, E. G., 536
M'Naghten Rule, 695
Modeling, 54–55, 128
Model Penal Code Test, 695
Monoamine oxidose (MAO), 27, 509
Montiel, Miguel, 281
Mood, 94
Moore, Joan, 711
Moos, R., 386
Moral Development, Theory of, 62, 63, 80,
    96
Morales, Armando, 277
Morales v. Turman (1974), 694
Moral standards, 707–9
Morbid anxiety, 381
Morbidity, 244
Mordkoff, A., 386
Moreno, Joseph, 335
Mormons, 280, 287
Mortality, 244
Mosley, Doris, 113
Motivation, 61, 91, 193
    Maslow's Theory of, 66–68, 80
Motor dysfunctions, 663
Mourning, 235, 237–42, 243, 256–57
Mowrer, O., 389
Multidisciplinary team approach, 129
Multiple Affect Adjective Check List, 405
Multiple personality, 455
Murillo-Rhode, Iidaura, 113
Murphy, Donna, 119
Murphy, Lois, 407
Murray, Ruth, 256
Music therapy, 129, 755
Myers, J. K., 507
Myths, 7–8

Nadar, P., 670
Nadelson, C. C., 259

Naftidrofuge (Praxilene), 590
Nagy, Joseph, 714
Narcissism, 533, 560, 634
Narcotics, 490
Natapoff, Janet, 373
Nathanson, A., 373
National Conference for Nursing Diagnosis,
    602
National Institute of Mental Health, 110
National Mental Health Act of 1946, 110
Nations, Wanda, 706
Natural disasters, 242–43, 262–63
Navajo Indians, 283
Nazarene Church, 288
Needs, 66–68, 80, 91–93
Negative reinforcement, 34
Negligence, 696–97
Neo-Analytic Theory, 37, 38, 45–53
Neo-behaviorism, 28, 29
Neuman, 66
Neurochemistry, 26–27
Neurophysiological factors, behavior and, 27
Neurosis, 40, 533–34
    comparison between psychosis and,
        439–40
    general symptoms and signs of, 439
    historical perspective of, 436–37
    meaning of, 438
    prevalence of, 437
    stress and, 438
Nevill, Dorothy, 643
Ney, G. Phillip, 209
Nicotine, 462, 494
Night hospital, 755
Nightingale, Florence, 109, 114
Nihilistic delusions, 512
Nonadrenalin, 26
Nonbarbiturate sedatives, 520, 521
Nonreversible (chronic) cognitive impair-
    ment, 580, 583–84, 589–90
Nonverbal behavior, 158–61, 165
Norepinephrine, 26, 27, 509
Norris, Catherine, 111, 419
Northrop, Cynthia, 707
Notman, M. T., 261
Nuclear family, 288
Nurse-client relationship, 721
    identification phase of, 204
    maintenance phase of, 206
    orientation phase of, 203–4
    termination phase of, 206–7
    working phase of, 205–6
    (*See also* Helping relationship)
Nurse therapist, 126
Nursing diagnosis, 121–22
    abusive behavior, 602–4
    alcoholism, 478
    anorexia nervosa, 672–73
    anxiety, 440–41
    change process and, 226
    child abuse, 677
    childhood psychosis, 659–60

cognitive impairment, 586
conversion symptoms, 450–51
crisis intervention, 246–47
depression, 518–19
dissociation, 455–56
drug abuse, 489
family and, 321–22
hyperchondriasis, 452–53
learning disabled child, 664
mental retardation, 668
obesity, 499
obsessive-compulsive behavior, 445–47
paranoia, 566
phobias, 449
schizophrenia, 542
school phobia, 670
sexual role conflicts, 645–46
stress, 406
Nursing process, 105–48
    components of (*See* Assessment; Evalua-
        tion; Intervention; Nursing diagnosis)
    definitions of, 107–8
    history of psychiatric, 108–13
    models for, 113–17
    philosophy of, 132–33, 731
    roles, 125–30, 185
    Standards of Psychiatric Nursing Practice,
        131–32
    (*See also* Change process; Crisis interven-
        tion; Helping relationship)
Nutrition, 416, 519–20, 587
    (*See also* Obesity)

Obesity, 462
    assessment of, 498–99
    definition of, 494
    eating characteristics, 497–98
    evaluation, 501–2
    intervention, 499–501
    scope of, 494
    stigma of, 497
    theories of causation, 495–97
Objectivity, 94
Observation, 5, 121, 156–58
Observer, 349, 355
Obsession, 439, 442, 445–48
Occupational and recreational therapy,
    755
Occupational health, 749–51
Occupational nurse, 649
Occupational therapist, 129
O'Connor v. Donaldson (1975), 693
Oedipal Conflict, 44, 70, 634, 636
Olson, Robert J., 714
Omnipotence, feeling of, 197–98
O'Morrow, G., 129
One Genus Postulate, 45, 77, 195
O'Neill, Maureen, 643
Openness, 345–46
Open systems, 75
Operant conditioning, 34–36, 76–77, 419,
    640, 665